HAIR

TRANSPL

HAIR
TRANSPLANTATION

2ND EDITION

Editor-in-Chief

Venkataram Mysore
MBBS DVD DNB MD DipRCPath (London) FRCP (Glasgow) FISHRS
Hair Transplant Surgeon, Dermatologist, Dermatopathologist, and
Director
Venkat Charmalaya—Centre for Advanced Dermatology and
Postgraduate Training Centre
Bengaluru, Karnataka, India
Accredited to Rajeev Gandhi University of Helath Sciences for Post Doctoral Fellowship
Email: *mnvenkataram@gmail.com*

Corresponding Editor

Kumaresan M

Co-Editors

Sandeep Sattur
Anil Kumar Garg
Kapil Dua
Narendra Patwardhan

Assistant Editors

Deepti M
Pooja Kanumuru
Anuradha Jindal
Govind Mittal
Madhulika Mhatre
Madura C
Aman Dua
Aniketh Venkataram
Sukhbir Singh
Mayank Singh
Kumaresan M
Mayank Singh

JAYPEE

JAYPEE BROTHERS MEDICAL PUBLISHERS
The Health Sciences Publisher
New Delhi | London

Jaypee Brothers Medical Publishers (P) Ltd

Headquarters
EMCA House
23/23-B, Ansari Road, Daryaganj
New Delhi 110 002, India
Landline: +91-11-23272143, +91-11-23272703
+91-11-23282021, +91-11-23245672
E-mail: jaypee@jaypeebrothers.com

Corporate Office
Jaypee Brothers Medical Publishers (P) Ltd.
4838/24, Ansari Road, Daryaganj
New Delhi 110 002, India
Phone: +91-11-43574357
Fax: +91-11-43574314
E-mail: jaypee@jaypeebrothers.com

Overseas Office
JP Medical Ltd.
83, Victoria Street, London
SW1H 0HW (UK)
Phone: +44-20 3170 8910
Fax: +44(0)20 3008 6180
E-mail: info@jpmedpub.com

Website: www.jaypeebrothers.com
Website: www.jaypeedigital.com

Inquiries for bulk sales may be solicited at: jaypee@jaypeebrothers.com

Hair Transplantation / Venkataram Mysore

First Edition: 2016

Second Edition: **2024**

ISBN: 978-93-5696-441-9

Printed at: Samrat Offset Pvt. Ltd.

Editors

Editor-in-Chief

Venkataram Mysore MBBS DVD DNB MD DipRCPath (London) FRCP (Glasgow) FISHRS
Hair Transplant Surgeon, Dermatologist, Dermatopathologist, and
Director
Venkat Charmalaya—Centre for Advanced Dermatology and
Postgraduate Training Centre
Bengaluru, Karnataka, India
Accredited to Rajeev Gandhi University of Helath Sciences for Post Doctoral Fellowship
Email: *mnvenkataram@gmail.com*

Corresponding Editor

Kumaresan M MD Dipl ABHRS
Consultant Dermatologist
CUTIS Skin Clinic and Hair Transplant Center
Coimbatore, Tamil Nadu, India
Email: *dr_kumaresh@yahoo.co.in*

Co-Editors

Sandeep Sattur MBBS MS (General Surgery)
MCh (Plastic Surgery)
Consultant Plastic and Hair Restorative Surgeon
Hairrevive—Center for Hair Restoration
Mumbai, Maharashtra, India
Email: *drsattur@hairrevive.com*

Anil Kumar Garg MS (General Surgery)
MCh (Plastic Surgery) FISHRS ABHRS
Consultant Plastic Surgeon, Director and CEO
Rejuvenate Hair Transplant Centre
Indore, Madhya Pradesh, India
Past President, AHRS (India)
Fellow ISHRS (USA), AAHRS (Asia), AHRS India
Member, WSRM, ISRM, APSI
Cosmetic, Hair Transplant and Microvascular Surgeon
Fellow, Microsurgery Taipei, Taiwan
Fellow, Peripheral Nerve Surgery, USA
Email: *anil@anilgarg.com*

Kapil Dua MBBS MS (ENT) Dip (ABHRS, USA)
Diplomate of American Board of Hair Restoration Surgery
Chairman and Chief Hair Transplant Surgeon
Honorary President, ISHRS (USA)
Past President, AHRS (India)
Board Member, AASHRS Asia and ABHRS (USA)
AK Clinics, New Delhi and Ludhiana
Ludhiana, Punjab, India
Email: *drkapildua@akclinics.com*

Narendra Patwardhan MD DV (London) DVD
Consultant Dermatologist and Hair Transplant Surgeon
Shreeyash Hospital
Pune, Maharashtra, India
Ex President AHRS India
Ex Vice President IADVL
Ex President IADVL (Maharashtra)
Ex President ACSI
Email: *ngpatwardhan@gmail.com*

Assistant Editors

Deepti M MD DVL FRGUHS (Aesthetic Dermatology)
Consultant Dermatologist
Venkat Center for Skin ENT and Plastic Surgery
Bengaluru, Karnataka, India
Email: *deepu85derma@gmail.com*

Pooja Kanumuru MBBS MD FRGUHS (Aesthetic Dermatology)
Consultant Dermatologist
Venkat Center for Skin ENT and Plastic Surgery
Bengaluru, Karnataka, India
Email: *pooja.kanumuru@gmail.com*

Anuradha Jindal MBBS MD Dermatology FRGUHS (Aesthetic Dermatology)
Consultant Dermatologist
Skin Win Clinic
Udupi, Karnataka, India
Email: *dr.anu17@gmail.com*

Govind Mittal MD FRUGHS (Dermatosurgery)
Consultant Dermatologist and Dermatosurgeon
Therepia Clinic
Bengaluru, Karnataka, India
Email: *govindmittal@gmail.com*

Madhulika Mhatre MBBS MD FRGUHS
Consultant Dermatologist and Cosmetologist
Wockhardt Hospital
Mumbai, Maharashtra, India
Email: *dr.madhulika@hotmail.com*

Madura C MBBS MD FRGUHS (Dermatosurgery)
Consultant Dermatologist and Dermatosurgeon
CUTIS Academy of Cutaneous Sciences
Bengaluru, Karnataka, India
Email: *maduradr@gmail.com*

Aman Dua MBBS MD (Dermatology)
Honorary President and Founder Member
Association of Hair Restoration Surgeons of India
Member, ISHRS, AAHRS
Managing Director and Hair Transplant Surgeon
AK Clinics, New Delhi and Ludhiana
Ludhiana, Punjab, India
Email: *dramandua@yahoo.co.in*

Aniketh Venkataram MS Mch FDAFPRAS FASAPS
Consultant Plastic, Aesthetic and Hair Transplant Surgeon
Venkat Center For Skin ENT and Plastic Surgery
Bengaluru, Karnataka, India
Email: *anikethv@gmail.com*

Sukhbir Singh MBBS MS (Surgery) DNB (Plastic Surgery)
Senior Consultant Plastic and Cosmetic Surgeon
Resplendent the Cosmetic Studio
New Delhi, India
Email: *sukhi21278@gmail.com*

Mayank Singh MS MCh (Plastic Surgery)
Diplomate of American Board of Hair Restoration Surgery
Vice President Association of Hair Restoration Surgeons of India
Member ISHRS, AAHRS, AHRS, APSI, IAAPS
Founder and Chief Hair Transplant Surgeon
CROWN: The Hair Transplant Experts
New Delhi, India
Email: *drmayanksingh@yahoo.in*

Kumaresan M MD Dipl ABHRS
Consultant Dermatologist
CUTIS Skin Clinic and Hair Transplant Center
Coimbatore, Tamil Nadu, India
Email: *dr_kumaresh@yahoo.co.in*

Contributors

Aman Dua MBBS MD (Dermatology)
Honorary President and Founder Member, Association of Hair Restoration Surgeons of India
Member, ISHRS, AAHRS
Managing Director and Hair Transplant Surgeon
AK Clinics, New Delhi and Ludhiana
Ludhiana, Punjab, India
Email: *dramandua@yahoo.co.in*

Amit Kerure MBBS MD (DVL)
Consultant Dermatologist and Hair Transplant Surgeon
Dr Amit Kerure Skin Clinic
Navi Mumbai, Maharashtra, India
Email: *amitkerure@gmail.com*

Anchal Shah MBBS MD DNB ABHRS
Dermatologist and Hair Transplant Surgeon, Dr Shalini Malhotra's Hair Restoration and Aesthetic Clinic
Delhi, India
Email: *dranchalshah@gmail.com*

Aniketh Venkataram MBBS MS (General Surgery) MCh (Plastic Surgery)
Consultant Plastic Surgeon
Venkat Center for Skin ENT and Plastic Surgery
Bengaluru, Karnataka, India
Email: *anikethv@gmail.com*

Anil Kumar Garg MS (General Surgery) MCh (Plastic Surgery) FISHRS ABHRS
Consultant Plastic Surgeon
Director and CEO
Rejuvenate Hair Transplant Centre
Indore, Madhya Pradesh, India
Past President, AHRS (India)
Fellow ISHRS (USA), AAHRS (Asia), AHRS India
Member, WSRM, ISRM, APSI
Cosmetic, Hair Transplant and Microvascular Surgeon
Fellow, Microsurgery Taipei, Taiwan
Fellow, Peripheral Nerve Surgery, USA
Email: *anil@anilgarg.com*

Anuradha Jindal MBBS MD Dermatology FRGUHS (Aesthetic Dermatology)
Consultant Dermatologist
Skin Win Clinic
Udupi, Karnataka, India
Email: *dr.anu17@gmail.com*

Anvitha C MBBS MD
Consultant Dermatologist
Nanjappa Multi-Speciality Hospital
Shivamogga, Karnataka, India
Email: *dranvithachidanand@gmail.com*

Aparna Acharya MS (General Surgery)
Member AHRS
Founder and Chief Hair Transplant Surgeon
Hair Plus Clinic
Pune, Maharashtra, India
Email: *draparnaacharya@gmail.com*

Balachandra S Ankad MD
Professor and Head
S Nijalingappa Medical College
Bagalkot, Karnataka, India
Email: *drbsankad@gmail.com*

Bhavni Oberoi MD DNB MRCP (SCE)
Head, Department of Dermatology
INHS Kalyani
Visakhapatnam, Andhra Pradesh, India
Email: *bhavni.oberoi@gmail.com*

Bhawna Bhardwaj MBBS DDVL (Dermatology)
Consultant Dermatologist and Hair Transplant Surgeon
AK Clinics
New Delhi, India
Email: *drbhawna@akclinics.com*

Bishan Mahadevia MS MCh (Plastic Surgery)
Consultant Plastic and Hair Transplant Surgeon
Dr M Hair Transplant Clinic
Ahmedabad, Gujarat, India
Email: *b6747717@hotmail.com*

BS Chandrashekar MD DNB
Chief Dermatologist and Medical Director
CUTIS Academy of Cutaneous Sciences
Bengaluru, Karnataka India
Email: *cutisclinic@gmail.com*

Deeksha Rao Venkataram MBBS MS (ENT)
Consultant ENT Surgeon
Venkat Center for Skin ENT and Plastic Surgery
Bengaluru, Karnataka India
Email: *drdeeksharv@gmail.com*

Dhanashree Bhide MD DNB
Consultant
KEM Hospital and Deenanath Mangeshkar Hospital
Pune, Maharashtra, India
Email: *dsbhide@gmail.com*

Diwaker Sharma MBBS MD
Consultant Dermatologist
Dr Shalini Malhotra's Hair Restoration and Aesthetic Clinic
Delhi, India
Email: *diwakersharmamd@gmail.com*

HM Omprakash MBBS DVD
Consultant Dermatologist
Samastha Skin Clinic
Mysuru, Karnataka, India
Email: *drhmomprakash@yahoo.com*

Indira Potthuri MBBS MD DNB FRGUHS
Fellow in Aesthetic Dermatology
Venkat Center for Skin, ENT and Plastic Surgery
Bengaluru, Karnataka India
Email: *indirapotthuri@gmail.com*

Indu S Sattur MBBS DA
Co-founder, Medical Director and Consultant Hair Restorative Surgeon
Hairrevive—Center for Hair Restoration
Mumbai, Maharashtra, India
Email: *drsattur@hairrevive.com*

Jisha Pillai MBBS MD
Consultant Dermatologist
Lilavati Hospital and Research Centre
Mumbai, Maharashtra, India
Email: *jishapillai86@gmail.com*

Kapil Dua MBBS MS (ENT) Dip (ABHRS, USA)
Diplomate of American Board of Hair Restoration Surgery Chairman and Chief Hair Transplant Surgeon
Honorary President, ISHRS (USA)
Past President, AHRS (India)
Board Member, AASHRS Asia and ABHRS (USA)
AK Clinics, New Delhi and Ludhiana
Ludhiana, Punjab, India
Email: *drkapildua@akclinics.com*

Kavish Chouhan MD (Dermatology) (AIIMS)
Director, Chief Consultant
Hair Transplant Surgeon and Dermatologist
DermaClinix
New Delhi, India
Email: *kavish_chouhan@yahoo.com*

KH Satyanarayana Rao MBBS MD PGDMLE PGDHHM Dip (STD/AIDS) (Bangkok)
Consultant Dermatologist
Central Government Health Scheme Polyclinic
Bengaluru, Karnataka, India
Email: *konanurrao@gmail.com*

Komal Ahuja MBBS DDV
Consultant Dermatologist
Dr Amit Kerure Skin Clinic
Navi Mumbai, Maharashtra, India
Email: *komal.w.1990@gmail.com*

Kuldeep Saxena MBBS DDV DAM (USA)
Medical Director
Cosmazone Pvt Ltd
Gwalior, Madhya Pradesh, India
Email: *saxenadrkuldeep@gmail.com*

Kuldeepsinh P Atodaria MD
Fellow
Tower Health Hospital, Reading
PA, USA
Email: *kuldeep.atodaria @yahoo.com*

Kumaresan M MD Dipl ABHRS
Consultant Dermatologist
CUTIS Skin Clinic and Hair Transplant Center
Coimbatore, Tamil Nadu, India
Email: *dr_kumaresh@yahoo.co.in*

Madhulika Mhatre MD FRGUHS (Aesthetic Dermatology) FIADVL (Trichology)
Director
Skin Saga Centre for Dermatology
Mumbai, Maharashtra, India
Email: *dr.madhulika@hotmail.com*

Madura C MBBS MD (FRGUHS Dermatosurgery)
Consultant Dermatologist
Chief Dermatosurgeon
Chief Hair Transplant Surgeon
CUTIS Academy of Cutaneous Sciences
Bengaluru, Karnataka, India
Email: *maduradr@gmail.com*

Manjot Marwah MBBS MD (Dermatology)
Dermatologist and Hair Transplant Surgeon
National Hair Clinic
Hamirpur, Himachal Pradesh, India
Email: d*rmanjotmarwah@hotmail.com*

Manoj Khanna MBBS MS MCh DNB FICS
Chairman and Managing Director
Enhance Clinic
Kolkata, West Bengal, India
National Secretary of India, ISAPS 2015–2023
President IAAPS 2015–2016
President AHRS-India 2012–2013
Email: *drmkhanna@gmail.com*

Mayank Singh MS MCh (Plastic Surgery)
Diplomate of American Board of Hair Restoration Surgery
Vice President Association of Hair Restoration Surgeons of India
Member ISHRS, AAHRS, AHRS, APSI, IAAPS
Founder and Chief
Hair Transplant Surgeon
CROWN: The Hair Transplant Experts
New Delhi, India
Email: *drmayanksingh@yahoo.in*

Deepti M MD DVL FRGUHS (Aesthetic Dermatology)
Consultant Dermatologist
Venkat Center for Skin and Plastic Surgery
Bengaluru, Karnataka, India
Email: *deepu85derma@gmail.com*

Megha Chandrashekar MBBS MD (FRGUHS Trichology)
Consultant Dermatologist
Hair Transplant Surgeon
CUTIS Academy of Cutaneous Sciences
Bengaluru, Karnataka, India
Email: *drmeghacs@gmail.com*

Megha Tandon MD (Dermatology)
Consultant Dermatologist
DermaClinix
New Delhi, India
Email: *tan.megha1993@gmail.com*

Mrinal Gupta MD DNB (Dermatology)
Consultant Dermatologist
Treatwell Skin Center
Jammu, Jammu and Kashmir, India
Email: *drmrinalgupta@yahoo.com*

Mukta Tulpule MBBS DDV
Consultant Dermatologist
Department of Skin and VD
Mai Mangeshkar Hospital
Pune, Maharashtra, India
Email: *tulpule.mukta@gmail.com*

Murali Chakravarthy MD DA DNB
Director
Department of Anesthesia
Critical Care and Pain Relief
Director
Clinical Affairs
Fortis Hospitals
Bengaluru, Karnataka, India
Email: *mailchakravarthy@gmail.com*

Narendra Patwardhan MD DV (London) DVD
Consultant Dermatologist and Hair Transplant Surgeon
Shreeyash Hospital
Pune, Maharashtra, India
Ex President AHRS India
Ex Vice President IADVL
Ex President IADVL (Maharashtra)
Ex President ACSI
Email: *ngpatwardhan@gmail.com*

Navjot Kaur MBBS MD (Dermatology)
Consultant Dermatologist and Hair Transplant Surgeon
AK Clinics
Ludhiana, Punjab, India

Neha Taneja MD (Dermatology) (AIIMS)
Consultant Dermatologist
DermaClinix
New Delhi, India
Email: *taneja.neha2908@gmail.com*

Nirmal B MD FRGUHS (Dermatosurgery)
Consultant Dermatologist and Head
Department of Dermatology
Meenakshi Mission Hospital and Research Institute and
DERMAL SQUARE—skin.hair.nail.clinic
Madurai, Tamil Nadu, India
Email: *nimu2swash@yahoo.co.in*

Nitika Deshmukh Wagh MBBS MD (Dermatology)
Consultant Dermatologist and Hair Transplant Surgeon
Dr Nitika Wagh Clinic and Deenanath Mangeshkar Hospital
Pune, Maharashtra, India
Email: *nitika4187@gmail.com*

Nitin Barde MD FRUGHS (Dermatosurgery)
Consultant Radiance Skin Antiaging and Hair Transplant Clinic
CUTIS Academy of Cutaneous Sciences
Bengaluru, Karnataka, India
Email: *nitinbarde@gmail.com*

Nivedita Sashidhar MD DVL FRGUHS (Aesthetic Dermatology)
Fellow in Aesthetic Dermatology
Venkat Center for Skin and Plastic Surgery
Bengaluru, Karnataka, India
Email: *dr.niveditasashidhar90@gmail.com*

Pooja Kanumuru MBBS MD FRGUHS (Aesthetic Dermatology)
Consultant Dermatologist
Venkat Center for Skin, Hair Plastic Surgery
Bengaluru, Karnataka, India
Email: *pooja.kanumuru@gmail.com*

Pradipkumar R Atodaria MS MCh (Plastic Surgery)
Cosmetic Surgeon
Atodaria Hair Transplant and Cosmetic Surgery Center
Surat, Gujarat, India
Email: *dratodaria@gmail.com*

Prashant K Palwade MBBS MD (Dermatology)
Consultant Dermatologist
Satej Skin, Hair and Laser Centre
Aurangabad, Maharashtra, India
Email: *prashantpalwade@gmail.com*

Pratik Thacker MBBS MD
Consultant Dermatologist
CODE (Centre of Dermatology Excellence)
Mumbai, Maharashtra, India
Email: *pratikthacker@outlook.com*

Pravin Bharatia MD (Skin and VD)
Associate Consultant
Department of Skin and VD
KEM Hospital
Pune, Maharashtra, India
Email: *pravin_bharatia@yahoo.com*

Priya Dsouza MD
Consultant Dermatologist
CUTIS Academy of Cutaneous Sciences
Bengaluru, Karnataka India
Email: *dsouzapriya66@gmail.com*

Radhika V Kaujalgi MD
Consultant Dermatologist
Venkat Center for Skin and Plastic Surgery
Bengaluru, Karnataka, India
Email: *radhu0253@gmail.com*

Rajesh Rajput Hair Restore MS MCh Honored to be Fellow ISHRS (USA)
Aesthetic and Hair Transplant Surgeon
Hair Restore
Mumbai, Maharashtra, India
Email: *drrajeshrajput@gmail.com*

Ram Chandran MS MCH
Consultant Plastic Surgeon
Apollo Hospital
Chennai, Tamil Nadu, India
Email: *ram.maha@gmail.com*

Ravina Surve MBBS MD (DVL) DNB (DVL)
Senior Resident
Kanachur Institute of Medical Sciences
Mangaluru, Karnataka, India

R Sri Satya MD DVL
Consultant Dermatologist
Skin Clinic
Visakhapatnam, Andhra Pradesh, India
Email: *sri.munni25@gmail.com*

Ruhi Uttamani-Sangle MBBS DDVL FRGUHS (Trichology)
Consultant Dermatologist and Trichologist
CUTIS Academy of Cutaneous Sciences
Bengaluru, Karnataka, India
Skinnovative Skin Clinic
Ahmednagar and Ulhasnagar
Maharashtra, India
Email: *ruhi.uttamani91@gmail.com*

Sajin Alexander MBBS MD (DVL) FRGUHS (Aesthetic Dermatologist)
Consultant Dermatologist
St Martha's Hospital
Bengaluru, Karnataka, India
Email: *drsajinalexander@gmail.com*

Sandeep Sattur MBBS MS (General Surgery) MCh (Plastic Surgery)
Consultant Plastic and Hair Restorative Surgeon
Hairrevive—Center for Hair Restoration
Mumbai, Maharashtra, India
Email: *drsattur@hairrevive.com*

Sanjay Parashar DNB (Plastic Surgery) MCh (Plastic Surgery) FICS (Plastic Surgery) MS (General Surgery) Fellowship Craniofacial Surgery (AU)
Educator and Consultant Plastic Surgeon, Cocoona Centre for Aesthetic Transformation
Cocoona Day Surgery Centre
Dubai, UAE
Email: *sanjay@cocoona.ae*

Sanjeev Aurangabadkar MBBS MD
Consultant Dermatologist
Dr Aurangabadkar's Skin and Laser Clinic
Hyderabad, Telagana, India
Email: *sanjeev.aurangabadkar@gmail.com*

Sayyad Ajara T Hamid DVL (Dermatology)
Consultant Dermatologist
DermaClinix
New Delhi, India
Email: *drtabassumsayyad@gmail.com*

Seema Garg MBBS MSc FISHRS ABHRS
Consultant Hair Transplant Surgeon
Diplomate of American Board of Hair Restoration Surgeons
Fellow: ISHRS
Member: ISHRS (USA), AHRS (India), ASI
Director: Rejuvenate Hair Transplant Centre
Indore, Madhya Pradesh, India
Email: *seema@anilgarg.com*

Shalini Malhotra ABHRS
Hair Transplant Surgeon and Consultant Dermatologist
Diplomate of American Board of Hair Restoration Surgery
Member, ISHRS, AHRS
SM Hair Restoration and Aesthetic Clinic
New Delhi, India
Email: *shalini15m@yahoo.com*

Shivani SR MBBS MD DNB
Fellow In Aesthetic Dermatology
Venkat Center for Skin and Plastic Surgery
Bengaluru, Karnataka, India
Email: *shivanisr3394@gmail.com*

Shuken Dashore MBBS (AIIMS, New Delhi) MD (Skin and VD) DNB
Consultant Dermatologist
Dr Dashore's DHL Centre
Indore, Madhya Pradesh, India
Email: *shukenadashore@gmail.com*

Sonia Sabhandasani Nanavati MBBS MD-DVL
Consultant Dermatologist and Hair Transplant Surgeon
Department of Dermatology
Dr Amit Kerure Skin Clinic
Navi Mumbai, Maharashtra, India
Email: *soniasabhandasani.92@gmail.com*

Sqn Ldr (Dr) Aseem Sharma MD DNB MBA FAGE IFAAD
Chief Dermatologist
Skin Saga Centre for Dermatology
Mumbai, Maharashtra, India
Ex-Assistant Professor of Dermatology, LTMMC & GH, Mumbai
Email: *aseemsharma082@gmail.com*

Sukhbir Singh MBBS MS (Surgery) DNB (Plastic Surgery)
Senior Consultant Plastic and Cosmetic Surgeon
Plastic and Cosmetic Surgery
Resplendent the Cosmetic Studio
New Delhi, India
Email: *sukhi21278@gmail.com*

Suneet Soni MCh (Plastic Surgery) FCLS (Mumbai) VSPMRS (Taiwan)
Plastic, Cosmetic and Microvascular Surgeon
Member-ISHRS, ISAPS, AHRS
Director
MEDISPA Laser and Cosmetic Surgery Center
Jaipur, Rajasthan, India
MEDISPA Hair Transplant Center
New Delhi, India
Ex Visiting Consultant
Fortis Escort Hospital, Jaipur
Email: *drsuneetsoni@gmail.com*

Syed Mubashir MD (Dermatology) FRUGHS (Dermatosurgery)
Professor and Head
Department of Dermatology
Government of Medical College
Baramulla, Jammu and Kashmir, India
Email: *syedmubashir2006@gmail.com*

TP Afra MD DNB
Consultant Dermatologist
Dr Afraz Ziva Skin and Hair Clinic and Baby Memorial Hospital
Kannur, Kerala, India
Email: *afrazain88@gmail.com*

Vaishalee Kirane DVD DNB (Skin)
Dermatologist and Trichologist
Dr Vaishalee's Skin and Hair Clinic
Joshi and Aditya Birla Hospitals
Pune, Maharashtra, India
Email: *vaishaleepk@gmail.com*

Venkataram Mysore MBBS DVD DNB MD DipRCPath (London) FRCP (Glasgow) FISHRS
Hair Transplant Surgeon
Dermatologist, Dermatopathologist and Director
Venkat Charmalaya—Centre for Advanced Dermatology and Postgraduate Training Centre
Bengaluru, Karnataka, India
Accredited to Rajeev Gandhi University of Helath Sciences for Post Doctoral Fellowship
Email: *mnvenkataram@gmail.com*

Viral Desai MCh DNB (Cosmetic and Plastic Surgery)
Aesthetic, Plastic, Hair Transplant Surgeon
Medical Director, Founder
Pioneer—CPLSS, DHI India, DHV-LLP
SKINVIBES LLP
Mumbai, Maharashtra, India
Email: *drviral@drviraldesai.com*

Vivek M Pai MBBS MD (Dermatology)
Consultant Dermatologist and Hair Transplant Surgeon
AK Clinics
Bengaluru, Karnataka, India

Vrushali Maisekar BAMS DNHE
Associate Resident Officer
Department of Dermatology
KEM Hospital
Pune, Maharashtra, India
Email: *pitakev@yahoo.com*

Yatra Kavadya Jain MD DNB
Consultant Dermatologist
NH MMI Narayana Superspeciality Hospital
Raipur, Chhattisgarh, India
Email: *yatrajain9@gmail.com*

Preface to the Second Edition

All great things are a series of small things together.

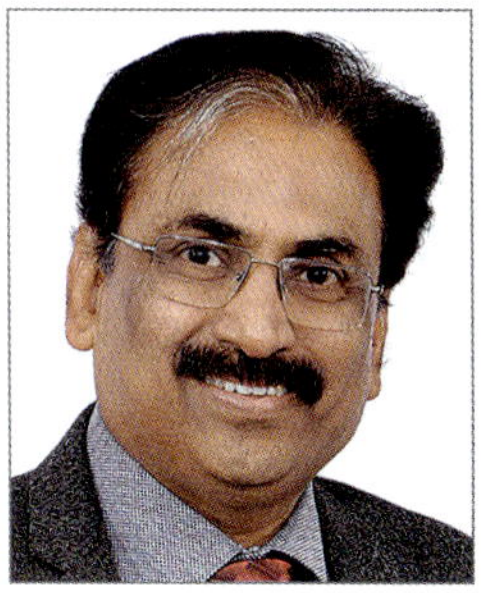

While much has changed and advanced in the field of hair restoration, this sentence from the previous edition holds good still, perhaps with greater relevance. Since the release of the first edition, there have been many new advances meriting a thorough revision and addition of several new chapters. These include advances in medical field such as oral minoxidil, new antiandrogens, procedures such as scalp micropigmentation, platelet-rich plasma and regenerative therapy, refinement of techniques and technology in follicular unit excision (FUE), and newer indications for FUE. Our understanding of the "*conundrum of hair loss in the naked ape*" has improved. Increasing popularity of the procedure has meant greater presence, in social media resulting in greater influence of digital marketing. There have been downsides to this too—quackery and blackmarketing have proliferated and misinformation has abounded. Concerningly, complications including death have occurred leading to a demand for regulation. It is therefore of satisfaction that the legal system, the National Medical Council, and the government have acted and formulated guidelines on the subject.

The result is there for the reader to see—the total number of chapters has increased to nearly 103! Every chapter has been thoroughly revised and new authors have been drafted to author the new chapters. The format remains the same, and the emphasis is on reader friendliness. This is an Indian book but written with a global perspective. It is earnestly hoped that the book will be received well by readers around the world.

I convey my gratitude to all the authors, for completing their chapters and making an important contribution. I thank my co-editors—Dr Sandeep Sattur, Dr Anil Kumar Garg, Dr Kapil Dua and Dr Narendra Patwardhan—who have contributed several chapters and also reviewed others; their experience and expertise have been indeed a great help in completing this book. Of course, my team of young section editors—Dr Deepti M, Dr Pooja Kanumuru, Dr Anuradha Jindal, Dr Govind Mittal, Dr Madhulika Mhatre, Dr Madura C, Dr Aman Dua, Dr Aniketh Venkataram, Dr Sukhbir Singh, Dr Mayank Singh, and Dr Kumaresan M—were immensely helpful in editing the drafts and correcting the proofs—in addition to helping me write several chapters. It has indeed been a privilege and a delight to work with young talent—my sincere thanks to all of them. My special thanks to Dr Kumaresan M who toiled hard as the communicating editor besides contributing important chapters.

A work of this type needs support from family, and I have received them in full measure, for this book, as for my previous books, from my wife Dr Jayashree Venkataram, son Dr Aniketh Venkataram, daughter Ankitha Venkataram, and daughter-in-law Dr Deeksha Venkataram. Needless to say, without their support, the book would not have been possible.

Venkataram Mysore

Preface to the First Edition

All great things are a series of small things together.

This applies succinctly to hair transplantation—and just as aptly to this book on hair transplantation.

Hair transplantation has come of age and is becoming increasingly popular, with greater acceptance from patients and physicians alike. A number of advances starting from the follicular unit concept, strip dissection, use of stereomicroscopy, dense packing, use of magnification, follicular unit extraction, body hair transplantation and now to automation and robotics have been responsible for this resurgence of hair transplantation—the past two decades has seen them all.

To those of us who have witnessed these developments and have been privileged to be a part of them, it has been an exhilarating and enriching journey—we have been part of history in the making. And now when the surgery has seen a boom in the country, the time is just right for an "Indian" book on hair transplantation.

A book on hair transplantation is different from others—so much that is practiced, is surgeon oriented and surgeon specific; so many of the techniques differ from one surgeon to another. So much of the information is new! So much continues to evolve and change! So there is no one way of doing! Afterall, hair transplantation is science and art—there is more art, more varieties of art than perhaps in most other surgeries; so many of the procedures and practices do not have evidence in the conventional definition of the term—there are a few publications in peer-reviewed journals. *To paraphrase Shakespeare, what is a paradox today may be provided proof tomorrow, by time.*

Therefore, what has been done is to document the practices of the surgeon, and wherever necessary, the editor has striven to point out the variations and other opinions. This has meant some repetitions of discussions, some of it at variance with others but the editor believes that they add value and variety. Afterall, *a surgeon needs to learn the art in all its variations and forms* and then decide on what he thinks best suits him. References are provided where they exist; in other places, a bibliography is provided.

Hair transplantation is unique in yet another way. It is practiced by a wide variety of specialists—some without full knowledge of hair and some without full background of surgery! So, there is an extensive discussion on trichology in addition to trichosurgery.

Lastly, this is also a field where there is not just science and art—there is also so much commerce! There have been a few ominous signs on the horizon with all and sundry getting into the practice, placing business ahead of medical practice, commerce before science and art. This has necessitated inclusion of chapters on setting up practice, marketing, and medicolegal issues and ethics.

This is an Indian book—and hence it has been a matter of great satisfaction that we could find talent among Indian hair transplant surgeons to write on all topics—and hence project an Indian perspective. Of course, most of what is presented is relevant to any patient anywhere and hence useful to a surgeon in any part of the world. It is earnestly hoped that the book will be received well by readers around the world.

I convey my gratitude to all the authors, for completing their chapters and making an important contribution. I thank my co-editors—Dr Sandeep Sattur, Dr Anil Kumar Garg, Dr Kapil Dua, and Dr Narendra Patwardhan, who have contributed several chapters and also reviewed others; their experience and expertise have been indeed a great help in completing this book. Of course, my team of young assistant editors—Dr Madura C, Dr Aniketh Venkataram, Dr Kumaresan M, Dr Manjoth Marwah, Dr Madhulika Mhatre, Dr Vani Yepuri, and Dr Vaishalee Kirane—were immensely helpful in editing the drafts and correcting the proofs—in addition to helping me write several chapters. It has indeed been a privilege and a delight to work with young talent—my sincere thanks to all of them.

A work of this type needs support from family, and I have received them in full measure, for this book, as for my previous books, from my wife Dr Jayashree Venkataram and daughter Ankitha Venkataram. Needless to say, without their support, the book would not have been possible.

Venkataram Mysore

Contents

PART B: Clinical Trichology

PART C: Investigations

SECTION 2: HAIR TRANSPLANTATION

PART A: Basic Sciences

SECTION

1

Trichology

PART A: Basic Sciences

SECTION OUTLINE

CHAPTER 1

Evolution of Baldness

Prashant K Palwade

Key Message

This chapter highlights evolution of humans and human hair. As per research data, there has been no evolution in hair structure in last 200,000 years. However, the distribution of hair has changed tremendously. Understanding the factors responsible for this evolution helps us by giving a direction toward future research topics in the field of trichology.

INTRODUCTION

Hair forms an integral part of the human body. It is a defining characteristic of mammals.[1] There are 193 species of monkeys and apes. 192 of them are covered with hair. The exception is naked ape called *Homo sapiens*.[2] In most of these species functions of hair include retention of heat, sexual dimorphism, attraction of mates, protection of skin, and reflection (or absorption) of sunlight. Before understanding various theories of hair evolution let us first take a quick look at milestones in evolution of planet earth and human being.

EVOLUTION OF LIFE ON EARTH AND HUMAN EVOLUTION

Formation of earth and starting point of life on earth is still a great mystery. There are many milestones in this process. Human evolution starts as early as 55 million years ago (MYA) in the form of appearance of primates on earth and goes through various stages to the formation of *Homo sapiens* 200,000 years ago. This process in addition to other aspects involved transition of hairy primates into less hairy modern human being **(Table 1 and Fig. 1)**.

TABLE 1: Evolution of life on earth.[3]

Timeline	Event
4600 million years ago (MYA)	Earth forms
2300 MYA	Oxygen levels start rising (great oxidation event)
550 MYA	Oxygen levels rise again substantially
545 MYA	Hard-shelled mollusks appear
530 MYA	Earliest vertebrates appear
450 MYA	Plants take roots
370 MYA	Amphibians emerged from water
330 MYA	Coal forming swamp forest start to flourish
300 MYA	Earliest reptiles started crawling
260 MYA	Reptiles take over
250 MYA	Planet suffers largest extinction ever
240 MYA	Dinosaurs take first step
200 MYA	Small furry mammals evolved, Dinosaurs dominate earth
150 MYA	Birds take first wing
65 MYA	Dinosaurs go extinct
60 MYA	Mammals take on

Continued

A gene called *FGF5* studied in animal models inhibits hair growth. Single mutation in *FGF5* promoted hair growth.

Human head hair might also keep growing because it has become insensitive to growth inhibitory factors produced by *FGF5* or similar genes.[14]

There are 10 main genes for the hair keratin, 9 of these are almost identical in humans, chimps, and gorillas. The 10th, *phihHaA*, is notably different. It is a pseudogene. This mutation occurred some 240,000 years ago. This is a time when humans acquired head hair that continues to grow.[15]

Why do Pubic Hairs Standout Prominently?

Humans are the only mammals with prominent pubic hair. Pubic hair indicates prospective sexual partners and mating with that individual could be potentially a fruitful exercise. Pubic hair would have arisen only after we became "naked apes", causing it to Standout so vividly against the backdrop of an otherwise hairless body says Robin Weiss, a virologist from University College, London in an article published in Journal of Biology.[16] Pubic hair during evolution has become bushy and prominent and acquired a new role as a prominent sexual ornament, a visual signal of sexual maturity and possibly a reservoir for sexual pheromones.

Evolution of Male Pattern Baldness

Pattern baldness is associated with senescence. It may signal social maturity, a nonthreatening form of dominance associated with wisdom and nurturance. There is very little published literature on the possible evolution of baldness as a sociosexual signal. Guthrie speculated that selection pressures operated upon males such that a receding hairline became a signal of threat, dominance, and age-related status.[17] Guthrie proposed that the loss of scalp hair may have allowed for an increase in the visual area for the intimidation display of reddening color during anger. He also suggested that the expanding areas of the forehead served as a threat display area for the oily, coarse skin particularly characteristic of the adult male. Keating, Mazur, and Segall[18] and Keating and Bai[19] presented some cross-cultural evidence that a receding hairline may convey a message of maturity and social dominance. Hankins, McKinnie, and Bailey[20] found that a bald head, relative to a condition of full cranial hair, did not affect subject's ratings of the target on job-related behaviors such as assertiveness. However, Roll and Verinis[21] found that balding figures, relative to nonbalding figures, were rated as least potent, least active, and least attractive. These perceptions suggest that baldness signals low dominance. Sigelman, Dawson, Nitz, and Whicker[22] examined the relationship between baldness, impression formation, and electability to public office in two studies. They found that Caucasian males who held high public offices exhibited significantly less hair loss than would be expected of a similar group of men their age in the general population. This finding is quite inconsistent with the idea that balding is a signal of age-related status and dominance. The empirical literature does not provide strong support for Guthrie's hypothesis that baldness signals aggressive dominance. It is suggested that male pattern baldness evolved as a signal of senescence and social maturity.[23] The senescence feature of male pattern baldness may be an advertisement of social maturity. Social maturity includes enhanced social status but decreased physical threat, increased approachability, and a propensity to nurture. Nurturance includes providing information, guiding, and instructing younger group members. The effect of the receding hairline, which shifts appearance from dominant-aggressive male to dominant-nurturing male, may account for the nearly universal tendency for male baldness to be associated with male philosophers, teachers, and priests.[24] Balding may have evolved through tertiary selection, through its contribution to kin selection altruism. That is, males may have conducted all of their social and sexual competition before they became bald. The baldness may not have aided in sexual attraction, but instead contributed to the bald male's survival against young male competitors, and gave the bald males more opportunity to engage in nurturance of their offspring and relatives. Such outcomes may have increased the fitness of their kin who carried the genes for baldness.[25]

WHAT'S NEXT?

There are two possibilities; either we will retain hair or we will not. As far as pubic hair is concerned, it is an ornament, worn or shed off depending on mood of the day. Possibility is that it may continue to evolve with evolving sex life.

As far as body hair is concerned, everyone likes it clean. Excess body hair is being disliked and many seek treatments to get rid of it. Possibility is that future generations will have less of body hair.

Scalp hair is the most sought-after thing and is influenced by many genetic and environmental factors. A lot of research is currently being directed at stem cell research and other areas, which can help retain the god-gifted crown on human being. Time will only tell what future holds for us, but for today, the scalp hair loss is causing a great concern in masses and will continue to do so in years to come.

SUMMARY

- Hair structure is not undergoing evolution, but hair distribution is.
- Body hair will diminish in the coming years with human evolution.
- Pubic hair is ornamental and may or may not be affected by evolution.
- Scalp hair has been affected tremendously by recent environmental and genetic changes and alopecia is developing in a larger population at an earlier age. Only time ahead and future genetic research will answer fate of human scalp hair in future evolution.

REFERENCES

1. Denton M (Ed). Evolution: A Theory in Crisis. New York: Adler & Adler; 1986.
2. Morris D (Ed). The Naked Ape. New York; McGraw-Hill; 1967.
3. Unmasking Evolution. [online] Available from www.unmaskingevolution.com. [Last accessed September, 2023].
4. Wong K, Simmons N. What is the difference between hair and fur? Sci Am. 2001.
5. Wells HG, Huxley JS, Wells GP. The science of life. New York: Doubleday; 1931.
6. Maderson PFA. When? Why? and How?: Some speculations on the evolution of the Vertebrate Integument. Am Zoologist. 1972;12:150-71.
7. Rowe TB, Macrini TE, Luo ZX. Fossil evidence on origin of the mammalian brain. Science. 2011;332(6032):955-7.
8. Darwin C. The decent of man, and selection in relation to sex. London: John Murray; 1871.
9. Schwartz GG, Rosenblum LA. Allometry of primate hair density and the evolution of human hairlessness. Am J Phys Anthropol. 1981;55(1):9-12.
10. Cooper W. Hair. New York: Stein and Day; 1971.
11. Bhattacharya S. Early humans lost hair to beat bugs. London: New Scientist; 2003.
12. Khumalo NP. African hair morphology: macrostructure to ultrastructure. Int J Dermatol. 2005;44:10-2.
13. Loussouarn G, El Rawadi C, Genain G. Diversity of Hair Growth Profiles. Int J Dermatol. 2005;44:6-9.
14. Higgins CA. FGF5 is a crucial regulator of hair length in humans. Proc Natl Acad Sci USA. 2014;111(29):10648-53.
15. Winter H. Human type I hair keratin pseudogene phihHaA has functional orthologs in the chimpanzee and gorilla: evidence for recent inactivation of the human gene after the Pan-Homo divergence. Hum Genet. 2001;108(1):37-42.
16. Weiss RA. Apes, lice and prehistory. J Biol. 2009;8(2):20.
17. Guthrie RD. Evolution of human threat display organs. In: Dobzhansky T, Hecht MK, Steers WC (Eds). Evolmionary Biology, Volume 4. New York: Appleton-Century-Crofts; 1970. pp. 257-302.
18. Keating CF, Mazur A, Segall MH. A cross-cultural exploration of physiognomic traits of dominance and happiness. Ethol Sociobiol. 1981;2(1):41-8.
19. Keating CF, Bai DL. Children's attributions of social dominance from facial cues. Child Development. 1986;57:1269-76.
20. Hankins NE, McKinnie WT, Bailey RC. Effects of height, physique, and cranial hair on job related attributes. Psychological Reports. 1979;45:853-4.
21. Roll S, Verinis JS. Stereotypes of scalp and facial hair as measured by the semantic differential. Psychological Reports. 1971;28:975-80.
22. Sigelman L, Dawson E, Nitz M, Whicker ML. Hair loss and electability: the bald truth. J Nonv Beh. 1990;14:269-83.
23. Frank Muscarella, Michael R. Cunningham. The evolutionary significance and social perception of male pattern baldness and facial hair. Ethol Sociobiol. 1996;17(2):99-117.
24. Vallis CP. Hair Transplantation for the Treatment of Male Pattern Baldness. Springfield, IL: Charles C. Thomas; 1982.
25. Bernstein IS. Dominance, aggression and reproduction in primate societies. J Theor Biol. 1976;60(2):459-72.

CHAPTER 2

Naked Ape

Anvitha C, Venkataram Mysore

Key Messages

- Human beings are the only primates without thick body hair.
- Evolution has played its part in reducing the thickness and density of body hair from our prime ancestors.
- It is indeed intriguing that while nature prefers the *Homo sapiens* to be relatively naked and hairless, the *Homo sapiens* is so obsessively fascinated with the preservation of persistence of hair.
- Understanding of the journey might help us in the preservation of hair in generations to come. These issues are indeed very relevant for all physicians who treat hair, such as dermatologists and hair transplant surgeons.

INTRODUCTION

Homo sapiens, having evolved from apes, exhibits many dissimilarities from their ancestors, with nakedness being the most prominent. It is evident that the main difference does not just lie in the quantity of hair, but also in the quality of it.

There are several theories for human hairlessness.

Aquatic ape theory contributes to the understanding of human nakedness.[1,2] According to this theory, the change in body hair was secondary to prolonged exposure to an aquatic environment. In ancient times, our ancestors were ridden with external parasites. Hence, Pagel and Bodmer[3] suggested that human nakedness came into existence to rid the former of these parasites.

Another reason for human nakedness could have been a way of dealing with excessive heating, according to some other theories.[4] The excessive heating might have been due to a change of diet (meat) and place. No substantial evidence is available to suggest a change of diet.[5] Harris[6] was of the opinion that parents were happier with hairless babies as compared to hairy ones (who were abandoned or killed).

Darwin's[7] theory introduced the idea that human nakedness evolved as a sexual feature where males were aroused by the lack of hair in females. However, this does not explain why the females denounced a hairy body. The above theories cannot explain the complete reason for the evolution of the feature of lack of hair.

Three major human characteristics, which have a bearing on the puzzle of nakedness of humans, need to be explained:

1. *Upstanding hominid*:[8] Upright bipedalism appears to be a significant characteristic that separates it from other primates. The turning point for the primates to evolve into humans is the ability to walk on two legs. No concrete theory has been put forth to explain the genesis of bipedalism. A lot of theories were introduced to explain the need for humans to adapt to walking on two legs and standing up straight. Here are a few:
   a. It helped them to keep away from wild animals and protect themselves.
   b. It helped them to rummage for food.
   c. It helped them to preserve their energy when compared to walking on four legs.[8]

   The ability to walk on two legs and stand up straight might have been triggered by a single mutation, which might have also been responsible for the loss of human body hair.[9]
2. *Reduction of body hair*:[8] The major function of body hair in primates was for the baby to hold on to the mother when she moved around.[8] The evolved bare

humans were forced to hold the baby with both hands as there was no hair for the baby to hold onto. Based on these observations, it can be postulated that the changes that happened were interdependent.[8]

3. *Concept of family*: One more unique characteristic feature of hairless humans was the introduction of the concept of society, family, etc. It is possible that the genesis of this feature is connected to the origin of others, i.e., standing up straight, walking on two legs, and having a hairless body.[9] The primates were polygamous, lacked a social mindset, and had intercourse only during a specific time of the female menstrual cycle. But with humanization, the social and reproductive unit of family was introduced, which slowly led to the formation of society. The males in the newfound society were monogamous and did not restrict intercourse only for reproduction.[8]

It is a common understanding that humans originally came from Africa.[10,11] The first few ancestors belonged to the genus *Ardipithecus* that mainly lived in forest areas.[12] The descendants of the former, called hominids belonging to the genus *Australopithecus*, inhabited different kinds of territories while their origin was still limited to Africa.[13] According to some studies made by paleontologists, it can be postulated that the ice age began on this earth 26 lakh years ago, which significantly altered the living conditions of the hominids.[14] In accordance to the change in the living conditions, the hominids learned to make tools and weapons out of rocks in order to slay animals.[14] In order to hunt the animals which were the only and richer source of nutrients, the descendants of the hominids that belong to the genus *Homo* developed ways of walking and running long distances through the development of a present human-like skeletal structure.[15] As a consequence of long-distance walking came excessive sweating, which resulted in overheating and the need for reducing body temperature. From the above observations, it was apparent that walking on two legs increased its efficiency in moving faster and using tools. 16 lakh years ago, it was found that *Homo erectus* was the earliest hominid to have long limbs that helped them to move better. Around the same time, human nakedness set in which helped reduce the body temperature.[4]

Hairlessness and melanin: The development of human nakedness led to some disadvantages like the loss of protection against sunlight, which was a great disadvantage as the hominids inhabited regions receiving high ultraviolet (UV) radiation, i.e., the Savannahs.[16] The loss of hair led to the damage of skin due to a drier environment. The higher exposure to UV radiation led to cutaneous malignancies and malfunctioning of the epidermal layer of the skin, which in turn led to an increased need of vitamins such as folic acid.[16] Folic acid is required for the repair and production of deoxyribonucleic acid (DNA) and for the formation of blood cells.[16] But this folic acid disintegrates on exposure to UV radiation as demonstrated in patients of Fitzpatrick skin types 1 and 2. Hence, evolution resulted in the formation of melanin.[17]

As humans migrated away from the equator, the intensity of the UVB rays reduced and this led to insufficient production of vitamin D.[16] Melanin, when present in higher concentration, led to slower production of vitamin D and thus insufficient production of vitamin D, leading to rickets. Rickets is a condition in which there is insufficient mineralization of the bone, leading to malformed bones, a serious complication of which was unsuccessful birth of babies.[16] In 1930, there was a health drive that underlined the importance of vitamin D in the diet, which proved to be important, as a study done in 1956 showed that 14% of the women had deformed pelvises due to vitamin D deficiency.[18] The death rate of the fetus and the maternal mortality rate had increased due to the increased occurrence of the deformed pelvis.[18] During pregnancy and lactation, the requirement for vitamin D increased, which evolutionarily encouraged a lighter skin tone among females.[17] Another reason that led to the amplification of vitamin D deficiency was the introduction of clothes. The behavior of head lice and body lice has helped us to estimate the initial use of clothing. These two lice resemble each other structurally but feed on different body parts. Head lice that live on the scalp feed more when compared to body lice that happen to feed less due to the obstruction caused by clothing.[19] Initially, only the head lice were present, which inhabited the scalp. But due to the introduction of clothing,[20] it restricted the surface of the body for feeding, which led to the evolution of lice into two types: Body and hair lice.[21] Hence, the evolution of human nakedness, in part, led to this emergence of two different types of lice.[22]

There was another theory put forward by Belt[23] that introduced the idea that human nakedness happened to diminish the load of parasites that inhabited the human body surface. Since humans had settled down in fixed places and lived in groups, the chances of ectoparasite infestation were very high. Thus, hairlessness helped them identify the parasite on their skin and aided in their removal.[23]

Persistence of hair in some places: The plausible reasons for persistence of hair in some places on the human body are worth pondering over. It was postulated that areas such as armpit and pubis required more moisture during movement as they were prone to friction.[4] However, this was not convincing as hair in these areas grow only on the onset of puberty, while children up to that age tend to do quite well without the same. This theory also does not hold good in regards to the location of pubic hair, i.e., on and around the genitalia but not in between the legs.[24]

Thus arises the question about the more probable function of this hair, which may be to hold on to the secretion of the glands of the areas. Wyatt[25] proposed that pubic and underarm hair served the function of differentiating between individual and prospective mate selection.

The other location of interest is the scalp hair. It appears that scalp hair protects the top of our head from extreme heat. Considering this, it is difficult to explain the incidence of androgenetic alopecia (AGA). It is also difficult to correlate the varying lengths of hair in males and females with this scalp hair function. Considering that scalp hair was preserved for body temperature regulation, the patient suffering from male pattern baldness does not seem to suffer from overheating. AGA seems to be increasing in incidence and prevalence. Female pattern baldness is, however, not as common as AGA. This variation is probably because scalp hair may be more of a feature of sexuality. The supporting factor for the same is the presence of beard and mustache hair in males, which is linked to male sexuality. It appears that the increased length of hair in females is akin to that of a belted kingfisher and can be primarily considered as a sexual feature. Since long hair was preferred in females and was genetically selected, it may have passed on to the males through genetics and leaves as much function as the nipples in males.

The enigma that is pattern baldness—AGA: The etiology of AGA remains a mystery till date, despite much research. Various hypotheses have been proposed.

Androgenetic alopecia seems to be more of a hormone-related condition. The hormone is most probably dihydrotestosterone (DHT). This hormone gets collected within the hair follicles of the scalp. Testosterone is converted to DHT by the enzyme 5-alpha-reductase (5a-R). This accumulation of DHT causes the hair to miniaturize over subsequent hair growth cycles,[26] probably by reducing blood flow to the hair follicle.[27] Over time, this leads to balding. The genetic role seems to be prominent in AGA, and quite a few genes have been labeled as the cause of the same. They include *STU1*[28] (receptor gene), 5a-R types 1 and 2 (*SRD5A1* and *SRD5A2*, respectively),[29] *CYP1744*, etc.

Another hypothesis has been put forward for the causation of AGA, called the skull expansion hypothesis. It proposes that a few specific parts of the cranium do not stop their growth even in adults prone to AGA. According to this, miniaturization of terminal hair in AGA is a result of decreased blood flow and nutrients to the frontal and parietal areas of the scalp as a direct consequence of the narrowing capillary blood vessels serving the areas, due to the progressive stretch on the scalp tissue, imposed on it by the frontal and parietal bones.[30] It also links the role of androgens to bone modeling. Androgens, including DHT, act to increase male bone deposition during the growth phase. The triggering of the new bone to grow and expand in the skull happens in the individuals prone to AGA.[30] Osteoblasts and osteocytes contain androgen receptors and 5α-R enzymes. Consequently, DHT triggers the multiplication of osteoblasts, which in turn leads to the formation of new bone.[31] The frequency of AGA in females is lesser when compared to males. This can be attributed to the fact that females have higher estrogen levels and lower testosterone levels.[32] Estrogen, unlike testosterone, decreases bone resorption.[33] As with all other bones, the parietal and frontal bones will be smaller in females, compared to males.[34] In a healthy premenopausal female, the estrogen level exceeds that of testosterone, and hence there are lower chances of skull expansion. But in cases where estrogen levels are low [e.g., polycystic ovarian disease (PCOD), menopause], male pattern baldness may be seen.[35] The shape of the skull and its potential to grow and expand are all genetically determined. Those who have a genetic predisposition toward AGA[26] will have greater potential for skull expansion. In patients who have AGA, this new bone growth, when triggered by increased levels of DHT, will expand the skull far beyond the ability of bone resorption.[30] The shape of the cranium and the ability for growth of the bone can explain the differences in the location of baldness happening on the frontal and parietal areas of the scalp.

Occipital sparing in AGA: The variation of hair over different parts of the scalp is dependent on hormone-related properties and differing structure of the scalp in patients having AGA.[36,37] The hair follicles in the occipital area of the scalp respond poorly to testosterone-related cellular response.[37,38] The concentration of androgen receptors and 5a-R enzyme is more in the frontal area of the scalp as compared to the occipital area for males and females.[39-42] Studies have also demonstrated higher levels of the enzyme aromatase, which is responsible for converting testosterone to estrogen in the occipital area in both genders.[36,39,43] The above qualities of the occipital area are because of its embryological origin. The embryological origin of a large part of the head in vertebrates is of the neural crest, while the posterior part of the head containing the occipital region originates from the mesoderm.[44] This may explain the different behavior of occipital scalp hair.

SUMMARY

What does this change in the thickness and length of hair signify? What is its role in the process of evolution? Does it imply that the future generations will have thinner and shorter hair and eventually none of it? It is crucial to understand the theories of hairlessness and ponder on their implications.

REFERENCES

1. Hardy A. Was man more aquatic in the past? New Scientist. 1960;7:642-5.
2. Morgan E. The Aquatic Ape Hypothesis. London: Souvenir Press; 1997.
3. Pagel M, Bodmer W. A naked ape would have fewer parasites. Proc R Soc Lond B. 2003;270:S117-9.
4. Jablonski NG. The naked truth. Sci Am. 2010;302:42-9.
5. Boesch C, Boesch H. Mental map in wild chimpanzees: an analysis of hammer transports for nut cracking. Primates. 1984;25:160-70.
6. Harris JR. Parental selection: a third selection process in the evolution of human hairlessness and skin color. Med Hypotheses. 2006;66:1053-9.
7. Darwin C. The Descent of Man, and Selection in Relation to Sex, Vol. 2. London: John Murray; 1871.
8. Sutou S. The hairless mutation hypothesis explains not only the origin of humanization from the human/ape common ancestor but also immature baby delivery. Human Genet Embryol. 2013;3:111.
9. Sutou S. Hairless mutation: a driving force of humanization from a human-ape common ancestor by enforcing upright walking while holding a baby with both hands. Genes Cells. 2012;17:264-72.
10. Stringer C. Human evolution: out of Ethiopia. Nature. 2003;423:692-3.
11. Stringer C. Modern human origins: progress and prospects. Philos Trans R Soc Lond Ser B Biol Sci. 2002;357:563-79.
12. White TD, Lovejoy CO, Asfaw B, Carlson JP, Suwa G. Neither chimpanzee nor human, Ardipithecus reveals the surprising ancestry of both. Proc Natl Acad Sci USA. 2015;112:4877-84.
13. Meindl RS, Chaney ME, Lovejoy CO. Early hominids may have been weed species. Proc Natl Acad Sci USA. 2018;115:1244-9.
14. Semaw S, Renne P, Harris JW, Feibel CS, Bernor RL, Fesseha N, et al. 2.5-million-year-old stone tools from Gona, Ethiopia. Nature. 1997;1:333-6.
15. Leakey R, Walker A, Brown FH, McDougall I, Feibel CS, Harris JM, et al. In: Walker A, Leakey RE (Eds). The Nariokotome Homo Erectus Skeleton. Cambridge, MA: Harvard University Press; 1993.
16. Jarrett P, Scragg R. Evolution, prehistory and vitamin D. Int J Environ Res Public Health. 2020;17(2):646.
17. Jablonski NG, Chaplin G. The evolution of human skin coloration. J Hum Evol. 2000;39:57-106.
18. Neer RM. The evolutionary significance of vitamin D, skin pigment, and ultraviolet light. Am J Phys Anthropol. 1975;43:409-16.
19. Reed DL, Smith VS, Hammond SL, Rogers AR, Clayton DH. Genetic analysis of lice supports direct contact between modern and archaic humans. PLoS Biol. 2004;2:e340.
20. Light JE, Smith VS, Allen JM, Durden LA, Reed DL. Evolutionary history of mammalian sucking lice (Phthiraptera: Anoplura). BMC Evol Biol. 2010;10:292.
21. Li W, Ortiz G, Fournier PE, Gimenez G, Reed DL, Pittendrigh B, et al. Genotyping of human lice suggests multiple emergencies of body lice from local head louse populations. PLoS Negl Trop Dis. 2010;4:e641.
22. Toups MA, Kitchen A, Light JE, Reed DL. Origin of clothing lice indicates early clothing use by anatomically modern humans in Africa. Mol Biol Evol. 2011;28:29-32.
23. Belt T. The Naturalist in Nicaragua. London: J. M. Dent & Sons; 1911.
24. Kasai K. Nihon Josei no Gaiseishokuki (External Genitalia of Japanese Females). Tokyo: Free Press; 1995.
25. Wyatt D. Pheromones and Animal Behaviour: Communication by Smell and Taste. Cambridge: Cambridge University Press; 2003.
26. Whiting DA. Male pattern hair loss: current understanding. Int J Dermatol. 1998;37(8):561-6.
27. Mellin TN, Busch RD, Rasmusson GH. Azasteroids as inhibitors of testosterone 5 alpha-reductase in mammalian skin. J Steroid Biochem Mol Biol. 1993;44(2):121-31.
28. Ellis JA, Stebbing M, Harrap SB. Polymorphism of the androgen receptor gene is associated with male pattern baldness. J Invest Dermatol. 2001;116:452-5.
29. Ellis JA, Stebbing M, Harrap SB. Genetic analysis of male pattern baldness and the 5alpha-reductase genes. J Invest Dermatol. 1998;110:849-53.
30. Taylor PJ. Big head? Bald head! Skull expansion: alternative model for the primary mechanism of AGA. Med Hypotheses. 2009;72:23-8.
31. Abu EO, Horner A, Kusec V, Triffitt JT, Compston JE. The localization of androgen receptors in human bone. J Clin Endocrinol Metab. 1997;82(10):3493-7.
32. Riedel-Baima B, Riedel A. Female pattern hair loss may be triggered by low oestrogen to androgen ratio. Endocr Regul. 2008;42(1):13-6.
33. Kumar PJ, Clark ML (Eds). Clinical Medicine. Edinburgh: W.B. Saunders; 1998. pp. 502-3.
34. Gori F, Hofbauer LC, Conover CA, Khosler S. Effects of androgens on the insulin-like growth factor system in an androgen-responsive human osteoblastic cell line. Endocrinology. 1999;140(12):5579-86.
35. Spano F, Donovan JC. Alopecia areata: Part 1: pathogenesis, diagnosis, and prognosis. Can Fam Physician. 2015;61(9):751-5.
36. Suchonwanit P, Triyangkulsri K, Ploydaeng M, Leerunyakul K. Assessing biophysical and physiological profiles of scalp seborrheic dermatitis in the Thai population. Biomed Res Int. 2019;2019:5128376.

37. Chanprapaph K, Sutharaphan T, Suchonwanit P. Scalp biophysical characteristics in males with androgenetic alopecia: a comparative study with healthy controls. Clin Interv Aging. 2021;16:781-7.
38. Suchonwanit P, McMichael AJ. Alopecia in association with malignancy: a review. Am J Clin Dermatol. 2018;19:853-65.
39. Sawaya ME, Price VH. Different levels of 5alpha-reductase type I and II, aromatase, and androgen receptor in hair follicles of women and men with androgenetic alopecia. J Invest Dermatol. 1997;109:296-300.
40. Suchonwanit P, Iamsumang W, Leerunyakul K. Topical finasteride for the treatment of male androgenetic alopecia and female pattern hair loss: a review of the current literature. J Dermatolog Treat. 2022;33:643-8.
41. Hibberts NA, Howell AE, Randall VA. Balding hair follicle dermal papilla cells contain higher levels of androgen receptors than those from non-balding scalp. J Endocrinol. 1998;156:59-65.
42. Chanprapaph K, Mahasaksiri T, Kositkuljorn C, Leerunyakul K, Suchonwanit P. Prevalence and risk factors associated with the occurrence of autoimmune diseases in patients with alopecia areata. J Inflamm Res. 2021;14:4881-91.
43. Suchonwanit P, Triamchaisri S, Wittayakornrerk S, Rattanakaemakorn P. Leprosy reaction in Thai population: a 20-year retrospective study. Dermatol Res Pract. 2015;2015: 253154.
44. Noden DM, Trainor PA. Relations and interactions between cranial mesoderm and neural crest populations. J Anat. 2005; 207:575-601.

CHAPTER 3

Hair Anatomy

Kumaresan M

Key Messages

- Recognition of hair anatomy is important for proper understanding of all aspects of pathophysiology and treatment of different hair problems, particularly androgenetic alopecia (AGA).
- There are important structural differences between hairs in different regions of the body.
- The concept of follicular unit forms the basis of different methods of transplantation.

INTRODUCTION

Hair follicle consists of three parts: (1) *infundibulum* from the opening to sebaceous gland—this part generally behaves like the epidermis; (2) *isthmus* from sebaceous gland downward to arrectores pilorum—this is the most vital part as it harbors the bulge stem cells; and (3) *inferior segment* from arrectores down to bulb—the part which disappears in telogen and is therefore temporary **(Fig. 1)**.

EMBRYOLOGY

Hair follicles are derived from a complex interplay of ectoderm and mesoderm. While most of the scalp dermis is derived from mesoderm, occipital mesoderm is derived from neuroectoderm.[1] This difference is thought to explain the reason why occipital scalp is androgen resistant and behaves differently in AGA as permanent hair. This forms the basis for the choice of occipital hair as donor hair in hair transplantation.

Hair follicles first appear at the end of second month on the eyebrows, eyelids, upper lip, and chin. Most, if not all, hair follicles are present by fifth month, and *it is believed that new hair follicles do not form after birth.* Eruption of hairs follows a cephalocaudal distribution. About 5 million hair follicles develop in both males and females. Scalp develops about 100,000 follicles. The differences between the two sexes in the distribution of various kinds of hairs are caused by different concentrations of circulating sex steroid hormones.

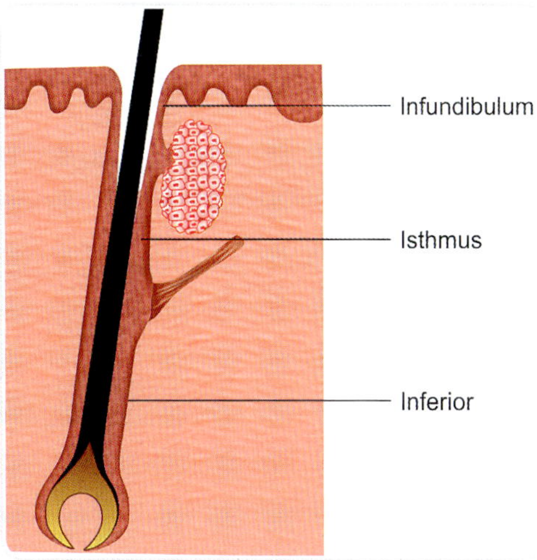

FIG. 1: Structure of hair follicle.

Morphogenesis of Hair (Figs. 2A and B)

The first dermal signaling occurs around 10 weeks of gestation, leading to formation of epithelial placode. This process is being controlled by *BOX gene*. This is also called the pregerm stage.

Stage 1: Hair Germ Stage

The hair follicle first appears as a small concentration of ectodermal cells, called a hair germ or hair bud, in the basal layer of the primitive, two-layered epidermis. The hair germ recruits the dermal cells to form a dermal condensate that promotes further differentiation of hair germ.

Stage 2: Hair Peg

Hair germ proliferates to form a rod-like hair peg that pushes down the dermis. The tip of the hair peg expands to form a bulbous hair peg called hair bulb.

Stage 3: Bulbous Hair Peg

Three areas of swelling appear along the hair peg as the column extends downward. The most superior swelling

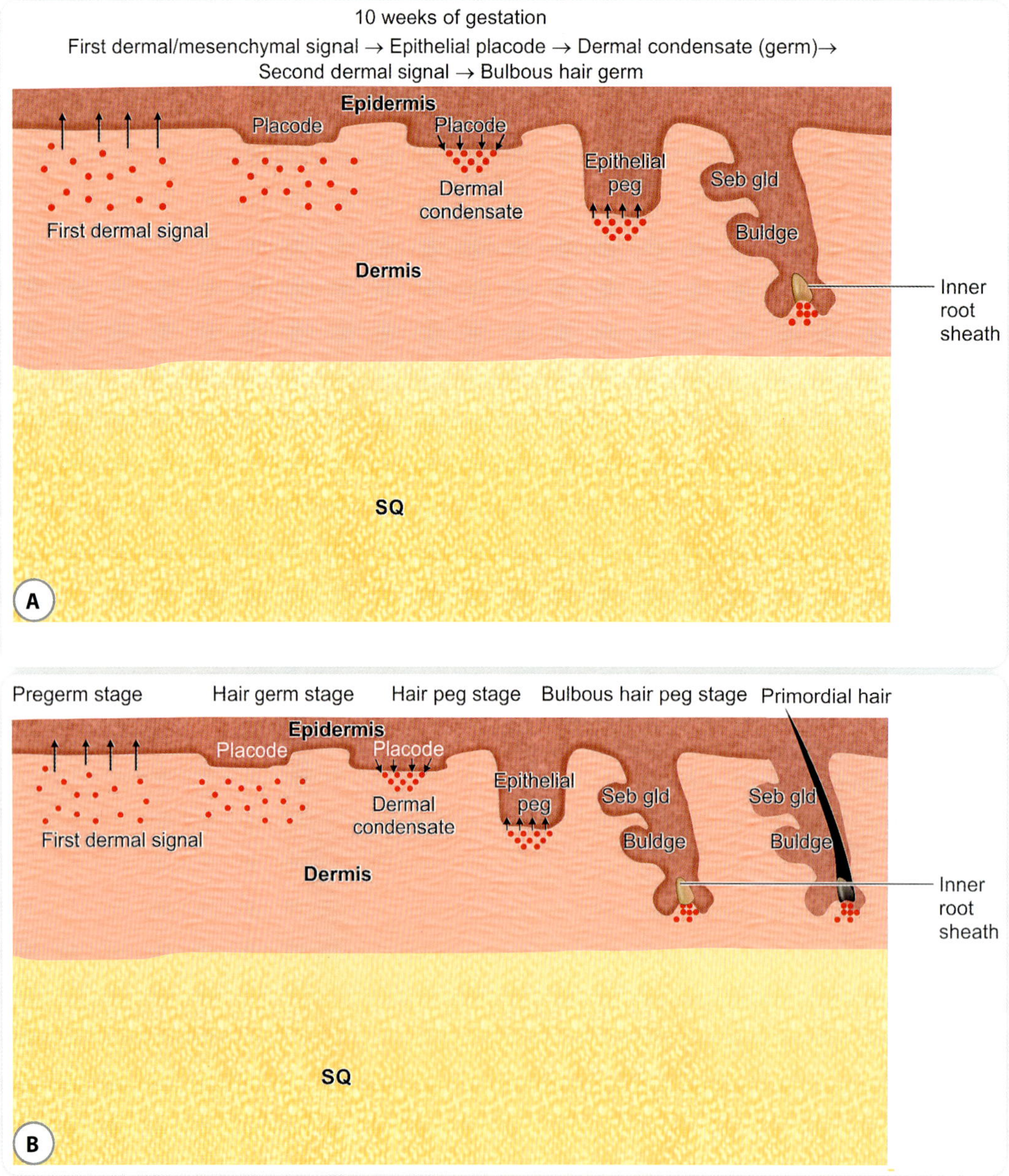

FIGS. 2A AND B: Embryological development of hair.
(Seb gld: sebaceous gland)

will become the apocrine gland, the middle swelling develops into sebaceous gland, and the lowest becomes the bulge area to which the arrector pili (AP) will attach. Dermal cells beneath the tip of the bulb proliferate to form dermal papilla (DP) and invaginate into the hair bulb. The epithelial cells of the hair bulb constitute the germinal matrix, which later will give rise to the hair.

Stage 4: Primordial Hair

As the cells of the germinal matrix, in the center of the hair follicles, proliferate, they are pushed upward and become keratinized forming the hair shaft. The peripheral cells of the developing hair follicle form the epithelial root (hair) sheath. The surrounding mesenchymal cells differentiate into the dermal (connective tissue) root sheath. Melanoblasts invade the hair bulb and form melanocytes. They produce melanin, which is transferred to the hair-forming cells in the germinal matrix before birth. Dermal root sheath gets associated with a bundle of smooth muscle cells called AP, except on the eyebrow and eye lashes.

Hair Cycle[2,3]

The hair follicle is a highly sensitive miniorgan whose cyclic transformations from phases of rapid growth (anagen), via apoptosis-driven regression (catagen) to relative quiescence (telogen) are profoundly influenced by numerous growth factors, cytokines, hormones, and neuropeptides **(Fig. 3)**. Synchronized fetal hair follicle cycling becomes asynchronous soon after birth, when each hair follicle starts to follow its own mosaic cycling pattern. In addition to the hair follicle epithelium, the mesenchyme, the extracellular matrix, vasculature and nerve innervations, and the hair follicle-associated cell populations also undergo dramatic transformations.

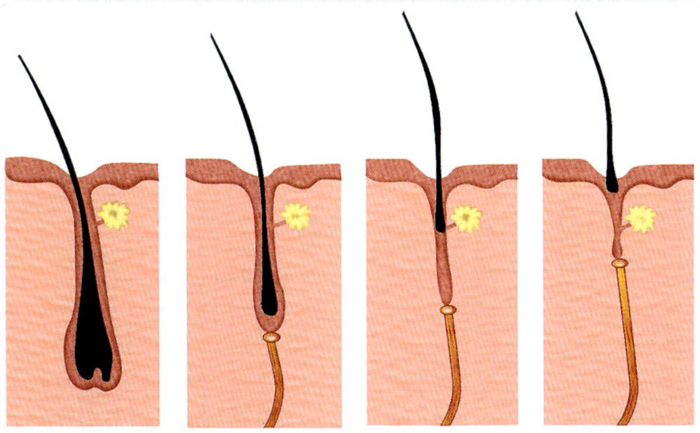

FIG. 3: Hair growth cycle.

Neighboring hairs within a follicular unit may be in different stages.

Anagen

The anagen phase experiences the active growth of hair. Duration of anagen is genetically predetermined, varies with the size of the hair follicle, and part of the body where it is located. Anagen phase may last several years on the scalp or for just a few weeks on the extremities—particularly on the legs. Anagen stage is further subdivided into six stages:

- *Anagen I*: DP is round and located in the dermis.
- *Anagen II*: DP is enlarged and partially surrounded by the keratinocytes.
- *Anagen IIIa*: Appearance of inner root sheath (IRS).
- *Anagen IIIb*: Newly formed hair shaft reaches the middle of the follicle, melanin formation begins.
- *Anagen IV*: Bulb reaches the subcutis, hair shaft reaches the hair canal.
- *Anagen V*: Hair follicle is fully formed.
- *Anagen VI*: Tip of the hair emerges through the epidermis.

Catagen

The anagen is followed by a short catagen phase in which the hair follicle regresses and dismantles the hair-growing part of the hair follicle. Duration of this stage lasts from 2 to 4 weeks. This phase can be divided into eight subphases starting with late anagen and ending in early telogen. Massive apoptosis in the bulbar, transient portion of the hair follicle contributes to regression of the hair follicle and the formation of a fibrous streamer in the skin. Catagen is the first component of the initial hair cycle occurring after first morphogenesis of the hair follicle.

Telogen

Telogen is the resting stage of hair follicle. Telogen hair follicle has regressed to about half of its previous size and does not extend beyond the upper dermis and are fully surrounded by interfollicular dermal fibroblasts. They do not display any part of the IRS, and the compact ball-shaped DP is closely attached to a small cap of secondary hair germ keratinocytes. The epithelial cells of the lower telogen follicle are characterized by the absence of DNA or RNA synthesis. There is also no trace of any synthesis of proteins characteristic of the anagen follicle, such as trichohyalin and the hair cortical keratins. DP cells become relatively quiescent having scant cytoplasm. The telogen hair shaft, the club hair, can be retained for months in this epithelial sac. The duration of telogen is generally 3 months. With each additional cycle telogen duration expands, and hair follicle cycling slows down considerably.

Exogen[4,5]

During exogen phase the hair shaft is actively shed from the follicle. The first morphologic sign of exogen is thinning of the rounded telogen shaft base. With time the lower telogen follicle base cells receive a signal, or series of signals that initiate exogen and the shaft separates from the sheath, its base becomes sculpted ("nibbled") and shed from the follicle. In the human scalp, the actual timing of exogen in relation to the activity of the hair follicle is less clear. In the majority of follicles, exogen is believed to occur before or during the transition from telogen to anagen.[1,2]

Kenogen[6,7]

Kenogen phase refers to the emptiness of the follicle after shedding of the hair shaft (teloptosis). It is normal to observe kenogen in healthy skin. During kenogen, the hair follicle rests physiologically, but duration and frequency are greater in AGA, possibly accounting for baldness. In addition to the classical cycle, the hair follicle may follow an alternative route during which the telogen phase, not accompanied by a coincident new early anagen, ends with teloptosis leaving the follicle empty.

TYPES OF HAIR

Classification of Hair (on the Basis of Shaft Thickness)[1]

- *Terminal hair*: More than 70 μ
- *Intermediate hair*: Between 30 and 70 μ
- *Vellus hair*: Less than 30 μ

In a true vellus hair, the thickness of outer root sheath (ORS) is equal to that of IRS **(Table 1)**. However, in a vellus-like hair, the thickness of ORS is more than that of IRS. Also vellus hairs do not possess arrectores muscle.

TABLE 1: Characteristics of vellus and terminal hair.

Characteristics	Vellus hair	Terminal hair
Consistency	Soft	Coarse
Pigmentation	Hypopigmented	Pigmented
Medulla	Absent	Present
Diameter	<0.03 mm	>0.06 mm
Length	<1 cm	>1 cm
Location of bulb	Upper dermis	Lower dermis/ subcutaneous tissue

Vellus hair replaces lanugo hair in postnatal life. Indeterminate hairs have characteristics intermediate between vellus and terminal hair.

Gross Anatomy of Terminal Hair[8]

The terminal hair is divided into an upper infundibulum, middle isthmus, and a lower segment region. The infundibulum and isthmus constitute the upper permanent region, and the lower segment region is transient and undergoes cyclical regeneration **(Fig. 1)**.

Infundibulum

It extends from the surface of skin to the point of opening of the sebaceous gland into the hair canal. It contains the fully formed hair shaft exiting from the surface. The upper portion called acroinfundibulum is lined by completely differentiated epidermis and the lower portion called infrainfundibulum is lined by undifferentiated cells.

Isthmus

The isthmus is the shortened segment of the hair follicle, extending from the attachment of the erector pili muscle (bulge region) into the entrance of the sebaceous gland duct. The hair shaft is fully mature at this stage and the IRS begins to disintegrate. The inferior most portion of the isthmus contains the bulge area of the hair follicle. *The bulge is composed of a biochemically distinct population of keratinocytes that possess the characteristics of epithelial stem cells. Some stem cells are found in ORS also.* Keratinocytes in the bulge area are relatively undifferentiated structurally and are multipotent, giving rise to several different cell types including epidermal keratinocytes, sebaceous gland cells, and at least seven different types of epithelial cells in the lower follicle. Although the bulge area is cylindrical and often difficult to identify in adult anagen hair follicles, it becomes quite prominent during the telogen phase of the hair cycling process. Bulge area is inundated with nerve endings and Merkel cells. *This network might play a role in providing signals for hair growth and cycling. In many ways, this is the most important part of the hair follicle.*

Inferior or Lower Segment

The lower segment consists of two parts:

1. *Stem*: The part of the follicle above the keratinous zone (Adamson's fringe) up to the insertion of arrector pilorum. The hair shaft and IRS are keratinized at this level. IRS maintains close contact with the hair cuticle.
2. *Bulb*: The bulb is the deep, bulbous portion of the follicle that surrounds the DP. While the DP is

responsible for directing and dictating the embryonic generation of a hair follicle, the bulb is the structure of actively growing cells, which eventually produce the long fine cylinder of a hair. The bulb of the hair follicle can be divided into two regions: (1) A lower region of undifferentiated cells, and (2) an upper region in which the cells become differentiated to form the inner sheath and the hair. A line across the widest part of the bulb separates the two regions at the critical level, and it is known as the line of Auber. Below the critical level lies the matrix, or germination center of the follicle, where every cell is mitotically active. From the matrix, cells move to the upper part of the bulb, where they increase in volume and become elongated vertically. Some of the cells in the upper bulb still show some mitotic activity, but these are too few to account for much of the growth of the hair.

Sebaceous Glands

These are unilobular or multilobular structures that connect to the hair follicle by a squamous epithelial duct. Each lobule consists of a peripheral cuboidal or flattened germinative cell layer. These cells give rise to a central, lipid-laden, vacuolated cell population with characteristic clear to foamy cytoplasm. Sebaceous glands are positioned in the mid-dermis adjacent to the hair shaft and empty by a holocrine mechanism into the hair follicle through a duct located where the IRS terminates. Sebum, a complex lipid mixture, acts as an emollient to the hair and skin and may have a protective function. Sebaceous glands are part of the pilosebaceous unit and so are found wherever hair follicles are located.

Sebaceous glands enlarge and become functionally active during puberty. They are found everywhere on the body, except the palms and soles, and are most abundant on the face and scalp. Sebum secretion is largely controlled by androgens and is associated with acne.

Histology of Terminal Hair

Dermal Papilla (Fig. 4)

The growth and unique cycling activities of the hair follicle is largely controlled by a group of specialized mesenchymal cells, located in a structure termed as DP. Hair bulb encloses the DP, which is continuous with the fibrous dermal sheath (DS) that surrounds the follicle. DP is a reservoir of cells with the potential to differentiate into a range of cell types that are of potential therapeutic importance.[9] *DP cells regulate the hair matrix cell division and the caliber of hair produced through various growth factors and growth factor receptors.*[10,11] Androgen receptors, growth factor receptors, have been demonstrated in DP.[9] DP cell numbers fluctuate over the hair cycle, and androgenetic hair loss is associated with gradual depletion/atrophy of DP cells.[10] A subset of DS cells is retained following each hair cycle, exhibit self-renewal, and repopulate the DS and the DP with new cells.[2]

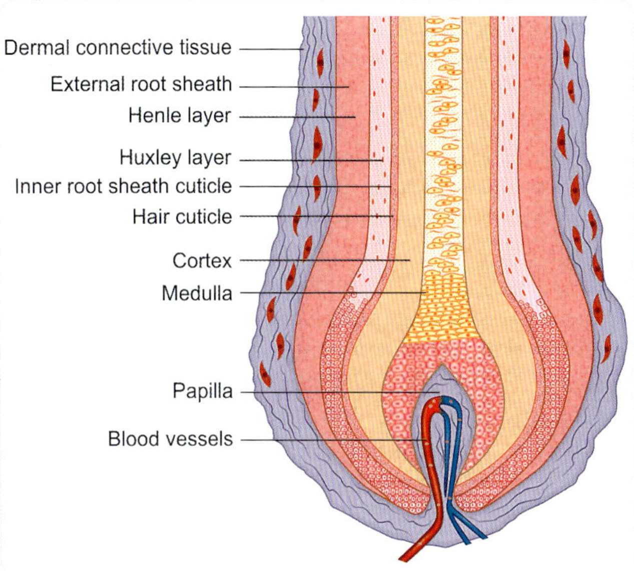

FIG. 4: Structure of hair follicle—longitudinal section.

Germinal Matrix

The germinal matrix is an area of reproducing cells situated around the papilla at the base of the hair bulb. It is the source of hair growth and is involved in transferring melanin to hair to give pigmentation.[8] During the active hair growth phase, cells in the matrix rapidly grow and differentiate, into the shaft, ORS and IRS, causing the hair to elongate. *Matrix cells are immunologically privileged.*

Dermal Sheath

The lower part of the follicle is surrounded by a collagenous layer known as the dermal or connective tissue sheath. Above the level of insertion of AP muscle the DS becomes less distinct and merges with the interfollicular dermis. The DS contains progenitor cells that maintain and regenerate the DP and can induce the formation of new hair follicles.[12] *The fibroblasts in DS are specialized, they can become wound healing fibroblasts and perform an important function in the repair of skin dermis after injury.*[12] The DS has close developmental and anatomical parallels with follicle ORS, the epithelial component that contains the stem cells responsible for replacing skin epidermis.[12]

Inner Root Sheath

The IRS of the hair follicle is a layered structure that extends from the base of the bulb to the isthmus. *IRS is present only in the inferior segment.* Beyond the point of insertion of AP the IRS disintegrates and replaced by the keratin of ORS. IRS is composed of three distinct layers of epithelial cells, which are Henle's layer, Huxley's layer, and the IRS cuticle (from outermost to inner most). The cells of the IRS are interlocked with those of the cuticle of the hair, firmly anchoring the hair in the follicle. The IRS must grow at the same rate as the hair, or faster as it molds and guides the shaft in its passage outward. Racial differences in cross section and size are determined by the IRS.[8]

Outer Root Sheath

Outer root sheath surrounds the hair follicle like a sleeve all the way to the bulb, and is distinct from other epidermal components of the hair follicle. The ORS is essentially a stratified epithelium that is contiguous with the epidermis. ORS is thinnest at the level of the bulb and thickest in the isthmus.[8] The cells of the ORS contain clear vacuolated cytoplasm because of the presence of large amounts of glycogen. Stem cells for various epithelial cell populations of the skin are located in the ORS tissue.[8] ORS cells can contribute to the regeneration of the epidermis. The ORS contains melanocytes, Merkel cells, and Langerhans cells.[13,14]

Companion Layer

The companion layer is the innermost layer of the ORS, and is more prominent in some follicles (especially of the beard) compared with others.[8] It contains cells that are morphologically and biochemically different from the IRS and ORS.[8] The cells of the companion layer are more flattened than the other cells of the ORS and do not contain glycogen.[8]

Hair Shaft[8,14]

The hair fiber or the hair shaft is the portion of hair that projects out of the skin of the scalp. It is a cylindrical, keratinized, and often pigmented filament. The hair shaft structure consists of dead cells that have been filled with hard keratins and binding materials, combined with small amounts of water. It is made of three components—the outer cuticle, cortex, and the inner medulla. The cuticle of hair shaft protects the inner, softer tissue the cortex. A healthy cuticle, other than being a protective layer, also controls the water content of the hair fiber and imparts a shining glossy appearance to the hair. Cortex lies in the middle of the hair shaft. These cortical cells give bulk, shape, elasticity and curl to the hair. Medulla is the inner most layer, composed of large, loosely connected keratinized cells. The composition of the medulla can vary even within the same hair. In human hair, the medulla may be as much as one-third of the diameter of the hair fiber. The formation of medulla cells can be continuous, discontinuous, or fragmental. In coarse hairs it is usually continuous or fragmental, whereas in fine hairs it appears discontinuous or it may be absent altogether. Large intra- and intercellular air spaces in the medulla to some extent determine the sheen and color tones of the hair. That is why there is a difference in the hair color when viewed under sunlight.[8]

Arrector Pili[15,16]

The AP muscle is a smooth muscle bundle that attaches to the external root sheath of the follicle and extends obliquely to its superior attachment site just below the epidermis **(Fig. 5)**. At the lower end of the isthmus, the large AP fascicles disintegrate into smaller fascicles and fibers, to closely encircle the entire circumference of the hair follicles at the bulge region. At the distal end, the AP shows extensive splaying into multiple branches in order to increase contact between the extracellular matrix and the smooth muscle cells. The only function attributed to this muscle is the elevation of the hair shaft, but the significance of the muscle goes beyond this function. By keeping the bulge regions close to each other, the AP muscles might contribute to create this well-protected area where the stem cells are maintained in a common appropriate microenvironment. *Attachment of arrectores to the bulge area is concave and one arrectores is associated with each hair follicle—this attachment is lost in AGA, and*

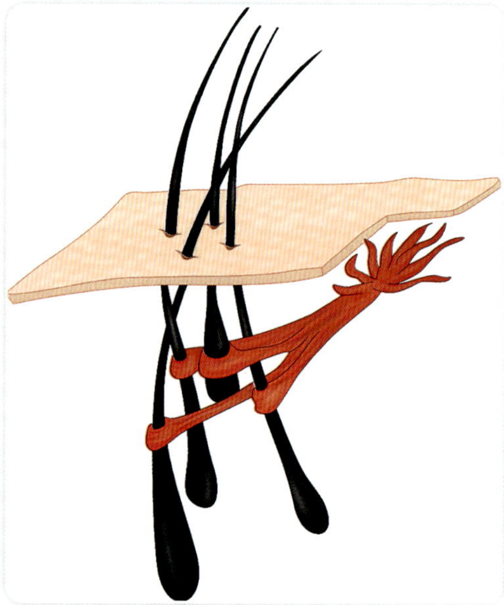

FIG. 5: Arrector pili and its insertion into the hair follicle.

this fact may be important in substance of stem cells and their subsequent loss in AGA. The fact that arrectores folds the hairs together in the follicular unit is a pivotal feature which is responsible for the logic of follicular unit extraction (FUE) as will be explained in chapter 49 Follicular Unit Extraction: Logic, Case Selection, and Indications.

Follicular Units (Fig. 6)

Hair shaft exits the scalp as groups or bundles. Each of this group represents a well-defined, histological structure called as follicular unit. *The concept of follicular unit was first recognized in a land mark paper by Headington in 1984, who studied transverse sections of scalp biopsies. He defined follicular units as groups of 1–4 hair follicles, their arrectores, sebaceous glands, surrounding connective tissue, nerve fibers, and vessels.*[17] The grouping is more pronounced in the region above the insertion of AP muscles.[18] Each follicular unit may contain 1–5 terminal hairs, but majority are composed of two or three terminal hairs.

The distribution of natural hair groupings in each follicular unit determines the person's hair density, and this has important bearing on the outcome of hair restoration.[18] Follicular unit density is the number of follicular unit per cm^2. Hair density is number of hairs per cm^2 (2.5–3 times the follicular unit density).

Individuals with normal follicular unit density may have a low hair density, the reason being that single hair follicular unit is more than the multiple hair follicular unit. There are significant racial differences in follicular unit and hair density **(Table 2)**.[19,20]

In India, while no studies exist on the type and density of follicular units, the author has observed that people of Tamil Nadu and Kerala have greater hair density but less follicular unit density, while people from north India resemble the caucasian pattern more.

Pyramid of Follicular Unit Splay[21]

Follicular groupings tend to exit the scalp similarly to flowers out of the neck of a vase. The follicles are closer together on the surface of the skin, but progressively farther apart as they move toward their position in the adipose tissue. This movement away from one another is termed follicle splay and individual variation is possible. In some, splay is minimal, whereas in others it can be significant **(Figs. 6 and 7)**. In a few, most follicles follow a similar direction, whereas one or two follicles in the same surface grouping diverge in a different direction. The degree and type of splay can affect the transection rate of follicles during FUE. Using a larger punch often accommodates splay. At other times, the physician might use a smaller punch and target only a few hairs within the larger follicular cluster.

TABLE 2: Average follicular unit and hair density in various races.

	Follicular unit density/cm^2	Hair density/cm^2
Caucasians	60–100	260 ± 30
Asians	100	170
Africans	60	160

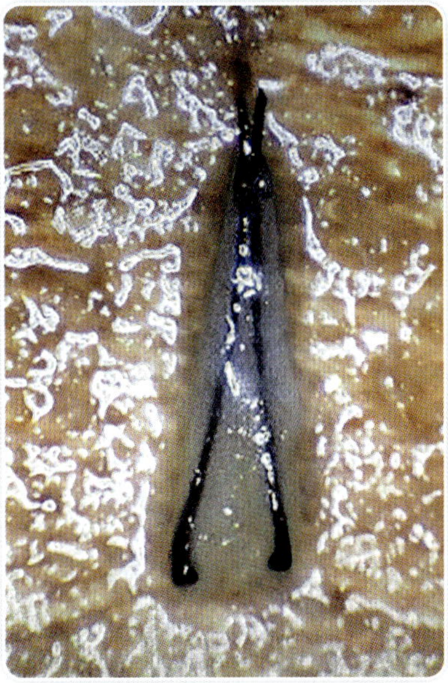

FIG. 6: Follicular unit with two hair and splay.

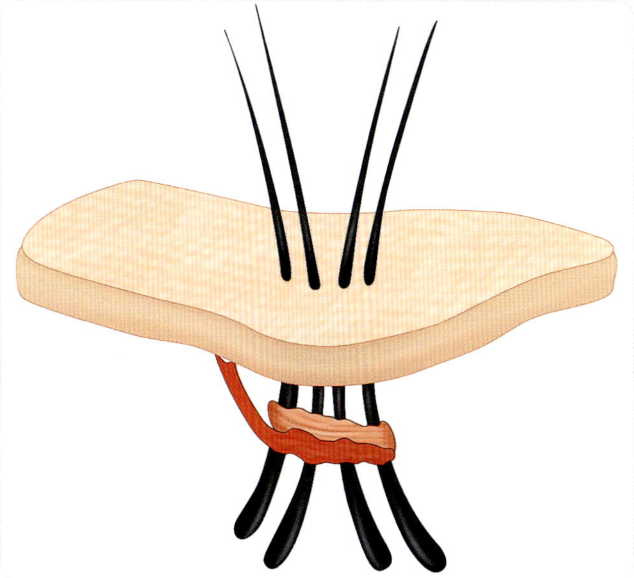

FIG. 7: Follicle splay.

Nerve Supply

The hair follicle is richly innervated by sensory and autonomic nerve fibers **(Fig. 8)**. Nerve fibers that innervate hair follicles form two networks: Around the distal ORS in the subepidermal dermis (follicular network A) and around the ORS between the sebaceous gland and the insertion point of the AP muscle (follicular network B).[22-24] The follicular network A consists of unmyelinated C-fibers expressing such neuropeptides as substance P, calcitonin gene-related peptide, peptide-histidine-methionine (PHM), and the enzymes choline acetyltransferase and tyrosine hydroxylase.[23,24] Follicular network B consists of a collar of longitudinal and circular nerve fibers arranged in the manner of a palisade around the ORS of the hair follicle. Substance P-positive nerves are also found in the DP.[24]

Vascular Supply (Fig. 9)

Hair follicles are surrounded by a dense and continuous plexus of capillaries. The lower third of anagen hair follicle is surrounded by dense network of parallel vessels connected cross hunts from the area above the bulb to the point of insertion of sebaceous glands; the cross shunts drop out and the follicle is surrounded by parallel vessels at the level of sebaceous gland; the vessels form a network around the gland and then terminate in a loose network at the surface of the skin.[25] Telogen follicles are surrounded by a palisade of capillaries connected by short, transverse vessels. Vellus follicles are surrounded by a simple capillary network.

Paul Kemp recently hypothesized that the scalp may contain four types of cells:[26]

- *Type 1*: Hair follicles containing dihydrotestosterone (DHT)-insensitive DP cells that will not miniaturize
- *Type 2*: Hair follicles containing DHT-sensitive DP cells that are not miniaturizing yet but probably will in the future
- *Type 3*: Hair follicles containing DHT-sensitive DP cells that are actively miniaturizing but can be rejuvenated
- *Type 4*: Hair follicles containing DHT-sensitive DP cells that have miniaturized too far that cannot be rejuvenated

SUMMARY

- Neighboring hairs within a follicular unit may be in different hair cycle stages.
- DP cell numbers fluctuate over the hair cycle, and hair loss is associated with gradual depletion/atrophy of DP cells.
- Isthmus is the most important part of hair follicle.
- Companion layer is seen in the beard hair ORS.
- AP is not present in eyebrow and eyelash hairs.

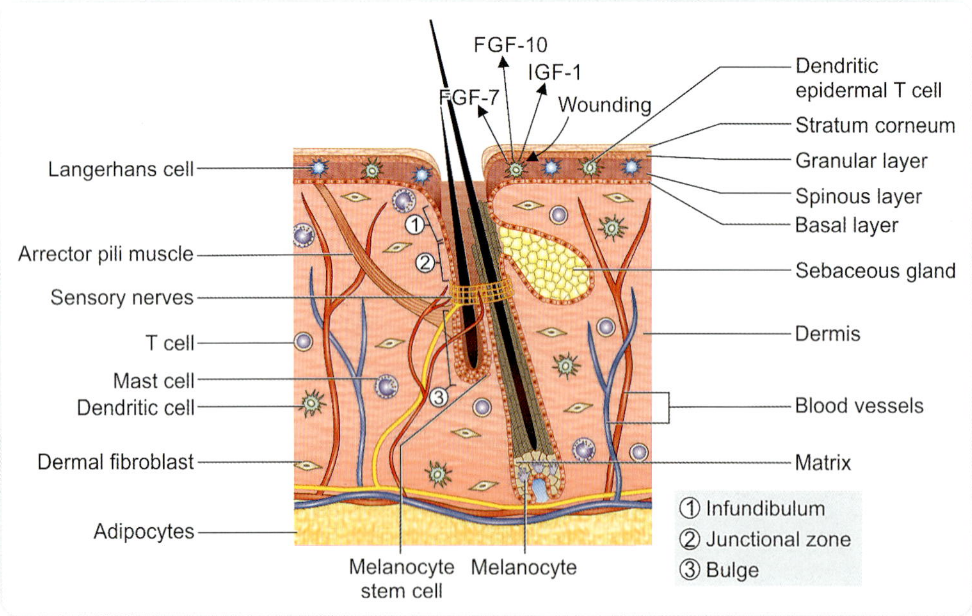

FIG. 8: Innervations of the hair follicle.
(IGF: insulin-like growth factor; FGF: fibroblast growth factor)

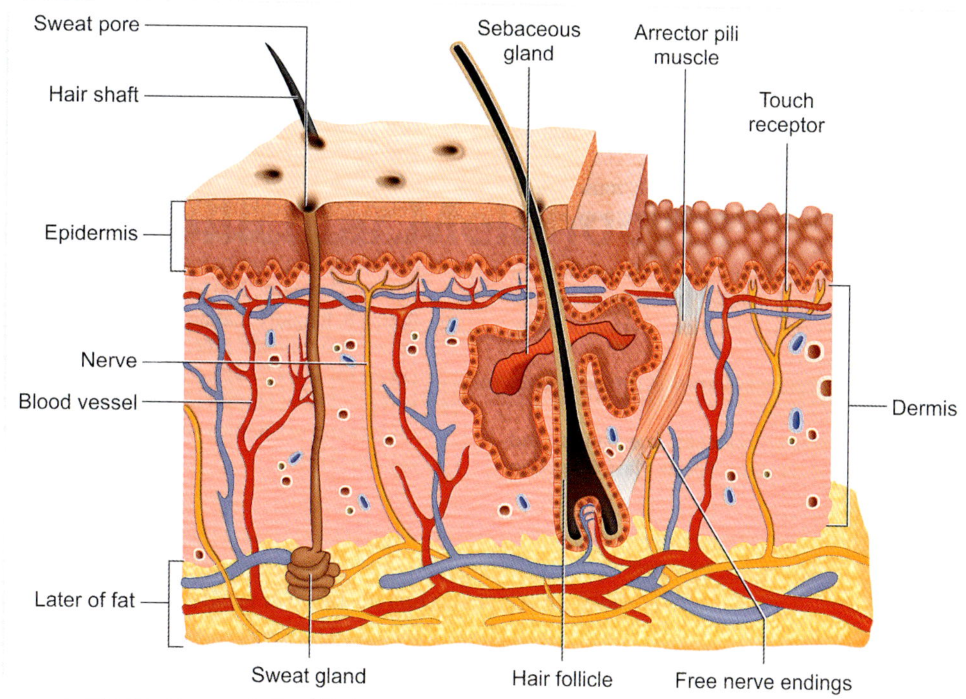

FIG. 9: Blood supply to hair follicle.

- Hair shaft exits the scalp as groups called follicular units.
- Individuals with normal follicular unit density may have low hair density.
- Follicles are closer together on the surface of the skin, but progressively farther apart as they move toward their position in the adipose called splay.

REFERENCES

1. Bleyl SB, Braver PR, Francis-West PH. Development of skin and its derivatives. In: Schoenwolf GC (Ed). Larsen's Textbook of Embryology, 4th edition. Philadelphia: Churchill Livingston Elsevier; 2009. pp. 202-5.
2. Müller-Röver S, Handjiski B, van der Veen C, Eichmüller S, Foitzik K. A comprehensive guide for the accurate classification of murine hair follicles in distinct hair cycle stages. J Invest Dermatol. 2001;117:3-15.
3. Schneider MR, Schmidt-Ullrich R, Paus R. The hair follicle as a dynamic miniorgan. Curr Biol. 2009;10:132-42.
4. Milner Y, Sudnik J, Filippi M, Kizoulis M, Kashgarian M, Stenn K. Exogen, shedding phase of the hair growth cycle: characterization of a mouse model. J Invest Dermatol. 2002;119:639-44.
5. Higgins CA, Westgate GE, Jahoda CA. From telogen to exogen: mechanisms underlying formation and subsequent loss of the hair club fiber. J Invest Dermatol. 2009;129:2100-8.
6. Rebora A, Guarrera M. Kenogen—a new phase of the hair cycle? Dermatology. 2002;205:108-10.
7. Bernard BA. The human hair follicle, a bistable organ? Exp Dermatol. 2012;21:401-3.
8. Messenger AG, de Berker DA, Sinclair RD. Disorders of hair. In: Burns T, Breathnach S, Cox N, Griffiths C (Eds). Rook's Textbook of Dermatology. Sussex: Wiley Blackwell; 2010. pp. 66.1-66.11.
9. Hsu CL, Liu JS, Lin AC, Yang CH, Chung WH, Wu WG. Minoxidil may suppress androgen receptor-related functions. Oncotarget. 2014;30:2187-97.
10. Rahmani W, Abbasi S, Hagner A, Raharjo E, Kumar R, Hotta A, et al. Hair follicle dermal stem cells regenerate the dermal sheath, repopulate the dermal papilla, and modulate hair type. Dev Cell. 2014;31:543-58.
11. Chi W, Wu E, Morgan BA. Dermal papilla cell number specifies hair size, shape and cycling and its reduction causes follicular decline. Development. 2013;140:1676-83.
12. Jahoda C, Reynolds AJ. Hair follicle dermal sheath cells: unsung participants in wound healing Lancet. 2001;358:1445-8.
13. Kumar A, Mohanty S, Sahni K, Kumar R, Gupta S. Extracted hair follicle outer root sheath cell suspension for pigment cell restoration in vitiligo. J Cutan Aesthet Surg. 2013;6:121-5.
14. Rose PT, Shapiro R, Morgan M, Patel NS. Hair anatomy and histology. In: Unger WP, Shapiro R, Unger R, Unger M (Eds). Hair transplantation. London: Informa Healthcare; 2011. pp. 2-8.
15. Clifton MM, Mendelson JK, Mendelson B, Montague D, Carter C, Smoller BR, et al. Immunofluorescent microscopic investigation of the distal arrector pili: a demonstration of the spatial

frontal scalp compared to the occipital region.[15] The level of aromatase is much higher in the occipital scalp than the frontal scalp.

Dihydrotestosterone can stimulate the growth of hair follicles on the face, chest, and genital area while inhibiting the growth of hair on the scalp.

Role of Aromatase

Aromatase cytochrome P-450, located in the outer sheath of the hair root, which catalyzes the conversion of androstenedione to estrone and testosterone to estradiol, also plays an important role in pattern hair loss as it results in lower circulating and tissue levels of testosterone and DHT. There are significant differences in the concentration and distribution of this enzyme between men and women:

- The concentration of aromatase in women is 2–5 times higher in the skin of the scalp as compared to men.[14]
- It is also higher, particularly in the frontal region, in women, which probably determines the retention of hairline in FPHL.
- In men, occipital levels of aromatase are higher than the frontal levels, thus explaining the persistence of occipital hairs.

These differences explain the different manifestations in male pattern hair loss and FPHL and also why the occipital scalp does not undergo miniaturization.

More comprehensive studies and understanding are required to establish a proper relation of various hormones to hair loss or growth, thus facilitating better treatments in poorly controlled hair disorders such as hirsutism and alopecia. **Table 1** enlists various hormonal drugs used in the treatment of AGA, FPHL and hirsutism, and their mechanism of action. Further details regarding these can be found in the respective chapters.

TABLE 1: Drugs used in androgenetic alopecia (AGA), female pattern hair loss (FPHL), and hirsutism.

Hormonal drug	Activity
Finasteride	Type II 5α-reductase enzyme inhibitor
Dutasteride	Types I and II 5α-reductase enzyme inhibitor
Flutamide	Androgen receptor inhibitor
Bicalutamide	Androgen receptor inhibitor
Spironolactone	Androgen receptor inhibitor, progestogenic action
Cyproterone acetate	Blocks androgen receptors (ARs) and inhibits gonadotropin-releasing hormone
Oral contraceptives (OCPs)—combination of estrogen and progesterone	• Reduction in gonadotropin secretion with a resultant drop in production of ovarian androgen • Decreasing levels of free testosterone by increasing the levels of sex hormone-binding globulin (SHBG) • Inhibiting the production of adrenal androgen

SUMMARY

- Response of hair follicles to androgens is varied in selective body sites and also in both genders.
- DHT is a potent androgen, binds to androgen receptors, and causes miniaturization of hair follicles.
- In men, type II 5AR activity is more, whereas in women, type I 5AR is more.
- Aromatase enzyme results in lowering DHT levels.
- Higher levels of aromatase in females, particularly in the frontal region, prevent from complete baldness.
- Similarly, higher levels of aromatase in the occipital region in men explain the retention of hairs in that area for a longer duration.

REFERENCES

1. Camacho-Martinez FM. Hair loss in women. Semin Cutan Med Surg. 2009;28:19-32.
2. Singal A, Sonthalia S, Verma P. Female pattern hair loss. Indian J Dermatol Venereol Leprol. 2013;79:626-40.
3. Vincent M, Yogiraj K. A descriptive study of alopecia patterns and their relation to thyroid dysfunction. Int J Trichol. 2013;5:57-60.
4. Church RE. Hypothyroid hair loss. Br J Dermatol. 1965;77:661-2.
5. Zaki SA, Lad V. Hypertrichosis due to congenital hypothyroidism. Int J Trichol. 2011;3:38-9.
6. Blok GJ, de Boer H, Gooren LJ, van der Veen EA. Growth hormone substitution in adult growth hormone-deficient men augments androgen effects on the skin. Clin Endocrinol (Oxf). 1997;47:29-36.
7. Horton R, Pasupuletti V, Antonipillai I. Androgen induction of steroid 5 alpha-reductase may be mediated via insulin-like growth factor-I. Endocrinology. 1993;133:447-51.
8. Signorelloa LB, Wuu J, Hsieh Cc, Tzonou A, Trichopoulos D, Mantzoros CS. Hormones and hair patterning in men: a role for insulin-like growth factor 1? J Am Acad Dermatol. 1999;40:200-3.
9. Kvedar JC, Gibson M, Krusinski PA. Hirsutism: evaluation and treatment. J Am Acad Dermatol. 1985;12:215-25.
10. Farthing MJ, Mattei AM, Edwards CR, Dawson AM. Relationship between plasma testosterone and dihydrotestosterone concentrations and male facial hair growth. Br J Dermatol. 1982;107:559-64.

11. Whiting DA. Possible mechanisms of miniaturization during androgenetic alopecia or pattern hair loss. J Am Acad Dermatol. 2001;45(3 Suppl.):S81-6.
12. Sawaya ME, Somani N. Antiandrogens and androgen inhibitors. In: Wolverton SE (Ed). Comprehensive Dermatologic Drug Therapy, 2nd edition. Philadelphia: Saunders; 2007. pp. 417-35.
13. Choudhry R, Hodgins MB, Van der Kwast TH, Brinkmann AO, Boersam WJ. Localization of androgen receptors in human skin by immunohistochemistry: implications for the hormonal regulation of hair growth, sebaceous glands and sweat glands. J Endocrinol. 1992;133:467-75.
14. Urysiak-Czubatka I, Kmieć ML, Broniarczyk-Dyła G. Assessment of the usefulness of dihydrotestosterone in the diagnostics of patients with androgenetic alopecia. Postepy Dermatol Alergol. 2014;31(4):207-15.
15. Randall VA. Androgens and hair growth. Dermatol Ther. 2008;21:314-28.

PART B: Clinical Trichology

SECTION OUTLINE

CHAPTER 7

Hair Loss and Causes: An Overview

Pooja Kanumuru, Venkataram Mysore

Key Messages

- Hair loss can be localized or generalized; scarring or nonscarring.
- Nonscarring alopecia includes androgenetic alopecia, telogen effluvium, and alopecia areata.
- Scarring type includes postburn traumatic scars, discoid lupus erythematosus, lichen planus pseudopelade, and localized scleroderma.
- Differentiation between the types is important from the point of view of prognosis.
- Hair transplant surgeon needs to be aware of these conditions.

INTRODUCTION

Hair loss is a common problem which causes anxiety in men and women. Correct diagnosis of hair disorders is complex and requires evaluation of clinical presentation, history, physical examination, and laboratory tests. Hair loss may be clinically categorized broadly into hair shaft abnormalities, scarring alopecia, or nonscarring alopecia. Nonscarring alopecia, the most common type, includes androgenetic alopecia, telogen effluvium, and alopecia areata **(Box 1)**. The hallmark of this group is the possibility of complete regrowth with adequate treatment. This chapter gives an overview of hair loss to give an introduction to the different conditions.

Androgenetic alopecia (pattern hair loss)[1-5] is by far the most common type of hair loss in both sexes **(Figs. 1 and 2)**. Male pattern hair loss is a genetically determined trait. It is characterized by a progressive decline in the duration of anagen, an increased duration of telogen, and miniaturization of scalp hair follicles leading to follicular regression. A detailed discussion on androgenetic alopecia is covered in subsequent chapters.

TELOGEN EFFLUVIUM[6]

Telogen effluvium is one of the most common hair fall conditions presented to a trichologist or hair transplant surgeon. Patients complain of increased shedding of hair which is associated with diffuse alopecia and reduced hair volume over the scalp. This excess shedding is the result of alterations of hair growth cycle with premature conversion of anagen follicles to telogen follicles, which represents a shift of 7% up to 25% of anagen follicles to telogen (which normally is <7%).

The primary insult is to the dermal papillae of the anagen follicle, which induces an early shunt to telogen. Causes for telogen effluvium are shown in **Box 2**.

Clinical Features

Clinically, telogen effluvium has been described as having at least three different clinical scenarios. It can be acute (<6 months), chronic (>6 months), and chronic repetitive.

At the onset, the patient perceives loss >100 scalp hairs. The shedding results in diffuse loss with a more prominent central and frontal scalp loss. The patient

BOX 1 Classification of causes for hair loss according to clinical pattern.[1]

- *Localized nonscarring*:
  - Alopecia areata
  - Trichotillomania
  - Trauma
  - Infection
- *Localized scarring*:
  - Lichen planopilaris (LPP)
  - Discoid lupus erythematosus
  - Frontal fibrosing alopecia
  - Pseudopelade of Brocq
  - Graham–Little syndrome
  - Central centrifugal cicatricial alopecia
  - Morphea/Scleroderma
  - Alopecia mucinosa
  - Folliculitis decalvans
  - Acne keloidalis
  - Infectious
  - Trauma/Traction alopecia
  - Neoplastic
  - Developmental defects
- *Diffuse, nonscarring*:
  - Androgenetic alopecia
  - Telogen effluvium
  - Alopecia areata
  - Anagen effluvium
- *Diffuse, hair shaft abnormalities*:
  - Structural defects with increased fragility
    - Monilethrix (beading of hair)
    - Pseudomonilethrix pili torti (twisting of hair)
    - Trichorrhexis nodosa
    - Trichothiodystrophy
    - Trichorrhexis invaginata (bamboo hair)
  - Structural defects without increased fragility
    - Pili annulati (ringed hair)
    - Woolly hair
    - Uncombable hair syndrome
    - Loose anagen hair syndrome

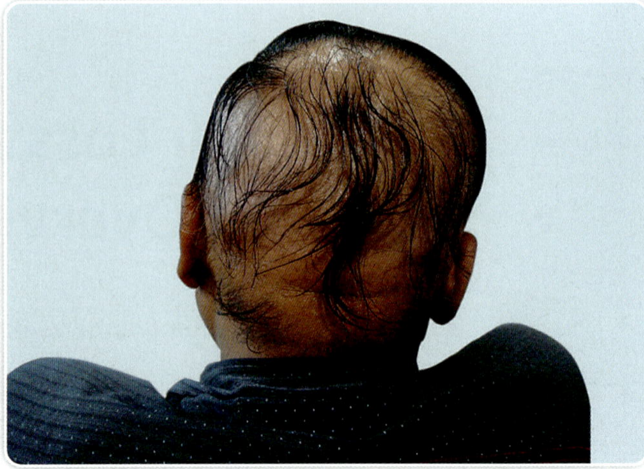

FIG. 1: Extensive alopecia areata.

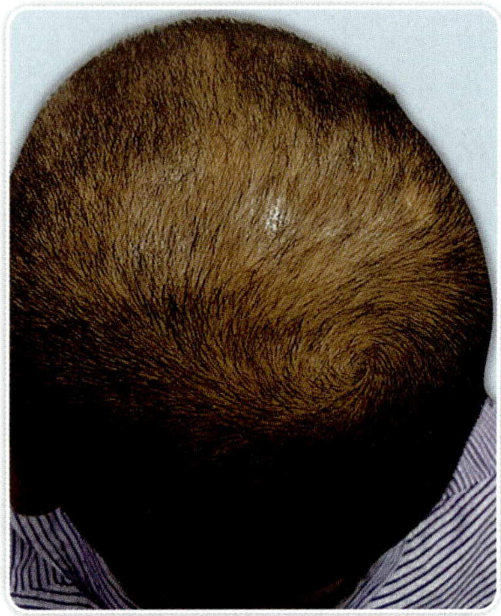

FIG. 2: Diffuse pattern alopecia (DPA).

usually relates loss of body hair to a diminished rate of hair growth. Nutritional causes are one of the major reasons for telogen effluvium. Nonanemic iron deficiency can also lead to this condition, which normalizes on correction of iron status.[7-9]

Diagnostic Techniques

The following laboratory tests are often useful when a nonandrogenetic cause for diffuse hair loss is suspected: Complete blood count, serum iron, serum ferritin, total iron-binding capacity, serum vitamin B12 level, triiodothyronine, thyroxine, and thyroid-stimulating hormone.

It is important to distinguish this pattern of hair loss as it needs medical management according to the etiology and cannot be benefited by hair transplantation.

ALOPECIA AREATA[1,2,6]

Alopecia areata is a complex genetic, autoreactive T-cell-mediated nonscarring disease that targets actively growing anagen hair follicles. It presents with one of the four major patterns:

1. Round or oval patches of hair loss
2. Alopecia totalis (loss of all scalp hair plus eyebrows, eyelashes, beard, axillary hair, and pubic hair)
3. Alopecia universalis (loss of all scalp and body hair)
4. Ophiasis pattern or sisaipho (involving hairlines)

BOX 2 Causes of telogen effluvium.

- *Nutritional*:
  - Rapid weight loss (crash diet)
  - Chronic iron deficiency
  - Protein or calorie deprivation
  - Excessive vitamin A ingestion
- *Stressful events*:
  - Febrile illnesses or chronic illnesses
  - Major surgery or trauma
  - Psychological stress
- *Endocrine*:
  - Hypo- or hyperthyroidism
  - Childbirth, miscarriage, or abortion
  - Discontinuation of estrogen-containing drugs
- *Drugs*:
  - Beta-blocker (propranolol)
  - Cholesterol-lowering agents
  - Captopril
  - Colchicine
  - Retinoids
  - Valproate
  - Selective serotonin reuptake inhibitors (SSRIs)
- *Inflammatory*:
  - Seborrheic dermatitis

Occasionally, a diffuse pattern is also seen causing confusion with androgenetic alopecia.

Pathogenesis

Anagen follicles are attacked by inflammatory T-cell infiltrate and then they move prematurely into catagen, followed by telogen, and then enter a dystrophic anagen status. Most follicles may continue to cycle but, while the disease remains active, are unable to progress beyond an early stage of anagen development and thus do not produce normal hair shafts. An important feature of the pathology is that hair follicles are not destroyed in alopecia areata because the disease spares the follicular stem cell compartment in the mid-outer root sheath region.

Clinical Features

Alopecia areata typically presents with round patches of hair loss, which may be single or multiple or may be coalescing. Scalp is usually normal unlike cicatricial alopecia in which scalp skin is scarred or hardbound with loss of follicular ostia **(Figs. 1 to 5)**. Typical "exclamation mark" hairs, which are short broken hair whose distal ends are broader than the proximal ends, may be present at the periphery of areas of hair loss. White or graying hairs are frequently spared. It can also affect other body hair, e.g., eyebrows, eyelashes, beard, and mustache.

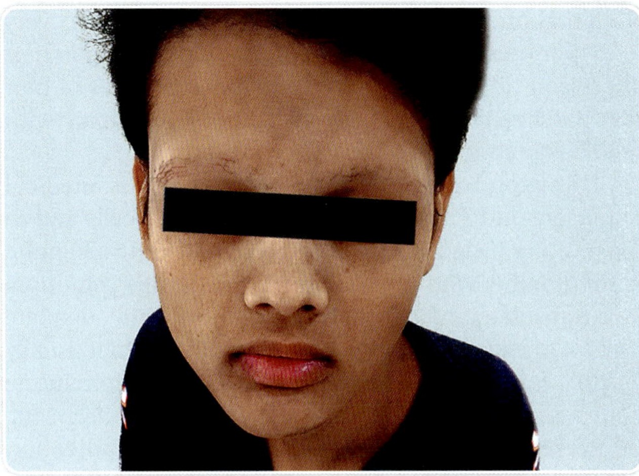

FIG. 3: Alopecia areata causing loss of hair from eyebrow, eyelashes, beard, and mustache.

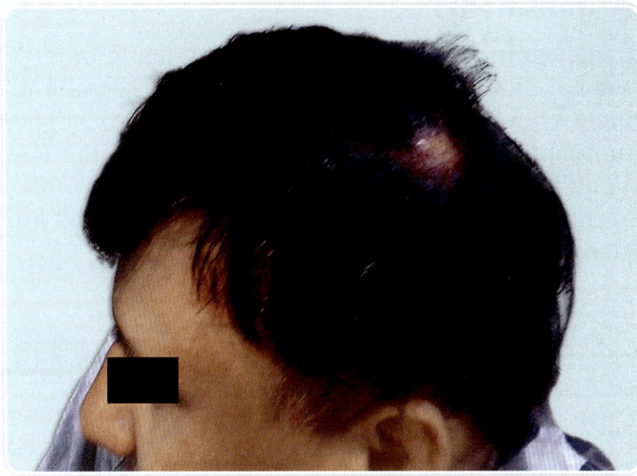

FIG. 4: Alopecia areata—spontaneous hair regrowth after nonsurgical management.

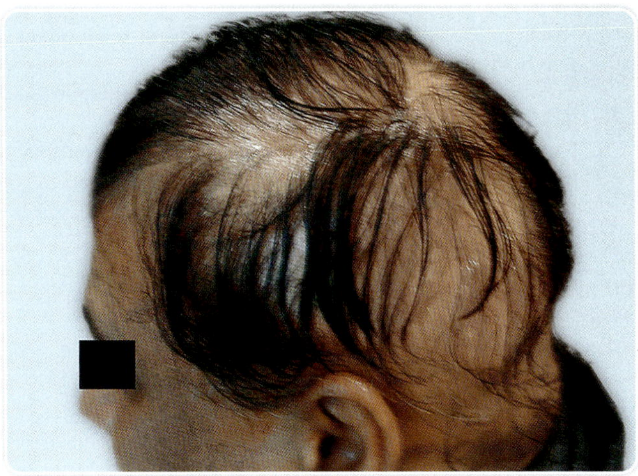

FIG. 5: Alopecia areata before medical management.

It may present with intermittent spontaneous recovery with periodic exacerbations of the hair loss patches. There can be a past history of such occurrences of hair loss patches in childhood with complete recovery with medical treatment.

This group of hair loss conditions needs medical management to suppress the autoreactive T cells and in most of the instances, hair regrows upon controlling the autoimmunity with medical treatment. In this condition, hair transplant should not be considered until adequate trials of medical treatment are given. Surgery is not usually feasible for alopecia areata because of the autoimmune nature and unpredictability of the course of alopecia areata.

Presence of alopecia areata is a contraindication to take up a case for surgery for androgenetic alopecia. Hence, a search should be made for the presence of small lesions indicative of alopecia areata.

Treatment

Treatment includes steroids—topical, systemic, or intralesional; immunomodulatory agents, e.g., tacrolimus, pimecrolimus; and counterirritants, e.g., phenol, topical immunotherapy with diphencyprone, phototherapy, steroids.

Scarring Alopecia **(Fig. 6)** is dealt with in detail in a later chapter 10.

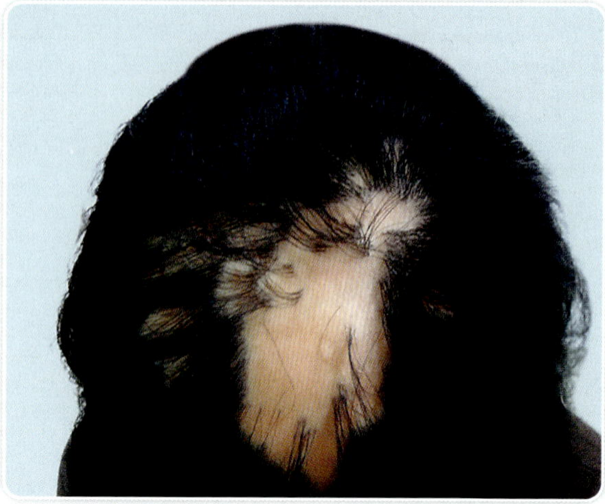

FIG. 6: Cicatricial alopecia—lichen planopilaris.

SUMMARY

A hair transplant surgeon needs to be aware of different causes for hair loss, which need to be managed appropriately.

This is particularly important because many hair transplant surgeons are not dermatologists.

Referral to the dermatologist is necessary in such cases.

REFERENCES

1. Paus R, Oslen EA, Messenger AG. Hair growth disorders. Wolff K, Goldsmith L, Katz S, Gilchrest BA, Paller AS, Leffell DJ (Eds). Fitzpatrick's Dermatology in General Medicine. New York: McGraw Hill; 2008. pp. 753-77.
2. de Berker DAR, Messenger AG, Sinclair RD. Disorders of hair. In: Burns T, Breathnach S, Cox N, Griffiths C (Eds). Rook's Textbook of Dermatology. Massachusetts: Blackwell Science Ltd.; 2004. p. 63(1-120).
3. Hamilton JB. Patterned loss of hair in man; types and incidence. Ann N Y Acad Sci. 1951;53:708-28.
4. Norwood OT. Male pattern baldness: classification and incidence. South Med J. 1975;68:1359-65.
5. Bernstein R. Avoiding pitfalls in planning a hair transplant. Expert Rev Dermatol. 2008;3(4):501-8.
6. Bergfeld WF. Telogen effluvium. McMichael AJ, Hordinsky MK (Eds). Hair and Scalp Disease. New York: Informa Healthcare; 2008. pp. 119-35.
7. Hard S. Non-anemic iron deficiency as an etiologic factor in diffuse loss of hair of the scalp in women. Acta Derm Venereol. 1963;43:562-9.
8. Trost LB, Bergfeld WF, Calogeras E. The diagnosis and treatment of iron deficiency and its potential relationship to hair loss. J Am Acad Dermatol. 2006;54(5):824-44.
9. Olsen EA, Reed K, Cacchio P, Caudill L. Iron deficiency in female pattern hair loss, chronic telogen effluvium, and control groups. J Am Acad Dermatol. 2010;63:991-9.

CHAPTER 8

Telogen Effluvium

Deepthi M

Key Messages

- Telogen effluvium (TE) was first described by Kligman in 1961.
- It is the most common cause of diffuse hair loss—nonscarring.
- It can be acute (<6 months) or chronic (>6 months).
- The causes may be stress, fever and infection, nutritional deficiency, thyroid disorders, systemic illness, etc.
- Careful history, scalp examination, hair pull test, modified wash test, and TrichoScan help in its diagnosis.
- In most instances, it is self-remitting, once the trigger is identified and corrected.
- Chronic telogen effluvium (CTE) is an idiopathic condition with a short anagen phase mainly affecting women of 30–60 years.

INTRODUCTION

Telogen effluvium is one of the most common causes of hair loss. It is characterized by nonscarring diffuse hair loss due to various stressors. The term "telogen effluvium" was coined by Kligman in 1961.[1] The word "effluvium" means "flow out" and TE represents the fall of telogen (club) hair. TE can be acute (<6 months) or chronic (>6 months).

EPIDEMIOLOGY

The incidence of TE among the general population is exactly unknown as many cases are not reported clinically.[2] TE can be noted among all ages, though it is seen more in the elderly (women).[3] Children also can present with TE; its prevalence varies from region to region.[4] Men and women both are affected; however, women may seek medical attention more commonly than men as they have long hair and are more concerned about hair fall.[5]

ETIOPATHOGENESIS

Telogen effluvium is characterized by increased shedding of club-shaped hair than normal due to some trigger which changes the dynamics of hair cycle. Each hair follicle undergoes different phases like anagen, catagen, and telogen in its life cycle. The anagen phase (growing phase) on scalp hair lasts for 3–8 years after which it enters the catagen phase. The catagen phase (involution phase) involves programmed cell death (apoptosis) and lasts for a short time, i.e., 3–4 weeks. After catagen, the hair enters the telogen phase (resting phase) during which the hair assumes club shape and lasts for 3–5 months, after which the hair falls off. At any time on the normal healthy scalp, anagen hair constitutes 80%, catagen hair 1%, and telogen hair 10–15%.[2,6,7] If telogen hair percentage increases, then it results in increased hair fall.

Headington proposed five mechanisms to explain TE.[8] They are as follows:

1. *Immediate anagen release*: When the anagen duration is shortened, the hair prematurely enters the telogen phase resulting in hair fall. For example: Drug-induced hair loss, stress, malnutrition.
2. *Delayed anagen release*: Hair stays for a longer duration in the anagen phase, followed by synchronous telogen shedding. For example: Postpartum TE.
3. *Short anagen syndrome*: This is characterized by shortening of the anagen phase (idiopathic anagen

shortening), leading to persistent TE. For example: Hair growth disorder in children,[9] CTE in women.[10]

4. *Immediate telogen release*: This is a shortened telogen phase resulting in immediate release of telogen hair with premature reentry of hair into anagen. For example: After topical minoxidil application.
5. *Delayed telogen release*: This is a prolonged telogen phase and a delayed transition to anagen phase.

The causes of TE can be drugs, stress, loss of weight, fever, etc., as listed in **Table 1**.

CLINICAL PRESENTATION

Acute Telogen Effluvium

Acute telogen effluvium (ATE) is characterized by sudden, abrupt diffuse hair loss that typically starts 2–3 months after an insult and usually recovers within 6 months once the trigger is removed. If ATE is not spontaneously remitting even after the identified stressor removal, then suspect early androgenetic alopecia (AGA) or diffuse alopecia areata. A trichoscopy examination helps in such scenario.

Chronic Telogen Effluvium

Chronic telogen effluvium (CTE) is characterized by diffuse hair loss lasting >6 months without widening of partition or miniaturization of hair. It was first described by David Whiting in 1996.[23] The etiology maybe idiopathic with shortening of the anagen phase.[24] It is now considered a different condition from chronic diffuse hair loss (CDHL). It is seen in women of 30–60 years of age.[25] There may/may not be a triggering factor to initiate hair loss in these patients. Examination reveals short regrowing hair in frontal and bitemporal areas with normal thickness. It is differentiated from ATE due to its prolonged hair loss and fluctuant course for many years. Reassurance is needed that the condition is not baldness as the patients fear baldness.

DIAGNOSIS

A thorough history, appropriate laboratory investigations, clinical examination of scalp, hair pull test, trichoscopy, and modified wash test help in diagnosing the condition. A scalp biopsy is rarely needed in order to differentiate it from other causes of diffuse hair loss, for example, diffuse alopecia areata and AGA.

Clinical History

A thorough history of any illness, fever, nutrition, stress, drug history, and personal history including any change in residence or work environment should be taken.[19]

Trichodynia is an important but nonuniform symptom associated with patients with TE or both TE and AGA.[26] The patient complains of pain, paresthesia, or discomfort in the skin of scalp. The exact cause of it is unknown but may correlate with the emotional stress of the patient.[27,28]

TABLE 1: Causes of telogen effluvium.

Type	Causes	Remarks
Acute telogen effluvium	Effluvium of newborn	Starts within 4 months and completes by 6 months
	Emotional stress	Change in work, residence, close kin loss,[11] etc.
	Fever	Viral, typhoid, COVID-19,[12] etc. infections
	Hospitalization and surgery	
	Pregnancy	2–5 months postpartum[13]
	Medications	Anticonvulsants, antithyroid, antihypertensives, oral retinoids, minoxidil, HRT, hypolipidemic, anticoagulants[14]
	Seasonal	Actinic effluvium due to sunlight, especially UV light (July to October)[15]
	Weight loss	Fasting or weight loss diets[16]
Chronic telogen effluvium	Nutritional deficiencies	Severe Zn, iron, protein, vitamin D deficiencies[17]
	Chronic starvation	Anorexia nervosa[18]
	Chronic systemic illness	SLE, dermatomyositis, IBD, malignancies[19,20]
	Endocrine	Thyroid (hypo and hyper)[19,20]
	Infections	Syphilis[21] and HIV[22]

(HIV: human immunodeficiency virus; HRT: hormone replacement therapy; IBD: inflammatory bowel disease; SLE: systemic lupus erythematosus; UV: ultraviolet)

Clinical Examination of Scalp

Careful examination of the scalp should be done to look for signs of inflammation such as erythema, scaling, hair shaft shape, length variation, density, and pattern of hair loss, and whether there is widening of hair partition or temporal recession.

Hair pull test:[29] About 50–60 hairs are grasped between the index and thumb fingers and the hairs are pulled away from the scalp slowly and firmly. Usually, two to three hairs are pulled out. More than 10% of pulled-out hair in four different quadrants indicates a positive test, provided the patient did not wash the hair for at least 24 hours prior to the test. It is an unreliable and less-sensitive test.[22]

Modified hair wash test:[30,31] The patient is advised to not wash scalp hair for 5 days and asked to wash the hair in a basin with a drain. The hair that is collected in the drain is collected and measured.

- *TE*: >100 shed hair, <10% vellus
- *AGA*: <100 shed hair, >10% vellus
- *Association of TE and AGA*: >100 shed hair, >10% vellus
- *Normal or remitting TE*: <100 shed hair, <10% vellus

Laboratory Investigations

Routine blood investigations such as complete blood counts (rule out anemia), thyroid profile, and advanced investigations to rule out deficiencies like liver function tests (protein), serum ferritin and total iron-binding capacity, serum zinc, and vitamin D can help in identifying the underlying cause.[11]

Trichoscopy[32]

Most cases have cut down the need for scalp biopsy to diagnose TE. TE shows decreased hair density globally on the scalp, empty hair follicles, and absence of miniaturized hair (<20% hair follicle size variability). Absence of hair diameter variation and pearly white dots (papules representing sebaceous gland hyperplasia) and involvement of scalp globally than in a pattern, differentiates TE from AGA.

Scalp Biopsy

It is suggested in patients with CDHL of >6 months' duration, especially in women to differentiate from female pattern hair loss (FPHL). Horizontal sectioning with a 5-mm punch biopsy at the level of reticular dermis and subcutaneous tissue is helpful. TE shows an increase in telogen ratio, normal hair diameter, and lack of inflammatory cells/fibrosis. In CTE, the anagen-to-telogen ratio is 8:1 when compared to normal scalp 14:1. The terminal-to-vellus hair ratio in CTE is more than 8:1 and it is less than 4:1 in FPHL patients.[33] Sometimes, a single biopsy is inconclusive and hence multiple biopsies may be needed for better diagnosis.

DIFFERENTIAL DIAGNOSIS

Telogen effluvium should be differentiated from other causes of diffuse hair loss such as patterned hair loss, trichotillomania, diffuse alopecia areata, psychogenic pseudoeffluvium, and anagen effluvium. The differences between pattern hair loss and TE are mentioned in **Table 2**.

Telogen gravidarum: Women experience a sudden abrupt diffuse nonscarring hair loss 2–5 months postpartum that stops within 6 months spontaneously. This is due to the drop in female hormones postpartum, especially estrogen as during the pregnancy it prolongs the anagen phase. It is usually self-remitting and does not require active management.[34]

TABLE 2: Differences between androgenetic alopecia (AGA) and telogen effluvium (TE).

	TE	Female pattern hair loss (FPHL)
Onset of hair fall	Abrupt sudden severe hair loss	Gradual onset
History	Preceded by trigger	Family history of baldness
Distribution	Diffuse sparsity of hair globally	Usually widened partition
Hair pull test	Hair pull test positive	Usually negative
Trichoscopy		
Empty hair follicles Miniaturization >20% Upright regrowing hair Peripilar sign	Present Absent Present Present	Present Present Absent Common
Scalp biopsy		
Terminal:velus hair	>8:1	<4:1

MANAGEMENT

The management involves understanding the distress of the patient, identifying the cause, and proper counseling. In most of the cases of TE, once the stressor is identified and addressed, the shedding of hair will be stopped within 6 months with regrowth of hair. Patients should be assured that regrowth is usually complete. Underlying disorders such as thyroid and anemia should be addressed.

Oral Nutrition Supplements

All patients of TE should be advised a balanced diet. Protein supplements can be advised in patients deficient in protein, for example, pure vegan diet. Nutritional supplements such as multivitamins, amino acids, iron, calcium, zinc, B12, folic acid, copper, and selenium can have an important role in the treatment of TE as they help in promoting hair growth and maintenance of hair structure.[11,17] Vitamin D and iron supplementation helps in patients with underlying deficient states and should be advised for at least a period of 3–6 months till the deficiencies are corrected.[35,36] Iron supplements should not be prescribed for a longer period, otherwise it leads to hemochromatosis. Oral biotin supplements can be advised within recommended dietary allowance (RDA), i.e., 30 µg. Biotin is a part of B vitamin complex and is water soluble. Anything in excess is excreted in urine. There is no evidence to suggest that higher doses of biotin help in hair loss patients.[37]

Topical Growth Serums with Peptides

Many peptides and growth serums are available in the market. There is varied evidence for their role in the management of hair loss. Probable mechanisms include improving vascularity, increasing anagen duration, decreasing inflammation and may help in hair growth in TE patients.[38] They can be combined with topical minoxidil preparations in CTE patients.[11]

Topical Minoxidil

Topical minoxidil is a potassium channel opener, causes vasodilatation, and helps to prolong the anagen phase. It may help in cases of CTE by prolonging the anagen phase.[39] 2% minoxidil in female patients and 5% in male patients is usually advised. Patients should be warned that there may be more hair loss initially when they start the treatment. It is not recommended in ATE patients as in most cases, it is self-remitting. Oral minoxidil is also tried in CTE patients where they could not tolerate topical minoxidil solution.[40]

Platelet-rich Plasma

In contrast to patterned hair loss patients, platelet-rich plasma (PRP) has little evidence in the management of TE patients. It may be tried in patients with CDHL who show early changes of AGA.[41]

Role of Mesotherapy

Mesotherapy with various cocktail solutions such as biotin, plant extracts, vitamins, minoxidil, and finasteride has been tried in the past. Except for minoxidil and finasteride, there is no clinical evidence or literature to support their efficacy in hair loss management.[42]

Oils and Shampoos

Patients need to be educated that oils and shampoos do not promote hair growth. Oils act only as lubricants and provide preconditioning to hair by smoothening the cuticle. Oils like coconut/almond can be applied 30–60 minutes prior to hair wash to the hair shaft. Patients are advised to thoroughly rinse shampoo and avoid aggressive rubbing of hair during shampooing to avoid friction-induced hair loss.

SUMMARY

Telogen effluvium is a nonscarring diffuse hair loss condition which is usually self-remitting. Reassurance that the condition can recover and it is not baldness should be emphasized. Identifying the trigger and correcting it are enough in most instances. Active management may be advised in patients where hair loss prolongs beyond 6 months or there are early signs of miniaturization.

Tips and Pearls

- TE in most instances is a self-remitting condition.
- Identifying trigger by proper history is essential.
- ATE may require removal of trigger and nutritional supplements and topical growth peptides.
- CTE requires thorough investigations, correction of deficiency if any, topical peptides, and topical 2% minoxidil lotion.
- Trichoscopy has reduced the necessity of scalp biopsy in differentiating CTE from other diffuse hair loss like diffuse alopecia areata and early FPHL.

REFERENCES

1. Kligman AM. Pathologic dynamics of human hair loss. I. Telogen effluvium. Arch Dermatol. 1961;83:175-98.
2. Harrison S, Sinclair R. Telogen effluvium. Clin Exp Dermatol. 2002;27(5):389-95.
3. Sulzberger MB, Witten VH, Kopf AW. Diffuse alopecia in women. Its unexplained apparent increase in incidence. Arch Dermatol. 1960;81:556-60.
4. Al-Refu K. Hair loss in children: common and uncommon causes; clinical and epidemiological study in Jordan. Int J Trichology. 2013;5(4):185-9.
5. Grover C, Khurana A. Telogen effluvium. Indian J Dermatol Venereol Leprol. 2013;79(5):591-603.
6. Kligman AM. The human hair cycle. J Invest Dermatol. 1959;33:307-16.
7. Lindner G, Botchkarev VA, Botchkareva NV, Ling G, van der Veen C, Paus R. Analysis of apoptosis during hair follicle regression (catagen). Am J Pathol. 1997;151(6):1601-17.
8. Headington JT. Telogen effluvium. New concepts and review. Arch Dermatol. 1993;129(3):356-63.
9. Trueb RM. Diffuse hair loss. In: Blume-Peytavi U, Tosti A, Whiting DA, Trueb R (Eds). Hair Growth and Disorders. Berlin: Springer; 2008. pp. 259-72.
10. Gilmore S, Sinclair R. Chronic telogen effluvium is due to a reduction in the variance of anagen duration. Australas J Dermatol. 2010;51(3):163-7.
11. Mysore V, Parthasaradhi A, Kharkar RD, Ghoshal AK, Ganjoo A, Ravichandran G, et al. Expert consensus on the management of Telogen Effluvium in India. Int J Trichology. 2019;11(3):107-12.
12. Inamadar AC. Covid Induced Telogen Effluvium (CITE): an insight. Indian Dermatol Online J. 2022;13(4):445-8.
13. Rebora A, Guarrera M, Drago F. Postpartum telogen effluvium. J Eur Acad Dermatol Venereol. 2016;30:518.
14. Tosi A, Misciali C, Piraccini BM, Peluso AM, Bardazzi F. Drug-induced hair loss and hair growth. Incidence, management and avoidance. Drug Saf. 1994;10(4):310-7.
15. Piérard-Franchimont C, Peérard GE. L'effluvium télogène actinique: une facette de la chronobiologie humaine. Int J Cosmet Sci. 1999;21(1):15-21.
16. Goette DK, Odom RB. Alopecia in crash dieters. JAMA. 1976;235(24):2622-3.
17. Guo EL, Katta R. Diet and hair loss: effects of nutrient deficiency and supplement use. Dermatol Pract Concept. 2017;7(1):1-10.
18. Strumia R. Skin signs in anorexia nervosa. Dermatoendocrinol. 2009;1:268-70.
19. Harrison S, Bergfeld W. Diffuse hair loss: its triggers and management. Cleve Clin J Med. 2009;76(6):361-7.
20. Sperling LC. Hair and systemic disease. Dermatol Clin. 2001;19(4):711-26, ix.
21. Kennedy C. Syphilis presenting as hair loss. Br Med J. 1976;2:854.
22. Barcaui CB, Gonçalves da Silva AM, Sotto MN, Genser B. Stem cell apoptosis in HIV-1 alopecia. J Cutan Pathol. 2006;33:667-71.
23. Whiting DA. Chronic telogen effluvium. Dermatol Clin. 1996;14(4):723-31.
24. Gilmore S, Sinclair R. Chronic telogen effluvium is due to a reduction in the variance of anagen duration. Australas J Dermatol 2010;51:163-7.
25. Shrivastava SB. Diffuse hair loss in an adult female: approach to diagnosis and management. Indian J Dermatol Venereol Leprol. 2009;75:20-7.
26. Kivanç-Altunay I, Savaş C, Gökdemir G, Köşlü A, Ayaydin EB. The presence of trichodynia in patients with telogen effluvium and androgenetic alopecia. Int J Dermatol. 2003;42:691-3.
27. Grimalt R, Ferrando J, Grimalt F. Trichodynia. Dermatology. 1998;196:374.
28. Rebora A. Trichodynia: a review of the literature. Int J Dermatol. 2016;55(4):382-4.
29. Chong AH, Wade M, Sinclair RD. The hair pull test and the hair pluck for analysis of hair abnormalities. Modern Med Australia. 1999;42:105-10.
30. Guarrera M, Fiorucci MC, Rebora A. Methods of hair loss evaluation: a comparison of TrichoScan(®) with the modified wash test. Exp Dermatol. 2013;22(7):482-4.
31. Asghar F, Shamim N, Farooque U, Sheikh H, Aqeel R. Telogen effluvium: a review of the literature. Cureus. 2020;12(5):e8320.
32. Inui S. Trichoscopy: a new frontier for the diagnosis of hair diseases. Expert Rev Dermatol. 2012;7:429-37.
33. Eudy G, Solomon AR. The histopathology of noncicatricial alopecia. Semin Cutan Med Surg. 2006;25:35-40.
34. Rebora A, Guarrera M, Drago F. Postpartum telogen effluvium. J Eur Acad Dermatol Venereol. 2016;30(3):518.
35. Moeinvaziri M, Mansoori P, Holakooee K, Safaee Naraghi Z, Abbasi A. Iron status in diffuse telogen hair loss among women. Acta Dermatovenerol Croat. 2009;17(4):279-84.
36. McMichael A. Approach to office visits for hair loss in women. Cutis. 2011;87(1):8-9.
37. Trüeb RM. Serum biotin levels in women complaining of hair loss. Int J Trichology. 2016;8:73-7.
38. Sadgrove NJ, Simmonds MSJ. Topical and nutricosmetic products for healthy hair and dermal antiaging using "dual-acting" (2 for 1) plant-based peptides, hormones, and cannabinoids. FASEB Bioadv. 2021;3(8):601-10.
39. Buhl AE, Waldon DJ, Baker CA, Johnson GA. Minoxidil sulfate is the active metabolite that stimulates hair follicles. J Invest Dermatol. 1990;95(5):553-7.
40. Perera E, Sinclair R. Treatment of chronic telogen effluvium with oral minoxidil: a retrospective study. F1000Res. 2017;6:1650.
41. Garg S, Manchanda S. Platelet-rich plasma-an 'elixir' for treatment of alopecia: personal experience on 117 patients with review of literature. Stem Cell Investig. 2017;4:64.
42. Mysore V. Mesotherapy in management of hairloss—is it of any use? Int J Trichology. 2010;2(1):45-6.

CHAPTER 9

Alopecia Areata

Radhika V Kaujalgi

Key Messages

- Alopecia areata is the most common type of nonscarring alopecia seen in both children and adults.
- Etiopathogenesis is discussed here with respect to genetic, environmental, and immunologic factors.
- Clinical presentation and various patterns are explained in detail along with associated conditions.
- Various treatments in the form of topical, intralesional and systemic corticosteroids, systemic Janus kinase (JAK) inhibitors, and topical minoxidil are discussed.

INTRODUCTION

Alopecia areata (AA) is a common, chronic, inflammatory, nonscarring type of hair loss. AA can present in many ways, ranging from small, well-circumscribed patches of hair loss to a complete absence of scalp and body hair. Patients affected by AA comprise all age groups, sexes, and ethnicities. Patients with AA frequently experience marked impairment in psychological well-being and self-esteem and may be more likely to suffer from psychiatric comorbidities.[1]

EPIDEMIOLOGY

Both sexes are equally affected by AA, affecting individuals of all ages and accounts for 0.1–0.2% of the general population.[1] AA is predicted to have a cumulative lifetime incidence of 2% in the US population and a prevalence of 0.1–0.2%. 60% of patients present with the first patch before 20 years of age.

ETIOPATHOGENESIS

During a typical growth cycle, the hair follicle goes through three phases: Anagen, catagen, and telogen. The longest phase, known as the anagen phase (2–6 years), is regarded as the growth phase. Hair growth is halted during the catagen phase (2–4 weeks), during which keratinocyte apoptosis takes place. The hair progressively starts to fall out during the telogen phase (2–3 months), which is followed by the start of a new growth cycle. Hair loss in AA patients may result from a disruption in one of these follicle growth phases, such as an early change from the anagen to catagen or anagen to telogen phase. AA is caused by genetic, immunologic, and environmental factors.[1]

Environmental factors: Stress and psychological problems can be the causes that lead to the development of AA. Food, chemicals, and infections have all been suggested as potential disease triggers. A diet rich in soy may control inflammatory activity and hence prevent AA.

Immunologic factors: Although the anagen hair follicle is typically an immune-privileged location, AA disrupts this. These modifications improve hair follicle cell's ability to deliver antigens and the movement of T lymphocytes toward hair follicles in AA lesions.

Autoimmune Hypothesis

Invading autoreactive T lymphocytes spare the stem cell compartment and enter the hair follicle. Disease severity and CD8+ T-cell density are correlated. Autoantigens produced by hair follicles may be at play. A "swarm of bees," or a concentration of inflammatory cells (mainly T cells), toward the bulb region of hair follicles, was the first indication of autoimmunity in AA toward hair follicles. An important percentage of the infiltration is made up of CD8+ T cells and CD4+ T cells, and antigen-presenting cells such as Langerhans cells are more prevalent than usual.

Genetic factors: A lot of AA instances are sporadic. Three different types of studies have been used to support assertions that strongly link genetic variables to the onset of the condition: (1) Family based connections, (2) studies based on heredity in first-degree relatives, where a positive familial incidence of 10–42% for AA has been documented, and (3) studies in monozygotic twins, where a concordance of 50% of getting the condition has been seen. Additionally, AA is polygenic in origin. To comprehend the immunological mechanisms connected to AA, genome-wide association studies (GWAS) are carried out. Stress-induced compounds known as natural killer group 2 member D (NKG2D) ligands function as danger signals for immune cells by interacting with the NKG2D receptor. A function for CD8+ NKG2D+ cytotoxic T cells in AA is supported by the fact that NKG2D+ cells are CD8+ T cells.[2] AA has an increased Janus kinase (JAK)/signal transducers and activators of transcription pathway but normal hair follicles do not. JAK1/2 is signalled by interferon gamma (IFN-γ), whereas JAK1/3 is signalled by interleukin 15 (IL-15). JAK inhibitors, including tofacitinib, ruxolitinib, and baricitinib, target the IFN-γ and IL-15 pathways. The mechanism is explained in **Figure 1**.

ASSOCIATED CONDITIONS

Atopy (including atopic dermatitis, asthma, and allergic rhinitis) and other autoimmune disorders may increase

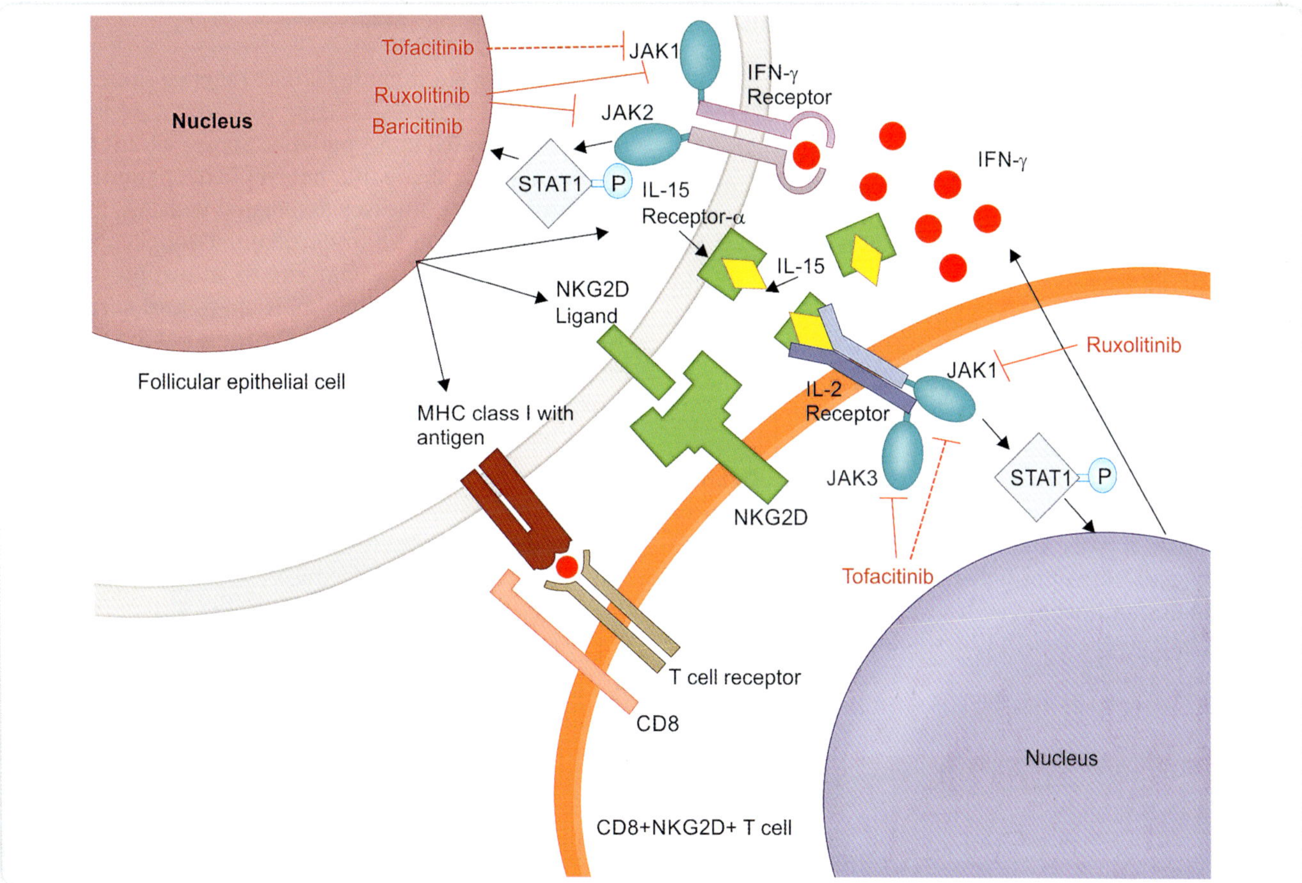

FIG. 1: Interferon-gamma (IFN-γ), which signals through Janus kinases 1 (JAK1) and JAK2 to increase production of interleukin-15 (IL-15), is produced by CD8+ T cells in alopecia areata. When IL-15 and the IL-15 receptor (also known as the chaperone protein) connect to the surface of CD8+ T cells, JAK1 and JAK3 are signalled, which increases the production of IFN-γ. The JAK inhibitors tofacitinib, ruxolitinib, and baricitinib have been found to have an impact on this pathway.

(MHC: major histocompatibility; NKG2D: natural killer group 2 member D)

Source: Reproduced from Strazzulla et al. (2018).[1]

the risk of developing AA. Multiple autoimmune illnesses, including thyroid disease (8–11.8%), psoriasis, and vitiligo (4.1%), have been linked to AA. Diabetes mellitus (3.2%), Down's syndrome, Addison's disease, autosomal recessive polyglandular syndrome, systemic lupus erythematosus, celiac disease, ulcerative colitis, multiple sclerosis, rheumatoid arthritis (0.9%), and pernicious anemia (10–60%) are other linked disorders. Mood and anxiety disorders are widespread in AA and can have a severe impact on one's quality of life. In 40–50% of AA patients, early cataract, fundus abnormalities, and punctate lens opacities may arise.[3]

CLINICAL PRESENTATION

Alopecia areata most typically manifests as well-defined areas of nonscarring, inflammatory hair loss that can spread to include the entire scalp, eyebrows, eyelashes, beard, and body hairs. Exclamation mark hairs are visible within or around the borders of the patches. These are short, broken hairs with proximal tapering near the scalp and distal thickening and broadening. The presence of exclamation mark hairs near the border indicates that the patch is active and progressing. The diagnosis is clinical in the majority of the cases. In uncertain circumstances, dermoscopy can be helpful. AA can develop to encompass all scalp hairs [alopecia totalis (AT)] or all scalp and body hairs [alopecia universalis (AU)] in severely affected patients.[1] AT/AU could develop in 5% of patchy AA. AA regrowth is typically white at first, followed by repigmentation.

Nail abnormalities that may be seen include geometric pitting (multiple, small, superficial pits regularly distributed along transverse and longitudinal lines), geometric punctate leukonychia (multiple white spots in a grill pattern), brittleness, striations, longitudinal ridging, Beau's nails, trachyonychia (sandpaper nails), onychorrhexis, onychomadesis, koilonychia, and red lunula. Males and people with severe AA are more likely to have nail alterations.[3] Classification of alopecia is mentioned in **Table 1**.

TABLE 1: Classification of alopecia.

Based on extent	New variants
Patchy alopecia, alopecia totalis, alopecia universalis	Acute and diffuse total alopecia
Based on pattern	**Unusual patterns**
• Reticular • Ophiasis • Sisaipho	• Perinevoid alopecia • Linear

CLINICAL SUBTYPES

Patients with the ophiasis subtype of AA exhibit band-like alopecia that commonly starts at the occipital hairline and spreads to the temples, or it can start at the frontal hairline. The sisaipho subtype has the reverse distribution, causing hair loss at the frontal, temporal, and parietal scalp but sparing hairs at the scalp's margin and looking similar to androgenetic alopecia. Furthermore, a "sudden graying" or "white overnight" type of AA causes pigmented hair loss. Perinevoid AA refers to hair loss that occurs around pigmented nevi, but removing the nevi has no effect on the hair loss.[3] Acute diffuse and complete alopecia is a more recently characterized form that causes diffuse and sudden hair loss, usually in women, and lasts around 3 months before regrowth, though recurrence is a possibility. Another unique presentation is the hair loss at the bitemporal area, which may be the only feature of AA.[4] An image of patchy AA is shown in **Figure 2**.

INVESTIGATIONS

Biomarkers of AA include IL-6, C-reactive protein (CRP), and vitamin D levels. Serum IL-6 and CRP levels are markedly elevated in AA patients. Serum vitamin D levels, on the other hand, are much lower in AA patients. To rule out autoimmune illnesses associated with AA, laboratory investigations may be undertaken. Trichoscopy should be performed on the patient to allow for a deeper examination of the follicle, hair shaft, and surrounding skin, as well as to help choose the ideal patch to acquire a biopsy specimen for the most accurate result. Black dots, broken hairs, tapering hair (exclamation marks), and short vellus hairs are trichoscopic features of AA. The presence

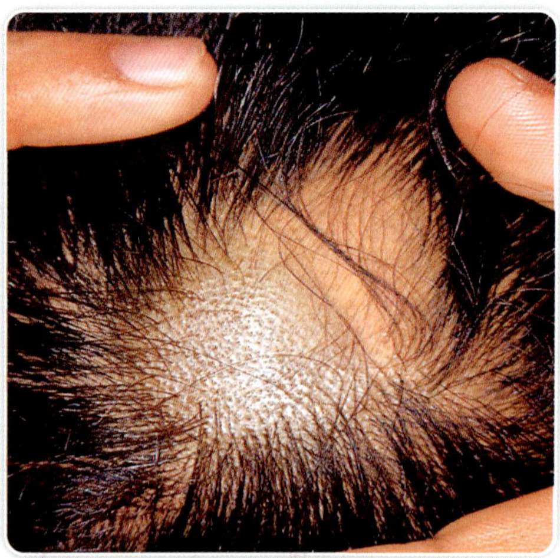

FIG. 2: Patchy alopecia areata on the scalp.

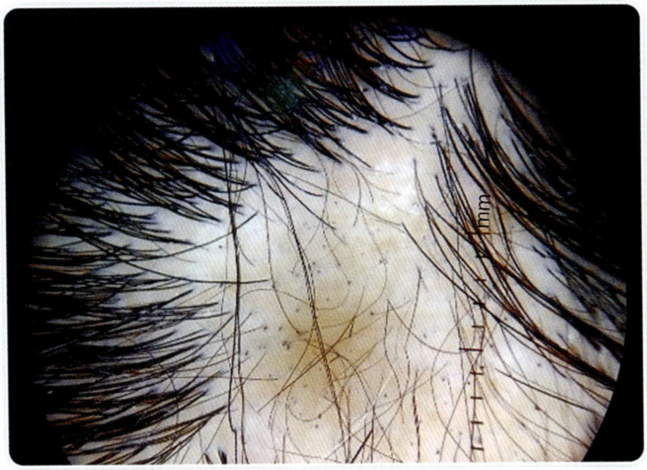

FIG. 3: Dermoscopy showing exclamation mark hair, short vellus hairs, black dots.

of black dots, broken hair, and tapering hair indicates the presence of active disease. Black and yellow spots are proportionate to the severity of AA, while tapering hair has no link with severity. Cadaverized hairs are hairs that have been fragmented before emerging from the scalp and can be seen in AA.[3] An image of dermoscopy is shown in **Figure 3**.

A Severity Alopecia Tool (SALT) score can be calculated by visually assessing the degree of terminal hair loss in four different perspectives of the scalp (top, posterior, right side, and left side of the scalp) and can be used to track the response to therapy. The SALT score can be used to determine the quantitative assessment of scalp hair loss.[5]

TREATMENT

Alopecia areata is mostly an aesthetic issue that causes greater emotional concerns, particularly in children and women. Proper counselled and explaining potential true expectations of various treatments are critical. **Table 2** lists the recommended therapy options. **Table 3** discusses the treatment plan.

Corticosteroids

Because of their anti-inflammatory properties, corticosteroids have been the basis of AA treatment. They are used topically, orally, and parenterally.

Topical steroids are used with varying degrees of efficacy. Desowen lotion 0.1%, fluocinolone acetonide 0.025% cream, 0.1% lotion, 0.05% betamethasone dipropionate lotion, and 0.05% clobetasol propionate lotion have all been used. Salicylic acid is used in combination with clobetasol propionate. It is advised to apply 1 cm beyond the affected area. Because of their ease of use, topical steroids are the preferred first-line treatment for AA.

TABLE 2: Treatment options for alopecia areata.

First-line therapies	
	Corticosteroids, intralesional
Corticosteroids, topical	Minoxidil
Second-line therapies	
Anthralin	Contact immunotherapy
Prostaglandin analogs	
Corticosteroids, systemic	Antihistamine
Cryotherapy, superficial	Platelet-rich plasma
Excimer laser	Tretinoin
	Capsaicin
	Azelaic acid
	Antidepressant
Garlic gel	Calcipotriol
Onion juice	PUVA
Third-line therapies	
JAK/STAT inhibitor	Sulfasalazine
Cyclosporine	Azathioprine
Methotrexate	IL-12/IL-23p40 blocker

(IL: interleukin; JAK/STAT: Janus kinase/signal transducer and activator of transcription; PUVA: psoralen with ultraviolet A)

TABLE 3: Alopecia areata treatment plan.

	>10 years	
<10 years	**<50%**	**>50%**
Topical steroid Topical anthralin JAK inhibitors	Topical steroid Topical minoxidil Intralesional steroids Topical anthralin	Topical steroid Topical minoxidil Topical immunotherapy Topical anthralin Systemic PUVA Systemic cyclosporine Scalp prosthesis

(PUVA: psoralen with ultraviolet A)

Intralesional corticosteroids have been used in the treatment of AA since 1958, and it is the therapy of choice for people with patchy AA (50%) with success rates of 60–75%. Immunosuppression is the primary mode of action. It is preferable to use triamcinolone acetonide.[6] It should be injected once every 4–6 weeks into the deep dermis or upper subcutaneous tissue with a 0.5-inch long 30-gauge needle at various locations 1 cm apart and 0.1 mL into each site. Different concentrations (2.5–10 mg/mL) are employed, with 10 mg/mL favored for the scalp and 2.5 mg/mL preferred for the eyebrows and face (beard area).

Systemic corticosteroids are given in daily, weekly, and monthly pulses with good results in patchy AA but less so in ophiasis, AT, and AU. There has been effectiveness with oral dexamethasone 0.5 mg/kg/day and injectable triamcinolone acetonide 40 mg/month. Use 40–60 mg of prednisone per day and taper by 5 mg/wk for active disease involving >50% of scalp area. Steroids can be used for 1–6 months, but longer periods should be avoided. To avoid the negative effects, pulse treatments are being investigated. Oral pulse therapy is more effective and tolerable, with fewer adverse effects. Contraindications and side effects should be discussed with the patients, and those should be identified by the practitioner at the right time.[3,7]

Minoxidil

Minoxidil is a biologic response modulator that promotes hair growth. It is used twice a day, in the morning and evening, and a 5% solution is more effective than a 2% solution. The first signs of hair regeneration appear after 12 weeks. Younger individuals respond more quickly than elderly patients. Minoxidil gives good results when combined with topical or intralesional steroids or anthralin. At night, use betamethasone dipropionate cream alone or in conjunction with salicylic acid to the patchy area. This combination therapy is ineffective in AT/AU patients.[8,9]

Role of JAK/STAT Inhibitors in Alopecia Areata

JAK/STAT (signal transducer and activator of transcription) signaling is a distinct intracellular signaling mechanism. When external ligands bind to intracellular JAK proteins, they become activated and phosphorylate STAT proteins, which dimerize and then translocate into the nucleus to regulate gene expression directly. JAKs are classified into four types: JAK1, JAK2, JAK3, and TYK2. The Food and Drug Administration has approved two JAK inhibitors for use in the United States (ruxolitinib and tofacitinib). Tofacitinib is a JAK inhibitor licensed by the Food and Drug Administration that inhibits JAK1, JAK2, and JAK3, but primarily JAK3. It can be taken once or twice a day in 5-mg/11-mg doses. Prior to starting tofacitinib, investigations such as complete blood count, liver function tests, renal function tests, Mantoux test, chest X-ray, Quantiferon Gold test, and a complete lipid profile must be performed. The most common side effects of tofacitinib are bacterial, mycobacterial, fungal, and viral infections, a rise in serum creatinine, anemia, neutropenia, thrombocytopenia, hypercholesterolemia, and pulmonary tuberculosis reactivation.[10]

Treatment of Children with Alopecia Areata

Children's therapeutic alternatives are limited due to lower tolerance and probable side effects. The first line of therapy is moderate corticosteroids. Topical minoxidil in children >10 years and topical immunotherapy are the other options. Systemic JAK inhibitors (tofacitinib) in children >2 years old are used, in a dosage of 5 mg once daily for a period ranging from 1 to 6 months depending upon the degree of improvement. Psychological issues in children are a key worry, and they should be addressed with good counselled for both the parents and the child. Systemic cyclosporine can be used in older children >14 years.[11]

SUMMARY

Alopecia areata is a prevalent type of hair loss that has a negative impact on the quality of life for many. The primary etiologies are genetic vulnerability, environmental factors, and autoimmunity. The main genes revealed by GWAS have paved the way for a better understanding of the pathogenesis of AA. There is a scarcity of controlled trials on successful AA treatments. Corticosteroids are the cornerstone of AA treatment. Minoxidil, immunotherapy, and psoralen with ultraviolet A (PUVA) are the additional options. T-cell pathways and NK-cell stimulating ligands are the focus of newer therapeutics.

Tips and Pearls

- Thyroid abnormalities are the most common associated conditions seen in alopecia areata.
- Poor prognostic factors in alopecia areata include early age at onset, positive family history, severe disease, and history of atopy.
- Patchy alopecia areata shows 50–80% spontaneous recovery in 1 year.
- Systemic JAK inhibitors are among the newest treatments in treating alopecia totalis/alopecia universalis.

REFERENCES

1. Strazzulla LC, Wang EHC, Avila L, Sicco KL, Brinster N, Christiano AM, et al. Alopecia areata: disease characteristics, clinical evaluation, and new perspectives on pathogenesis. J Am Acad Dermatol. 2018;78(1):1-12.
2. Juárez-Rendón KJ, Rivera Sánchez G, Reyes-López MA, García-Ortiz JE, Bocanegra-García V, Guardiola-Avila I, et al. Alopecia areata. Current situation and perspectives. Arch Argent Pediatr. 2017;115(6):e404-11.
3. Seetharam KA. Alopecia areata: an update. Indian J Dermatol Venereol Leprol. 2013;79(5):563-75.
4. Meah N, Wall D, Trindade de Carvalho L, Sinclair R. Bitemporal alopecia areata. Australas J Dermatol. 2020;61(3):263-5.
5. Olsen EA, Hordinsky MK, Price VH, Roberts JL, Shapiro J, Canfield D, et al. Alopecia areata investigational assessment guidelines—part II. National Alopecia Areata Foundation. J Am Acad Dermatol. 2004;51(3):440-7.
6. Lee S, Lee WS. Management of alopecia areata: updates and algorithmic approach. J Dermatol. 2017;44(11):1199-211.
7. Messenger AG, McKillop J, Farrant P, McDonagh AJ, Sladden M. British Association of Dermatologists' guidelines for the management of alopecia areata 2012. Br J Dermatol. 2012;166(5):916-26.
8. Madani S, Shapiro J. Alopecia areata update. J Am Acad Dermatol. 2000;42(4):549-66.
9. Garg S, Messenger AG. Alopecia areata: evidence-based treatments. Semin Cutan Med Surg. 2009;28(1):15-8.
10. Wang EHC, Sallee BN, Tejeda CI, Christiano AM. Montagna Symposium 2017 - Janus Kinase inhibitors for treatment of alopecia areata. J Invest Dermatol. 2018;138(9):1911-6.
11. Peloquin L, Castelo-Soccio L. Alopecia areata: an update on treatment options for children. Paediatr Drugs. 2017;19(5):411-22.

CHAPTER 10

Scarring Alopecia

Madhulika Mhatre, Bhavni Oberoi

Key Messages

- Scarring alopecia, also known as cicatricial alopecia, refers to a collection of hair loss disorders that may be diagnosed in up to 3% of hair loss patients.
- It is characterized by potentially permanent and irreversible destruction of hair follicles and their replacement with scar tissue.
- In primary cicatricial alopecias, the pathology starts at the hair follicle level and is classified based on the type of inflammatory infiltrate.
- In case of secondary cicatricial alopecias, it is prudent to identify the cause and treat it.
- Early intervention in the course of the disease may halt its progression and reverse the alopecia, but burnt-out cases with frank cicatrization may need surgical intervention in the form of scalp reduction or hair transplantation.

INTRODUCTION

Cicatricial alopecia (CA) or scarring alopecia is a troublesome group of inflammatory alopecias that are characterized by irreversible destruction of the hair follicles. These are clinically characterized by the loss of visible follicular ostia over the area of scarring and histopathologically as fibrous tracts that replace the pilosebaceous structures.[1] The current treatment modalities are targeted on halting the disease progression; however, a large group of patients present when the disease is already burnt out and damage has occurred. Hair transplant seems to be the only plausible treatment for this group of patients. This territory has hardly been explored, and a lot of questions need to be answered such as when to operate, what technique to use, and how to ensure viability of the grafted follicles in the scarred area. This chapter shall bring to light what has been done and can be done for the same.

Cicatricial alopecias can be broadly classified into primary cicatricial alopecia (PCA), secondary cicatricial alopecia (SCA), and developmental/hereditary CA.[2] In PCA, the primary site of inflammation is the hair follicles where the stem cells in the bulge area get targeted due to the destructive inflammatory process and result in irreversible hair loss from the affected site on the scalp[3] whereas, in SCA, the hair follicles are secondarily damaged as a result of a more generalized destructive process in the body or within the skin, which ultimately leads to the destruction of the hair follicle stem cells.[4] A few examples include trauma (burns, radiation, traction), any infiltrative processes (morphea, scleroderma, sarcoidosis, neoplasias), and infections (bacterial, fungal, viral, mycobacterial).[5] A brief classification of the important causes based on the clinical presentation and histopathology has been summarized in **Box 1**.

COMMON PRIMARY CICATRICIAL ALOPECIAS

Chronic Cutaneous Lupus Erythematosus

Chronic cutaneous lupus erythematosus (CCLE) primarily affects White and African American women, typically between the ages of 20 and 40 years. It manifests

BOX 1 Classification of cicatricial alopecia.[6]

Primary cicatricial alopecia

Lymphocyte-associated:

- Chronic cutaneous lupus erythematosus
- Lichen planopilaris (LPP)—classical type, frontal fibrosing alopecia, Graham–Little syndrome
- Classic pseudopelade (Brocq)
- Central centrifugal cicatricial alopecia
- Alopecia mucinosa
- Keratosis follicularis spinulosa decalvans

Neutrophil-associated:

- Folliculitis decalvans
- Dissecting cellulitis/folliculitis (perifolliculitis abscedens et suffodiens)

Mixed inflammatory infiltrate:

- Folliculitis (acne) keloidalis
- Folliculitis (acne) necrotica
- Erosive pustular dermatosis
- Nonspecific

Secondary cicatricial alopecia

Infections:

- Bacterial
- Viral
- Fungal

Immunological:

- Sarcoidosis
- Necrobiosis lipoidica
- Morphea
- Graft-versus-host disease

Neoplasms:

- Alopecia mucinosa
- Lymphoproliferative

Exogenous:

- Burns
- Surgical and traumatic scars

Dermatoses:

- Psoriasis
- Immunobullous disorders

Hamartomas:

- Organoid nevus
- Miscellaneous

as well-circumscribed, round/oval erythematous, infiltrative scaly plaques on sun-exposed areas and the scalp. CCLE lesions exhibit follicular plugging, telangiectasias, atrophy, and pigment changes.[7] While localized CCLE is not often associated with systemic involvement, the generalized form may exhibit systemic symptoms and laboratory abnormalities.

DERMOSCOPY

Dermoscopic findings include follicular plugging, starburst pattern, follicular red dots and rosettes in the early stages of the disease. Large yellow dots with radial, thin arborizing vessels emerging from the dot can be seen (also known as "red spider in yellow dot"). In the later stages structureless whitish areas and telangiectasia can be seen.

Treatment options include hydroxychloroquine, chloroquine, quinacrine, oral and intralesional corticosteroids, isotretinoin, acitretin, dapsone, thalidomide, methotrexate, azathioprine, cyclosporine, ustekinumab, and other experimental therapies. Protection from ultraviolet (UV) light is crucial, with hats and broad-spectrum sunscreen recommended. Hydroxychloroquine is the primary treatment, with dose adjustments based on seasons. Oral prednisolone may be considered for severe or refractory cases. Adding second antimalarial or oral retinoids may be necessary in resistant cases. Additional treatments include azathioprine, mycophenolate mofetil, and thalidomide. Smoking can reduce hydroxychloroquine efficacy, emphasizing the importance of smoking cessation. CCLE patients may experience regrowth with early aggressive treatment. Telogen effluvium may occur with oral retinoid use.

Lichen Planopilaris

Lichen planopilaris (LPP) is a hair disorder characterized by progressive alopecia, pruritus, and scaly skin. It primarily affects women and presents with follicular plugging, atrophy, and pigment changes. Dermoscopy reveals perifollicular erythema, follicular scales, and reduced follicular ostia. Histopathologically, LPP shows a lymphocytic infiltrate around hair follicles, leading to destruction and scarring.

The treatment of LPP involves a combination of topical, intralesional, and systemic therapies. Topical corticosteroids provide relief from itching and burning. Intralesional corticosteroid injections at sites of active inflammation can stop hair loss. Systemic therapy is often required, with antimalarials such as hydroxychloroquine being the first-line treatment, typically administered below 6.5 mg/kg or 400 mg/day.[8] Oral corticosteroids are reserved for rapidly progressing or severely symptomatic cases. Other options include oral retinoids, doxycycline, and mycophenolate.

Besides classic LPP, there are two main clinical variants, namely frontal fibrosing alopecia (FFA) and Graham–Little–Piccardi–Lasseur syndrome, with the former presenting with a progressing band of alopecia of the hairline in postmenopausal women and the latter being characterized by the triad of scarring patchy alopecia of the scalp, nonscarring alopecia of the axillae/pubic region, and spinous follicular papules of the trunk/limbs.

- FFA is a specific subtype of scarring alopecia that primarily affects the frontal hairline and eyebrows. It was first described in the 1990s and has since become increasingly recognized. FFA predominantly affects postmenopausal women but can also occur in premenopausal women and men. Based on histological findings, FFA is thought to be a possible clinical variant of LPP.

Signs and Symptoms

Frontal fibrosing alopecia typically presents with a gradual recession of the frontal hairline, which may also involve the temporal areas. The hair loss often appears as a band-like pattern along the frontotemporal hairline with a pseudofringe appearance in a few. The "lonely hair" sign, which was seen in 25% of the patients, must not be regarded as pathognomonic for FFA as it also occurs in other forms of CA. It does, however, enable the distinction from nonscarring forms such as traction alopecia.

In addition to the scalp, FFA may cause eyebrow loss, including the outer third or complete loss of the eyebrows. Other signs and symptoms may include the following:

- *Perifollicular erythema*: Redness and inflammation around the hair follicles, particularly near the frontal hairline
- *Perifollicular scaling*: Presence of fine scales around the affected hair follicles
- *Hair follicle miniaturization*: Affected hair follicles may become progressively smaller and thinner over time
- *Itching and burning sensation*: Some individuals with FFA experience itching or a burning sensation in the affected areas.

Dermoscopy Findings

Dermoscopy, a noninvasive technique that magnifies the skin surface, can aid in the diagnosis of FFA. Common dermoscopy findings associated with FFA include:

- *Perifollicular erythema*: Redness surrounding the affected hair follicles
- *Perifollicular scaling*: Presence of fine, white scales around the follicular openings
- *Follicular pore loss*: Loss of visible openings of hair follicles within the affected area
- *"Empty" hair follicles*: Hair follicles that appear devoid of hair shafts
- *Fibrotic white dots*: Small white dots scattered within the affected area, representing areas of fibrosis and scarring

Management Options

The management of FFA aims to slow down disease progression, alleviate symptoms, and potentially promote hair regrowth. While there is no definitive cure for FFA, several treatment options have shown varying degrees of success:

- *Topical corticosteroids*: High-potency topical corticosteroids, such as clobetasol propionate, can be applied to the affected areas to reduce inflammation and halt disease progression. However, long-term use may have side effects, and response rates can vary.
- *Systemic treatment*: In cases where topical treatments are insufficient, systemic medications, such as hydroxychloroquine or finasteride, may be prescribed to control inflammation and potentially promote hair regrowth. These medications should be used under medical supervision due to possible side effects. Recent research suggests a potential role of peroxisome proliferator-activated receptor γ agonist medications, such as pioglitazone hydrochloride, in refractory LPP treatment.[9]
- *Laser therapy*: Low-level laser therapy (LLLT) has been explored as a potential treatment for FFA. It involves the use of laser devices to stimulate hair follicles and promote regrowth. However, further research is needed to establish its effectiveness.
- *Surgical interventions*: Hair transplantation may be considered for individuals with stable disease and sufficient donor hair. Transplanting healthy hair follicles from unaffected areas to the frontal hairline can help restore the hairline. However, scarring from FFA may pose challenges to achieving optimal results.
- *Supportive measures*: In addition to medical interventions, supportive measures, such as cosmetic camouflage techniques, wigs, or eyebrow microblading, can help improve cosmetic appearance and boost self-confidence.

Early diagnosis and appropriate management are crucial to slow down disease progression and alleviate symptoms.

Pseudopelade of Brocq (Synonyms: Alopecia Cicatrisata, Alopecia Atrophicans)

Pseudopelade of Brocq, also known as idiopathic scarring alopecia, is a rare form of CA characterized by the gradual development of patchy hair loss with little or no accompanying symptoms. This condition primarily affects middle-aged individuals, with a slight female predilection.

Clinical Features

Pseudopelade of Brocq typically presents as discrete, well-defined patches of hair loss that may resemble other forms of scarring alopecia or alopecia areata. The patches of hair loss usually have an irregular shape and are commonly found on the vertex or crown of the scalp. The affected areas appear smooth and atrophic, often described as "cicatricial," and the scalp may have a shiny appearance. Unlike other forms of scarring alopecia, patients with pseudopelade of Brocq usually do not experience symptoms such as itching, pain, or inflammation.

Histopathological examination of affected scalp biopsies typically reveals a variable degree of lymphocytic inflammation around the hair follicles, often accompanied by fibrosis (scarring). The hair follicles may show miniaturization, which refers to a decrease in hair follicle size. The extent of inflammation and fibrosis can vary among individuals and throughout the course of the disease.

Dermoscopy

In pseudopelade of Brocq, dermoscopy findings can vary but commonly include:

- *Tapering hairs*: Hairs that appear thin and tapered toward the distal end within the affected area
- *White dots*: Small white dots scattered throughout the patches of hair loss
- *Follicular ostia*: Absence of visible follicular openings in the affected areas
- *Perifollicular erythema*: Redness surrounding the hair follicles may be present in some cases.

Management

The management of pseudopelade of Brocq is challenging as the underlying cause is unknown, and there is currently no definitive cure. Treatment aims to slow down disease progression, alleviate symptoms, and potentially promote hair regrowth. Management options may include the following:

- *Topical corticosteroids*: High-potency topical corticosteroids may be prescribed to reduce inflammation and potentially halt disease progression. However, the response to treatment can vary among individuals.
- *Intralesional corticosteroids*: In some cases, injecting corticosteroids directly into the affected areas may be considered to target inflammation.
- *Systemic treatment*: Systemic medications, such as hydroxychloroquine or methotrexate, may be prescribed for individuals with a more extensive or progressive disease to control inflammation.
- *Supportive measures*: Supportive measures include gentle hair care practices, using camouflage techniques to improve cosmetic appearance, and seeking psychological support.
- *Surgical options*: Hair transplantation or scalp reduction may be considered once the disease is in the burnt-out stage.

Alopecia Mucinosa

Alopecia mucinosa, also known as follicular mucinosis, is a rare inflammatory disease characterized by the deposition of mucopolysaccharides (mucin) in the pilosebaceous units. It can present as a primary disorder or as a secondary disorder associated with other benign or malignant diseases.

It commonly affects the face, head, and neck, presenting as localized lesions. It can occur in children and young adults as a remitting or chronic relapsing type, while older adults may experience a chronic relapsing course. The lesions tend to resolve within 2 months to 2 years.

Histopathology is characterized by the presence of mucin deposits within the follicular epithelium. There are mixed cell infiltrates in the perivascular and interstitial areas. Pautrier microabscesses are not typically observed, and significant plasma cells or eosinophil-containing infiltrates are usually absent.

The treatment of idiopathic follicular mucinosis is not well defined. Various treatment options have been reported, including topical, intralesional, and systemic corticosteroids, dapsone, antimalarials, isotretinoin, indomethacin, minocycline, interferon, and photodynamic therapy.[10] However, specific treatment recommendations for idiopathic cases are lacking. Regular follow-up is essential to monitor the resolution of lesions or the progression of associated diseases.

Central Centrifugal Cicatricial Alopecia

Central centrifugal cicatricial alopecia primarily affects women of African descent and typically starts at the crown of the scalp, spreading centrifugally. Symptoms include progressive hair loss, scarring, and sometimes scalp tenderness.

Dermoscopy may show perifollicular erythema, perifollicular scale, and areas of hypopigmentation.

Histopathological examination reveals inflammation around hair follicles and destruction of hair follicles.

Management involves discontinuing harmful hairstyling practices, using topical or systemic corticosteroids, and adopting gentle hair care routines.

PART C: Investigations

SECTION OUTLINE

CHAPTER 11

Investigations in Hair Loss

Dhanashree Bhide, Pravin Bharatia, Mukta Tulpule, Ruhi Uttamani-Sangle

Key Messages

- This chapter covers most of the semi-invasive and noninvasive tests that can be performed in hair loss patients.
- In modern days, sophisticated investigations such as trichoscopy have become a necessity in hair clinics.
- These tests need to be interpreted properly so as to confirm the clinical diagnosis.
- In problematic situations such as diffuse hair thinning in females, these tests can aid in identifying the etiology.

INTRODUCTION

In dermatology clinics, some patients present with hair fall and some with hair loss, meaning thereby reduction of scalp hair volume without noticeable hair fall. In a few patients, female pattern hair loss and telogen effluvium can coexist. As a hair restoration surgeon, the doctor has to mainly deal with patients with androgenetic alopecia and scarring alopecias. The diagnosis in both these situations is clinical. Male pattern hair loss usually does not require any investigations. However, especially in women, the situation can be tricky as sometimes female pattern hair loss can mimic telogen effluvium, loose anagen syndrome, and diffuse alopecia areata. Hence, investigations are required to pinpoint the cause. Besides biochemical investigations, tests such as KOH (potassium hydroxide) mount, Wood's lamp examination, trichoscopy, phototrichogram, and light microscopy are useful tools to diagnose various dermatological conditions leading to hair fall or hair loss. In recent years, with advancement in trichoscopy and easy availability of good handheld devices, it has become an essential tool in trichology practice. A hair restoration surgeon should be aware of these diagnostic tests so as to reach a conclusion in difficult situations. In this chapter, these tests will be covered from a practical point of view avoiding long exhaustive lists of various etiologies.

CLINICAL TESTS

Other than detailed history and photographic documentation, certain clinical tests are extremely helpful in clinical evaluation in cases of alopecia **(Table 1)**.

Besides these clinical tests, in certain situations, especially if infective etiology is suspected, the following tests are beneficial.

KOH Mount

Apparatus: 10% KOH, light microscope, burner, glass slide, artery forceps, and blade to collect the specimen.

Method and Collection[1-3]

Clean the area with spirit. Lusterless hair and stubs, which include roots, should be plucked with sterile artery forceps. Wood's lamp guidance may be taken to collect the specimen. Scrape the skin from the scalp with the blunt edge of scalpel. For facilitating easy removal of scales, the area should be made wet with normal saline. For a better yield, epilate short hair stubs. Scrape crusts along the edges of suspected area.

Method of 10% KOH Mount[4,5]

Ten percent KOH drop is kept on a clean, grease-free glass slide. The hair sample is placed in the KOH drop and slide passed through a burner flame to hasten keratolysis.

TABLE 1: Clinical tests in the evaluation of cases of alopecia.

Jaquet's or fold sign	Fold an area of the scalp between the two thumbs. If skin folds are formed easily, the test is considered positive and indicates an absence of hair fibers	To differentiate between noncicatricial and cicatricial alopecia
Hair pull test	Approximately 20–60 hairs are grasped between thumb and fingers from the base of the hairs near the scalp and firmly, but not forcefully, tugged away from the scalp. If >10% hairs are pulled away from the scalp, the test is positive	Positive test indicates active hair shedding and helps in diagnosing active alopecia areata
Hair card test	Simple examination technique performed using a small white card for pigmented hair and a black card for white hair	To differentiate newly growing hair from broken hair
Hair growth window test	A 1–2 cm area of hair is shaven or clipped as close to the scalp as possible, and the length of the hair that regrows is measured after a week. The normal hair growth rate is 2.5 mm a week (1 cm a month)	Used to measure hair growth and, more importantly, to convince patients that their hair are growing well
Daily scalp hair counts	Patients are instructed to collect hairs shed in 1 day, count them, and place them in plastic bags. Daily hair counts for 7 days are maintained. If the patient is losing >100 hairs per day, the hair should be examined microscopically to detect the pathology in hair bulb and hair shaft abnormalities	To diagnose telogen effluvium and disorders in hair bulbs and shafts that present with excessive hair shedding
Standardized wash test	The patient refrains from shampooing for 5 days and then shampoos and rinses the hair in the basin. The hairs remaining in the water and the gauze are collected and sent for examination	This is an important technique to differentiate telogen effluvium from female pattern hair loss

After the sample is softened, a clean glass coverslip is kept and pressed, preventing the formation of air bubbles. The sample is kept in KOH for a variable duration ranging from 5 to 30 minutes before examination.

Advantages

Potassium hydroxide examination of hair is simple to perform, rapid, and inexpensive. It does not require sophisticated gadgets or infrastructure, but interpretation requires some experience.

Wood's Lamp Examination of Hair

Apparatus: Wood's lamp **(Fig. 1)**

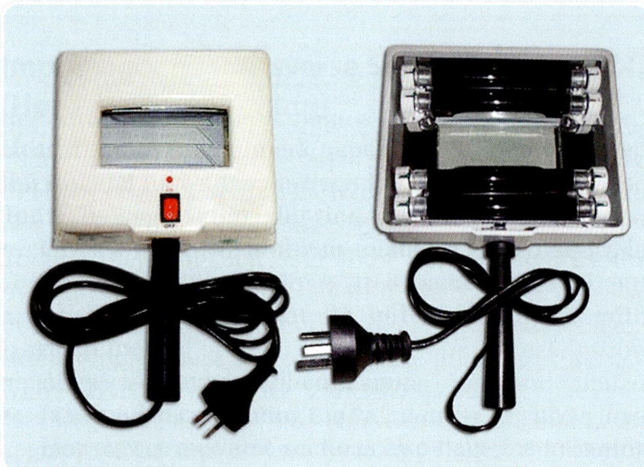

FIG. 1: Wood's lamp.

Method and Prerequisites[6]

The skin of the affected area should be clean as exudates, tetracycline in sweat, hair gels, serum, oil, soap residue, and other cosmetics may fluoresce and interfere with interpretation. Wait for 1 minute to allow the lamp to warm up. The examination room should be totally dark with black occlusive shades. The examiner should get dark-adapted to see the contrast better. The light source should be held 4-5 inches from the lesion. Head bath on the day of examination should not be allowed as it may dilute the pigment.

In day-to-day practice, Wood's lamp is useful to diagnose infective causes of hair fall, especially tinea capitis **(Table 2)**.

TABLE 2: Fluorescence characteristics of various species of tinea capitis.[7,8]

Organism	Color of fluorescence
Microsporum audouinii *Microsporum canis* *Microsporum ferrugineum* *Microsporum distortum*	Blue–green
Microsporum gypseum	Dull yellow
Trichophyton schoenleinii	Dull blue

However, Wood's lamp findings should be confirmed by other methods such as fungal culture.

Light Microscopic Examination of Hair

Apparatus: Light microscope **(Fig. 2)**, glass slide, and cello tape

Method[9,10]

Light microscopy is performed in the diagnosis of various hereditary and congenital abnormalities of hair shaft, which may produce intrinsic and extrinsic changes. To demonstrate intrinsic changes, proximal 1–2 cm of plucked hair is examined.

For examination, two types of mounts can be prepared:
1. Dry mount—may cause scattering of light
2. Wet mount—with KOH

This method helps to distinguish between various infections and infestations, diagnose various hair shaft abnormalities and genodermatoses, and identify the changes in various nutritional and metabolic causes. It is a useful tool to identify primary hair disorders as well as other disorders affecting hair secondarily. The findings of light microscopy can be confirmed by advanced techniques such as polarized microscopy, confocal scanning microscopy, phototrichogram, TrichoScan, and trichoscopy **(Tables 3 and 4)**.

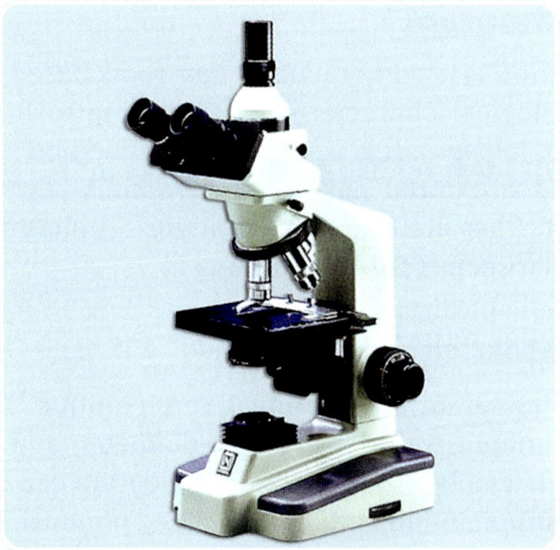

FIG. 2: Light microscope.

Trichoscopy

Apparatus: Trichoscope

Method[13,14]

Dermatoscopic examination of hair and scalp is called trichoscopy. The examination of hair and scalp disorders was time-consuming in the past. Methods such as light microscopy required plucking of hair and sampling, which led to delay in the diagnosis. With the advent of trichoscopy, which is a noninvasive method, focal affected areas can be easily examined. It is also possible to screen eyebrows and eyelashes along with the entire scalp in a short span of time.

Some shaft abnormalities, such as pili torti, cannot be diagnosed on light microscopy but can be easily diagnosed in outpatient department (OPD) by using trichoscopy. With the advent of trichoscopy, scalp biopsy is very rarely required as a diagnostic tool. Phototrichogram and automated phototrichogram (TrichoScan and Folliscope) are other sophisticated methods for this purpose.

Trichoscope: A trichoscope functions like a magnifying lens with add-on features. The conventional handheld device has magnification of 10×. Many new models are smartphone- and tablet-compatible devices that allow the user to store images. Trichoscopy has various illumination options such as visible light, ultraviolet light, and polarized light. Nonpolarized dermoscopy requires direct contact with skin and is more useful to visualize

TABLE 3: Comparison of light microscopy with other microscopy techniques.[10-12]

	Light microscopy	Polarized microscopy	Confocal scanning microscopy
Principle	Use of visible light and mirrors for improving resolution	Use of polarized light in which all rays vibrate in one plane	Optical imaging technique by adding spatial pinhole placed at the confocal plane of the lens to eliminate out-of-focus light
Resolution	0.2 μm	0.2 μm	200 μm
Key feature	Hair shaft abnormalities	Double refractile object appears illuminated against a dark background, e.g., trichothiodystrophy "tiger-tail appearance"	Projects three-dimensional (3D) optical images of a transverse section of skin and hair in real time
Advantage	Easy, inexpensive	No scattering of light, hence deeper penetration	3D imaging and newer technology
Disadvantage	Low resolution	Limited usage in dermatology	Expensive, high expertise level required

TABLE 4: Latest dermoscopes.

Devices	DermLite DL5	Heine Delta 30	Illuco IDS-1100
Magnification	True 10×	10×	10×
Optics	32 mm 16× white, 4× UV (365 nm), 4× PigmentBoost, 1 torch LED	32-mm lens with 30-mm view	25 mm with 22 mm-view 32 LED
Smartphone compatibility	Yes	Yes	Yes
Camera compatibility	Yes	Yes	Yes
Wood's mode	Yes	No	No
Polarization	Polarized, cross-polarized, parallel polarized	Polarized and nonpolarized	Polarized light contact dermoscopy, polarized light noncontact dermoscopy, nonpolarized light contact dermoscopy, nonpolarized light noncontact dermoscopy

(LED: light-emitting diode)

Note: We thank all the above dermoscope companies for device specifications obtained from respective websites.

superficial structures in the epidermis such as scales. Polarized dermoscopy does not require direct contact with the skin and is better to view deeper dermal structures, pigmentation, and blood vessels. Hybrid dermoscopes can switch between polarized and nonpolarized modes.[20]

To aid the diagnosis of fungal infections, UV light-enhanced trichoscopy (UVET) may be more useful, which covers the wavelength of Wood's lamp.[21,22] It is also possible to adjust the magnification, and one can view structures up to the reticular dermis. Trichoscopy should always be started on dry scalp first to assess scales and casts and then contact trichoscopy with immersion fluids such as alcohol or spring water spray if required. In trichoscopic evaluation, one should look for follicular openings or dots, interfollicular structures, and various hair signs. The hair follicular openings may be normal, empty, fibrotic, or containing biological material. To help differentiate between androgenetic alopecia and telogen effluvium, the trichoscopic characteristics of hair diameter diversity, vellus hair, focal atrichia, and predominance of abnormalities in the frontal area should be observed. These findings are present only in androgenetic alopecia. The trichoscopic features of empty hair follicles with yellow dots, peripilar sign, regrowing hair, and honeycomb presentation are present in both androgenetic alopecia and telogen effluvium.[20,23]

Trichoscopy with video attachment is called videotrichoscopy and has magnification from ×20 to ×160. It is equipped with software which can help in automated assessing hair number and diameter.[24-26]

Hair shaft thickness may be roughly estimated with a handheld dermoscope (thin, normal, thick). Videodermoscopes-based software allows a detailed assessment of hair shaft thickness in micrometers. Although precise measurement of hair shaft thickness is not essential for diagnosis, it may be useful for monitoring treatment efficacy and in clinical trials.

Trichogram

Trichogram is used to quantify hair roots based on their morphological characteristics according to hair cycle (anagen, telogen). It is a semi-invasive method requiring plucking of 50–100 hairs from two sites—frontal and occipital. They are examined after glass mounting under light microscopy **(Table 5 and Box 1)**.

Phototrichogram[27-29]

Phototrichogram is a noninvasive technique. By using this technique, hair density, hair diameter, and stage of hair cycle can be studied. Phototrichogram can be automated or nonautomated. In automated phototrichogram, TrichoScan and Folliscope are two options available.

Nonautomated Phototrichogram[30]

A specific area of 1 cm^2 is marked with a permanent marker, and hair is first clipped as close to the scalp surface as possible. Then, a dry mount is prepared, and they are examined with 40× magnification under a microscope. The scalp is also photographed with a digital camera. Variables such as light condition and distance are kept fixed during this process. Images are recorded on day 0 and day 2 without shampooing the hair in between.

Automated Phototrichogram[31]

In this method, both quantitative and qualitative assessment of hair can be done using specialized software. TrichoScan and Folliscope are the two methods of performing automated phototrichogram.

TABLE 5: Trichoscopic features of various hair disorders.[23,35-41]

Hair disorder	Trichoscopic feature
Cicatricial alopecia	Milky red/ivory white areas lacking follicular openings
Noncicatricial alopecia	Presence of empty follicular openings
Alopecia areata	Black dots, micro exclamation mark tapered hair (suggests disease activity)
Alopecia areata incognito	Yellow dots and presence of short miniaturized regrowing hair
Telogen effluvium	Uniform hair shaft thickness, absence of vellus hair, changes not restricted to frontal area, upright regrowing hair more marked
Lichen planus pigmentosus	Perifollicular inflammation, tubular perifollicular scaling, elongated concentric blood vessels, white dots merging to form white areas
Frontal fibrosing alopecia	Mild perifollicular scaling and erythema, absence of vellus hair
Fibrosing alopecia in pattern distribution	Heterogeneous hair shaft thickness, perifollicular scaling, white dots merging to form white areas
Folliculitis decalvans	Tufted hair, follicular pustules with emerging hair shafts, perifollicular starburst pattern with hyperplasia
Dissecting cellulitis of scalp	3D yellow dots imposed over dystrophic hair, large yellow amorphous areas, pinpoint white dots with whitish halo
Discoid lupus erythematosus	Large arborizing vessels, large hyperkeratotic follicular dots
Psoriasis	Regularly distributed, twisted and lace-like blood vessels
Seborrheic dermatitis	Thin arborizing vessels
Tinea capitis	Comma, corkscrew and zig-zag hair

BOX 1 Trichoscopic features of androgenetic alopecia.[42]

Male pattern hair loss (MPHL) **(Figs. 3 and 4)**

Early MPHL:

- Increased hair shaft diameter variability (diversity > 20% is diagnostic)
- Circle or pigtail hairs
- Presence of wavy hair, which is regrowing and appears thin and isolated, coils surrounded by other normal hair

Moderate MPHL:

- Many small yellow dots show the presence of keratotic material and are devoid of hair shafts
- The large yellow dots are caused by sebaceous debris around terminal hairs

Severe MPHL:

- Short vellus hair and peripilar sign
- Brownish halo around terminal hair
- Honeycomb pattern due to scalp pigmentation
- Pinpoint white dots

Female pattern hair loss (FPHL) **(Figs. 5 and 6)**

Major criteria:

- Frontal area has more than four yellow dots in four fields
- Average hair thickness is lower in frontal area than occiput (calculated with 50 hair from each area)
- >10% of frontal area has thin hair (below 0.3 mm)

Minor criteria:

- Ratio of single hair unit follicles in the frontal area to ones in the occiput is greater than 2:1
- The ratio of vellus hair present in the frontal area to occiput is greater than 1.5:1

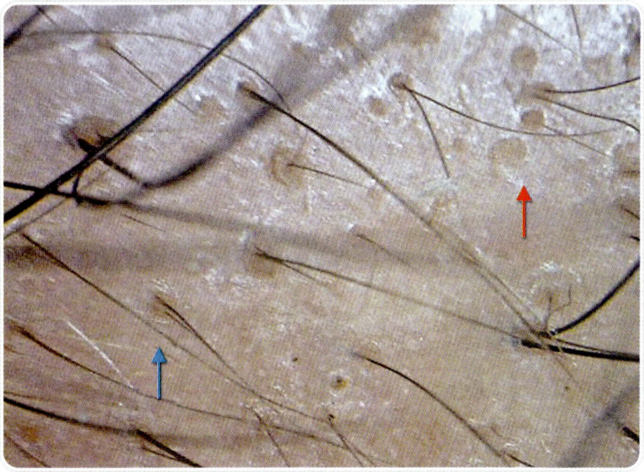

FIG. 3: Advanced androgenetic alopecia showing sparse hair follicles, empty hair follicles, yellow dots (red arrow), and hair shaft diameter variation (blue arrow).

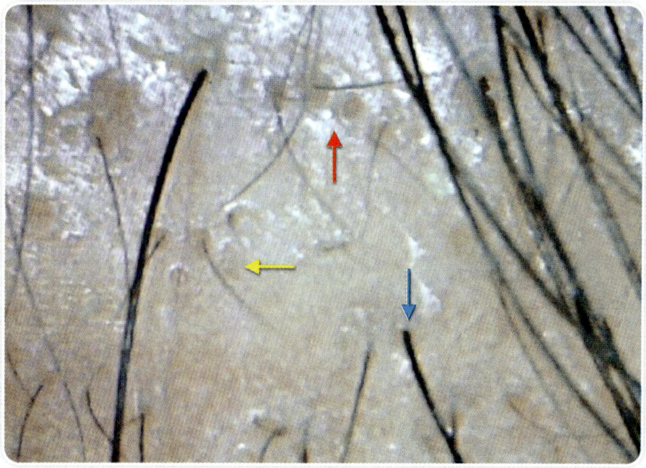

FIG. 4: Androgenetic alopecia showing predominance of single hair-bearing follicles (blue arrow), vellus hair transformation (yellow arrow), and peripilar sign (red arrow).

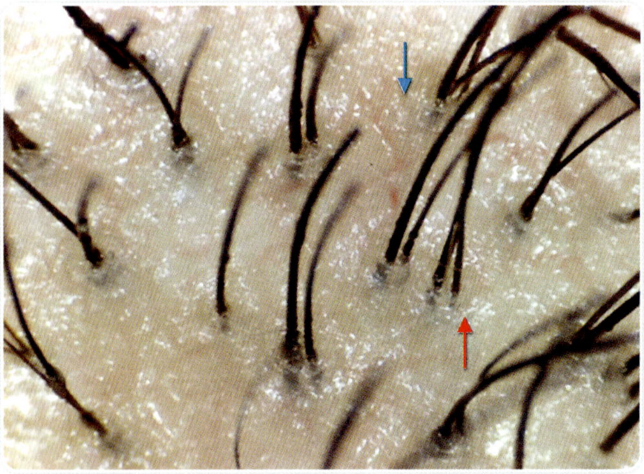

FIG. 5: Normal scalp showing interfollicular simple red loop pattern (blue arrow) and follicles with two to three terminal hair of the same diameter (red arrow).

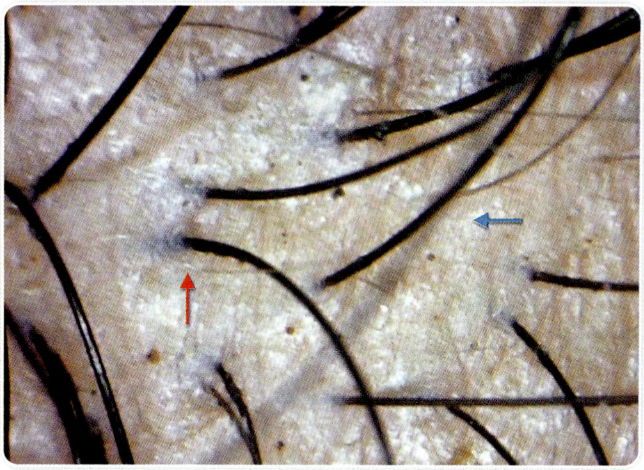

FIG. 6: Female pattern hair loss. Single hair follicular units (red arrow) and anisotrichosis (blue arrow).

TrichoScan (Fig. 7)[32,33]

TrichoScan has a digital camera with automated digital image analysis software.

Method: 1 cm^2 area from the crown is marked. Hair is clipped to 1 mm length. Trichoscope is pressed against hair to flatten the fibers. Magnification of image taken is 20×, and the same procedure is repeated after 3 days.

Parameters such as density, thickness, anagen:telogen ratio, and length are automatically analyzed with the software.

Folliscope[34]

Folliscope is a USB connection-based device that can be connected to a computer; it has a high-definition microscopic camera. It automatically measures various

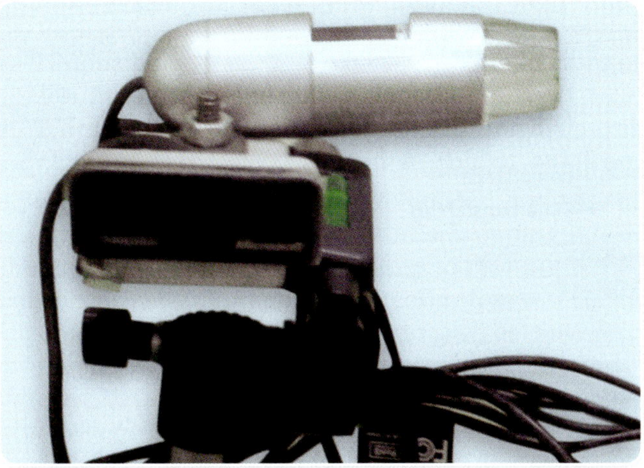

FIG. 7: TrichoScan.

trichological parameters. The advantage of this system is that it does not require plucking or trimming and can be performed on dry scalp **(Tables 6 and 7)**.

Cross-section Trichometry[43]

Cross-section trichometry is a noninvasive device that can measure hair mass and changes in it. Hair mass is affected by the density and the diameter of the hair. The Haircheck® is a commercial device that helps us to assess changes in hair mass caused by thinning, shedding, breakage, or growth in males and females with progressive alopecia or those receiving alopecia treatment.

Scalp Biopsy

This section has been discussed further in later chapters.

TABLE 6: Specific appearances of hair shaft disorders.[13-19]

Hair disorder	Trichoscopic appearances
Monilethrix	Beaded appearance
Loose anagen syndrome	Rumpled/floppy sock appearance
Alopecia areata	Exclamation mark appearance, tapered hair, black dots, yellow dots
Pili torti	Twisted appearance
Trichorrhexis invaginata	Bamboo appearance (the split hair shaft appears as two paint brushes aligned in opposition)—diagnostic of Netherton's syndrome. When hair shaft breaks at the site of this abnormality, the distal end of broken hair will have a concave, cupped appearance, which is called "golf tee" hair because it resembles the plastic tee used to support a golf ball. In the absence of typical bamboo hair, trichorrhexis invaginata may be diagnosed based on golf tee hairs only
Trichotillomania	Broken hair, coiled hair, tulip hair, broom hair, flame hair, black dots
Tinea capitis	Comma hair, corkscrew hair, zigzag or Z-hair, morse code hair, block hair, and i-hair

TABLE 7: Comparison table of hair investigation methods.[28,29]

	Trichoscopy	Trichogram	Phototrichogram	Automated phototrichogram
Key feature	Visualization of hair and scalp with a dermoscope	Visualization of hair and hair follicle at high magnification	Light microscopy of plucked hair and sequential photographs of a selected scalp area mounted on a glass slide with a digital camera	Similar to a phototrichogram but it is automated, software based
Modifications	Polarized and nonpolarized trichoscopy, UVET		Contrast-enhanced phototrichogram—hair dye makes better contrast	
Advantages	• Requires only dermoscope • Helps in diagnosing hair bulb disorders and hair shaft disorders • Suitable in clinical practice	• Does not require sophisticated equipment • Cost-effective and fast • Helps in detecting hair shaft disorders, hair loss of infectious etiology • Best suited for clinical practice	• Digital photographs taken to maintain record • Hair shaft diameter can be measured along with the hair density, hair length, and linear growth rate • Suitable for research trials	• Automated assessment of parameters such as hair length, density, anagen:telogen ratio, growth rate, Hamilton–Norwood grade, and thickness • Fast • Best suitable for research trials

Continued

Continued

	Trichoscopy	Trichogram	Phototrichogram	Automated phototrichogram
Disadvantages	Cannot determine hair density, anagen:telogen ratio, growth rate, etc.	Cannot determine hair density, anagen:telogen ratio, growth rate, etc.	• Hair shaving required for consistent results, reduces patient compliance • Time-consuming	• Expensive equipment and expertise required • Results may be inconsistent for different areas • Hair shaving reduces patient compliance

(UVET: UV light-enhanced trichoscopy)

SUMMARY

It may be time-consuming to perform these procedures during busy OPD hours. However, they are useful diagnostic tools, and proper understanding of the findings on trichoscopy or phototrichogram can certainly help in better understanding of the problem. In an institution-based practice, they can be used for research purpose. In spite of some drawbacks, they still are important diagnostic procedures in trichology.

Tips and Pearls

- Of all investigations, in the modern hair clinic, trichoscopy is the most useful tool.
- It helps to easily differentiate between scarring and nonscarring alopecias.
- Easy diagnosis of infective and hair shaft disorders is also possible.
- Disease activity of conditions such as alopecia areata can be monitored.

REFERENCES

1. Mubki T, Rudnicka L, Olszewska M, Shapiro J. Evaluation and diagnosis of the hair loss patient: part I. History and clinical examination. J Am Acad Dermatol. 2014;71:415.e1-5.
2. Chaya AK, Pande S. Methods of specimen collection for diagnosis of superficial and subcutaneous fungal infections. Indian J Dermatol Venereol Leprol. 2007;73(3):202-5.
3. Kurade SM, Amladi SA, Miskeen AK. Skin scraping and a potassium hydroxide mount. Indian J Dermatol Venereol Leprol. 2006;72(3):238-41.
4. Fonseka S, Lim CSH, Bandara UN, Dissanayake M. New contrast stain for the rapid diagnosis of dermatophytosis and pityriasis versicolor. Lab Med. 2011;42:649-52.
5. Asawanonda T, Taylor CR. Wood's light in dermatology. Int J Dermatol. 1999;38:801-7.
6. Gupta LK, Singhi MK. Wood's lamp. Indian J Dermatol Venereol Leprol. 2004;70:131-5.
7. Diagnostic and therapeutic techniques. In: Arndt K, Hsu J, Alam M, Bhatia A, Chilukuri S (Eds). Manual of Dermatologic Therapeutics, 8th edition. A Lippincott Manual. Alphen aan den Rijn: Wolters Kluwer; 2014. pp. 380-96.
8. Singh S, Beena PM. Comparative study of different microscopic techniques and culture media for the isolation of dermatophytes. Indian J Med Microbiol. 2003;21:21-4.
9. Hainer BL. Dermatophyte infections. Am Fam Physician. 2003; 67(1):101-5.
10. Maguire Jr HC, Kligman AM. Hair plucking as a diagnostic tool. J Invest Dermatol. 1964;42:77-9.
11. Hair and scalp disorders. In: Sacchidanand S, Oberoi C, Inamdar AC (Eds). IADVL Textbook of Dermatology, 4th edition. New Delhi: Bhalani Publishing House; 2015. pp. 1468-588.
12. Barth JH. Investigation of hair, hair growth and hair follicle. In: Rook A, Dawber R (Eds). Diseases of Hair and Scalp, 2nd edition. Oxford: Blackwell Scientific; 1991. pp. 588-606.
13. Adya KA, Inamadar AC, Palit A, Shivanna R, Deshmukh NS. Light microscopy of the hair: a simple tool to "untangle" hair disorders. Int J Trichol. 2011;3(1):46-56.
14. Jain N, Doshi B, Khopkar U. Trichoscopy in alopecias: diagnosis simplified. Int J Trichol. 2013;5(4):170-8.
15. de Berker DA, Paige DG, Ferguson DJ, Dawber RP. Golf tee hairs in Netherton disease. Pediatr Dermatol. 1995;12(1):7-11.
16. Slowinska M, Rudnicka L, Schwartz RA, Kowalska-Oledzka E, Rakowska A, Sicinska J, et al. Comma hairs: a dermatoscopic marker for tinea capitis: a rapid diagnostic method. J Am Acad Dermatol. 2008;59(5 Suppl):S77-9.
17. Sandoval AB, Ortiz JA, Rodriguez JM, Vargas AG, Quintero DG. Dermoscopic pattern in tinea capitis. Rev Iberoam Micol. 2010;27(3):151-2 [in Spanish].
18. Hughes R, Chiaverini C, Bahadoran P, Lacour JP. Corkscrew hair: a new dermoscopic sign for diagnosis of tinea capitis in black children. Arch Dermatol. 2011;147(3):355-6.
19. Rudnicka L, Olszewska M, Rakowska A, Slowinska M. Trichoscopy update 2011. J Dermatol Case Rep. 2011;5(4):82-8.
20. Neema S. Basic Principles of Dermoscopy in IADVL Atlas of Dermoscopy. New Delhi: Jaypee Brothers Medical Publishers Pvt. Ltd; 2022. pp. 7-8.
21. Khopkar U. Dermoscopy and Trichoscopy in Diseases of the Brown Skin. New Delhi: Jaypee Brothers Medical Publishers Pvt. Ltd; 2012. pp. 169-81.
22. Mubki T, Shamsaldeen O, McElwee KJ, Shapiro J. An update on diagnosis and treatment of female pattern hair loss. Expert Rev Dermatol. 2013;8(4):427-36.

23. Rebora A, Guarrera M, Baldari M, Vecchio F. Distinguishing androgenetic alopecia from chronic telogen effluvium when associated in the same patient: a simple noninvasive method. Arch Dermatol. 2005;141:1243-5.
24. Rakowska A. Trichoscopy (hair and scalp videodermoscopy) in the healthy female. Method standardization and norms for measurable parameters. J Dermatol Case Rep. 2009;3:14-19.
25. Ross EK, Vincenzi C, Tosti A. Videodermoscopy in the evaluation of hair and scalp disorders. J Am Acad Dermatol. 2006;55:799-806.
26. Dhurat R. Phototrichogram. Indian J Dermatol Venereol Leprol. 2006;72:242-4.
27. Ueki R, Tsuboi R, Inaba Y, Ogawa H. Phototrichogram analysis of Japanese female subjects with chronic diffuse hair loss. J Investig Dermatol Symp Proc. 2003;8:116-20.
28. Rushton DH, de Brouwer B, de Coster W, van Neste DJ. Comparative evaluation of scalp hair by phototrichogram and unit area trichogram analysis within the same subjects. Acta Derm Venereol. 1993;73:150-3.
29. Saraogi PP, Dhurat RS. Automated digital image analysis (TrichoScan®) for human hair growth analysis: ease versus errors. Int J Trichol. 2010;2(1):5-13.
30. Van Neste D, Trüeb RM. Critical study of hair growth analysis with computer-assisted methods. J Eur Acad Dermatol Venereol. 2006;20:578-83.
31. Aktan S, Akarsu S, Ilknur T, Demirtaşoğlu M, Ozkan S. Quantification of female pattern hair loss: a study in a Turkish population. Eur J Dermatol. 2007;17:321-4.
32. Lee BS, Chan JY, Monselise A, McElwee K, Shapiro J. Assessment of hair density and caliber in Caucasian and Asian female subjects with female pattern hair loss by using the Folliscope. J Am Acad Dermatol. 2012;66(1):166-7.
33. D'Amico D, Vaccaro M, Guarneri F, Borgia F, Cannavo S, Guarneri B. Phototrichogram using videomicroscopy: a useful technique in the evaluation of scalp hair. Eur J Dermatol. 2001;11:17.
34. Neste DJ. Contrast enhanced phototrichogram (CE-PTG): an improved non-invasive technique for measurement of scalp hair dynamics in androgenetic alopecia—validation study with histology after transverse sectioning of scalp biopsies. Eur J Dermatol. 2001;11:326-31.
35. Inui S, Nakajima T, Itami S. Scalp dermoscopy of androgenetic alopecia in Asian people. J Dermatol. 2009;36(2):82-5.
36. de Moura LH, Duque-Estrada B, Abraham LS, Barcaui CB, Sodre CT. Dermoscopy findings of alopecia areata in an African-American patient. J Dermatol Case Rep. 2008;2:52-4.
37. Wallace MP, de Berker DA. Hair diagnoses and signs: the use of dermatoscopy. Clin Exp Dermatol. 2010;35:41-6.
38. Tosti A. Dermoscopy of Hair and Scalp Disorders with Clinical and Pathological Correlations. Bologna, Italy: Informe Healthcare; 2007.
39. Canfield D. Photographic documentation of hair growth in androgenetic alopecia. Dermatol Clin. 1996;14:713-21.
40. Dhurat R, Saraogi P. Hair evaluation methods: merits and demerits. Int J Trichol. 2009;1(2):108-19.
41. Rakowska A, Slowinska M, Kowalska-Oledzka E, Rudnicka L. Trichoscopy in genetic hair shaft abnormalities. J Dermatol Case Rep. 2008;2:14-20.
42. Kim GW, Jung HJ, Ko HC, Kim MB, Lee WJ, Lee SJ, et al. Dermoscopy can be useful in differentiating scalp psoriasis from seborrhoeic dermatitis. Br J Dermatol. 2011;164:652-6.
43. Wikramanayake TC, Mauro LM, Tabas IA, Chen AL, Llanes IC, Jimenez JJ. Cross-section trichometry: a clinical tool for assessing the progression and treatment response of alopecia. Int J Trichol. 2012;4(4):259-64.

CHAPTER 12

Histopathology of Hair Loss

Venkataram Mysore

Key Messages

- Histopathology provides qualitative and quantitative assessment of hair follicles.
- Two 4-mm punch biopsy samples for horizontal and vertical section are essential for proper diagnosis.
- Hematoxylin and eosin stains are the primary stains. Direct immunofluorescence (DIF) can help in selected diseases such as discoid lupus erythematosus (DLE) and lichen planopilaris (LPP).

INTRODUCTION

Histopathology is an important tool for the diagnosis of different types of alopecia. While dermoscopy has decreased the need for biopsy, histopathology remains the only method of conclusively establishing the etiology in many cases.

BIOPSY

Indications of Biopsy[1-3]

From the point of view of hair transplantation (HT) surgery, biopsy in androgenetic alopecia (AGA) is indicated in the following situations:

- In cases of diffuse AGA to rule out alopecia areata
- In cases of female pattern hair loss to distinguish it from other diagnoses such as chronic telogen effluvium
- Scarring alopecias to confirm disease activity
- In cases of subtle scarring alopecias, which mimic AGA

All such cases need to be referred to a dermatologist for a biopsy and further interpretation.

Punch biopsy is performed under local anesthesia. Two punch biopsies are obtained, of 4 mm each—one for horizontal and one for vertical section **(Fig. 1)**. If direct immunofluorescence (DIF) is planned, an additional biopsy may be needed.

Importance of Transverse Sections (Horizontal Sectioning)

Headington, in a landmark paper in 1984, demonstrated the value of transverse sections in biopsies in alopecias.[4] The technique has the following advantages:

- Gives a better idea of hair follicle cycle dynamics in nonscarring alopecias
- Allows measurement of follicle diameter with micrometer
- Allows the study of follicular units
- Is helpful in calculating the hair density in a given area

However, transverse sections also have the following limitations:

- Multiple levels have to be studied and hence are more difficult and expensive.
- Epidermal changes are not well appreciated.

Sections are cut perpendicular to the direction of hair as they emerge on the epidermal side; if no hairs can be seen, section at 15° to epidermis.

- Mark with India ink at each level: Two levels are cut. One at the lower dermis, one at the upper dermis.

Vertical sections are preferred for alopecia associated with epidermal changes, such as lupus erythematosus.

Hematoxylin and eosin are the primary stains. Elastic tissue stains, periodic acid-Schiff (PAS), and mucin stains are optional.

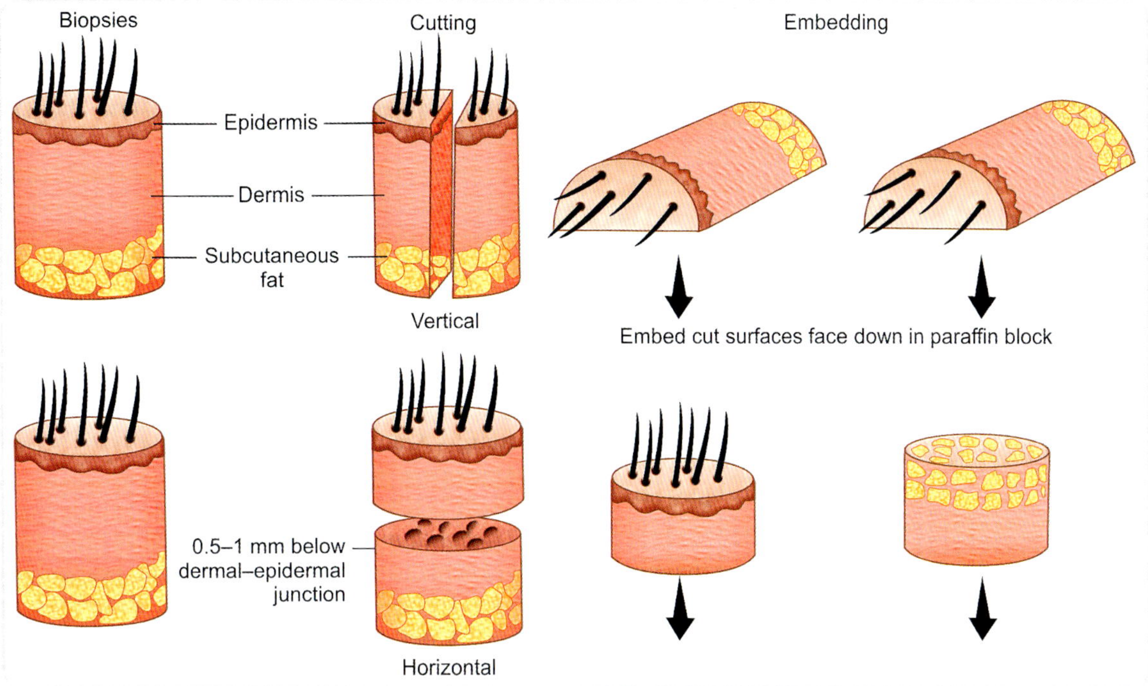

FIG. 1: Vertical versus horizontal sections.

DEFINITION OF THE FOLLICULAR UNIT

- It has been demonstrated that hair follicles, sebaceous glands, arrectores pilorum muscles, and the surrounding connective tissue occur in specialized anatomical units called the "follicular units." The follicular unit consists of:
- One to four terminal follicles
- One, or rarely two, vellus follicles
- Associated sebaceous lobules and insertions of the arrector pili
- Perifollicular vascular plexus and neural network
- Perifollicular collagen

This concept of follicular unit has now become the cornerstone of recent techniques in HT.

CLASSIFICATION

Traditionally, alopecias have been classified into nonscarring and scarring types. **Box 1** shows the different nonscarring alopecias.[1,2]

BOX 1 Nonscarring alopecia.

- Congenital alopecias
- Premature catagen/telogen—Telogen effluvium
- Premature telogen with anagen arrest (alopecia areata)
- Miniaturization and vellus follicle formation (androgenetic alopecia)
- Anagen effluvium
- Hair shaft abnormalities

Alopecia Areata[5] (Fig. 2)

Representative features are seen in early lesions, in middermis.

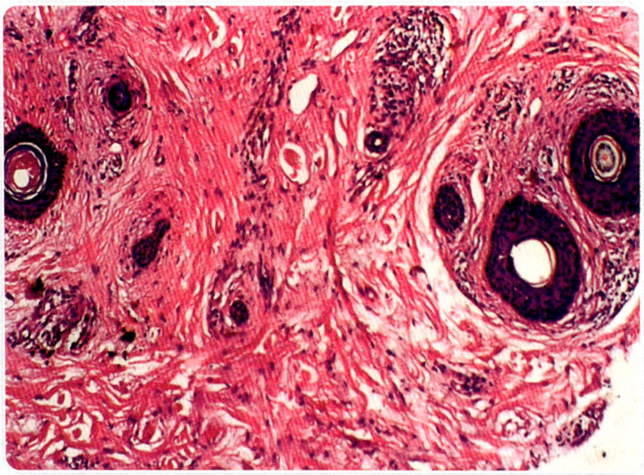

FIG. 2: Alopecia areata.

Even though clinical and dermoscopic features are fairly diagnostic, biopsy is needed and can be helpful in selected cases. Biopsy shows a lichenoid histopathology characterized by dense inflammatory lymphocytic infiltrate involving the isthmus and infundibulum of the hair follicles, apoptotic cells in the external root sheath, and a concentric fibrosis surrounding the hair follicles.[10] Association of FFA with lichen planus also has been reported.

Central Centrifugal Cicatricial Alopecia

It is a newly described entity characterized by hair loss starting in the central scalp and progressing centrifugally. It has been previously referred to by other terms such as follicular degeneration syndrome and hot-comb alopecia.

- The earliest observable histological abnormality is the premature desquamation of the inner root sheath.
- In severely affected follicles, this is followed by complete follicular degeneration.

Folliculitis Decalvans

- Polymorphonuclear cells within hair follicle.
- Chronic inflammatory infiltrate of plasma cells and lymphocytes around appendages.
- Presence of scarring in dermis.

Alopecia Mucinosa

Alopecia mucinosa can be idiopathic or associated with mycosis fungoides.

- Hair follicles appear vacuolated, cystic, and empty.
- Alcian blue stain demonstrates this vacuolation to be due to acid mucopolysaccharide.
- Dense lymphocytic infiltration surrounding and permeating into the hair follicle.
- In alopecia mucinosa associated with mycosis fungoides, atypical lymphocytes are seen.

APPROACH TO DIAGNOSIS OF ALOPECIAS

Any interpretation of skin biopsy in alopecia should answer the following questions:

- Is it scarring or nonscarring alopecia?
- If nonscarring—which type?
- If scarring, which type?
- Is there a possibility of hair growth?

TABLE 1: Summary of findings in alopecias.

Infundibular level	
Lichenoid reaction (interfollicular epidermis)	Lupus erythematosus Lichen planopilaris (one-third of cases)
Lymphocytic infiltrate ± fibrosis	• Lupus erythematosus • Lichen planopilaris • Pseudopelade (in middle third)
Neutrophilic infiltrate ± fibrosis, with lymphocytes and plasma cells	• Dissecting cellulitis of the scalp • Folliculitis decalvans • Acne keloidalis • Infectious folliculitis
Miniature hair shafts	Androgenic alopecia
Melanin casts	Trichotillomania/traumatic alopecia
Isthmus level	
Lymphocytic infiltrate ± fibrosis	• Lupus erythematosus • Lichen planopilaris • Pseudopelade
Miniature bulbs and follicles of varying diameter without inflammation	Androgenic alopecia
Miniature bulbs with swarm of bees cells	Alopecia areata
Loss of internal root sheath	Follicular degeneration syndrome
Melanin casts/trichomalacia	Trichotillomania/traumatic alopecia
Hair bulb level	
Fibrous tract and reduced number of follicles	• Alopecia areata • Lupus erythematosus • Lichen planus • Androgenic alopecia
Inflamed hair bulbs ("swarm of bees")	Active alopecia areata
"Torn" catagen follicles ± hemorrhage	Trichotillomania

Biopsy is the most important investigation in alopecias **(Table 1)**. It allows:

- *Qualitative interpretation*: Morphology of follicles, inflammation, fibrosis, etc.
- *Quantitative information*: Size, number, and follicular phase

Much of this data can only be obtained from transverse sections.

SUMMARY

- Histopathology is a valuable investigation in cases of scarring alopecia and diffuse alopecia.
- Biopsy should be performed for DIF for diagnosis of lupus erythematosus and to rule it out from pseudopelade.
- It is of value when planning HT in cases of scarring alopecia.
- Frontal fibrosing alopecia needs to be kept in mind as a differential diagnosis of AGA.

REFERENCES

1. Yeliur IK, Tirumalae R. Histopathologic approach to alopecia. Indian J Dermatopathol Diagn Dermatol. 2018;5(2):79.
2. Mysore V. Fundamentals of Pathology of Skin, 4th edition. Delhi: Wolters Kluwer; 2015. pp. 6-20.
3. Knopp E. The scalp biopsy for hair loss and its interpretation. Semin Cutan Med Surg. 2015;34:57-66.
4. Headington JT. Transverse microscopic anatomy of the human scalp. A basis for a morphometric approach to disorders of the hair follicle. Arch Dermatol. 1984;120:449-56.
5. Werner B, Mulinari-Brenner F. Clinical and histological challenge in the differential diagnosis of diffuse alopecia: female androgenetic alopecia, telogen effluvium and alopecia areata—part II. An Bras Dermatol. 2012;87:884-90.
6. Whiting DA. Histopathologic features of alopecia areata: a new look. Arch Dermatol. 2003;139:1555-9.
7. Muller SA. Trichotillomania: a histopathologic study in sixty-six patients. J Am Acad Dermatol. 1990;23:56-62.
8. Sperling LC, Solomon AR, Whiting DA. A new look at scarring alopecia. Arch Dermatol. 2000;136:235-42.
9. Hordinsky M. Cicatricial alopecia: discoid lupus erythematosus. Dermatol Ther. 2008;21:245-8.
10. Zinkernagel MS, Trueb RM. Fibrosing alopecia in a pattern distribution: patterned lichen planopilaris or androgenetic alopecia with a lichenoid tissue reaction pattern? Arch Dermatol. 2000;136:205-11.

CHAPTER 13

Trichoscopy for the Hair Transplant Surgeon

Balachandra S Ankad

INTRODUCTION

Trichoscopy, the dermoscopy of hair and scalp, is a diagnostic method in which analysis of scalp and hairs is performed using an instrument called dermoscope. Dermoscope, which is analogous to ophthalmoscope or otoscope, uses a light source to enable the clinician to visualize surface and subsurface structures in skin. Trichoscopy gives an account of hair shaft abnormalities, follicular openings, scalp vasculature, and interfollicular area. It has proven to be a good diagnostic adjunct in inflammatory, infective, and tumorous dermatoses of the scalp.[1]

INSTRUMENT[2]

Dermoscope consists of *light-emitting diodes (LED)* as light source that are both polarized and nonpolarized modes and *magnifying achromatic lens* that magnifies from 10–16 to 20–220-fold. It also includes *battery* for power supply and *facility* to capture the images **(Fig. 1)**.

Types of Dermoscope

- Handheld manual dermoscope with 10–16 magnification, which requires external source (smartphone or dedicated camera) to visualize and capture the images **(Fig. 1)**.
- Videodermoscope, with magnification range between 20 and 220-fold, to be attached to a monitor or a desktop to display and save images **(Fig. 2)**.

Physics of Dermoscope

Why are our eyes unable to see the underneath structures of skin? The factors are as follows: (1) Incident light is reflected, scattered, refracted, and absorbed; (2) difference between the refractive indices of stratum corneum (1.55) and air (1.0). To attenuate these factors, achromatic lens (with a refractive index of 1.52) in dermoscope, interface medium, and polarization are utilized. Thereby, there is reduction in the reflective glare, and light penetrates deeper, which helps in the visualization of deep structures. Polarized and nonpolarized lights assist in the visibility of deeper and superficial structures, respectively. Scales, milia-like cysts, comedo-like openings, and skin furrows are better seen with nonpolarized light, while pigment, vessels, and collagen are demonstrated well with polarized lights.[3]

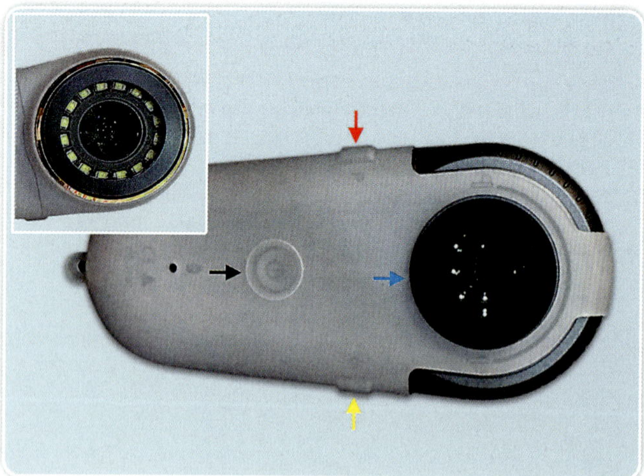

FIG. 1: Parts of a handheld dermoscope. Power button (black arrow), a button for polarized and nonpolarized modes (red arrow), and magnet ring facility around the eyepiece for smartphone attachment (blue arrow). Note the button for brightness variation (yellow arrow). *Inset*: Achromatic lens with light-emitting diodes.

Source: With permission from Ankad BS, Mukherjee SS, Smitha SV. Trichoscopy in hair disorders in darker skin: an approach to diagnosis. Clin Dermatol Rev. 2020;4:102-14.

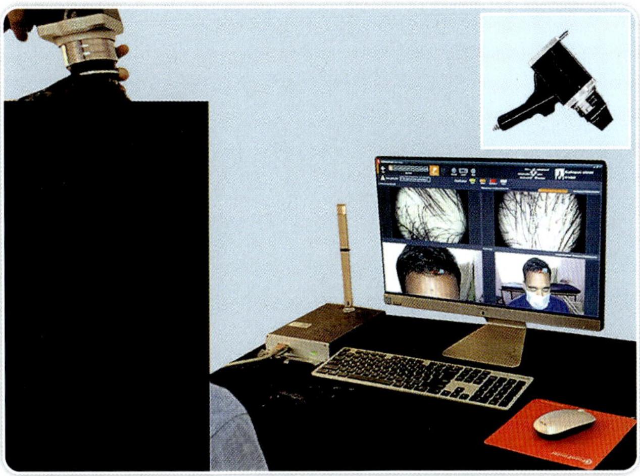

FIG. 2: Videodermoscope with display of clinical image of scalp and trichoscopy as well. *Inset*: FotoFinder Medical 1000 videodermoscope.

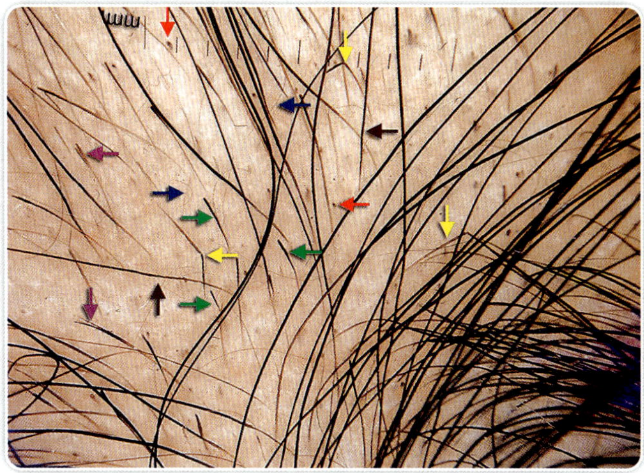

FIG. 3: Trichoscopy of alopecia areata showing exclamation mark hairs (green arrows) and tapered hairs (maroon arrows). Note the coudability hairs (yellow arrows), short vellus hairs (blue arrows), and trichoptilosis (purple arrows).

Source: With permission from Ankad BS, Mukherjee SS, Smitha SV. Trichoscopy in hair disorders in darker skin: an approach to diagnosis. Clin Dermatol Rev. 2020;4:102-14.

STEPWISE APPROACH TO TRICHOSCOPY

Trichoscopy is practiced by a definite protocol to make sure to include all structures of the scalp and hair. One should examine a given scalp dermatosis in the following pattern:[4]

1. Hair shaft abnormalities
2. Follicular changes
3. Interfollicular area (for pigment changes)
4. Vascular structures

In detail, *hair shaft abnormalities* result from congenital and acquired dermatoses that cause twisting, curving, narrowing, and breakage of hair shaft. Examples of narrowing of shaft include exclamation mark hairs, tapered hairs **(Fig. 3)**, monilethrix hairs, Pohl-Pinkus constrictions **(Fig. 4)**, and tulip hairs. Broken hairs and circle (pigtail) hairs **(Fig. 5)**, comma hairs and coiled hairs **(Fig. 6)**, zig-zag hairs **(Fig. 7)**, and flame hairs constitute examples of hair shaft abnormalities.

The *follicular changes* include black dots, yellow dots, white dots, and red dots. Black dot is the remnant of hair shaft that is cut at scalp surface **(Fig. 5)**. Yellow dot represents dilated infundibulum with sebum and/or keratin **(Fig. 8)**. White dot is due to either hair follicle opening or eccrine opening. Follicular white dots vary in size and shape, whereas eccrine white dots are uniform in size and shape **(Fig. 4)**. Red dots are seen exclusively (until now) in discoid lupus erythematosus (DLE) due to extravasation of erythrocytes around the follicle **(Fig. 9)**. The other follicular changes include follicular keratotic plugs, wherein keratin mass plugs the follicular openings.

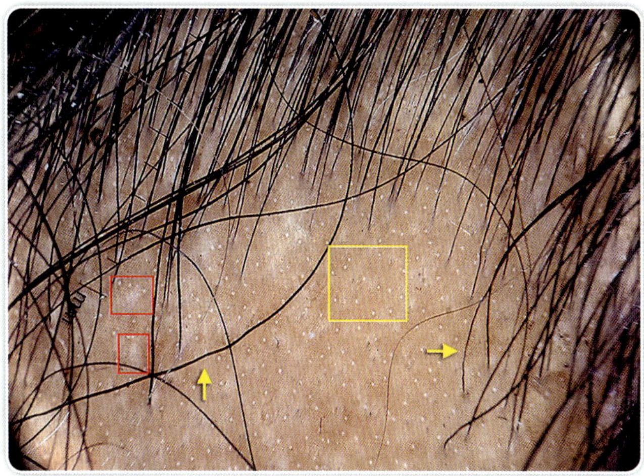

FIG. 4: Trichoscopy of alopecia areata showing Pohl-Pinkus constrictions (yellow arrows) and white dots of eccrine (yellow box) and follicular openings (red boxes).

The *interfollicular area* shows blue-gray dots, white areas, scales, and pigmentation. Blue-gray dots represent dermal melanin/melanophages seen in the perifollicular position in lichen planopilaris (LPP), giving a "targetoid pattern." In contrast, they are situated in interfollicular and perifollicular areas, showing a scattered pattern. White areas are due to fibrosis and are typically seen in cicatricial alopecia **(Fig. 10)**. Reticular/honeycomb pigmentation is characteristically seen as a normal phenomenon in skin of color. It is due to increase in the melanin after sun

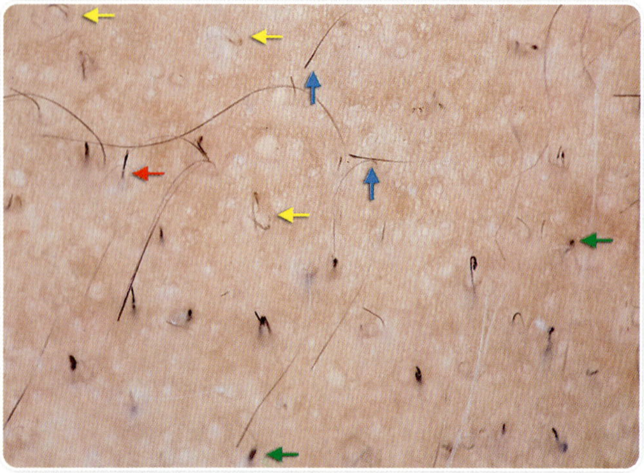

FIG. 5: Trichoscopy of alopecia areata showing broken hairs (red arrow), pigtail hairs (yellow arrows), and black dots (green arrows). Note the exclamation mark hairs (blue arrows).

Source: With permission from Ankad BS, Mukherjee SS, Smitha SV. Trichoscopy in hair disorders in darker skin: an approach to diagnosis. Clin Dermatol Rev. 2020;4:102-14.

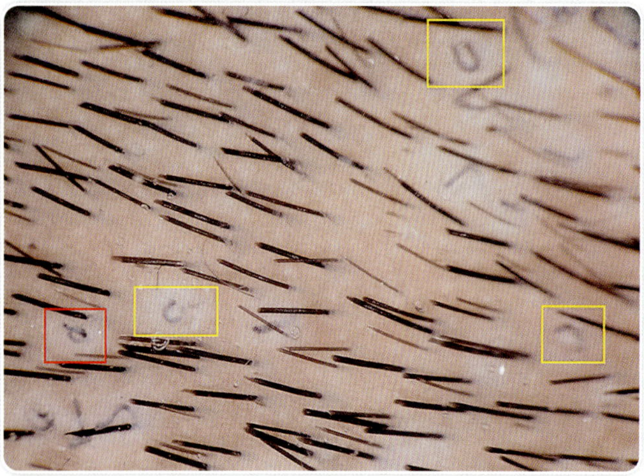

FIG. 6: Trichoscopy of tinea capitis showing comma hairs (yellow boxes) and coiled hair (red box).

exposure to the bald scalp **(Fig. 5)**. Scales are located either in perifollicular **(Fig. 7)** or in interfollicular **(Fig. 9)** area. They are of white, yellow, and brown color. They are focal and/or diffuse in arrangement. Few other changes include brown area—postinflammatory pigmentation, yellow area—serous discharge, and red area—dilated vessels.

Vascular structures on the scalp consist of simple loop vessels, which are normally seen, twisted red loops that are noted in both seborrheic dermatitis and psoriasis, and thick arborizing vessels in DLE **(Fig. 11)**. In few instants, concentric perifollicular vessels are noted in LPP and frontal fibrosing alopecia.

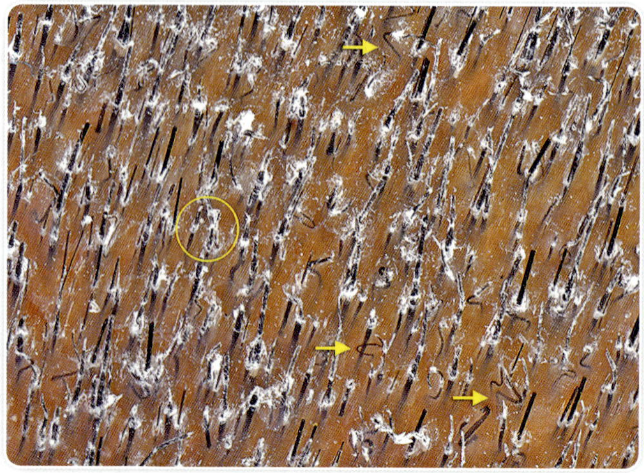

FIG. 7: Trichoscopy of tinea capitis showing zig-zag hairs (yellow arrows) and perifollicular scale (yellow circle).

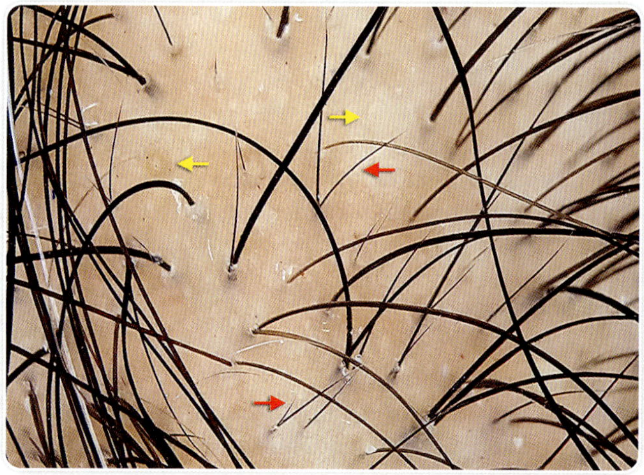

FIG. 8: Trichoscopy showing yellow dots (yellow arrows) and upright regrowing hairs (red arrows).

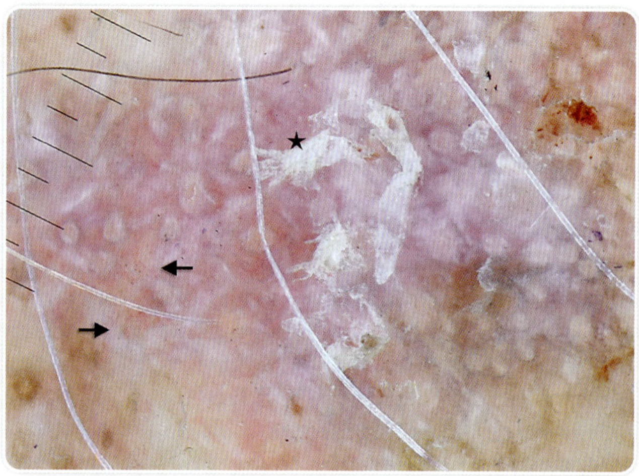

FIG. 9: Trichoscopy of discoid lupus erythematosus showing perifollicular red dots (black arrows) and scales in the interfollicular area (black star).

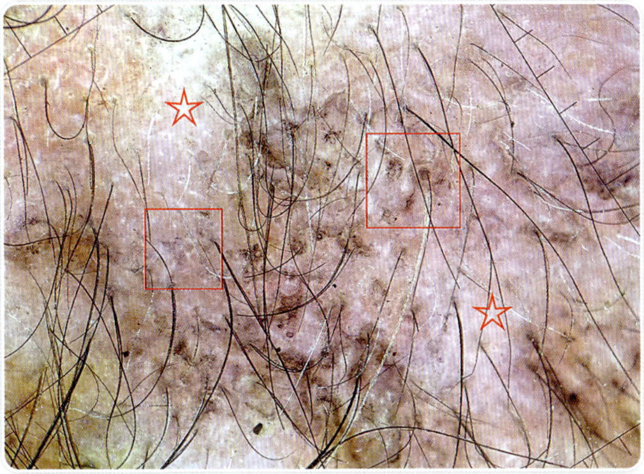

FIG. 10: Trichoscopy of discoid lupus erythematosus showing scattered pattern of blue–gray pigment globules (red boxes) and white areas (red stars).

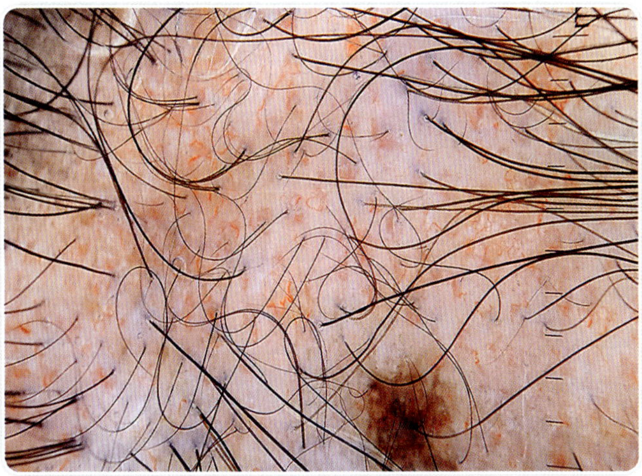

FIG. 11: Trichoscopy of discoid lupus erythematosus showing thick arborizing vessels.

TRICHOSCOPY IN THE PERSPECTIVE OF HAIR TRANSPLANTATION

Generally, hair transplantation is performed in patterned hair loss, and rarely it is done in other causes of hair loss. Trichoscopy is crucial for transplantation, not only as a preoperative tool to assess the donor area but also to recognize other causes of hair loss. It determines hair density and number of follicular units in donor area. It demonstrates specific trichoscopic features in patterned hair loss. Furthermore, it distinguishes the mimickers such as alopecia areata incognito (AAI) and fibrosing alopecia in patterned distribution (FAPD).[5]

Before we proceed for transplantation, it is prudent to know trichoscopy of normal scalp. In healthy individuals, normal scalp demonstrates two types of hairs, namely terminal hairs and vellus hairs. The former appear as properly pigmented with uniformly thick hair and the latter hairs are poorly pigmented with reduced diameter and length **(Fig. 12)**. Accordingly, the thickness and color are uniform in >80% of the hairs, which are terminal hairs. Thin hairs with reduced pigment constitute up to 20% of the hairs. Follicular units are grouped with single to four hairs.[6]

In androgenetic alopecia, there is hair diameter diversity (anisotrichosis) with reduced terminal hairs with miniaturization and vellus hair formation, in both male pattern and female pattern hair loss **(Fig. 13)**. In addition, yellow dots, peripilar sign, and single follicular units are characteristically found. Yellow dots **(Fig. 13)** are commonly observed in frontal area as compared to occipital scalp. Two types of peripilar signs are present. Early in the disease process, brownish discoloration of perifollicle area is termed "brown peripilar sign" **(Fig. 14)**. In the late stage, it becomes white, which is referred to as "white peripilar sign" **(Fig. 15)**. These two features are suggestive of impending perifollicular fibrosis.

As mentioned above, AAI is typified by numerous yellow dots on the entire scalp. They vary in size. Other features include upright regrowing hairs, tapered terminal hairs, and circle (pigtail) hairs. Occasional black dots are seen **(Fig. 16)**. It should be noted that AAI is late in onset and it affects parieto-occipital scalp.[7] It is noteworthy that

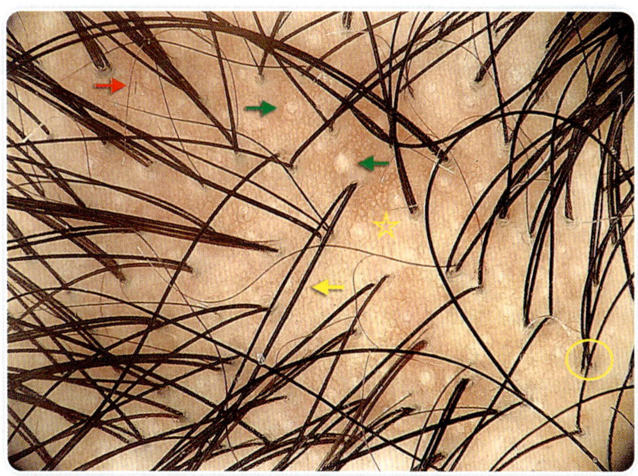

FIG. 12: Trichoscopy of normal scalp showing terminal hair (yellow arrow) and vellus hairs (red arrow) with follicular unit (yellow circle). Note the eccrine and follicular openings (green arrows) and honeycomb pigmentation (yellow star).

Source: With permission from Ankad BS, Mukherjee SS, Smitha SV. Trichoscopy in hair disorders in darker skin: an approach to diagnosis. Clin Dermatol Rev. 2020;4:102-14.

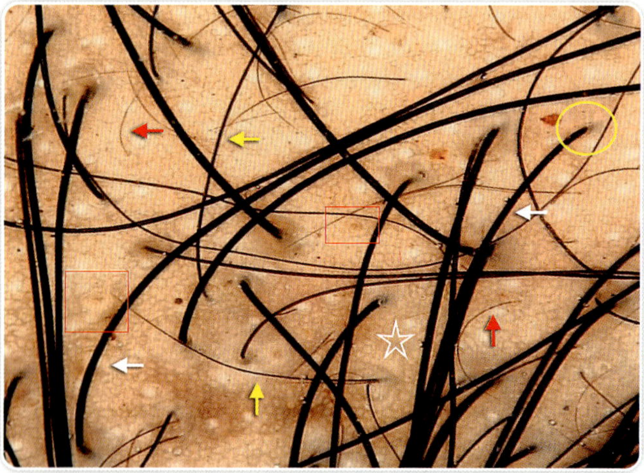

FIG. 13: Trichoscopy of androgenetic alopecia showing terminal hairs (white arrows), miniaturized hairs (yellow arrows), and vellus hairs (red arrows). Yellow dots (red boxes), pigment network (white star), and single hair follicular unit (yellow circle) are well appreciated.

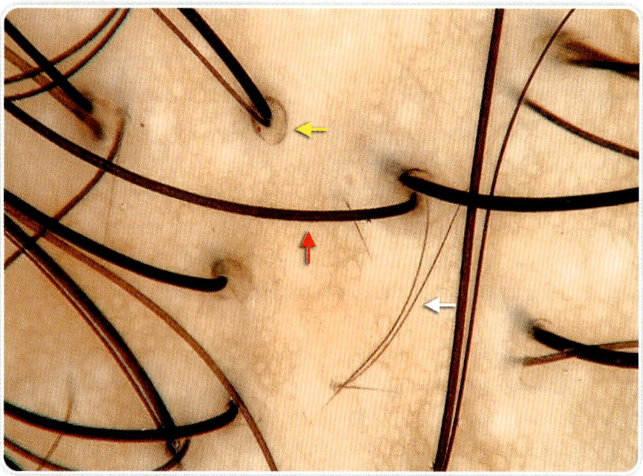

FIG. 14: Trichoscopy of androgenetic alopecia showing brownish pigmentation around follicles termed "brown peripilar sign" (yellow arrow), terminal hairs (red arrow), and vellus hairs (white arrow).

a yellow dot would appear as whitish-yellow dots in skin of color. It is mandatory that the mimickers of patterned hair loss should be differentiated before advocating hair transplantation. Since AAI is treatable with topical steroids with full response, the diagnosis of patterned hair should be ascertained by trichoscopy. If trichoscopy is doubtful, one may take a call for histopathological confirmation. Follicular units and hair density are determined by recent technology such as FotoFinder Trichoscale **(Fig. 2)**. A hair transplant surgeon can utilize these facilities for identification of anisotrichosis and calculate hair density in donor area.

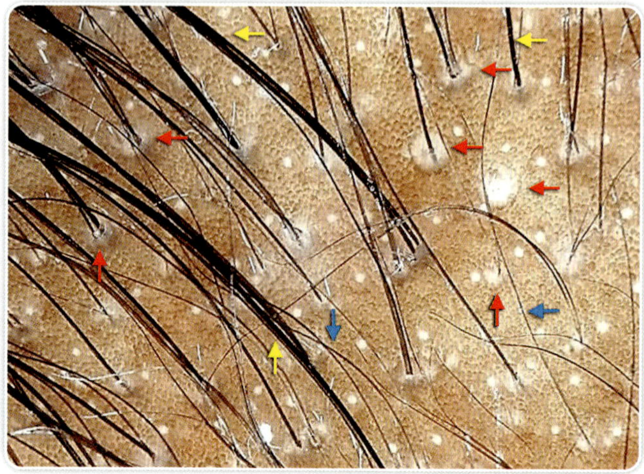

FIG. 15: Trichoscopy of androgenetic alopecia in an advanced stage shows peripilar white halo (red arrows), numerous miniaturized hairs (blue arrows), and terminal hairs (yellow arrows). Note the honeycomb pigmentation, hair diameter diversity, and pinpoint white dots.

Source: With permission from Ankad BS, Mukherjee SS, Smitha SV. Trichoscopy in hair disorders in darker skin: an approach to diagnosis. Clin Dermatol Rev. 2020;4:102-14.

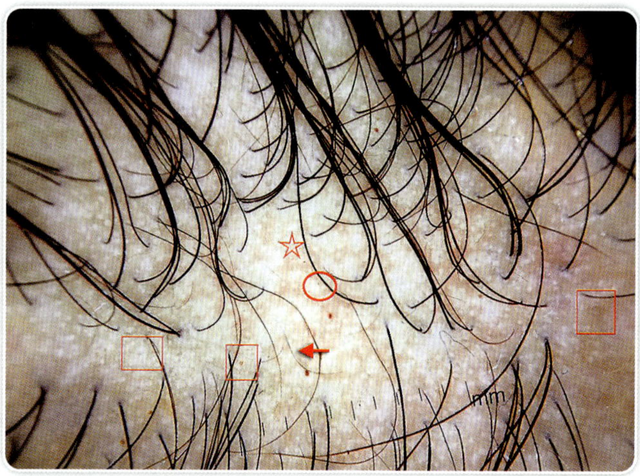

FIG. 16: Trichoscopy of alopecia areata incognito shows yellow dots (red boxes), upright regrowing hairs (red arrow), and black dots (red circle). Note the honeycomb pigmentation (red star).

Courtesy: Dr Chetan Rajput, Professor, SBH Govt. Medical College Dhule, Maharashtra.

SUMMARY

Hence, trichoscopy is an in vivo method that assists in identification of patterned hair loss, and preoperative assessment of donor area is possible as well. Finally, there is a learning curve in trichoscopy; one should perform it to master it.

REFERENCES

1. Rudnicka L, Rakowska A, Olszewska M. Trichoscopy: how it may help the clinician. Dermatol Clin. 2013;31:29-41.
2. Adya KA. Dermoscopy: an overview of the principles, procedure and practice. In: Ankad BS, Mukherjee SS, Nikam BP (Eds). Dermoscopy-Histopathology Correlation. Singapore: Springer Nature; 2021. pp. 1-14.
3. Benvenuto-Andrade C, Dusza SW, Agero AL, Scope A, Rajadhyaksha M, Halpern AC, et al. Differences between polarized light dermoscopy and immersion contact dermoscopy for the evaluation of skin lesions. Arch Dermatol. 2007;143:329-38.
4. Lacarrubba F, Micali G, Tosti A. Scalp dermoscopy or trichoscopy. Curr Probl Dermatol. 2015;47:21-32.
5. Issa NT, Tosti A. Trichoscopy for the hair transplant surgeon-assessing for mimickers of androgenetic alopecia and preoperative evaluation of donor site area. Indian J Plast Surg. 2021;54(4):393-8.
6. Rakowska A, Olszewska M, Rudnica L, Slowwinska M, Czuwara J, Rusek M, et al. Hair shafts. In: Rudnica L, Olszewska M, Rakowska A (Eds). Atlas of Trichoscopy. London: Springer; 2012. pp. 25-8.
7. Alessandrini A, Starace M, Bruni F, Brandi N, Baraldi C, Misciali C, et al. Alopecia areata incognita and diffuse alopecia areata: clinical, trichoscopic, histopathological, and therapeutic features of a 5-year study. Dermatol Pract Concept. 2019;9(4):272-7.

PART D: Pattern Hair Loss

SECTION OUTLINE

CHAPTER 14

Classification of Pattern Hair Loss*

Mrinal Gupta, Venkataram Mysore

Key Messages

- Currently, the Hamilton–Norwood classification system for males and the Ludwig system for females are the most commonly used systems to describe patterns of hair loss. However, these systems have limitations.
- Numerous classification systems have been proposed by various researchers for grading purposes.
- Basic and specific (BASP) classification takes care of some of the limitations but is more complex.

INTRODUCTION

Patterned hair loss is the most common cause of hair loss seen in both sexes after puberty, typically presenting with progressive thinning, miniaturization, and loss of hair at the affected sites. Hair loss varies in extent and severity, and numerous stages exist between the stages of early frontotemporal recession to the stage of residual occipital hair. Several classification systems for pattern hair loss in both males and females have been proposed.[1,2]

The ideal classification of hair loss should have the following characteristics:

- It should be simple.
- It should be easy to apply.
- It should incorporate all the evolutionary stages of hair loss.
- It should include the rarer hair loss patterns.
- It should be applicable to all racial groups.
- A single classification system should include both male and female pattern hair loss.
- It should help in defining the indication for surgical treatment and in deciding the type of surgery.
- Various classification systems for pattern hair loss described in the literature are reviewed.

CLASSIFICATIONS OF MALE PATTERN HAIR LOSS

Beek (1950): Beek evaluated 1,000 Caucasian males with pattern hair loss and classified them into two types—(i) frontal and (ii) frontovertical baldness, based on the stage of evolution.[1] It was a simple classification that described only two stages of hair loss and did not take into account the various evolutionary stages but is important as this was the first attempt to classify hair loss.

Hamilton (1951): Hamilton, an anatomist, studied >300 males with hair loss and proposed a detailed classification system based on frontoparietal and frontal recession and frontal thinning, which consisted of eight evolutionary aspects and three subgroups. The various categories of hair loss described by Hamilton include (A) *scalps which are not bald* (types I–III) and (B) *scalps which are bald* (types IV–VIII), which are defined as follows **(Fig. 1)**:[3]

- *Type I*: The absence of bilateral recessions along the anterior border of the hairline in the frontoparietal regions. In this, there is a variant form in which the entire anterior border of the hairline lies high on the forehead, which is referred to as type IA.

*The content of this chapter was published in a review article in Journal of Cutaneous and Asthetic Surgery. Classification of patterened hair loss: a review. 2016;9(1):1-55.

The authors gratefully acknowledge the permission received from the journal for reproducing the content in this chapter.

the entire top of the scalp. The various grades of hair loss described by Norwood include the following **(Fig. 3)**:[6]

- *Type I*: Minimal or no recession of the hairline
- *Type II*: Triangular, usually symmetrical, areas of recession at the frontotemporal hairline
- *Type III*: This represents the minimal extent of hair loss sufficient to be considered as baldness according to Norwood. There are deep symmetrical recessions at the temples that are bare or only sparsely covered by hair. In type III vertex, the hair loss is primarily from the vertex with limited recession of the fronto-temporal hairline that does not exceed the degree of recession seen in type III.
- *Type IV*: The frontotemporal recession is more severe than in type III, and there is sparse hair or no hair on the vertex. The two areas of hair loss are separated by a band of moderately dense hair that extends across the top. This band connects with the fully-haired fringe on the sides of the scalp.

Norwood's classification for male pattern hair loss: Norwood's classification system is widely used for male pattern hair loss and defines various stages of hair loss progression. Here are the different stages described in the classification:

- *Type I*: Minimal or no recession of the hairline
- *Type II*: Slight recession of the hairline at the temples
- *Type III*: Frontotemporal recession starts, creating an M-shaped hairline.
- *Type III Vertex*: Hair loss extends to the vertex (crown) of the scalp.

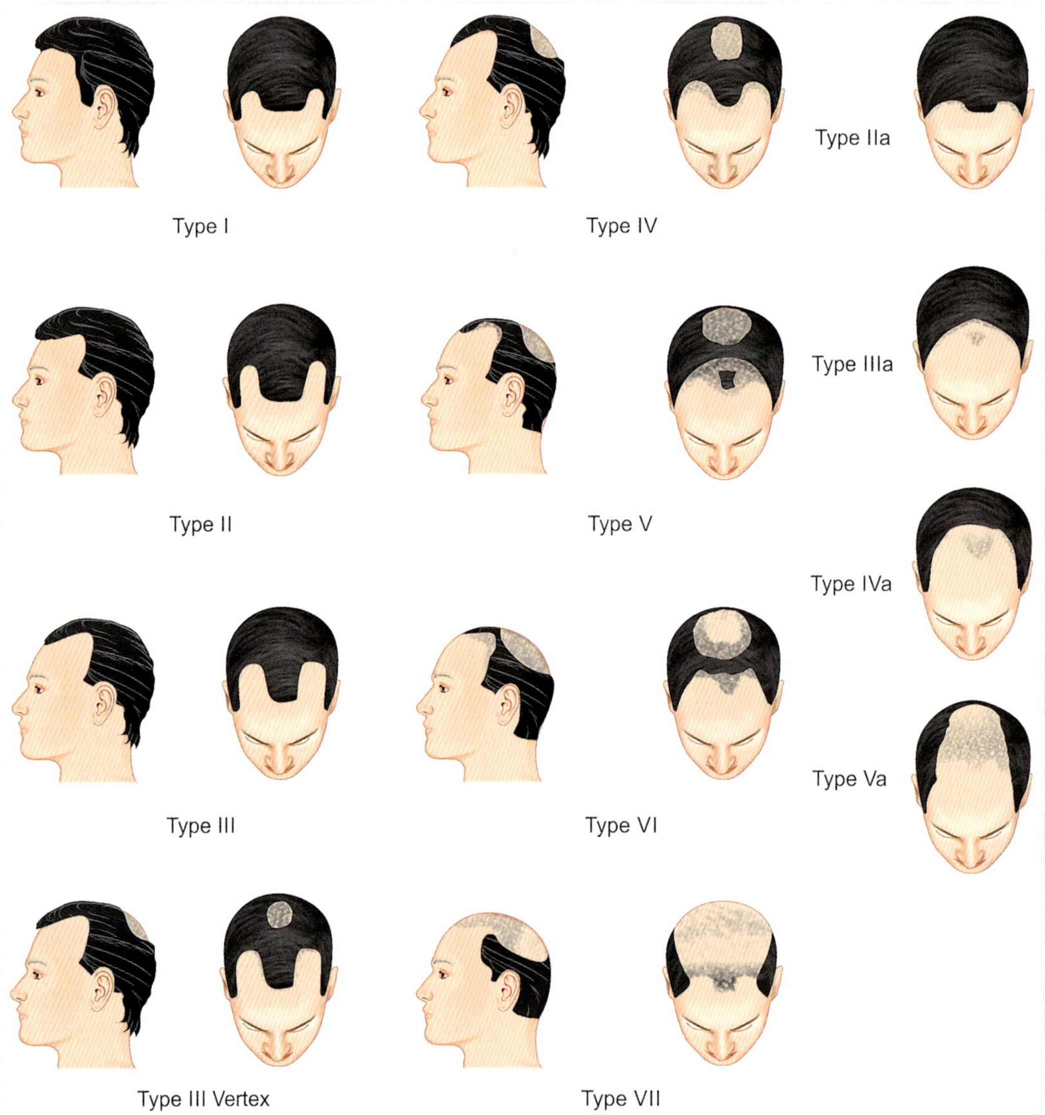

FIG. 3: Norwood's classification of male pattern hair loss.

- *Type IV*: Further frontal and temporal recession; vertex loss more pronounced
- *Type V*: Vertex and frontotemporal regions of hair loss are connected; the bridge of hair on the crown narrows.
- *Type VI*: Bridge of hair on the crown disappears, frontotemporal and vertex regions merge.
- *Type VII*: Most severe form, only a narrow horseshoe-shaped band of hair remains on the sides and back of the scalp.

  Norwood also introduced a type A variant that involves continuous frontal hairline recession without leaving an island of hair in the midfrontal region. Various type A variants were described based on specific features.

Advantages of Norwood's classification: Detailed and includes various rarer patterns of hair loss not described by previous classifications.

Disadvantages of Norwood's classification: Does not address diffuse hair loss or specific variations, such as balding patches on the vertex or occiput with a preserved anterior hairline, and does not describe the disappearance of the temporal hump in some patients.

Bouhanna (1976): Based on observations in European Caucasians, Bouhanna designed a much simplified male pattern baldness classification system in 1976, which included just three basic hair loss presentations with two variants as follows **(Fig. 4)**:

- *Stage 1*:
  - Type a: Symmetric recession of the frontal margin forming two temporal areas of recession of varying depth
  - Type b: Sparseness at the cranial summit or vertex
- *Stage 2*:
  - Type a: Uniform recession of the frontal margin as far as the cranial summit
  - Type b: With associated vertex
- *Stage 3*:
  - The ultimate stage of alopecia, with only a remnant temporo-occipital crown[7]

Advantages: Bouhanna's classification was a simplified classification system based on the extent of hair loss and allowed a precise evaluation of surgical indication of hair transplantation.

Disadvantages: This classification is a simple classification that does not include the complete evolutionary staging of hair loss and is also not helpful in deciding about the type of surgical procedure required, which was later addressed by Bouhanna himself in a multifactorial classification.

Dynamic classification of Dardour and Bouhanna (1996): They proposed a classification system that included all the

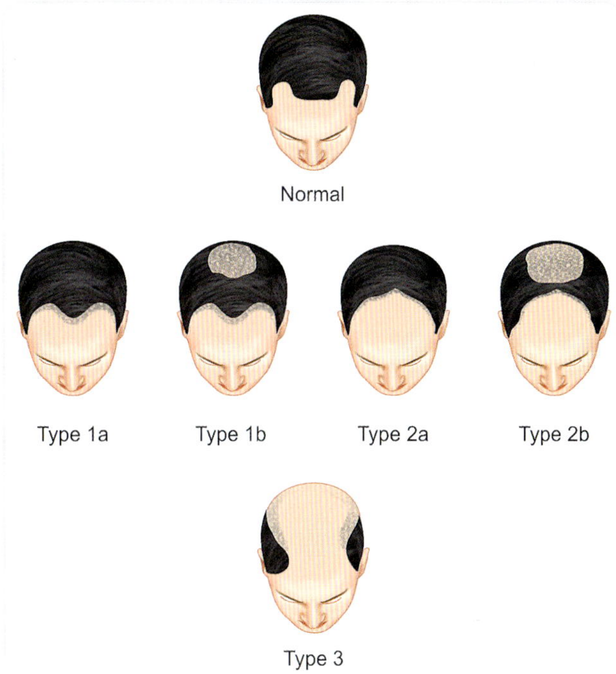

FIG. 4: Bouhanna's classification of male hair loss.

parameters, both morphological and dynamic, that affects the scalp and the hair itself. This classification includes for each heading a symbol followed by a number, which indicates its situation. The various parameters included in this system include the stage of hair loss, density of hair, laxity of the scalp, aspect of hair, color and thickness of hair, and rate of hair growth.[8]

Advantages: This classification was more detailed than the previously described systems, and it took into account various parameters that were not considered by Hamilton such as the covering power of hair, density in each region, and rate of growth of hair.

- *Stage 1:*
  - Type a: Symmetric recession of the frontal margin resulting in two temporal areas of varying-depth recession
  - Type b: Sparseness at the cranial summit or vertex
- *Stage 2*:
  - Type a: Uniform recession of the frontal margin extending to the cranial summit
  - Type b: Accompanied by vertex involvement
- *Stage 3*:
  - Represents the ultimate stage of alopecia, characterized by a remaining temporo-occipital crown

Advantages: Bouhanna's classification provides a simplified approach based on the extent of hair loss, facilitating accurate assessment of the need for surgical hair transplantation.

Disadvantages: This classification lacks a comprehensive evolutionary staging of hair loss and does not guide the selection of surgical procedures. Bouhanna himself addressed this limitation by developing a multifactorial classification.

Dynamic classification of Dardour and Bouhanna (1996): Their proposed system incorporates a comprehensive set of parameters affecting the scalp and hair, including both morphological and dynamic factors. Each parameter is represented by a symbol followed by a number indicating its status. Parameters encompass hair loss stage, hair density, scalp laxity, hair appearance, color, thickness, and growth rate.

Advantages: This detailed classification considers various factors previously unaccounted for, such as hair covering power, regional density, and hair growth rate, offering a more comprehensive assessment compared to earlier systems.

Disadvantages: It is too complicated and difficult to apply in routine practice as it involves a large number of measurements and parameters.

Koo (2000): As the Norwood's classification method is too detailed and complicated to be used for various surgical operations and also does not list some peculiar types of baldness, it is not very helpful in determining the surgical procedures. Koo et al. studied >1,700 Korean males with patterned hair loss and proposed a new, simpler classification method. In this classification, the male pattern baldness is classified into six subtypes by the English alphabetical letter shape of the bald area. The various subtypes in this classification include the following **(Figs. 5A to F)**:

- *Type M*: When both sides of the frontotemporal hairlines look triangular or like the letter M
- *Type C*: When the anterior hairline looks like a half-circle or the letter C. M and C types of male pattern baldness do not have hair loss on the vertex.
- *Type O*: When there is a round or ovoid bald patch on the vertex or occiput while the anterior hairline is well preserved.
- *Type U*: When the recession of the anterior hairline progresses over the vertex, which looks like a horse-shoe or the letter U.
- *Types MO and CO*: When recession of the fronto-temporal hairline exists, with a bald patch on the vertex, as combined patterns, these are types MO and CO, according to the shape of the recession of the anterior hairline.[9]

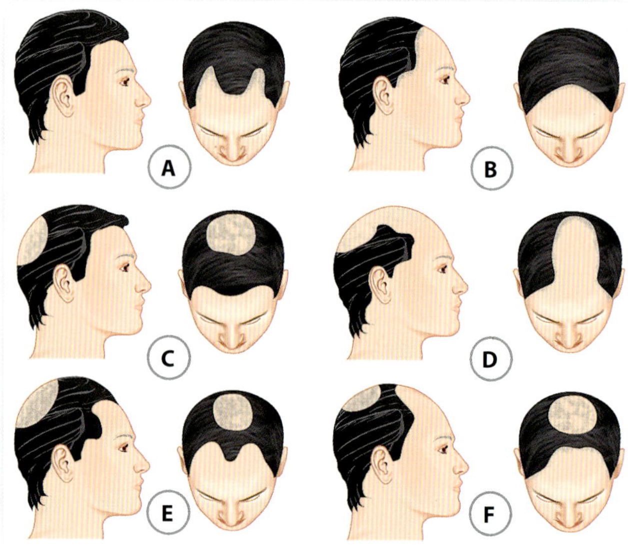

FIGS. 5A TO F: Koo's classification of male pattern hair loss. (A) M type; (B) C type; (C) O type; (D) U type; (E) MO type; (F) CO type.

Advantages: This classification system has advantages over the previous classification as it is simpler, easy to apply, does not require complex measurements, and is useful in planning surgery.

Disadvantages: *Diffuse hair loss mimicking female pattern hair loss*: This classification does not describe diffuse hair loss mimicking female pattern hair loss, unlike most other classifications except for the Bouhanna revised classification.

CLASSIFICATIONS OF FEMALE PATTERN HAIR LOSS

Ebling and Rook (1975): They developed a five-stage classification system for female pattern baldness: The first two stages are the same as the Ludwig system. Type I shows perceptible thinning of the hair on the crown. Type II shows pronounced rarefaction of the hair on the crown within the area seen in type I. Type III shows continued diffuse hair loss in the region defined in types I and II, but also the initial loss of hair from the frontotemporal hairline. Type IV shows a continuation of this diffuse loss and frontotemporal recession, and in type V, there is complete loss of hair on the top of the scalp resembling a male pattern of baldness **(Fig. 6)**.[10]

Advantages: Ebling and Rook took into account that women could have both a diffuse form of alopecia and also a male pattern with a recession of the frontotemporal hairline.

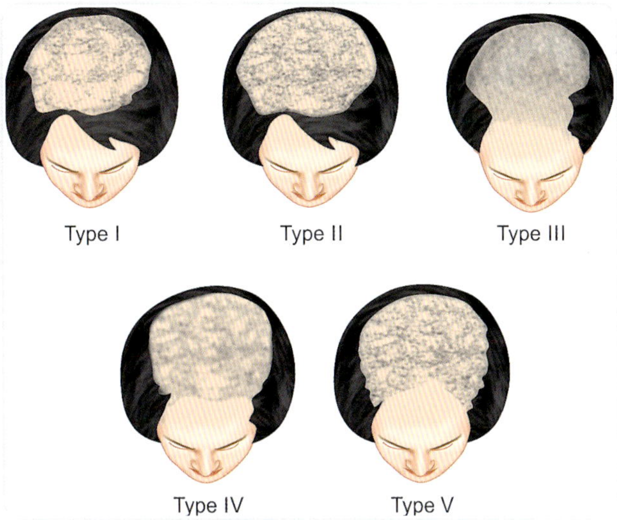

FIG. 6: Ebling and Rook's classification of female hair loss.

Disadvantages: This classification did not incorporate the accentuation of frontovertical alopecia, which was later included by Olsen.

Ludwig (1977): Ludwig observed 468 females with hair loss and proposed a classification based on the stage of evolution. The classification consisted of three grades of hair loss which include the following **(Fig. 7)**:

- *Grade I*: Perceptible thinning of the hair on the crown, limited in the front by a line situated 1–3 cm behind the frontal hairline
- *Grade II*: Pronounced rarefaction of the hair on the crown within the area seen in grade I
- *Grade III*: Full baldness (total denudation) within the area seen in grades I and II[10]

Advantages: Ludwig classification is a simple, easy-to-use classification system, which also emphasized the preservation of the frontal fringe despite progressive centrifugal loss over the top of the scalp.

Disadvantages: Ludwig did not incorporate the accentuation of frontovertical alopecia, which was later on included by Olsen. Moreover, the females with male pattern hair loss also could not be classified with this system.

Savin (1992): Savin came up with nine computer images, which are now typically referred to as the Savin scale, as a pictorial classification scale to quantify pattern hair loss clinically in women which into eight stages of increasing crown balding, in addition to a special subcategory to detect frontal anterior recession **(Fig. 8)**.[11]

Advantages: These staged illustrations provided a finer visual gradient of hair loss pattern and density than the previous classification scale for women with pattern baldness. The Savin scale is a simple and useful tool for assessing degrees of hair loss in women, which is fairly consistent between different investigators using the same scale which adds degrees of hair loss that were missing in the Ludwig grading.

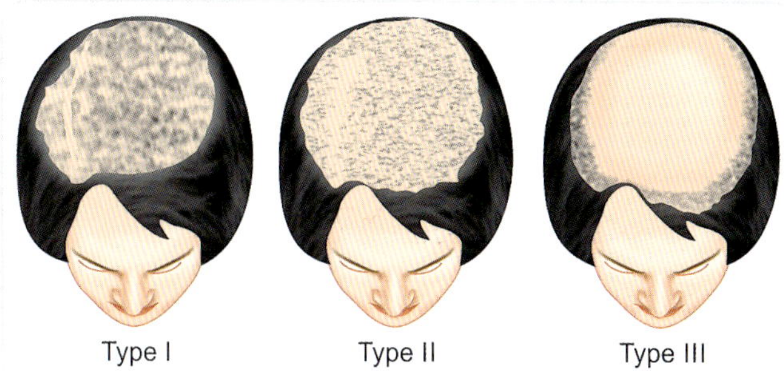

FIG. 7: Ludwig's classification of female pattern hair loss.

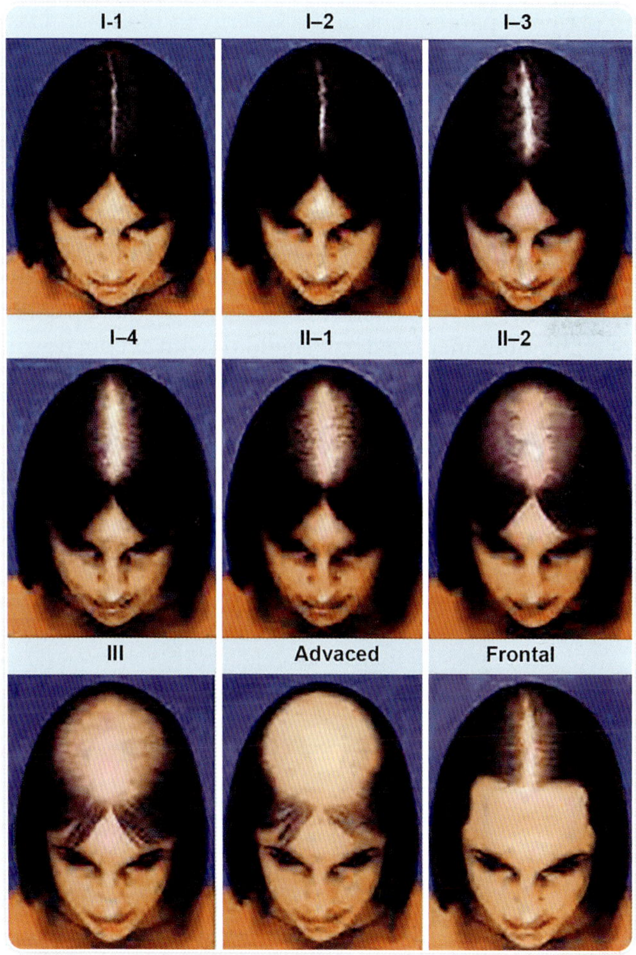

FIG. 8: Savin's pictorial classification of female pattern hair loss.

Disadvantages: This system also did not address the progressive frontal hair loss (Christmas tree pattern).

Olsen (1994): Olsen proposed a classification that was similar to Ludwig's classification but incorporated the accentuation of frontovertical alopecia, which has a triangular or "Christmas tree" pattern. Olsen observed that hair loss in women may occur in a subtle pattern of loss that is only apparent when one performs a midline part, where there is often a progressive decrease in hair density from the vertex to the front of the scalp, which he described as a "Christmas tree" distribution of loss. This pattern is visible both in the early as well as the advanced stages of hair loss.[12]

Sinclair (2004): It is a self-report photographic measure of patients' perceptions of the severity of their hair loss, which comprises five color photographs of women's scalps with the hair parted centrally. The first photograph is of a normal scalp and photographs 2–5 are of scalps of women with increasingly severe hair loss. The photographs are numbered from 1 to 5 and respondents are required to circle the number of the photograph that they feel most closely resembles the appearance of their own hair when parted in the center **(Fig. 9)**. Women with stages 1 and 2 hair loss tend to present with either episodic or continuous increased hair shedding with a reduction in the volume of the hair when held in a ponytail. Women with stages 3, 4, and 5 hair loss may present with either loss of volume of hair over the scalp with widening of the central part, episodic increased hair shedding, or continuous hair shedding.[13]

Advantages: Sinclair grading is a simple grading system and can be used with ease both by the clinicians and the patients alike for defining the extent of hair loss and for assessing the response to treatment.

CLASSIFICATION FOR PATTERN HAIR LOSS: IRRESPECTIVE OF SEX

Bouhanna (2000): Bouhanna proposed a multifactorial classification for both male and female pattern hair loss, integrating several parameters, which included extension of bald and hair-bearing areas, elasticity and density of the scalp, and hair characteristics such as diameter, length, shape, and color, which contribute to the covering power of the hair. This classification has proved useful in assessing the changes in hair parameters during the course of medical treatment and also in deciding the indication of hair transplantation for surgical management.[14]

The various parameters included by Bouhanna in his classification are as follows:

- *Extent of bald and hairy areas*: The extent of bald and hairy areas was assessed by using the following different parameters:
  - Median sagittal distance: It is the distance between the edge of the frontal hairline and the lower occipital ridge. In males, this distance is 34–37 cm, while in females, it is 30–34 cm.

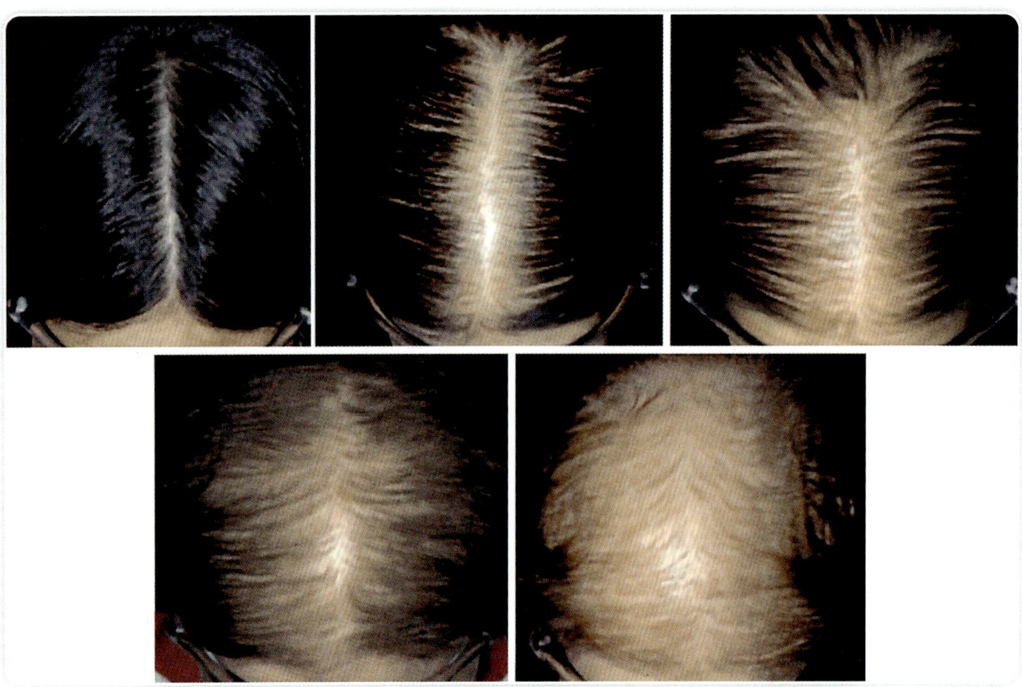

FIG. 9: Sinclair's five-point visual analog scale for female hair loss.

- Left and right sagittal paramedian distances: It is the distance between the bottom of the left or right frontal recession and the lower occipital line. In males, this distance is 33–36 cm, while in females, it is 30–33 cm.
- Transverse supra-auricular distance: It is the distance between the two left and right supra-auricular hairlines. In males, it is 30–34 cm, while in females, it is 28–32 cm.
- Temporal anterior spacing distance: It is the distance between the two most proximal anterior temporal lines. In males, this distance is 34–40 cm, while in females, it is 30–36 cm.
- Stage of maximal balding: In males, 5 cm is considered as the stage of maximal balding, while in females, it cannot be measured as the hair loss is diffuse.
- Mobility of the scalp: It is graded from 0 to 3, where 0 = 0 folds, 1 = 1–2 folds, 2 = 3–4 folds, and 3 ≥5 folds, which are determined by bimanual compression of the scalp.
- Thickness of the scalp: It is determined by inserting a subcutaneous needle vertically till it reaches galea and the inserted portion is measured with a micrometer measuring device. It is graded from 0 to 3, where 0 ≤2 mm (very thin), 1 = 2–5 mm (thin), 2 = 5–8 mm (medium), and 3 ≥8 mm (thick).

- *Covering power of hair*: It is determined by evaluating various parameters, which are as follows:
  - Hair density: It is graded from 0 to 3, where 0 ≤50 hairs/cm^2 (poor), 1 = 50–100 hairs/cm^2 (medium), 2 = 100–200 hairs/cm^2 (good), and 3 ≥200 hairs/cm^2 (very good).
  - Hair diameter: It is assessed by microscopic measurement of hair shaft diameter and is graded from 0 to 3, where 0 = vellus hair (<40 μm), 1 = small caliber (40–60 μm), 2 = medium caliber (60–80 μm), and 3 = big caliber (>80 μm).
  - Shape of hair shaft: The hair shaft has been classified as straight, wavy, curly, and frizzy.
  - Hair length: It is graded from 0 to 3, where ≤1 cm, 1 = 1–2 cm, 2 = 3–5 cm, and 3 ≥5 cm.
  - Growth rate of hair: It is also graded on a scale of 0–3, where 0 ≤0.2 mm/day, 1 = 0.2–0.3 mm/day, 2 = 0.3–0.4 mm/day, and 3 ≥0.4 mm/day.
  - Hair color: Four hair colors were proposed, which include black, blonde, red, and white.

Advantages: This classification system is a detailed classification system taking into consideration different parameters that could be quantified and computerized. Moreover, this classification could help in determining the indication and type of surgery required.

Disadvantages: The inclusion of numerous parameters and measurements also makes it time consuming and difficult to apply in routine practice.

BASIC AND SPECIFIC CLASSIFICATION (2007)[2]

The basic and specific (BASP) classification is a novel stepwise and universal classification system for patterned hair loss, regardless of sex. This system is based on observed patterns of hair loss, including the shape of the anterior hairline and the density of hair on the frontal and vertex areas. Lee et al. evaluated >2,200 subjects with patterned hair loss using this classification system, which consists of the basic (BA) type and the specific (SP) type.

The BA type signifies the shape of the anterior hairline, while the SP type indicates the density of hair on distinct areas (frontal and vertex). There are four basic types (L, M, C, and U) and two specific types (F and V), each of which is further subdivided into three or four grades (subtypes) based on their severity **(Fig. 10)**. The final type is determined by the combination of the determined BASP types. The various types of hair loss according to BASP classification include the following discussed here.

Basic Types

- *Type L*: No recession is observed along the anterior border in the frontotemporal region resembling a linear line and usually indicates no hair loss.
- *Type M*: Recession in the frontotemporal hairline is more prominent than the midanterior hairline, and the hairline resembles the letter M. It is further divided into four subtypes depending on the severity of baldness.
  - Type M0: The original hairline is preserved, and no hair loss has occurred.
  - Type M1: Frontotemporal recession extends posteriorly but not beyond the anterior third of a virtual line connecting the original hairline and the top of the vertex.
  - Type M2: Frontotemporal recession extends further posteriorly but not beyond the middle third of a virtual line connecting the original hairline and the top of the vertex.
  - Type M3: Frontotemporal recession extends beyond the middle third section into the posterior third of the area of a virtual line connecting the original hairline and the top of the vertex.
- *Type C*: Recession in the midanterior hairline is more prominent than the frontotemporal hairline.

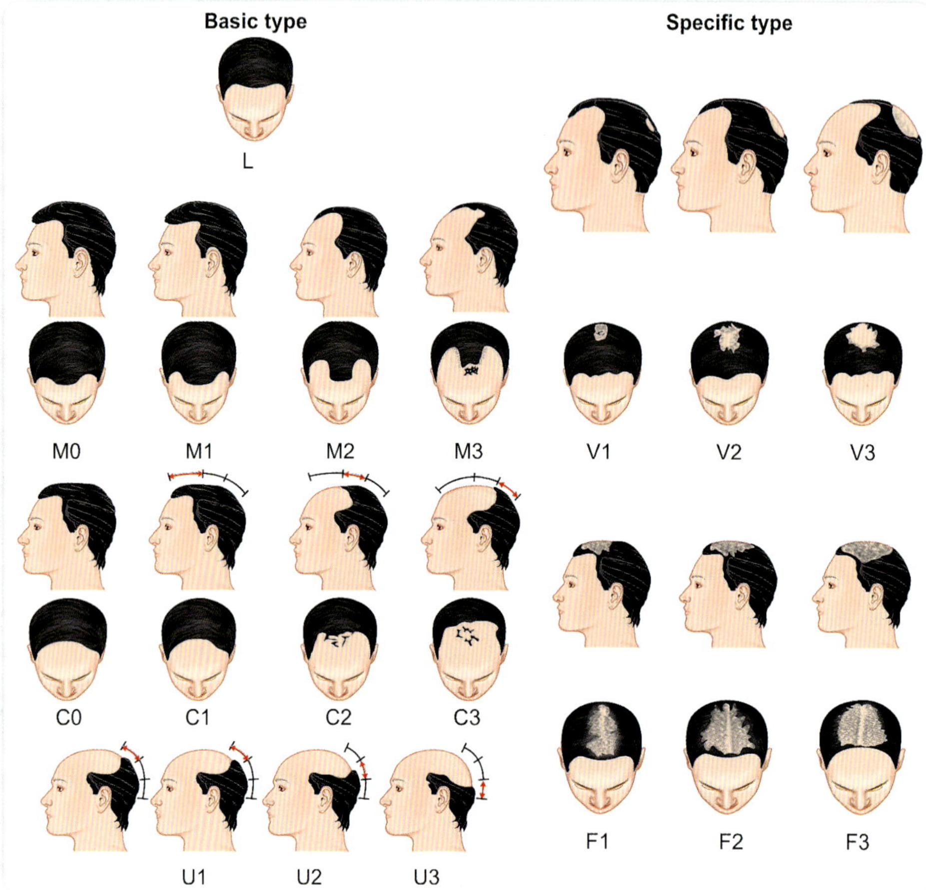

FIG. 10: Basic and specific classification of hair loss.

The entire anterior hairline regresses posteriorly in the shape of a half-circle, resembling the letter C. It is further divided into four subtypes depending on the severity.

- Type C0: The original anterior hairline is preserved, and no hair loss is visible.
- Type C1: The midanterior hairline recedes to the anterior one-third of the virtual line connecting the original hairline and the top of the vertex.
- Type C2: The midanterior hairline recedes to the middle one-third of the virtual line connecting the original hairline and the top of the vertex.
- Type C3: The midanterior hairline recedes to the posterior one-third of the virtual line connecting the original hairline and the top of the vertex.

- *Type U*: The anterior hairline recedes posteriorly beyond the vertex forming a horseshoe shape resembling the letter U. It is the most severe type of hair loss. It is further divided into three subtypes, depending on the severity of baldness.
  - Type U1: The anterior hairline recedes to lie within the superior one-third of the virtual line connecting the vertex and the posterior occipital protuberance.
  - Type U2: The anterior hairline recedes to lie within the middle one-third of the virtual line connecting the vertex and the posterior occipital protuberance.
  - Type U3: The anterior hairline recedes to lie within the inferior one-third of the virtual line connecting the vertex and the posterior occipital protuberance.

Specific Types

- *Type F*: It represents a general decrease in the density of hair over the entire top of the scalp, regardless of the anterior hairline, and is usually more marked over the frontal area of the scalp.
  - Type F1: Thinning of the hair on the crown is perceptible (mild change).
  - Type F2: Thinning of the hair on the crown is pronounced (moderate change).
  - Type F3: The hair on the crown is very sparse or absent (severe change).

- *Type V*: The hair around the vertex is notably sparser, and hair loss is seen more distinctly in the vertex than in the frontal area.
  - Type V1: Thinning of the hair around the vertex is perceptible (mild change).
  - Type V2: Thinning of the hair around the vertex is pronounced (moderate change).
  - Type V3: Thinning of the hair around the vertex is very sparse or absent (severe change).

The final type is decided by a combination of the BASP type, e.g., basic type (C1) + specific type (V1) denotes the final type C1V1.[2]

Advantages: This classification system offers numerous advantages over the preexisting systems as it is more comprehensive and systematic and can be used irrespective of gender. It also takes care of the diffuse thinning pattern. Moreover, this system is easy to memorize and practice and has better reproducibility and repeatability than the previous classifications in routine clinical practice.[15] Hence, in our opinion, this is perhaps the most useful and relevant classification for pattern hair loss.

However, still the classification has not achieved popularity as the Hamilton–Norwood classification is etched in the memory of physicians.

SUMMARY

Various classification systems have been proposed to classify male and female pattern hair loss.

For male pattern hair loss, notable classifications include the following:

- *Beek (1950)*: It is a simple classification with two types—(i) frontal and (ii) frontovertical baldness.
- *Hamilton (1951)*: It is a detailed classification with eight evolutionary aspects and three subgroups.
- *Ogata (1953)*: It is classified into 15 subtypes based on Japanese men.
- *Setty (1953)*: It simplified Hamilton's classification into three subtypes for white and black males.
- *Norwood (1975)*: It is the most widely used classification, with seven types and type A variants.

Although a large number of classification systems are available today, all of them have certain limitations as either they do not describe the complete evolutionary stages of hair loss or are too detailed for practical use. The Norwood-Hamilton system is the most widely used while the BASP classification is a more detailed and practical system, but still the most ideal classification is yet to be found.

REFERENCES

1. Beek CH. A study on extension and distribution of the human body-hair. Dermatologica. 1950;101:317-31.
2. Lee WS, Ro BI, Hong SP, Bak H, Sim WY, Kim DW, et al. A new classification of pattern hair loss that is universal for men and women: basic and specific (BASP) classification. J Am Acad Dermatol. 2007;57:37-46.
3. Hamilton JB. Patterned loss of hair in man; types and incidence. Ann N Y Acad Sci. 1951;53:708-28.
4. Ogata T. Development of patterned alopecia. Sogo Rinsho. 1953;2:101-6.
5. Setty LR. Hair patterns of scalp of white and Negro males. Am J Phys Anthropol. 1970;33:49-56.
6. Norwood OT. Male pattern baldness: classification and incidence. South Med J. 1975;68:1359-65.
7. Bouhanna P, Nataf J. A propos des transplantations de cuir chevelu: critiques et propositions. Rev Chir Esthet. 1976;7:17-23.
8. Bouhanna P, Dardour JC. Male baldness: dynamic classification of Dardour and Bouhanna. In: Bouhanna P, Dardour JC (Eds). Hair Replacement Surgery. Berlin: Springer-Verlag; 1996. pp. 33-4.
9. Koo SH, Chung HS, Yoon ES, Park SH. A new classification of male pattern baldness and a clinical study of the anterior hairline. Aesth Plast Surg. 2000;24:46-51.
10. Ludwig E. Classification of the types of androgenetic alopecia (common baldness) occurring in the female sex. Br J Dermatol. 1977;97:247-54.
11. Savin RC. A method for visually describing and quantitating hair loss in male pattern baldness [abstract]. J Invest Dermatol. 1992;98:604.
12. Olsen EA. Androgenetic alopecia. In: Olsen EA (Ed). Disorders of Hair Growth: Diagnosis and Treatment. New York: McGraw-Hill; 1994. pp. 257-83.
13. Sinclair R, Jolley D, Mallari R, Magee J. The reliability of horizontally sectioned scalp biopsies in the diagnosis of chronic diffuse telogen hair loss in women. J Am Acad Dermatol. 2004;51:189-99.
14. Bouhanna P. Multifactorial classification of male and female androgenetic alopecia. Dermatol Surg. 2000;26:555-61.
15. Hong H, Ji JH, Lee Y, Kang H, Choi GS, Lee WS. Reliability of the pattern hair loss classifications: a comparison of the basic and specific and Norwood-Hamilton classifications. J Dermatol. 2013;40:102-6.

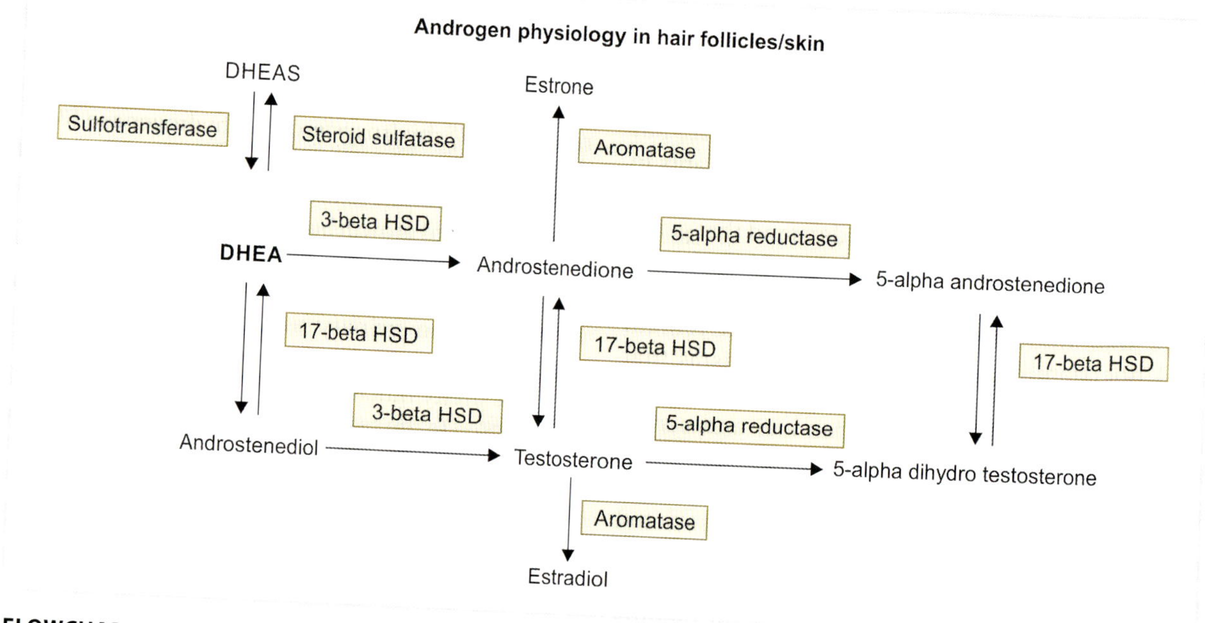

FLOWCHART 2: Androgen metabolism.

(DHEAS: dehydroepiandrosterone sulfate; HSD: hydroxysteroid dehydrogenase)

in dermal papilla (DP) and sebaceous glands but not in the ORS, hair bulb, and bulge and the bulge area.[27] AR is one of the key molecules that regulate androgen sensitivity in DP, considering that studies have shown increased expression of AR in balding follicles of MPHL subjects as well as in the beard follicles.[27]

Androgen Pathway

Circulating androgens enter the hair follicle via the capillaries of the DP at the base of the follicle and bind to the AR.[33] Once the ligand (T or DHT) binds on the ligand-binding domain, the androgen and AR complex translocates to the nucleus, where it binds to the androgen response elements (AREs) within the classical target genes to activate or repress the target genes.[1,27,32,33] Embryonic induction of hair follicles and maintaining the functional integrity of adult follicles through hair cycles is governed by the interaction between DP and follicular epithelium, possibly through paracrine mediators, which may work as coactivators/integrators or corepressors.[1,14,27] AR coactivators like Hic-5/ARA55 are highly expressed in DP of balding follicles as well as in beard follicles, playing a role in enhancing androgen sensitivity, while another AR coactivator ARA70β/ELE1β is expressed much less in balding follicles compared to nanbalding occipital follicles, which may play a role in the development of MPHL **(Flowchart 3)**.[27,33]

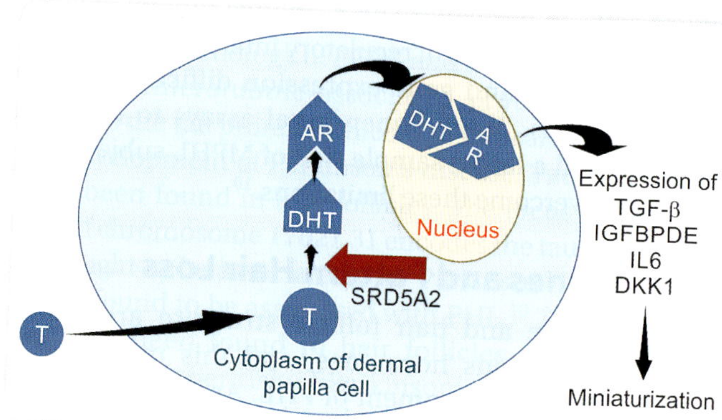

FLOWCHART 3: Possible mechanism of androgen action on hair follicle.

(AR: androgen receptor; DHT: dihydrotestosterone; IL: interleukin; TGF: transforming growth factor)

In MPHL, the postulated mechanism for growth inhibition by androgens is that androgen/AR complex may directly repress the production/secretion of mitogenic substances or may induce factors that can then trigger the growth inhibition of keratinocytes.[1] Studies looking at gene expression between cells of DP from frontal, occipital, and beard hair follicles identified the androgen-inducible hair growth inhibitors like TGF-β1 and 2, dickkopf1 (DKK1), and interleukin-6 (IL-6), which help us understand the pathways of androgen action in hair growth as well as MPHL.[27,33] In hair development and cycling, several master regulatory genes have been recognized. For anagen induction and development and regeneration of follicles in vivo, the WNT gene signaling pathway and insulin-like growth factors (IGFs) are essential, while the TGF-β pathways promote catagen and are responsible for apoptosis.[1,27,33] All these factors have autocrine effect on the DPCs and paracrine effect on the keratinocytes.[14] The androgen paradox to some extent can be explained by the gene expression. Growth-promoting WNT receptor genes, including EDA2R, IGF, and IGF-binding proteins, are overexpressed in beard DP cells. Growth inhibiting TGF-β and IGF-binding protein degrading enzymes IL-6 and DKK1 are predominantly expressed in DP of the frontal follicles. DKK1 is a WNT antagonist and is responsible for keratinocyte growth inhibition, while TGF-β2 is one of the most important catagen induction signals, and EDA2R induces anagen and causes hair growth.[33] This pattern of gene expression in DPCs of frontal and beard follicles could be the basis of the androgen paradox. The frontal DPCs also produced many stress proteins, including heat shock proteins. This could be a factor in premature (before the androgen hormone stimulation) senescence and severe cellular stress in the frontal DPCs.[33]

The WNT signaling pathway is crucial for the development and regeneration of hair follicles in vivo as well as for maintaining the integrity of the hair growth cycle. In MPHL, the DP, under the action of androgens, secretes paracrine and autocrine factors that promote catagen entry in hair follicles. This molecular crosstalk between AR signaling and WNT/β-catenin pathways influences androgen action on hair growth.[27,34,35]

Estrogens

There are three major forms of physiological estrogens in females: Estrone (E1), estradiol (E2 or 17β-estradiol), and estriol (E3), and E2 is the most potent and the major product of estrogen biosynthesis.[36] Though there are limited studies of estrogen's action on hair follicle, controversy regarding estrogen's inhibitory and stimulatory influence on the hair follicle comes from a host of publications citing rodent (murine) and human results.[37] Estrogen signaling is primarily mediated through estrogen receptors (ERs), estrogen receptor alpha and estrogen receptor beta, which are encoded by separate genes (ESR1 and ESR2, respectively) located on different chromosomes.[36] The recently discovered G protein-coupled estrogen receptor (GPR30 or GPER) and the orphan receptor, estrogen-related receptor (ERR), may be additional receptors through which estrogens may influence hair characteristics.[36,37] Though immunolocalization studies identified ESR2 as the major ER, genetic studies have revealed a greater role for ESR1 in the pathogenesis of PHL.[11] ESR1 is coexpressed with AR in the DP and is also the dominant ER in undifferentiated adipocytes, which may influence hair cycle changes in PHL through the adipogenesis pathway.[11,37,38] Based on in vitro and murine studies, it could be speculated that estrogens may work as androgen antagonists, but this will need more in-depth studies. Considering that the androgens play a pivotal role in MPHL development and intricate relation of androgen and estrogen metabolism (through aromatase), the evidence from the recent molecular genetic studies tends to only confirm the influence of genetic variation in the ER pathway to MPHL development.[11]

Progesterone

Progesterone can impact androgen signaling centrally by inhibiting luteinizing hormone (LH) secretion and locally by inhibiting 5-alpha reductase activity, thereby preventing the conversion of testosterone to DHT. But, the exact role in PHL is not clear.[26]

Prolactin

Prolactin, also known as luteotropin, is a polypeptide hormone that is involved not only in hair development but also in lactation, reproduction, angiogenesis, and osmoregulation.[26,39] It is central neurohormone of the hypothalamic–pituitary axis (HP axis) encoded by the PRL gene on chromosome 6 and is produced in the anterior pituitary gland.[11,26] It has been long recognized as a powerful seasonal hair cycle regulator, but now, studies have revealed that it has variable sex and site-specific differences in gene expression. In murine studies, PRL appears to operate primarily as a potent hair growth inhibitor, and in human hair follicle culture of male occipital follicles, it is a catagen promoter.[40] However, in hair follicle organ culture experiment using female frontotemporal scalp hair follicles, PRL significantly promoted hair shaft elongation as well as hair matrix keratinocyte proliferation in situ in serum-free hair follicle organ culture, which was reversed by PRL antagonist.[11,41] The seemingly conflicting effects reported in the literature may well be reconciled if one interprets them as representations of site- and/or gender-dependent hair follicle responses to PRL. Given this sexual dimorphism, it could be speculated that PRL may have an inhibitory effect on stem cell function in male hair follicles, which could result in the stalled growth observed in miniaturized follicles seen in MPHL.[11,41]

Melatonin

Melatonin is secreted mainly by the pineal gland and is responsible for the diurnal rhythm of a variety of physiological systems. Apart from being a free radical scavenger and inducing DNA repair, the highly active anagen hair bulb is thought to use melatonin synthesis on-site as a self-protective strategy.[26,39,42,43] Evidence for melatonin involvement in MPHL biology comes from the GWAS studies, which recognized genes encoding molecules relevant to melatonin signaling and degradation at a minimum of six genetic risk loci.[8] One of the loci maps RORA (RAR-related orphan receptor A) gene, which encodes for the nuclear mediator of melatonin signaling, RORα (retinoid-related orphan receptor alpha).[11] Melatonin can have receptor-dependent and receptor-independent actions on the hair follicles, which are mediated by interacting with androgen and estrogen pathways.[43] It counteracts the anagen-shortening effects of androgens by negative regulation of ER expression; this could also explain the clinically observed anti-hair loss effect in PHL.[11,43] The in vitro effects of melatonin on human hair follicles are conflicting, but one study of topical melatonin application gave credence to its stimulatory effect on hair follicles.[43] Another aspect of melatonin's impact on hair follicles is the effect on hair pigmentation, where it may have a role in the transformation of pigmented terminal hair follicles into unpigmented vellus hair follicles.[11]

Melanocortin

Melanocortins act on epidermal and hair follicle melanocytes and have long been documented as major stimulators of pigmentation.[25] Melanocortin-1 receptor (MC-1R), MC-4R, and prohormone proopiomelanocortin (POMC) are all expressed in human DPCs, and GWAS has identified MC-1R as a candidate gene for PHL. MC-1R encodes the receptor for the melanocortins α-melanocyte-stimulating hormone (α-MSH) and adrenocorticotropic hormone (ACTH), which are derived from the POMC.[11,25,44,45] How these elements contribute to PHL is still a matter of research. The plausible theories are based on the finding that MC-1R was upregulated in balding hair follicles compared to nonbalding hair follicles, and since melanocortins are implicated in melanogenesis, they may play a role in terminal to unpigmented vellus hair transformation.[11] The sex hormones (testosterone and estrogen) and paracrine factors tend to regulate expression of MC-1R.[46]

Thyroid Gland Hormones

Hypothalamic-pituitary-thyroid axis controls many metabolic processes, including those in the hair follicle cells.[26] Thyroid gland secretes thyroid hormones—thyroxine (T4) and triiodothyronine (T3). Thyroid hormones act by binding to nuclear receptors [thyroid hormone receptors (TRs)], which are encoded by different genes—TR alpha and TR beta, which are expressed in the hair follicles.[26,47] Studies have shown that thyroid hormones demonstrate that T3 and/or T4 directly target the hair follicle and control multiple hair biology parameters, ranging from hair follicle cycling to pigmentation.[48] In addition, thyroid hormones play a significant role in influencing mitochondria, whose activity controls human energy metabolism and homeostasis. Hair follicle growth is an energy-consuming process, which is regulated by the hormones of the hypothalamic-pituitary-thyroid axis with T3 and T4 specifically stimulating the keratinocytes to induce mitochondrial activity.[26] Relevance of thyroid hormones to PHL is not very clear. In women with PHL, thyroid disorders may be incidental or may represent a pathogenic loop.[49] The evidence linking MPHL and hypothyroidism is very limited with studies suggesting that MPHL of this type (with hypothyroidism) might be a surrogate marker of response to thyroid hormone replacement.[49]

Corticotropin- and Gonadotropin-releasing Hormone

Hair follicles are prominent targets of prototypic stress mediators [such as corticotropin-releasing hormone (CRH), ACTH, cortisol, catecholamines, PRL, substance P, and nerve growth factor] as well as potent sources of these key mediators of systemic stress responses as they are enabled with a fully functional peripheral hypothalamic-pituitary-adrenal (HPA) axis.[11,42] One of the earliest identified autosomal risk loci was at 17q21.31. The important variant is located in the gene that encodes the G protein-coupled receptor CRHR1 (corticotropin-releasing hormone receptor 1), which binds neuropeptides of the CRH family.[11] Ex vivo human hair follicle organ cultures have shown that CRH induces premature catagen-like state by inhibiting keratinocyte proliferation and differentiation. Microdissected anagen hair follicles and full-thickness scalp skin, when treated with CRH, showed mast cell maturation and degranulation in the human hair follicle connective tissue sheath, which is like perifollicular microinflammation seen in actively progressing hair loss.[50] Increased expression of CRH in hair follicles of aged versus younger individuals could signify premature catagen entry of follicles as one ages in genetically predisposed individuals.[11,26] Another endocrine pathway is the GnRH pathway which is a component of the hypothalamus-pituitary-gonadal axis. GnRH could possibly mediate MPHL because its rise coincides with puberty as well as early onset of MPHL.[41,51]

Parathyroid Hormone-like Hormone

The parathyroid hormone-like hormone (PTHLH) gene located on chromosome12p11.22 has been identified as a candidate gene for MPHL in several GWAS studies.[8,9,42] The PTHLH is like the parathyroid hormone, and PTHLH is expressed in balding and nonbalding scalp hair follicles, whereas parathyroid hormone-releasing hormone receptor 1 (PTH1R) is expressed in the surrounding mesenchyme. It is possible that PTH signaling and PTHLH may act as negative regulators of hair growth and promote anagen shortening/premature catagen entry via PTHLH/PTHR1 and cAMP/PKA/PKC during MPHL pathogenesis.[11,52,53]

Insulin-like Growth Factor Signaling

Associations between PHL and insulin metabolism were initially noticed in epidemiological studies, which were later substantiated in genome-wide studies.[12] Apart from genes in insulin receptor signaling and insulin-like growth factor 1 receptor (IGF1R) signaling, studies have implicated insulin-like growth factor binding protein 3 (IGFBP3), which is located on chromosome 7p12.3, as a candidate gene.[11] IGF1, which controls cellular proliferation and helps anagen maintenance and sustains immune privilege, is itself regulated by androgens and growth hormone.[11,54] Hair follicle regression and catagen induction are influenced by IGFBP3, while IGF-I signaling works as mitogenic and morphogenetic regulator in hair follicle biology.[11]

Prostaglandins

Prostaglandins are unsaturated carboxylic acids synthesized from arachidonic acid by cyclooxygenase (COX) enzyme. They are signaling molecules observed in most tissues and represent inflammatory response.[55] Many studies have linked expression levels of PGs with hair growth.[55-59] Four major PGs that are expressed in hair follicles and play a role in hair loss are prostaglandin D2 (PGD2), prostaglandin I2 (PGI2), prostaglandin E2 (PGE2), and prostaglandin F2 alpha (PGF2α).[55] Biopsies from balding scalps in MPHL showed significant upregulation of PGD2 and its PGD2 enzyme synthase and reduced expression of PGE2 and PGF2α alluding that PGE2 and PGF2α are pro hair growth while PGD2 impedes hair growth.[56] Maintenance of precise balance between these four PGs is the key factor for maintaining hair growth.[57] The difference in phenotypes of FPHL and MPHL could, to some extent, be explained by the finding that hair follicles in female scalps express more of PGE2 and PGF2α than in the males. However, the expression of PGD2 and PGI2 receptors is similar (low) in the nonbald regions in men and women, and PGE2 and PGF2α receptor levels are significantly high compared to bald areas in both men and women. PG may represent a final common pathway, even if PHL in females may not be androgen-mediated.[58] Studies have shown that PGD2 influences the conversion of androstenedione to testosterone in human keratinocytes and also increases the reactive oxygen species (ROS). The addition of *N*-acetyl cysteine-reduced testosterone production in these keratinocytes implies crosstalk between PGD2–ROS axis and testosterone production.[59] PGD2 has been shown to promote AR and AKT (protein kinase B) signal via prostaglandin D2 receptor 2 (DP2) in human DPCs, thus playing an important role in AR expression. These findings support an additional explanation for the development of PHL involving PGD2-DP2 (prostaglandin D2 receptor) in human DPCs.[57] PGs may play differing roles in PHL development depending on the stage of hair loss, and more studies are essential to clarify the precise functional roles and the details of underlying signaling mechanism of PGs in hair follicles.

Peroxisome Proliferator-activated Receptor Pathway

Though androgen signaling is a prominent cause of PHL, drugs that block the T/DHT pathway, like finasteride, are not effective in a significant number of patients. This points to the possible presence of additional/alternative pathways, more so in women in whom androgens may not play a significant role.[60] One of the possible mechanisms investigated is the PPAR pathway. PPARs are nuclear hormone receptors that regulate gene transcription either negatively or positively.[61,62] Research has revealed that dysregulation of PPARs is connected to the development of a wide range of human diseases, including athero-sclerosis, obesity, T2DM, and many others.[62] A full transcriptome profile analysis comparing the hair bulb region of normal and miniaturized hair follicles from vertex and occipital region in males with and without PHL showed the relevance of the retinoid receptor, particularly the PPAR pathway (other than AR), in causation of progressive hair miniaturization.[60] Of all the PPAR isoforms, PPAR-γ (PPAR gamma) is prominently expressed in the human pilosebaceous unit (PSU), which likely incorporates—besides the hair follicle, sebaceous gland, and APM—also perifollicular adipocytes and the eccrine gland.[62] Genes in the energy metabolism pathway, induced during exercise and well characterized in high-energy consumption tissues such as muscle, heart, and brain, are regulated by interaction of peroxisome proliferator-activated receptor gamma coactivator 1-alpha (PPARGC1 alpha or PGC1a), a transcriptional coactivator and PPAR gamma.[60] In studies on mice hair, the dynamic expression of PGC1a in the differentiating zone of mouse hair during anagen suggests it may be involved in orchestrating energy metabolism via mitochondrial biogenesis as mitochondrial activity is found to peak during hair growth, where oxidative phosphorylation predominates over aerobic glycolysis in the proliferating and differentiating cells of the hair follicle.[60,62] Its ability to bind to large array of genes, such as retinoid X receptor alpha (RXRa), ERs, and AR, plays a role in interactions between AR, PPAR, and retinoid pathways in hair differentiation.[60] Transcriptome profiling on extracted follicular units of patients with MPHL showed upregulation of PGC1a in cells of the inner root sheath (IRS) and ORS along with upregulation of AR protein in miniaturized hair follicles. The role of PPAR-gamma signaling comes from these findings along with the observation that miRNA profiling showed targeting of genes involved in PPAR signaling in miniaturized hair.[60,62] Apart from this, PPAR gamma also impacts androgen synthesis by decreasing the activity of 17,20-lyase of cytochrome P450c17 and 3β-HSD activity, two key enzymes in the androgen pathway, leading to lower androgen levels. These actions of the PPAR pathway could be a basis for formulating drugs that could modulate PPAR activity.[62]

Arrector Pili Muscle

The APM plays a role in thermal regulation and sebum production, and it inserts at the level of the bulge (which is the epithelial stem cell niche).[63] Loss of progenitor cells, which are responsible in maintaining both the APM and the DP, reflects as gradual loss of muscle volume in the APM with fat infiltration, as shown by computer-generated three-dimensional reconstructions of scalp biopsy specimens from MPHL.[63] Moreover, bulge stem cells act as tendon cells, providing a physical connection to the APM, creating a smooth muscle cell niche via nephronectin expression (upregulated by Wnt/β-catenin activation, directly or via inhibition of BMP signaling).[64] The stability of bulge stem cell compartment assures that APM attachment is firm regardless of the stage of the hair growth cycle. It is theorized that the interaction between the mesoderm-derived APM and ectoderm-derived follicle bulge epithelium is essential for the maintenance of the PSU, very much in the same way as the interaction between the mesoderm-derived DP and the ectoderm-derived epithelial hair follicle matrix **(Figs. 2 and 3)**.[63]

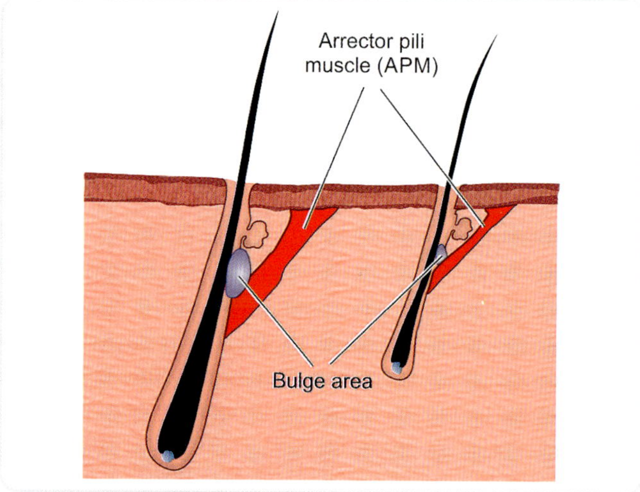

FIG. 2: Interaction between arrector pili muscle (APM) and follicular bulge epithelium.

Note: Loss of a progenitor cell population in the bulge area in pattern hair loss (PHL) leads to progressive muscle volume loss and fat infiltration of the APM.

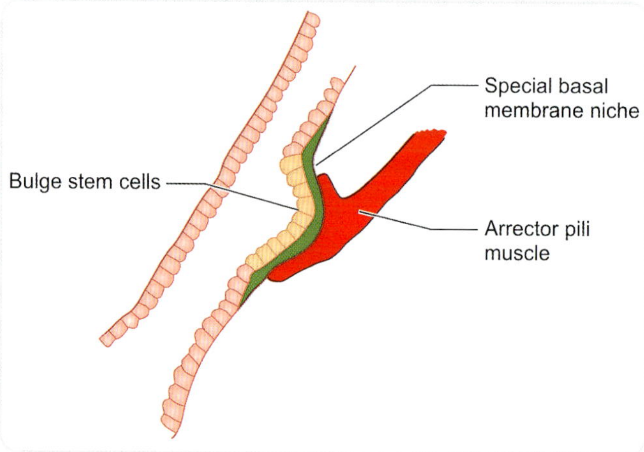

FIG. 3: Bulge cells provide anchorage to arrector pili muscle (APM).

Vascularity/Hypoxia

The scalp is known to have a robust blood supply originating in the subcutaneous tissue. It has been assumed that decreased blood flow in the scalp might contribute to or cause hair loss, which was based on the study using 133Xe washout method to measure the subcutaneous blood flow (SBF) in patients with early male pattern baldness. The results clearly showed a reduced SBF in patients with early male pattern baldness.[65] Another study measured the transcutaneous oxygen saturation (PO_2) of the scalp to determine if there was a relative microvascular insufficiency and associated tissue hypoxia in areas of hair loss in male pattern baldness. Transcutaneous PO_2 was found to be lower in bald areas of the scalp compared to the hairy areas creating a situation of relative hypoxia. Relative microvascular insufficiency has been observed in the regions of the scalp that lose hair in male pattern baldness.[66] SBF is thought to be influenced by the lipid content in the subcutaneous tissue and the surface temperature of the scalp skin. As a result, the relevance of reduced SBF to etiology of MPHL is inconclusive.[65] Also, this does not explain why there is selective vascular insufficiency in the frontal area and not in the occipital area if one looks at the pattern of hair loss in MPHL or FPHL.

The vasculature system is a critical component of the stem cell niche in many models, and the HFSC are no exception.[65] Another recent study, using transcriptome analysis, studied the microvasculature of the DP. AR-mediated paracrine signaling, mainly TGF-beta signaling, from DPCs induced apoptosis of microvascular endothelial cells in the DP of the balding scalp of MPHL was observed. These findings define a role of AR-mediated regression of blood vessels in DP in MPHL and support the notion that early anti-AR treatment is better than late treatment.[67] This study shows that reduced vascularity to the follicle is a result of the biomechanisms leading to PHL rather than the cause of it.

Interestingly, low-oxygen environment increases the expression of hypoxia-inducible factor-1 (HIF-1), which is a key transcription factor for oxygen sensing and oxygen-related signal transduction.[68] Three-dimensional cell culture is used to maintain hair inductivity in order to understand molecular mechanisms in DPCs, and studies on DPCs using this technology have shown that hypoxia exposure in DPCs triggers a rise in proliferation. This is thought to be due to the modulation of lactate dehydrogenase activity. Apart from increased proliferation, hypoxia also increases hair inductivity through paracrine effects by release of growth factors and hypoxia-induced ROS generation.[68] Informatic analysis showed that HIF1A was found to be downregulated in MPHL tissues, and HIF1A expression levels favorably correlated with hair inductivity-related genes.[69] Transcriptome changes in hair follicles from MPHL patients showed that the HIF-1 pathway genes, EGLN1 and EGLN3 (egl-9 family hypoxia-inducible factor 1 and 3), as well as WNT pathway inhibitors SERPINF1 (serpin family F member 1) and SFRP2 (secreted frizzled-related protein 2), may play important roles and may serve as important targets for therapy in PHL.[69]

Oxidative Stress

Reactive oxygen species are usually formed as byproducts of the normal metabolism of oxygen in aerobic cells.[70] ROS signaling leads to various deleterious effects, including melanocyte apoptosis in hair graying and skin cancer.[71] Studies have shown that cultured DPCs from hair follicles in the balding area showed flattened morphology and a significant reduction in mobility, population doubling, increased levels of ROS, and senescence-associated β-Gal activity, all suggestive of a role for oxidative stress in PHL.[72] This oxidative stress is thought to be a factor in premature senescence of DPCs, which compromises hair follicle epithelial–mesenchymal interaction underlying hair cycling.[73] There are also several literature reports that attempt to link PHL to increased oxidative stress. PHL was associated with increased risk factors for cardiovascular disease and with increased presence of inflammation.[74] The study assessing the plasma levels of stress markers showed increased MDA (malondialdehyde) level, a marker of lipid peroxidation, together with a decreased TEAC (Trolox equivalent antioxidant capacity) in the plasma of the patients with PHL suggesting that an increased oxidative stress was present in these patients.[74] This study also showed significantly decreased SOD (superoxide dismutase) activity but no change in catalase, glutathione peroxidase, nonprotein thiols level, and total antioxidant activity in erythrocytes, suggesting the presence of a compensatory mechanism for SOD dysfunction in red blood cells of patients with androgenetic alopecia.

Original understanding that ROS is toxic and responsible for DNA damage, protein oxidation, and lipid peroxidation may not be entirely true. ROS was recently shown to work as a second messenger for a variety of signaling pathways that modulate proliferation, differentiation, and senescence of cells and support stem cell self-renewal.[70] Zhao et al. in their study on mice found that oxidative stress progressively elevated in HFSCs during telogen to catagen, and this leads to FOXP1 (forkhead box protein 1) relocating from the nucleus to the cytoplasm of HFSC. This FOPXp1 movement out of the nucleus causes deficiency of FOXp1 in the hair follicles, which leads to reduced ROS buildup and increased HFSC proliferation.[70] The quantum of ROS generation decides the impact on HFSCs. ROS generated basically during normal cellular metabolism is thought to drive the progression of hair follicle cycle. It does this by controlling DNA damage and repair, hair follicle apoptosis, and macrophage polarization sequentially to help the hair follicle cycle. However, studies have not been able to determine the critical levels of ROS between helping cell proliferation and causing apoptosis in hair follicles.[75] Additional studies will be required to understand the impact of ROS signaling, which may be physiologically linked to other pathways that govern hair growth and regeneration. Another important point here is the use of nutritional supplements/antioxidants to suppress the oxidative stress leading to hair loss.[76] Though the control of oxidative stress using antioxidants has been shown to be beneficial in many animal models, the inference from human studies remains controversial.[77] The probable cause for this could be that blanket suppression of ROS could disrupt important ROS-mediated cellular signaling and hence may not be desirable or effective. Also, the nutritional status of patients will impact the efficacy of antioxidant supplementation. The question being whether these supplements will be effective in those patients who are not deficient in these nutrients.[77]

CONNECTING THE DOTS

Differing presentations of PHL spatiotemporally have patterning as a common feature with involvement of frontal, mid-scalp, and crown regions with sparing of the occipital regions. The nonaffected areas have thick and pigmented terminal hair, which gradually change to a fine, nonpigmented vellus state through a process known as miniaturization. This is the appearance in almost 90% of patients with PHL with reduction in caliber (qualitative) but no real change in the number of follicles (quantitative).[78] Reduced scalp coverage seems to stem from a combination of altered hair cycle dynamics and follicular miniaturization, leading to a reduction in the length and diameter of hairs. The exact contribution of these two elements is variable. The exact molecular basis of regional predilection is not clear. Some events at molecular and cellular level can be theorized, but the final biological pathway still remains elusive. Moreover, the normal process of aging will also impact the changes in the hair follicle, but this impact may or may not add up to the key role of hormonal factors.

Though epidermal and mesodermal tissue types give rise to the human hair follicle, there is significant interaction of the hair follicle cells with the surrounding cells such as adipocytes, immune cells, and neural crest-derived cells (melanocytes). The signaling pathways between epithelial hair follicle stem cells (eHFSCs) located in the bulge area and the mesenchyme represented by the DP and the dermal sheath (DS) are required to create, sustain, and renew the continuously cycling hair follicle to produce the keratinized hair shaft. The DP and DS, on the other hand, play an important role in differentiating the pattern of overlying epithelial cells.

The various phases that the follicular hair cycle goes through in the lifetime change the morphology of the DP, form a new hair shaft, and shed the old hair shaft. Anagen or the growth phase is characterized by the multiplication and differentiation of epithelial cells, arising directly or indirectly from the bulge, that go on to form the follicle and eventually the hair itself.[78] During this phase, the morphology and volume of DPCs and bulbs become larger. Catagen (regression phase/involution phase) is a 2–4-week period characterized by involution and preplanned apoptosis. By the end of the catagen stage, the hair follicles have shrunken, and the DPCs have begun to shrink and ascend to below the bulge area.[78-80] Telogen (resting phase) is a 2–4-month period when the biological activity of the hair follicle is the feeblest.[78,80] During telogen, there is direct interaction between DPCs, which have ascended to below the bulge and stem cells of the bulge. This interaction between DPCs and bulge stem cells is vital for the activation of stem cells and the initiation of new hair cycles.[79] Exogen (shedding phase) is the phase attributed to the release of the hair shaft from the follicle where the hair shaft is actively shed.[78] Kenogen (latent lag phase) refers to a lag phase, or a follicle in telogen which has lost its club hair (exogen) prior to re-entry into anagen. This phase is not observed in all follicles but is increased in PHL.[78]

Hair shaft diameter is directly proportional to the size of the DP, and a densely populated DP along with a large volume DP translates into a thicker hair shaft. In PHL, the proportions of the DP are reduced, which is imitated as miniaturization with reduced hair shaft thickness. The initial theory of miniaturization occurring over several hair cycles is now challenged with studies showing that miniaturization can occur as an abrupt large-step process during one cycle transition instead of over several cycles.[78] Morphological development and cycling of hair follicles are tightly regulated by signaling pathways such as WNT, BMP, EDAR, and sonic hedgehog (Shh).[79] During catagen, the DP becomes less populated with DPCs migrating out of the DP into the DS, which is largely degraded. In telogen, only a small number of hair follicle dermal stem cells (hfDSCs) surrounding the DP are left. In normal circumstances, the DP is completely repopulated to the previous anagen state via proliferation and migration of these hfDSCs into the DP. Miniaturization is thought to be caused by increased effluence of DP cells during anagen-to-catagen transition and/or, conjointly, hfDSCs not adequately replenishing the DP during the telogen-to-anagen transition.[78] The issue of miniaturization and hair loss in PHL is not only due to the loss of cells from DP but also the loss of stem cells from the epithelial portion of the hair follicle. In MPHL, global gene expression studies have revealed the preservation of KRT15+ (intermediate filament protein keratin 15) epithelial stem cells with reduction of the more dynamic progenitor stem cells (CD200hi ITGA6hi and CD34hi). Therefore, it appears that rather than a disorder of stem cells, MPHL may be a dysregulation of stem cell to progenitor cell transition, either due to an independent defect or an inability to respond to signaling initiating the transition.[64,78,81] It is also possible that the signaling from DP, which initiates the conversion of bulge cells into progenitors, may be altered or weakened.[78] As mentioned earlier, observational studies on the APM attachment and MPHL observed that APM of miniaturized follicles within a follicular unit are replaced by fat. The integrity of the APM is maintained in alopecia areata, and hence, miniaturization is thought to be reversible in this condition. Studies have revealed signaling that exists between the cells of the bulge and APM, with bulge cells expressing nephronectin, provides a space for smooth muscle cells of APM to act as tendon cells for the APM.[82] This puts a question of whether the change in APM is a cause of miniaturization or an effect of it.

The cellular biomechanism behind miniaturization is not very clear, but the presence of androgens is essential to the process, at least in most men and in some women. Both DS and DP express AR, which is a ligand-activated transcription factor.[78] By virtue of available data pointing to genetic variability in AR being essential for the development of early onset of MPHL, androgens have been strongly associated with MPHL. Other potential loci have been identified in subsequent genetic studies.[8-23] Recent GWAS evaluating MPHL recognized 71 possibly causative loci linked particularly with three pathways: The pathway involving WNT signaling, the apoptosis pathway, and the AR signaling pathway.[20] In balding, the most powerful androgen to bind the AR is DHT, which is a metabolite of testosterone by conversion with SRD5A2 in the follicular mesenchyme. The capacity of the hair follicle to convert testosterone depends on the expression of the enzyme SRD5A2, and it is known that the balding scalp expresses higher levels of SRD5A2. The differences in the expression of SRD5A2 enzyme and AR are responsible for the pattern of hair loss. The differing responses in beard hair follicles, which are stimulated to grow, and scalp hair follicles, which miniaturize, come from local microenvironment factors that include the receptors, hormone metabolism, and hair follicle properties.[81] The DHT/AR complex, which inhibits growth in scalp hair follicles, is thought to be due to upregulation of apoptotic factors such as TGF-β1, TGF-β2, IL-6, and Dkk1, and the suppression of growth-promoting factors such as WNT5A, WNT10B, and BMP2.[27,81]

Currently, finasteride is one of the therapeutic options, which inhibits SRD5A2 enzyme and targets the specific pathway. But studies and clinical experience have taught us that it is not effective in all patients with PHL, and that means there is more than one pathway operating. In summary, if we are to identify more therapeutic targets and treat PHL effectively, we need to understand the different molecular and cellular processes, which lead to PHL. PHL is a progressive disease that tends to worsen with time, and that is one factor, which is confounded by changes in the follicle caused by aging. Usually, when the genetic risk loci are identified for a particular condition, the underlying biomechanisms are also mapped out. Though many genetic risk loci for PHL have been identified in the last decade, the underlying biological pathways are still elusive. Though genome-wide studies have already revealed and are expected to further reveal unexpected associations of PHL with medical conditions and traits, a clear understanding of the pathobiology of PHL should be the objective of further genetic and molecular research.

REFERENCES

1. Olsen E. Pattern hair loss in men and women. In: Olsen Elise (Ed). Disorders of Hair Growth: Diagnosis and Treatment, 2nd edition. New York: McGraw-Hill; 2003.
2. Otberg N, Shapiro J. Current views on pattern hair loss in chapter 2. Male and female pattern hair loss. In: Unger WP, Shapiro R, Unger R, Unger M (Eds). Hair Transplantation, 5th edition. Boca Raton: CRC Press; 2011.
3. Osborn D. Inheritance of baldness. J Hered. 1916;7:347-55.
4. Küster W, Happle R. The inheritance of common baldness: two B or not two B? J Am Acad Dermatol. 1984;11(5 Pt. 1):921-6.
5. Hamilton JB. Patterned loss of hair in man; types and incidence. Ann N Y Acad Sci. 1951;53:708-28.
6. Hamilton JB. Male hormone stimulation is prerequisite and an incitant in common baldness. Am J Anat. 1942;71:451-80.
7. Ayob SM, Messenger AG. Androgens, hair loss and eugenics: a tale of discovery and American social history. Exp Dermatol. 2015;24(6):412-3.
8. Heilmann-Heimbach S, Herold C, Hochfeld L, Hillmer AM, Nyholt DR, Hecker J, et al. Meta-analysis identifies novel risk loci and yields systematic insights into the biology of male-pattern baldness. Nat Commun. 2017;8:14694.
9. Hagenaars SP, Hill WD, Harris SE, Ritchie SJ, Davies G, Liewald DC, et al. Genetic prediction of male pattern baldness. PLoS Genet. 2017;13(2):e1006594.
10. Heilmann-Heimbach S, Hochfeld LM, Paus R, Nöthen MM. Hunting the genes in male-pattern alopecia: how important are they, how close are we and what will they tell us? Exp Dermatol. 2016;25:251-7.

11. Heilmann-Heimbach S, Hochfeld LM, Henne SK, Nöthen MM. Hormonal regulation in male androgenetic alopecia—sex hormones and beyond: evidence from recent genetic studies. Exp Dermatol. 2020;29:814-27.
12. Pirastu N, Joshi PK, de Vries PS, Cornelis MC, McKeigue PM, Keum N, et al. GWAS for male-pattern baldness identifies 71 susceptibility loci explaining 38% of the risk. Nat Commun. 2017;8:1584.
13. Richards JB, Yuan X, Geller F, Waterworth D, Bataille V, Glass D, et al. Male-pattern baldness susceptibility locus at 20p11. Nat Genet. 2008;40(11):1282-4.
14. Lolli F, Pallotti F, Rossi A, Fortuna MC, Caro G, Lenzi A, et al. Androgenetic alopecia: a review. Endocrine. 2017;57(1):9-17.
15. Brockschmidt FF, Heilmann S, Ellis JA, Eigelshoven S, Hanneken S, Herold C, et al. Susceptibility variants on chromosome 7p21.1 suggest HDAC9 as a new candidate gene for male-pattern baldness. Br J Dermatol. 2011;165(6):1293-302.
16. Puc J, Kozbial P, Li W, Tan Y, Liu Z, Suter T, et al. Ligand-dependent enhancer activation regulated by topoisomerase-I activity. Cell. 2015;160(3):367-80. [Erratum: Cell. 2015;163(2):520-2.]
17. Hoi CS, Lee SE, Lu SY, McDermitt DJ, Osorio KM, Piskun CM, et al. Runx1 directly promotes proliferation of hair follicle stem cells and epithelial tumor formation in mouse skin. Mol Cell Biol. 2010;30(10):2518-36.
18. Choi BY. Targeting Wnt/β-catenin pathway for developing therapies for hair loss. Int J Mol Sci. 2020;21:4915.
19. Redler S, Messenger AG, Betz RC. Genetics and other factors in the aetiology of female pattern hair loss. Exp Dermatol. 2017;26:510-7.
20. Heilmann S, Kiefer AK, Fricker N, Drichel D, Hillmer AM, Herold C, et al. Androgenetic alopecia: identification of four genetic risk loci and evidence for the contribution of WNT signaling to its etiology. J Invest Dermatol. 2013;133(6):1489-96.
21. Koellner CM, Mensink KA, Highsmith WE. Chapter 5—basic concepts in human molecular genetics. In: Coleman WB, Tsongalis GJ (Eds). Essential Concepts in Molecular Pathology, 2nd edition. Cambridge: Academic Press; 2020. pp. 81-99.
22. Hochfeld LM, Bertolini M, Broadley D, Botchkareva NV, Betz RC, Schoch S, et al. Evidence for a functional interaction of WNT10A and EBF1 in male-pattern baldness. PLoS One. 2021;16(9):e0256846.
23. Xu Y, Xu Y, Liao L, Zhou N, Theissen SM, Liao XH, et al. Inducible knockout of Twist1 in young and adult mice prolongs hair growth cycle and has mild effects on general health, supporting Twist1 as a preferential cancer target. Am J Pathol. 2013;183(4):1281-92.
24. Redler S, Brockschmidt FF, Tazi-Ahnini R, Drichel D, Birch MP, Dobson K, et al. Investigation of the male pattern baldness major genetic susceptibility loci AR/EDA2R and 20p11 in female pattern hair loss. Br J Dermatol. 2012;166(6):1314-8.
25. Yap CX, Sidorenko J, Wu Y, Kemper KE, Yang J, Wray NR, et al. Dissection of genetic variation and evidence for pleiotropy in male pattern baldness. Nat Commun. 2018;9:5407.
26. Grymowicz M, Rudnicka E, Podfigurna A, Napierala P, Smolarczyk R, Smolarczyk K, et al. Hormonal effects on hair follicles. Int J Mol Sci. 2020;21(15):5342.
27. Inui S, Itami S. Androgen actions on the human hair follicle: perspectives. Exp Dermatol. 2013;22:168-71.
28. Sawaya ME, Price VH. Different levels of 5alpha-reductase type I and II, aromatase, and androgen receptor in hair follicles of women and men with androgenetic alopecia. J Invest Dermatol. 1997;109:296-300.
29. McEwan IJ, Brinkmann AO. Androgen physiology: receptor and metabolic disorders. In: Feingold KR, Anawalt B, Blackman MR, Boyce A, Chrousos G, Corpas E, et al., (Eds). Endotext [Internet]. South Dartmouth (MA): MDText.com, Inc.; 2000.
30. Zahi M. The Role of 5-alpha Reductase 3 in Steroid Metabolism. Texas: The University of Texas MD Anderson Cancer Center UT Health Graduate School of Biomedical Sciences Dissertations and Theses (Open Access); 2016. p. 661.
31. Azzouni F, Godoy A, Li Y, Mohler J. The 5 alpha-reductase isozyme family: a review of basic biology and their role in human diseases. Adv Urol. 2012;2012:530121.
32. Davey RA, Grossmann M. Androgen receptor structure, function and biology: from bench to bedside. Clin Biochem Rev. 2016; 37(1):3-15.
33. Kim MK, Kim JC. 1H differences in gene expression in bald and non-bald dermal papillae in chapter 1. Basic science. In: Unger WP, Shapiro R, Unger R, Unger M (Eds). Hair Transplantation, 5th edition. Boca Raton: CRC Press; 2011.
34. Itami S, Inui S. Role of androgen in mesenchymal epithelial interactions in human hair follicle. J Investig Dermatol Symp Proc. 2005;10(3):209-11.
35. Premanand A, Reena Rajkumari B. Androgen modulation of Wnt/β-catenin signaling in androgenetic alopecia. Arch Dermatol Res. 2018;310(5):391-9.
36. Cui J, Shen Y, Li R. Estrogen synthesis and signaling pathways during aging: from periphery to brain. Trends Mol Med. 2013;19(3):197-209.
37. Lephart ED. Human scalp hair: modulation by various factors and hormones do estrogens inhibit or stimulate—a perplexing perspective. J Cosmet Dermatol. 2019;18(6):1860-5.
38. Thornton MJ, Taylor AH, Mulligan K, Al-Azzawi F, Lyon CC, O'Driscoll J, et al. The distribution of estrogen receptor β is distinct to that of estrogen receptor α and the androgen receptor in human skin and the pilosebaceous unit. J Investig Dermatol Symp Proc. 2003;8(1):100-3.
39. Hasan R, Juma H, Eid FA, Alaswad HA, Ali WM, Aladraj FJ. Effects of hormones and endocrine disorders on hair growth. Cureus. 2022;14(12):e32726.
40. Foitzik K, Krause K, Conrad F, Nakamura M, Funk W, Paus R. Human scalp hair follicles are both a target and a source of prolactin, which serves as an autocrine and/or paracrine promoter of apoptosis-driven hair follicle regression. Am J Pathol. 2006;168(3):748-56.
41. Langan EA, Ramot Y, Goffin V, Griffiths CME, Foitzik K, Paus R. Mind the (gender) gap: does prolactin exert gender and/or site-specific effects on the human hair follicle? J Invest Dermatol. 2010;130(3):886-91.
42. Paus R. Frontiers in the (neuro-)endocrine controls of hair growth. J Investig Dermatol Symp Proc. 2007;12(2):20-2.
43. Fischer TW, Slominski A, Tobin DJ, Paus R. Melatonin and the hair follicle. J Pineal Res. 2008;44:1-15.
44. Böhm M, Eickelmann M, Li Z, Schneider SW, Oji V, Diederichs S, et al. Detection of functionally active melanocortin receptors and evidence for an immunoregulatory activity of alpha-melanocyte-stimulating hormone in human dermal papilla cells. Endocrinology. 2005;146(11):4635-46.
45. Wolf Horrell EM, Boulanger MC, D'Orazio JA. Melanocortin 1 receptor: structure, function, and regulation. Front Genet. 2016;7:95.

46. Scott MC, Suzuki I, Abdel-Malek ZA. Regulation of the human melanocortin 1 receptor expression in epidermal melanocytes by paracrine and endocrine factors and by ultraviolet radiation. Pigment Cell Res. 2002;15:433-9.
47. Contreras-Jurado C, Lorz C, García-Serrano L, Paramio JM, Aranda A. Thyroid hormone signaling controls hair follicle stem cell function. Mol Biol Cell. 2015;26(7):1263-72.
48. Van Beek N, Bodó E, Kromminga A, Gáspár E, Meyer K, Zmijewski MA, et al. Thyroid hormones directly alter human hair follicle functions: anagen prolongation and stimulation of both hair matrix keratinocyte proliferation and hair pigmentation. J Clin Endocrinol Metab. 2008;93(11):4381-8.
49. Popa A, Carsote M, Cretoiu D, Dumitrascu MC, Nistor CE, Sandru F. Study of the thyroid profile of patients with alopecia. J Clin Med. 2023;12(3):1115.
50. Ito N, Sugawara K, Bodó E, Takigawa M, van Beek N, Ito T, et al. Corticotropin-releasing hormone stimulates the in situ generation of mast cells from precursors in the human hair follicle mesenchyme. J Invest Dermatol. 2010;130(4):995-1004.
51. Livadas S, Chrousos GP. Control of the onset of puberty. Curr Opin Pediatr. 2016;28(4):551-8.
52. Skrok A, Bednarczuk T, Skwarek A, Popow M, Rudnicka L, Olszewska M. The effect of parathyroid hormones on hair follicle physiology: implications for treatment of chemotherapy-induced alopecia. Skin Pharmacol Physiol. 2015;28(4):213-25.
53. Cho YM, Woodard GL, Dunbar M, Gocken T, Jimènez JA, Foley J. Hair-cycle-dependent expression of parathyroid hormone-related protein and its type I receptor: evidence for regulation at the anagen to catagen transition. J Invest Dermatol. 2003;120(5):715-27.
54. Horesh EJ, Chéret J, Paus R. Growth hormone and the human hair follicle. Int J Mol Sci. 2021;22(24):13205.
55. Shin DW. The physiological and pharmacological roles of prostaglandins in hair growth. Korean J Physiol Pharmacol. 2022;26(6):405-13.
56. Garza LA, Liu Y, Yang Z, Alagesan B, Lawson JA, Norberg SM, et al. Prostaglandin D2 inhibits hair growth and is elevated in bald scalp of men with androgenetic alopecia. Sci Transl Med. 2012;4(126):126ra34.
57. Jeong KH, Jung JH, Kim JE, Kang H. Prostaglandin D2-mediated DP2 and AKT signal regulate the activation of androgen receptors in human dermal papilla cells. Int J Mol Sci. 2018;19(2):556.
58. Chovarda E, Sotiriou E, Lazaridou E, Vakirlis E, Ioannides D. The role of prostaglandins in androgenetic alopecia. Int J Dermatol. 2021;60(6):730-5.
59. Mantel A, McDonald JT, Goldsborough K, Harvey VM, Chan J. Prostaglandin D2 uses components of ROS signaling to enhance testosterone production in keratinocytes. J Investig Dermatol Symp Proc. 2017;18:S81-4.
60. Ho BS, Vaz C, Ramasamy S, Chew EGY, Mohamed JS, Jaffar H, et al. Progressive expression of PPARGC1α is associated with hair miniaturization in androgenetic alopecia. Sci Rep. 2019;9(1):8771.
61. Hihi A, Michalik L, Wahli W. PPARs: transcriptional effectors of fatty acids and their derivatives. Cell Mol Life Sci. 2002;59:790-8.
62. Ramot Y, Bertolini M, Boboljova M, Uchida Y, Paus R. PPAR-γ signalling as a key mediator of human hair follicle physiology and pathology. Exp Dermatol. 2020;29:312-21.
63. Sinclair R, Torkamani N, Jones L. Androgenetic alopecia: new insights into the pathogenesis and mechanism of hair loss. F1000Res. 2015;4(F1000 Faculty Rev):585.
64. Garza LA, Yang CC, Zhao T, Blatt HB, Lee M, He H, et al. Bald scalp in men with androgenetic alopecia retains hair follicle stem cells but lacks CD200-rich and CD34-positive hair follicle progenitor cells. J Clin Invest. 2011;121(2):613-22.
65. Klemp P, Peters K, Hansted B. Subcutaneous blood flow in early male pattern baldness. J Invest Dermatol. 1989;92(5):725-6.
66. Goldman BE, Fisher DM, Ringler SL. Transcutaneous PO2 of the scalp in male pattern baldness: a new piece to the puzzle. Plast Reconstr Surg. 1996;97(6):1109-16; discussion 1117.
67. Deng Z, Chen M, Liu F, Wang Y, Xu S, Sha K, et al. Androgen receptor-mediated paracrine signaling induces regression of blood vessels in the dermal papilla in androgenetic alopecia. J Invest Dermatol. 2022;142(8):2088-99.e9.
68. Seo J, Yan L, Kageyama T, Nanmo A, Chun YS, Fukuda J. Hypoxia inducible factor-1α promotes trichogenic gene expression in human dermal papilla cells. Sci Rep. 2023;13(1):1478.
69. Liu Q, Tang Y, Huang Y, Wang J, Yang K, Zhang Y, et al. Insights into male androgenetic alopecia using comparative transcriptome profiling: hypoxia-inducible factor-1 and Wnt/β-catenin signalling pathways. Br J Dermatol. 2022;187(6):936-47.
70. Zhao J, Li H, Zhou R, Ma G, Dekker JD, Tucker HO, et al. Foxp1 regulates the proliferation of hair follicle stem cells in response to oxidative stress during hair cycling. PLoS One. 2015;10(7):e0131674.
71. Upton JH, Hannen RF, Bahta AW, Farjo N, Farjo B, Philpott MP, et al. Oxidative stress-associated senescence in dermal papilla cells of men with androgenetic alopecia. J Invest Dermatol. 2015;135:1244-52.
72. Huang WY, Huang YC, Huang KS, Chan CC, Chiu HY, Tsai RY, et al. Stress-induced premature senescence of dermal papilla cells compromises hair follicle epithelial-mesenchymal interaction. J Dermatol Sci. 2017;86:114-22.
73. Prie BE, Iosif L, Tivig I, Stoian I, Giurcaneanu C. Oxidative stress in androgenetic alopecia. J Med Life. 2016;9(1):79-83.
74. Carrasco E, Calvo MI, Blázquez-Castro A, Vecchio D, Zamarrón A, de Almeida IJD, et al. Photoactivation of ROS production in situ transiently activates cell proliferation in mouse skin and in the hair follicle stem cell niche promoting hair growth and wound healing. J Invest Dermatol. 2015;135(11):2611-22.
75. Liu M, Liu X, Wang Y, Sui Y, Liu F, Liu Z, et al. Intrinsic ROS drive hair follicle cycle progression by modulating DNA damage and repair and subsequently hair follicle apoptosis and macrophage polarization. Oxid Med Cell Longev. 2022;2022:8279269.
76. Almohanna HM, Ahmed AA, Tsatalis JP, Tosti A. The role of vitamins and minerals in hair loss: a review. Dermatol Ther (Heidelb). 2019;9(1):51-70.
77. Wang W, Kang PM. Oxidative stress and antioxidant treatments in cardiovascular diseases. Antioxidants (Basel). 2020;9(12):1292.
78. Pantelireis N, Higgins CA. A bald statement—current approaches to manipulate miniaturisation focus only on promoting hair growth. Exp Dermatol. 2018;27:959-65.
79. Lin X, Zhu L, He J. Morphogenesis, growth cycle and molecular regulation of hair follicles. Front Cell Dev Biol. 2022;10:899095.
80. Schwartzenfeld DM, Karamikian J. Chapter 18—hair transplantation. In: Weinzweig J (Ed). Plastic Surgery Secrets Plus, 2nd edition. Missouri: Mosby; 2010. pp. 123-7.
81. Yue Z, Yang F, Zhang J, Li J, Chuong CM. Regulation and dysregulation of hair regeneration: aiming for clinical application. Cell Regen. 2022;11(1):22.
82. Fujiwara H, Ferreira M, Donati G, Marciano DK, Linton JM, Sato Y, et al. The basement membrane of hair follicle stem cells is a muscle cell niche. Cell. 2011;144(4):577-89.

CHAPTER 17

Genetics of Androgenetic Alopecia

Manjot Marwah, Venkataram Mysore

Key Messages

- Androgenetic alopecia (AGA) has multifactorial and polygenic inheritance.
- The androgen receptor (AR) gene on the X chromosome is the most important gene in AGA; hence, maternal influence is stronger in AGA.
- The more the number of family members affected, the higher the chances of developing AGA.
- The deoxyribonucleic acid (DNA) sequencing in AR gene has multiple variants, and their study holds the secret toward future diagnostic tests and treatments in AGA.

BACKGROUND

Francis Crick, who along with Watson unraveled the mystery of the nuclear thread of life deoxyribonucleic acid (DNA), said "Almost all aspects of life are engineered at the molecular level and without understanding molecules we can only have a sketchy understanding of life itself." He was of course referring to the gene.[1] Despite this understanding, most of the studies on androgenetic alopecia (AGA) are focused on the role of environmental factors and androgen metabolism, while the genetic predisposition to AGA remains poorly understood. This genetic involvement in AGA is clearly seen by the marked racial differences in prevalence of AGA, such as non-Caucasians often exhibit significantly lesser balding. Of the few studies done in this field over the past two decades, most of them have been contradicting, till recent times where a more generalized theory on polymorphism of the androgen receptor (AR) gene has been accepted. This chapter focuses on the journey of discovering the different genes involved in AGA and their influence in male and female pattern baldness.

INTRODUCTION

The earliest theory proposed in this field was by Osborn in 1916.[2] She suggested that pattern baldness was inherited by the Mendelian trait. She believed that balding men would be either heterozygous (Bb) or homozygous (BB), whereas balding women would be homozygous (BB). This gave rise to widely accepted opinion that AGA is caused by an autosomal dominant gene with reduced penetrance in women. This theory was contradicted by Kuster and Happle in 1984 by presenting five arguments favoring a polygenic inheritance of the trait:[3] (1) The high prevalence of the trait; (2) the distribution of balding patterns in the general population along a Gaussian curve of variation; (3) the fact that the risk increases with the number of relatives already affected; (4) the slightly increased risk of relatives of severely affected women as compared to the relatives of mildly affected women, and (5) the fact that a predisposition inherited from an affected mother is of greater importance than that inherited from an affected father. They concluded that the simple Mendelian model of Bb and BB can no longer be upheld.

GENES AFFECTING ANDROGENETIC ALOPECIA

Over the past few decades, it has been accepted that we are dealing with a polygenic inheritance and various genes have been discovered in association with AGA. Out of these AR gene is the most important, and its variants

TABLE 1: Studies on genes in androgenetic alopecia from 1999 to 2010.[4]

No.	Study	Population	Gene studied
1.	Sawaya et al. 1998	Male and female	AR gene
2.	Ellis et al. 2001	Male	Polymorphism of AR gene (*StuI* restriction site)
3.	Westeberg et al. 2001	Female	AR and ERB gene
4.	Hillmer et al. 2005	Male	AR gene
5.	Levy–Nissenbaum et al. 2005	Male	AR gene (*StuI* restriction site)
6.	Hillmer et al. 2008	Male	3q26 locus on X-chromosome
7.	Richards et al. 2008	Male	20q11.22 locus on X-chromosome
8.	Prodi et al. 2008	Sardinians	EDA2R gene
9.	All et al. 2008	Female	AR gene
10.	Brockschmidt et al.[5] 2011	Male	7p21.1

(AR: androgen receptor; ERB: estrogen receptor B; EDA2R: ectodermal dysplasia A2 receptor; StuI: *Streptomyces tubercidicus I*)

have been widely studied. **Table 1** gives us a brief outlook of the genes studied till date.

Recently, chromosome 7 has also been proved to have a role in AGA. Susceptibility variants on chromosome 7p21.1 suggest histone deacetylase 9 (HDAC9) is a new candidate gene for male pattern baldness.[5] Several other genes where associations could not be proved conclusively include 5α reductase, aromatase, estrogen receptor-α, and insulin-like growth factor 2 (IGF-2) genes. The role of Y chromosome needs further comprehensive examination of the genome.[6]

ANDROGEN RECEPTOR GENE

Nearly two decades after Kuster and Happle's study, several candidate gene and genome-wide studies unequivocally identified this gene on the X chromosome as the first gene contributing to the development of AGA.[6,7] The AR protein is a member of the nuclear receptor super family and mediates the effects of androgens. A functional AR and circulating androgens are essential requirements for the development of AGA. There is three times more AR in frontal hair than occipital hair.[4]

- *Polymorphism of the AR gene*: Variation in the DNA sequencing of AR gene has caused a surge of research in this field.[6] It has been observed that the aminoterminal domain of AR gene, which contains a region encoded by CAG repeats, is required for transcription activation. The number of AR repeats is inversely proportional to the androgen levels in men and women. Hence, men with high number of androgen repeats get bald, and similarly this presents with hirsutism, acne, polycystic ovary syndrome (PCOS) and baldness in women.[8] The length of the CAG repeats was also proved to be related to androgen expression, such as shorter length showing greater androgen activity. There are three gene polymorphisms of particular interest:[6]
  i. The *Streptomyces tubercidicus I (StuI)* restriction fragment
  ii. The CAG triplet repeat length
  iii. The GCC triplet repeat lengths
- *Role of AR gene in pathogenesis*:[9] The current mechanism for androgen action in balding follicles involves intracellular metabolism of testosterone to the more potent 5α-dihydrotestosterone (DHT) inside the cells of the regulatory dermal papilla. DHT binds with AR genes to form a gene transcriptional regulator complex that interacts with genomic DNA to alter gene expression. Altered transcription of autocrine factors causing increased secretion of inhibitory factors and/or reduced secretion of stimulatory factors will reduce hair follicle activity causing balding. Such alterations have been shown in AGA using cultured dermal papilla cells, and changes in several genes have been detected including those for autocrine factors transforming growth factor-β (TGF-β) and stem cell factor (SCF).

Isolated hair follicles from balding scalp also express less hepatocyte growth factor (HGF) and macrophage-stimulating protein (MSP) and some of their receptors c-Met and receptor originated from nantes (RON). All these factors secreted from the dermal papillae have great influence on the hair cycle. Vascular endothelial growth factor controls hair growth and follicle size through angiogenesis. HGF is involved in the cyclic growth of hair follicles. Platelet-derived growth factor induces and maintains the anagen phase of hair follicles. IGF-1 controls the hair growth cycle and differentiation of hair shafts.

There is a complex interplay of different signaling systems such as Wnt signaling pathways, IGFs which cause anagen induction with inhibitory pathways such as TGF-β, which induce catagen progression. A genome-wide association study (GWAS) suggested that Wnt10A is the gene responsible for effect on cr2q35. A reduction in Wnt10A expression leads to shortening of anagen phase, as observed in AGA hair follicles.[10]

APPLICATION IN DIAGNOSTICS AND TREATMENT

Understanding the genetics of hair loss has practical implications on both the diagnosis and treatment of baldness.

Early diagnosis: Identify those at high risk of becoming bald, before it is clinically apparent, so that hair loss can be treated in its earliest stages where medications have the greatest chance of being successful.

- A new screening test (Hairdx.com) can now test people who are at a risk to develop AGA in future. This test is different in men and women due to the difference in pathogenesis. In men, it tests 8 variants on AR gene, with the *StuI* variant being the most common. A positive test indicates a 70% chance of developing AGA in future. In women, the test detects the length of CAG and GGC repeats within the AR gene. For example, if the length of repeats is <15, then the woman has a 97.3% chance to develop patterned hair loss in future.[11]
- Hillmer et al. have identified a second contributing genetic locus on chromosome 20p11 with no obvious connection to the androgen pathway. They have proposed a newer test for screening in AGA and have demonstrated that this test allows a better risk prediction than the currently available tests.[12]

Gene therapy: Fortunately, the scalp is readily accessible to topical therapies as it allows direct penetration of a drug to a target area. It is theoretically possible to introduce genetic material directly into cells using liposome-DNA mixtures that carry the missing gene(s) to generate new hair. The recent discovery of a gene Lhx2 which leads to more hair growth raises exciting possibilities of treating baldness in the next decade. This gene is active during the anagen, and it is turned off during the telogen.[13]

SUMMARY

- Androgenetic alopecia has multifactorial and polygenic inheritance.
- The AR gene on the X chromosome is the most important gene in AGA; hence, maternal influence is stronger in AGA.
- The more the number of family members affected, the higher the chances of developing AGA.
- The DNA sequencing in AR gene has multiple variants, and their study holds the secret toward future diagnostic tests and treatments in AGA.

REFERENCES

1. Yesudian P. Genes matter! Int J Trichol. 2010;2:1.
2. Osborn D. Inheritance of baldness. J Hered.1916;7(8):347-5.
3. Küster W, Happle R. The inheritance of common baldness: two B or not two B?. J Am Acad Dermatol. 1984;11(5 Pt 1):921-6.
4. Boychenko O, Bernstein RM. Update on the pathogenesis, genetics and medical treatment of patterned hair loss. Schweiger ES1. J Drugs Dermatol. 2010;9(11):1412-9.
5. Brockschmidt FF, Heilmann S, Ellis JA, Eigelshoven S, Hanneken S, Herold C, et al. Susceptibility variants on chromosome 7p21.1 suggest HDAC9 as a new candidate gene for male-pattern baldness. Br J Dermatol. 2011;165:1293-302.
6. Ellis JA, Harrap SB. The genetics of androgenetic alopecia. Clin Dermatol. 2001;19:149-54.
7. Hillmer AM, Hanneken S, Ritzmann S, Becker T, Freudenberg J, Brockschmidt FF, et al. Genetic variation in the human androgen receptor gene is the major determinant of common early-onset androgenetic alopecia. Am J Hum Genet. 2005;77:140-8.
8. Sawaya ME, Shalita AR. Androgen receptor polymorphisms (CAG repeat lengths) in androgenetic alopecia, hirsutism, and acne. J Cutan Med Surg. 1998;3(1):9-15.
9. Li J, Jiang TX, Chuong CM. Many paths to alopecia via compromised regeneration of hair follicle stem cells. Semin Cutan Med Surg. 2012;31(4):258-66.
10. Heilmann S, Kiefer AK, Fricker N, Drichel D, Hillmer AM, Herold C, et al. Androgenetic alopecia: identification of four genetic risk loci and evidence for the contribution of WNT signaling to its etiology. J Invest Dermatol. 2013;133(6):1489-96.
11. Demuro-Mercon C, Rhodes T, Girman CJ, Vatten L. Male-pattern Hair Loss in Norwegian Men: a Community-based Study. Dermatology. 2000;200:219-22.
12. Hillmer AM, Brockschmidt FF, Hanneken S, Eigelshoven S, Steffens M, Flaquer A, et al. Susceptibility variants for male-pattern baldness on chromosome 20p11. Nat Genet. 2008;40(11): 1279-81.
13. Törnqvist G, Sandberg A, Hägglund AC, Carlsson L. Cyclic expression of Lhx2 regulates hair formation. PLoS Genet. 2010;6(4):e1000904.

CHAPTER 18

Smoking and Hair Loss

Nivedita Sashidhar, Yatra Kavadya Jain, Venkataram Mysore

Key Messages

- Tobacco smoking has sustained its popularity despite its association with ill health.
- Smoking is known to be detrimental to skin and hair growth.
- There are several plausible mechanisms of action for hair loss, such as vasoconstriction, deoxyribonucleic acid (DNA) damage, free radical generation, and hormonal effects.
- There is a significant positive association between the duration and severity of smoking.
- It highlights the need to spread awareness about this preventable, important environmental factor.

INTRODUCTION

Tobacco smoking and exposure to environmental tobacco smoke are considered risk factors for carcinomas and cardiovascular and respiratory diseases, and the health effects of tobacco smoke have become a serious global health problem. Smoking is not only a preventable cause of significant systemic disease, but its role in skin aging and hair loss has also been a great topic of interest and research in recent times. It has generally been considered inimical to hair growth, and its role in hair loss affects the follicular growth cycle. Chemical components found in tobacco smoke, such as nicotine, are capable of accumulating in hair and have become reliable biomarkers for detecting smoke exposure.[1,2]

COMPOSITION OF TOBACCO SMOKE

Tobacco smoke has both a solid particulate phase and a volatile gas phase.[3] The main contents of solid phase include nicotine, phenol, catechol, quinolone, aniline, toluidine, nickel, *N*-nitrosodimethylamine, benzanthracene, benzopyrenes, and 2-naphthylamine. The main toxic contents of the gas phase include carbon monoxide, carbon dioxide, nitrogen oxides, acetone, hydrogen cyanide, acrolein, ammonium, pyridine, 3-vinylpyridine, formaldehyde, *N*-nitrosodimethylamine, and *N*-nitrosopyrrolidine.[4]

HAIR AS A BIOMARKER OF NICOTINE EXPOSURE

Nicotine and other metabolites enter the body through ingestion, inhalation, transdermal patches, topical cream, etc. Nicotine can enter hair by either absorption through blood[5-9] or from exposure to environmental smoke.[10-12]

It is believed that nicotine moves by passive diffusion from the bloodstream into the growing hair cells at the base of the follicle and then becomes tightly bound in the interior of the hair shaft during subsequent keratogenesis. Therefore, nicotine incorporation in hair is dependent on the average concentration in the blood over time, which, in turn, depends on the dose inhaled or ingested.

Knowing the rate at which hair grows and the distance of the analyzed hair section from the scalp, levels in hair may then be related to exposure levels (whether active or passive) in a time-dependent manner.[9] Nilsen et al. found concentration of nicotine more in the distal end of hair as compared to the proximal end, which was attributed to longer exposure of the distal hair to environmental smoke.[12] Based on this, studies have suggested that the level of nicotine in hair can be a possible marker of long-term smoke exposure.

It has been suggested that there is a difference in the metabolism of nicotine between smokers and nonsmokers; the conversion of nicotine to cotinine and its elimination in urine can be more rapid among smokers than nonsmokers.[9]

Cotinine is present in hair but in much lower concentrations than nicotine. This may reduce detection of tobacco exposure, thus explaining the relatively poor correlation with the history of exposure among nonsmokers in several studies.[13-16] It seems that cotinine is not distributed through the body in exactly the same manner as nicotine.

MECHANISMS OF SMOKING LEADING TO HAIR LOSS

The mechanisms of action by which smoking causes hair loss are multifactorial **(Box 1)** and are further elaborated as follows:

Vasoconstrictor Effect

Vasoconstriction of cutaneous microvasculature by nicotine metabolites is an important effect of acute and chronic smoking. Nicotine acts by neither amplifying the vasoconstrictor effect of norepinephrine nor attenuating acetylcholine-induced endothelium-dependent skin vasodilation.[17]

BOX 1 Mechanisms of action by which smoking causes hair loss.

- Vasoconstrictor action by smoke metabolites
- Retention of DNA adducts causing DNA damage
- Smoke-induced imbalance in the follicular protease/antiprotease systems
- Oxidative stress and disequilibrium of antioxidant system
- Sustained microinflammation causing perifollicular fibrosis
- Desensitization of nicotinic acetylcholine receptors
- Androgen-dependent hair thinning

(DNA: deoxyribonucleic acid)

Treatment Pearl

It is now a routine advice to patients to stop smoking before hair transplantation, even though studies specifically in hair transplantation are lacking.

Effect on Deoxyribonucleic Acid

Cigarette smoking results in the retention of deoxyribonucleic acid (DNA) adducts, which can cause DNA damage to both nuclear and mitochondrial DNA.[18] Cigarette smoke induces imbalance in protease/antiprotease systems, which play an important role in extracellular matrix remodeling during hair follicle regression (catagen phase), thus affecting hair follicle growth cycle.[19]

Effect on Free Radicals and Antioxidants

Smoke metabolites can induce oxidative stress by generation of free radicals, in particular reactive oxygen species (ROS), and interact with nucleic acids (both in the mitochondria and in the nucleus), resulting in mutation predisposing DNA strands to break.[20] It may cause early apoptosis of the hair follicle, resulting in early catagen phase. Naito et al. using TUNEL staining found that lipid peroxides can induce apoptosis of hair follicle cells and human epidermal keratinocytes by up-regulating apoptosis-related genes.[21] They also observed that the topical application of linolein hydroperoxides, one of the lipid peroxides, causes early catagen phase in the murine hair cycle.

Oxidation of lipids by ROS can also cause premature cell death by damaging phospholipid cellular membranes, thus affecting hair follicle molecular balance. Smoking results in an imbalance of the antioxidant systems, which may cause follicular keratinocytes to release immunomodulatory cytokines such as interleukin (IL)-1 α, IL-1 β, and tumor necrosis factor -alpha (TNF-α) which are potent inhibitors of hair follicle growth.[21]

Smoking may Enhance Senescence

Bahta et al. cultured dermal hair papilla cells (DPCs) from balding and nonbalding scalp and demonstrated that balding DPCs grew slower in vitro than nonbalding DPCs.[22] The finding of premature senescence of balding DPCs along with the expression of oxidative stress markers and DNA damage in vitro suggests that balding DPCs are sensitive to environmental stress.

Nicotine can cause sustained microinflammation of the hair follicle, inflammatory cell infiltrate, connective tissue remodeling, and interplay of collagenases, culminating into perifollicular fibrosis.[23] Nicotine can cause overstimulation of cellular nicotinic acetylcholine receptors, leading to their desensitization of receptors. This leads to hair follicle destruction by activation of programmed cell death pathways present in keratinocytes.[1]

■ Hormonal Effects

Smoking may lead to an increase in androgen-dependent hair thinning. The hypoestrogenic state may be due to increased hydroxylation of estradiol and inhibition of the enzyme aromatase.[24]

> **■ Treatment Pearl**
>
> *Smoking may cause increased levels of androgens, so the possibility of androgenetic alopecia (AGA) can be correlated with increased testosterone levels.*[25]

EFFECTS OF SMOKING ON HAIR LOSS

There have been several animal and human studies with many favoring the view that smoking induces hair loss, while others have not supported this view. There are studies that have found association with the following:

- Positive smoking history contributed to the early onset of AGA
- Greater number of cigarettes smoked directly proportional to the severity of AGA
- Increased smoking duration associated with increased severity of AGA
- Gender, pattern of AGA, and associated factors such as obesity

The first to report a significant relationship between smoking and hair loss in humans was a study by Mosley and Gibbs in the United Kingdom.[26] A review of literature published in 2020 regarding the relationship between smoking, premature graying of hairs, and alopecia, both androgenic alopecia and frontal fibrosing alopecia, concluded a positive correlation between the length of smoking and alopecia severity in patients with AGA.

However, it is important to note that there is no scientific evidence demonstrating an improvement in hair growth after the cessation of smoking. Furthermore, while patients undergoing hair transplant are routinely advised to stop smoking before hair loss, there are no studies documenting the effect of smoking on hair growth after hair transplantation **(Table 1)**.

SUMMARY

While genetic factors play an integral role in alopecia, environmental factors, particularly smoking, must be taken into consideration. *There is evidence to support a relation between the amount of smoking and the severity of baldness and also the age of onset of AGA through a number of plausible mechanisms.* In view of the immense psychological impact of hair loss on both men and women and increasing awareness of the detrimental effects of smoking, *the onus lies with the dermatologist to advise patients of AGA to stop smoking.*

> ***Tips and Pearls***
>
> - Educate the patient and counsel about ill effects of smoking and hair loss.
> - All patients undergoing hair transplantation are routinely advised to cut down/eventually quit smoking.
> - It is known to improve the rate of graft survival due to restored normal blood supply.
> - However, there are no studies documenting the effect of smoking on hair growth after hair transplantation.
> - Positive association between the duration and severity of smoking and hair loss emphasizes on the need to curtail the same.
> - As AGA is a continuous process, patients have to be forewarned about the need for compliance with treatment/ lifestyle modifications for sustainable results.

TABLE 1: Studies demonstrating positive association between smoking and hair loss.

Author	Place of study	Year	Study design	Sample size	Duration of study	Study subject details	Smoking status	Observation and results
Mosley and Gibbs[26]	United Kingdom	1996	Controlled retrospective trial	$n = 606$ (male = 268, female = 338)	3 months	Age group > 30 years: 152 males and 152 females were smokers. Hamilton baldness scale, category III and above regarded as bald. Bald smokers: male: 103; female: 2 Bald nonsmokers: male: 63, female: 2	Not included	Odds ratio for the association of smoking and baldness in men was 1.93 (95% confidence interval 1.13–3.28). While for females, corresponding calculation was not performed
Su and Chen[27]	Taiwan	2007	Uncontrolled retrospective trial	$n = 740$	2 months (April 2005–June 2005)	Mean age of 65 years. Norwood and Ludwig classification system. In age group 40–49, 50–59, 60–69, and >70 years, the age-specific prevalence of Norwood type A variant was 5.1, 1.1, 8.1, and 7.4%, respectively, and those of female pattern AGA were 0.0, 2.1, 1.6, and 2.4%, respectively	Smoking status categorized as never, quit, current smoker of <20 cigarettes and smokers of >20 cigarettes a day	Smokers had an increased risk of moderate or severe AGA (Norwood type 4) and smoking status (OR, 1.77; 95% CI, 1.14–2.76), current cigarette smoking of 20 cigarettes or more per day (OR, 2.34; 95% CI, 1.19–4.59), and smoking intensity (OR, 1.78; 95% CI, 1.03–3.07)
Gatherwright et al.[28]	Ohio	2012	Controlled retrospective trial	$n = 98$ (female)	2 years (2009–2011)	98 female identical twins (49 sets). Mean age: 53 years	Not included	Frontal hair loss noted less in twins who had never smoked ($p = 0.021$; $n = 8$). Increased frontal hair thinning was also significant in smokers. Temporal hair loss greater in smokers ($p = 0.096$, $n = 10$)
Gatherwright et al.[29]	Ohio	2013	Controlled retrospective trial	$n = 92$ (male)	2 years (2009–2011)	92 male identical twins (46 sets). Mean age: 52 years	Not included	Increased duration of smoking and frontal hair loss showed positive correlation ($p < 0.001$), but the quantity of smoking was not statistically significant. Twins who smoked had more vertex hair loss than their nonsmoking siblings ($p = 0.047$, $n = 20$)
Park et al.[30]	Korea	2016	Controlled retrospective trial	$n = 1,884$ (male = 915, female = 969)	2 years (October 2012–December 2014)	Mean age: 56.6 years. 991 subjects had AGA (613: Males and 378: Females). BASP classification was used and classified as follows, 443 subjects: Mild AGA, 381: Moderate AGA, and 167: Severe AGA	Divided as presence or absence of smoking	Smokers in AGA group 334/991 (33.7%) were higher than the non-AGA group 214/892 (24%) ($p = 0.0000$). Subjects with more smoking had more severe form of AGA [mild: 125/443 (28.2%), moderate: 143/381 (37.5%), severe: 66/167 (39.5%) ($p = 0.004$)]

Continued

Continued

Author	Place of study	Year	Study design	Sample size	Duration of study	Study subject details	Smoking status	Observation and results
Fortes et al.[31]	Italy	2017	Uncontrolled retrospective trial	$n = 351$ (237 males, 114 females)	1 year (2010–2011)	Mean age: 35 years. Male: 133 subjects with mild (Hamilton–Norwood classifications I–III) and 104 subjects with moderate and severe (Hamilton–Norwood classification IV–VII). Female: 104 subjects with mild (Ludwig type 1) and 10 subjects with moderate/severe (Ludwig types II and III)	Subjects categorized as never, quit, current smokers of <10 cigarettes and smokers of >10 cigarettes per day	Subjects with severe AGA smoked more as compared to less severe AGA (17.5% vs. 7.6%, $p = 0.05$). Furthermore, AGA subjects who were heavy smokers had almost three times an increased risk of having a moderate/severe alopecia in comparison to those who never smoked
Vora et al.[32]	Gujarat, India	2019	Controlled prospective trial	$n = 100$ (male)	2 years (June 2014–May 2016)	50 subjects with AGA and 50 age-matched control subjects were included with a mean age of 29.32 and 31.5 years, respectively. The degree of AGA was based on the Norwood scale (3–7). AGA developing before 36 years of age and reaching at least stage 3 of the Hamilton–Norwood classification is termed as early onset AGA	Not included	The prevalence of smoking was more in male patients with early onset AGA, 26 (52%) as compared to controls 11 (22%) ($p = 0.002$)
Salem et al.[33]	Egypt	2021	Controlled prospective trial	$n = 1,000$ (smokers 500; nonsmokers 500)	1 year 6 months (January 2018–September 2019)	Mean age: 25 years of smokers group. 235 (47%) had grade 3 AGA and 120 subjects (24%) had grade 4 AGA. In the nonsmokers group, 100 subjects (20%) had grade 2 AGA and 50 subjects (10%) had either grade 3 or 4 AGA	Smokers were who smoked >10 cigarettes over >1 year	Majority of smokers (425) had a form of AGA, while only (200) nonsmokers had a degree of AGA ($p < 0.01$)

(AGA: androgenetic alopecia; BASP: basic and specific; CI: confidence interval; OR: odds ratio)

REFERENCES

1. Babadjouni A, Pouldar Foulad D, Hedayati B, Evron E, Mesinkovska N. The effects of smoking on hair health: a systematic review. Skin Appendage Disord. 2021;7(4):251-64.
2. Belli AA, Etgu F, Ozbas Gok S, Kara B, Dogan G. Risk factors for premature hair graying in young Turkish adults. Pediatr Dermatol. 2016;33(4):438-42.
3. Kavadya Y, Mysore V. Role of smoking in androgenetic alopecia: a systematic review. Int J Trichology. 2022;14(2):41-8.
4. Ortiz A, Grando SA. Smoking and the skin. Int J Dermatol. 2012;51:250-62.
5. Nafstad P, Botten G, Hagen JA, Zahlsen K, Nilsen OG, Silsand T, et al. Comparison of three methods for estimating environmental tobacco smoke exposure among children aged between 12 and 36 months. Int J Epidemiol. 1995;24:88-94.
6. Eliopoulos C, Klein J, Koren G. Validation of self-reported smoking by analysis of hair for nicotine and cotinine. Ther Drug Monit. 1996;18:532-6.
7. Nilsen T, Nilsen OG. Accumulation of nicotine in human hair during long-term controlled exposure to a low concentration of nicotine vapour. Pharmacol Toxicol. 1997;81:48-52.
8. Pichini S, Altieri I, Pellegrini M, Pacifici R, Zuccaro P. The analysis of nicotine in infants' hair for measuring exposure to environmental tobacco smoke. Forensic Sci Int. 1997;84:253-8.
9. Al-Delaimy WK. Hair as a biomarker for exposure to tobacco smoke. Tob Control. 2002;11:176-82.
10. Zahlsen K, Nilsen OG. Nicotine in hair of smokers and non-smokers: sampling procedure and gas chromatographic/mass spectrometric analysis. Pharmacol Toxicol. 1994;75:143-9.
11. Baumgartner WA, Hill VA. Sample preparation techniques. Forensic Sci Int. 1993;63:121-35.
12. Nilsen T, Zahlsen K, Nilsen OG. Uptake of nicotine in hair during controlled environmental air exposure to nicotine vapour: evidence for a major contribution of environmental nicotine to the overall nicotine found in hair from smokers and non-smokers. Pharmacol Toxicol. 1994;75:136-42.
13. Kintz P, Tracqui A, Mangin P. Detection of drugs in human hair for clinical and forensic applications. Int J Legal Med. 1992;105:1-4.
14. Kintz P, Ludes B, Mangin P. Evaluation of nicotine and cotinine in human hair. J Forensic Sci. 1992;37:72-6.
15. Kintz P. Gas chromatographic analysis of nicotine and cotinine in hair. J Chromatogr. 1992;580:347-53.
16. Dimich-Ward H, Gee H, Brauer M, Leung V. Analysis of nicotine and cotinine in the hair of hospitality workers exposed to environmental tobacco smoke. J Occup Environ Med. 1997;39:946-8.
17. Black CE, Huang N, Neligan PC, Levine RH, Lipa JE, Lintlop S, et al. Effect of nicotine on vasoconstrictor and vasodilator responses in human skin vasculature. Am J Physiol Regul Integr Comp Physiol. 2001;281:R1097-104.
18. Liu CS, Kao SH, Wei YH. Smoking-associated mitochondrial DNA mutations in human hair follicles. Environ Mol Mutagen. 1997;30:47-55.
19. Trüeb RM. Association between smoking and hair loss: another opportunity for health education against smoking? Dermatology. 2003;206:189-91.
20. Wu D, Cederbaum AI. Alcohol, oxidative stress, and free radical damage. Alcohol Res Health. 2003;27:277-84.
21. Naito A, Midorikawa T, Yoshino T, Ohdera M. Lipid peroxides induce early onset of catagen phase in murine hair cycles. Int J Mol Med. 2008;22:725-9.
22. Bahta AW, Farjo N, Farjo B, Philpott MP. Premature senescence of balding dermal papilla cells in vitro is associated with p16(INK4a) expression. J Invest Dermatol. 2008;128:1088-94.
23. Mahé YF, Michelet JF, Billoni N, Jarrousse F, Buan B, Commo S, et al. Androgenetic alopecia and microinflammation. Int J Dermatol. 2000;39:576-84.
24. Kaufman KD. Androgen metabolism as it affects hair growth in androgenetic alopecia. Dermatol Clin. 1996;14:697-711.
25. Nargis T, Beja V, Pinto M, Shenoy MM. Early onset androgenetic alopecia in men and associated risk factors: a hospital based study. Int J Res Dermatol. 2017;3:267-71.
26. Mosley JG, Gibbs AC. Premature grey hair and hair loss among smokers: a new opportunity for health education? BMJ. 1996;313:1616.
27. Su LH, Chen TH. Association of androgenetic alopecia with smoking and its prevalence among Asian men: a community-based survey. Arch Dermatol. 2007;143:1401-6.
28. Gatherwright J, Liu MT, Gliniak C, Totonchi A, Guyuron B. The contribution of endogenous and exogenous factors to female alopecia: a study of identical twins. Plast Reconstr Surg. 2012;130:1219-26.
29. Gatherwright J, Liu MT, Amirlak B, Gliniak C, Totonchi A, Guyuron B. The contribution of endogenous and exogenous factors to male alopecia: a study of identical twins. Plast Reconstr Surg. 2013;131:794e-801e.
30. Park SY, Oh SS, Lee WS. Relationship between androgenetic alopecia and cardiovascular risk factors according to BASP classification in Koreans. J Dermatol. 2016;43:1293-300.
31. Fortes C, Mastroeni S, Mannooranparampil TJ, Ribuffo M. The combination of overweight and smoking increases the severity of androgenetic alopecia. Int J Dermatol. 2017;56:862-7.
32. Vora RV, Kota RK, Singhal RR, Anjaneyan G. Clinical profile of androgenic alopecia and its association with cardiovascular risk factors. Indian J Dermatol. 2019;64:19-22.
33. Salem AS, Ibrahim HS, Abdelaziz HH, Elsaie ML. Implications of cigarette smoking on early-onset androgenetic alopecia: a cross-sectional study. J Cosmet Dermatol. 2021;20:1318-24.

CHAPTER 19

Psychological Aspects of Hair Loss

Manjot Marwah, Venkataram Mysore, Pooja Kanumuru

Key Messages

- Hair loss causes psychological disability, often out of proportion to the physical impact.
- Proper understanding and empathy are vital to manage patients with hair loss.
- A detailed history, particularly with respect to underlying psychological factors, and appropriate psychological counseling, if necessary, by an expert are needed.
- This is particularly relevant for patients seeking surgical management.

"Ugly is a field without grass, a plant without leaves, or a head without hair."

—Ovid "The Silent Woman"

INTRODUCTION

Scalp hair never fails to turn heads and make a bold statement. Society perceives hair as a sign of youthfulness, vigor, and success. Loss of hair at an early age results in patients feeling physically and socially less attractive, less virile, less likable, and having low self-esteem. A patient with hair loss goes through multiple feelings and emotions due to this personal and societal pressure. Common emotional aspects linked to this include self-consciousness, embarrassment, frustration, and jealousy. This could lead to psychological stress that is out of proportion to the problem. This is worsened by excessive advertising of hair treatments and camouflage techniques on television, newspapers, and social media sites.

This often results in unrealistic aspirations and expectations. Women with acute telogen effluvium or active scarring alopecia often opt for surgery as a cure. It is not uncommon to get patients with grade 6 alopecia, coming with their past photos or pictures of movie stars and asking for hairlines like theirs. Frequently, we also get a patient who quotes a study on stem cells under trial and asks, "Doctor, can you do this for me?" Hence, each patient approaches with different psychology and emotion—a factor that needs to be always taken into consideration in a hair loss patient consultation.

In many patients, these emotions are so overwhelming that they start affecting the patient's daily lifestyle—limiting social activities, avoiding family occasions, and spending an enormous amount of time and money on hair grooming. This behavioral impact is noticed not only in men but in women too. Surveys have shown that around 40% of women with alopecia have had marital problems, and around 63% claimed to have career-related problems.[1] The same grade of alopecia may trigger different psychological responses in different patients; some may be physiologically normal responses while some are borderline psychosomatic disorders; rarely a typical case of an underlying psychological disorder precipitated by alopecia may be encountered. To substantiate this further, clinical studies have also shown that borderline personality disorder (BPD) and body dysmorphic disorder (BDD) are the two most significant conditions in relation to cosmetic surgery, occurring in approximately 10–15% of individuals seeking cosmetic procedures.[2] Such patients need to be treated psychologically too along with their

BOX 1 Factors responsible for increasing demand in hair transplant surgeries.

- Increased longevity
- Changing tastes and attitudes
- Media hype
- Increased awareness
- Increased affordability
- Demand for longer-lasting drastic results
- Impatience and distrust of medical treatments
- Hassle-free one-time treatment option

hair treatments, to get satisfying results. Hence, clinicians managing hair loss patients must grasp the psychological impact of hair loss. Identifying patients with body dysmorphic syndrome is vital to prevent adverse outcomes and facilitate proper management. This enables clinicians to provide counseling, refer patients if necessary, and occasionally assume the role of a psychotherapist.

CURRENT SCENARIO

According to the International Society of Hair Restoration Surgery (ISHRS) 2022 Practice Census, the global hair transplant industry is thriving as evidenced by a 10% increase in size since 2016.[3] ISHRS 2020 census analysis shows that surgical hair restoration is chosen by 37% of people worldwide to enhance their social life.[4] Several other factors have also led to this changing trend and increasing demand in hair transplant surgeries **(Box 1)**.

Paradoxically, coinciding with the demand for procedures, there is an increasing fear of side effects and a demand for simpler and safer procedures. Often in the same patient, one sees an obsessive urge for the procedure and also a paranoid fear of side effects—the twin demands of providing "guaranteed efficacy with absolutely no side effects" is one of the challenges of hair transplant surgery.

Disease versus Desire

As a result, trichology, as in cosmetology, is changing from a disease-oriented specialty to a desire-satisfying specialty, where a patient demands a procedure for a perceived problem. This has led to a debate as to whether such patients are indeed patients or there should be another term such as clients.

The differences between a patient and a client are given in **Table 1**.

TABLE 1: Patient versus client.

Patient	Client
Has a disease	Has a desire
Mostly needs medical treatment; occasional surgical treatment	Mostly needs a procedural treatment
Fear of consequences of disease, fear of infection, fear of spread	Well aware; often has read well; often knows what treatment is needed
Accepts treatments willingly	Wants options—safe options
Easier to counsel about side effects	Paranoid about side effects
Respectful toward doctor; doctor is dominant	Demands an equal relationship
Easier to handle if there is a side effect	Demanding; can be aggressive; greater potential for a medicolegal situation

Being a successful hair transplant surgeon is always a multifaceted job. It involves being a director, an organizer, a marketing salesman, an entrepreneur, a surgeon, a clinician, and yes, a psychologist **(Box 2)**. If one patient has had a bad experience while undergoing a hair transplant, he not only gives the doctor a bad reputation but also discourages other patients from thinking about a hair restoration surgery as the results are visible for all to see. Hence, making sure that the patient has a pleasant experience and understanding their feelings at every step comprise a crucial part of this job. No wonder, *hair transplantation has been referred to as a "psychiatric surgery."*

BOX 2 Characteristics of a good hair transplant surgeon.

- Emphasis on treatment
- Emphasis on information and education
- Emphasis on results—from different modalities including drugs
- Emphasis on safety
- Emphasis on a plan that includes managing the treatment for future hair loss
- Emphasis on patient satisfaction
- Emphasis on a comfortable and joyful experience
- Emphasis on empathy and being nonjudgmental

ASSESSMENT OF THE PSYCHOLOGY OF A HAIR LOSS PATIENT

In 1818, Heinroth described the term "psychosomatic," referring to the influence of the mind on the body. The easiest way for a physician of a nonpsychiatric background to assess the psychology or thinking of the patient is via a good doctor–patient relationship. This is easier said than done. It is a fact that even the best medical education and training do not confer good communication and interpersonal skills—these are acquired through great experience and observation—though they may come naturally to some. Only a doctor with good communication skills will be able to handle all types of patients and also segregate the cases that need psychotherapy.

The most important aspect while evaluating a patient's psychology is to give the patient adequate consultation time. A minimum of 15 minutes per consultation is a must. It is often worthwhile to give a questionnaire asking the patient to fill it out. A counselor or a junior doctor can also screen the patient first. It is important that the patient is provided an opportunity to vent out their feelings.

The following points give a stepwise guideline on evaluating a patient's psychology when they enter an aesthetic clinic.

1. *General observation*: Assessment of the patient should start from the minute the patient enters the clinic. Subtle signs such as who is accompanying the patient, is the patient's dressing sense loud or subtle, is the patient maintaining eye contact, or who is talking more during the visit—the patient or the accompanying person should be looked for.

   Being anxious, nervous, and self-conscious is a normal feeling while visiting a doctor, and hence it is important to make the patient feel comfortable during the visit.
2. *Clinical observation*: Notice if the patient has exaggerated frown lines or glabellar lines, indicating stress. Any sign of a past cosmetic procedure carried out? Early signs of aging? Any sign of depression, such as hesitation marks?
3. *Ambience and courtesy:* To make the patient comfortable, greet the patient by their name and get them seated comfortably. This helps in relieving the initial anxiety too. Notice if the patient is quiet most of the time or talkative, reluctant in mentioning the complaints, or overzealous and demanding.
4. *Questioning:* Ask the patient about their concerns—what is bothering them? How much is it bothering? Are they socializing? Are they trying to hide the hair loss? Are they considering surgical options? Did anyone else tell them to get the surgery? For how long have they wanted to get this surgery? Asking open-ended questions helps in allowing the patient to talk more and open up.

   Ask for details about the expectations; ask, what and how much would satisfy them. Is there any minimum that they expect? Show them photos of the results that can be achieved and then ask whether they will be happy with such results.
5. *Medical history:* History of any sleep disturbances, alcohol consumption or smoking, appetite loss, or weight gain gives a hint about physical and mental well-being. Family history regarding relations may be asked indirectly, such as recent divorce or marriage, which gives a hint on interpersonal relationships. The patient's work type tells about their job satisfaction. Any hesitation to answer a question may also indicate a stress factor and should be noted.[5]

TYPES OF EMOTIONS IN ALOPECIA

The difference between emotions and psychology is that emotions are what a patient feels or experiences and psychology is how the doctor perceives these emotions. The patient may feel sad and rejected but diagnosing him with depression is the doctor's job.

- *Denial:* Few patients are in denial about their hair loss. This is seen in men who usually comb their hair over the bald patch to create the illusion of a full hairy head. A woman having a receding hairline will usually change her hairstyle and start keeping a fringe. Such patients usually approach a doctor late and suffer due to poor treatment choices.
- *Panic*: Anxiety and panic are some of the common feelings seen in younger patients suffering from hair loss. The fear of looking old and unattractive and the inability to style hair are especially high in women. Women are used to styling hair, curling it, straightening it, and when they are unable to do it due to excessive hair thinning, they have trouble dealing with it.
- *Dissatisfaction with appearance*: Living with alopecia can be difficult in a culture that views hair as a sign of youth and good health. Feelings of low self-esteem can be seen with any grade of alopecia but are more common with men experiencing profound alopecia.[5] This study also showed that this effect was seen more in younger males comparatively.
- *Rejection*: The majority of people suffering from higher grades of alopecia have experienced social teasing and humiliation. Those who cannot deal with it usually start avoiding social functions. This may cause introversion and shyness, and in extreme cases, it may result in depression.[6]
- *Fixation*: Alopecia leads to obsession in a few patients. They get fixated on their loss, and it can lead to an obsessive-compulsive disorder in severe cases. Continuously fidgeting with their hair and looking in the mirror for long hours are a few of the hints pointing toward fixation.

UNDERSTANDING THE PSYCHOLOGY BEHIND THE EMOTION

Not all patients have an underlying psychological issue. However, all patients do have an underlying emotion or motive behind getting a hair transplant surgery. Most of the reasons are purely physiological or due to an "*ideal*" self-image built by the person; rarely do we encounter patients with psychosomatic causes asking for a surgery. These are the patients who need to be segregated.

- *"Ideal" self-image*: Every decision an individual makes, as per his choice of clothes, house, or car, is based on a self-image that he considers ideal for him. Similarly, patients usually have an ideal image in their minds when they approach for hair transplantation. There is a goal, an "ideal" self-image they imagine; this determines the patient's behavior and their obsession and demands. This is the most common reason patients get the procedure and if the patient has realistic expectations and is self-motivated, the procedure is going to benefit the patient not only physically, but also emotionally.
- *Psychosomatic causes:* One-third of the patients visiting a dermatologist have associated emotional and psychosomatic factors. Only treating the physical aspect in these patients is not going to yield proper results; the psychological factor needs to be resolved too.[7] The most common presentation of these factors seen in an aesthetic clinic is in cases of BDD and depression.

BODY DYSMORPHIC DISORDER

Body dysmorphic disorder has been defined as a preoccupation with an imagined or slight defect in appearance that leads to significant impairment in functioning. It usually starts during adolescence, with 16 years old as the average age of diagnosis. It has been reclassified and considered as a type of obsessive-compulsive disorder.[8] **Box 3** gives a list of screening questions to be asked during history taking.

After the screening, BDD can be confirmed by a simple tool—the Visual Analog Scale (VAS). The doctor and the patient independently rate disfigurement and record severity on the optical VAS using values between 0 and 10 (with 0 meaning "no disfigurement" and 10 meaning "most severe disfigurement"). When a discrepancy of >4 points on the VAS occurs, BDD is highly suspicious.

Etiology

Poot et al. have tried to simplify the factors behind psychosomatic disorders in **Figure 1**.[9]

BOX 3 **List of screening questions in body dysmorphic disorder (BDD).**

- Do you believe that your alopecia (hair loss) is abnormal for your age?
- Have you ever been very concerned about your appearance?
- Do you often and carefully view yourself in the mirror? How much time do you spend doing so?
- Do you attempt to hide your hair loss with caps, scarves, or camouflage?
- Does your preoccupation with appearance affect your life in the areas of your profession, social contacts, and partnerships? Have you neglected normal activities because of the defect?

↓

If the answer to these five questions is "*yes*," it is highly likely that the patient has BDD, and elective aesthetic surgery should not be performed.

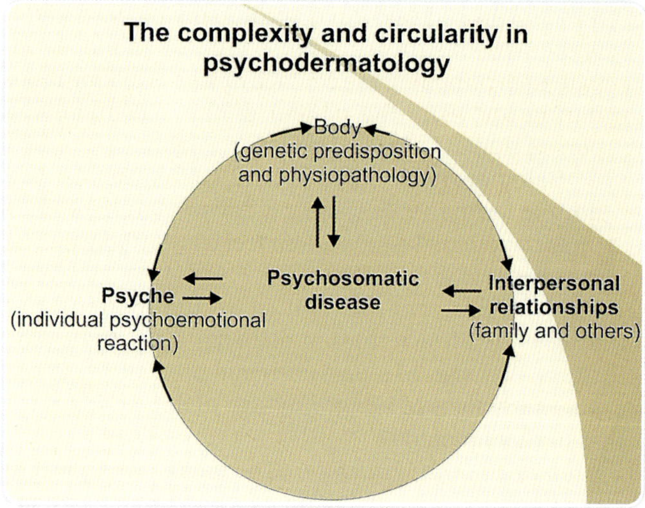

FIG. 1: Factors responsible for psychosomatic disorders.

Interpersonal Relationships

Rejection or neglectful nature of family may lead to BDD in the patients.[10] Teasing in schools may lead to BDD in young adolescents too. Careful social history taking is important in such cases.

Studies have proven that 9–15% of the patients visiting a dermatologist for aesthetic procedures suffer from BDD.[11] This emphasizes the need for aestheticians to be aware of this condition and its presentation in the cosmetic patient population. A quality of life index questionnaire followed by the authors is provided in the Annexure.

Intervention and Decision to do the Procedure

An ideal case to perform a procedure is one with no obvious psychopathology, clearly defined areas of dissatisfaction, realistic expectations, and self-motivation. Contradictorily, aesthetic procedures should be avoided in patients with major depression, signs of self-mutilation, troubled or agitated on the day of surgery, or on antipsychotics.[12,13] Depending on the assessment of the patient, if the physician feels that there are no psychosomatic factors behind the patient's demand for the surgery, he should go ahead. Borderline cases or mild cases of obsessive-compulsive disorder or BDD also benefit from cosmetic procedures or a combination of psychiatric and cosmetic treatment.[9] BDD patients believe that they have a "defective appearance," and despite undergoing a surgery, they will feel that it still looks defective; hence, they are always dissatisfied. Research findings indicate that almost 98% of patients diagnosed with BDD reported perceiving no change after elective treatment, while 16% believed that cosmetic procedures actually worsened their appearance.[14,15] They usually have a tendency to get multiple surgeries. Such patients also refuse to get psychiatric help initially. Counseling and communication skills are of utmost importance in such instances. It is the dermatologist's responsibility to act like a psychotherapist and explain the complexity of the condition to the patient. Only after the patient has an insight will they be willing to accept change. Such patients should not be accepted for surgery on the first visit. Occasionally, a patient may need to be referred to a psychiatrist or at least an opinion on the telephone is sought. The doctor should work in a formalized collaboration with a psychiatrist so that it is easier for the patient to open up to psychiatric therapy without much resistance.[16] Occasionally, a dermatologist may also have to prescribe selective serotonin reuptake inhibitors, such as fluoxetine, sertraline, or escitalopram, in case the patient is extremely reluctant to visit a psychiatrist.

Doing a procedure on a patient with BDD may have dire consequences too as patients may occasionally turn violent. There are two cases of murder of surgeons by patients showing symptoms of BDD.[17] Surveys according to the literature show that 2% of plastic surgeons have experienced physical threats from patients with BDD, while 10% havc faced threats of violence and legal action.[17,18]

Warning Signs for When not to do Procedures

It is important for a dermatologist not just to know when to do and how to do, but also when not to do. Tips that can be of help in identifying such patients are listed in **Box 4.**

T explain such patients in a practical aspect, some personal examples of patients encountered by the author are as follows:

BOX 4 Tips for when not to do procedures in confused patients.

- A patient who is obsessively concerned
- A patient who wants 100% guarantee
- A patient who wants absolute safety
- A patient who demands multiple procedures
- *A patient who says*: I want to look like that person or that film star
- A patient who has visited several doctors for the same indication previously
- A patient who comes for the same problem repeatedly without ever deciding

- A young girl was brought in by her father for hair loss, demanding hair transplantation. However, she had a full head of hair, and attempts to convince her otherwise failed. Biopsy and trichoscopy were performed to demonstrate that everything was normal, but she refused to agree. One day, she was brought in as an "emergency," claiming that she had lost 90% of her hair, but upon examination, she still had a full head of hair. At this point, a psychiatric component was suspected, and she was asked to see a psychiatrist. The father, who was a doctor, agreed, only to return a week later, requesting that the drugs prescribed by the psychiatrist be given on a dermatologist's prescription to avoid appearing psychiatric. After consulting with a psychiatrist, a prescription was given. However, this request was repeated multiple times, and finally, the author refused to provide any further prescriptions until a psychiatrist gave their opinion. The psychiatrist intervened and diagnosed schizophrenia, and surprisingly, the father had known it all along but had refused to accept it.
- A patient requested hair transplantation over their beard despite having a good beard.
- A patient who was obsessed about their donor scar after hair transplantation (strip surgery) kept calling and questioning the possibility of a scar. Eventually, the patient was not considered a good candidate due to unrealistic expectations.

SUMMARY

Only a psychologically fit patient will be satisfied with surgery. The doctor should not be trained only in aesthetics but also in psychotherapy and should know the basics of pharmacology behind psychology. The judgment of making a decision in such patients depends totally on the physician's knowledge and experience in dealing with psychological conditions. **Annexure 1** shows a quality of life questionnaire for a hair loss patient.

ANNEXURE 1: A Quality of Life Index Questionnaire.

1.	How upset or embarrassed you are with respect to your hair problem?	Very much A lot A little Not at all	☐ ☐ ☐ ☐
2.	How much has your hair problem been interfering with your social activities?	Very much A lot A little Not at all	☐ ☐ ☐ ☐
3.	How often do you try to change your hairstyle or try to conceal your hair problem?	Very often Often Seldom Not at all	☐ ☐ ☐ ☐
4.	How frequently do your friends or relatives comment about your hair problem?	Very often Often Seldom Not at all	☐ ☐ ☐ ☐
5.	How much has your hair problem affected your performance at school/college or job prospects?	Very much A lot A little Not at all	☐ ☐ ☐ ☐
6.	How much has your hair problem affected your marriage prospects or marital life?	Very much A lot A little Not at all	☐ ☐ ☐ ☐
7.	How much applying creams, sprays, and shampoos for hair care has been time-consuming for you?	Very much A lot A little Not at all Not applicable	☐ ☐ ☐ ☐ ☐
8.	How frequently do you search online or read about your hair problem and the treatments available?	Very often Often Seldom Not at all	☐ ☐ ☐ ☐
9.	How frequently do you consult a doctor regarding your hair problem?	Very often Often Seldom Not at all	☐ ☐ ☐ ☐
10.	How much have the side effects of the hair treatments/cost of the treatments concerned you?	Very much A lot A little Not at all	☐ ☐ ☐ ☐

Scoring

Very much/very often: 3

A lot/often: 2

A little/seldom: 1

Not at all: 0

Not applicable: 0

Question unanswered: 0

Maximum: 30

Minimum: 0

0–1: No effect at all on patient's life

2–5: Small effect on patient's life

6–10: Moderate effect on patient's life

11–20: Very large effect on patient's life

21–30: Extremely large effect on patient's life

Questions 1, 8, 9—feelings and anxiety: Score maximum 9

Question 2—leisure: Score maximum 3

Question 3—daily activities: Score maximum 3

Questions 6, 4—personal relationships: Score maximum 6

Question 5—work and school: Score maximum 3

Questions 7, 10—treatments: Score maximum 6

If one question is left unanswered, this is scored 0 and the scores are summed and expressed as usual out of a maximum of 30. If two or more questions are left unanswered, the questionnaire is not scored.

Tips and Pearls

- Establish rapport with the patient—understand not only his indications but also reasons for indications.
- Be empathetic; spend time with the patient—avoid doctor's ego.
- Know not only when to do and how to do, but also when not to do.
- Learn to say no.
- Always underpromise but overdeliver.
- If there is a side effect, be prepared for an aggressive reaction.

REFERENCES

1. Hunt N, McHale S. The psychological impact of alopecia. BMJ. 2005;331:951-3.
2. Wever CCC, Wever AMEA, Constantian M. Psychiatric disorders in facial plastic surgery. Facial Plast Surg Clin North Am. 2020;28:451-60.
3. International Society of Hair Restoration Surgery: 2022 Practice Census Results. (2022). [online] Available from https://ishrs.org/wp-content/uploads/2022/04/Report-2022-ISHRS-Practice-Census_04-19-22-FINAL.pdf. [Last accessed September, 2023].
4. ISHRS Practice Census Infographic. [online] Available from https://ishrs.org/2020/06/09/ishrs-practice-census-infographic/. [Last accessed September, 2023].
5. Girman CJ, Rhodes T, Lilly FR, Guo SS, Siervogel RM, Patrick DL, et al. Effects of self-perceived hair loss in a community sample of men. Dermatology. 1998;197:223-9.
6. Williamson D, Gonzalez M, Finlay AY. The effect of hair loss on quality of life. J Eur Acad Dermatol Venereol. 2001;15:137-9.
7. Gupta MA, Gupta AK. Psychodermatology: an update. J Am Acad Dermatol. 1996;34:1030-46.
8. Phillips KA, McElroy SL, Hudson JI, Pope Jr HG. Body dysmorphic disorder: an obsessive-compulsive spectrum disorder, a form of affective spectrum disorder, or both? J Clin Psychiatry. 1995;56:41-51.
9. Poot F, Sampogna F, Onnis L. Basic knowledge in psychodermatology. J Eur Acad Dermatol Venereol. 2007;21:227-34.
10. Phillips KA. Body dysmorphic disorder: the distress of imagined ugliness. Am J Psychiatry. 1991;148:1138-49.
11. Uzun O, Başoğlu C, Akar A, Cansever A, Ozşahin A, Cetin M, et al. Body dysmorphic disorder in patients with acne. Compr Psychiatry. 2003;44:415-9.
12. Elsaie ML. Psychological approach in cosmetic dermatology for optimum patient satisfaction. Indian J Dermatology. 2010;55(2):127-9.
13. Koblenzer CS. Psychocutaneous disease. Orlando: Grune and Stratton; 1987.
14. Sarwer DB. Awareness and identification of body dysmorphic disorder by aesthetic surgeons: results of a survey of American Society for Aesthetic Plastic Surgery members. Aesthetic Surg J. 2002;22:531-5.
15. Bowyer L, Krebs G, Mataix-Cols D, Veale D, Monzani B. A critical review of cosmetic treatment outcomes in body dysmorphic disorder. Body Image. 2016;19:1-8.
16. Joseph AW, Ishii L, Joseph SS, Smith JI, Su P, Bater K, et al. Prevalence of body dysmorphic disorder and surgeon diagnostic accuracy in facial plastic and oculoplastic surgery clinics. JAMA Facial Plast Surg. 2017;19:269-74.
17. Sweis IE, Spitz J, Barry Jr DR, Cohen M. A review of body dysmorphic disorder in aesthetic surgery patients and the legal implications. Aesthetic Plast Surg. 2017;41:949-54.
18. Wang Q, Cao C, Guo R, Li X, Lu L, Wang W. Avoiding psychological pitfalls in aesthetic medical procedures. Aesthetic Plast Surg. 2016;40:954-61.

CHAPTER 20

Nutrition and Androgenetic Alopecia

Rajesh Rajput

Key Messages

- Nutrition has received increasing attention in recent research in pathophysiology of different types of alopecia.
- Androgenetic alopecia, though thought to be androgen mediated, may involve other factors.
- Correction of nutrition is an important part of the management of alopecia.

INTRODUCTION

Recent advancements in cellular metabolism and molecular biology have revealed various androgenetic alopecia (AGA) phenotypes: Acellular aging and senescence phenotype,[1] a slow metabolism quiescence phenotype,[2] a microinflammation and altered immunity, immune senescence and inflammaging phenotype,[3,4] a reactive oxygen species (ROS) induced oxidative stress phenotype,[5] and a lifestyle- and environment-generated epigenetic phenotype.[6] These phenotypes are often intertwined in simultaneous, progressive pathologies. Hair follicles, being synchronous individual mini organs, react with variable responses, creating combinations and distributions of temporary or progressive hair loss, presenting as resolving telogen effluvium, continuing chronic telogen effluvium, diffuse hair loss, AGA, alopecia areata, scarring alopecia, combined cicatricial pattern hair loss,[7] or fibrosing alopecia in pattern distribution.[8] All these phenotypes arise from cellular dysfunction. Nutrients can counter aging, prevent inflammation, build immunity, neutralize oxidative stress, and protect against epigenetic changes.

NUTRIENTS ESSENTIAL FOR CELLULAR FUNCTION

Nutrients are required for the generation of energy, neutralization and elimination of toxins, repair of cellular organelles, repair of deoxyribonucleic acid (DNA), replacement of damaged cells, and achieving rapid cell division for hair growth. Nutrients are also responsible for the secretion of hormones, neurotransmitters, chemical mediators, regulators of cell function, defense, and immunity. The inability to keep up with these functions manifests as oxidative stress, compromised immune response, inability to counter inflammation, cellular aging, and senescence. Hair being a tissue with a high metabolic rate, even a modest imbalance affects the growth cycle converting mitosis to apoptosis. AGA, once classified to be noninflammatory, now has evidence of inflammation. Follicles with microinflammation fail to respond to standard minoxidil treatment.[9] Long-term finasteride studies had 48% nonresponders and 17% who deteriorated despite taking finasteride 1 mg/day for 1 year.[10] Follicles cannot respond unless the internal cellular environment has been corrected to have proper redox balance, energy generation, repair of cellular damage, and well-regulated cellular function to meet the high mitotic and metabolic demand.[11] Clinically, nutrition has been reported to achieve hair growth with consistent results.[12-18]

NUTRIENTS, CELL SYSTEMS, AND DEOXYRIBONUCLEIC ACID DAMAGE

Nutrient deficiencies of vitamins B6, B12, C, and E, folic acid, iron, and zinc can cause single- and double-strand DNA breakage, which mimics radiation damage.[19]

Even modest nutrient deficiencies cause gradual mitochondrial decay and molecular aging, which can be prevented with optimal availability of nutrients.[19,20]

Endogenous as well as exogenous DNA damage can be protected by provitamin A, carotenoids, carotenes, β-cryptoxanthin, and nonvitamin A carotenoids such as lycopene, lutein, astaxanthin, and zeaxanthin.[21] Selenium acts on endocrine systems, modifying the expression of at least 30 selenoproteins. While selenoenzymes are the family of glutathione peroxidases (GSH-Px), thioredoxin reductases and iodothyronine deiodinases capable of modifying cell functions as antioxidants for redox balance and thyroid metabolism. Selenium is involved in cell growth, apoptosis, cell signaling, and transcription factors.[22] Biotin and biotin metabolites affect the transcription of genes encoding cytokines, oncogenes, glucose metabolism, and cellular homeostasis.[23]

LIFESTYLE, EPIGENETIC DEOXYRIBONUCLEIC ACID METHYLATION, AND NUTRIENTS

Lifestyle and epigenetic factors include stress, physical activity, sleep, behavior, obesity, smoking, alcohol, tobacco, food habits, sleep, night shifts, exposure to pollution, ultraviolet (UV) rays, and endocrine-disrupting chemicals (EDCs).[24] Epigenetic mechanisms, including DNA methylation and histone modification, influence gene expression without altering the DNA sequence, creating an acquired phenotype different from the inherited genotype.[25]

Nutrients with one carbon metabolism, vitamins B12, B6, folate, riboflavin, methionine, choline, betaine, and bioactive compounds such as retinoic acid, resveratrol, curcumin, sulforaphane, and tea polyphenols, can modulate epigenetic patterns by regulating universal methyl donor and enzymes that catalyze DNA methylation and histone modifications.[25]

Deoxyribonucleic acid methylation provides a measure for biological aging, detected during major surgery, pregnancy, coronavirus disease 19 (COVID-19), stress, lifestyle, environment, etc., and is reversible with antiaging nutrients.[24] ROS are involved in the mechanism of senescence and altered gene expression, which can be prevented and reversed with antioxidants and micronutrients.[26] Nutrient deficiencies detected in AGA are summarized in **Table 1**.

ACQUIRED ANDROGEN SENSITIVITY FROM CONTINUED EXPOSURE TO NONANDROGENIC FACTORS

Clinical incidence and progress of hair loss could never be linked to raised androgens or dihydrotestosterone (DHT).[38,39] AGA is described as the prolongation of telogen and shortening of anagen. Clinically, every alopecia begins as simple hair fall or telogen effluvium. This telogen effluvium is caused by nonandrogenic factors such as fever, stress, lifestyle, pollution, epigenetics, environmental factors, sleep, alcohol, smoking, and diet. Continued exposure to these nonandrogenic factors promotes gradual cellular dysfunction and accumulation

TABLE 1: Nutrient deficiencies detected in androgenetic alopecia.

Deficiencies detected	Published studies
Low levels of zinc, copper, iron, and manganese were detected with hair, serum, and urine analysis in male androgenetic alopecia	Jin et al.[27]
Low serum zinc, copper, and ferritin	Deshwali et al.[28]
Iron deficiency	Rushton et al.[29]
Lower copper and zinc in frontal hair compared to unaffected occipital hair, deficiencies of manganese, selenium, and zinc	Skalnaya and Tkachev[30]
Deficiencies of Cu, Zn, amino acids lysine, histidine, isoleucine, leucine, alanine, and cysteine	Gowda et al.[31]
Vitamin D deficiency	Zubair et al.[32]
Zinc and micronutrient deficiency compromising thyroid function. Nutrients are interdependent on each other for biological action	Ambooken et al.[33]
Iron, zinc, and micronutrient deficiencies compromising erythropoiesis which affects hair growth	Kelkitli et al.[34]
Anemia from vitamin A deficiency which affects hair growth	Semba and Bloem[35]
Deficiencies of Zn, Cu, Mg, Se, vitamins B12, E, D, and folic acid	Kondrakhina IN et al.[36]
Low vitamins D, B12, and ferritin	Öner Ü et al.[37]

of ROS, which are proven to increase the sensitivity of androgen receptors (ARs), making them hypersensitive to normal circulating androgens.[40] ROS also trigger the release of inflammatory cytokines, which further augment various AR-sensitive pathways.[40] Thus, the follicles have now become sensitive to normal androgens and DHT due to relentless exposure to nonandrogenic factors. The predisposition to androgen sensitivity, if not genetic, is now acquired. The understanding explains the common clinical presentation of hair loss with normal DHT and without any family history. The effects of these nonandrogenic factors can be countered with nutrients to neutralize ROS, repair and restore cellular function, and achieve hair growth. Early intervention in telogen effluvium with nutritional supplements is recommended. Researchers in nutrition and cell metabolism have established theories that can explain the dysfunction of hair growth cycles.

GAP THEORY OF METABOLIC STEPS

Cell division progresses with feedback through "check gaps" in four steps: Gap 1 (check), initiate synthesis, gap 2 (check), and proceed to mitosis. Cell status is checked for feedback from the environment, surrounding cells, metabolic modulators, and availability of glucose, amino acids, iron, zinc, vitamins B12, A, D, and folic acid before determining the progress or arrest of cell mitosis and growth.[41]

TRIAGE AND MARGINAL MICRONUTRIENT DEFICIENCY

In conditions of nutrient deficiencies, the body prioritizes short-term survival over long-term health through physiological triage. This is evident in the redistribution of blood flow to the vital organs during low oxygen pressure or shock. Triage prioritizes adenosine triphosphate (ATP) synthesis over DNA repair, erythrocyte function over leukocytes, and neuroendocrine functions over liver enzymes.[42] The high metabolic demand of the hair follicle is subject to triage even under marginal nutrient deficiencies. Hair growth is compromised to divert nutrients toward more important systems. This diversion maintains normal nutrient levels in circulation by compensating the deficiencies and masking their detection on laboratory tests until the point of extreme failure.

Pietrzik's concept of marginal micronutrient deficiency (1985) states that subclinical deficiencies prevail and progress in incremental steps before clinical manifestation.[43] Nonavailability of one nutrient interrupts the biological actions. Mitochondrial heme synthesis could be arrested due to deficiency of any nutrient, such as iron, copper, zinc, biotin, riboflavin, pyridoxine, or pantothenate, leading to mitochondrial decay, leakage of oxidants, and DNA damage.[42] Failure of one metabolic step cascades over multiple other systems, causing progressive derangement, degenerative changes, and aging.[42] Present nutritional recommendations are focused on the prevention of disorders from deficiencies and not on the optimum requirement for cellular function or homeostasis.[42] Chronic diet is described as restricted eating to control average or below-average weight with prolonged suboptimal cell functions with no threat to survival,[43] prevailing long before the manifestation of deficiency disorders.

Kantor's threshold hypothesis states that low iron levels decrease the threshold for the development of various alopecias.[44] Gradual subclinical covert deficiencies develop from restricted eating, improper processing of nutrients, malabsorption, smoking, alcohol, coffee, rushed meals, increased demand in stress, pregnancy, lactation, and exercise with the intention to burn out and control weight. Nutritionists term the deficit from consumption of foods without meeting the nutrient requirements as hidden hunger.[45] Micronutrient deficiencies are common and remain unnoticed. The consequences are visible early in high metabolic tissues, such as the hair follicles.

ROLE OF MITOCHONDRIAL METABOLISM

Mitochondria, which generate energy and regulate apoptosis, play a crucial role in hair growth. Hair loss may have a maternal genetic influence due to the inheritance of mitochondrial DNA solely from the mother.[46] Mitochondrial respiratory chain, cytochrome enzymes, and ATP generation depend on nutrient availability and redox balance.[19,47] Oxidative stress can disrupt mitochondrial function, mitosis, cell proliferation, and differentiation.[48] Optimum nutrients can delay mitochondrial degeneration and aging.[20]

Oxidative Stress, Apoptosis, and Reactive Oxygen Species

Cells function in an equilibrium of antioxidant defenses. Even a modest rise in ROS can influence genetic expression,[49] creating the oxidative stress hair loss phenotype.[5]

Reactive oxygen species, generated internally through cellular metabolism and externally by pollution, UV rays, or scalp microbes, can lead to cellular damage and aging.[50-52] ROS directly influence hair follicle stem cells and cause senescence of the dermal papilla cells.[53,54]

Reactive oxygen species are essential for cell cycle progression, cellular signaling pathways, and immunity. However, raised ROS causes active damage to proteins, nucleic acids, lipids, and lipid peroxidation of cell membranes and cell organelles, leading to activation of apoptosis.[55] Mitochondria and the endoplasmic reticulum regulate apoptosis through ROS.[56] Antioxidants and nutrients are crucial for maintaining redox homeostasis, neutralizing ROS, and promoting hair growth.[57,58]

Reactive oxygen species are mediators for DHT and stress-induced hair loss.

In 1942, Hamilton suggested that hair loss in males was caused by testosterone.[59] Later, it was known that the conversion of testosterone to DHT caused hair loss. Further studies recognized that DHT releases transforming growth factor-beta (TGF-β), which is responsible for miniaturization. Now we know that the release of TGF-β is mediated by ROS.[60,61] Latent TGF-β in the extracellular matrix is also activated by ROS.[62] Experiments have revealed that using a free radical scavenger to neutralize the ROS can block the release of TGF-β, thus countering the action of DHT.[61] Stress-induced hair loss is mediated by substance P, which is known to act through ROS.[63] Antioxidants can counteract the effects of ROS and mitigate hair loss.

ROLE OF AUTOPHAGY

Programmed breakdown of intracellular organelles is executed under deficiency states to retrieve nutrients and conserve nutritional balance.[64] The process termed autophagy is triggered by reduced oxygenation, low levels of growth factors, insulin, amino acids, low calories, and nutrient deprivation, sensed by adenosine monophosphate (AMP)-activated protein kinases. It can be inactivated by the restoration of the same factors. Stress induces substance P and ROS inhibit hair cycles by autophagy through raised lipid peroxidation and suppressing superoxide dismutase (SOD) and GSH-Px, which have become markers of autophagy. These events can be countered with antioxidants.[65] Autophagy has a prime role in maintaining anagen. It regulates keratinization of the hair shaft and ensures the removal of inflammasomes, protein aggregates, and metabolic endotoxins, initiating the renewal, repair, and replacement of aging cells. The availability of nutrients and antioxidants regulates autophagy.[66]

Nutritional deficiencies of zinc, copper, iron, manganese, amino acids, and vitamin D are summarized in **Table 1**. Multiple nutrient deficiencies affecting thyroid function and erythropoiesis also affect hair loss.[67,27-35]

SPECIFIC NUTRIENTS HAVE A DIRECT ROLE IN HAIR GROWTH

Vitamin D has a direct growth-inducing action on the dermal papilla.[68] Omega-3 fatty acids are anti-inflammatory and immune modulatory.[69] Low-dose gamma-linolenic acid (GLA) is a 5α-reductase inhibitor, while arachidonic acid promotes angiogenesis and mitosis of keratinocytes.[70,71] GLA, activated dihomo-gamma-linolenic acid (DGLA), and arachidonic acid are precursors to prostaglandins PGE1 and PGE2, which regulate inflammation and immunity. Vitamins A, C, E, β-carotene, and selenium prevent lipid peroxidation of the fatty acids and facilitate prostaglandin synthesis.[72] A combination of α-tocopherol and tocotrienol improved hair counts by 34% through the inhibition of lipid peroxidation.[73] Zinc has multiple actions as an immune modulator, inhibitor of catagen, and regulator of apoptosis, preventing follicle regression and accelerating anagen recovery.[74] Iron in addition to oxygen delivery is required for the conversion of the storage form of thyroxin T4 to the active hormone T3. Iron is an essential regulator of DNA synthesis and repair.[75,76] Vitamin A α-retinoid nuclear receptor forms a dimer with vitamin D receptor for controlling anagen initiation and regulation of the hair growth cycles.[77] The role of individual nutrients, the recommended daily allowance (RDA), and sources are enlisted in **Table 2**.

CLINICAL TRIALS

A host of controlled clinical trials and placebo-controlled double-blind trials have reported the benefits of nutrients in hair loss management. A controlled clinical trial showed control of hair loss in 4–6 weeks, average improvement in density 18% at 2 months and 30% in 4 months, and improvement in caliber 9% at 2 months and 21% in 4 months, with no nonresponders.[12] Other trials with vitamins, nutrients, iron, zinc, and trace elements have also reported clinical improvement in the management of AGA with nutritional supplements.[13-18]

SUMMARY

The interruption of anagen and dysregulation of the hair growth cycle can be traced back to the loss of internal cellular environment, homeostasis, and derangement of cellular function. Nutrients can restore the hair cycles. Nonandrogenic factors cause the generation of ROS, which activate ARs, creating acquired sensitivity, without a genetic predisposition. Early intervention with nutritional support should be encouraged for restoration of hair growth.

TABLE 2: Hair growth nutrients, RDA, source, and action.

	Men RDA	Women RDA	Plant source	Animal source	Action in hair growth
Thiamine Vitamin B1	1.2 mg	1.1 mg	Fortified foods, breakfast cereals, energy bars, seeds, legumes, rice	Pork	Production of adenosine triphosphate (ATP), which provides energy for all cellular functions, can improve growth of cultured keratinocytes
Riboflavin Vitamin B2	1.3 mg	1.1 mg	Fortified foods, spirulina, flours from teff, millet, chestnut, buckwheat, and amaranth are sources of B-group vitamins	Lamb liver,	Coenzyme for the production of ATP, cellular respiration, conversion of amino acid tryptophan to niacin (B3), conversion of vitamin A, retinol to active retinoic acid, and synthesizing active form of folate essential for hair metabolism
Niacin Vitamin B3	16 mg	14 mg	Fortified food and beverages, baker's yeast, rice bran, peanuts	Meat	Anti-inflammatory, boosts circulation, improves sheen, smoothness, supple texture, repairs keratin damage, improves hair length
Pantothenic acid Vitamin B5	5 mg	5 mg	Fortified food and beverages, dried shiitake mushrooms, rice bran	Beef liver	Synthesis of coenzyme A (CoA) essential for energy and metabolism of protein, carbohydrates, and fat. Dexpanthenol is a widely used natural humectant in hair care products for thinning and hair loss
Pyridoxine Vitamin B6 up to 50 years	1.3 mg	1.3 mg	Fortified food and beverages, rice bran, fortified margarines, ground sage, bananas, chickpeas, potatoes, pistachios	Pork, turkey, beef	Prevents anemia and water retention, reduces stress, improves blood flow and carbohydrate and protein metabolism, counters hair loss due to smoking and pollution
Vitamin B6 beyond 50 years	1.5 mg	1.7 mg			
Biotin Vitamin B7 or H	30 µg	30 µg	Seeds, nuts, corn, soy meal, widely in all foods, secreted by gut microbes	Organ meats, eggs, fish, meat	Sulfur content helps hair growth, prevents dry skin, regulates blood sugar, improves glucose, amino acid, and fat metabolism, has a role in histone modification, cell signaling, and gene regulation
Folic acid Vitamin B9	400 µg	400 µg	Fortified food and beverages, baker's yeast, green leafy vegetables	Poultry liver	Prevents megaloblastic anemia, required for DNA synthesis, cellular metabolism, premature graying
Cyanocobalamin Vitamin B12	2.4 µg	2.4 µg	Fortified food and beverages	Shellfish, clams, oysters, beef, animal liver, lean meat, herring, crab	Corrects anemia, essential for formation of RBCs and oxygenation, DNA repair, cell proliferation, hair growth, autoimmune disorders, serotonin formation
Vitamin D3	600 IU	800 IU	Mushrooms (if exposed to UV light)	Cod liver oil, fortified milk and dairy products, halibut, mackerel, salmon, fatty fish	Calcium metabolism, immune regulator, anti-inflammatory, direct action on dermal papilla, growth differentiation of keratinocytes, premature graying. Directly induces action of dermal papilla cells for hair growth

Continued

Continued

	Men RDA	Women RDA	Plant source	Animal source	Action in hair growth
Vitamins K1 and K2	120 µg	90 µg	Leafy green vegetables such as spinach, Swiss chard, lettuce, parsley, chard, cabbage, kale, cauliflower, broccoli, brussels sprouts	Eggs, dairy, meat, fermented foods such as cheese and yogurt. Vitamin K2 is secreted by gut microbes and works with vitamin D	Blood coagulation, regulates bone and calcium metabolism along with vitamin D. Vitamin K1 is available from food while vitamin K2 can be synthesized by gut microbes. It can reverse hair loss caused by blood thinners
Vitamins as antioxidants					
Vitamin A/β-carotene	900 µg	700 µg	Red sweet peppers, veal, carrots, yellow deep orange vegetables and fruits, collard greens, kale, spinach, carrots, sweet potatoes, pumpkins, melon, and apricots represent some good sources of β-carotene	Fish liver oil, liver, egg yolk, butter, and cream, cod liver oil, liver are sources of vitamin A	Antioxidant, regulates sebum, iron metabolism, thyroid hormones, cell growth, differentiation, keratinization, immunity
Vitamin C	90 mg	75 mg	Citrus fruits, bell peppers, kiwis, berries, broccoli, tomato juice, and other green and yellow vegetables, sweet peppers, raw acerola, dried chives and coriander, rose hips		Antioxidant, collagen synthesis, iron absorption, oxidative stress, pollution, prevents dryness, spilt ends, boosts immunity
Smokers add	35 mg	35 mg			
Vitamin E	15 mg	15 mg	Fortified food and beverages, wheat germ oil, hazelnut oil, fortified peanut butter, chili powder, vegetable oils, specifically wheat germ, soybean, and safflower nuts and seeds		Protects cell membrane from free radicals, autoimmunity, emotional and environmental stress, improves frizzy hair, damaged hair, restores shine, regulates sebum, lipid peroxidation, antioxidant
Minerals					
Iron	18 mg	18 mg	Nuts, dried fruit, fortified bread and breakfast cereal, legumes, beans, lentils, chickpeas, dark leafy green vegetables, spinach, silver beet, broccoli, oats, tofu, thyme	Red meats, beef, lamb, pork, liver, kidney, poultry, eggs, shellfish, tuna, salmon, sardines, heme iron from animal source is absorbed better	Component of cellular proteins, enzymes, cofactors, respiration, energy metabolism, immune function, collagen synthesis, glucose metabolism, antibody production, drug detoxification, conversion of β-carotene to active vitamin A. Essential redox cofactor in DNA metabolism, DNA repair, regulating cell cycles and ribonucleotide reductase, a rate-limiting step in DNA synthesis. Nonavailability of iron promotes DNA damage, prevents cell proliferation, and creates genome instability

Continued

Continued

	Men RDA	Women RDA	Plant source	Animal source	Action in hair growth
Iron beyond 50 years	8 mg	8 mg			
Calcium	1000 mg	1200 mg	Fortified cereals, beverages, tofu, energy bars, basil, sesame, poppy, chia seeds, almonds, rhubarb, amaranth, edamame, figs, soy, lentils, winged beans, spinach, bok choy, as well as turnip, mustard, collard, okra, kale, cabbage, broccoli, and brussels sprouts	Sardines, salmon, whey, cheese, yogurt, milk powder	Structural integrity of the bones and hair. Calcium maintains ionic balance, buffers blood pH, helps in neurotransmission, muscle contraction, heart rhythm, blood clotting, and action of cellular enzymes
Zinc	11 mg	8 mg	Wheat germ, sesame, poppy, alfalfa, celery, mustard, beans, nuts, almonds, whole grains, pumpkin seeds, sunflower seeds, black currant, all based on content in the soil	Oysters, lobster, red meats, beef, lamb, liver have the highest bioavailability of zinc	Cell proliferation, collagen formation, repairs oxidative damage, sebum regulation, prevents catagen apoptosis, promotes anagen, immunomodulator
Iodine	150 µg	150 µg	Iodized salt, kelp, seaweed	Cod, oyster, shellfish, egg, liver, Greek yogurt	Functional element in thyroid hormone which regulates energy utilization, oxygen consumption, protein synthesis, mitosis, growth, differentiation, significantly enhancing hair growth when normal and retarding it in hypothyroid states
Copper	900 µg	900 µg	Seaweed products, dried shiitake mushrooms, oysters, sesame seeds, cocoa powder, cashews, sunflower seeds	Animal liver	Hair elasticity, pigmentation and skin tone, formation of RBC
Selenium	55 µg	55 µg	Brazil nuts and mixed nuts	Animal kidneys, oysters, cod	Rapidly absorbed antioxidant, elasticity, UV damage and aging, thyroid function, hair shaft strength, premature graying
Sulfur—methylsulfonylmethane			Ensured by adequate protein intake		Prevents brittle and dry hair
Silica or silicon RDA not defined					Silicon provides strength to the cell walls and structural integrity. Required for synthesis of collagen, elastin, strength, and growth of the connective tissue, skin, hair, nail, and bone
Individual nutrients with benefits in hair growth					
L-tyrosine					Accelerates hair growth, strengthens hair shaft, prevents graying, improves thyroid function
L-lysine					Hair growth in telogen effluvium, improves iron uptake
L-ornithine					DNA and protein synthesis
L-arginine					Rapid cell division, repair, endothelial stability
Glycine					Precursor to biosynthesis of various proteins, collagen, restores hair health

Continued

Continued

	Men RDA	Women RDA	Plant source	Animal source	Action in hair growth
Coenzyme Q10					Rapid energy for growing cells, reduces oxidative stress, builds immunity, anti-inflammatory, antiaging, gene expression
Omega-3					Anti-inflammatory, improves gene expression
Gamma-linolenic acid					Anti-inflammatory, prostaglandin E2 precursor
Manganese sulfate					Accelerates hair growth and prevents UV damage
Magnesium hydroxide					Calcium, potassium, parathyroid, insulin metabolism, requirement raised in stress
Para-aminobenzoic acid					Prevents premature graying of hair
Inositol					Prevents hair thinning
Vanadium sulfate					Insulin-like anabolic, Na and K transport
Chromium polynicotinate					Cellular metabolism and energy utilization
Molybdenum					Assists use of iron stores, fat burning
Green apple extract, proanthocyanidin					Flavonoid and free radical scavenger. Selective protein kinase C (PKC) inhibitor, procyanidin B-2, promote hair epithelial cell growth and stimulate anagen induction
Green tea extract, EGCG, or epigallocatechin-3-gallate, polyphenol					Antioxidant and protection from UV damage. Stimulates growth of cultured dermal papilla cells through proliferative and antiapoptotic effects

REFERENCES

1. Ji J, Ho BS, Qian G, Xie XM, Bigliardi PL, Bigliardi-Qi M. Aging in hair follicle stem cells and niche microenvironment. J Dermatol. 2017;44(10):1097-104.
2. Piccini I, Sousa M, Altendorf S, Jimenez F, Rossi A, Funk W, et al. Intermediate hair follicles from patients with female pattern hair loss are associated with nutrient insufficiency and a quiescent metabolic phenotype. Nutrients. 2022;14(16):3357.
3. Lee YI, Choi S, Roh WS, Lee JH, Kim TG. Cellular senescence and inflammaging in the skin microenvironment. Int J Mol Sci. 2021;22(8):3849.
4. Xia S, Zhang X, Zheng S, Khanabdali R, Kalionis B, Wu J, et al. An update on inflamm-aging: mechanisms, prevention, and treatment. J Immunol Res. 2016;2016:8426874.
5. Trüeb RM. Oxidative stress in ageing of hair. Int J Trichology. 2009;1(1):6-14.
6. Koyama T, Kobayashi K, Wakisaka N, Hirayama N, Konishi S, Hama T, et al. Eleven pairs of Japanese male twins suggest the role of epigenetic differences in androgenetic alopecia. Eur J Dermatol. 2013;23:113-5.
7. Olsen EA. Female pattern hair loss and its relationship to permanent/cicatricial alopecia: a new perspective. J Investig Dermatol Symp Proc. 2005;10(3):217-21.
8. Zinkernagel MS, Trüeb RM. Fibrosing alopecia in a pattern distribution: patterned lichen planopilaris or androgenetic alopecia with a lichenoid tissue reaction pattern? Arch Dermatol. 2000;136:205-11.
9. Whiting DA. Diagnostic and predictive value of horizontal sections of scalp biopsy specimens in male pattern androgenetic alopecia. J Am Acad Dermatol. 1993;28(5 Pt 1):755-63.
10. Kaufman KD, Olsen EA, Whiting D, Savin R, DeVillez R, Bergfeld W, et al. Finasteride in the treatment of men with androgenetic alopecia. Finasteride Male Pattern Hair Loss Study Group. J Am Acad Dermatol. 1998;39(4 Pt 1):578-89.
11. Ruiz-Tagle SA, Figueira MM, Vial V, Espinoza-Benavides L, Miteva M. Micronutrients in hair loss. Our Dermatol Online. 2018;9(3):320-8.
12. Rajput RJ. Controlled clinical trial for evaluation of hair growth with low dose cyclical nutrition therapy in men and women without the use of finasteride. Plast Aesthet Res. 2017;4:161-73.
13. Ablon G. A 6-month, randomized, double-blind, placebo-controlled study evaluating the ability of a marine complex supplement to promote hair growth in men with thinning hair. J Cosmet Dermatol. 2016;15(4):358-66.
14. Farris PK, Rogers N, McMichael A, Kogan S. A novel multi-targeting approach to treating hair loss, using standardized nutraceuticals. J Drugs Dermatol. 2017;16(11):s141-8.
15. Trost LB, Bergfeld WF, Calogeras E. The diagnosis and treatment of iron deficiency and its potential relationship to hair loss. J Am Acad Dermatol. 2006;54(5):824-44.
16. Karashima T, Tsuruta D, Hamada T, Ono F, Ishii N, Abe T, et al. Oral zinc therapy for zinc deficiency-related telogen effluvium. Dermatol Ther. 2012;25(2):210-3.
17. Ring C, Heitmiller K, Correia E, Gabriel Z, Saedi N. Nutraceuticals for androgenetic alopecia. J Clin Aesthet Dermatol. 2022;15(3):26-9.
18. Kondrakhina IN, Zatevalov AM, Gatiatulina ER, Nikonorov AA, Deryabin D, Kubanov A. Evaluation of the effectiveness of personalized treatment of trace element and vitamin status in men with initial stages of androgenic alopecia treated with conservative therapy. Ann Russ Acad Med Sci. 2021;76(6):604-11.
19. Ames BN. A role for supplements in optimizing health: the metabolic tune-up. Arch Biochem Biophys. 2004;423(1):227-34.
20. Ames BN. Optimal micronutrients delay mitochondrial decay and age-associated diseases. Mech Ageing Dev. 2010;131(7-8):473-9.
21. Azqueta A, Collins AR. Carotenoids and DNA damage. Mutat Res. 2012;733(1-2):4-13.
22. Beckett GJ, Arthur JR. Selenium and endocrine systems. J Endocrinol. 2005;184(3):455-65.
23. Rodriguez-Melendez R, Zempleni J. Regulation of gene expression by biotin (review). J Nutr Biochem. 2003;14(12):680-90.
24. Park LK, Friso S, Choi SW. Nutritional influences on epigenetics and age-related disease. Proc Nutr Soc. 2012;71(1):75-83.
25. Poganik JR, Zhang B, Baht GS, Tyshkovskiy A, Deik A, Kerepesi C, et al. Biological age is increased by stress and restored upon recovery. Cell Metab. 2023;35(5):807-820.e5.
26. Dröge W. Free radicals in the physiological control of cell function. Physiol Rev. 2002;82(1):47-95.
27. Jin W, Zhu Z, Wu S, Zhang X, Zhou X. Determination of zinc, copper, iron and manganese contents in hair for MPA patients and healthy men. Guang Pu Xue Yu Guang Pu Fen Xi. 1998;18(1):91-3.
28. Deshwali S, Kare PK, Agrawal BK, Alex A. Study of serum zinc, copper and ferritin levels in alopecia patients. Int J Adv Res Biol Sci. 2015;2(7):94-6.
29. Rushton DH, Bergfeld WF, Gilkes JJ, Van Neste D. Iron deficiency and hair loss: nothing new? J Am Acad Dermatol. 2011;65(1):203-4.
30. Skalnaya MG, Tkachev VP. Trace elements content and hormonal profiles in women with androgenetic alopecia. J Trace Elem Med Biol. 2011;25:50-3.
31. Gowda D, Premalatha V, Imtiyaz D. Prevalence of nutritional deficiencies in hair loss among Indian participants: results of a cross-sectional study. Int J Trichol. 2017;9(3):101-4.
32. Zubair Z, Kantamaneni K, Jalla K, Renzu M, Jena R, Jain R, et al. Prevalence of low serum vitamin D levels in patients presenting with androgenetic alopecia: a review. Cureus. 2021;13(12):e20431.
33. Betsy A, Binitha MP, Sarita S. Zinc deficiency associated with hypothyroidism: an overlooked cause of severe alopecia. Int J Trichology. 2013;5(1):40-2.
34. Kelkitli E, Ozturk N, Aslan NA, Kilic-Baygutalp N, Bayraktutan Z, Kurt N, et al. Serum zinc levels in patients with iron deficiency anemia and its association with symptoms of iron deficiency anemia. Ann Hematol. 2016;95(5):751-6.
35. Semba RD, Bloem MW. The anemia of vitamin A deficiency: epidemiology and pathogenesis. Eur J Clin Nutr. 2002;56(4):271-81.
36. Kondrakhina IN, Verbenko DA, Zatevalov AM, Gatiatulina ER, Nikonorov AA, Deryabin DG, et al. A cross-sectional study of plasma trace elements and vitamins content in androgenetic alopecia in men. Biol Trace Elem Res. 2020;199(9):3232-41

37. Öner Ü, Akdeniz N. Nonscarring scalp alopecia: which laboratory analysis should we perform on whom? Turk J Med Sci. 2022;52(1):188-94
38. Sreekumar G, Pardinas J, Wong CQ, Whiting D, Katz HI, Price V, et al. Serum androgens and genetic linkage analysis in early onset androgenetic alopecia. J Invest Dermatol. 1999;113: 277-9.
39. Vierhapper H, Nowotny P, Maier H, Waldhäusl W. Production rates of dihydrotestosterone in healthy men and women and in men with male pattern baldness: determination by stable isotope/dilution and mass spectrometry. J Clin Endocrinol Metab. 2001;86:5762-4.
40. Mondal D, Narwani D, Notta S, Ghaffar D, Mardhekar N, Quadri SSA. Oxidative stress and redox signaling in CRPC progression: therapeutic potential of clinically-tested Nrf2-activators. Cancer Drug Resist. 2021;4(1):96-124.
41. Bohnsack BL, Hirschi KK. Nutrient regulation of cell cycle progression. Annu Rev Nutr. 2004;24:433-53.
42. Ames BN. Low micronutrient intake may accelerate the degenerative diseases of aging through allocation of scarce micronutrients by triage. Proc Natl Acad Sci U S A. 2006;103(47): 17589-94.
43. Huskisson E, Maggini S, Ruf M. The role of vitamins and minerals in energy metabolism and well-being. J Int Med Res. 2007;35:277-89.
44. Kantor J, Kessler LJ, Brooks DG, Cotsarelis G. Decreased serum ferritin is associated with alopecia in women. J Invest Dermatol. 2003;121:985-8.
45. Muthayya S, Rah JH, Sugimoto JD, Roos FF, Kraemer K, Black RE. The global hidden hunger indices and maps: an advocacy tool for action. PLoS One. 2013;8(6):e67860.
46. Sato M, Sato K. Maternal inheritance of mitochondrial DNA by diverse mechanisms to eliminate paternal mitochondrial DNA. Biochim Biophys Acta. 2013;1833(8):1979-84.
47. Ames BN, Atamna H, Killilea DW. Mineral and vitamin deficiencies can accelerate the mitochondrial decay of aging. Mol Aspects Med. 2005;26(4-5):363-78.
48. Chew EGY, Lim TC, Leong MF, Liu X, Sia YY, Leong ST, et al. Observations that suggest a contribution of altered dermal papilla mitochondrial function to androgenetic alopecia. Exp Dermatol. 2022;31(6):906-17.
49. Tang Y, Luo B, Deng Z, Wang B, Liu F, Li J, et al. Mitochondrial aerobic respiration is activated during hair follicle stem cell differentiation, and its dysfunction retards hair regeneration. PeerJ. 2016;4:e1821.
50. Turpaev KT. Reactive oxygen species and regulation of gene expression. Biochemistry (Mosc). 2002;67(3):281-92.
51. Jun MS, Kwack MH, Kim MK, Kim JC, Sung YK. Particulate matters induce apoptosis in human hair follicular keratinocytes. Ann Dermatol. 2020;32(5):388-94.
52. Sebetić K, Sjerobabski Masnec I, Cavka V, Biljan D, Krolo I. UV damage of the hair. Coll Antropol. 2008;32(Suppl 2):163-5.
53. Schwartz JR, Henry JP, Kerr KM, Mizoguchi H, Li L. The role of oxidative damage in poor scalp health: ramifications to causality and associated hair growth. Int J Cosmet Sci. 2015;37(Suppl 2): 9-15.
54. Tan DQ, Suda T. Reactive oxygen species and mitochondrial homeostasis as regulators of stem cell fate and function. Antioxid Redox Signal. 2018;29(2):149-68.
55. Upton JH, Hannen RF, Bahta AW, Farjo N, Farjo B, Philpott MP. Oxidative stress-associated senescence in dermal papilla cells of men with androgenetic alopecia. J Invest Dermatol. 2015;135:1244-52.
56. Baker K, Staecker H. Low dose oxidative stress induces mitochondrial damage in hair cells. Anat Rec (Hoboken). 2012;295(11):1868-76.
57. Redza-Dutordoir M, Averill-Bates DA. Activation of apoptosis signalling pathways by reactive oxygen species. Biochim Biophys Acta. 2016;1863(12):2977-92.
58. He L, He T, Farrar S, Ji L, Liu T, Ma X. Antioxidants maintain cellular redox homeostasis by elimination of reactive oxygen species. Cell Physiol Biochem. 2017;44(2):532-53.
59. Hamilton JB. Male hormone stimulation is prerequisite and an incitant in common baldness. Am J Anat. 1942;71:451-80.
60. Inui S, Fukuzato Y, Nakajima T, Yoshikawa K, Itami S. Identification of androgen-inducible TGF-beta1 derived from dermal papilla cells as a key mediator in androgenetic alopecia. J Investig Dermatol Symp Proc. 2003;8(1):69-71.
61. Shin H, Yoo HG, Inui S, Itami S, Kim IG, Cho AR, et al. Induction of transforming growth factor-beta 1 by androgen is mediated by reactive oxygen species in hair follicle dermal papilla cells. BMB Rep. 2013;46(9):460-4.
62. Barcellos-Hoff MH, Dix TA. Redox-mediated activation of latent transforming growth factor-beta 1. Mol Endocrinol. 1996;10(9):1077-83.
63. Liu N, Wang LH, Guo LL, Wang GQ, Zhou XP, Jiang Y, et al. Chronic restraint stress inhibits hair growth via substance P mediated by reactive oxygen species in mice. PLoS One. 2013;8(4):e61574.
64. Russell RC, Yuan HX, Guan KL. Autophagy regulation by nutrient signaling. Cell Res. 2014;24(1):42-57.
65. Wang L, Guo LL, Wang LH, Zhang GX, Shang J, Murao K, et al. Oxidative stress and substance P mediate psychological stress-induced autophagy and delay of hair growth in mice. Arch Dermatol Res. 2015;307(2):171-81.
66. Sukseree S, Karim N, Jaeger K, Zhong S, Nagelreiter IM, Gruber F, et al. Autophagy controls the protein composition of hair shafts. J Invest Dermatol. 2023;143(5):S245.
67. Ozturk P, Kurutas E, Ataseven A, Dokur N, Gumusalan Y, Gorur A, et al. BMI and levels of zinc, copper in hair, serum and urine of Turkish male patients with androgenetic alopecia. J Trace Elem Med Biol. 2014;28(3):266-70.
68. Aoi N, Inoue K, Chikanishi T, Fujiki R, Yamamoto H, Kato H, et al. 1α,25-dihydroxyvitamin D3 modulates the hair-inductive capacity of dermal papilla cells: therapeutic potential for hair regeneration. Stem Cells Transl Med. 2012;1(8):615-626.
69. Simopoulos AP. Omega-3 fatty acids in inflammation and autoimmune diseases. J Am Coll Nutr. 2002;21(6):495-505.
70. Liang T, Liao S. Inhibition of steroid 5 alpha-reductase by specific aliphatic unsaturated fatty acids. Biochem J. 1992;285(Pt 2): 557-62.
71. Munkhbayar S, Jang S, Cho A-R, Choi SJ, Shin CY, Eun HC, et al. Role of arachidonic acid in promoting hair growth. Ann Dermatol. 2016;28(1):55-64.
72. Das UN. Nutrients, essential fatty acids and prostaglandins interact to augment immune responses and prevent genetic damage and cancer. Nutrition. 1989;5(2):106-10.

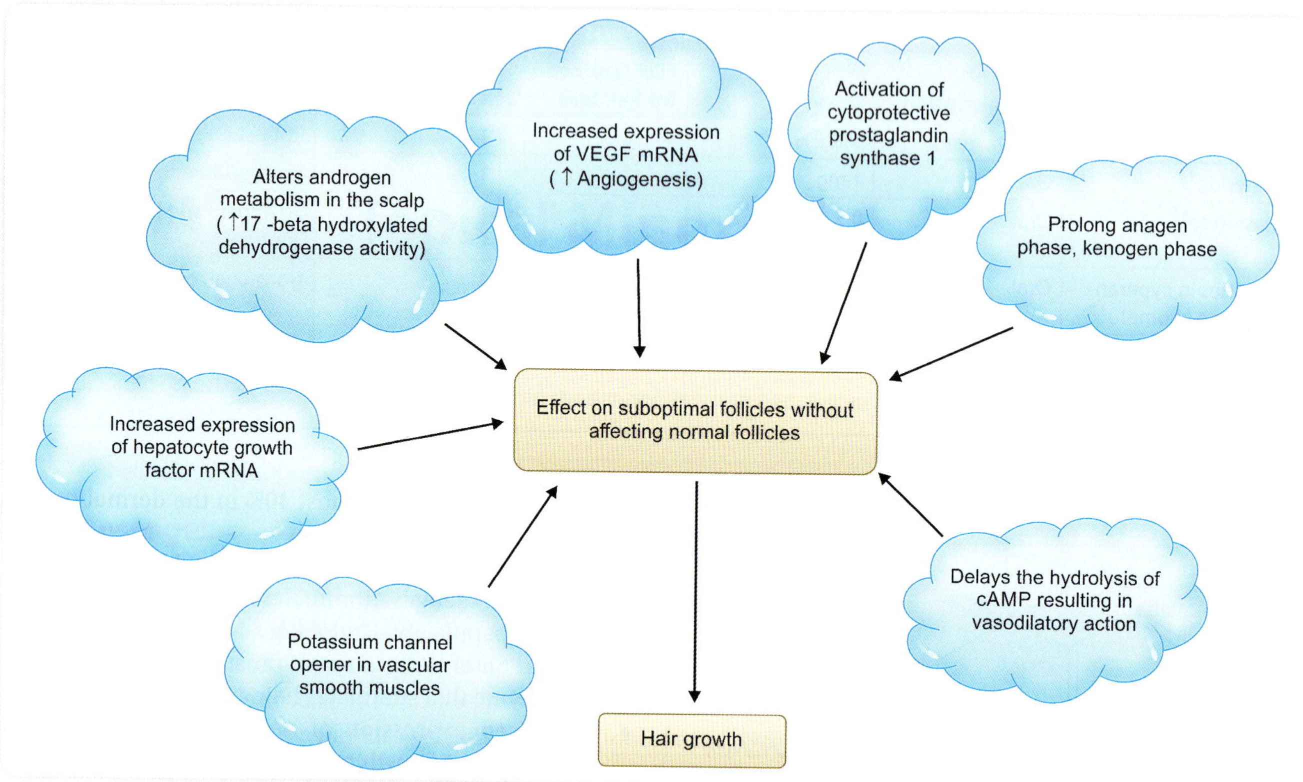

FIG. 2: Mechanism of action of minoxidil in hair growth.
(cAMP: cyclic adenosine monophosphate; mRNA: messenger ribonucleic acid; VEGF: vascular endothelial growth factor)

Efficacy

Apart from the 2 and 5% concentrations that are most commonly used, concentrations ranging from 2 to 15% are available in the market.[12] 2% concentration is preferred in female pattern hair loss (FPHL).[9] Compared to 5% solution, it has been found that a twice-daily application of 2% is preferred due to less adverse effects and better compliance.[12] Compared to 3%, 2% minoxidil was found to be equal or better in the treatment of male pattern hair loss (MPHL), with twice-daily application showing better hair growth in the frontotemporal and vertex areas.[13] Having said that, 5% minoxidil foam is USFDA approved for FPHL and has been found to be as efficacious as twice daily application of 2% minoxidil. Fewer side effects and only once a day application tips the scales in favor of the former formulation compared to the latter.[5,12] Another study comparing 5 and 10% minoxidil found 5% to be better than 10%. Almost 10% minoxidil was associated with increased irritation and lower compliance in patients.[6] Another observation was that 5% once-daily application was comparable in efficacy to 2% twice-daily application in FPHL.[3] **Table 2** shows the level of evidence of different formulations

TABLE 2: Different formulations available in the treatment of patterned hair loss.

Formulation of minoxidil	Concentration	Frequency	Level of evidence
Solution (males)[3]	5%	Twice daily	1
Solution (males)[3]	2%	Twice daily	1
Foam (males)[3]	5%	Twice daily	1
Solution (females)[3]	2%	Twice daily	1
Foam (females)[3]	5%	Once daily	1
0.5% minoxidil solution + 0.025% tretinoin solution[12,14]	0.5% + 0.025%	–	2
5% minoxidil solution + 0.01% tretinoin solution[12,15,16]	5% + 0.01%	Once daily	2
5% minoxidil solution + 1% zinc pyrithione shampoo[12,17]	5% + 1%	–	2
2–5% minoxidil solution + finasteride 1 mg/day + 2% ketoconazole shampoo[12,18]	2–5% + 1 mg/day + 2%	–	2

in the treatment of AGA. Effects of topical application should be assessed by 6 months, and if improvement is noticed, it should be continued to maintain the results.[3]

INDICATIONS

Food and Drug Administration-Approved Indications

- AGA
- FPHL[5]

Off-label Indications of Topical Minoxidil

- Alopecia areata
- Beard enhancement
- Central centrifugal cicatricial alopecia
- Chemotherapy-induced alopecia
- Eyebrow enhancement
- Frontal fibrosing alopecia
- Monilethrix
- Loose anagen hair syndrome
- Telogen effluvium[5]

Minoxidil Combinations

Other preparations in combination with minoxidil are also available. These may be used in cases not responding to conventional minoxidil preparations. A few are as below and are shown in **Table 3**:

- *Minoxidil sulfate-based formulations*: These can be used in patients not responding to conventional preparations with reduced levels of sulfotransferase enzymes and have shown better effects.[5,8,19]
- *Combined with tretinoin*: Improved response has been noticed with this preparation as tretinoin facilitates better percutaneous absorption of minoxidil and can be useful in nonresponders by upregulating follicular sulfotransferase enzymes.[16,20] Here, once-a-day application was equal in efficacy compared to twice-a-day application of 5% minoxidil-only preparation.[16]
- *Other combinations with caffeine, curcumin, melatonin, azelaic acid, 2% ketoconazole shampoo, and 1% pyrithione zinc* are also available in the literature and have been found to be superior to minoxidil-alone preparations in the treatment of MPHL.[21]
- *Combined with 0.25% finasteride*, it has been shown to be useful.[22,23]

TABLE 3: Mechanism of action of different agents used along with minoxidil to increase efficacy.

Preparation	Mechanism of action	Effects
Curcumin[21]	• Active chemical of turmeric ○ Downregulates cyclooxygenase-2, lipoxygenase, inducible nitric oxide synthetase enzymes ○ Inhibits nuclear factor-κB signaling ○ Decreased proinflammatory cytokines such as tumor necrosis factor (TNF)-α and interleukin (IL)-1	• Anti-inflammatory, antimicrobial, antineoplastic, antiandrogenic • Reduction in follicular regression
Caffeine[21]	• Phosphodiesterase inhibition ○ Expression of insulin-like growth factor (IGF)-1 ○ It downregulates: – Testosterone-induced transforming growth factor (TGF)-β1 expression, which is a growth inhibitor – The inhibitory effects of testosterone on hair growth	• Promotes cellular proliferation • Promotes hair shaft elongation • Promotes anagen duration • Hair matrix keratinocyte proliferation
Melatonin[21]	Stimulates extra-pineal melatonin receptors present in anagen hair follicles, leading to hair growth	Antioxidant, hair growth
Azelaic acid[24]	5-alpha-reductase inhibitor	Hair growth
Ketoconazole shampoo 2%[12,25]	–	• Anti-inflammatory • Antimicrobial • Reduces inflammation typical of androgenetic alopecia (AGA) and improves the hair status
1% pyrithione zinc[12,14]	Inhibits 5-α-reductase enzyme in vitro	• Antimicrobial • Anti-inflammatory • Antioxidant

ADVERSE EFFECTS

Minoxidil is generally considered safe, but some adverse effects may occur as follows:

- *Irritant contact dermatitis*: The most common adverse effect, manifesting as itching and scaling, is mainly due to propylene glycol (PG) contained in minoxidil solutions.[5,12]
- *Paradoxical hair shedding*: It results from the stimulation of exogen as telogen follicles reenter anagen.[3]
- *Allergic contact dermatitis*: It is uncommonly seen. It occurs as a reaction to the vehicle, PG, or minoxidil itself. Allergic reactions to minoxidil are rare; however, a patch test can help identify the causative agent.[5]
- *Facial hypertrichosis*: It is seen more in females than males and is dependent on the concentration, with topical minoxidil 5% having the highest incidence of unwanted hair growth. It can occur in distant sites but most commonly occurs as a result of improper application.[5,11]

  Oral consumption of minoxidil solution (accidental or otherwise) can be life-threatening, manifesting in adults as refractory shock, tachycardia, fluid retention, rarely as pulmonary edema, and papilledema without overt raised intracranial pressure, while in children, it presents with serious cardiovascular effects.[26,27]
- *Headache*: It is a common initial complaint. Usually, it subsides with the continuation of treatment. It can also exacerbate migraines and, in some cases, may need stoppage of treatment.[13]
- *Cardiovascular adverse effects*: Chest pain (most common),[28,29] palpitations, sinus tachycardia, paroxysmal atrial fibrillation, and sinus arrhythmias are other not-so-common cardiac adverse effects (0.1–1%).[28-30]

BOX 1 **Adverse effects of topical minoxidil.**

- *Common*:
  - Paradoxical hair shedding[3]
  - Irritant contact dermatitis[5,12]
  - Allergic contact dermatitis[5]
  - Facial hypertrichosis[5,11]
  - Headache[13]
- *Uncommon*:
  - Chest pain, palpitations, sinus tachycardia, paroxysmal atrial fibrillation, sinus arrhythmias[28-30]
  - Scalp comedones[31]
  - Burning sensation, erythema/skin rashes, itching[5,6,32,33]
  - Increased hair loss[7]
  - Edema of the face[32]
  - Changes in vision/blurred vision[34]
  - Dizziness, fainting[31,32]
  - Flushing, numbness/tingling of hands, feet, or face[11,32]
  - Rapid weight gain[11]
  - Polymenorrhea[6]

Box 1 shows the different adverse effects associated with topical minoxidil use.

CONTRAINDICATIONS

- Hypersensitivity to the drug
- Enough studies are not available to warrant its use in pregnancy and lactation.[3]

CONCLUSION

Proven efficacy and few side effects have made minoxidil important in the management of hair loss. Its availability, in combination with other potent medications in the market, has made it one of the most indispensable management options today and in the days to come.

Tips and Pearls

- Always explain the process, the effects, and the results of topical minoxidil beforehand to the patient.
- Remind the patient that increased hair shedding during the first month of therapy is only temporary while also reminding that the discontinuation can also lead to hair fall.
- Advise the application of 1 mL of the solution or half a cup of the foam twice daily over the scalp for best results.
- Even application of the preparation over the scalp is advised.
- Care while applying is recommended to reduce unwanted runoff of preparation to neighboring areas and thus undesirable hair growth.

REFERENCES

1. Harth W, Blume-Peytavi U. Psychotrichology: psychosomatic aspects of hair diseases. J Dtsch Dermatol Ges. 2013;11(2):125-35.
2. Hadshiew IM, Foitzik K, Arck PC, Paus R. Burden of hair loss: stress and the underestimated psychosocial impact of telogen effluvium and androgenetic alopecia. J Invest Dermatol. 2004;123(3):455-7.
3. Kanti V, Messenger A, Dobos G, Reygagne P, Finner A, Blumeyer A, et al. Evidence-based (S3) guideline for the treatment of androgenetic alopecia in women and in men—short version. J Eur Acad Dermatol Venereol. 2018;32(1):11-22.
4. Adil A, Godwin M. The effectiveness of treatments for androgenetic alopecia: a systematic review and meta-analysis. J Am Acad Dermatol. 2017;77(1):136-41.e5.
5. Wolff H, Fischer TW, Blume-Peytavi U. The diagnosis and treatment of hair and scalp diseases. Dtsch Arztebl Int. 2016;113(21):377-86.
6. Suchonwanit P, Thammarucha S, Leerunyakul K. Minoxidil and its use in hair disorders: a review. Drug Des Devel Ther. 2019;13:2777-86.
7. Ghonemy S, Alaraw A, Bessar H. Efficacy and safety of a new 10% topical minoxidil versus 5% topical minoxidil and placebo in the treatment of male androgenetic alopecia: a trichoscopic evaluation. J Dermatolog Treat. 2019;32(2):236-41.
8. Goren A, Castano JA, McCoy J, Bermudez F, Lotti T. Novel enzymatic assay predicts minoxidil response in the treatment of androgenetic alopecia. Dermatol Ther. 2014;27(3):171-3.
9. Goren A, Shapiro J, Roberts J, McCoy J, Desai N, Zarrab Z, et al. Clinical utility and validity of minoxidil response testing in androgenetic alopecia. Dermatol Ther. 2015;28(1):13-6.
10. Goren A, Mccoy J, Kovacevic M, Situm M, Chitalia J, Dhurat R. The effect of topical minoxidil treatment on follicular sulfotransferase enzymatic activity. J Biol Regul Homeost Agents. 2018;32(4):937-40.
11. Mysore V. Chapter 11. Minoxidil. Hair Transplantation, 1st edition. New Delhi: Jaypee Brothers Medical Publishers Pvt. Ltd; 2016. pp. 71-3.
12. Varothai S, Bergfeld WF. Androgenetic alopecia: an evidence-based treatment update. Am J Clin Dermatol. 2014;15(3): 217-30.
13. Katz HI, Hien NT, Prawer SE, Goldman SJ. Long-term efficacy of topical minoxidil in male pattern baldness. J Am Acad Dermatol. 1987;16(3 Pt. 2):711-8.
14. Berger RS, Fu JL, Smiles KA, Turner CB, Schnell BM, Werchowski KM, et al. The effects of minoxidil, 1% pyrithione zinc and a combination of both on hair density: a randomized controlled trial. Br J Dermatol. 2003;149:354-62.
15. Bazzano GS, Terezakis N, Galen W. Topical tretinoin for hair growth promotion. J Am Acad Dermatol. 1986;15:880-3, 890-3.
16. Shin HS, Won CH, Lee SH, Kwon OS, Kim KH, Eun HC. Efficacy of 5% minoxidil versus combined 5% minoxidil and 0.01% tretinoin for male pattern hair loss: a randomized, double-blind, comparative clinical trial. Am J Clin Dermatol. 2007;8(5):285-90.
17. Khandpur S, Suman M, Reddy BS. Comparative efficacy of various treatment regimens for androgenetic alopecia in men. J Dermatol. 2002;29:489-98.
18. Tsuboi R, Arano O, Nishikawa T, Yamada H, Katsuoka K. Randomized clinical trial comparing 5% and 1% topical minoxidil for the treatment of androgenetic alopecia in Japanese men. J Dermatol. 2009;36:437-46.
19. Dias PCR, Miot HA, Trüeb AM, Ramos PM. Use of minoxidil sulfate versus minoxidil base in androgenetic alopecia treatment: friend or foe? Skin Appendage Disord. 2018;4(4):349-50.
20. Sharma A, Goren A, Dhurat R, Agrawal S, Sinclair R, Trüeb RM, et al. Tretinoin enhances minoxidil response in androgenetic alopecia patients by upregulating follicular sulfotransferase enzymes. Dermatol Ther. 2019;32(3):e12915.
21. Hosking AM, Juhasz M, Atanaskova Mesinkovska N. Complementary and alternative treatments for alopecia: a comprehensive review. Skin Appendage Disord. 2019;5(2): 72-89.
22. Suchonwanit P, Srisuwanwattana P, Chalermroj N, Khunkhet S. A randomized, double-blind controlled study of the efficacy and safety of topical solution of 0.25% finasteride admixed with 3% minoxidil vs. 3% minoxidil solution in the treatment of male androgenetic alopecia. J Eur Acad Dermatol Venereol. 2018;32(12):2257-63.
23. Chen L, Zhang J, Wang L, Wang H, Chen B. The efficacy and safety of finasteride combined with topical minoxidil for androgenetic alopecia: a systematic review and meta-analysis. Aesthetic Plast Surg. 2020;44(3):962-70.
24. Gugle AS, Jadhav VM, Kote RP, Deshmukh MD, Dalvi AV. Comparative study of efficacy of topical minoxidil 5% and combination of topical minoxidil 5%, topical azelaic acid 1.5% and topical tretinoin 0.01% on the basis of dermoscopic analysis in androgenetic alopecia. MVP J Med Sci. 2015;2(2):90-9.
25. Piérard-Franchimont C, De Doncker P, Cauwenbergh G, Piérard GE. Ketoconazole shampoo: effect of long-term use in androgenic alopecia. Dermatology. 1998;196(4):474-7.
26. Shashikala TP, Singh R, Muthukrishnan J. Refractory shock following ingestion of topical minoxidil solution. Med J Armed Forces India. 2016;72(Suppl. 1):S133-4.
27. Claudet I, Cortey C, Honorat R, Franchitto N. Minoxidil topical solution: an unsafe product for children. Pediatr Emerg Care. 2015;31(1):44-6.
28. Karam P. Topical minoxidil therapy for androgenic alopecia in the Middle East. The Middle-Eastern Topical Minoxidil Study Group. Int J Dermatol. 1993;32(10):763-6.
29. AliKhan FS, Maibach H. Topical absorption and systemic toxicity. Cutan Ocul Toxicol. 2011;30(3):175-86.
30. Olsen EA, Dunlap FE, Funicella T, Koperski JA, Swinehart JM, Tschen EH, et al. A randomized clinical trial of 5% topical minoxidil versus 2% topical minoxidil and placebo in the treatment of androgenetic alopecia in men. J Am Acad Dermatol. 2002;47(3):377-85.
31. Stern RS. Topical minoxidil: a survey of use and complications. Arch Dermatol. 1987;123(1):62-5.
32. Kubba R. Topical minoxidil in androgenetic alopecia, how good is it? Indian J Dermatol Venereol Leprol. 1990;56:187-92.
33. Olsen EA, DeLong ER, Weiner MS. Long-term follow-up of men with male pattern baldness treated with topical minoxidil. J Am Acad Dermatol. 1987;16(3 Pt. 2):688-95.
34. Aktas H, Alan S, Türkoglu EB, Sevik Ö. Could topical minoxidil cause non-arteritic anterior ischemic optic neuropathy? J Clin Diagn Res. 2016;10(8):WD01-2.

CHAPTER 22

Oral Minoxidil

Sajin Alexander, Venkataram Mysore

Key Messages

- Oral minoxidil (OM) can be used as an alternative to topical minoxidil.
- It undergoes hepatic sulfonation.
- The most common dosage is 0.25–5 mg.
- The higher the dose, the more the adverse effects.
- Pregnancy category C drug

INTRODUCTION

The discovery of hair growth as an adverse reaction to oral minoxidil (OM) paved the way to an alley of topical preparations of immeasurable opportunities in the field of trichology. This accidental realization ushered in an era where topical minoxidil grew into one of the most significant and indispensable forms of therapy in any and every management approach for hair loss. However, intolerance, incompliance, and ineffectiveness in some patients have led many to look closely at the original molecule for answers and, as a result, have made many dermatologists worldwide to take a second look at its oral preparation.

Relevance and Significance

There are only two Food and Drug Administration (FDA)-approved medications for the treatment of androgenetic alopecia (AGA).[1] Effective alternatives are lacking. In cases of adverse reactions to topical minoxidil as well as nonresponders, OM can be used as another option.[2]

DISCUSSION

History

Developed by the Upjohn Company (now Pfizer) in the 1960s, OM was approved by FDA for the treatment of treatment-resistant hypertension in the 1970s. Soon, its popularity soared among doctors and patients alike, leading to rampant use of the drug and for longer durations. This resulted in a peculiar observation of hypertrichosis as an adverse effect. This prompted further study of this drug topically and in the year 1988, 2% minoxidil solutions were approved for the treatment of male AGA. In 1991, 5% was approved for male pattern hair loss (MPHL) and 2% for female pattern hair loss (FPHL). 5% lotion and foam formulations received approval for MPHL in 1997 and 2006, respectively.[3]

Mechanism of Action

Little is known about the effects of OM on hair growth as the majority of the literature available propounded the action and response regarding topical minoxidil.[4]

But before we dive into its possible mechanism, one has to answer the question, *"what causes nonresponse to topical minoxidil?"*

Minoxidil is a prodrug and requires sulfotransferase enzyme for the conversion into its active form, minoxidil sulfate. This enzyme, present in the outer root sheath (ORS) of the hair follicle, is responsible for this conversion with regard to topical minoxidil. In nonresponders to topical minoxidil, this enzyme is found to be in low levels in the ORS. Measuring the levels found that ORS sulfotransferase levels of <0.4 optical density (OD) 405 were noticed in nonresponders.[5]

In OM, this conversion into minoxidil sulfate occurs in the presence of enzyme sulfotransferase (phenol sulfotransferase) via hepatic sulfonation.[6] In fact, recently it has been shown that ORS sulfotransferase enzyme measurement can be an enzymatic assay to identify nonresponders to OM too. Values of <0.254 OD405 are considered here.[7]

The various mechanisms postulated to promote hair growth are as follows:

- Relaxation of vascular smooth muscle through the opening of sarcolemmal adenosine triphosphate 2 (ATP2)-dependent potassium channels (the major mechanism in resolving high blood pressure)[8]
- Entry into G1 phase of the cell cycle from latent post-telogen phase as a result of potassium channel activity leading to prolongation of the kenagen phase
- Hyperpolarization of the cell membrane and inhibition of calcium entry due to potassium channel opening, thereby affecting smooth muscles of the peripheral artery
- Delay in the hydrolysis of cyclic adenosine monophosphate (cAMP) leading to vasodilatory action by inhibiting phosphodiesterase **(Flowchart 1)**[3,9]

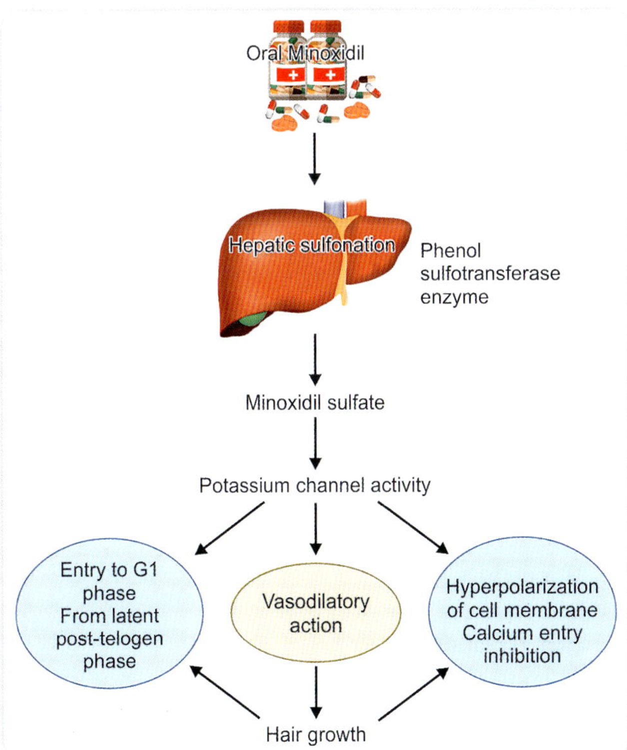

FLOWCHART 1: Mechanism of action of oral minoxidil in hair growth.

HEMODYNAMIC EFFECTS

Once administered, OM gets absorbed almost completely (95%) from the gastrointestinal tract (GIT) and becomes apparent in plasma in 15–30 minutes. The plasma half-life of OM is 4 hours, and peak concentration is noticed in 30–60 minutes. It does not cross the blood–brain barrier. Chronic administration of the drug does not lead to an adaptive increase in drug metabolism, and 7–10 days is considered the whole body clearance rate of OM. More than 90% of the drug and its metabolite are excreted in urine as such and a glucuronide conjugate metabolite in a span of 4 days.[10]

EFFICACY

Oral minoxidil is given a grade D recommendation by the Japanese Dermatological Association due to its side effect profile and lack of clinical trials.[11,12] Even though it is US FDA approved for the treatment of hypertension, it is not approved for hair loss.[2] However, an increasing number of papers published are giving evidence of its potential benefits in the treatment of alopecia.[2,13-17]

Current available data advocates a low-dose OM regimen in the treatment of AGA. This is to mitigate the known adverse reactions associated with this drug. Dosages ranging from 0.25 to 5 mg have been used, with the majority of these studies advising doses <2.5 mg **(Table 1)**.

One observation that can be made in the available data is the preference of lower doses and the same is preferred in females compared to males in patterned hair loss. This may perhaps be to avoid untold adverse effects such as hypertrichosis in women. Doses ranging from 0.25 to 1.25 mg have been used in women with better results reported compared to men. Higher doses were required for a better outcome in men.[13,15,18,27] A single dose of 5 mg or divided over a day led to a dramatic response in AGA but with more adverse reactions. This may be far more common in comparison to lower doses but is not severe and is reversible and tolerable.[14,16]

But the golden question is, "How does it fair with regards to topical minoxidil?"

The following points help answer the above question:

- *Better efficacy*: 1 mg OM compared to 5% topical minoxidil by Ramos et al. and 5 mg OM versus 5% topical minoxidil by Fiedler-Weiss et al. found OM to be superior.[20,21]
- *More accessible and practical*: Oral consumption is easier than the topical application of lotions.
- *Cheaper*: When compared for the same period
- Better compliance

TABLE 1: Various dosages of oral minoxidil (OM) used in published data.

Study	OM dose (mg)	Combination drug used	Sample size
Sinclair[13]	0.25	Tab. spironolactone 25 mg	100
Jimenez-Cauhe et al.[14]	–2.5 –5	–	16
Beach[15]	1.25	–	16
Lueangarun et al.[16]	5	–	30
Pirmez and Salas-Callo[18]	0.25	–	25
Therianou et al.[19]	0.5	–	9
Ramos et al.[20]	1	–	52
Fiedler-Weiss et al.[21]	10	–	65
Perera and Sinclair[22]	0.25–2.5	–	36
Yang and Thai[23] (case report)	1	–	1
Sinclair[24] (case series)	• Case 1: 0.25 • Case 2: 0.25–0.5	–	2
Cranwell and Sinclair[25]	0.5	–	1
Wambier et al.[26]	• Females: 2.5 • Males: 5	Oral tofacitinib 10 mg	12
Vano-Galvan et al.[27]	• Males: 2.5 • Females: 1	–	51
Olamiju and Craiglow[28]	2.5	–	6
Beach et al.[29]	1.25	–	51
Sanabria et al.[30]	0.5–5	–	435
Panchaprateep and Lueangarun[31]	5	–	30
Vastarella et al.[32]	1.25	–	12
Jha et al.[33]	1.25	–	32
Rodrigues-Barata et al.[34]	0.25–2	–	148
Jha et al.[35]	Group A: 1.25 Group B: 2.5	• Group A: Platelet-rich plasma • Group B: Platelet-rich plasma	• A = 47 • B = 48

- *Increased tolerability*: With regard to the side effect profile
- *Increased flexibility*: As one can combine other treatment options (such as commercial fibers) to improve hair fullness in bald areas with ease[15]

Sublingual Minoxidil

Sublingual low-dose minoxidil of 0.25 mg is available and has been found to be safer and more effective than conventional low-dose OM. This is based on the principle that it has lesser side effects and has better bioavailability as it bypasses the hepatic first-pass metabolism as compared to orally administered minoxidil. Even though this preliminary report is encouraging, further studies on larger sample sizes are required before consecrating this conclusion.[36]

INDICATIONS

FDA approved

- Treatment-resistant hypertension[2]

Off-label indications:

- AGA[37]
- Alopecia areata[21,26]
- Telogen effluvium[22]
- Monilethrix[24]
- Loose anagen hair syndrome[25]
- Lichen planopilaris[27,29]
- Traction alopecia[29]
- Central centrifugal cicatricial alopecia[29]
- Chemotherapy-induced alopecia[23,29]
- Frontal fibrosing alopecia[29,38] **(Table 2)**

TABLE 2: Indications other than androgenetic alopecia (AGA).

Studies	Indications	Dose (mg)	Results
Fiedler-Weiss et al.[21]	Alopecia areata	10	80%—improvement
Wambier et al.[26]		• Males: 5 • Females: 2.5	93%—median regrowth
Perera and Sinclair[22]	Telogen effluvium	0.25–2.5	92%—improvement
Yang and Thai[23]	Chemotherapy-induced alopecia	1	• Significant regrowth of hair • Patient satisfaction—good
Beach et al.[29]		1.25	• 65%—hair regrowth • 27%—reduced hair fall
Sinclair[24]	Monilethrix	0.25–0.5	Significant hair regrowth and reduced hair breakage
Cranwell and Sinclair[25]	Loose anagen hair syndrome	0.5	Exceptional improvement in hair density and length
Vano-Galvan et al.[27]	Lichen planopilaris (LPP)	• Males: 2.5 • Females: 1	• 39%—improvement of hair thickness • Better results—diffuse > patchy type LPP
Beach et al.[29]		1.25	• 65%—hair regrowth • 27%—reduced hair fall
Beach et al.[29]	Frontal fibrosing alopecia	1.25	• 65%—hair regrowth • 27%—reduced hair fall
Pirmez and Abraham[38]		0.5–2.5	Cosmetically acceptable regrowth
Beach et al.[29]	Traction alopecia	1.25	• 65%—hair regrowth • 27%—reduced hair fall
Beach et al.[29]	Central centrifugal cicatricial alopecia	1.25	

ADVERSE EFFECTS

- *Major*:
  - Weight gain as a result of sodium and water retention, which rarely can worsen to congestive cardiac failure
  - Tachycardia and increased cardiac output
  - Pulmonary hypertension
  - Pericardial effusion
- *Minor*:
  - Hypertrichosis
  - Itchy eyes
  - Headache
  - Skin rashes
  - Polymenorrhea[39]

Table 3 show studies done on oral minoxidil and the adverse effects reported.

A dose-dependent relation has been noticed with regard to adverse effects, with side effects more common with doses of ≥5 mg and least in lesser dosages.[13-16,18]

The most common side effect with OM is hypertrichosis. The risk is 4% at doses of 0.25 mg, 37.5% at 1.25 mg, and 93% at 5 mg.[13,15,16] Discontinuation of the drug can reverse the effects. The sequence in which this hair growth is noticed first is on the temple followed by the glabella, forehead, or over the skin infront of the ears and is reversible on discontinuation.[34,35]

Hypotension is another adverse effect noticed.[13,27] However, doses ranging from 2.5 to 10 mg were found to have minuscule effects in normotensive subjects. Though considered safe, measurement of baseline blood pressure (BP) in subjects planning to be started on OM is advised. In the event of BP values < 90/60 mm Hg, addition of 50 mg of sodium chloride to the dose can be considered.[13,40]

Swelling of the feet, lower legs, hands, face, or rapid weight gain can occur in some due to salt and water retention.[41] The risk varies with dose, with 4% at doses of 0.25 mg to 10% at doses of 5 mg. Oral spironolactone 25 g can be added to OM to lessen this burden while potentiating the effects of minoxidil.[8,13]

Rare cases of T-wave flattening or inversion, T-wave alterations, and other ST-wave changes have been noticed on electrocardiogram (ECG). Withdrawal of the drug within a day has shown to reverse these effects.[3,16,28]

Drug reaction in the form of Stevens-Johnson syndrome and toxic epidermal necrolysis has also been reported in few studies. However, these patients were treated with OM for hypertension on higher doses and had underlying chronic renal impairment. The cause of

TABLE 3: Adverse effects of low-dose oral minoxidil.

Study	Dose	Sample size	Adverse effects
Sinclair[13]	0.25 mg + tab. spironolactone 25 mg	100	• Mild • Urticaria—2%, hypotension—2%, facial hypertrichosis—4%
Jimenez-Cauhe et al.[14]	2.5 mg 5 mg	16	• Mild—29.3% • Hypertrichosis—24.3%, pedal edema—4.8%, hair shedding—2.4%
Beach[15]	1.25 mg	16	• Mild • Hypertrichosis—37.5%
Lueangarun et al.[16]	5 mg	30	Hypertrichosis—93%, pedal edema—10%, ECG alteration—10%
Pirmez and Salas-Callo[18]	0.25 mg	25	Hypertrichosis—20%, hair shedding—16%, pedal edema—4%
Therianou et al.[19]	0.5 mg	9	Two cases of mild hypertrichosis
Ramos et al.[20]	1 mg	52	Pretibial edema—4%, hypertrichosis—27%
Fiedler-Weiss et al.[21]	5 mg twice daily	65	Hypertrichosis—17%, fluid retention, headache, depression
Perera and Sinclair[22]	0.25–2.5 mg	36	Facial hypertrichosis—39%, transient postural, dizziness—5.6%, ankle edema—2.8%
Yang and Thai[23] (case report)	1 mg	1	No adverse effects noticed after 1 year of therapy
Sinclair[24] (case series)	• Case 1: 0.25 mg • Case 2: 0.25–0.5 mg	2	• Case 1: No adverse effects noticed after 2 years of therapy • Case 2: No adverse effects noticed after 18 months of therapy
Cranwell and Sinclair[25]	0.5 mg	1	No adverse effects mentioned
Vano-Galvan et al.[27]	• Males: 2.5 mg • Females: 1 mg	51	• Adverse effects: Mild—37% • Hypertrichosis—27.5%, postural hypotension—5.9%, tachycardia—3.9%, weight gain—1.9%
Olamiju and Craiglow[28]	2.5 mg	6	None—treatment was well tolerated and without any adverse effects
Beach et al.[29]	1.25 mg	51	Lightheadedness—4, palpitations—2, ankle edema—1, hypertrichosis—22, skin urticaria—1, other paresthesia—1
Sanabria et al.[30]	0.5–5 mg	435	Hypertrichosis—54%, headache—10%, insomnia—7%, edema—9%, dizziness—7%, palpitations—4%, facial edema—1%
Panchaprateep and Lueangarun[31]	5 mg	30	Hypertrichosis—93%, ECG findings—20%—premature ventricular contraction (occasional), T-wave inversion, pedal edema—10%
Vastarella et al.[32]	1.25 mg	12	Mild hypertrichosis—25%, postural hypotension—8.3%, peripheral edema—25%
Jha et al.[33]	1.25 mg	32	Hypertrichosis and peripheral edema in 1 patient

such a reaction has been explained as due to the immune response triggered by the defective detoxification products of minoxidil sulfate which accumulate due to inadequate clearance, which in turn intensifies the immune reaction further.[39,42-45]

CONTRAINDICATIONS

- Pheochromocytoma
- Previous hypersensitivity reactions to ingredients, hypotension
- Cardiac comorbidities
- Pregnancy (category C) or breastfeeding.[17]

PRECAUTIONS

- Always take a detailed history along with blood pressure and ECG in patients with suspicious history.
- Inform the patient regarding all facets of the therapy for better compliance.
- Begin therapy with the lowest dose.
- Always advise taking the tablet at night.

- Counsel the patient regarding adverse effects and the symptoms to watch out for.
- Recommend the use of a digital watch for detecting any pulse variation.
- Avoid treatment in pregnant and lactating women.

SUMMARY

Oral minoxidil in lower doses appears to be bearable and devoid of any major side effects[33,34] and can be considered as an effective replacement for topical minoxidil in allergic and nonresponding patients. Having said that, evidence supporting OM is low and concerns over systemic side effects remain, and therefore larger studies are required to correctly ascertain the value of this drug.

Tips and Pearls

- *Get your basics right!*
  - Detailed history
  - Record the data
  - Do the relevant investigations
- Choose your patient wisely
- Do the basic investigations and record BP and ECG
- Begin treatment with the lowest dose
- Do not exceed 5 mg
- Advise taking the drug only at night
- Recommend timely follow-ups and visits
- Advise regarding the side effects and get an informed consent—*can't be too careful these days!*

REFERENCES

1. Adil A, Godwin M. The effectiveness of treatments for androgenetic alopecia: a systematic review and meta-analysis. J Am Acad Dermatol. 2017;77:136-41.e5.
2. Almohanna HM, Perper M, Tosti A. Safety concerns when using novel medications to treat alopecia. Expert Opin Drug Saf. 2018;17:1115-28.
3. Kumaresan M. Minoxidil In: Mysore V (Ed). Hair Transplantation. New Delhi: Jaypee Brothers Medical Publishers; 2016. pp. 71-3.
4. Messenger AG, Rundegren J. Minoxidil: mechanisms of action on hair growth. Br J Dermatol. 2004;150:186-94.
5. Goren A, Castano JA, McCoy J, Bermudez F, Lotti T. Novel enzymatic assay predicts minoxidil response in the treatment of androgenetic alopecia. Dermatol Ther. 2014;27:171-3.
6. Falany CN, Kerl EA. Sulfation of minoxidil by human liver phenol sulfotransferase. Biochem Pharmacol. 1990;40:1027-32.
7. Ramos PM, Goren A, Sinclair R, Miot HA. Oral minoxidil bio-activation by hair follicle outer root sheath cell sulfotransferase enzymes predicts clinical efficacy in female pattern hair loss. J Eur Acad Dermatol Venereol. 2020;34:e40-1.
8. Pindado-Ortega C, Saceda-Corralo D, Vañó-Galván S. RF-Oral minoxidil for female pattern hair loss and other alopecias. Actas Dermosifiliogr (Engl Ed). 2019;110:861-2.
9. Goren A, Shapiro J, Roberts J, McCoy J, Desai N, Zarrab Z, et al. Clinical utility and validity of minoxidil response testing in androgenetic alopecia. Dermatol Ther. 2015;28:13-6.
10. Lowenthal DT, Affrime MB. Pharmacology and pharmacokinetics of minoxidil. J Cardiovasc Pharmacol. 1980;2 (Suppl. 2):S93-106.
11. Shao S, Zhang X, Duan L, Fang H, Rao S, Liu W, et al. Lysyl hydroxylase inhibition by minoxidil blocks collagen deposition and prevents pulmonary fibrosis via TGF-β_1/Smad3 signaling pathway. Med Sci Monit. 2018;24:8592-601.
12. Manabe M, Tsuboi R, Itami S, Osada SI, Amoh Y, Ito T, et al. Guidelines for the diagnosis and treatment of male-pattern and female-pattern hair loss, 2017 version. J Dermatol. 2018;45:1031-43.
13. Sinclair RD. Female pattern hair loss: a pilot study investigating combination therapy with low-dose oral minoxidil and spironolactone. Int J Dermatol. 2018;57:104-9.
14. Jimenez-Cauhe J, Saceda-Corralo D, Rodrigues-Barata R, Hermosa-Gelbard A, Moreno-Arrones OM, Fernandez-Nieto D, et al. Effectiveness and safety of low-dose oral minoxidil in male androgenetic alopecia. J Am Acad Dermatol. 2019;81:648-9.
15. Beach RA. Case series of oral minoxidil for androgenetic and traction alopecia: tolerability & the five C's of oral therapy. Dermatol Ther. 2018;31:e12707.
16. Lueangarun S, Panchaprateep R, Tempark T, Noppakun N. Efficacy and safety of oral minoxidil 5 mg daily during 24-week treatment in male androgenetic alopecia. J Am Acad Dermatol. 2015;72:AB113.
17. Gomolin A, Litvinov IV, Netchiporouk E. Oral minoxidil: a possible new therapy for androgenetic alopecia. J Cutan Med Surg. 2020;24 (Suppl. 3):88-9.
18. Pirmez R, Salas-Callo CI. Very-low-dose oral minoxidil in male androgenetic alopecia: a study with quantitative trichoscopic documentation. J Am Acad Dermatol. 2020;82:e21-2.
19. Therianou A, Vincenzi C, Tosti A. How safe is prescribing oral minoxidil in patients allergic to topical minoxidil? J Am Acad Dermatol. 2020;86:429-31.
20. Ramos PM, Sinclair RD, Kasprzak M, Miot HA. Minoxidil 1 mg oral versus minoxidil 5% topical solution for the treatment of female-pattern hair loss: a randomized clinical trial. J Am Acad Dermatol. 2020;82:252-3.
21. Fiedler-Weiss VC, Rumsfield J, Buys CM. Evaluation of oral minoxidil in the treatment of alopecia areata. Arch Dermatol. 1987;123:1488-90.
22. Perera E, Sinclair R. Treatment of chronic telogen effluvium with oral minoxidil: a retrospective study. F1000Res. 2017;6:1650.
23. Yang X, Thai KE. Treatment of permanent chemotherapy-induced alopecia with low dose oral minoxidil. Australas J Dermatol. 2016;57:e130-2.
24. Sinclair R. Treatment of monilethrix with oral minoxidil. JAAD Case Rep. 2016;2:212-5.
25. Cranwell WC, Sinclair R. Loose anagen hair syndrome: treatment with systemic minoxidil characterised by marked hair colour change. Australas J Dermatol. 2018;59:e286-7.

26. Wambier CG, Craiglow BG, King BA. Combination tofacitinib and oral minoxidil treatment for severe alopecia areata. J Am Acad Dermatol. 2021;85:743-5.
27. Vañó-Galván S, de Carvalho LT, Saceda-Corralo D, Rodrigues-Barata R, Kerkemeyer KL, Sinclair RD, et al. Oral minoxidil improves background hair thickness in lichen planopilaris. J Am Acad Dermatol. 2020;84:1684-6.
28. Olamiju B, Craiglow BG. Combination oral minoxidil and spironolactone for the treatment of androgenetic alopecia in adolescent girls. J Am Acad Dermatol. 2021;84:1689-91.
29. Beach RA, McDonald KA, Muylaert Barrett B. Low-dose oral minoxidil for treating alopecia: a 3-year North American retrospective case series. J Am Acad Dermatol. 2021;84:761-3.
30. Sanabria B, Vanzela TN, Miot HA, Ramos PM. Adverse effects of low-dose oral minoxidil for androgenetic alopecia in 435 patients. J Am Acad Dermatol. 2021;84:1175-8.
31. Panchaprateep R, Lueangarun S. Efficacy and safety of oral minoxidil 5 mg once daily in the treatment of male patients with androgenetic alopecia: an open-label and global photographic assessment. Dermatol Ther (Heidelb). 2020;10:1345-57.
32. Vastarella M, Cantelli M, Patrì A, Annunziata MC, Nappa P, Fabbrocini G. Efficacy and safety of oral minoxidil in female androgenetic alopecia. Dermatol Ther. 2020;33:e14234.
33. Jha AK, Sonthalia S, Zeeshan MD, Vinay K. Efficacy and safety of very-low-dose oral minoxidil 1.25 mg in male androgenetic alopecia. J Am Acad Dermatol. 2020;83:1491-3.
34. Rodrigues-Barata R, Moreno-Arrones OM, Saceda-Corralo D, Jiménez-Cauhé J, Ortega-Quijano D, Fernández-Nieto D, et al. Low-dose oral minoxidil for female pattern hair loss: a unicenter descriptive study of 148 women. Skin Appendage Disord. 2020;6:175-6.
35. Jha AK, Zeeshan M, Singh A, Roy PK. Platelet-rich plasma with low dose oral minoxidil (1.25mg versus 2.5mg) along with trichoscopic pre- and post-treatment evaluation. J Cosmet Dermatol. 2021;20:3220-6.
36. Sinclair R, Trindade de Carvalho L, Ferial Ismail F, Meah N. Treatment of male and female pattern hair loss with sublingual minoxidil: a retrospective case-series of 64 patients. J Eur Acad Dermatol Venereol. 2020;34(12):e795-6.
37. Shashikala TP, Singh R, Muthukrishnan J. Refractory shock following ingestion of topical minoxidil solution. Med J Armed Forces India. 2016;72(Suppl. 1):S133-4.
38. Pirmez R, Abraham LS. Eyebrow regrowth in patients with frontal fibrosing alopecia treated with low-dose oral minoxidil. Skin Appendage Disord. 2021;7:112-4.
39. Suchonwanit P, Thammarucha S, Leerunyakul K. Minoxidil and its use in hair disorders: a review. Drug Des Devel Ther. 2019;13:2777-86.
40. Fleishaker JC, Andreadis NA, Welshman IR, Wright CE 3rd. The pharmacokinetics of 2.5- to 10-mg oral doses of minoxidil in healthy volunteers. J Clin Pharmacol. 1989;29:162-7.
41. Pathomvanich D. Hair restoration surgery in Asians. In: Pathomvanich D, Imagawa K (Eds). Is There a Place for Oral Minoxidil? An Overview. Tokyo: Springer; 2010. pp. 73-7.
42. Karaoui LR, Chahine-Chakhtoura C. Fatal toxic epidermal necrolysis associated with minoxidil. Pharmacotherapy. 2009;29:460-7.
43. Halstenson CE, Opsahl JA, Wright CE, Fleishaker JC, Andreadis NA, Sobieraj J, et al. Disposition of minoxidil in patients with various degrees of renal function. J Clin Pharmacol. 1989;29:798-802.
44. DiSantis DJ, Flanagan J. Minoxidil-induced Stevens-Johnson syndrome. Arch Intern Med. 1981;141:1515.
45. Callen EC, Church CO, Hernandez CL, Thompson ED. Stevens-Johnson syndrome associated with oral minoxidil: a case report. J Nephrol. 2007;20:91-3.

CHAPTER 23

Finasteride

Anuradha Jindal, Madhulika Mhatre, Venkataram Mysore

Key Messages

- Finasteride is the only Food and Drug Administration (FDA)-approved oral medication for androgenetic alopecia (AGA).
- It is a type II 5-alpha reductase inhibitor and hence affects the androgen-mediated miniaturization process.
- It is shown to be effective with level A evidence in the management of AGA in males with a dose of 1 mg/day.
- The side effect profile, which includes sexual side effects, has caused much adverse publicity to the drug among patients, which affects patient compliance.

INTRODUCTION

Finasteride is the only oral Food and Drug Administration (FDA)-approved medication for use in men with androgenetic alopecia (AGA).[1] Finasteride is a competitive inhibitor of type II 5-alpha reductase (5αR) and inhibits the conversion of testosterone to dihydrotestosterone (DHT).[2,3]

The chemical name of finasteride is *N*-tert-butyl-3-oxo-4-aza-5α-androst-1-ene-17β-carboxamide. The empirical formula of finasteride is $C_{23}H_{36}N_2O_2$, and its molecular weight is 372.55 g/mol **(Fig. 1)**.

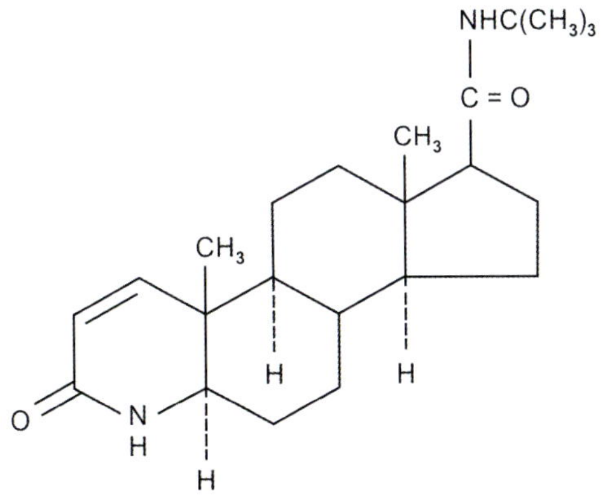

FIG. 1: Structure of finasteride.

MECHANISM OF ACTION OR PHARMACOLOGY

Androgen receptors play an important role in promoting the expression of inducible transcription factors for hair growth and regulation.

There are three types of 5αR receptors isoenzymes recognized:

1. *Type I 5αR*—present in sebaceous glands, sweat glands, dermal papillae, epidermal and follicular keratinocytes. They play an important role in sebum regulation.
2. *Type II 5αR*—in outer root sheaths of hair follicles, epididymis, vas deferens, seminal vesicle, and prostate.
3. *Type III 5αR*—in peripheral tissues.

Finasteride, a synthetic 4-azasteroid compound, is a specific inhibitor of type II and type III 5αR, an intracellular enzyme that converts testosterone to DHT.[4,5] Finasteride does not have any hormonal properties in itself. By inhibiting type II 5αR, it blocks the peripheral conversion of testosterone to DHT, resulting in significant decrease in serum and tissue DHT levels.[6-9] **Figure 2** shows the mechanism of action of finasteride.

A study by Drake et al.[10] showed that scalp DHT levels decreased by 13% with placebo and by 64.1 and 69.4% with 1 and 5 mg of finasteride, respectively, after 42 days of treatment. Serum levels decreased by 71.4 and 72.2%

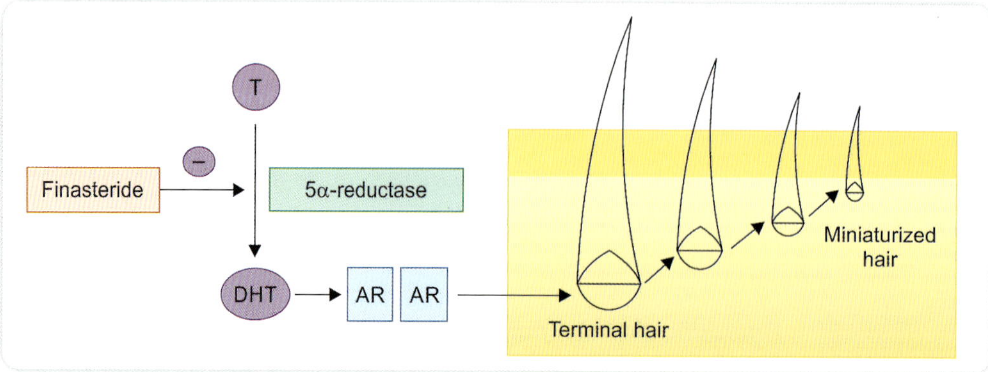

FIG. 2: Mechanism of action of finasteride.
(AR: androgen receptor; DHT: dihydrotestosterone; T: testosterone)

with 1 and 5 mg on the same schedule. These authors also showed that dosages as low as 0.2 mg daily decreased scalp and serum DHT levels, and further studies are needed to find the minimal efficacious dosage.[10-12]

Finasteride also inhibits the conversion of progesterone to 5α-dihydroprogesterone (DHP) and deoxycortisone to dihydrocortisone. It further inhibits the subsequent conversion of DHP and dihydrocortisone to tetrahydroprogesterone and isopregnanolone, respectively. These neurosteroids (isopregnanolone and tetrahydroprogesterone) exerts anticonvulsant, anti-depressant, and anxiolytic effects in our body. Alterations in the levels of the neurosteroids are said to be the reason for depression, anxiety, mood disturbances, and suicidal thoughts as reported in reports.

The rationale for the use of finasteride to treat male pattern hair loss is based on the long established evidence of the role of androgens, the absence of AGA in men with congenital deficiency of type II 5αR, and the presence of increased 5αR activity and DHT levels in hair follicles of men with balding scalps.[2,6-9,13-15] Finasteride rapidly lowers serum and scalp DHT levels by >60%.

Pharmacokinetics

Finasteride is well absorbed in the gastrointestinal tract, metabolized in the liver by cytochrome P450 3A4 (CYP3A4) enzyme subfamily, and excreted in urine and feces. The oral bioavailability of finasteride is 80% and is not influenced by food intake. Finasteride crosses the blood–brain barrier but is insignificantly distributed into cerebrospinal fluid.

Dihydrotestosterone levels return to pretreatment levels after approximately 14 days of cessation of therapy. The serum half-life is 5–6 hours. Minute quantities (nanogram levels) are detectable in semen.

INDICATIONS

Food and Drug Administration-Approved Indication

The FDA approved finasteride in the United States (US) in 1997 at a dosage of 1 mg/day for use in men with AGA. Multiple clinical studies demonstrated responsiveness to finasteride treatment among men with AGA, those with mild-to-moderate degrees of hair loss in the vertex and frontal areas. From studies by Leydon et al. and Kaurman, it can be concluded that finasteride can stabilize hair loss in 80% of patients with vertex hair loss and in 70% of patients with frontal hair loss.[16,17] Mild-to-moderate regrowth was seen in 61% on the vertex and 37% on the frontal area. Continued daily use of 1 mg oral finasteride may be needed for sustained benefit. Finasteride treatment increases the total hair count by increasing actively growing anagen hair. The ratio of anagen to telogen hairs was also shown to increase progressively over 48 weeks of finasteride treatment.[18]

A response to finasteride may be seen after 4 months, but patients should be encouraged to continue the treatment for at least 24 months before it can be finally evaluated. If successful, the treatment should be continued indefinitely as the balding process continues once treatment is stopped. The rapid hair fall that is noticed on stopping minoxidil does not occur with finasteride.

Other Dermatological Uses

Female Pattern Androgenetic Alopecia

The data regarding the use of finasteride in female pattern hair loss (FPHL) is conflicting. Large-scale studies on its efficacy are currently limited with one large multicenter randomized placebo-controlled trial failing to find any change in hair growth or progression of hair loss with finasteride 1 mg/day in postmenopausal women with FPHL over a 1 year follow-up period.[19] However, smaller case reports and case series have demonstrated efficacy for finasteride 1.25 mg/day in four cases of FPHL in both pre- and postmenopausal women with hyperandrogenism, finasteride 2.5 mg/day in five cases of FPHL in postmenopausal women without hyperandrogenism, and finasteride 5 mg/day in one case of FPHL in a postmenopausal woman without hyperandrogenism.[20-22]

Yeon et al. conducted a nonrandomized, uncontrolled trial including 87 pre- and postmenstrual normoandrogenic females treated with high dose of finasteride, and the patients reported good clinical improvement.[23] Another study conducted by Oliveira-Soares et al. conducted a study including 86 pre- and postmenstrual females with FPHL, who were treated with 5 mg/day finasteride. At 12 months, phototrichograms showed significantly increased hair density by 18.9% and hair diameter by 9.4% compared to baseline. Global photographic assessment showed clinical improvement in 81% patients.[24]

Finasteride does appear to be successful in some patients, but further large-scale studies are required to determine optimal dosing regimens.

Hirsutism

As increased 5αR activity is considered a pathogenetic mechanism of hirsutism, selective enzyme inhibition has been proposed as a rational medical approach to this condition. Consistently, finasteride has been tried in hirsute women, but the drug is yet to find a place in routine management of hirsutism.[25-27]

Acne Vulgaris

In a comparative study with flutamide and cyproterone acetate (CPA), finasteride 5 mg daily was found to be less beneficial in the treatment of acne in hyperandrogenic females.[28]

Further studies for evaluating finasteride for these disorders of androgen excess are in order.

CONTRAINDICATIONS

- Hypersensitivity to finasteride or any component of the product
- Use in children
- Finasteride is classified as pregnancy category X and is contraindicated in women who are or may get pregnant. It can cause feminization of the fetus.
- Blood donation is contraindicated in those who are currently on finasteride and up to 6 months following the last dose of finasteride.

ADVERSE EFFECTS

The most common adverse events noticed with the use of finasteride are sexual or psychiatric, which occur due to the suppression of peripheral androgens or change in levels of central neurogenic steroids.

Effect on sexual function: A number of studies have analyzed and studied the side effects caused by finasteride. These studies reveal that sexual adverse effects occur at the rate of 2.1–3.8%, erectile dysfunction (ED) being the most common followed by ejaculatory dysfunction, loss of libido, and gynecomastia. These effects seem to occur early in the therapy and return to normal on stopping the drug or over a time on continuous use of the drug. The only causal relation between finasteride and sexual adverse effects is decreased ejaculatory volume because of predominant action of DHT on prostate.[29] A long-term study showed that drug-related sexual side effects such as decreased libido, ED, and ejaculatory disorders occurred in <2% of men. The incidence of each side effect mentioned decreased to ≤0.3% by the 5 years of treatment with finasteride.[18] Moreover, in many cases, the side effects have been attributed to the nocebo effect. Nocebo effect refers to an adverse effect that results from the psychological awareness of the possibility of the side effects, but is not a direct result of the specific pharmacological action of the drug.[30,31]

In addition, many practitioners feel that in patients who are apprehensive about the side effects, it is worthwhile considering administration of lower daily doses or staggered pulse doses of the drug to enhance patient compliance. Plasma half-life of finasteride is 6–8 hours, and tissue binding is 4–5 days. Doses of 0.2 mg are adequate to suppress both scalp skin and serum DHT levels. While 0.2 mg caused 55% DHT suppression, 5 mg/day achieved 69% DHT suppression. The drug may be, therefore, initially administered at 0.5 mg daily or one tablet alternate days to gain confidence of the patient, and the 1 mg/day dosage may be restored once the patient is comfortable with the drug.[30]

Postfinasteride syndrome: Postfinasteride syndrome, also called 5αR inhibitor syndrome, describes persistent sexual, neurological, and physical adverse reactions in patients who have taken finasteride. This has been a greatly debated concept and as yet has no published evidence of its existence, and hence the matter needs proper research. Symptoms start to manifest within weeks of quitting the drug, when testosterone levels begin to drop. The most common persistent side effects of finasteride are loss of libido, ED, depression, suicidal ideation, anxiety, panic attacks, Peyronie's disease, penile shrinkage, gynecomastia, muscle atrophy, cognitive impairment, insomnia, severely dry skin, and tinnitus.

Teratogenicity: Finasteride has teratogenic effects in animals, causing genitourinary abnormalities in male offspring. It is, therefore, advised that pregnant females or those of childbearing potential should not take finasteride or handle crushed or broken tablets. The risk of teratogenicity in humans has not been evaluated, but finasteride may cause hypospadias in the developing male fetus. Exposure to semen of men who are taking finasteride does not pose a real risk to the pregnant woman's male fetus.[29]

Effect on immunity: Most recent studies have suggested that finasteride may be potentially involved in altering immune surveillance against cancer in aging males, since androgens are now thought to modulate immune response such as the Th1/Th2 cell balance.[32]

Psychiatric side effects: Depression, anxiety, panic attacks, insomnia, and fatigue are predominant reported side effects with finasteride; decreased levels of neurosteroids.

Other side effects: Other side effects reported in literature include dry skin, headaches, and gastrointestinal upset.[33] A few studies have suggested that finasteride might induce depressive symptoms, and therefore, this medication should be prescribed cautiously for patients with high risk of depression.[34-36]

The USFDA has instructed to add suicidal ideation and depression as adverse reactions on Propecia (finasteride) labels.

Carcinoma breast: Finasteride, by causing inhibition of DHT production, alters the estrogen-to-androgen ratio and may also increase the risk of gynecomastia and male breast cancer.[35]

Role in prostate cancer: The Prostate Cancer Prevention Trial (PCPT) reported a decreased incidence of prostate cancer overall but an increase in the incidence of high-grade prostate cancer with finasteride compared with placebo. It also said that the effects of finasteride on prostate volume and selective inhibition of low-grade cancer, rather than effects on tumor morphology, may have contributed to the increase in high-grade cancers with finasteride.[36-38]

DRUG INTERACTIONS

Finasteride shows significant interaction with erythromycin, isoniazid, and carbamazepine. Dose adjustment is not required for chronic kidney disease, but the dose has to be reduced in hepatic abnormalities.

No significant drug interactions of clinical importance have been demonstrated with finasteride.

MONITORING GUIDELINES

No specific laboratory monitoring guidelines are required for patients on finasteride. However, it is well known that DHT enlarges the prostrate, and therefore, men taking finasteride should be aware that prostate-specific antigen (PSA) levels will be reduced. Although not mandatory, a baseline PSA value for older patients should be done before starting finasteride in elderly population. Studies have revealed that men aged >50 years and taking finasteride for benign prostatic hyperplasia (BPH) had a 50% reduction in PSA levels, whereas younger men, ages 18–40 years, taking finasteride for AGA had an approximate 20–30% reduction. To interpret PSA levels in men treated with finasteride, it is necessary to take the reduction into account.[39]

Blood donation is also contraindicated for patients on finasteride for at least a 6-month period after the last dose to prevent blood donation to a pregnant female transfusion recipient, which may harm the male fetus.

TOPICAL FINASTERIDE

It was postulated that the adverse effects of oral finasteride could be reduced if finasteride was applied topically to the affected scalp. This approach was studied by Mazzarella and coresearchers who treated 52 patients with AGA, both male and female, with topical finasteride 0.005% solution in a single-blind, placebo-controlled manner. Treatment efficacy was assessed from both scalp photography and hair loss counts after washing. After 16 months, 73% subjects of the finasteride groups have experienced a slight reduction of the balding area compared with none in the placebo group. Monthly hair loss in the finasteride group was approximately 60% less than that of the placebo group ($p < 0.001$). Further trials are required in order to confirm these early results.[40]

SUMMARY

5α-reductase inhibitors were developed approximately 20 years ago. Finasteride was the first highly specific inhibitor of the human type II 5αR enzyme developed for clinical use. Accumulated data from various clinical trials have established finasteride's importance as a treatment for androgen-dependent disorders, including AGA. Moreover, finasteride is not a new drug, and worldwide experience with a higher dose of finasteride over many years in the treatment of men with BPH confirms the long-term safety of the compound. The side effect profile is summarized in **Box 1**. In view of increasing reluctance on the part of patients to take this drug, it has been recommended that the drug be administered at a reduced dose of 0.5 mg daily

BOX 1 Side effect profile of finasteride.

- *Sexual*:
  - Erectile dysfunction
  - Loss of libido
  - Genital shrinkage
- *Physical*:
  - Weight gain
  - Gynecomastia
  - Muscle weakness and atrophy
- *Metabolic*:
  - Osteoporosis
  - Anemia
  - Hot flushes
  - Hypertension, diabetes, heart disease, lipid abnormalities
- *Emotional/cognitive*:
  - Depression
  - Emotional lability
- *Systemic*:
  - Fatigue
  - Lack of energy

initially to ensure patient acceptance.[41] Later, once the patient is comfortable, a standard dose of 1 mg daily may be ensured.

Tips and Pearls

- Finasteride is a USFDA-approved, effective, and vital drug in the management of patterned hair loss.
- Proper counseling of the patient is required before starting finasteride.
- Nocebo effect is a well-known effect with finasteride.
- No specific monitoring or blood test is required while starting the patient on finasteride, although a baseline PSA would be advisable to do at baseline in elderly males.
- The USFDA has advised to label suicide ideation and depression as side effects on the label of Propecia (finasteride).
- Sexual side effects are usually reported in <2% of cases, usually at higher dose (>5 mg/day) with finasteride and are reversible after stopping the medicine.
- Starting at lower dose or alternate days therapy and then shifting to full dose of 1 mg/day would be a better approach to gain the confidence of the patient.

REFERENCES

1. Sawaya ME. Antiandrogens and androgen inhibitors. In: Wolverton SE (Ed). Comprehensive Dermatologic Drug Therapy, 2nd edition. Philadelphia: Saunders; 2007. pp. 417-35.
2. Rittmaster RS. Finasteride. N Engl J Med. 1994;330:120-5.
3. Liang T, Heiss CE, Cheung AH, Reynolds GF, Rasmusson GH. 4-Azasteroidal 5 alpha-reductase inhibitors without affinity for the androgen receptor. J Biol Chem. 1984;259:734-9.
4. Shapiro J, Price VH. Hair regrowth: therapeutic agents. Dermatol Clin. 1998;16(2):341-56.
5. Sawaya ME. Novel agents for the treatment of alopecia. Semin Cutan Med Surg. 1998;17(4):276-83.
6. Stoner E. The clinical development of a 5 alpha-reductase inhibitor, finasteride. J Steroid Biochem Mol Biol. 1990;37:375-8.
7. Imperato-McGinley J, Guerrero L, Gautier T, Peterson RE. Steroid 5α-reductase deficiency in man: an inherited form of male pseudohermaphroditism. Science. 1974;186:1213-5.
8. Walsh PC, Madden JD, Harrod MJ, Goldstein JL, MacDonald PC, Wilson JD. Familial incomplete male pseudohermaphroditism, type 2. Decreased dihydrotestosterone formation in pseudovaginal perineoscrotal hypospadias. N Engl J Med. 1974;291:944-9.
9. Griffin JE, Wilson JD. The androgen resistance syndromes: 5α-reductase deficiency, testicular feminization, and related disorders. In: Scriver CR, Beaudet AL, Sly WS, Valle D (Eds). The Metabolic Basis of Inherited Diseases, 6th edition. New York: McGraw-Hill; 1989. pp. 1919-44.
10. Drake L, Hordinsky M, Fiedler V, Swinehart J, Unger WP, Cotterill PC, et al. The effects of finasteride on scalp skin and serum androgen levels in men with androgenetic alopecia. J Am Acad Dermatol. 1999;41(4):550-4.
11. Imperato-McGinley J, Miller M, Wilson JD, Peterson RE, Shackleton C, Gajdusek DC. A cluster of male pseudohermaphrodites with 5α-reductase deficiency in Papua New Guinea. Clin Endocrinol (Oxf). 1991;34:293-8.
12. Gormley GJ, Stoner E, Bruskewitz RC, Imperato-McGinley J, Walsh PC, McConnell JD, et al. The effect of finasteride in men with benign prostatic hyperplasia. N Engl J Med. 1992;327:1185-91.
13. Kaufman K. Androgen metabolism as it affects hair growth in androgenetic alopecia. Dermatol Clin. 1996;14:697-711.
14. Whiting DA. Diagnostic and predictive value of horizontal sections of scalp biopsy specimens in male pattern androgenetic alopecia. J Am Acad Dermatol. 1993;28:755-63.
15. Dallob AL, Sadick NS, Unger W, Lipert S, Geissler LA, Gregoire SL, et al. The effect of finasteride, a 5 alpha-reductase inhibitor, on scalp skin testosterone and dihydrotestosterone concentrations in patients with male pattern baldness. J Clin Endocrinol Metab. 1994;79:703-6.
16. Leyden J, Dunlop F, Miller B, Winters P, Lebwohl M, Hecker D, et al. Finasteride in the treatment of men with frontal male pattern hair loss. J Am Acad Dermatol. 1999;40(6):930-7.
17. Kaurman K. Treatment with finasteride 1 mg per day in men with male pattern hair loss. Australas J Dermatol. 1997;38:20.
18. Van Neste D, Fuh V, Sanchez-Pedreno P, Lopez-Bran E, Wolff H, Whiting D, et al. Finasteride increases anagen hair in men with androgenetic alopecia. Br J Dermatol. 2000;143(4):804-10.
19. Price VH, Roberts JL, Hordinsky M, Olsen EA, Savin R, Bergfeld W, et al. Lack of efficacy of finasteride in postmenopausal women with androgenetic alopecia. J Am Acad Dermatol. 2000;43 (5 Pt 1):768-76.

20. Shum KW, Cullen DR, Messenger AG. Hair loss in women with hyperandrogenism: four cases responding to finasteride. J Am Acad Dermatol. 2002;47(5):733-9.
21. Trüeb RM, Swiss Trichology Study Group. Finasteride treatment of patterned hair loss in normoandrogenic postmenopausal women. Dermatology. 2004;209(3):202-7.
22. Thai KE, Sinclair RD. Finasteride for female androgenetic alopecia. Br J Dermatol. 2002;147(4):812-3.
23. Yeon JH, Jung JY, Choi JW, Kim BJ, Youn SW, Park KC, et al. 5 mg/day finasteride treatment for normoandrogenic Asian women with female pattern hair loss. J Eur Acad Dermatol Venereol. 2011;25(2):211-4.
24. Oliveira-Soares R, E Silva JM, Correia MP, Andre MC. Finasteride 5 mg/day treatment of patterned hair loss in normo-androgenetic postmenopausal women. Int J Trichol. 2013;5(1):22-5.
25. Moghetti P, Castello R, Magnani CM, Tosi F, Negri C, Armanini D, et al. Clinical and hormonal effects of the 5α-reductase inhibitor finasteride in idiopathic hirsutism. J Clin Endocrinol Metab. 1994;79:1115-21.
26. Wong IL, Morris RS, Chang L, Spahn M, Stanczyk FZ, Lobo R. A prospective randomized trial comparing finasteride to spironolactone in the treatment of hirsute women. J Clin Endocrinol Metab. 1995;80:233-8.
27. Castello R, Tosi F, Perrone F, Negri C, Muggeo M, Moghetti P. Outcome of long-term treatment with the 5α-reductase inhibitor finasteride in idiopathic hirsutism: clinical and hormonal effects during a 1-year course of therapy and 1-year follow-up. Fertil Steril. 1996;66:734.
28. Carmina E, Lobo RA. A comparison of the relative efficacy of antiandrogens for the treatment of acne in hyperandrogenic women. Clin Endocrinol (Oxf). 2002;57(2):231-4.
29. Mysore V. Finasteride and sexual side effects. Indian Dermatol Online J. 2012;3(1):62-5.
30. Mondaini N, Gontero P, Giubilei G, Lombardi G, Cai T, Gavazzi A, et al. Finasteride 5 mg and sexual side effects: how many of these are related to a nocebo phenomenon? J Sex Med. 2007;4:1708-12.
31. Price VH. Treatment of hair loss. N Engl J Med. 1999;341(13):964-73.
32. Palusiński R, Barud W. Proscar and propecia—a therapeutic perspective. J Clin Endocrinol Metab. 2004;89(12):6359.
33. Bayram F, Müderris II, Guven M, Kelestimur F. Comparison of high-dose finasteride (5 mg/day) versus low-dose finasteride (2.5 mg/day) in the treatment of hirsutism. Eur J Endocrinol. 2002;147(4):467-71.
34. Rahimi-Ardabili B, Pourandarjani R, Habibollahi P, Mualeki A. Finasteride induced depression: a prospective study. BMC Clin Pharmacol. 2006;6:7.
35. Altomare G, Capella GL. Depression circumstantially related to the administration of finasteride for androgenetic alopecia. J Dermatol. 2002;29(10):665-9.
36. Römer B, Gass P. Finasteride-induced depression: new insights into possible pathomechanisms. J Cosmet Dermatol. 2010;9(4):331-2.
37. Lee SC, Ellis RJ. Male breast cancer during finasteride therapy. J Natl Cancer Inst. 2004;96(4):338-9.
38. Lucia MS, Epstein JI, Goodman PJ, Darke AK, Reuter VE, Civantos F, et al. Finasteride and high-grade prostate cancer in the Prostate Cancer Prevention Trial. J Natl Cancer Inst. 2007;99(18):1375-83.
39. Guess HA, Heyse JF, Gormley GJ, Stoner E, Oesterling JE. Effect of finasteride on serum PSA concentration in men with benign prostatic hyperplasia. Results from the North American phase III clinical trial. Urol Clin North Am. 1993;20(4):627-36.
40. Mazzarella GF, Loconsole G, Cammisa GA, Mastrolonardo GM, Vena G. Topical finasteride in the treatment of androgenic alopecia. Preliminary evaluations after a 16-month therapy course. J Dermatol Treat. 1997;8:189-92.
41. Mysore V, Shashikumar BM. Guidelines on the use of finasteride in androgenetic alopecia. Indian J Dermatol Venereol Leprol. 2016;82(2):128-34.

CHAPTER 24

Dutasteride

Deepthi M

Key Messages

- Dutasteride is a dual inhibitor of 5α-reductase enzyme (types 1 and 2).
- It is a potent inhibitor, 100 times for type 1 and almost 3 times for type 2, of 5α-reductase enzyme.
- It is 90% more effective in suppressing serum dihydrotestosterone (DHT) levels compared to 70% with finasteride.
- It is approved by Food and Drug Administration (FDA) only for benign prostatic hyperplasia.
- Off-label, it has been tried for androgenetic alopecia (AGA), female pattern hair loss (FPHL), frontal fibrosing alopecia, hormonal acne, and hirsutism.
- Similar to finasteride, it also helps in inhibiting androgen-mediated miniaturization of scalp hair.
- Its side effect profile is similar to finasteride which includes sexual side effects such as decreased libido and erectile dysfunction, which are temporary and are reversed once medication is stopped.
- It is pregnancy category X.

INTRODUCTION

Dutasteride is a Food and Drug Administration (FDA)-approved medication for use in men with benign prostatic hyperplasia (BPH). It is a competitive inhibitor of both isoenzymes types 1 and 2—5α-reductase that inhibits the conversion of testosterone to dihydrotestosterone (DHT).

PHARMACOLOGY

Dutasteride has a similar structure to finasteride except at the 21 carbon position, there is a trifluorophenyl group, which makes it highly electronegative **(Fig. 1)**. Due to this structure, probably, dutasteride can inhibit both isoenzymes and has longer elimination half-time. The elimination half-time of dutasteride is very long, 4–5 weeks, in contrast to 5–6 hours for finasteride. Due to its long half-time, it can be administered on a once-weekly regimen. It is metabolized by CYP3A4 and may have interactions with drugs metabolized by it. Oral dutasteride is available as soft gelatin capsules in a dosage of 0.5 mg in India.

MECHANISM OF ACTION

Testosterone is converted into more potent DHT by the 5α-reductase enzyme, which has two isoenzymes, types 1 and 2. Type 1 is present in the pilosebaceous unit (hair follicle and sebaceous gland), adrenal, liver, and

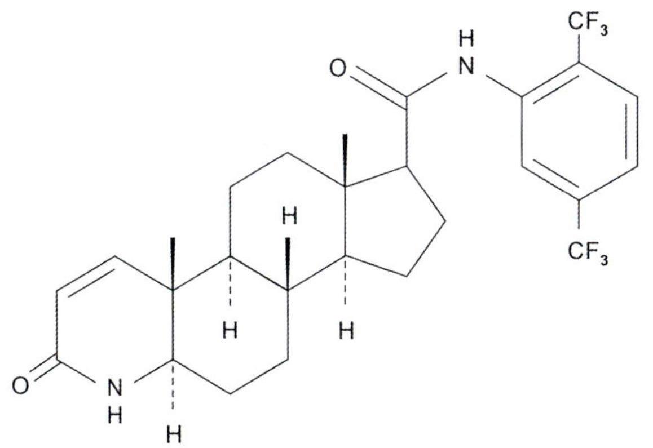

FIG. 1: Structure of dutasteride.

placebo-controlled study of dutasteride versus finasteride. J Am Acad Dermatol. 2006;55(6):1014-23.
11. Zhou Z, Cui Y, Wu J, Jin H. Efficacy and safety of dutasteride compared with finasteride in treating males with benign prostatic hyperplasia: a meta-analysis of randomized controlled trials. Exp Ther Med. 2020;20(2):1566-74.
12. Sánchez-Meza E, Ocampo-Candiani J, Gómez-Flores M, Herz-Ruelas ME, Ocampo-Garza J, Orizaga-Y-Quiroga TL, et al. Microneedling plus topical dutasteride solution for androgenetic alopecia: a randomized placebo-controlled study. J Eur Acad Dermatol Venereol. 2022;36(10):e806-8.
13. Saceda-Corralo D, Rodrigues-Barata AR, Vañó-Galván S, Jaén-Olasolo P. Mesotherapy with dutasteride in the treatment of androgenetic alopecia. Int J Trichol. 2017;9:143-5.

CHAPTER 25

Overview and Approach to Medical Management of Male Pattern Hair Loss

BS Chandrashekar, Priya Dsouza, Madura C

Key Messages

- Minoxidil and finasteride are the only evidence-based drugs till date for the management of androgenetic alopecia (AGA).
- Early recognition and intervention are key to stopping progression.
- Recent understanding of pathogenesis of AGA has led to emergence of multiple therapies with promising results, but still awaiting evidence.

INTRODUCTION

Androgenetic alopecia (AGA) without treatment is progressive. The timely onset of therapy can delay the progression of hair loss and thereby improve the quality of life of the affected people. Various myths regarding hair growth exist, which have aided quackery in the management. Proper knowledge of management with topical and systemic medications is essential. Camouflaging in the form of wigs can be used during therapy, and many patients might ultimately need to resort to hair transplantation.

MEDICAL MANAGEMENT

The choice of therapy in the management of AGA is based on the efficacy, practicability, ease of application, risk–benefit ratio, affordability, comorbidities, and side effect profile of the drugs. Currently, the Food and Drug Administration (FDA) recommends two drugs for the management of AGA, mainly topical minoxidil (TM) in the concentration of 2% and 5% and oral finasteride 1 mg orally.

Topical Minoxidil

Oral minoxidil (OM) has been used to treat hypertension since the 1960s.[1] Hypertrichosis because of minoxidil treatment was observed shortly thereafter and has been said to occur in 100% of users.[2,3] These observations led to the development of TM preparations, which were approved by the FDA in 1984. Both 2 and 5% solutions are currently in use for treatment in males; the 5% minoxidil solution has shown higher efficacy than the 2% solution. The drug is a vasodilator and has several mechanisms of action **(Fig. 1)**, which may lead to hair growth.[4-6] Details of the drug can be found in chapters 21 and 22 on Minoxidil.

The 5% minoxidil solution is more effective, and the standard formulation [with propylene glycol (PG)] is preferred. Patients should be informed of telogen shedding, which is usually seen in the first 8 weeks of therapy. The response to treatment should be assessed ideally at the end of 6 months.

Minoxidil preparations are available in various forms such as gel, lotion, foam, and spray. To overcome challenges such as reduced drug penetration, increased loss of minoxidil, scalp sensitivity, pruritus, irritation, and crystallization of minoxidil due to evaporation of ethanol and to enhance minoxidil absorption or to overcome the problem of nonresponders to conventional treatment, newer formulations/minoxidil boosters can be implicated.[8] Advantages of foam over standard formulation are that it is PG free (used in patients with allergic to PG), thermolabile (breaks down rapidly as soon as it meets the skin), there is little or no residue when it encounters skin, and it has the ability to deliver

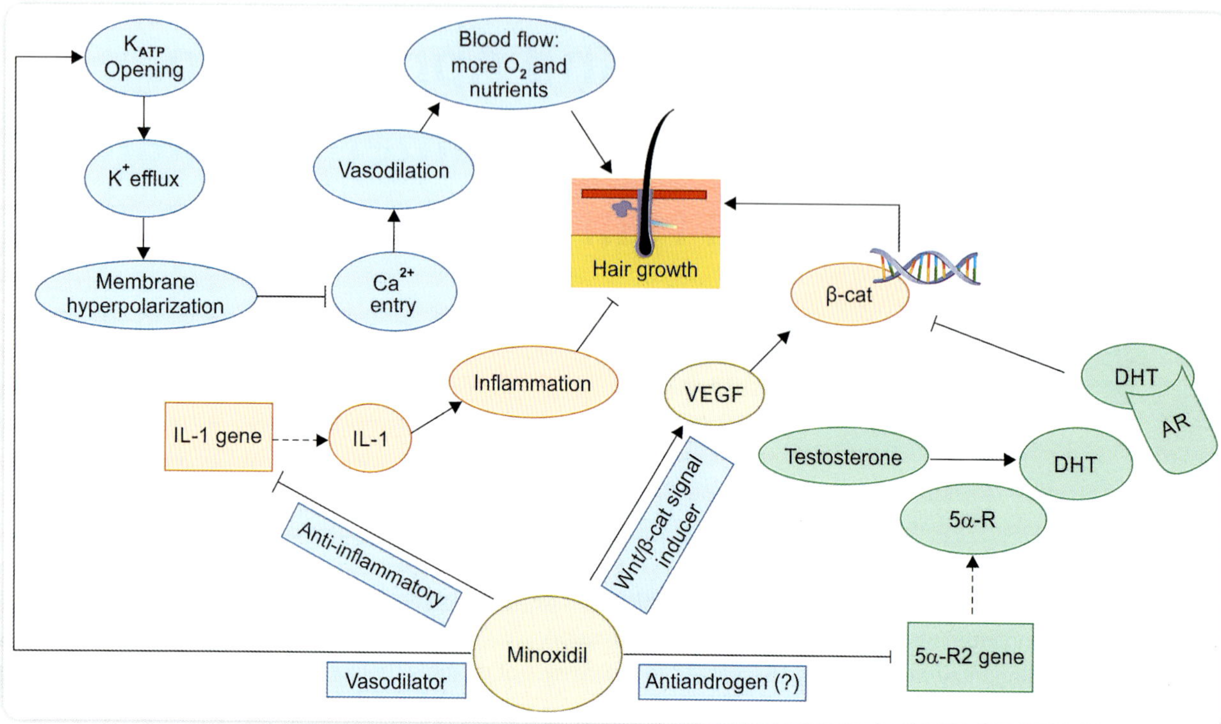

FIG. 1: Mechanism of action of minoxidil: Works through multiple pathways.[7]

(5α-R: 5 alpha-reductase; AR: androgen receptor; ATP: adenosine triphosphate; β-cat: beta-catenin; Ca: calcium; DHT: dihydrotestosterone; IL: interleukin; K: potassium; O_2: oxygen; VEGF: vascular endothelial growth factor; Wnt: wingless-related integration site)

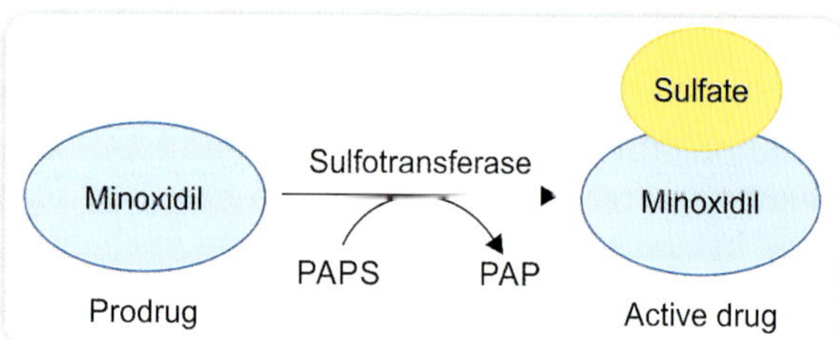

FIG. 2: Sulfotransferase converts minoxidil to minoxidil sulfate.[7]

(PAPS: 3′-phospho-5′-adenylyl sulfate; PAP: 3′-phospho-adenosine-5′-phosphate)

a greater amount of the active drug at an increased rate compared to other vehicles.[9]

Higher dose of TM like 10% can be used in patients who are low metabolizers to 5% and in nonresponders for better clinical response but not as a first line of treatment.[10]

Oral Minoxidil

Oral minoxidil remains an off-label therapy. Minoxidil is converted to its active form, minoxidil sulfate, in the outer root sheath (ORS) of the hair follicle by endogenous sulfotransferase enzymes **(Fig. 2)**. Sulfotransferases are xenobiotic metabolizing enzymes expressed in many tissues with the highest expression found in the human liver. Hair follicle ORS cells also express sulfotransferase, and ORS sulfotransferase activity predicts TM therapeutic response. Given orally, OM would be converted also by liver (SULT2A1) and platelet sulfotransferase and might reach a higher follicular accumulation. Expression of sulfotransferase in the scalp varies greatly between individuals, and this difference in expression explains the varied response to minoxidil treatment. Weak hair growth due to low follicular SULT1A1 can be overcome with OM through dose escalation.[7]

Conventionally, low-dose oral minoxidil (LDOM) refers to any dose below 5 mg. The hypotensive effect of OM occurs at dosages above 10 mg daily. The dose of OM in men is 2.5–5 mg/day, and the dose of 0.25 mg had the lowest incidence of hypertrichosis (<10% of patients). Gupta et al.[11] performed a network meta-analysis by comparing the effect on the change in terminal hair count after 24 weeks in male pattern hair loss (MPHL) and found that LDOM at a 5 mg/day dose was significantly more efficacious than 0.25 mg/day, topical 5% minoxidil foam/solution, and 5ARIs (5-alpha reductase inhibitors).

Major adverse effects of OM are sodium and fluid retention, cardiac effects, and hypertrichosis. Electrocardiogram (ECG) monitoring is required with a standard dose of OM. In a multicentric study of 1,404 patients, it is suggested that baseline ECG is unnecessary when doses of minoxidil ≤5 mg are administered; however, this should be assessed on a case-by-case basis.[12]

Clinical trials and studies have been conducted for sublingual minoxidil, and adverse effects observed were less compared to OM (mild hypertrichosis, mild postural dizziness, and peripheral edema). The rationale for use of sublingual minoxidil is to reduce the hemodynamic side effects, increasing the follicular minoxidil sulfate bioavailability.[13]

Low-dose oral minoxidil is an effective and safe treatment in healthy patients, having difficulties with TM preparation and those where TM is not effective due to deficiency of follicular sulfotransferase enzyme.

Minoxidil response test: Clinical response to 5% TM for the treatment of AGA is typically observed after 3–6 months. A prevalence of 40% individuals expresses low sulfotransferase enzyme. Two studies have previously reported that sulfotransferase enzyme activity in plucked hair follicles predicts a patient's response to TM therapy. The study of Goren et al. yielded an accuracy of 95.9% in ruling out nonresponders to TM for the treatment of AGA, thus demonstrating the clinical utility of minoxidil response testing prior to initiating prolonged therapy for AGA and switching to OM or 5ARIs in case of nonresponders to TM.[14]

Side Effect Profile

Itching of the scalp, increased dandruff, and erythema are commonly reported. Contact allergic dermatitis to minoxidil can occur and could be either to minoxidil itself or, more commonly, to PG or other constituents in the vehicle.[15] Patch testing is worthwhile in differentiating the cause of contact dermatitis, and the new minoxidil preparation that does not contain PG is an alternative in these patients. Hypertrichosis on the face and hands is a side effect observed in some people after TM.

5α-Reductase Inhibitors

The enzyme 5α-reductase converts testosterone to its active form dihydrotestosterone (DHT), and inherited sensitivity of the hair follicles to DHT is one of the etiological factors in AGA. Two types of 5α-reductase are seen in humans. Type I is seen mainly in the liver, skin, and scalp, while type II predominates in the prostate, genitourinary tract, and hair follicle.

Finasteride

Finasteride is a 5α-reductase type II inhibitor that acts by reducing scalp DHT levels. The optimal dose of finasteride in the treatment of AGA is 1 mg/day. Placebo-controlled studies have shown that finasteride significantly increases hair count after 1–2 years of therapy, and the effect is sustained after 5 years of therapy.[16,17] Oral finasteride 1 mg/day is recommended to improve or to prevent progression of AGA in male patients above 18 years with mild-to-moderate AGA. The response to treatment should be assessed at 6 months, although in some men, it may not become evident until 12 months. The rapid hair loss noted, with TM, after stopping does not happen with oral finasteride. According to Kaufman et al.,[16] the effect of oral finasteride is much better than the placebo group in 2 years, and reversal of hair density after withdrawal of oral finasteride after a year was noted. This was because of the increased levels of DHT once finasteride had been stopped. Studies in both humans and animals have shown that the combination of minoxidil 2% and finasteride 1 mg is superior to finasteride or minoxidil monotherapies.[18,19]

Topical finasteride, currently used as an off-label drug, when combined with TM yields promising results compared to minoxidil monotherapy.[20] Combination is considered beneficial to maintain hair density after achieving initial improvement with oral finasteride **(Figs. 3A to D)**, thereby obviating the use of oral finasteride indefinitely.[21] No systemic sexual side effects are noted. Patient compliance is better as there is no psychological fear of taking systemic medications and related side effects. A study conducted to compare the efficacy of oral versus topical finasteride by Hajheydari et al.[22] says that the efficacy of topical finasteride was at par with that of oral finasteride. However, the penetration of topical finasteride is of concern; hence, when combined with TM (vasodilator and potassium channel opener), it aids in better absorption. It is available as a combination of 2%, 3%, 5%, or 10% minoxidil with 0.1% finasteride.

Side Effects

Decreased libido, erectile dysfunction, and ejaculatory problems have been reported in around 3–5% of men.[23]

Gynecomastia, exfoliative dermatitis, testicular pain, and depressive mood changes have been observed in rare cases.[24] If treatment is started after the age of 45 years, monitoring of the prostate-specific antigen (PSA) level should be considered. The PSA levels may need to be taken as double the estimated baseline value to compensate for the reduction due to finasteride, resulting in an interpretation of the test remaining accurate.

Dutasteride

Dutasteride has similar characteristics to finasteride but is more potent in reducing scalp DHT. It inhibits both type I and II 5α-reductase enzymes. Dutasteride is FDA approved for the treatment of benign prostatic

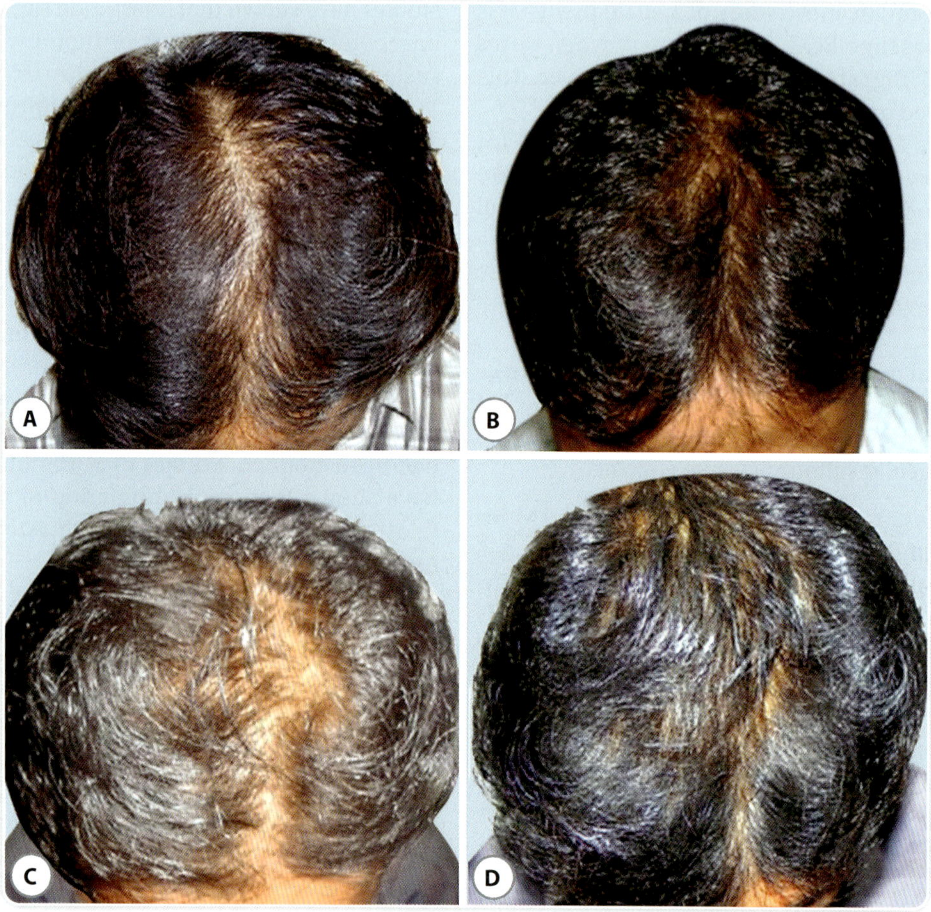

FIGS. 3A TO D: (A) Initial phase before starting treatment; (B) Improvement noticed after oral finasteride treatment; (C) Decline in hair density after stopping the treatment for a period of 8 months; (D) Good improvement in hair density after restarting topical medication (minoxidil with finasteride).[21]

hyperplasia (BPH). A randomized controlled trial (RCT) by Olsen et al.[25] demonstrated a dose-dependent increase in hair growth, and the efficacy of dutasteride 0.5 and 2.5 mg/day was superior to finasteride 5 mg/day. The mean reduction in DHT with finasteride was 70% and with dutasteride was >90%. Twin studies showed that dutasteride 0.5 mg/day for 1 year resulted in significantly more hair growth than placebo.[26] A retrospective Spanish study demonstrated no side effects with patients receiving low-dose dutasteride (0.5 mg one to three times weekly), and 66% of those in monotherapy presented with some degree of improvement.[27]

Despite being an off-label treatment, dutasteride is safe to assume according to the available evidence and demonstrates better efficacy with similar adverse effects profile than finasteride in MPHL.

Saceda-Corralo et al.[28] performed a multicentric retrospective study including 541 patients; in a first-year treatment with dutasteride (0.01% solution), mesotherapy was conducted once in 3 months' interval. International observer assessment improved in 89% patients. Eighty-six patients received dutasteride mesotherapy as monotherapy, response was assessed after 1 year, and clinical improvement could be observed in two-thirds of patients and one-third presented a marked improvement.

Dutasteride mesotherapy in combination with LDOM was seen to be more effective than LDOM as monotherapy. There were no statistical differences seen in the clinical response of the frontal area between both groups, but the combination group had significant clinical response in the vertex area.[29] Treatment algorithm has been proposed in the management of male pattern hair loss. Kindly refer to **Flowchart 1**.

Camouflage

Wigs, Prostheses, and Hair Extensions

Many men prefer wigs to scalp surgery. Wigs can either be interwoven with existing hair or worn over the top of existing hair. Interwoven wigs, also known as hair

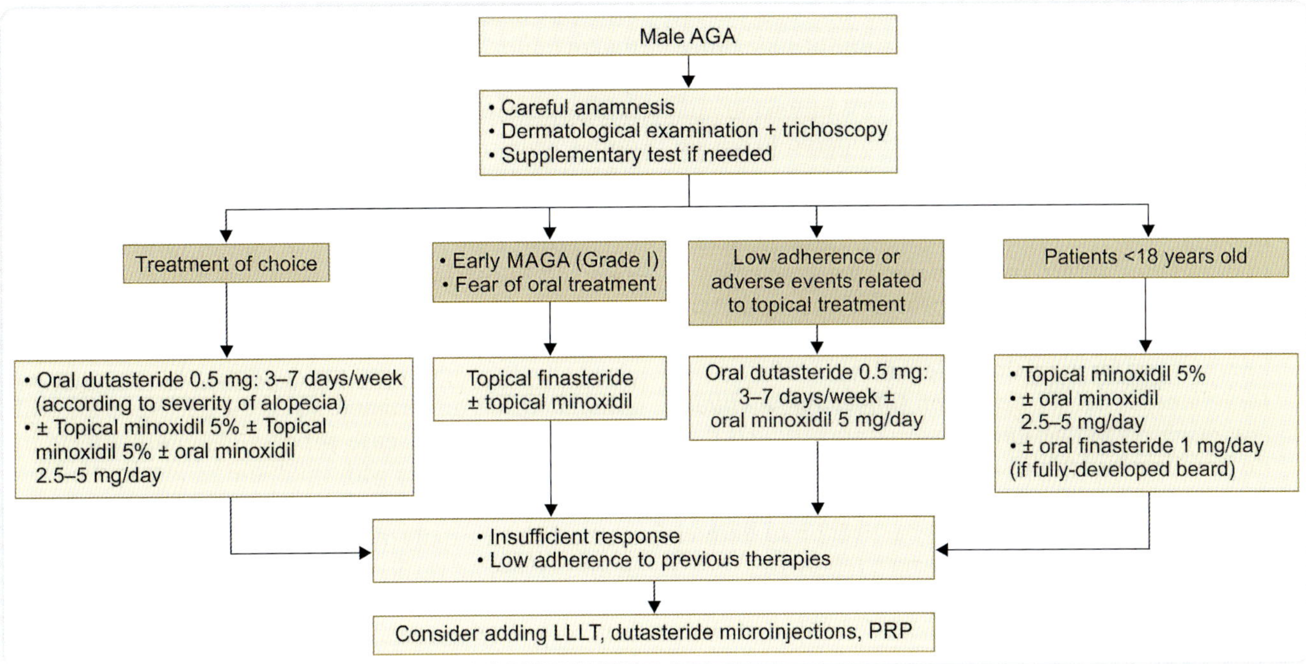

FLOWCHART 1: Treatment algorithm proposed in the management of male pattern hair loss.[27]
(AGA: androgenetic alopecia; LLLT: low-level laser therapy; PRP: platelet rich plasma)

extensions, tend to lift as the hair beneath grows and requires adjustment every few weeks; this may add considerably to the expense. Hair-thickening fibers create an illusion of thicker and fuller hair. These fibers bind to existing hair by static electricity as the positively charged wool keratin is attracted to negatively charged terminal and vellus hair of scalp.[30] The major disadvantage is the limited utility of these fibers in areas of complete baldness. Prosthetic hair implantation using synthetic hair is no longer recommended, mainly because of the high incidence of adverse effects.[31,32]

Scalp micropigmentation (SMP) uses a tattoo in a stippling pattern that mimics hair follicles that are cut close to the scalp. The process involves insertion of microdroplet of pigment into the dermis via skin. This method is helpful in men who do not qualify for hair transplantation, or in whom hair transplants have failed to achieve the density expected. It can help to disguise scalp scars post hair transplantation. SMP is a skill that needs to be acquired; otherwise, it can lead to pigment bleeding, color changes from poor choice of pigments, and poor procedure follow-up.[30]

EMERGING THERAPIES IN THE MANAGEMENT OF ANDROGENETIC ALOPECIA

The quest for better therapies with faster results, better compliance, and low side effect profile is never ending. There are thousands of unproven claims and products to help with hair regrowth. Some of the newer therapies which have been introduced are as follows:

- *Caffeine complex:* Caffeine enhances hair shaft elongation, prolongs anagen duration, and stimulates hair matrix keratinocyte proliferation. A topical combination of caffeine, niacinamide, panthenol, dimethicone, and an acrylate polymer (CNDPA) has been shown to improve hair fiber diameter, thus helping in enhancing the cosmetic appearance of patients with thinning hair.[33]
- *Platelet-rich plasma:* Hair follicle growth cycle is regulated by many growth factors such as vascular endothelial growth factor (VEGF), epidermal growth factor (EGF), insulin-like growth factor (IGF-1), and fibroblast growth factor (FGF). These factors help in transforming the dormant state stem cell follicle into an active state, thereby leading to hair growth.
- *Mesotherapy with growth factors:* Mesotherapy employs injections of pharmaceutical medications into the intradermal tissue. The mechanism of action could be explained by probable binding of growth factors to their own cellular receptors, resulting in activation of cell proliferation and/or differentiation. The efficacy of the modality lacks evidence.
- *Microneedling:* Microneedling has been hypothesized to produce hairs through microinjury.
- *Absorbable threads:* Insertion of different types of absorbable threads such as polydioxanone and poly-

L-lactic acid (PLLA) can increase the expression of hair-related genes and stimulation of hair bulge stem cells. Khattab et al. found 27.1% increase in hair density with combination therapy (2% minoxidil and one session of threads therapy), compared to a 5.4% in a 2% minoxidil-only group.[34]

- Various researches have demonstrated the underlying importance of Wnt proteins and wound growth factors in stimulating dermal papilla-associated stem cells.
- *Low-level laser therapy:* It is promoted as a safe and effective way for augmentation of hair growth, with low evidence for the claimed benefit
- *Miscellaneous agents: Bergamot, Ginkgo biloba, hibiscus, raspberry ketone, and adenosine* are products that do not have a definite scientific basis and evidence. The proposed mechanisms of actions have been:[32]
    - Promotion of hair growth by activation of dermal papillae and induction of anagen regrowth
    - Improvement of perifollicular vascularization
    - Inhibition of 5α-reductase and reduction of DHT activity
    - Anti-inflammatory effect
    - Improvement of hair follicle nutrition

A further extensive list of additional medications used in the treatment of AGA is explained in **Table 1**. *It is further clarified here that evidence for these modalities is either weak or nonexistent.*

DILEMMAS AND CONCERNS IN THE MANAGEMENT OF ANDROGENETIC ALOPECIA

Very often in our day-to-day clinical practice, we come across young men in their late teens or early twenties coming with the complaints of hair loss. Often, the physician's first reaction may be that the hair loss may be insignificant or the patient may just be showing exaggerated concern. However, proper understanding is needed to handle these cases. A young man with early baldness can have either apparent reduction in density of hair with increased daily hair loss or thinning and softness of existing hair or history of balding either on maternal or on paternal side. Trichoscopy can help in detecting miniaturization. The initial treatment can be TM in low concentration (3–5%) starting initially as twice-daily application with slow tapering to once-daily application. In these cases, a shampoo containing ketoconazole can be initiated daily or thrice weekly on an alternate-day basis. Ketoconazole is known to have a weak DHT-blocking effect and anti-inflammatory effect and also may be equivalent to causing hair growth similar to that of minoxidil 2%.[18]

Not uncommonly, we see a middle-aged man with diffuse loss of hair over the scalp progressing over a period of few years. Many times, they also have comorbidities such as hypothyroidism, other coexisting skin conditions, or chronic disorders such as hypertension and diabetes.

Diffuse hair loss can be a sign of diffuse alopecia areata, diffuse unpatterned hair loss, or chronic telogen effluvium. The essential step lies in confirming the diagnosis by dermoscopy or biopsy of the scalp, which also helps in prognosis of the condition. When treatment is initiated, it is important to stress the need for a full scalp treatment as the disease process generally affects the entire scalp. Patients with mild and moderate hair loss can be managed with TM 5% or TM 5% with finasteride 0.1% on a twice-daily basis for approximately 3–4 months before assessing response. In severe hair loss, oral finasteride or oral dutasteride remains a viable option along with topical 5% minoxidil solution.

Androgenetic alopecia being a chronic and progressive condition, compliance becomes a matter of question in these patients. The first step in managing a case of patterned hair loss is developing a rapport with the patient and having an open-ear approach to their doubts and fears to gain the confidence and instill faith, thereby removing the myths, false beliefs, and fears regarding their concern. Counseling the patient with respect to the disease process, possible effects, and adverse effects of the medications along with the probable expected outcome plays a vital role. Citing day-to-day chronic medical problems such as hypertension and diabetes may further help in explaining the chronicity of the problem and stress on the importance of continued medications. Reassuring the patient that after a while he can be maintained on mild and minimum required medication also adds on to the compliance and motivates the patient to continue therapy. Good quality pre- and post-treatment photographic records help in demonstrating visible improvement of the condition. In case of unsatisfactory results, add-on therapies such as low-level laser therapy, platelet-rich plasma, peptides, and advanced hair nutritional therapy can be considered.

Proper counseling and explaining regarding the possible side effects of oral finasteride may help in removing the phobia regarding the same.[54] Allowing a choice of medications after giving informed options also helps in improving compliance and sustaining therapy.

In many patients, response to drugs, particularly minoxidil, reaches a stage of plateau after about

TABLE 1: Summary of evidence for the use of miscellaneous agents in the treatment of androgenetic alopecia.

Molecule	Mechanism of action	Mode of administration
Caffeine[33]	Promotion of hair regrowth by activation of the dermal papillae and induction of anagen hair regrowth	Topical 0.001% and 0.005%
Adenosine[32]	Adenosine upregulates the expression of vascular endothelial growth factor and fibroblast growth factor-7 in cultured dermal papilla cells	Topical
Ginkgo biloba[32]	Activation of dermal papillary cells	Topical
Melatonin[35]	Counters the oxidative stress, antiapoptotic effect	Topical
Prostaglandins[36]	Inhibition of the activity of PTGDS (prostaglandin synthetase), PGD2, or GPR44	Topical
Proanthocyanidins[37]	Gets converted to proanthocyanins which have antioxidative potential	Topical
Retinoids[38]	Tretinoin has been shown to promote and regulate cell proliferation and differentiation in the epithelium and may promote vascular proliferation	Topical
Aminexil[39]	Antifibrotic and increases vascular circulation	Topical
Apigenin[40]	Increases capillary microcirculation	Topical
Botulinum toxin[41]	Decompression of the perforating blood vessels through relaxation of the investing musculature with concomitant increase in oxygen delivery to the coronal and frontal areas of the scalp. A secondary effect would be a reduction in the concentration of dihydrotestosterone (DHT) which is implicated as a primary factor in androgenic alopecia	Intradermal injections
Saw palmetto[42]	Weak inhibition of DHT activity	Oral, topical
Ketoconazole[43]	Inhibition of DHT activity	Topical
Zinc pyrithione[44]	Anti-inflammatory	Topical
Vitamin D[45]	Vitamin D receptor directly or indirectly regulates the expression of genes required for hair follicle cycling, including the Hedgehog signaling pathway	Oral
Platelet-rich plasma[46]	Increases blood circulation, growth factors are known to activate the proliferative phase and transdifferentiation of hair and stem cells and produce new follicular units. bFGF is reported to promote the in vitro proliferation of papilla cells and thereby plays a key role in elongating hair shaft	Injectable
Micronutrients and minerals[47,48]	Hair nutrition, sustenance, and vitality of hair follicle	Oral
Topical 1% Cetirizine[49]	Cetirizine is a second-generation H1 blocker. It inhibits the action of PGD2 (inhibitory effect on hair cycle) and promotes PGE2 (stimulatory effect on hair cycle)	Topical
Setipiprant[50]	PGD2 inhibits hair growth and hair lengthening, Setipiprant is a selective PGD2R antagonist. The first clinical study was conducted in AGA men with the dose 1,000 mg BID being generally safe and well tolerated but did not demonstrate statistically significant efficacy differences from placebo. Further studies are required to establish its potential	Oral
Pyrilutamide[51]	Androgen receptor antagonist (phase 3 clinical trial in China and USA)	Topical
Clascoterone[52]	Direct androgen receptor inhibitor. Recently approved by FDA for acne vulgaris. In phase 2 clinical trial for MPHL, target area hair growth as well as hair growth assessment scores increased when comparing it to vehicle	Topical
SAMiRNA-AR68[53]	Self-assembled Michelle inhibitory RNAs can decrease the androgen receptor levels via RNA interference. It has been tested topically in a clinical trial with the highest dose of 5 mg/mL once weekly in male and female patients; they showed an average increase in hair growth of 1.3–1.9 hairs/cm^2 per month, which could be comparable to oral finasteride	Topical

(AGA: androgenetic alopecia; bFGF: basic fibroblast growth factor; FDA: Food and Drug Administration; MPHL: male pattern hair loss; PGD2: prostaglandin D2; RNA: ribonucleic acid)

3–4 years of treatment, where the improvement in the condition may not be appreciated by the patient. This puts them in a scenario where they feel that the condition is not improving further, and doubts regarding therapy may set in which can lead to dropouts.

Demonstration of photographic records showing sustained improvement while on treatment motivates the patient to continue therapy. Buying time from the patient by explaining the hair cycle and hair remodeling process gives him time to accept and understand the disease process and see visible results of the treatment.

Many of these patients may discontinue all allopathic medications because of fear of side effects and in a desire to seek better results may resort to alternative therapies or in some cases they may be so satisfied with the results that they may discontinue the medical line of management without consulting the treating physician. It becomes imperative on the part of the treating doctor to reinforce the need for continued therapy when they return.

Maintaining photographic records helps in assessing the deterioration of the condition and in further current assessment and grading. Handheld dermoscopy can be a useful tool in assessing the perifollicular fibrosis and predicting response to treatment as well as for choosing the molecule for therapy. Based on the current grading of the condition, therapy can be restarted, and add-on therapies may be considered.

Considering the multipronged approach that we need to follow with both oral medications and topical applications in an advanced grade of hair loss, the patients are always concerned regarding the side effects and adverse effects of the same. Moreover, increased awareness through various sources such as peers and the Internet regarding the possible side effects of the medications always poses a concern in their minds. The most common phobia encountered in the practice of trichology is finasteride phobia. Acknowledging and addressing the concerns of a patient of finasteride phobia are of prime importance. Citing examples of evidence-based studies may help in satisfying the doubts of the patient.[36] Explaining the role of the drug in androgenetic hair loss with emphasis on benefits of the molecule if taken and outcome if not taken must be mentioned. While the patient is on medications, it is important to bring to his notice that side effects generally occur within 6–8 weeks of instillation of therapy which are usually reversible within 4–6 months of stopping therapy. Also, the dose and frequency of the medication can be altered and modulated based on the response, and a start-stop-start therapy may be considered to show the beneficial effects of the medication.

Combination therapies may be chosen in the following scenarios:

- Norwood–Hamilton grade IV onward
- Diffuse unpatterned hair loss
- Coexistent diffuse alopecia areata

Finasteride side effects: Although uncommon, every trichologist at some point of time has encountered patients who presented with side effects from the ongoing medications of AGA. Thorough knowledge of the side effects, the probable time frame within which it may occur, and the ways to tackle it are important and save the patient a lot of stress.

The most common side effects encountered with oral finasteride are listed below:

- Decreased ejaculatory volume
- Thinning of the ejaculated fluid
- Decrease in sperm count
- Impotence
- General weakness
- Myalgia

The first step of counseling involves reinforcing the fact that all side effects are likely to be reversible within 4–6 months after stopping therapy. For the concerns regarding the first three side effects, a semen analysis may be ordered for. If the side effects do not subside after discontinuation of therapy, an opinion of the uroandrologist may be sought.

SUMMARY

Treating a patient of hair loss is an art that requires gathering of data, building up of expertise, and practicing experience and evidence-based medicine to give the best possible outcome with minimum possible side effects.

Tips and Pearls

- Treatment is always tailored to the needs of the patient, physician's grading of AGA, and with proper counseling on treatment duration.
- The treatment must be a multipronged approach in advanced grade of hair loss.
- Maintaining photographic records helps in assessing the deterioration of the condition and in further current assessment and grading.
- Explaining the evidence of oral finasteride and especially its possible side effects, helps patients in removing the drug phobia and to be compliant.

REFERENCES

1. Kosman ME. Evaluation of a new antihypertensive agent: minoxidil. JAMA. 1980;244:73-5.
2. Devine BL, Fife R, Trust PM. Minoxidil for severe hypertension after failure of other hypotensive drugs. Br Med J. 1977;2: 667-9.
3. Jacobs D, Buttigieg CF. Minoxidil experience in Australia 1974–1980. Med J Aust. 1981;1:477-8.
4. Wester RC, Maibach HI, Guy RH, Novak E. Minoxidil stimulates cutaneous blood flow in human balding scalps: pharmacodynamics measured by laser Doppler velocimetry and photopulse plethysmography. J Invest Dermatol. 1984;82:515-7.
5. Lachgar S, Charveron M, Gall Y, Bonafe JL. Minoxidil upregulates the expression of vascular endothelial growth factor in human hair dermal papilla cells. Br J Dermatol. 1998;138:407-11.
6. Buhl AE, Conrad SJ, Waldon DJ, Brunden MN. Potassium channel conductance as a control mechanism in hair follicles. J Invest Dermatol. 1993;101:148s-52s.
7. Gupta AK, Talukder M, Venkataraman M, Bamimore MA. Minoxidil: a comprehensive review. J Dermatolog Treat. 2022; 33(4):1896-906.
8. Lopedota A, Cutrignelli A, Denora N, Laquintana V, Lopalco A, Selva S, et al. New ethanol and propylene glycol free gel formulations containing a minoxidil-methyl-β-cyclodextrin complex as promising tools for alopecia treatment. Drug Dev Ind Pharm. 2015;41(5):728-36.
9. Gogtay JA, Panda M. Minoxidil topical foam: a new kid on the block. Int J Trichol. 2009;1(2):142.
10. McCoy J, Goren A, Kovacevic M, Shapiro J. Minoxidil dose response study in female pattern hair loss patients determined to be non-responders to 5% topical minoxidil. J Biol Regul Homeost Agents. 2016;30(4):1153-5.
11. Gupta AK, Charrette A. Topical minoxidil: systematic review and meta-analysis of its efficacy in androgenetic alopecia. Skinmed. 2015;13(3):185-9.
12. Jimenez-Cauhe J, Saceda-Corralo D, Rodrigues-Barata R, Moreno-Arrones OM, Ortega-Quijano D, Fernandez-Nieto D, et al. Safety of low-dose oral minoxidil treatment for hair loss. A systematic review and pooled-analysis of individual patient data. Dermatol Ther. 2020;33(6):e14106.
13. Sinclair R, Trindade de Carvalho L, Ferial Ismail F, Meah N. Treatment of male and female pattern hair loss with sublingual minoxidil: a retrospective case-series of 64 patients. J Eur Acad Dermatol Venereol. 2020;34(12):e795-6.
14. Goren A, Shapiro J, Roberts J, McCoy J, Desai N, Zarrab Z, et al. Clinical utility and validity of minoxidil response testing in androgenetic alopecia. Dermatol Ther. 2015;28(1):13-6.
15. Friedman ES, Friedman PM, Cohen DE, Washenik K. Allergic contact dermatitis to topical minoxidil solution: etiology and treatment. J Am Acad Dermatol. 2002;46:309-12.
16. Kaufman KD, Olsen EA, Whiting D, Savin R, DeVillez R, Bergfeld W, et al. Finasteride in the treatment of men with androgenetic alopecia. J Am Acad Dermatol. 1998;39:578-89.
17. Finasteride Male Pattern Hair Loss Study Group. Long-term (5-year) multinational experience with finasteride 1 mg in the treatment of men with androgenetic alopecia. Eur J Dermatol. 2002;12:38-49.
18. Khandpur S, Suman M, Reddy BS. Comparative efficacy of various treatment regimens for androgenetic alopecia in men. J Dermatol. 2002;29:489-98.
19. Diani AR, Mulholland MJ, Shull KL, Kubicek MF, Johnson GA, Schostarez HJ, et al. Hair growth effects of oral administration of finasteride, a steroid 5 alpha-reductase inhibitor, alone and in combination with topical minoxidil in the balding stumptail macaque. J Clin Endocrinol Metab. 1992;74:345-50.
20. York K, Meah N, Bhoyrul B, Sinclair R. A review of the treatment of male pattern hair loss. Expert Opin Pharmacother. 2020; 21(5):603-12.
21. Chandrashekar BS, Nandhini T, Vasanth V, Sriram R, Navale S. Topical minoxidil fortified with finasteride: an account of maintenance of hair density after replacing oral finasteride. Indian Dermatol Online J. 2015;6(1):17-20.
22. Hajheydari Z, Akbari J, Saeedi M, Shokoohi L. Comparing the therapeutic effects of finasteride gel and tablet in treatment of the androgenetic alopecia. Indian J Dermatol Venereol Leprol. 2009;75:47-51.
23. Wilton L, Pearce G, Edet E, Freemantle S, Stephens MD, Mann RD. The safety of finasteride used in benign prostatic hypertrophy: a non-interventional observational cohort study in 14,772 patients. Br J Urol. 1996;78:379-84.
24. Rahimi-Ardabili B, Pourandarjani R, Habibollahi P, Mualeki A. Finasteride induced depression: a prospective study. BMC Clin Pharmacol. 2006;6:7.
25. Olsen EA, Hordinsky M, Whiting D, Stough D, Hobbs S, Ellis ML, et al. The importance of dual 5α-reductase inhibition in the treatment of male pattern hair loss: results of a randomized placebo-controlled study of dutasteride versus finasteride. J Am Acad Dermatol. 2006;55:1014-23.
26. Stough D. Dutasteride improves male pattern hair loss in a randomized study in identical twins. J Cosmet Dermatol. 2007;6:9-13.
27. Dominguez-Santas M, Diaz-Guimaraens B, Saceda-Corralo D, Hermosa-Gelbard A, Muñoz-Moreno Arrones O, Pindado-Ortega C, et al. The state-of-the-art in the management of androgenetic alopecia: a review of new therapies and treatment algorithms. JEADV Clin Pract. 2022;1:176-85.
28. Saceda-Corralo D, Moustafa F, Jaén-Olasolo P, Vañó-Galván S, Camacho FM. Mesotherapy with dutasteride for androgenetic alopecia: a retrospective study in real clinical practice. J Drugs Dermatol. 2022;21:742-7.
29. Villarreal-Villarreal CD, Boland-Rodriguez E, Rodríguez-León S, Le Voti F, Vano-Galvan S, Sinclair RD. Dutasteride intralesional microinjections in combination with oral minoxidil vs. oral minoxidil monotherapy in men with androgenetic alopecia: a retrospective analysis of 105 patients. J Eur Acad Dermatol Venereol. 2022;36:e570-2.
30. Saed S, Ibrahim O, Bergfeld WF. Hair camouflage: a comprehensive review. Int J Womens Dermatol. 2017;3(1 Suppl):S75-80.
31. Tsuboi R, Itami S, Inui S, Ueki R, Katsuoka K, Kurata S, et al. Guidelines for the management of androgenetic alopecia (2010). J Dermatol. 2012;39:113-20.
32. Lepaw MI. Therapy and histopathology of complications from synthetic fiber implants for hair replacement. A presentation of one hundred cases. J Am Acad Dermatol. 1980;3:195-204.

33. Davis MG, Thomas JH, van de Velde S, Boissy Y, Dawson TL, Iveson R, et al. A novel cosmetic approach to treat thinning hair. Br J Dermatol. 2011;165:24-30.
34. Khattab FM, Bessar H. Accelerated hair growth by combining thread monofilament and minoxidil in female androgenetic alopecia. J Cosmet Dermatol. 2020;19(7):1738-44.
35. Fischer TW, Trueb RM, Hanggi G, Innocenti M, Elsner P. Topical melatonin for treatment of androgenetic alopecia. Int J Trichol. 2012;4:236-45.
36. Blume-Peytavi U, Lonnfors S, Hillmann K, Garcia Bartels N. A randomized double-blind placebo-controlled pilot study to assess the efficacy of a 24-week topical treatment by latanoprost 0.1% on hair growth and pigmentation in healthy volunteers with androgenetic alopecia. J Am Acad Dermatol. 2012;66:794-800.
37. Kamimura A, Takahashi T, Watanabe Y. Investigation of topical application of procyanidin B-2 from apple to identify its potential use as a hair growing agent. Phytomedicine. 2000;7:529-36.
38. Bazzano GS, Terezakis N, Galen W. Topical tretinoin for hair growth promotion. J Am Acad Dermatol. 1986;15:880-93.
39. Camacho FM, Camacho-Serrano F, Moreno Gimenez JC, García HMJ, Polo PJ, Perea CM, et al. Treatment of alopecias of male and female patterns. Clinical efficacy of aminexil and SP94 in two surveys of 180 patients, men and women. Med Cutan Iber Lat Am. 2013;41:18-33.
40. Huh S, Lee J, Jung E, Kim SC, Kang JI, Lee J, et al. A cell-based system for screening hair growth-promoting agents. Arch Dermatol Res. 2009;301(5):381-5.
41. Freund BJ, Schwartz M. Treatment of male pattern baldness with botulinum toxin: a pilot study. Plast Reconstr Surg. 2010;126:246e-8e.
42. Rossi A, Mari E, Scarno M, Garelli V, Maxia C, Scali E, et al. Comparitive effectiveness of finasteride vs Serenoa repens in male androgenetic alopecia: a two-year study. Int J Immunopathol Pharmacol. 2012;25:1167-73.
43. Pierard-Franchimont C, De Doncker P, Cauwenbergh G, Pierard GE. Ketoconazole shampoo: effect of long-term use in androgenic alopecia. Dermatology (Basel, Switzerland). 1998;196:474-7.
44. Berger RS, Fu JL, Smiles KA, Turner CB, Schnell BM, Werchowski KM, et al. The effects of minoxidil, 1% pyrithione zinc and a combination of both on hair density: a randomized controlled trial. Br J Dermatol. 2003;149:354-62.
45. Rasheed H, Mahgoub D, Hegazy R, El-Komy M, Abdel Hay R, Hamid MA, et al. Serum ferritin and vitamin D in female hair loss: do they play a role? Skin Pharmacol Physiol. 2013;26(2):101-7.
46. Takikawa M, Nakamura S, Nakamura S, Ishirara M, Kishimoto S, Sasaki K, et al. Enhanced effect of platelet-rich plasma containing a new carrier on hair growth. Dermatol Surg. 2011;37:1721-9.
47. Floersheim GL. An examination of effect of biotin on alopecia and hair quality. Z Hautkrankheiten. 1992;67:246-52.
48. Pyo HK, Yoo HG, Won CH, Lee SH, Kang YJ, Eun HC, et al. The effect of tripeptide-copper complex on human hair growth in vitro. Arch Pharm Res. 2007;30:834-9.
49. Zaky MS, Abo Khodeir H, Ahmed HA, Elsaie ML. Therapeutic implications of topical cetirizine 1% in treatment of male androgenetic alopecia: a case-controlled study. J Cosmet Dermatol. 2021;20:1154-9.
50. DuBois J, Bruce S, Stewart D, Kempers S, Harutunian C, Boodhoo T, et al. Setipiprant for androgenetic alopecia in males: results from a randomized, double-blind, placebo-controlled Phase 2a trial. Clin Cosmet Investig Dermatol. 2021;14:1507-17.
51. National Library of Medicine (US). (2021, July–2021, August). Safety, tolerability and PK of KX-826 in healthy males with alopecia following topical multiple dose ascending. Identifier NCT04502901.
52. Cartwright M, Mazzetti A, Moro L, Rosette C, Gerloni M. A summary of in vitro, phase I, and phase II studies evaluating the mechanism of action, safety, and efficacy of clascoterone (cortexolone 17a propionate, CB-03-01) in androgenetic alopecia. J Am Acad Dermatol. 2019;81:AB13.
53. Yun SI, Lee SK, Goh EA, Kwon OS, Choi W, Kim J, et al. Weekly treatment with SAMiRNA targeting the androgen receptor ameliorates androgenetic alopecia. Sci Rep. 2022;12(1):1607.
54. Sato A, Takeda A. Evaluation of efficacy and safety of finasteride 1 mg in 3177 Japanese men with androgenetic alopecia. J Dermatol. 2012;39:27-32.

CHAPTER 26

Medical Management of Female Pattern Hair Loss

Manjot Marwah, Deepti M

Key Messages

- Management of female pattern hair loss (FPHL) is a difficult condition to treat due to its associated psychological impact and limited treatment options despite recent advances.
- Counseling is of utmost importance in this condition, and minoxidil 2% lotion topically remains the mainstay in all grades of FPHL.
- Different options, including medical, surgical, and camouflage, need to be used to provide benefits to the patients.

INTRODUCTION

Female pattern hair loss (FPHL) is one of the most challenging hair disorders to treat, due to its multifactorial etiology and associated psychological impact. The role of a genetic basis or androgenic nature has still not been clearly established, and the impact of iron deficiency and hypothyroidism is still debatable.[1-3] Multiple topical and oral medications targeting these etiologies have been tried; however, topical minoxidil has remained the mainstay in FPHL treatment, irrespective of the etiology. The role of antiandrogens has been proved successful in recent studies, especially in patients with hyperandrogenism.[4,5] Many newer modalities of treatment have also been introduced.[4]

Treatment for FPHL includes:

- Medical management
- Noninvasive or semi-invasive management
- Surgical management
- Cosmetic camouflage

COUNSELING

Irrespective of the grade of alopecia, all females with hair loss need good counseling. Patients should be explained the nature of their hair loss, the requirement of adequate investigations, and the necessity for long-term treatment and counseled regarding any unrealistic expectations. Stressing on these points helps in increasing patient compliance too. Making the patient aware of options such as surgical modalities and camouflage techniques helps decrease anxiety and depression in severely affected women.

MEDICAL MANAGEMENT

As the etiology of FPHL can be hormonal or nonhormonal, medical management is divided into the following groups:

- *Nonhormonal*:
  - Minoxidil 2% or 5% topically
- *Hormonal*:
  - *Antiandrogens*:
    - Antiandrogenic combination oral contraceptives [cyproterone acetate (CPA) and drospirenone]
    - Flutamide
    - Bicalutamide
    - Spironolactone
  - *5α reductase inhibitors*:
    - Finasteride
    - Dutasteride
- Miscellaneous adjuvant medications

Minoxidil

Minoxidil is the only US Food and Drug Administration (FDA)-approved topical agent for FPHL and can be used in FPHL in normoandrogenic and hyperandrogenic women.[6] Details are discussed in chapters 21 and 22 on Minoxidil.

Dosage

Topical minoxidil is the only FDA-approved treatment for FPHL. Minoxidil 2% lotion twice-daily (approved in 1991) and 5% foam once-daily application (approved in 2014) still are the mainstay treatment for FPHL. Although studies have claimed a better response to 5% lotion, the chances of side effects are higher with 5% lotion.[7] However, a study done by Blume-Peytavi et al. has shown that once-daily application of 5% foam causes lesser side effects and better compliance than 2% lotion twice daily with comparable efficacy.[8]

Side Effects

The side effects are minimal with 2% lotion. However, nonvirilizing hypertrichosis, irritant contact dermatitis (due to the propylene glycol vehicle), dryness, and deposition of the drug on the hair shaft mimicking dandruff are more with 5% lotion.[9] These effects are reversible on treatment break and reduction of concentration (within 4-6 months). The unsightly dandruff-like scaly appearance can be reduced by using shampoos with salicylic acid and/or zinc pyrithione (ZPTO).

Application

While prescribing, the following instructions are of utmost importance:

- The drug must be applied on a dry, nonoily scalp (as an oily scalp decreases absorption).
- Minoxidil should be applied as 1 mL of solution with a pipette twice daily or half a cap of foam once at night, gently massaged and left in place for at least 4 hours. When using the spray applicator, it has to be spread evenly over the affected scalp.
- Contamination of the pillow by trickling down of the lotion while sleeping can cause hypertrichosis of the face. Hence, patients should apply the drug at least 2 hours before going to bed.
- There is often an increase in hair shedding for the initial few weeks on starting minoxidil due to the anagen surge.[10]
- The efficacy of the drug should be decided only after 6 months.
- If the patient stops using minoxidil, she will lose only what she has gained over the last 3-4 months.[11]

Newer Formulations

Recently, gel and foam forms of minoxidil have been made available. Many minoxidil combinations with other formulations are available in the market.

Some newer combinations include the following:

- Tretinoin 0.05% or 0.01%, increases the absorption by three times, but the chance of irritation is greater with it.[12-15]
- Azelaic acid is also added to the combination occasionally.
- Redensyl has mainly four active ingredients: Dihydroquercetin glucoside, epigallocatechin gallate-glucoside (EGCG2), glycine, and zinc. Studies have shown that EGCG2 has anti-inflammatory properties by reducing interleukin (IL)-8 release from keratinocytes, stimulating dermal papilla fibroblasts, free radical action, and stimulating human hair follicle growth.[16-18]
- Procapil contains three active ingredients: Apigenin (vasodilatation), oleanolic acid (5α reductase 1 and 2 inhibitors), and histidine lysine peptides (promatrix metalloproteinase activity) and causes increased hair diameter, better hair anchorage, and hair growth.[16,17,19]
- Capixyl is a biomimetic peptide (acetyl tetrapeptide-3) known to increase hair density and hair width. In many preparations, it is added along with red clover extract, which acts as an inhibitor of 5α reductase 1 and 2.[16,19]
- Melatonin lotion may help in pattern hair loss patients by its melatonin receptor-mediated antiandrogen action and antioxidative effects.[20]
- Aminexil 1.5% is thought to reverse perifollicular fibrosis, but its superiority over minoxidil alone is not proved.
- Topical finasteride (no proven additional benefit).[21]

Antiandrogens

All antiandrogens act by inhibiting the binding of 5α-dihydrotestosterone (DHT) to androgen receptor. Due to this central action, all drugs in this category cause feminization of the male fetus, and hence oral contraceptive pills (OCPs) need to be administered along with them. Nowadays, many of these antiandrogens are synthetic progesterones and are given as combination OCPs.

Antiandrogenic Oral Contraceptive Pills

Antiandrogenic OCPs are the first-line therapy for women suffering from hair loss associated with polycystic ovarian syndrome (PCOS). PCOS being the most common cause of hormonal imbalance in premenopausal women these days, the importance of these drugs needs to be emphasized. Additionally, OCPs are also given along with antiandrogens; hence, selecting the right one is of utmost importance. An OCP contains estrogen and progesterone. The progesterone component can be proandrogenic or antiandrogenic. The third (norgestimate and desogestrel) and fourth (drospirenone) generation progesterones are considered least androgenic. Since the third-generation ones have higher thromboembolic properties, drospirenone is considered the safest and most antiandrogenic progesterone in combination OCPs.

The other newer synthetic progesterone with antiandrogenic properties is CPA.

Cyproterone Acetate

There is sufficient evidence to support the use of CPA benefiting FPHL associated with hyperandrogenism.[22-24]

Dosage regimens: In premenopausal women, cyclic antiandrogen therapy (CAT) is used globally, i.e., 100 mg/day of CPA on days 5–15 and 50 μg of ethinylestradiol on days 16–25 of the cycle.[25-27] In India, it is available as a combination of 2 mg CPA and 35 μg ethinylestradiol. It has been proved effective in FPHL along with additional 20 mg CPA on days 5–20.[28] In postmenopausal women, 50 mg/day of CPA daily is used.[29] CPA has not proved superior to spironolactone or topical minoxidil in FPHL, but one study has claimed it to be the best treatment option in FPHL.[30]

Side effects: Weight gain, menstrual irregularities, breast tenderness, nausea, decreased libido, and depression are few of the adverse effects. CPA is contraindicated in women with liver abnormalities due to its biliary secretion.

Drospirenone

Drospirenone is a 17α spironolactone derivative and has antiandrogenic, progestogenic, and antialdosteronic activities. It is used as an OCP at 3 mg/day with 30 μg of ethinylestradiol. Due to its antimineralocorticoid features, it has become the most widely used OCP as its dose does not cause any weight gain or fluid retention. However, the use of drospirenone simultaneously with spironolactone can increase the chances of hyperkalemia, though there are no studies to prove this theory.

Flutamide

Flutamide is a pure nonsteroidal antiandrogen and is approved in the USA only for prostate cancer. It has been considered as the treatment of choice for hair loss and hirsutism in PCOS and results in greater reduction in hair loss than any other antiandrogen or finasteride.[22,31,32]

Dosage

One study has proven that 250 mg/day for 1 year gives good results. However, to avoid the side effects, low doses (12.5–62.5 mg/day) along with OCPs can be administered and give satisfactory results in women with PCOS.[33]

Side Effects

At higher doses, hepatotoxicity is seen in 13% of patients and thus monitoring of liver transaminase is essential.[30] Increase in levels to more than twice the normal range should be an indication to stop the drug.[34] Since hepatotoxicity is so common and can be severe, this drug is not used frequently in the Indian scenario. Other common side effects are dry skin, lethargy, mood changes, decreased libido, and feminization of the male fetus.

Bicalutamide

Bicalutamide is a nonsteroid competitive inhibitor of androgens to the androgen receptor. It is metabolized in the liver and excreted in urine and feces. It has a longer elimination half-time (7 days), higher affinity to the androgen receptor, better tolerability, and less hepatotoxic when compared to flutamide. It is FDA approved for the management of prostate cancer. Due to its antiandrogen action, it can also be used for the management of FPHL, seborrhea, acne, hirsutism, and PCOS.

Dosage

Bicalutamide in doses of 10–50 mg/day has been tried in FPHL patients in few studies and showed good improvement in hair count with minimal adverse effects.[35-37]

Side Effects

The side effects include gastrointestinal upset, peripheral edema, menstrual irregularities, and reversible mild elevation of liver transaminases. Bicalutamide in combination with oral minoxidil helps in reducing the hypertrichosis associated with oral minoxidil. Bicalutamide is pregnancy category X and may cause feminization of the male fetus; hence, it is not advised in the reproductive age group.

Spironolactone

Spironolactone is approved in the USA for hypertension and in Australia for hirsutism. It is an antagonist of aldosterone with antiandrogenic action. Despite a lack of sufficient studies with an adequate cohort size, this drug is widely used in FPHL. There is no minimally effective dosage proved in the case of spironolactone.

Dosage

When used for 6 months at a dose of 50–200 mg/day, it can reduce the total testosterone level substantially.[38] Improvement is seen after 6 months of treatment.[39]

Side Effects

Spironolactone is a category C drug for pregnancy. The adverse effect of hyperkalemia is very rare in healthy women, but the physician must be aware of the risk and warn the patient from consuming excessive amount of bananas and/or coconut water. Other side effects such as lethargy, menorrhagia, and cutaneous side effects can occur. It can occasionally precipitate lupus-like eruptions and alopecia too.[40]

5α Reductase Inhibitors

There are two main drugs in this category that act on 5α reductase enzyme and block the conversion of testosterone to DHT, namely:

1. Finasteride
2. Dutasteride.

Finasteride

Finasteride exclusively acts on 5α reductase type 2 present in hair follicles and prostate and reduces systemic as well as peripheral follicular androgenic activity. It is the most commonly used oral drug in male androgenic alopecia at a dose of 1 mg/day and is US FDA approved for the same. It can be used in hyperandrogenic and normoandrogenic women too. Normoandrogenic women occasionally have high levels of 5α reductase; hence, they may tend to benefit from this drug.[41]

Dosage

In women, the dose requirement is higher. Studies have shown that a 5 mg/day dose is required in postmenopausal women with or without hyperandrogenism. In premenopausal women, it can be used along with an OCP at the same dose.[42] If the OCP is antiandrogenic, the dose of finasteride can be reduced to 2.5 mg/day.[43] Recently, it is also available as a topical agent; however, it did not have any advantage over minoxidil.[44]

Side Effects

Finasteride is a category X drug as it can cause feminization of the male fetus. It is generally well tolerated, and the adverse effects such as breast tenderness and decreased libido decrease after the first few months of therapy. It can be absorbed via the skin surface; however, the amount absorbed is too less to cause any effects. Nevertheless, it is advisable to inform the patient about this. Blood donations can be done after 1 month of stopping finasteride.

Dutasteride

Dutasteride acts on both type 1 and type 2 5α reductase. There are fewer reports of dutasteride in women. It is three times more potent inhibitor of type 2 enzyme than finasteride.[45] It can cause serious side effects on the fetus if used in a premenopausal female. It is not US FDA approved for hair loss.

Dosage

Due to the lack of studies, the same dose used in men is used in women, i.e., 2.5 mg/day.

A topical preparation used in mesotherapy has been shown to be effective in one study.[46]

Side Effects

The side effects of this drug are related to sexual performance and reproduction which are mainly seen in males.

Oral minoxidil: Oral minoxidil is not FDA approved for AGA. It is not used commonly for the management of AGA due to its side effects at a standard dose.[47] Recently, it has been tried in male pattern hair loss at a low dosage as most of the side effects are dose dependent and showed improvement in hair density and hair shedding. A study done by Sinclair with low-dose minoxidil 0.25 mg daily plus spironolactone 25 mg OD demonstrated minoxidil to be effective in FPHL and a safer alternative in women who cannot tolerate or are unwilling to use topical minoxidil.[48] However, larger studies are needed to study the efficacy and safety profile in FPHL. Side effects with oral minoxidil are water retention, hypertrichosis, postural hypotension, weight gain, and palpitations. Oral minoxidil is a pregnancy category C drug.

MISCELLANEOUS NUTRITIONAL AND ADJUVANT DRUGS

Various new studies have focused on different modalities of approach to hair loss in women and men. Newer target molecules and bioengineering have also been adopted in this field to overcome the limited treatment options. All these modalities work only as adjuvants and are still being researched. **Box 1** gives a brief list of a few of them, used in androgenic alopecia in men and women. They surely give us hope for newer more efficient drugs in the near future.

NONINVASIVE AND SEMI-INVASIVE MODALITIES

- Platelet-rich plasma (PRP) therapy is the newest adjuvant to all hair loss treatments and is being used worldwide; however, it does not work as an isolated treatment modality. Lack of sufficient studies and standardization in the methodology has raised questions on its efficacy.[49,50] Other forms of PRP, such as the use of human platelet lysate and growth factor concentrate, are also available commercially but are still under trial.

BOX 1 **Newer and alternative drugs used in the management of female pattern hair loss (FPHL).**

- *Iron supplements*: Extremely important in India, due to the high prevalence of iron deficiency anemia and proved association with hair loss[51]
- *Vitamin B12, folic acid, and biotin*: OCPs with CPA with ethinylestradiol can worsen B12 deficiency; hence, supplementation is required along with them[25]
- *Cysteine, histidine, copper, and zinc*: These amino acids and trace elements have been proved in a few studies to be beneficial. Copper peptides are nowadays one of the most marketed supplemental therapies[52]
- *Alfatradiol 0.025% solution*: Alfatradiol is a topical weak estrogen and 5α reductase inhibitor used in FPHL, but due to contrary results of the efficacy, the studies are insufficient[53]
- *Melatonin 0.1% solution topically*: Known to cause hormone alteration in DHT and testosterone, it has been tried in one study topically as 0.1% solution, leading to a significant increase in anagen hair[54]
- *Biomimetic peptides (trifolium pratense flower extract combined with acetyl tetrapeptide-3) used topically*: Its mode of action is by inhibition of 5α reductase activity, reduction of inflammatory reactions, and stimulation of ECM protein synthesis in the vicinity of the hair follicle[19]
- *Stemoxydine 5% solution*: It is a potent prolyl-4-hydroxylase competitive inhibitor, used topically to mimic hypoxic signals and maintain hair growth and cycling. In a single study, stemoxydine was applied once a day (6 mL), and at the end of 3 months of the trial, there was an increase of 4% in hair density. Currently, this molecule is patented by L'Oréal Research and Innovation, Clichy, France[55]
- *Valproic acid solution 8.3% topically*: Valproic acid (VPA), a widely used anticonvulsant, inhibits glycogen synthase kinase 3β and activates the Wnt/β-catenin pathway, which is associated with hair growth cycle and anagen induction[56]
- *Roxithromycin 5% solution used topically*: Roxithromycin increases hair elongation and inhibits catagen-like changes induced in vitro with IFN-gamma in murine and human hair follicles by its antiapoptotic activity to keratinocytes[57]

(CPA: cyproterone acetate; DHT: dihydrotestosterone; ECM: extracellular matrix; IFN: interferon; OCPs: oral contraceptive pills)

- Low-level laser and nonablative fractional lasers such as 1550-nm fractional erbium glass laser, 2940 erbium:YAG laser treatment in FPHL have been studied in very few studies; hence, their efficacy is questionable.[58-61]
- Another controversial therapeutic regimen that claims to improve androgenic alopecia by the improvement of vascularization and hair nutrition is mesotherapy. Vitamins, hormonally acting agents, etc., are intracutaneously injected, but there was no evidence of efficacy found.
- Botulinum toxin injection, in a dose of 150 U injected into the scalp muscles, may decrease the traction component by the pull of the muscle occipitofrontalis. This causes vasodilatation and an increase in the oxygen supply to the hair follicles. This may improve FPHL as low-oxygen environments favor the conversion of testosterone to DHT, while in high-oxygen environments, it is converted to estradiol. However, these studies still remain controversial due to lack of data.[62]
- *Microneedling*: This may work by the stimulation of dermal papillae stem cells and various hair growth-related genes and inducing activation of growth factors.[63]
- *Hair stimulating complex (HSC) (follistatin, Wnt 7a, and wound healing growth factors)*: Recently, bioengineered, nonrecombinant, human cell-derived formulation, termed hair stimulating complex, containing follistatin, Wnt 7a, and wound healing growth factors to promote hair growth activity in male pattern baldness, has been studied, with some promise. It is given as a single intradermal injection, with a 1-year follow-up.[64]
- *Dutasteride mesotherapy*: Dutasteride is a bigger molecule. Therefore, its efficacy is limited due to its penetration into the skin, and hence mesotherapy with dutasteride may provide better efficacy. This is demonstrated in the study done by Moftah et al.[65]
- *Monofilament threads* made of polydioxanone (PDO) and poly-L-lactic acid (PLLA) have been tried in small studies and showed improvement in hair count in FPHL patients.[66-68] Though the mechanism of action is not well elucidated, they may act on the same principle of microneedling by promoting constant connective tissue regeneration. A study by Khattab et al. showed that a combination of topical minoxidil with PLLA threads showed better improvement in terms of hair density, thickness, and appearance than topical minoxidil alone in FPHL patients.

SURGICAL MANAGEMENT

Nowadays, hair transplants are being attempted in women with a good donor area. Due to the chronicity of FPHL and scarce treatment options, most of the patients may already be applying minoxidil 2% lotion for 2–3 years prior to their consultation with no significant improvement and treatment failure. In such cases, to avoid frustration and depression in patients, surgery can be offered along with medical management.[69] This modality has been discussed in detail in the chapter 15 on Female Pattern Hair loss.

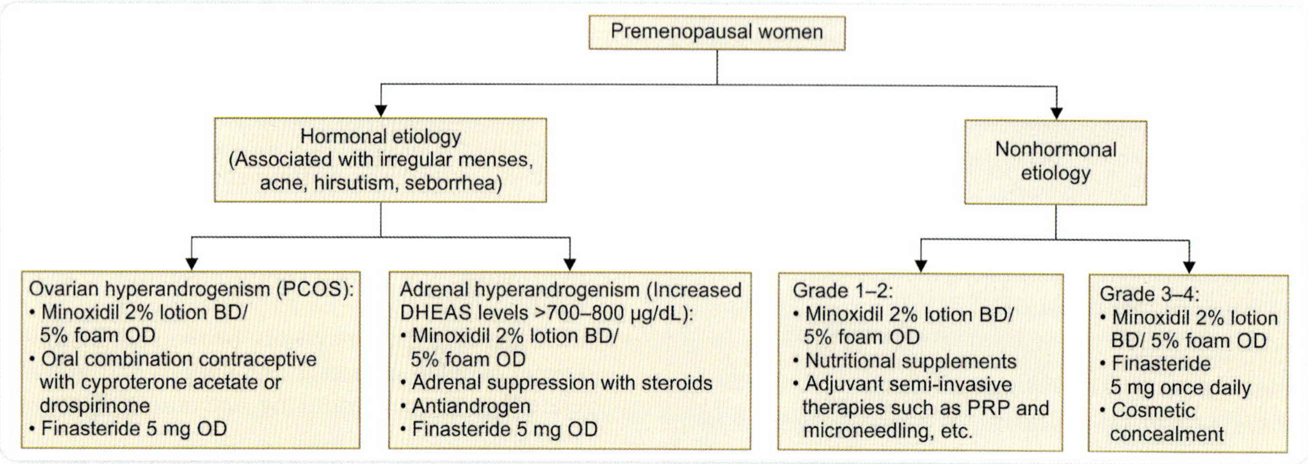

FLOWCHART 1: Algorithm to treat premenopausal women.

(DHEAS: dehydroepiandrosterone sulfate; FDA: Food and Drug Administration; OD: once daily; PCOS: polycystic ovarian syndrome; PRP: platelet-rich plasma)

COSMETIC CAMOUFLAGE

In severe cases, hairpieces and wigs are good camouflaging and concealment options. Mild grades of alopecia can be concealed with hair fibers and micropigmentation.

Scalp micropigmentation (SMP) is a new technique involving tattooing of the scalp in pinpoints giving an illusion of increased hair density. It has been discussed in detail in the chapter 33 on Hair Camouflage.

SUMMARY

Female pattern hair loss is a biological process that is multifactorial. Various medicines are used to treat it, few acting via a biological response to hormonal mechanism and few acting peripherally via nonhormonal mechanisms. Topical minoxidil (2% solution bid or 5% foam OD) is the only treatment approved by the US FDA, and it remains the mainstay in all treatment protocols for FPHL. However, the treatment approach of FPHL is changing with the recent trends. There are various medical, semi-invasive, surgical, and camouflage options available now. A newer approach combining all these modalities will give better patient compliance and more promising results. **Flowcharts 1 and 2** are algorithms to help formulate a treatment plan for patients suffering from FPHL.

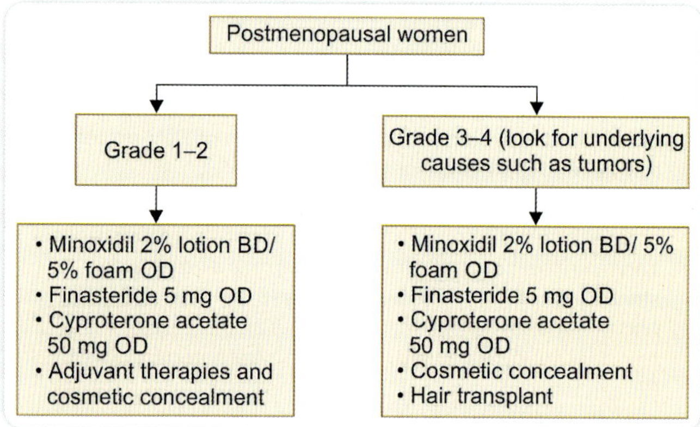

FLOWCHART 2: Algorithm to treat postmenopausal women.

Tips and Pearls

- Understanding the patient concerns and proper counseling for long-term treatment should be the first step in FPHL management.
- Topical 2% minoxidil twice daily or 5% foam application is the only FDA-approved medication in FPHL patients.
- Combination therapies of topical minoxidil with various plant-based products and topicals have been tried in few short studies with proven efficacy and hence can be tried.
- Antiandrogens such as spironolactone and bicalutamide have a role in female patients with other signs of hyperandrogenism, along with OCPs in the reproductive age group.
- Androgen inhibitors such as finasteride and dutasteride can be advised in postmenopausal women who reached a plateau phase with topical minoxidil or who are not responding with topical minoxidil lotion.
- Nonsurgical modalities such as monofilament threads and fractional nonablative lasers should be reserved for patients who are not responding to or who cannot be administered conventional therapies.
- Changing the hair style and using camouflage with microfibers and SMP can be suggested to willing patients in the early stages.

REFERENCES

1. Sinclair R. There is no clear association between low serum ferritin and chronic diffuse telogen hair loss. Br J Dermatol. 2002;147:982-4.
2. Kantor J, Kessler LJ, Brooks DG, Cotsarelis G. Decreased serum ferritin is associated with alopecia in women. J Invest Dermatol. 2003;121:985-8.
3. Messenger AG. Thyroid hormone and hair growth. Br J Dermatol. 2000;142:633-4.
4. Sawaya ME, Shapiro J. Alopecia: unapproved treatments or indications. Clin Dermatol. 2000;18:177-86.
5. Ludwig E. Classification of the types of androgenetic alopecia (common baldness) occurring in the female sex. Br J Dermatol. 1977;97:247-54.
6. Blumeyer A, Tosti A, Messenger A, Reygagne P, Del Marmol V, Spuls PI, et al. Evidence-based (S3) guideline for the treatment of androgenetic alopecia in women and in men. J Dtsch Dermatol Ges. 2011;9:S1-57.
7. Varothai S, Bergfeld WF. Androgenetic alopecia: an evidence-based treatment update. Am J Clin Dermatol. 2014;15(3): 217-30.
8. Blume-Peytavi U, Hillmann K, Dietz E, Canfield D, Garcia Bartels N. A randomized, single-blind trial of 5% minoxidil foam once daily versus 2% minoxidil solution twice daily in the treatment of androgenetic alopecia in women. J Am Acad Dermatol. 2011;65:1126-34.
9. Olsen EA. Pattern hairloss in men and women. In: Olsen EA (Ed). Hair Disorders: Diagnosis and Treatment. New York: McGraw-Hill; 2004.
10. Messenger AG, Rundegren J. Minoxidil: mechanisms of action on hair growth. Br J Dermatol. 2004;150(2):186-94.
11. Olsen EA, Weiner MS. Topical minoxidil in male pattern baldness: effects of discontinuation of treatment. J Am Acad Dermatol. 1987;17:97-101.
12. Bazzano GS, Terezakis N, Galen W. Topical tretinoin for hair growth promotion. J Am Acad Dermatol. 1986;15:880-3.
13. Savin RC, Atton AV. Minoxidil. Update on its clinical role. Dermatol Clin. 1993;16:188-92.
14. Camacho F, Mazuecos J. Advances in dermatologic therapy. Monogr Dermatol. 1994;7:211-35.
15. Yoo HG, Chang IY, Pyo HK, Kang YJ, Lee SH, Kwon OS, et al. The additive effects of minoxidil and retinol on human hair growth in vitro. Biol Pharm Bull. 2007;30(1):21-6.
16. Karaca N, Akpolat ND. A comparative study between topical 5% minoxidil and topical "redensyl, capixyl, and procapil" combination in men with androgenetic alopecia. J Cosmetol Trichol. 2019;5:1000140.
17. Park SY, Jeong YJ, Kim SH, Jung JY, Kim WJ. Epigallocatechin gallate protects against nitric oxide-induced apoptosis via scavenging ROS and modulating the Bcl-2 family in human dental pulp cells. J Toxicol Sci. 2013;38(3):371-8.
18. Kwon OS, Han JH, Yoo HG, Chung JH, Cho KH, Eun HC, et al. Human hair growth enhancement in vitro by green tea epigallocatechin-3-gallate (EGCG). Phytomedicine. 2007;14(7-8): 551-5.
19. Loing E, Lachance R, Ollier V, Hocquaux M. A new strategy to modulate alopecia using a combination of two specific and unique ingredients. J Cosmet Sci. 2013;64(1):45-58.
20. Fischer TW, Trüeb RM, Hänggi G, Innocenti M, Elsner P. Topical melatonin for treatment of androgenetic alopecia. Int J Trichology. 2012;4(4):236-45.
21. Sinclair RD, Dawber RPR. Androgenetic alopecia in men and women. Clin Dermatol. 2001;19:167-78.
22. Brzezińska-Wcisło L. Assessment of efficacy of Diane-35 in androgenetic feminine alopecia. Wiad Lek. 2003;56:202-5.
23. Singal A, Sonthalia S, Verma P. Female pattern hair loss. Indian J Dermatol Venereol Leprol. 2013;79:626-40.
24. Shrivastava SB. Diffuse hair loss in an adult female: approach to diagnosis and management. Indian J Dermatol Venereol Leprol. 2009;75:20-8.
25. Dawber RP, Sonnex T, Ralfs I. Oral antiandrogen treatment of common baldness in women. Br J Dermatol. 1982;107(Suppl): S20-21.
26. Vexiau P, Chaspoux C, Boudou P, Fiet J, Jouanique C, Hardy N, et al. Effects of minoxidil 2% vs. cyproterone acetate treatment on female androgenetic alopecia: a controlled, 12-month randomized trial. Br J Dermatol. 2002;146:992-9.
27. Hoedemaker C, van Egmond S, Sinclair R. Treatment of female pattern hair loss with a combination of spironolactone and minoxidil. Australas J Dermatol. 2007;48:43-5.
28. Peereboom-Wynia JD, van der Willigen AH, van Joost T, Stolz E. The effect of cyproterone acetate on hair roots and hair shaft diameter in androgenetic alopecia in females. Acta Derm Venereol. 1989;69:395-8.
29. Sinclair R, Wewerinke M, Jolley D. Treatment of female pattern hair loss with oral antiandrogens. Br J Dermatol. 2005;152: 466-73.
30. Camacho-Martínez FM. Hair loss in women. Semin Cutan Med Surg. 2009;28:19-32.
31. Martín-Hernández T, Jorquera E, Torres A, Camacho F, Herrera E. Effectiveness flutamide and cyproterone acetate in the treatment of hirsutism associated with polycystic ovary syndrome. Actas Dermosifiliogr. 1995;86:327-34.
32. Paradisi R, Porcu E, Fabbri R, Seracchioli R, Battaglia C, Venturoli S. Prospective cohort study on the effects and tolerability of flutamide in patients with female pattern hair loss. Ann Pharmacother. 2011;45:469-75.
33. Yazdabadi A, Sinclair R. Treatment of female pattern hair loss with the androgen receptor antagonist flutamide. Australas J Dermatol. 2011;52:132-4.
34. Dinh QQ, Sinclair R. Female pattern hair loss: current treatment concepts. Clin Interv Aging. 2007;2:189-99.
35. Carvalho RM, Santos LDN, Ramos PM, Machado CJ, Acioly P, Frattini SC, et al. Bicalutamide and the new perspectives for female pattern hair loss treatment: what dermatologists should know. J Cosmet Dermatol. 2022;21(10):4171-5.
36. Ismail FF, Meah N, Trindade de Carvalho L, Bhoyrul B, Wall D, Sinclair R. Safety of oral bicalutamide in female pattern hair loss: a retrospective review of 316 patients. J Am Acad Dermatol. 2020;83(5):1478-9.
37. Fernandez-Nieto D, Saceda-Corralo D, Jimenez-Cauhe J, Moreno-Arrones OM, Rodrigues-Barata R, Hermosa-Gelbard A, et al. Bicalutamide: a potential new oral antiandrogenic drug for female pattern hair loss. J Am Acad Dermatol. 2020;83(5): e355-6.

38. Neumann F, Schleusener A, Albring M. Pharmacology of antiandrogens. In: Hammerstein Androgenization in Women, Acne, Seborrhoea, Androgenetic Alopecia and Hirsutism: Lectures and Discussions of a Symposium, Berlin, February 23rd-24th, 1979. Bridgewater, NJ: Excerpta Medica; 1980. pp. 147-92.
39. Camacho F, Sánchez-Pedreño P. Spironolactone/in treating syndrome. Med Cut Iber Latin Am. 1993;21:107-14.
40. Georgala S, Katuolis AC, Georgala C, Moussatou V, Bozi E, Stavrianeas NG. Topical estrogen therapy for androgenetic alopecia in menopausal females. Dermatology. 2004;208:178-9.
41. Rogers NE, Avram MR. Medical treatment for male and female pattern hair loss. J Am Acad Dermatol. 2008;59:547-66.
42. Yeon JH, Jung JY, Choi JW, Kim BJ, Youn SW, Park KC, et al. 5 mg/day finasteride treatment for normoandrogenic Asian women with female pattern hair loss. J Eur Acad Dermatol Venereol. 2011;25:211-4.
43. Lorizzo M, Vinzenci C, Voudouris S, Piraccini BM, Tosti A. Finasteride treatment of female pattern hair loss. Arch Dermatol. 2006;142:298-302.
44. Lengg N, Heidecker B, Seifert B, Trüeb RM. Dietary supplement increases anagen hair rate in women with telogen effluvium: results of a double-blind placebo-controlled trial. Therapy. 2007;4:59-65.
45. Olsen EA, Hordinsky M, Whiting D, Stough D, Hobbs S, Ellis ML, et al. The importance of dual 5alpha-reductase inhibition in the treatment of male pattern hair loss: results of a randomized placebo-controlled study of dutasteride versus finasteride. J Am Acad Dermatol. 2006;55:1014-23.
46. Kohler C, Tschumi K, Bodmer C, Schneiter M, Birkhaeuser M. Effect of finasteride, 5 mg (Proscar) on acne and alopecia in female patients with normal serum levels of free testosterone. Gynecol Endocrinol. 2007;23:142-5.
47. Fabbrocini G, Cantelli M, Masarà A, Annunziata MC, Marasca C, Cacciapuoti S. Female pattern hair loss: a clinical, pathophysiologic, and therapeutic review. Int J Womens Dermatol. 2018;4(4):203-11.
48. Sinclair RD. Female pattern hair loss: a pilot study investigating combination therapy with low-dose oral minoxidil and spironolactone. Int J Dermatol. 2018;57:104-9.
49. Trost LB, Bergfeld WF, Calogeras E. The diagnosis and treatment of iron deficiency and its potential relationship to hair loss. J Am Acad Dermatol. 2006;54(5):824-44.
50. Morganti P, Fabrizi G, James B, Bruno C. Effect of gelatin-cystine and serenoa repens extract on free radicals level and hair growth. J Appl Cosmetol. 1998;16(3):59-64.
51. Wüstner H, Orfanos CE. Alopecia androgenetica and its local treatment with estrogen- and corticosteroid externa. Z Hautkr. 1974;49(20):879-88.
52. Fischer TW, Burmeister G, Schmidt HW, Elsner P. Melatonin increases anagen hair rate in women with androgenetic alopecia or diffuse alopecia: results of a pilot randomized controlled trial. Br J Dermatol. 2004;150:341-5.
53. Genty G, Lecardonel J, Bernard B, Rathman-Josserand M. P007: hypoxia and human hair follicle stem/progenitor cells. Int J Trichology. 2012;4(2):131-52.
54. Jo SJ, Shin H, Park YW, Paik SH, Park WS, Jeong YS, et al. Topical valproic acid increases the hair count in male patients with androgenetic alopecia: a randomized, comparative, clinical feasibility study using phototrichogram analysis. J Dermatol. 2014;41(4):285-91.
55. Ito T, Fukamizu H, Ito N, Seo N, Yagi H, Takigawa M, et al. Roxithromycin antagonizes catagen induction in murine and human hair follicles: implication of topical roxithromycin as hair restoration reagent. Arch Dermatol Res. 2009;301(5):347-55.
56. Marwah M, Godse K, Patil S, Nadkarni N. Is there sufficient research data to use platelet-rich plasma in dermatology? Int J Trichology. 2014;6:35-6.
57. Takikawa M, Nakamura S, Nakamura S, Ishirara M, Kishimoto S, Sasaki K, et al. Enhanced effect of platelet-rich plasma containing a new carrier on hair growth. Dermatol Surg. 2011;37:1721-9.
58. Leavitt M, Charles G, Heyman E, Michaels D. HairMax LaserComb laser phototherapy device in the treatment of male androgenetic alopecia: a randomized, double-blind, sham device-controlled, multicentre trial. Clin Drug Investig. 2009;29:283-92.
59. Lee GY, Lee SJ, Kim WS. The effect of a 1550 nm fractional erbium-glass laser in female pattern hair loss. J Eur Acad Dermatol Venereol. 2011;25:1450-4.
60. Ke J, Guan H, Li S, Xu L, Zhang L, Yan Y. Erbium: YAG laser (2,940 nm) treatment stimulates hair growth through upregulating Wnt 10b and β-catenin expression in C57BL/6 mice. Int J Clin Exp Med. 2015;8(11):20883-9.
61. Day D, McCarthy M, Talaber I. Non-ablative Er:YAG laser is an effective tool in the treatment arsenal of androgenetic alopecia. J Cosmet Dermatol. 2022;21:2056-63.
62. Freund BJ, Schwartz M. Treatment of male pattern baldness with botulinum toxin: a pilot study. Plast Reconstr Surg. 2010;126:246e-8e.
63. Dhurat R, Sukesh Ms, Avhad G, Dandale A, Pal A, Pund P. A randomized evaluator blinded study of effect of microneedling in androgenetic alopecia: a pilot study. Int J Trichology. 2013;5:6-11.
64. Zimber MP, Ziering C, Zeigler F, Hubka M, Mansbridge JN, Baumgartner M, et al. Hair regrowth following a Wnt- and follistatin containing treatment: safety and efficacy in a first-in-man phase 1 clinical trial. J Drugs Dermatol. 2011;10(11):1308-12.
65. Moftah N, Moftah N, Abd-Elaziz G, Ahmed N, Hamed Y, Ghannam B, et al. Mesotherapy using dutasteride-containing preparation in treatment of female pattern hair loss: photographic, morphometric and ultrustructural evaluation. J Eur Acad Dermatol Venereol. 2013;27(6):686-93.
66. Metwalli M, Khattab FM, Mandour S. Monofilament threads in treatment of female hair loss. J Dermatolog Treat. 2021;32(5):521-5.
67. Bharti J, Sonthalia S, Patil P, Dhurat R. Scalp threading with polydioxanone monofilament threads: a novel, effective and safe modality for hair restoration. J Eur Acad Dermatol Venereol. 2017;31(11):e492-3.
68. Khattab FM, Bessar H. Accelerated hair growth by combining thread monofilament and minoxidil in female androgenetic alopecia. J Cosmet Dermatol. 2020;19(7):1738-44.
69. Unger WP, Unger RH. Hair transplanting: an important but often forgotten treatment for female pattern hair loss. J Am Acad Dermatol. 2003;49:853-60.

PART F: Nonpharmacological Treatments

SECTION OUTLINE

CHAPTER 27

Microneedling in Androgenetic Alopecia

Madhulika Mhatre, Pratik Thacker

Key Messages

- Microneedling is a relatively new tool in the treatment of androgenetic alopecia, with multiple mechanisms of action being proposed.
- It stimulates hair growth by the local release of growth factors, increases angiogenesis, and upregulates Wnt proteins.
- Handheld dermarollers or motorized microneedling pens are commonly used with or without a meso-solution.
- Sessions can be done every 7–14 days for 2–4 months.
- Medical management needs to be continued simultaneously for long-lasting results.
- Safety and efficacy have been demonstrated in multiple studies, but standard guidelines have not yet been established.

INTRODUCTION

Microneedling is a minimally invasive procedure that creates multiple microinjuries on the skin surface using different handheld instruments, with the most common being dermarollers and motorized pens. It was first used in 1994 by Orentreich and Orentreich in the form of subcision and then by Camirand and Doucet for improving surgical scars using a tattoo gun without ink.[1] It has then been used extensively for facial rhytids, scars, and improving skin texture. Since the last decade, there has been a growing interest in the use of microneedling for promoting hair growth indifferent alopecias, especially androgenetic alopecia (AGA). In 2013, an Indian study by Dhurat et al. on 100 AGA subjects found that over a 12-week period, once-weekly microneedling combined with twice-daily 5% minoxidil increased hair counts significantly versus minoxidil monotherapy alone.[2] Since then, multiple studies have shown encouraging results using different protocols.

MECHANISM OF ACTION (FLOWCHART 1)

The following mechanisms of action have been accepted:

- *Increased production of growth factors and neovascularization*:[3,4] Microinjuries stimulate the dermal wound healing cascade. This leads to the local release of platelet-derived growth factor (PDGF), transforming growth factors alpha and beta (TGF-α and TGF-β), and fibroblast growth factor (FGF). Resultant fibroblast proliferation, in turn, leads to neovascularization and improved circulation. These together are believed to activate the stem cells in the hair bulge.
- *Upregulation of Wnt proteins*:[3,4] The activation of Wnt/β-catenin pathway plays a vital role in the transition of hair follicle from the telogen to anagen phase. This pathway is dysregulated in AGA-affected hair follicles, triggering apoptosis in dermal papilla. This leads to shortened anagen phase, depletion of papillary cells with each re-entry into the anagen phase, and hence progressive miniaturization of

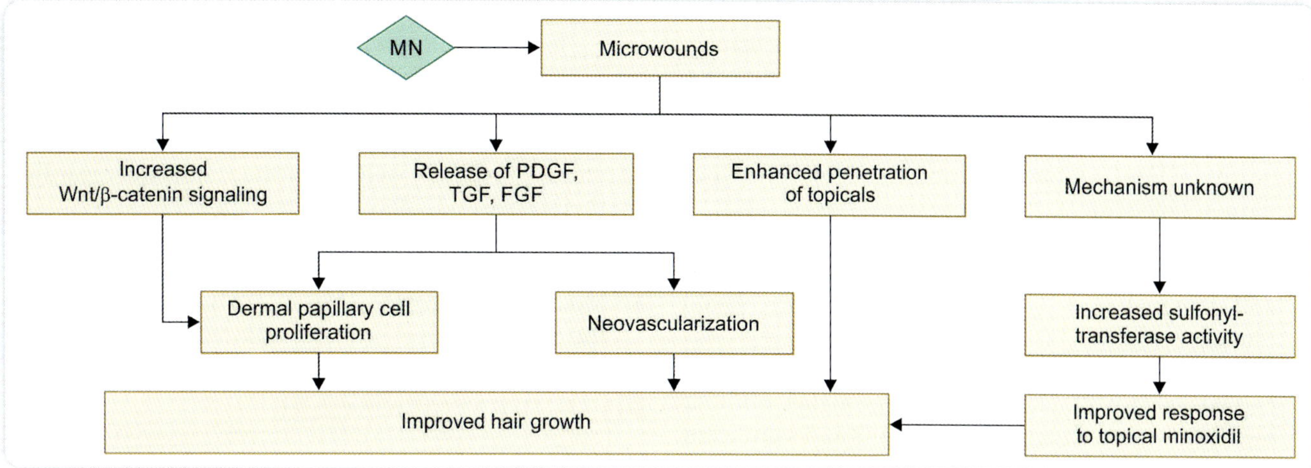

FLOWCHART 1: Mechanism of action.
(FGF: fibroblast growth factor; MN: microneedles; PDGF: platelet-derived growth factor; TGF: transforming growth factor)

hairs. Microneedling promotes anagen-initiating Wnt/β-catenin signaling and dermal papillae stem cell proliferation.

- *Overcoming topical minoxidil resistance*:[5] Sulfotransferase enzyme in the outer root sheath of hair follicles converts minoxidil from prodrug to active form, and its reduced activity leads to a poor response to topical minoxidil. Sharma et al. found that, over 21 days, once-weekly microneedling led to a median increase in sulfotransferase activity of 37.5% and hence achieved a better response compared to topical minoxidil used alone.
- *Improving transdermal penetration of topicals*:[6] Molecules > 500 kD do not penetrate the skin easily. Hence, microneedling has been used in many aspects of medicine to enhance the penetration of topically applied molecules. However, there are conflicting reports of the significance of topically applied mesotherapy solutions combined with microneedling, and its significance in AGA remains in question.

PATIENT SELECTION

Patients of any grade of AGA who are willing to follow-up regularly and can maintain good scalp hygiene before and after the procedure are selected. Among men, those with grades 3 and 4 are likely to respond the best.

- *Preprocedural evaluation*:
  - Rule out any inflammatory or infective scalp disorders.
  - Take a history ruling out any bleeding or clotting disorders.
  - Laboratory investigations are not needed for the procedure.

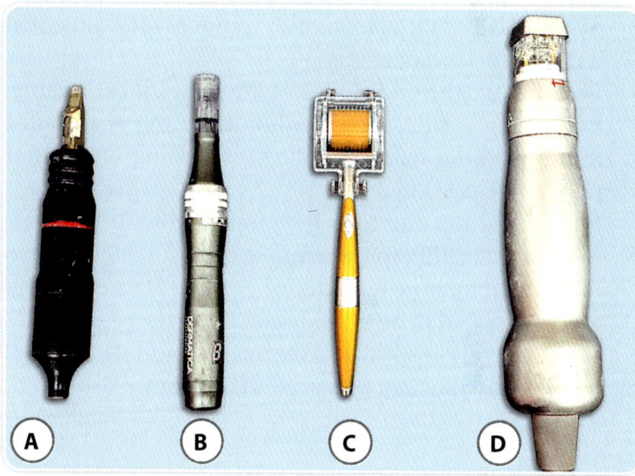

FIGS. 1A TO D: Various microneedling devices: (A) Tattoo device; (B) Microneedling pen; (C) Dermaroller; (D) Microneedling radiofrequency.

- *Microneedling devices* **(Figs. 1A to D)**:
  - Dermaroller
  - Microneedling pen
  - Tattoo machine
  - Microneedling radiofrequency

PRACTICAL GUIDELINES

Since there are no established best practices, the below guidelines are based on a compilation of studies and the author's practical experience:

- Ask the patient to have a shampoo wash before the appointment whenever possible. Additionally, cleanse the scalp with spirit and povidone iodine solution prior to the procedure.

- Anesthesia is generally not needed. Talkaesthesia and distraction devices such as a vibrator are usually sufficient. In overtly anxious patients, topical EMLA cream can be applied 1 hour before the procedure.
- Needle depth: Choose between 0.5 and 1.5 mm based on the patient's tolerability and the achievement of pinpoint bleeding.
- When using a dermaroller: Five to seven passes are generally needed, going along the vertical, horizontal, and diagonal axes. Apply moderate pressure. Avoid reusing dermarollers for multiple sessions.
- When using a motorized microneedling pen: Use cartridges with 12 needles or less, as higher number of needles cause entanglement of hairs and significant discomfort. Two to three passes are generally sufficient. Tips are not to be reused.
- When using a tattoo device, the authors use the round magnum 7 (RM7) needle cartridge **(Fig. 2)**.
- Rolling/gliding movements should be in the direction of the hair shafts to avoid unnecessary physical damage to the hair shafts.
- Even though the role of meso-solutions is questionable, massaging a cool, sterile solution on the scalp after microneedling has a significant soothing effect that patients appreciate.
- Microneedling can also be combined with platelet-rich plasma (PRP) in the same session since both have independent mechanisms of action. However, the following need to be considered:
  - When PRP is sprayed over microchannels, the PRP solution may not penetrate significantly.[6]
  - When injected, the pain of PRP injections or microneedling, whichever is done as a latter step, is significantly more.
- Microneedling can also be combined with synthetic growth factors or meso-solutions. However, their efficacy is still not well established, and data regarding their usage and safety is inadequate.
- Sessions can be repeated every 7–14 days for 8–12 sessions.
- Most studies have found results to be long-lasting with the continuation of proper medical therapy.

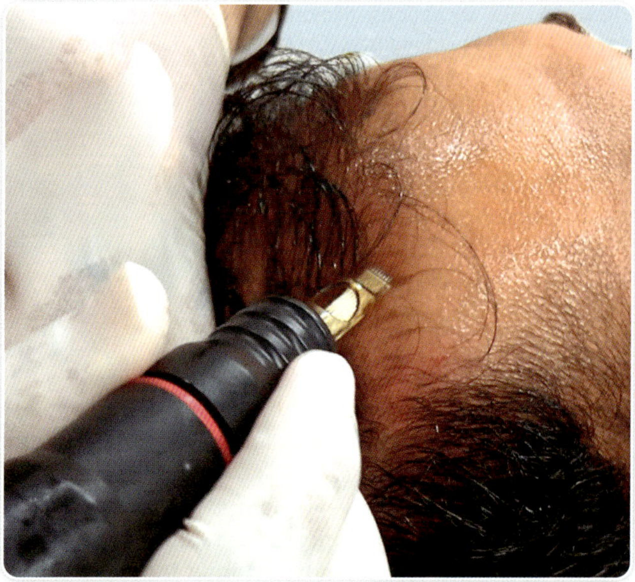

FIG. 2: Microneedling with a tattoo device.

POST-TREATMENT CARE

- Patients are asked to avoid excess sweating and dust exposure for 2 days after each session.
- Minoxidil applied on the same day, at night, is usually well tolerated. However, the patient may be asked to use it after 24 hours since the solution is likely to be nonsterile after few days of use.
- Hair wash with water can be allowed the next day and shampoo after 48 hours.
- Oral antibiotics are not needed. Topical antiseptics are usually not needed, and the decision to use them can be case-based.

Microneedling is a safe and a promising tool in hair stimulation for male and female AGA, with increasing support from the literature across the world.[7] The 2013 study by Dhurat et al. clearly showed that microneedling combined with twice-a-day topical minoxidil gave better results than topical minoxidil alone.[2] In 2016, Farid and Abdelmaksoud compared the results of microneedling combined with PRP versus topical minoxidil.[8] They established that without topical minoxidil, microneedling alone is clearly inferior to topical minoxidil alone, concluding that minoxidil monotherapy was more effective and should remain the first treatment option based on greater hair counts and faster hair growth time. However, they did recommend microneedling as an acceptable second-line treatment option for those who could not tolerate topical minoxidil. Lee et al. showed that microneedling with growth factor solution (FGF, vascular endothelial growth factor, insulin-like growth factor, keratinocyte growth factor, stem cell factor, superoxide dismutase, and Noggin) showed 10% higher hair counts compared to microneedling with isotonic saline at the end of 5 weeks.[9] This study included 11 women, and comparison was done on each half of the scalp in all women. A small sample size and a short follow-up period of just 5 weeks warrant more studies to establish the significance of topical growth factor solutions with mesotherapy. Modified microneedles are already being used to enhance drug delivery in other medical fields and may be the future in mesotherapy in AGA as well. These include coated microneedles, hollow microneedles, and dissolvable microneedles. Standard guidelines are yet to be established, and clinical best practices for now are largely anecdotal.

Tips and Pearls

- A significant number of patients getting PRP done drop out of treatment due to pain and discomfort. Pain of microneedling is much less making it the procedural therapy of choice for many AGA patients.
- Your intention while suggesting microneedling to your patient should be increasing hair density and not stopping acute episodes of hair fall. If hair fall exists due to a specific cause (e.g., recent illness or nutrition deficiency), it needs to be corrected first.
- Frequency and number of sessions may have a bigger impact on the outcome than the meso-solution used. Prioritize the patient's budget accordingly.
- Maintain good photographs and formulate a method to judge improvement objectively **(Figs. 3 and 4)**.
- Home-based dermarollers are a growing trend. These are 0.2–0.5-mm dermarollers and may not reach the desired dept in the dermis. Additionally, patients may not be efficient in cleaning and sanitizing dermarollers effectively before and after each use, leading to serious infection-related complications. There are no guidelines for their correct self-use.

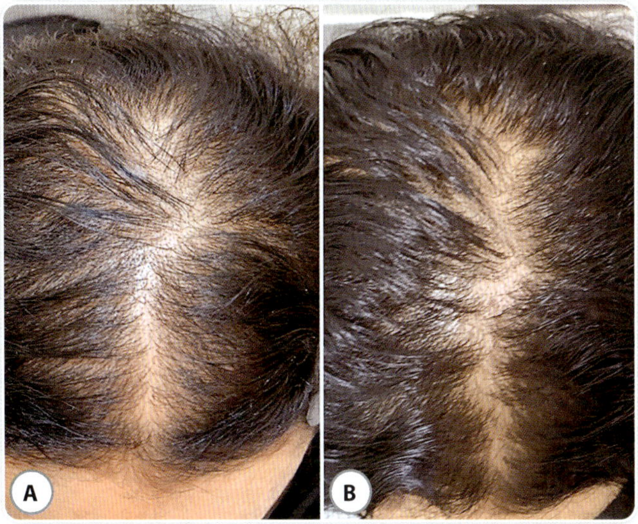

FIGS. 3A AND B: (A) Before and (B) after four sessions of microneedling with dermaroller.

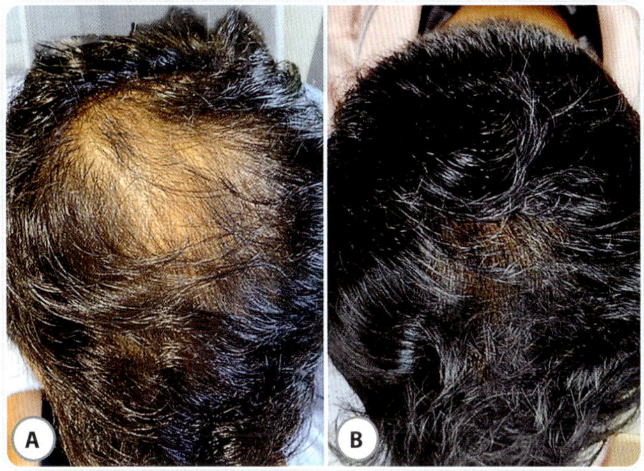

FIGS. 4A AND B: (A) Before and (B) after six sessions of microneedling with motorized microneedling device.

SUMMARY

- Microneedling is an emerging treatment in AGA. While early evidence shows promise, robust evidence is yet to be demonstrated for its use.
- Hence, it can be regarded as an additional option in the management of selected cases of AGA.

REFERENCES

1. Alster TS, Graham PM. Microneedling: a review and practical guide. Dermatol Surg. 2018;44(3):397-404.
2. Dhurat R, Sukesh M, Avhad G, Dandale A, Pal A, Pund P. A randomized evaluator blinded study of effect of microneedling in androgenetic alopecia: a pilot study. Int J Trichology. 2013;5:6-11.
3. Fertig RM, Gamret AC, Cervantes J, Tosti A. Microneedling for the treatment of hair loss? J Eur Acad Dermatol Venereol. 2018;32(4):564-9.
4. Schweiger ES, Boychenko O, Bernstein RM. Update on the pathogenesis, genetics and medical treatment of patterned hair loss. J Drugs Dermatol. 2010;9:1412-9.
5. Sharma A, Surve R, Dhurat R, Sinclair R, Tan T, Zou Y, et al. Microneedling improves minoxidil response in androgenetic alopecia patients by upregulating follicular sulfotransferase enzymes. J Biol Regul Homeost Agents. 2020;34(2):659-61.
6. Dhurat R, Sharma A, Goren A, Daruwalla S, Situm M, Kovacevic M. Mission impossible: dermal delivery of growth factors via microneedling. Dermatol Ther. 2019;32(3):e12897.
7. English RS, Ruiz S, Do Amaral P. Microneedling and its use in hair loss disorders: a systematic review. Dermatol Ther (Heidelb). 2022;12:41-60.
8. Farid CI, Abdelmaksoud RA. Platelet-rich plasma microneedling versus 5% topical minoxidil in the treatment of patterned hair loss. J Egypt Women's Dermatol Soc. 2016;13:29-36.
9. Lee YB, Eun YS, Lee JH, Cheon MS, Park YG, Cho BK, et al. Effects of topical application of growth factors followed by microneedle therapy in women with female pattern hair loss: a pilot study. J Dermatol. 2013;40:81-3.

CHAPTER 28

Regenerative Treatments in Androgenetic Alopecia: Overview

Aniketh Venkataram, Deeksha Rao Venkataram

Key Messages

- The pluripotent nature of stem cells underlies their vast potential for the treatment of androgenetic alopecia (AGA).
- The main sources for stem cells include bone marrow, adipose tissue, scalp tissue, and blood.
- Mechanical stromal vascular fraction (SVF) is currently the main source for adipose-derived stem cells (ADSCs). While promising, more research is needed.
- Hair follicle stem cells have the advantage of using the same surgical site; however, studies are in the phase of infancy.
- Such stem cell treatments should be used carefully, with proper consent and patient selection in a research setting.

INTRODUCTION

Regenerative medicine and the role of stem cells are being studied for applications in nearly every field of medicine. Hence, it was inevitable that they would be viewed through the lens of hair loss treatment too.

The pluripotent nature of stem cells underlies their vast potential for the treatment of androgenetic alopecia (AGA).[1] Add to this the attraction of using autologous tissue. However, traditional methods of obtaining stem cells were complicated, usually involving culturing. This meant that they were often expensive and could not be done in a single stage.

Several advances in recent years have heightened interest in this field. Chief among them are the evolution of simpler techniques to isolating regenerative elements and stem cells. These techniques are done in a single session with harvest, minimal manipulation (usually physical), and immediate injection. This reduces cost and eliminates regulatory issues with the use of stem cells.[2]

PHYSIOLOGY OF HAIR LOSS

Alopecia involves modifications to two types of stem cells: Hair follicle stem cells (HFSCs) and dermal papilla cells (DPCs). In scars, there is irreversible loss of these stem cells. But in AGA, these cells can be preserved till the late stage, which enables reversal.[3,4]

Hair follicle stem cells express markers including CD34, K15, K19, CD200, PHLDA1, and EpCAM/Ber-EP4. DPCs express alkaline phosphatase, alphaSMA, laminin, fibronectin, and CD133.[5,6] These markers are modified in disease states. CK15 and CD34 are both lower, especially in the frontal scalp in AGA. Stem cells in the bulge remain in the resting phase for the vast majority of their lives. They are influenced by the mesenchymal cells of the dermal papilla and appear to be key in hair growth signal transmission. Early techniques of stem cell treatment for AGA involved isolating these stem cells, culturing them, and then reinjecting them.

Stem cells are aimed at regenerating hair follicles through various methods:[7-9]

- Reversing pathological mechanisms
- Regenerating mature follicles from their parts, especially bulge cells
- Neogenesis of hair follicles in culture

The main sources for stem cells include:

- Bone marrow
- Adipose tissue
- Scalp tissue
- Blood

Bone marrow source is painful, expensive, and complicated.

ADIPOSE-DERIVED STEM CELLS

Normally, hair follicles encompassed by subcutaneous fat cells and the dermis shape an interfollicular dermal macroenvironment, which is imperative for maintaining the best possible growth of bulge and follicle cells.[10,11] Adipocytes emit BMP2 during the late catagen stage and early telogen stage, which supports the resting states in the niche, whereas emission of BMP2 is lessened toward the finish of the telogen stage, which bolsters the activation of hair follicle-derived mesenchymal stem cells (HF-MSCs). Thus, adipocytes have a critical role in extending the anagen stage.[11,12]

Adipose tissue contains numerous cells including adipocytes, adipose-derived stem cells (ADSCs), endothelial cells, fibroblasts, mural cells, and leukocytes.[13] The ADSCs have self-renewable capacity and display multilineage potential. The number of pluripotent cells contained in a cubic centimeter of adipose tissue is 100–1,000 times larger than the number of stem cells contained in bone marrow.[14] ADSCs also secrete various growth factors which have been shown to promote hair growth.[11,15-17] These growth factors include vascular endothelial growth factor (VEGF), hepatocyte growth factor (HGF), insulin-like growth factor-1 (IGF-1), platelet-derived growth factor (PDGF), keratinocyte growth factor (KGF), and fibroblast growth factors 1 and 2 **(Table 1)**.

TABLE 1: Role of growth factors.

Growth factors	Mechanism of hair stimulation
Vascular endothelial growth factor (VEGF)	Improves perifollicular vascularization, resulting in increased size of hair follicles and shafts[15]
Hepatocyte growth factor (HGF)	Delays transition from anagen to telogen, has mild anagen inducible property, promotes hair follicle growth, and elongates the hair length[16]
Platelet-derived growth factor (PDGF)	Induces and maintains the anagen phase of the hair cycle[17]
Insulin-like growth factor-1 (IGF-1)	Prolongs resting phase of the hair cycle and delays initiation of the new anagen phase. Promotes follicular proliferation and differentiation[11]
Keratinocyte growth factor (KGF) (fibroblast growth factor-10)	Stimulates proliferation and differentiation of early progenitor cells within the hair follicles. Induces anagen phase in resting hair follicles[18,19]
Fibroblast growth factor-1 (FGF-1), FGF-2	Induces anagen phase in resting hair follicles[19]

Adipose-derived stem cells-derived proteins improve hair growth and protect human DPCs against cytotoxic injury caused by androgen and reactive oxygen species. Moreover, adipose-derived stem cell-conditioned media (ADSC-CM) induces the anagen phase, promotes hair growth in mice, and enhances the elongation of hair shafts in ex vivo human hair organ cultures. ADSC-CM promotes hair growth in vitro, ex vivo, and in vivo.

Stromal Vascular Fraction

The stromal vascular fraction (SVF) refers to all the cellular elements of the adipose tissue, excluding adipocytes. It includes smooth muscle cells, endothelial cells, blood cells, stem cells, and extracellular matrix. Although adipocytes represent 80–90% of the volume of the harvested fat, they only represent 25% of the cell count. The remaining 75% is called the SVF **(Fig. 1)**.[18] The majority of the activity of SVF is attributable to ADSCs. However, evidence suggests that the presence of all the SVF cellular elements is helpful for ADSC activity. This phenomenon is attributed to the intercellular cross-talking and signaling between these cells.[19]

Mechanism of Isolation

Stromal vascular fraction is obtained by two methods: Chemical and mechanical. The goal in both these methods is to maintain the viability of stem cells and other nucleated cells of the SVF.

Chemical methods involve enzymatic digestion with collagenase, which is subsequently inactivated. The pool of mononuclear cells is then isolated through filtration and centrifugation. This chemical SVF can then be used to culture ADSCs. Hence, SVF can be an intermediate step in the preparation of ADSCs.[20]

Enzymatic techniques are superior in terms of their ability to concentrate the SVF. However, they are limited by the additional time and equipment required.

Mechanical methods use physical disruption, such as shaking, vortexing, and sonification, followed by washing and filtration. They contain fragments of extracellular matrix along with the cells.[21]

Mechanical SVF has found increasing popularity in the field of aesthetic regenerative therapy as follows:

- It is easier to perform.
- It requires less equipment.
- It can be done in one sitting along with the harvest.
- It does not require any regulatory oversight.

Analysis of Studies on Adipose Tissue as a Treatment for Hair Regeneration

Fat has been used in several ways for hair regeneration: Autologous fat transfer, nano fat, and adipose-derived stromal vascular fraction (ADSVF).

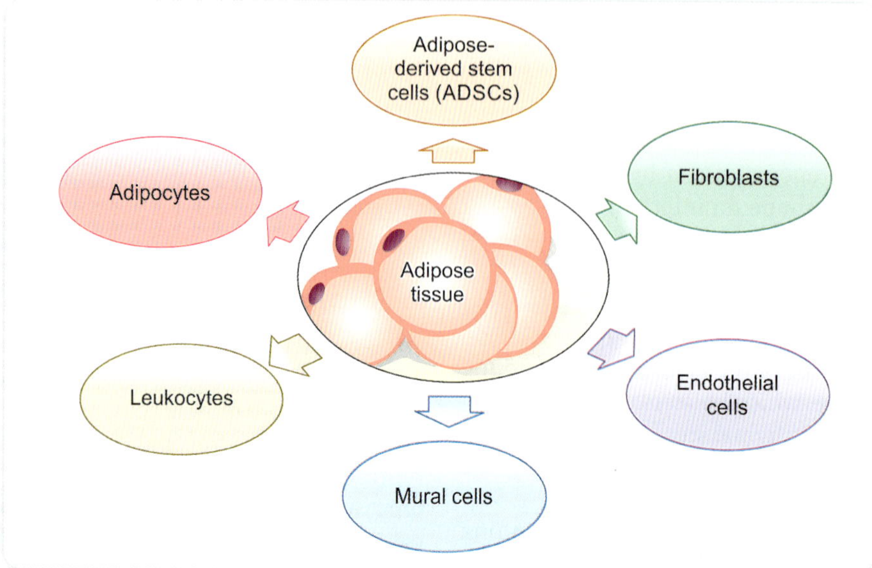

FIG. 1: Contents of stromal vascular fraction (SVF).

Autologous Fat

Dini et al. reported a case of a 25-year-old woman with alopecia areata of the left eyebrow with atrophy caused by intralesional steroid. After one session of autologous fat transplantation (AFT), not only was there an expected improvement in the atrophic scar, hair regrowth was observed in the lesion 3 months after the fat transfer.[22] Cho et al. reported a case of a 26-year-old woman with alopecia secondary to localized scleroderma which extended to the frontal scalp as an atrophic alopecic patch. Two sessions of AFT at 3-month intervals were performed. In addition to improvement in the atrophy and depression, regrowth of terminal hairs was observed at 3 months, which had further grown thicker and longer 3 months after the second AFT.[23]

Studies Using Nanofat

Nanofat is a form of mechanically emulsified SVF first described by Tonnard et al. in 2013.[24] Vestita et al. described a study using nanofat for androgenic alopecia in 12 cases.[25] Authors prepared nanofat using the Tonnard protocol, and a single session of nanofat injection was given. Each treated area showed an increase in the number and thickness of hair. Patient satisfaction was also found to have improved significantly after 6 months onward.[26]

Studies using Stromal Vascular Fraction

Shin et al. performed a retrospective observational study in 27 patients with female patterned hair loss (PHL) treated with ADSC-CM[20] [commercial ADSC-CM product called AAPE™ (advanced ADSC protein extract), Prostemics Co., Ltd., Seoul, South Korea].[25] After 12 weeks of treatment, mean hair density increased from 105.4 to 122.7 hairs/cm^2, representing an increase of 16.4%. Mean hair thickness increased from 57.5 to 64.0 μm, an increase of 11.3%. These improvements were statistically significant.

Fukuoka et al. published three studies[24,27,28] in which they evaluated the hair regenerative effects of AAPE™ in patients with male- and female PHL. All three of these studies showed statistically significant improvement in hair growth. However, while the authors performed three studies over 5 years, they seem to have recruited different patients in each study, and hence the follow-up period was not long in any of the studies.

Perez-Meza et al. performed an observational study on nine patients with female- and male PHL using a mixture of purified fat and SVF. A mean increase of 31 hairs/cm^2 of the scalp (23% relative percentage increase) was documented in five patients with proper follow-up. However, no statistically significant change was noted in cumulative thickness or percentage of hairs in the anagen or telogen phase.[29]

Such low-quality studies and lack of higher level of evidence are true of all new treatment modalities. But based on the above review, it can be said that adipose tissue and ADSCs may represent a new and promising therapy for hair regeneration, and physicians need to be aware of developments in this field. High-quality large randomized controlled trials (RCTs) are needed so that standardized and effective protocols can be made.

HAIR FOLLICLE

Zanzottera et al. reported a case series of three patients who underwent hair restoration surgery along with the application of ADSCs and growth factors. ADSC was obtained from hypodermis and adipose tissue discarded from the donor strip of the scalp, processed using the Rigenera system. The Rigenera device is a standardized sample preparation system for the automated mechanical disaggregation of cell population and yields a cellular suspension composed of erythrocytes, epithelial cells, ADSCs, and immature adipocytes. Cell suspension was injected subcutaneously into the recipient area on the frontal region of the scalp. Patients were evaluated after 5 days, 2 weeks, and 1 month based on photographs and patient's impressions. The authors reported that there was continuous growth of the transplanted hair as early as 2 months after the procedure, with shortening of the dormant phase.[30] However, there was no comparative group, and hence a definite conclusion is difficult to draw.

SUMMARY

Regenerative treatments in the management of hair loss have attracted great attention, both of doctors and of lay public. However, the evidence shows that the potential and promise are yet to be met. Till standardization is achieved, controlled trials establish the evidence, and long-term data are available, their routine use in clinical management is debatable. Evidence-based medicine demands that physicians adapt a questioning attitude and adhere to strict protocols while adapting such treatments. The following guidelines are recommended whenever physicians use such treatments:

- Use such treatments only when standard treatments fail.
- Full explanation should be provided to the patients about all aspects of the treatment and the available evidence, with a specific mention that adequate evidence is not yet available for the treatment, as part of informed consent.
- Proper documentation about efficacy and safety should be ensured.
- Cost of such treatments should be reasonable.
- There should be no advertisements for such treatments.

REFERENCES

1. Owczarczyk-Saczonek A, Krajewska-Włodarczyk M, Kruszewska A, Banasiak Ł, Placek W, Maksymowicz W, et al. Therapeutic potential of stem cells in follicle regeneration. Stem Cells Int. 2018;5:1049641.
2. Coelho MB, Cabral JM, Karp JM. Intraoperative stem cell therapy. Annu Rev Biomed Eng. 2012;14:325-49.
3. Ohyama M, Terunuma A, Tock CL, Radonovich MF, Pise-Masison CA, Hopping SB, et al. Characterization and isolation of stem cell-enriched human hair follicle bulge cells. J Clin Invest. 2006;116: 249-60.
4. Mohammadi P, Youssef KK, Abbasalizadeh S, Baharvand H, Aghdami N. Human hair reconstruction: close, but yet so far. Stem Cells Dev. 2016;25:1767-79.
5. Purba TS, Haslam IS, Poblet E, Jiménez F, Gandarillas A, Izeta A, et al. Human epithelial hair follicle stem cells and their progeny: current state of knowledge, the widening gap in translational research and future challenges. BioEssays. 2014;36:513-25.
6. Inoue K, Aoi N, Sato T, Yamauchi Y, Suga H, Eto H, et al. Differential expression of stem-cell-associated markers in human hair follicle epithelial cells. Lab Invest. 2009;89:844-56.
7. Gentile P, Scioli MG, Bielli A, Orlandi A, Cervelli V. Stem cells from human hair follicles: first mechanical isolation for immediate autologous clinical use in androgenetic alopecia and hair loss. Stem Cell Invest. 2017;4:58.
8. Asakawa K, Toyoshima KE, Ishibashi N, Tobe H, Iwadate A, Kanayama T, et al. Hair organ regeneration via the bioengineered hair follicular unit transplantation. Sci Rep. 2012;2:424.
9. Balañá ME, Charreau HE, Leiroós GJ. Epidermal stem cells and skin tissue engineering in hair follicle regeneration. World J Stem Cells. 2015;7:711-27.
10. Zhang P, Kling RE, Ravuri SK, Kokai LE, Rubin JP, Chai JK, et al. A review of adipocyte lineage cells and dermal papilla cells in hair follicle regeneration. J Tissue Eng. 2014;5:2041731414556850.
11. Festa E, Fretz J, Berry R, Schmidt B, Rodeheffer M, Horowitz M, et al. Adipocyte lineage cells contribute to the skin stem cell niche to drive hair cycling. Cell. 2011;146:761-71.
12. Yi R. Concise review: mechanisms of quiescent hair follicle stem cell regulation. Stem Cells. 2017;35:2323-30.
13. Eto H, Suga H, Matsumoto D, Inoue K, Aoi N, Kato H, et al. Characterization of structure and cellular components of aspirated and excised adipose tissue. Plast Reconstr Surg. 2009;124:1087-97.
14. Moseley TA, Zhu M, Hedrick MH. Adipose-derived stem and progenitor cells as fillers in plastic and reconstructive surgery. Plast Reconstr Surg. 2006;118:121S-8S.
15. Rehman J, Traktuev D, Li J, Merfeld-Clauss S, Temm-Grove CJ, Bovenkerk JE, et al. Secretion of angiogenic and antiapoptotic factors by human adipose stromal cells. Circulation. 2004;109:1292-8.
16. Suga H, Eto H, Shigeura T, Inoue K, Aoi N, Kato H, et al. IFATS collection: fibroblast growth factor-2-induced hepatocyte growth factor secretion by adipose-derived stromal cells inhibits postinjury fibrogenesis through a c-Jun N-terminal kinase-dependent mechanism. Stem Cells. 2009;27:238-49.

17. Won CH, Yoo HG, Kwon OS, Sung MY, Kang YJ, Chung JH, et al. Hair growth promoting effects of adipose tissue-derived stem cells. J Dermatol Sci. 2010;57:134-7.
18. Alexander RW. Understanding adipose-derived stromal vascular fraction (SVF) cell biology in reconstructive and regenerative applications on the basis of mononucleated cell components. J Prolother. 2013;10:15-29.
19. Banyard DA, Sarantopoulos CN, Borovikova AA, Qiu X, Wirth GA, Paydar KZ, et al. Phenotypic analysis of stromal vascular fraction after mechanical shear reveals stress-induced progenitor populations. Plast Reconstr Surg. 2016;138(2):237e-47e.
20. Oberbauer E, Steffenhagen C, Wurzer C, Gabriel C, Redl H, Wolbank S. Enzymatic and non-enzymatic isolation systems for adipose tissue-derived cells: current state of the art. Cell Regen. 2015;4:7.
21. van Dongen JA, Stevens HP, Harmsen MC, van der Lei B. Mechanical micronization of lipoaspirates: squeeze and emulsification techniques. Plast Reconstr Surg. 2017;139(6):1369e-70e.
22. Dini M, Mori A, Quattrini Li A. Eyebrow regrowth in patient with atrophic scarring alopecia treated with an autologous fat graft. Dermatol Surg. 2014;40:926-8.
23. Cho SB, Roh MR, Chung KY. Recovery of scleroderma-induced atrophic alopecia by autologous fat transplantation. Dermatol Surg. 2010;36:2061-3.
24. Tonnard P, Verpaele A, Peeters G, Hamdi M, Cornelissen M, Declercq H. Nanofat grafting: basic research and clinical applications. Plast Reconstr Surg. 2013;132:1017-26.
25. Vestita M, Filoni A, Bonamonte D, Elia R, Giudice G. Abstract: The Use of Nanofat in Androgenic Alopecia: a Prospective Blinded Study. Plast Reconstr Surg Global Open. 2017;5:90.
26. Shin H, Ryu HH, Kwon O, Park BS, Jo SJ. Clinical use of conditioned media of adipose tissue-derived stem cells in female pattern hair loss: a retrospective case series study. Int J Dermatol. 2015;54:730-5.
27. Fukuoka H, Suga H, Narita K, Watanabe R, Shintani S. The latest advance in hair regeneration therapy using proteins secreted by adipose-derived stem cells. Am J Cosmet Surg. 2012;29:273-82.
28. Fukuoka H, Suga H. Hair regeneration treatment using adipose-derived stem cell conditioned medium: follow-up with trichograms. Eplasty. 2015;15:e10.
29. Fukuoka H, Narita K, Suga H. Hair regeneration therapy: application of adipose-derived stem cells. Curr Stem Cell Res Ther. 2017;12:531-4.
30. Perez-Meza D, Ziering C, Sforza M, Krishnan G, Ball E, Daniels E. Hair follicle growth by stromal vascular fraction-enhanced adipose transplantation in baldness. Stem Cells Cloning. 2017;10:1-10.

CHAPTER 29

Platelet-rich Plasma in Hair Loss

Shuken Dashore

Key Messages

- Double-spin open method is the preferred method of preparation of PRP as it allows cost-effective preparation of PRP with the versatility of varying the volume of preparation. When using commercial kits, a narrow-neck tube method is the preferred method of preparation over gel separator tubes.
- ACD-A anticoagulant and microprocessor-controlled with brushless motors and swing-out rotors achieving 1–1.5 million platelets/cumm is the recommended method for preparation of PRP.
- PRP is advisable in AGA Norwood–Hamilton grades II–V patients with three to five sessions 1 month apart, in the dose of 1–1.5 mL/cm^2.
- Vibration pain relief and cryoanalgesia are the two most commonly perform methods to provide pain relief during PRP injection but ring block is ideal.
- Injection of platelet-rich plasma with 31g insulin syringe at the depth of 1.5 to 2.5 mm is recommended.

INTRODUCTION

Platelet-rich plasma (PRP) is a concentration of platelets derived from the centrifugation of whole blood (WB), which, when activated, releases numerous growth factors and cytokines instrumental in wound healing and tissue regeneration. Over the past few decades, the application of PRP has shown considerable promise in various medical and surgical fields. Recently, its role in the management of hair loss has garnered significant attention in the dermatological and cosmetic arenas.

Hair loss, or alopecia, represents a common dermatological issue, with androgenetic alopecia (AGA) being the most prevalent form affecting both males and females. It not only leads to physical changes but often has profound psychosocial implications, affecting individuals' self-esteem and quality of life.[1]

Platelet-rich plasma is posited to enhance hair growth by prolonging the anagen (growth) phase of the hair cycle and stimulating angiogenesis, collagen synthesis, and cell proliferation.

Despite the biological plausibility and promising early results, the application of PRP in hair loss is not without controversy. The literature showcases a considerable heterogeneity regarding PRP's preparation and administration protocols, dosing regimens, treatment intervals, and efficacy measures.[2]

This chapter aims to elucidate the role of PRP in the management of hair loss, focusing on the science underpinning its use, the evidence base supporting its application, the current challenges faced, and the future prospects. By amalgamating current knowledge and research, we seek to provide a comprehensive overview for clinicians and researchers interested in this exciting frontier of regenerative medicine.

HISTORY

The concept of utilizing PRP in healthcare can be traced back to the 1970s when hematologists began exploring its potential in transfusion medicine. The technique was primarily used to manage thrombocytopenia. However, it was not until the early 1990s that the term "platelet-rich plasma" was introduced by Ferrari et al. during a study on heart surgery. They demonstrated PRP's potential in improving wound healing and hemostasis.[3]

TABLE 2: Different growth factors and their mechanisms of action in hair growth.

Growth factor/cytokine	Source	Function
PDGF	Platelets in PRP	Initiates callus formation, promotes endothelial cell proliferation, involved in angiogenesis
TGF-β	Platelets in PRP	Regulates growth and differentiation of bulge cells
FGF-2	Platelets in PRP	Stimulates hair growth
VEGF	Platelets in PRP, dermal papilla (DP) cells	Involved in neovascularization, maintains hair follicle in the anagen phase
EGF	Platelets in PRP	Regulates growth and differentiation of bulge cells
IGF-1	Platelets in PRP, DP cells	Stimulates cell proliferation, induces and prolongs the anagen phase
GDNF	Platelets in PRP	Stimulates cell proliferation, protects hair follicle from premature catagen transition
FGF-7	DP cells	Maintains hair follicle in the anagen phase
Hepatocyte growth factor	DP cells	Maintains hair follicle in the anagen phase

(EGF: epidermal growth factor; FGF: fibroblast growth factor; GDNF: glial cell-derived neurotrophic factor; IGF: insulin-like growth factor; PDGF: platelet-derived growth factor; PRP: platelet-rich plasma; TGF: transforming growth factor; VEGF: vascular endothelial growth factor)

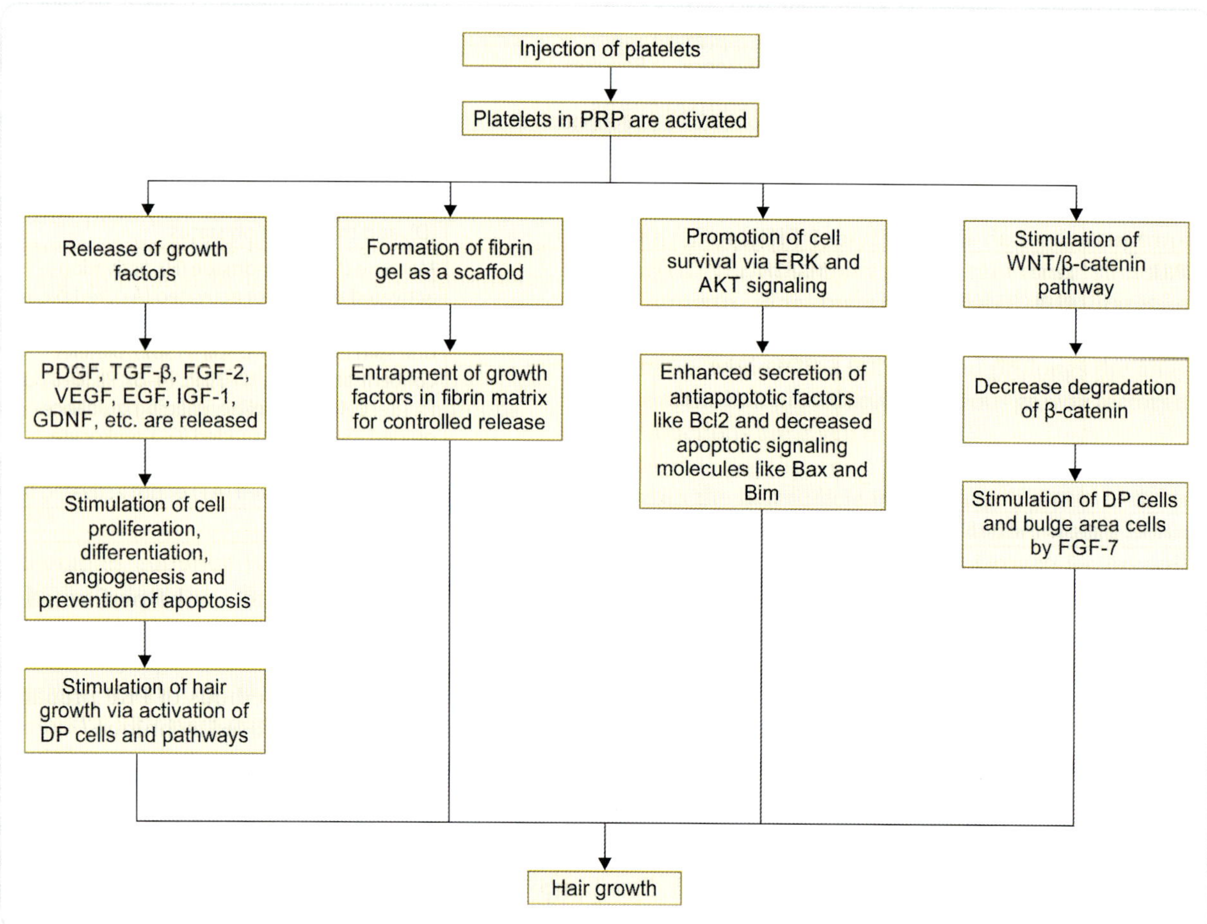

FLOWCHART 1: Different mechanisms of action of platelet-rich plasma (PRP) in hair growth.

(DP: dermal papilla; EGF: epidermal growth factor; FGF: fibroblast growth factor; GDNF: glial cell-derived neurotrophic factor; IGF: insulin-like growth factor; PDGF: platelet-derived growth factor; TGF: transforming growth factor; VEGF: vascular endothelial growth factor)

in the studies by Khatu et al. a
respectively.[19,20] *Most studies have r*
patient satisfaction and quality of
irrespective of clinical improvem
randomized controlled trial (RCT
efficacy of minoxidil foam versus PF
saw a much better quality of life in
patient satisfaction on the PRP si
to negligible improvement on the
Although assessment at 12 weeks r
for assessing the results of PRP, i
improvement is robust and is seen e

- *Histopathological examination*: Bi
treated with PRP revealed incre
thickness, fibroblast prolifera
deposition, and neoangiogenesis
vessels.[18] Furthermore, *increased*
the epidermis and hair follicular bul
decreased perifollicular fibrosis w
However, questions remain regarding
effects of PRP. Although it stimulate
collagen deposition, it also reduc
fibrosis. Additionally, the role of PRP i
the hair follicle apoptotic and perif
effects of TGF-β1, a known content
further exploration. Anitua et al. pr
complex milieu of growth factors in
action of TGF-β1 and prevents its ind
of fibroblasts to myofibroblasts.[24]
- *Studies with negative outcomes of*
results from two RCTs raised further
PRP's efficacy. Puig et al. and Mapar
studies with potential methodologic
highlighting the need for standardize
study designs in the field of PRP res
study assessed the results of PRP after
and the second one performed only t
examined the difference using a hand le
- *Adverse effects*: In terms of safety, PRP
not been associated with major side
blindness, scarring, worsening of hair l
However, minor side effects *such as*
itching, desquamation, transient ede
have been reported.[27]

While the therapeutic efficacy of P
largely substantiated by recent high-qualit
unresolved questions and methodological
necessitate further rigorous research for
PRP administration and exploring its com
hair follicular biology.

followed by another centrifugation to amass platelets suspended in the minimum final plasma volume. First, WB is collected in tubes containing anticoagulants. Centrifugation, operating at a steady acceleration, is carried out to segregate RBCs from the rest of the WB. Post the initial centrifugation, the WB is partitioned into three segments: A top layer mainly comprised of platelets and white blood cells (WBC), a middle layer—referred to as the buffy coat—abundant in WBCs, and a bottom layer primarily composed of RBCs. Subsequently, a second centrifugation is carried out. The "g" for the second spin should be just sufficient to facilitate the formation of pellets at the tube's base. The top portion of the volume, largely consisting of platelet-poor plasma (PPP), is then removed. The pellets are evenly mixed in the bottom third to formulate the PRP.[2]

Fukaya and Ito[16] proposed a novel and cost-effective technique for preparing PRP: *The syringe-only approach*. They advocate modifying a 5-mL syringe to allow it to be inserted into the centrifuge. The syringe is put into the centrifuge piston down. Following separation, the supernatant is delivered to a separate syringe for the second spin through a three-way cannula. This approach has the benefit of being a closed method in which the blood product remains inside readily accessible medical disposables such as three-way cannulas and syringes, which are even authorized for intravenous injections.

The turn-down turn-up approach is another innovative method reported in the literature. This approach takes only a single 10-mL syringe and two 8.5-mL vacutainers. It is a two-spin procedure in which vacutainers are inverted for the first spin and properly positioned for the second. However, this approach frequently produces PRP with a high hematocrit or RBC concentration. Machado et al. used this approach to generate a 4.17-fold increase in platelet concentration in their PRP.[17]

The closed technique involves the use of commercial devices or kits. Here, the blood or the PRP is not exposed to the environment during the process of preparation of PRP.[2]

Commercial kits for PRP preparation often use three basic methods: (1) Narrow-neck tube method, (2) gel separator method, or (3) automated cell separators.[2] There are other systems that use proprietary centrifuges along with tubes. These manufacturers name their products differently, but technically, they may be variants of basic forms of platelet concentrates; for example, autologous conditioned plasma by Arthrex® may be a variant of injectable-platelet-rich fibrin (i-PRF). **Table 3** lists common commercial kits that are available and their characteristics.

The *narrow-neck tube method* uses a special tube that has four parts: An extended top, a constricted center (or the narrow neck), an expanded bottom, and a turn screw. This method requires only a single spin and has been found to increase the platelet count by 2.5-fold.[2]

The *gel separation technique* is another commonly used method. These kits contain 1–2 mL of a thixotropic polymer gel in the blood collection tube. The gel has a specific gravity lower than RBCs and WBCs but more than

TABLE 3: Different commercially available kits and their methods of preparation of platelet-rich plasma (PRP).

Devices	Volume of blood collected in tube (mL)	Number of spins	Basic method used	Centrifuge type required
T-lab®	10	1	Buffy coat method	Any
Selphyl®	9	1	Gel separator	Any
Y-cell bio®	15	1	Narrow neck tube method	Any
PRGF Endoret®	9	1	Buffy coat method	Any
Cascade®	9	2	Gel separator	Any
Plateltex®	9	2	Double spin method	Any
Regenkit®	9	1	Gel separator	Any
ACP Arthrex®	15	1	Autologous conditioned plasma [similar to injectable-platelet-rich fibrin (i-PRF)]. No anticoagulant used. Double syringe system	Proprietary
GPS III®	30–60	1	Bouy-based separation system	Proprietary
Genesis®	12	1	Narrow neck tube method	Proprietary
Harvest SmartPrep 2®	20–60	1	Modified buffy coat method	Proprietary
Magellan®	30–60	Automated system	–	Proprietary
Angel®	40–180	Automated system	–	Proprietary

the platelets. On centrifugation, the plasma containing platelets ar below.[2]

Automated cell separators are systems. These machines can gi volume. They usually have a high high as 9.8%.

Key messages: Double-spin open method of preparation of PRP as preparation of PRP with the ve volume of preparation.

When using commercial kits method is the preferred method separator tubes.

MATHEMATICS OF PLATE PLASMA

The fundamental principles of ma play a role in PRP preparation, ai the process. There are three basic f dose of platelets, and platelet conc factor, which are crucial for gaug concentration of the PRP producec

It is important to know tha efficient. An optimal method sh platelet yield, ensuring both a concentration for effective treatn produce 5 mL of PRP with five-fold and assuming 80% yield, around 3 be drawn.[2]

Another aspect is platelet yield reveal that methods yielding high p be pure, and those producing pur yields. This can be due to varying affecting the centrifugation process

Centrifuge characteristics also tion. Relative centrifugal force measure as it remains constant acr types. It is important to use the sam (minimum, average, or maximum) a when calculating RCF for consist formula for RCF to rotations per mi on various websites.[2]

In most of the studies that are ra and blinded, which have demo outcome of PRP in AGA, the qua ranged from 0.05 to 0.1 mL for each we take into account that the typical on the scalp is around 150 cm² (as d the total amount of PRP needed wo 7.5 mL (calculated by multiplying

TABLE 1: Review of various trials in LLLT.

Study	Study group	Device used, parameters, and treatment	Results
Wikramanayake et al., 2012[16]	C3H/HeJ mice, alopecia areata	HairMax LaserComb 655 nm, 20 seconds daily, thrice weekly for 1–½ months	Increased hair regrowth
Shukla et al., 2010[17]	Swiss albino mice	HairMax LaserComb 632 nm, 1 and 5 J/cm² at 24-hour intervals for 5 days	Increase in the number of hair follicles treated
Lanzafame et al., 2013[18]	44 men (AGA)	Helmet (TOPHAT655) 655 nm, 67.3 J/cm², 25 minutes alternate days for 16 weeks	Greater hair count
Jimenez et al., 2014[19]	128 men and 141 women	HairMax LaserComb 655 nm, 3 times/week for 8–15 minutes for 26 weeks	Increased terminal hair density with overall improvement on thickness

(AGA: androgenetic alopecia)

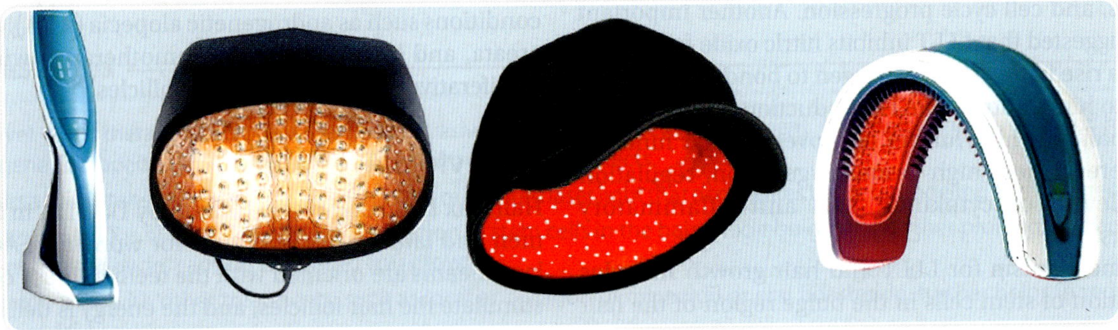

FIG. 2: Few devices in current use for low-level light therapy.

the scalp of the patients. Laser caps can be used at home as well. These caps offer full scalp coverage with uniform distribution of the energy.

Currently, LEDs have also been tested; however, further evidence is needed as studies are still lacking.

Few of the devices in current use are HairMax LaserComb, GrivaMax Laser Cap 272, HairMax LaserBand (Lexington, USA), TOPHAT 655, Capillus Laser Caps **(Fig. 2)**.

Usage

The most common devices use a light spectrum with wavelengths of 650–1,200 nm, fluences of 1–10 J/cm², and a power density of 3–90 mW/cm². The treatment typically ranges from 15 to 30 minutes with a frequency of three sessions a week for 6 months.

Efficacy in Androgenetic Alopecia

Low-level laser therapy is a newer, better, noninvasive, effective therapeutic option in promoting regrowth of hair in AGA. It mainly acts on the stem cells in the hair follicle epithelial matrix, which helps to prolong the duration of the anagen phase, leading to increased hair growth.

Few studies conducted in 2013 showed increased hair count, hair density, and hair diameter in men and women with AGA.[18,24] Another trial conducted among men with AGA documented an increase in hair density after laser therapy and greater patient compliance of 83%.[25]

The current level of evidence suggests that it can be only an ancillary therapy.

Safety and Side Effects

Patients have reported improved texture and quality of hair following LLLT. The only side effect reported was the temporary onset of telogen effluvium occurring in the first 1–2 months after commencing laser therapy[26] which would cease on consistent usage. Another study has suggested the possibility of dysplastic lesions on the scalp due to the proliferative effects of LLLT.[27]

OTHER LASERS FOR ANDROGENETIC ALOPECIA (TABLE 2)

Newer approaches in the form of nonablative and ablative fractional lasers have been recently employed in improving hair growth. The various lasers used for AGA are nonablative 1,550-nm erbium-glass;[24] 1,470-nm

TABLE 2: Summary of various studies of lasers in androgenetic alopecia.

Study	Study group	Devices used, parameters, and treatment regimen	Results
Day D, McCarthy M, Talaber I. Non-ablative Er:YAG laser is an effective tool in the treatment arsenal of androgenetic alopecia. J Cosmet Dermatol. 2022;21(5):2056-63[29]	16 patients (7 males and 9 females) with active androgenetic alopecia (AGA) in different stages	Nonablative erbium (Er):YAG laser (SMOOTH mode, 7-mm spot size, 7.00-J/cm^2 pulse fluence, 3.3-Hz frequency)	Decrease in AGA grade
Lee et al., 2011 [30]	27 patients completed a 5-month schedule of laser treatment	5–10-mm tip 6-mJ pulse energy 800-spots/cm^2 density static mode	A 1,550-nm fractional Er–glass laser irradiation may be an effective and safe treatment option for women with female pattern hair loss
Kim et al., 2011 [31]	20 participants were treated over five sessions at 2-week intervals	A fractional photothermolysis laser was used at the energy of 5 mJ and a total density of 300 spots/cm^2	This pilot study showed that a 1,550-nm fractional Er-glass laser might induce hair growth

thallium laser; and ablative 2,940-nm erbium:YAG[25] as well as ablative 10,600-nm CO_2 laser.[26]

Mechanism of Action

Induction of hair growth is through upregulation of the Wnt/β-catenin pathway and also through effective penetration of the scalp. Furthermore, the mechanism of action of such lasers on hair regrowth is not well documented; however, it has been proposed that wound healing stimulated by trauma plays an important role.

Hair follicle stem cells provide daughter cells that migrate to the epidermal defect and promote reepithelialization. This hypothesized wound healing process is more during the anagen phase of the hair cycle, and other hair follicles regrow after wounding.[27]

A combination of agents such as minoxidil and lasers has shown to produce a synergistic effect in enhancing hair growth.[28]

Human and animal studies have suggested the effectiveness and safety of the 1550-nm fractional erbium–glass laser; ablative fractional 2,940-nm erbium:YAG laser; and ablative fractional CO_2 laser on regrowth of hair.[29] It is particularly used to stimulate vellus to intermediate vellus hair with a session interval of about 2 weeks for about 5–6 sessions. However, more large-scale studies are required to prove their outcome and efficacy consistently.

SUMMARY

The advantages of LLLT are as follows:
- Noninvasive and safe
- Minimal side effects
- Convenient and accessible, can be used at home also
- Indicated in several hair loss conditions.
- Long-term maintenance to help preserve and optimize the results achieved
- Can be combined with medications such as minoxidil or finasteride or used in conjunction with hair transplant surgery to enhance results and promote postsurgical healing.
- However, at the current level of evidence, it can only be recommended as an ancillary therapy, particularly in patients who are apprehensive or cannot tolerate drugs.

REFERENCES

1. Mester E, Szende B, Gärtner P. The effect of laser beams on the growth of hair in mice. Radiobiol Radiother (Berl). 1968;9: 621-6.
2. Loevschall H, Arenholt-Bindslev D. Effect of low level diode laser irradiation of human oral mucosa fibroblasts in vitro. Lasers Surg Med. 1994;14:347-54.
3. Vink EM, Cagnic BJ, Cornelissen MJ, Declercq HA, Cambier DC. Increased fibroblast proliferation induced by light emitting diode and low power laser irradiation. Lasers Med Sci. 2003;18:95-9.
4. Avci P, Gupta GK, Clark J, Wikonkal N, Hamblin MR. Low-level laser (light) therapy (LLLT) for treatment of hair loss. Lasers Surg Med. 2014;46(2):144-151.

5. Gupta AK, Foley KA. A critical assessment of the evidence for low-level laser therapy in the treatment of hair loss. Dermatol Surg. 2017;43(2):188-97.
6. Ghanaat M. Types of hair loss and treatment options, including the novel low-level light therapy and its proposed mechanism. South Med J. 2010;103(9):917-21.
7. Conlan MJ, Rapley JW, Cobb CM. Biostimulation of wound healing by low-energy laser irradiation. A review. J Clin Periodontol. 1996;23(5):492-6.
8. Yu HS, Wu CS, Yu CL, Kao YH, Chiou MH. Helium-neon laser irradiation stimulates migration and proliferation in melanocytes and induces repigmentation in segmental-type vitiligo. J Invest Dermatol. 2003;120(1):56-64.
9. Lubart R, Eichler M, Lavi R, Friedman H, Shainberg A. Low-energy laser irradiation promotes cellular redox activity. Photomed Laser Surg. 2005;23:3-9.
10. Chung H, Dai T, Sharma SK, Huang YY, Carroll JD, Hamblin MR. The nuts and bolts of low-level laser (light) therapy. Ann Biomed Eng. 2012;40:516-33.
11. de Freitas LF, Hamblin MR. Proposed mechanisms of photobiomodulation or low-level light therapy. IEEE J Sel Top Quantum Electron. 2016;22:7000417.
12. Pillai JK, Mysore V. Role of low-level light therapy (LLLT) in androgenetic alopecia. J Cutan Aesthet Surg. 2021;14(4):385-91.
13. Sakurai Y, Yamaguchi M, Abiko Y. Inhibitory effect of low-level laser irradiation on LPS-stimulated prostaglandin E2 production and cyclooxygenase-2 in human gingival fibroblasts. Eur J Oral Sci. 2000;108:29-34.
14. Bjordal JM, Couppe C, Chow RT, Tuner J, Ljunggren EA. A systematic review of low level laser therapy with location-specific doses for pain from chronic joint disorders. Aust J Physiother. 2003;49(2):107-16.
15. Brosseau L, Welch V, Wells G, deBie R, Gam A, Harman K, et al. Low level laser therapy (classes I, II and III) in the treatment of rheumatoid arthritis. Cochrane Database Syst Rev. 2000;(2): CD002049.
16. Wikramanayake TC, Rodriguez R, Choudhary S, Mauro LM, Nouri K, Schachner LA, et al. Effects of the Lexington LaserComb on hair regrowth in the C3H/HeJ mouse model of alopecia areata. Lasers Med Sci. 2012;27:431-6.
17. Shukla S, Sahu K, Verma Y, Rao KD, Dube A, Gupta PK. Effect of helium-neon laser irradiation on hair follicle growth cycle of Swiss albino mice. Skin Pharmacol Physiol. 2010;23:79-85.
18. Lanzafame RJ, Blanche RR, Bodian AB, Chiacchierini RP, Fernandez-Obregon A, Kazmirek ER, et al. The growth of human scalp hair mediated by visible red light laser and LED sources in males. Lasers Surg Med. 2013;45:487-95.
19. Jimenez JJ, Wikramanayake TC, Bergfeld W, Hordinsky M, Hickman JG, Hamblin MR, et al. Efficacy and safety of a low-level laser device in the treatment of male and female pattern hair loss: a multicenter, randomized, sham device-controlled, double-blind study. Am J Clin Dermatol. 2014;15:115-27.
20. Cauwels RG, Martens LC. Low level laser therapy in oral mucositis: a pilot study. Eur Arch Paediatr Dent. 2011;12 (2):118-23.
21. Christie A, Jamtvedt G, Dahm KT, Moe RH, Haavardsholm EA, Hagen KB. Effectiveness of nonpharmacological and non-surgical interventions for patients with rheumatoid arthritis: an overview of systematic reviews. Phys Ther, 2007;87(12): 1697-715.
22. Jamtvedt G, Dahm KT, Holm I, Flottorp S. Measuring physiotherapy performance in patients with osteoarthritis of the knee: a prospective study. BMC Health Serv Res. 2008;8:145.
23. Joo HJ, Jeong KH, Kim JE, Kang H. Various wavelengths of light-emitting diode light regulate the proliferation of human dermal papilla cells and hair follicles via Wnt/β-catenin and the extracellular signal-regulated kinase pathways. Ann Dermatol. 2017;29(6):747-54.
24. Kim H, Choi JW, Kim JY, Shin JW, Lee SJ, Huh CH, et al. Low-level light therapy for androgenetic alopecia: a 24-week, randomized, double-blind, sham device-controlled multicenter trial. Dermatol Surg. 2013;39:1177-83.
25. Kim S, Park M, Lee C. Phototherapy of androgenetic alopecia with low level narrow band 655-nm red light and 780-nm infrared light. J Am Acad Dermatol. 2007;56:AB112.
26. Satino JL, Markou M. Hair regrowth and increased hair tensile strength using the HairMax LaserComb for low-level laser therapy. Int J Cosmet Surg Aesthet Dermatol. 2003;5:113-17.
27. Frigo L, Luppi JS, Favero GM, Maria DA, Penna SC, Bjordal JM, et al. The effect of low-level laser irradiation (In-Ga-Al-AsP—660 nm) on melanoma in vitro and in vivo. BMC Cancer. 2009;9: 404.
28. Ke J, Guan H, Li S, Xu L, Zhang L, Yan Y. Erbium: YAG laser (2,940 nm) treatment stimulates hair growth through upregulating Wnt 10b and β-catenin expression in C57BL/6 mice. Int J Clin Exp Med. 2015;8(11):208839.
29. Bae JM, Jung HM, Goo B, Park YM. Hair regrowth through wound healing process after ablative fractional laser treatment in a murine model. Lasers Surg Med. 2015;47(5):433-40.
30. Lee GY, Lee SJ, Kim WS. The effect of a 1550 nm fractional erbium-glass laser in female pattern hair loss. J Eur Acad Dermatol Venereol. 2011;25(12):1450–4.
31. Kim WS, Lee HI, Lee JW, Lim YY, Lee SJ, Kim BJ, et al. Fractional photothermolysis laser treatment of male pattern hair loss. Dermatol Surg. 2011;37(1):41-51.

CHAPTER 32

Synthetic Hair Fibers

Indira Potthuri, Venkataram Mysore

Key Messages

- The use of artificial hair fibers is controversial and is banned by the Federal Drug Administration due to its many disadvantages.
- Hence, it is important that the practitioners know about all the aspects of its use.
- Hair loss is a significant issue for patients, and treating hair loss can be challenging for medical professionals.

HISTORY OF ARTIFICIAL HAIR AND REGULATORY INDICATIONS

Artificial hair implantation was introduced in the 1970s as a new technique but because of unsuitable materials and techniques, frequent severe adverse events were seen and soon it was unpopular among different dermatologists and surgeons. As a result of numerous negative outcomes experienced, in 1983, the US Food and Drug Administration (FDA) outlawed implantation with industrial fibers such as monoacrylic, polyacrylic, polyester, and naturally processed human hair. With advancements in biomedical technology, many biocompatible inorganic materials have been used, which have been more successful and have resulted in lesser complications.

In 1993, biocompatible fibers—biocompatible artificial hair (Biofibre®, Medicap®, Carpi, Italy) were developed, and clinical trials were performed with encouraging results. Therefore, the Council Concerning Medical Devices in the European Union recognized the artificial hair implant technique as a medical act in 1996. They are also certified by the Therapeutic Goods Administration, Australia. Biofibre® has reapplied for FDA approval but is still banned in the USA. The International Society of Hair Restoration Surgery (ISHRS) does not provide an official stand about synthetic hair fibers.[1,2]

COMPOSITION

In the start, synthetic fibers made of monoacrylic, polyacrylic, polyester materials or natural fibers, including processed human hair and artificial fibers were used. The primary requirements are biocompatibility, traction resistance, lack of capillarity, physical-chemical stress resistance, low tissue trauma, and acceptable aesthetic attributes. Biocompatible fiber is a sterile, inert, and ultraviolet (UV)-resistant polyamide fiber, which is around 0.08–0.09 mm thick and 160–460 mm long, used for both males and females. The new fibers are considered to be safer, tolerable, and more biocompatible.

There are three various shapes of Biofibre® hair—straight, wave, and curly—as well as three different lengths—15, 30, and 45 cm. They are also categorized as lightweight regular fibers in the frontal area and high-density fibers in the crown area.[1,3]

INDICATIONS

Indications include androgenic alopecia, primary cicatricial alopecia (scarring alopecia due to innate hair follicle-directed causes), and secondary cicatricial alopecia (scarring alopecia due to incidental causes such as traumatic burns and surgical scarring).

The claimed advantage is an immediate aesthetic outcome and enough hair in a short amount of time without the need for a donor location through a simple office procedure.[1,4]

PATIENT SELECTION

Careful patient selection is necessary. There needs to be careful scalp examination to determine the cause of alopecia, exclusion of treatable conditions, and review of blood work and other appropriate investigations to rule out systemic and autoimmune diseases including human immunodeficiency virus (HIV), hepatitis, diabetes, and cardiac disease. Patients with diabetes mellitus, hepatitis A, B, and C, autoimmune disorders, chronic scalp diseases, severe psychosis, unstabilized alopecia areata, poor personal hygiene, or employment in dusty or polluted surroundings are not candidates for Biofibre® hair implants. Before beginning an implanted test, the patient must have a thorough examination that includes blood tests such as complete blood count, urea, creatinine, bilirubin (total and direct), gamma-glutamyl transferase (GGT), alanine aminotransferase (ALT), aspartate aminotransferase (AST), fibrinogen, treponema pallidum hemagglutination (TPH), anti-HIV, and hepatitis A, B, and C markers/hepatitis B surface antigen (HBsAg).

The patients are initially implanted with 100 fibers and examined every week for at least a month as part of a compatibility test, which is necessary to observe the tolerability of the implanted fibers. Additional implant sessions could be scheduled if the fibers are well tolerated and cause no adverse effects. A typical implantation treatment consists of three to four sessions and involves the insertion of about 1,000 fibers per session. Side effects such as mild inflammation and pustular lesions can be observed.[1]

IMPLANTATION TECHNIQUE

The use of biocompatible hair implant fibers, modern automatic equipment, careful selection of patients, and correct aftercare are essential requirements to achieve the expected results.

- The implant technique is a surgical technique, performed under local anesthesia by either a manual implanter or an automatic machine.
- A small hooking needle places the root of the fiber under the scalp at the galea level, where the root can be held by fibrous tissue. The root is a reversible knot that ensures the correct anchorage of the implant and allows total fiber extraction. This knot helps the fibers to anchor directly into the dermis and subcutaneous tissue of the scalp. Each fiber is placed 2 mm apart at an angle of 45°. This manual procedure is performed under local anesthesia and at a rate of around 600 fibers/hour, depending on the surgeon. The BiofibreVR automated implantation device was introduced by Medicap® in Italy in 2013.
- Automated implants reduce the trauma and complexity associated with the manual procedure and help in reaching the right depth at the site of implantation.

POSTPROCEDURE CARE

Systemic antibiotic coverage is advised for a week, with modifications to the course of treatment depending on the patient's medical history and specific local conditions. Head wash with ketoconazole shampoo is advised after 3 days. For the first 3 weeks until cicatrization occurs, the patient must refrain from participating in sports, using the sauna, and other activities that can make them sweat excessively. Additionally, for 1 week following the implant procedure, one should abstain from smoking and drinking alcohol. A 4-week break must be respected before starting the subsequent implant sessions.[1,3]

FOLLOW-UP CARE

The fibers can be washed like natural hair and combed carefully; however, patients should avoid hair treatments such as bleaching, styling, and heat curling *for few months*. The reversible knot at the root of the fibers allows for their removal from the scalp in case of severe complications.

With the appropriate traction, each fiber can be pulled out entirely with no residue in the scalp, if needed, in case of nontreatable side effects or unsatisfied results.

A number of habits, such as poor patient hygiene or a lack of asepsis during the procedure, excessive density or quantity of fibers implanted in one session, a traumatic implant procedure, a patient's intolerance to certain fibers, a poor choice of implant location, and failure in aftercare procedures, can result in side effects from the implant procedure.

DISADVANTAGES

The implanted "hair" will not grow, which is a drawback of this method. To maintain the desired aesthetic outcome, touchup sessions are necessary. Implants are not an option in areas such as the temples, low front line on the forehead, and over very thin or atrophic scalp.[4-6]

COMPLICATIONS

Since artificial hair fibers are foreign objects, they can cause cellular and tissue reactions. These include:[1,4,6]

- The possibility of an allergic reaction, granulomatous hypersensitivity
- Reactions to foreign bodies
- Acute and chronic inflammation
- Likelihood of fibrous encapsulation of the implanted material
- Risk of microbial infection through the portals created
- Recurrent folliculitis
- 15–20% annual hair fiber loss rate
- Contact dermatitis
- Fear about potential carcinogenicity
- Cicatricial alopecia
- Cyst formation

ARE SYNTHETIC HAIR FIBERS APPROPRIATE TO USE?

Artificial hair fibers are controversial. Because of their dubious history, being outlawed by the US FDA, and the possibility of side effects, they have not gained widespread acceptability. It is important to note that there are safe and effective treatment options for hair restoration such as follicular unit extraction and follicular unit transplantation. In the current state of hair restoration, with significant progress in different methods, the place for this modality is limited to rare cases with no donor and a willing patient with appropriate governmental permissions. It should be viewed as an experimental approach, acquire ethics committee approval, and follow all protocol requirements.[1,4,6]

SUMMARY

- Synthetic hairs have had a checkered history.
- When the donor area is exhausted or unsuitable for hair transplantation, artificial hair implantation can be thought of as an alternate treatment.
- The use of artificial hair implants is still debatable, especially since the US FDA has outlawed this practice.

REFERENCES

1. Roccia M, França K, Castillo D, Tchernev G, Wollina U, Tirant M, et al. Artificial hair: by the dawn to Automatic Biofibre® hair implant. Open Access Maced J Med Sci. 2017;6:156-62.
2. Gupta AK, Venkataraman M, Quinlan EM. Artificial hair implantation for hair restoration. J Dermatolog Treat. 2022;33(3):1312-8.
3. Satolli F, Rovesti M, Moran ABB, Griselli G, Agarwal M, Abdel-Hakim Rateb SA, et al. Biofibre® artificial hair implant: retrospective study on 1,518 patients with alopecia and present role in hair surgery. Dermatol Ther. 2019;32(4):e12985.
4. Mysore V. Controversy: synthetic hairs and their role in hair restoration? Int J Trichology. 2010;2:42-4.
5. Agrawal M. Modern artificial hair implantation: a pilot study of 10 patients. J Cosmet Dermatol. 2008;7:315-23.
6. Mysore V. Synthetic hairs: should they be used? Indian J Dermatol Venereol Leprol. 2006;72:5-7.

CHAPTER 33

Hair Camouflage

Vrushali Maisekar

Key Messages

- There is a need for alternative options for hair transplant.
- Hair camouflage can be as follows:
  - Nonsurgical hair replacement, including hair additions, hair wigs, natural hair, and artificial hair.
  - Hair camouflaging agents, including hair fibers, hairspray, scalp lotions, and scalp pigmentation.
- Knowledge of these options can be helpful in routine practice.

INTRODUCTION

While it is true that hair transplantation (HT) has become increasingly popular in recent years, there exists a section of the patient population who may either not be suitable or not want HT. Once permanent hair loss begins due to conditions such as cicatricial alopecia, there are very few options left. In such circumstances where the donor area has been impaired, the role of HT is also constrained. Alternative methods need to be offered to such patients, from temporary solutions such as hairpieces to more permanent ones such as scalp micropigmentation.[1,2]

This chapter discusses the topic of hair camouflage under the following heads:

- *Hair camouflage*:
  - History
  - Hair camouflage today: Hair additions, hair fibers
- *Hair additions*:
  - Components of hair additions
  - Methods to attach hair additions
  - Indications
  - Advantages and disadvantages
- Hair camouflaging agents

HAIR CAMOUFLAGE

History

Hair camouflaging is the simplest and the easiest way of dealing with baldness; this gives out the illusion of thick hair. Many people with hair loss and baldness tend to prefer this option as it appears easy to comply with.

Hair camouflage dates back to 2700 BCE when Egyptian wigs were constructed of human hair. Cheaper substitutes, such as palm leaves, fibers, and wool, were also used widely. They denoted social status, rank, and religious piety. The hair was gummed and powdered, and false curls and ringlets were worn. Sometimes, a complete head of false hair called "Perruque" was worn. French King Louis XIV used hairpieces to camouflage his thinning hair. In the 17th and 18th centuries, large full-bottomed expensive wigs marked the class and income of individuals in certain countries. Lucrative trade was constructed around their care and maintenance. Hair was harvested from heads of the rural working class. The hair market took a boom after 1968. Today, there is a mass production of wigs flooding the market with different styles, colors, and textures. The African population gives supreme importance to fashionable wigs without undergoing time-consuming and painful hair straightening.

Hair Camouflage Today

The present-day hair camouflages in vogue are:

- Hair additions
- Hair camouflaging agents

Indications

Nonsurgical hair replacement is recommended for individuals with:

- Extensive androgenetic alopecia (AGA) in men and women, which cannot be managed by either medical or surgical options, after full consultation and counseling
- Extensive hair loss due to chemotherapy in patients
- Ectodermal dysplasia
- Alopecia totalis
- Extensive pseudopelade
- Thin hair desiring fuller hair but do not wish to have medical or surgical options
- Celebrities and models use this for enhancing their glamour value.

Contraindications

A decision to undergo a hairpiece should be taken after proper thought, consultation, and counseling. Often, young men are misled into wearing wigs and then regret it. Individuals who are allergic to adhesives should not opt for an adhesive system. A test patch is usually recommended before this type of treatment. Allergy to the base of the piece is hardly seen.[2-4]

HAIR ADDITIONS

Hair additions are artificial hairs worn on a thinning or bald scalp. Hair additions can be readymade or customized. Readymade hair additions in the market have fixed and standard fit. They can give poor fitting, discomfort, and limited choice of style and color. Custom-made additions, on the other hand, are designed for comfort. The experts take exact measurements of the head and scalp to fit it perfectly. The density, color, and texture are decided in the design process.

Hair additions come in three types—wigs, weaves, or hair pieces and extensions. They have the following components.

Components of Hair Additions

- Base
- Hair
- Method of hair attachment to the base
- Accessories required

Base

Base is the main structural component of hair addition, giving it shape and contour **(Fig. 1)**. The base is made up of polyurethane and nylon. Older materials like natural fibers had a problem of natural body oil and moisture absorption.

Also, it did not retain the shape for a longer period of time. The most recent bases have an advantage of a natural looking frontline and hairline.

An individual's choice of a hairpiece depends on the type of hair and the base of the unit. The type of bases determines the life of the unit. It also gives a natural and artificial look to the work done. The different types include filamentous, front lace, and full lace patches. The thinner the base, the more adherent to the scalp, thus imparting a natural look.

Hair

Hair comes in two types:

1. Human or natural hair
2. Synthetic hair

Human or Natural Hair

Human hair further comes in three basic types:

1. European hair
2. Asian hair
3. Indian hair

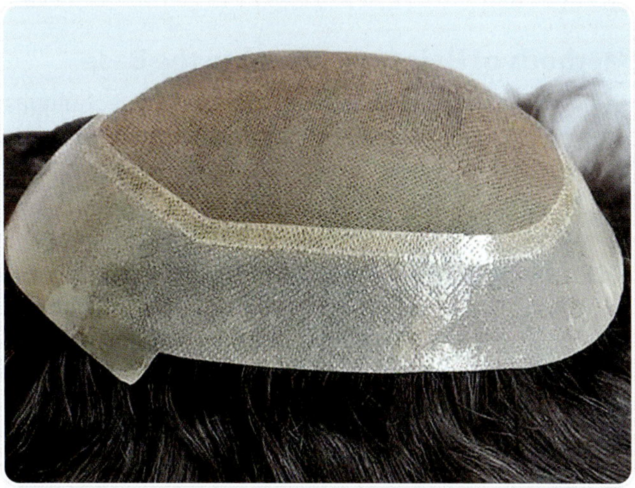

FIG. 1: The base of a hair addition.

TABLE 1: Differences between human and synthetic hair.

Human hair	Synthetic hair
Looks natural	Cheaper option
Humidity affects them, can go limp or curl	Humidity does not affect them
One needs to spend time styling the addition	Tend to lose luster if not properly cared
Less dense and more believable	Light in weight and easy to dry
Can be styled, colored, and curled	Should be worn with a wig cap
Short life	Hold curls for a longer period
	Longer life

European hair has the finest texture and comes in different colors. Indian hair is of medium texture and is used in most additions.

Hair obtained from humans is processed to make it tangle-free and attractive. Tangle-free hair is obtained by chemically removing the cuticles using an acid bath. This process reduces friction among hairs, leaving the hair tangle-free. In order to give the appearance of natural healthy hair, a laminate is applied to the hair to give it a shiny and silky look.

Synthetic Hair

It is made up of vinyl chloride and acrylonitrile, which together form modacrylic fibers. Synthetic fibers are lighter in weight and, hence, dry fast. It is generally assumed that human hair is better than synthetic hair. But the choice depends on what one expects from the hair. **Table 1** shows the differences between human hair and synthetic hair.

Methods of Hair Attachment to the Base

Individual fibers are attached to the base by techniques; they can be looped and sealed, hand-knotted, punched in, and machine-lifted.

Accessories Required

It is essential to understand the accessories as they can potentially cause discomfort or allergies after attachment. Glue/adhesives, glue removers, threads, adhesive tapes, clips, combs, fusion connectors, and electric combs are common accessories used.[2-4]

Methods to Attach Hair Additions

Two major attachment classifications are as follows **(Flowchart 1)**:

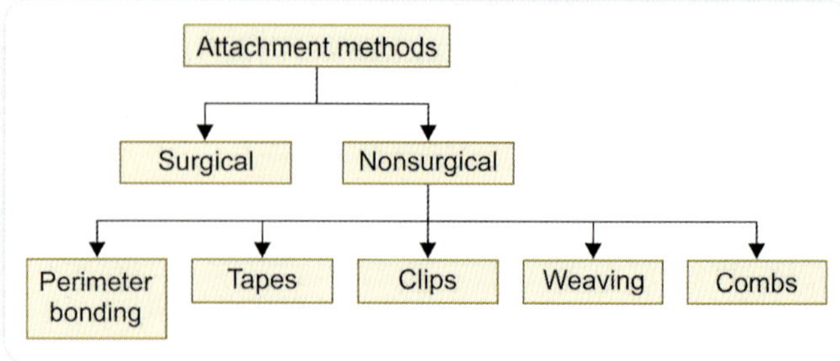

FLOWCHART 1: Different attachment methods.

1. Surgical attachments
2. Nonsurgical attachments—wigs, hair patches, and hair extensions

Surgical Attachments

- Two to three loops are surgically created using a skin graft from the patient's retroauricular area. Each loop is then used as an anchor point for a clip that is attached to the loop.
- *Suturing*: It is a permanent attachment technique that involves sewing the addition directly to the scalp.
  - *Disadvantages*: High rate of infection, cutting through, and permanent scar.

Nonsurgical Hair Replacement

Wigs

Wigs are full cap prosthesis designed to cover the entire head, preferred by people with hair loss of a major portion of the scalp, such as chemotherapy patients, alopecia totalis or universalis, and ectodermal dysplasia.

A wig is tailored after exact measurements such as the circumference of the head, ear to ear across the top of the head, and frontal hairline to the nape of the neck. Many wigs have an adjustable hook behind to adjust the fitting. Wearing a wig is as good as wearing a cap that can be removed easily. Adhesive tapes can be used to ensure adhesion to the scalp. Wigs include both medical and nonmedical wigs. Cranial prosthesis is the term used to describe a wig worn to cover alopecia due to various reasons such as medical conditions or chemotherapy. Maintenance of a wig is pretty easy as in regular brushing and washing once in 10–15 days with mild shampoos. A wig lasts for about 1–4 years, depending upon its make.

Hair Patch Fixing

Popular methods of hair patch fixing are discussed below **(Fig. 2)**.

Perimeter bonding: Today's most popular method of hair attachment is perimeter bonding. Adhesives are used

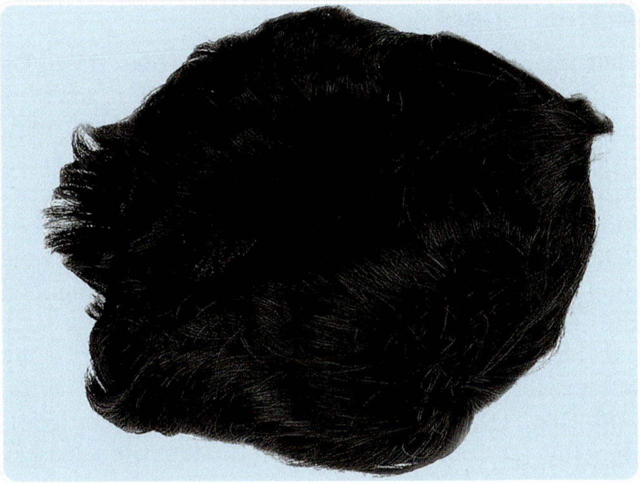

FIG. 2: Hair patch.

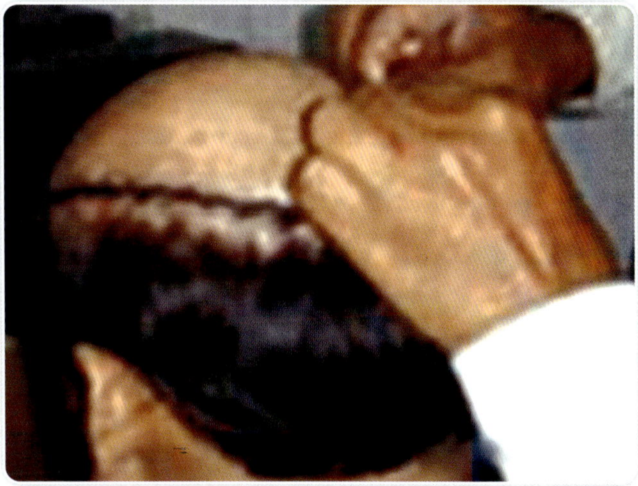

FIG. 3: Hairweaving.

to fix the hairpieces to the scalp. A hair patch is tailored according to the bald area and other specifications. The fringe of the perimeter of the bald head is first shaved to a length of 1/8 inch. Glue is then applied along this fringe. The hairpiece is then fixed onto the scalp. Daily activities such as hair wash, swimming, and riding a vehicle can be carried out as usual by the client after this.

Maintenance: The frequency of visits for maintenance depends on how fast the fringe of hair is growing. The patch remains affixed for approximately 4–5 weeks. As the fringe of hair grows, the patch becomes loose. The patch is then removed with adhesive removers. The scalp and the patch are thoroughly cleaned. The fringe of the hair is shaved again, and a haircut is given to the client for his original hair. The patch is then affixed again as before.

- *Disadvantages*: Allergic contact dermatitis may develop due to the adhesives. A patch test for a possible allergic reaction to the adhesive is advisable.

Weaving

Weaving involves the tight braiding of existing hair around the perimeter of the balding area **(Fig. 3)**. The hair patch is then sewn to the braids, which serve as an anchor. The procedure needs to be repeated after 4–6 weeks as the braided hair grows, hence making the braid attachment loose.

- *Disadvantages*: Tight braids can lead to traction alopecia.

Clipping

Clipping is popularly used by men and women as it is a user-friendly method of attachment. Small various-sized clips are attached to the underside of the hair addition. The addition is then clipped onto the existing hair and snapped close for security. In women, a patch of long hair is used to cover the thinned scalp, especially AGA type.

- *Disadvantage*: Though user-friendly, the clips can cause traction alopecia.

Fusion, beading, and micropoint linking are other methods of hair attachment but are not very popular.

BOX 1 Advantages and disadvantages of nonsurgical hair replacement.

Advantages:
- Procedure is fast and can have a full crop of hair very soon
- One gets an opportunity to try different colors, textures, and styles
- Procedure is noninvasive, painless, and less time consuming
- Initial investment is less

Disadvantages:
- Not permanent as it does not produce new hair
- Added hair may get damaged and dull with time
- Follow-up may be time-consuming
- Allergic dermatitis to adhesives, though rare, may happen

Hair Extension

Hair extensions are usually chosen by females to create a long-hair look; long strands of hair are attached to short-length existing hair with clips, cold fusion, or hot fusion methods.

The advantages and disadvantages of nonsurgical hair replacement are given in **Box 1**.

Demiwigs

Only the crown and, to a lesser degree, the vertex of the scalp are covered by a demiwig. It only covers the top of the scalp, leaving the patient's natural hair free to grow along the sides and back of the scalp.

Wiglets

A wiglet's flat or cone-shaped base can be used to conceal small patches of scalp baldness, making it effective for localized camouflage.[2,3,5-7]

HAIR CAMOUFLAGING AGENTS

Visibility of the scalp skin is the complaint that many men and women present with. The contrast between the hair and the scalp skin can be reduced by using camouflaging agents. Camouflaging agents available presently fall into six categories:

1. Hair fibers
2. Powder cakes
3. Scalp lotions
4. Scalp sprays
5. Hair crayons
6. Scalp tattooing (tricopigmentation/micropigmentation)

Hair Fibers

Hair fibers come as powders or sprays **(Figs. 4A to C)**. These are natural keratin protein hair fibers made of plant cellulose. They bind and statically cling to the negatively charged existing hair to hide any receding areas, providing considerable density, volume, and natural-looking coverage. The minimum hair length should be 0.5 inches when these fibers are used. They will not work on a shaved or totally bald head. These fibers remain on the head until the next shampoo.

The incidence of allergic or irritant dermatitis is not known. They contain FD&C (Food, Drugs, and Cosmetics) and D&C (Drugs and Cosmetics) dyes, dimethylol-dimethyl (DMDM) hydantoin (a formaldehyde releaser), iodopropynyl butylcarbamate (cosmetic preservative), etc.

Powder Cakes

Powder cakes come as circular disks. They are applied with a wet sponge applicator on washed and towel-dried hair.

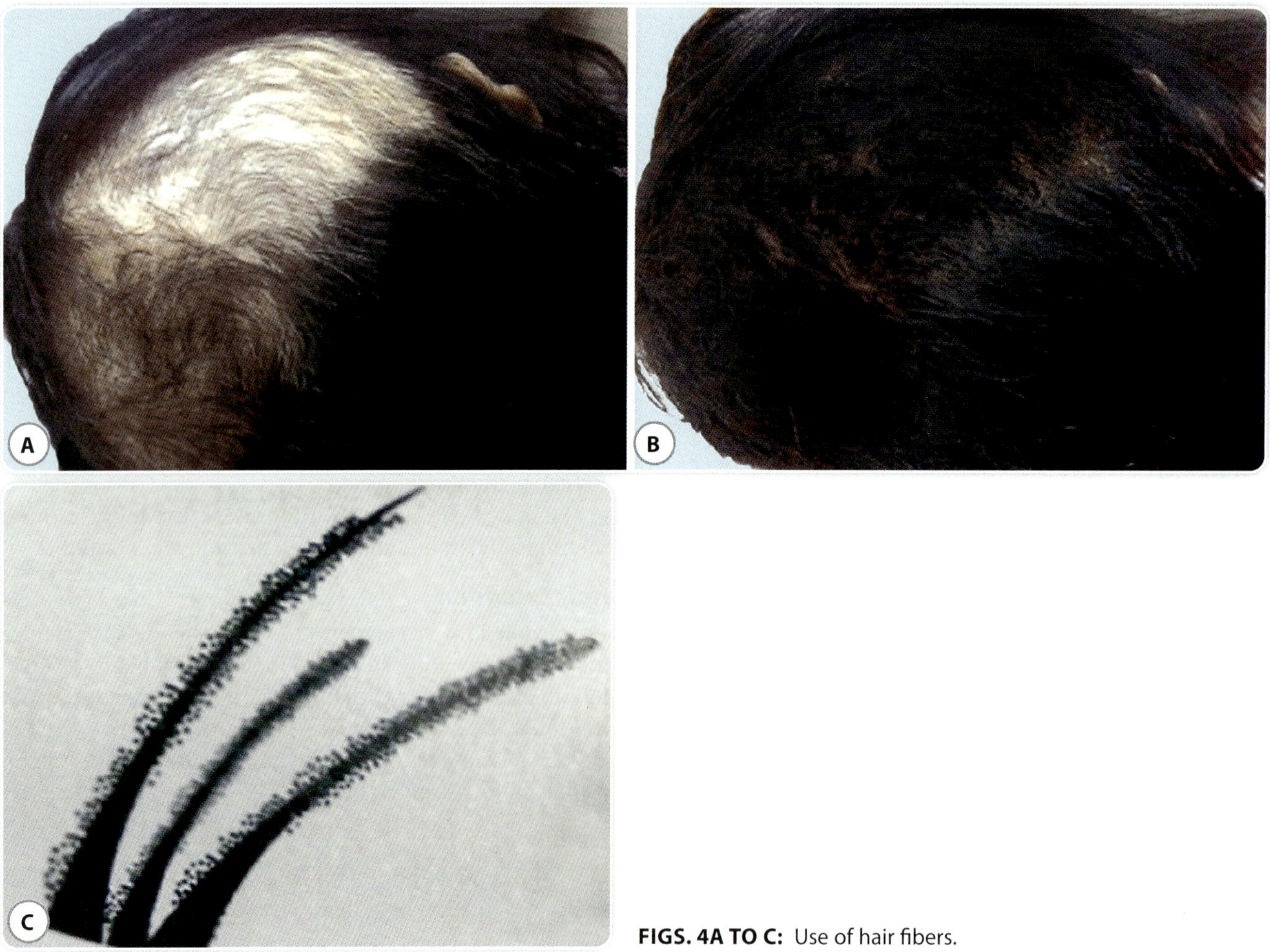

FIGS. 4A TO C: Use of hair fibers.

This not only coats the scalp but also thickens thinning vellus hair, making it appear thicker. After the application, the hair is brushed to evenly distribute the product throughout the thinning area. This product is water-resistant, allowing for safe swimming with it on the scalp. It can be washed out by shampooing. Allergies or irritant contact dermatitis are not common with this product. Potential allergens include ethylenediamine, propylene glycol, methyldibromo glutaronitrile, phenoxyethanol, methylparaben, fragrance, and FD&C and D&C dyes.

Scalp Lotions

- They work by eliminating the contrast between hair and scalp.
- Lotions are intended for men with significant thinning and are applied on the scalp. One can combine the lotion with fibers for a synergistic effect.
- To apply, the hair is combed away from the thinning area. The lotion is rubbed firmly and blended into the surrounding hair for a natural appearance.
- They are available in a tube packing with an applicator.
- They are waterproof and can be washed out with shampoo.

Scalp Spray

Scalp spray is an easy-to-comply method. Sprays are applied to dried hair. The spray is applied to styled hair 4–6 inches above the area to be camouflaged and allowed to dry for 30–60 seconds. This product is removed by shampooing. Potential allergens include propylene glycol and lanolin.

Hair Crayon

Hair crayon is rubbed onto the scalp and helps color the scalp and hair; it is used preferably on smaller areas. It can be used every day or after every shower.[2,3,6-8]

Table 2 summarizes the different camouflaging agents.

Scalp Tattooing (Tricopigmentation/ Micropigmentation)

Tiny pigments are deposited within the upper dermis of the scalp skin, designed to replicate an individual hair-shaven follicle. This creates a three-dimensional visual illusion of a full head of hair. It has a temporary version that lasts for 12–24 months. Here, an individual gets to know the look before committing to a long-term solution. One can proceed to permanent or long-term pigmentation later, which may last for many years or even decades. During the procedure, a microdroplet of pigment is inserted into the upper dermis through the skin using a standard tattoo instrument that can accommodate one to six needles cycling between 100 and 150 cycles/second.

TABLE 2: Camouflage agents.

Product	Packing	Water reaction	Allergy and potential allergen	Disadvantage
Powder cakes	Circular disk with a sponge applicator	Water-resistant, removed by shampooing	No incidence of allergy known. *Potential allergens*: • Ethylene diamine • Propylene glycol • Methyldibromo glutaronitrile • Phenoxyethanol • Methylparaben • Fragrance, D&C, DF&C dyes	Temporary camouflage
Scalp lotions	Lami tubes or bottled	Water-resistant, removed by shampooing	• Allergy not known • Propylene glycol • Triethanolamine • Fragrance • Imidazolidinyl, urea, paraben	Temporary
Scalp spray	Aerosol spray	Removed by shampooing	Propylene glycol, lanolin	Temporary
Hair fibers	Small drums with mesh on the top to deliver the powder	Washed out after washing with plain water	• FD&C, D&C dyes • DMDM hydantoin • Iodopropynyl butylcarbamate	Temporary

(D&C: Drugs and Cosmetics; DMDM: dimethylol-dimethyl; FD&C: Food, Drugs and Cosmetics)

Indications

- Replacement of lost density
- Hairline reconstruction
- Scar camouflage
- Alopecia correction
- Complimentary to hair transplant to give a fuller look
- In to donor scar, which is otherwise not amenable to repair

Disadvantages include allergic contact dermatitis, infection, granuloma formation, and color change over a period of time[3,4,8]

CAMOUFLAGE FOR THE LASH AND BROW

Artificial eyelashes are a type of temporary camouflage, whereas tattooing and microblading stay much longer. Lash singlets are a fairly simple fashion accessory that is simply adhered to the natural lashes. Demi lashes are lighter and have less hairs than a full set of lashes; they are also made to blend in with the natural lashes. Complete eyelashes can be used when there is a total loss of eyebrows. Wearing artificial eyelashes can irritate the eye, tarsal plate, and eyelid. The most well-known technique for cosmetic tattooing of the eyebrows is known as microblading. This type of semi-permanent tattooing uses tiny, fine-point needles that are combined with a handle to simultaneously scratch and deposit micropigment under the skin.[3,4,8]

INTEGRATING SCALP CAMOUFLAGING IN ROUTINE PRACTICE

These treatments can be used along with medical management. For individuals using minoxidil, it is important to note that minoxidil is applied first to the scalp and allowed to dry before any of the camouflaging agents. Also, the product needs to be removed before applying the next minoxidil application.

Individuals undergoing hair transplant can safely apply hair fibers as early as 2 weeks post-transplant. These products are useful to minimize the appearance of post-transplant.

SUMMARY

Hair camouflaging trend is on the rise worldwide. Various new options with cosmetic appeal are becoming available. It needs a scientific approach and standardized methods to ensure safety and uniformity across the world.

REFERENCES

1. Cash TF, Price VH, Savin RC. Psychological effects of androgenic alopecia on women: comparisons with balding men and with female control subjects. J Am Acad Dermatol. 1993;29:568-75.
2. Donovan JCH, Shapiro R, Shapiro P, Zupan M, Pierre-Louis M, Hordinsky MK. A review of scalp camouflaging agents and prostheses for individuals with hair loss. Dermatol Online J. 2012;18(8):1.
3. Harris J, Emanuel M. Cosmetic hair additions. In: The Hair Replacement Revolution: A Consumer's Guide to Effective Hair Replacement Techniques. New York: Square One Publishers; 2003. pp. 59-75.
4. Kobre SD. The Truth about Women's Hair Loss: What Really Works for Treating and Preventing Thinning Hair. New York: McGraw-Hill; 2000. pp. 94-6.
5. Art of Wigs. [online] Available from www.artofwigs.com. [Last accessed October, 2023].
6. Hair Fear. [online] Available from www.hairfear.com. [Last accessed October, 2023].
7. Sarangi K. Nonsurgical hair replacement. In: Sawant S (Ed). Textbook of Dermatosurgery Cosmetology, 2nd edition. Mumbai, India: ASCAD; 2005. pp. 437-42.

CHAPTER 34

Scalp Micropigmentation and Microblading

Aseem Sharma, Ravina Surve, Amit Kerure, Madhulika Mhatre

Key Messages

- *Scalp micropigmentation (SMP) and microblading (MB): Innovative solutions for hair and eyebrow concerns*:
  - SMP is a nonsurgical technique that uses specialized pigments to replicate the appearance of hair follicles, providing an effective solution for hair loss, alopecia, and thinning hair.
  - MB is a semipermanent eyebrow enhancement technique that uses fine incisions filled with pigment to create natural-looking eyebrows, addressing eyebrow-related concerns.
  - Dermatological expertise and safe practices are essential.
  - Dermatologists play a critical role in performing or supervising SMP and MB procedures, ensuring safe and effective outcomes.
  - Emphasize the importance of selecting qualified and experienced practitioners who adhere to strict hygiene standards and follow proper infection control protocols.
- *Managing expectations and realistic results*:
  - Dermatologists must educate patients about the achievable outcomes of SMP and MB procedures.
  - While SMP can create the illusion of a fuller head of hair, it does not stimulate hair growth, and MB enhances eyebrow appearance without altering natural growth patterns.
- *Post-procedure care and follow-up*:
  - Dermatologists should provide comprehensive aftercare instructions to promote proper healing and maintain the longevity of SMP and MB results.
  - Regular follow-up appointments are crucial for monitoring progress and addressing any concerns or touch-up requirements.
- *Psychological impact and patient satisfaction*:
  - Address the psychological and emotional impact of SMP and MB on patients' self-esteem and confidence, particularly for those struggling with hair loss or eyebrow issues. Discuss the potential benefits of these procedures in improving body image and enhancing overall well-being.
  - By focusing on these key messages, the dermatology Chapter on SMP and MB can provide valuable insights into both practitioners and patients, emphasizing the importance of expertise, safety, and managing expectations for successful outcomes.

INTRODUCTION

There is an array of options available to address the issue of hair loss in modern times. As hair thinning and loss progress, the contrast between the scalp and hair color becomes more pronounced, leading to visible scalp exposure.[1] This can often result in social anxiety and diminished self-esteem for affected individuals.

While oral and topical medications can assist with balding scalps, they may not always yield optimal results. Hair transplantation procedures have gained popularity recently, but many individuals may not feel comfortable undergoing such invasive treatments. For these patients, camouflage techniques offer a viable alternative to achieve a visually appealing look. Various methods, including hair biofibers, wigs, and concealers, can be employed as temporary solutions. Additionally, medical tattooing of the scalp, known as "scalp micropigmentation" (SMP) or scalp microblading, has gained popularity among individuals who are not inclined toward hair transplantation or those with scarring alopecia. During SMP, tattoo ink is delicately inserted into the upper dermis of the scalp in a stippling pattern, while scalp microblading involves creating natural-looking strokes to provide a fuller appearance to the scalp by reducing the contrast between the scalp skin and hair.

SCALP MICROPIGMENTATION

The practice of tattooing dates back to the Neolithic era and has experienced evolving perceptions throughout history. In recent times, tattooing has gained immense popularity, particularly among the adolescent population. Notably, SMP was first reported by Traquina, who performed micropigmentation procedures on 62 patients with scalp scars.[2] However, this early method was crude, resulting in inconsistent color uptake.

Fortunately, tattooing in the medical field has undergone significant advancements in technique and understanding, leading to improved outcomes. SMP involves the precise insertion of pigment in a stippling pattern within the dermis, acting as a permanent concealer. While the technique may seem straightforward, it requires customization for each individual patient, emphasizing the importance of having trained professionals perform the procedure.

Patient Selection/Indications

Preprocedure checklist for SMP and microblading:

1. Consultation and informed consent
2. *Medical history form*: Provision for a form to be filled out, including information about any medical conditions, allergies, skin sensitivities, and medications they are currently taking.
3. *Patch test (if applicable)*: 3–4 weeks prior to the actual procedure, if indicated
4. No prior investigations are needed to be performed.
5. *Avoidance*: Alcohol, aspirin, ibuprofen, and other rheologics for 72 hours prior to the procedure to reduce the risk of excessive bleeding.
6. *Sun protection*: Instructions to protect the treated area (scalp or eyebrows) from excessive sun exposure and avoid tanning beds for at least 2 weeks before the procedure. Sunburnt skin can lead to complications and affect pigment retention.
7. *Avoid chemical treatments*: Instructions to refrain from using hair dyes or undergoing any chemical treatments on their scalp or eyebrows for at least a week before and 3–4 weeks after the procedure.
8. Shaving or trimming (for SMP)
9. Preprocedure preparedness checklist:
   a. Color mixing, matching, and involving the patient in the decision-making process
   b. Sterile environment, standard cleansing-disinfection
   c. Fresh instruments (blade, pigment)
   d. Alcohol swabs and plain wipes
   e. Immediate postprocedure care

Patient/Indications

Scalp micropigmentation is ideal for patients with no grossly visible balding. It suits best for people in whom fullness of the scalp can be achieved, which can be camouflaged under normal hair.

- Patients with androgenetic alopecia in early stages
- Patients undergoing hair transplantation as an adjunctive treatment
- Patients with recalcitrant patchy alopecia
- Patients with scarring alopecias
- Patients with donor site scarring undergoing follicular unit transplantation
- Patients with linear traumatic scars

Materials Required

Pigments

Special tattoo pigments with nontoxic, nonallergenic, and inert properties are utilized for SMP. While both organic and inorganic pigments are available, inorganic pigments are predominantly used **(Box 1)**. Among the commonly employed pigments are iron oxides, titanium dioxide, and barium sulfate.[3]

BOX 1 Classification of pigments.

- *Organic pigments*:
  - Fruit, vegetable dyes—natural
  - Azo compounds
  - Dioxazine
  - Quinacridone
- *Inorganic pigments*:
  - Iron oxide
  - Titanium dioxide
  - Barium sulfate

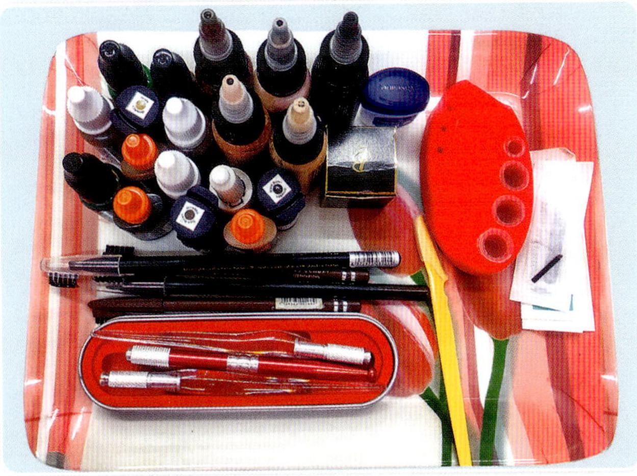

FIG. 1: Pigments used for micropigmentation—scalp micropigmentation and microblading.

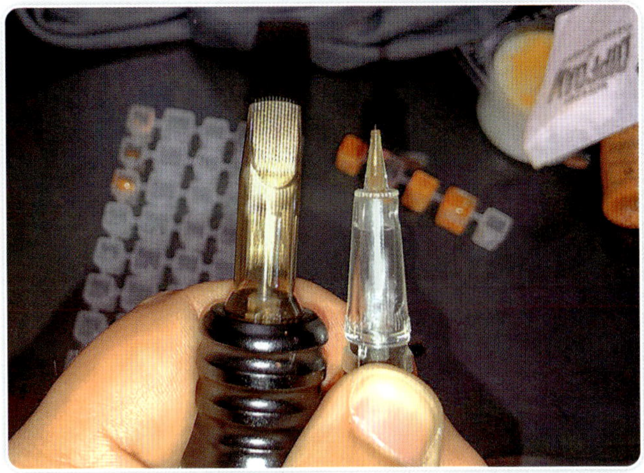

FIG. 2: Needles used for scalp micropigmentation—the difference between round liners and magnums.

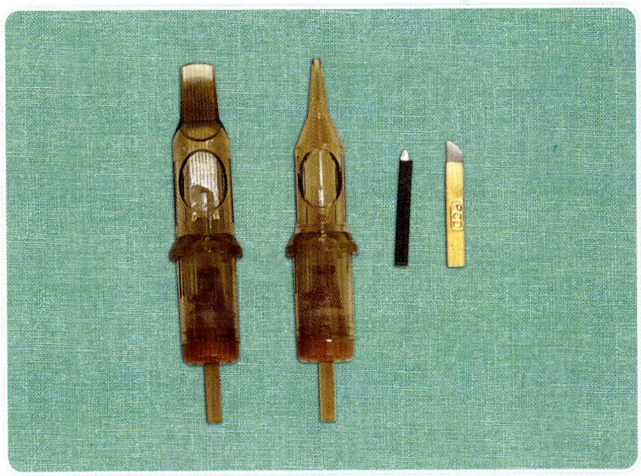

FIG. 3: Needles used for scalp micropigmentation and microblading.

The selection of pigment color should be based on the patient's skin type. Optimal results can be achieved by using a jet black color or a combination of jet black and brown pigments. The selection of pigments is based on the patient's skin type, keeping in mind that black pigments may result in a greenish-blue tinge.[4] Red or orange pigments might be used in corrective micropigmentation procedures to neutralize or balance out undesired colors from previous tattoos or permanent makeup, especially for lip micropigmentation, as it is a complementary color to brown— the color of one's skin. However, the same are not used routinely in SMP **(Fig. 1)**.

The synthetic inorganic pigments are longer lasting and more inert as compared to organic dyes. Allergic reactions are also less with synthetic inorganic pigments.

Color mixing is the most important part of medical tattooing, wherein the color wheel and an understanding of primary, secondary, and the concept of complementary and contrasting colors need to be understood.

Needles

Various needle options are available for SMP, including 1RL, 2RL, 3RL, and 5RL. For creating the appearance of fullness on the scalp, three-point needles are commonly used, while a 1RL needle is preferred for designing the hairline. For achieving a dense look on the scalp, a 3RL needle or a three-pronged needle is commonly used. Conversely, a one-pronged needle is preferred for creating a natural hairline anteriorly **(Figs. 2 and 3)**.

Machine

An electrically driven tattoo machine is employed for performing the SMP procedure. Machines could have a coil-based engine or rotary-based crank and shaft; the latter is also available as a "pen." The SMP procedure involves an electrically driven tattoo machine with a single-use disposable needle attached. The needle's vibratory up-and-down motion creates an alternating effect of pressure and suction, facilitating the deposition of pigment. The difference between rotary pens and tattoo machines lies in the technology used to drive the crankshaft and not the setting. Some pen machines, in fact, house more torque capability than coil-based tattoo machines. An ideal oscillatory speed would lie between 4,000 and 9,000 revolutions per minute for precision and good pigment deposition **(Fig. 4)**.

Miscellaneous Paraphernalia

Local anesthesia can be administered either through the application of an EMLA cream or by providing a field block.

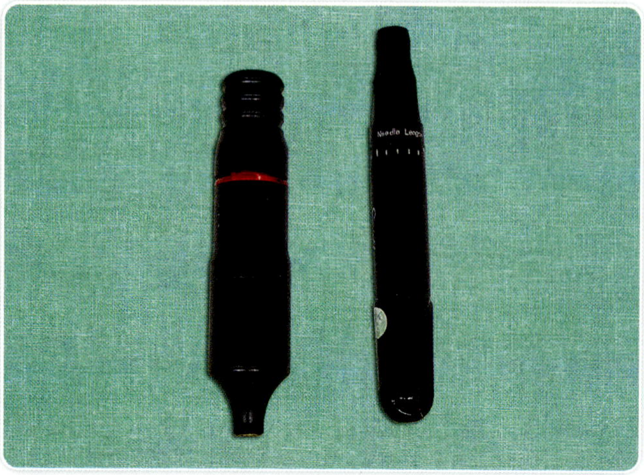

FIG. 4: Rotary pen machines commonly used by the authors for scalp micropigmentation.

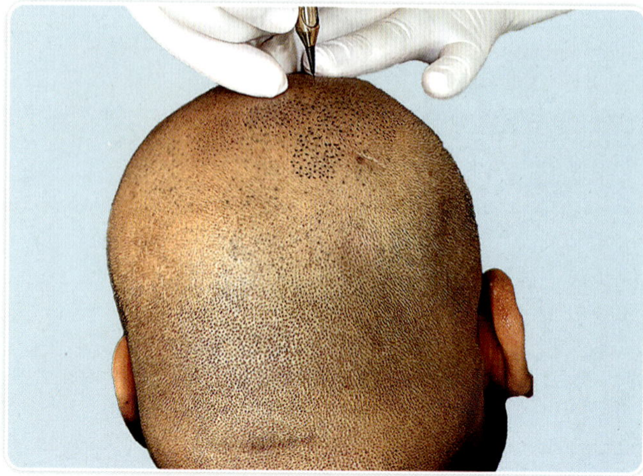

FIG. 5: 3RL needle used on the scalp vertex to create a random dot placement.

To prevent pigment contamination, it is essential to utilize small, disposable cup-shaped pigment holders. It is important to ensure that the needle does not touch the rim of the pigment holder to prevent needle blunting. Additionally, the viscosity of the pigment should be appropriate, as excessively watery consistency can lead to poor dye uptake.

Factors Influencing the Outcome of Scalp Micropigmentation

The outcome of a SMP procedure is influenced by several factors. To ensure a natural and optimal outcome in SMP, the following factors should be considered:

- *Technique and needle*: The angle, depth, and pattern of needle insertion, along with the contact time, size, and speed of the needle, all play a significant role.
- *Dye*: The color and viscosity of the dye used are crucial factors to consider.
- *Skin*: The resistance of the skin, particularly in cases of scarring alopecia, can impact the procedure's results.
- *Control of needle depth*: The depth of needle insertion is crucial in determining the pigment deposition in specific skin layers. If the needle is too superficial, the pigment may wash off within 4–6 weeks. Conversely, if the depth is too deep, the dye may spread and create an unnatural look. The ideal depth is up to the papillary dermis (up to 0.7 mm).
- *Speed and contact period*: The speed of the motor and the contact period of the needle with the scalp play significant roles. Higher motor speed is often necessary for patients with scarring alopecia to overcome increased resistance. The contact period of the needle should be at least 0.5–1 second for proper pigment diffusion.[1]

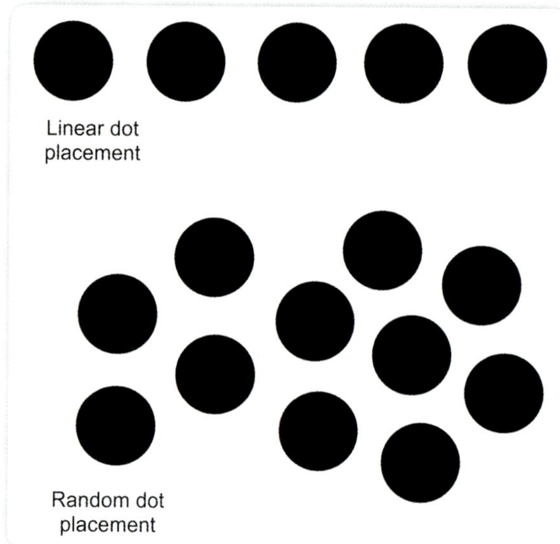

FIG. 6: Random dot placement, shown pictorially.

- *Random dot placement*: Dots should be placed randomly rather than in a linear fashion to achieve a natural appearance **(Figs. 5 and 6)**.
- *Angle of needle insertion*: The needle should be inserted perpendicular to the scalp surface, aligned with the direction of hair growth. This technique results in round dots, while an acute angle can lead to trailing of dye and an unnatural appearance **(Fig. 7)**.

Procedural Steps

- *Preprocedural preparation*:
    - Written informed consent is taken. Proper photos are taken with adequate lighting.
    - Patient should be asked about any prior allergies to local anesthetics or pigments. Patient should avoid

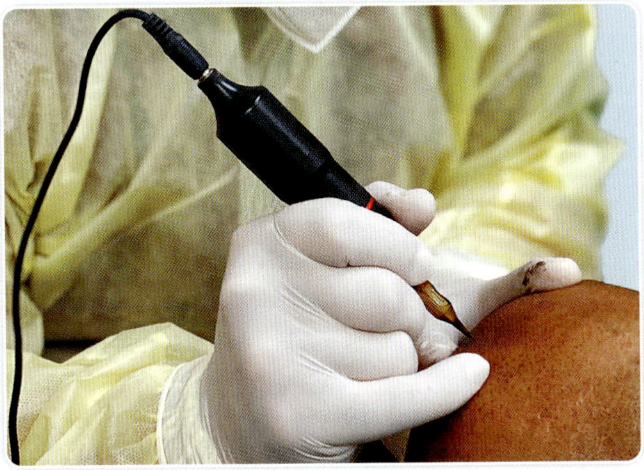

FIG. 7: Angle of insertion shown on the scalp during scalp micropigmentation.

taking ginkgo biloba, vitamin E supplements, and aspirin for at least 1 day prior to the procedure. Marking should be done to denote the area to be treated prior to starting the procedure so as to give a general idea to the patient about where the targeted response will be visible.

- *Procedural steps*:
  - Patient can be in prone or supine position, depending on which area of the scalp is to be treated.
  - Local anesthesia can be administered either through the application of an EMLA cream or by providing a field block.
  - Site to be treated is prepared, and the instruments required are made ready. On the tattoo machine, an appropriate-sized needle is attached, and pigment according to the patient's skin type and indication is chosen. To begin with, the motorized pen is started and the needle is dipped in pigment. To prevent pigment contamination, it is essential to utilize small, disposable cup-shaped pigment holders. It is important to ensure that the needle does not touch the rim of the pigment holder to prevent needle blunting. Additionally, the viscosity of the pigment should be appropriate, as excessively watery consistency can lead to poor dye uptake. The skin over the scalp is then stretched with two fingers to make the skin taut. The motorized pen is held in a pen-holding fashion and the needle is inserted on the scalp along the direction of the hair follicle.
  - Optimum pigment deposition can be achieved with 5,500–6,500 cycles per minute and a good skin contact for about 0.5–1 second. For cicatricial alopecia, a higher speed may be required to overcome the resistance of the scalp. To give a natural look, random dot placement should be done. Also, the dots should be neither too small nor too big and should mimic the size of the hair follicles of the patient.
- *Duration of procedure*: A full head SMP procedure may take approximately 5–6 hours to complete.

Post-treatment Care

- *Topical antibiotic cream*: After the procedure, a topical antibiotic cream is applied to the scalp.
- *Washing the scalp*: Patients can safely wash their scalp 24 hours after the procedure. They should continue applying the antibiotic cream for a period of 5 days.
- *Pain management*: Painkillers may be required for 2–3 days following the procedure to manage any discomfort.
- However, the patient should avoid hot, steamy showers, swimming in salty waters, or excessive sun exposure for a couple of weeks.
- *Follow-up*:
  - Immediate postoperative: Superficial pigment may wash off in 48 hours; also, over a period of few weeks, softening of scalp pigment will be noted. The patient should be checked for any signs of superficial skin infection.
  - Long postoperative follow-up appointments are scheduled at 3 and 6 months after the procedure to assess pigment uptake and overall results. If necessary, a touch-up session can be planned.
- *Duration of procedure*: A full-head SMP procedure may take approximately 5–6 hours to complete.

Tattoo fading and color selection: Over time, the tattoo effect may lighten due to epidermal turnover and shedding of pigment. Therefore, appropriate colors should be utilized. Patients with graying hair should be informed that they might need to dye their hair to reduce the contrast between the dye and the scalp.[5]

Potential for repeat session: In some cases, a repeat session may be required after 8–9 months to maintain the desired result. **Figures 8 and 9** show pre- and post-photos of SMP, respectively.

Precautions and Contraindications

Allergies: It is important to avoid the procedure if the patient has any known allergies to pigments used in SMP.

Scarring alopecias: In cases of scarring alopecias, a test patch can be performed beforehand to determine the appropriate parameters, such as motor rotations and needle depth, to achieve optimal results.

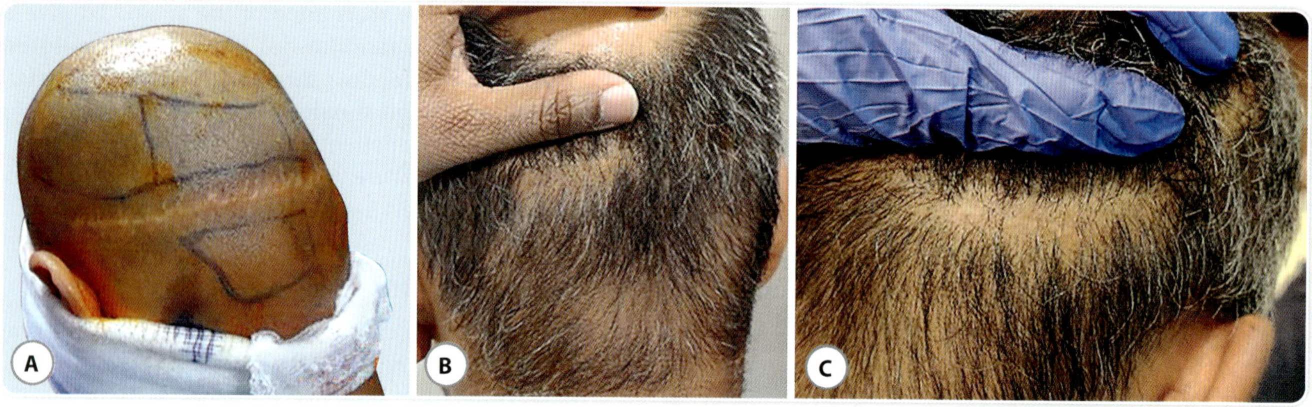

FIGS. 8A TO C: Prephotos of scalp micropigmentation (SMP) in a case of follicular unit transplantation (FUT) scar.

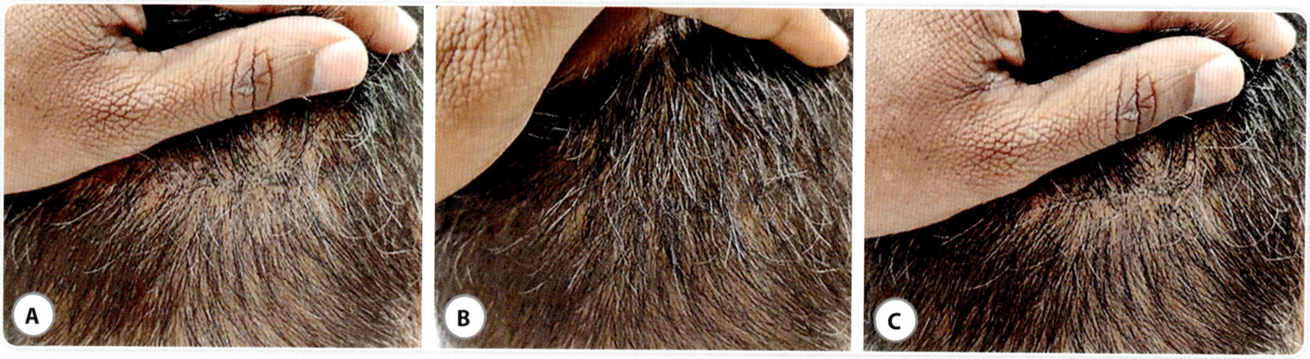

FIGS. 9A TO C: Post-photos of scalp micropigmentation in a case of follicular unit transplantation scar.

Supplements: Certain supplements such as ginkgo biloba, vitamin E supplements, nonsteroidal anti-inflammatory drugs (NSAIDs), and aspirin should be avoided for at least 1 day prior to the treatment.

There are no such contraindications to this procedure; however, it should be avoided in patients with keloidal tendency.

Side Effects

Allergic reactions: Although rare, allergic reactions to the pigments used may occur as a potential side effect.

Patient may develop certain milder side effects, such as pain and erythema over the scalp. Very rarely, if proper aseptic precautions are not taken, then superficial skin infection such as folliculitis may develop. If the pigment placement is not done properly or the plane of pigment placement is faulty, then cosmetically unpleasant-looking dotted appearance is seen on the scalp.

Scalp micropigmentation is a great camouflaging technique, though it is simple, it requires a proper understanding of the procedure and technique. It serves as an excellent adjuvant for patients with hair transplantation, since with hair transplantation, it is difficult to give original hair density. It is an indispensable tool for treating certain types of scarring alopecia, especially post strip follicular unit transplantation and linear traumatic scars on the scalp, where the scarred skin area is smaller and can be easily concealed by this technique. Also, in cases of recalcitrant patchy alopecia, it is a great procedure to boost patients' confidence. There are no side effects, and it is a relatively safer procedure. It may be combined with a hair transplant, where one would need a lower number of grafts to transplant, since the use of contrasting pigments would mitigate that. In the authors' experience, the ideal gap between SMP and hair transplant should be 45 days if SMP is performed before the transplant, and 6 months if follicular unit extraction (FUE) is done first.

SCALP MICROBLADING

Scalp microblading is a relatively new procedure that has gained popularity since 2015, particularly in Asian countries. Similar to eyebrow microblading, scalp microblading is an emerging technique used to enhance the appearance of the scalp, especially in the temporal region. This procedure involves the precise placement of pigments in linear strokes, creating the illusion of fuller hair and mimicking the natural hair pattern. It is not employed as much as brow microblading as SMP yields better aesthetic outcomes and a more natural-looking scalp.

Indications

- Temporal area hair thinning in males and females with androgenetic alopecia, restoring the hairline to give a youthful look
- To give a fuller/voluminous scalp look in patients with thin hair
- Scarring alopecia

Instruments Required

Microblading pen: This manual instrument consists of three parts: Handle, rotating adjuster, and grooved blade holder. Disposable needles are attached to the blade holder, which can be reused after autoclaving. Alternatively, single-use prefitted microblading pens are also available. Some practitioners use a motorized permanent makeup machine with adjustable speed for this procedure.

Blades: Blades used in scalp microblading contain multiple needles arranged in a row. Various blade options are available, such as 7, 9, or 12 needles, with needle thickness ranging from 0.4 to 0.16 mm. Beginners often prefer flexible needles, while experienced practitioners may opt for harder needles.[6]

Ink holders: Plastic or metal ring containers are used to hold the ink and prevent contamination **(Figs. 10 and 11)**.

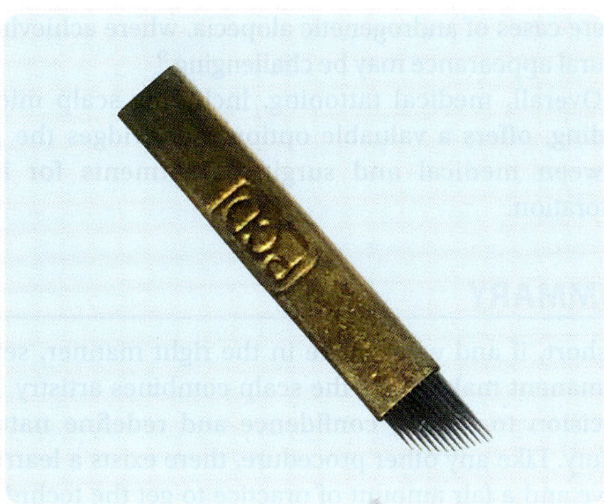

FIG. 10: A microblading needle.

Procedure

The procedure begins with the application of a topical anesthetic cream to numb the skin in the desired region. Aseptic precautions are taken to ensure a sterile environment. The microblading pen, equipped with a suitable needle, is used to create precise linear strokes that mimic natural hair. Proper stretching of the skin is necessary to ensure optimal pigment deposition. Selecting the appropriate color shade to match the patient's hair is crucial. The ideal depth of the needle should reach the papillary dermis, which can be identified by the presence of lymph exudate and pinpoint bleeding.

Two main types of strokes are typically employed: Main strokes, which are longer and more prominent, and supporting strokes that merge with the main strokes. All strokes are made at a 45° angle to simulate natural hair follicles.[6] After the procedure, the pigment can be gently smudged on the treated area for 5 minutes before being wiped away with normal saline.

Postprocedure

Patients should avoid excessive sweating, workouts, and contact with water for up to 48 hours following the procedure. They should also be aware that slight color

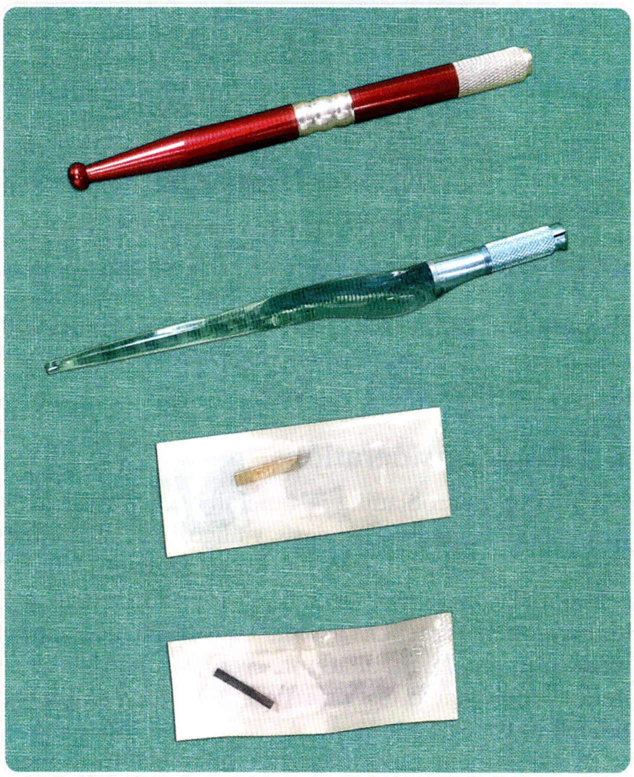

FIG. 11: Microblading pen holder with needles.

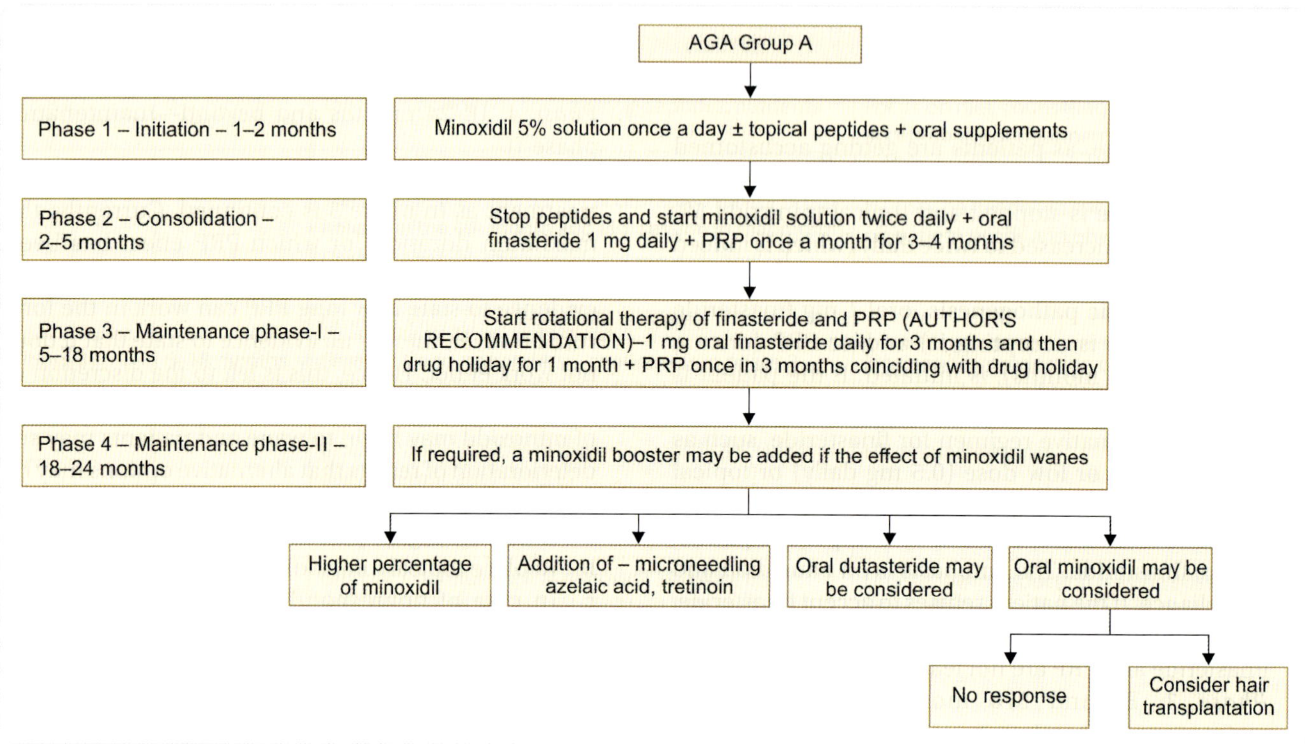

FLOWCHART 1: Algorithm for group A patients (patients who accept finasteride).
(AGA: androgenetic alopecia; PRP: platelet-rich plasma)

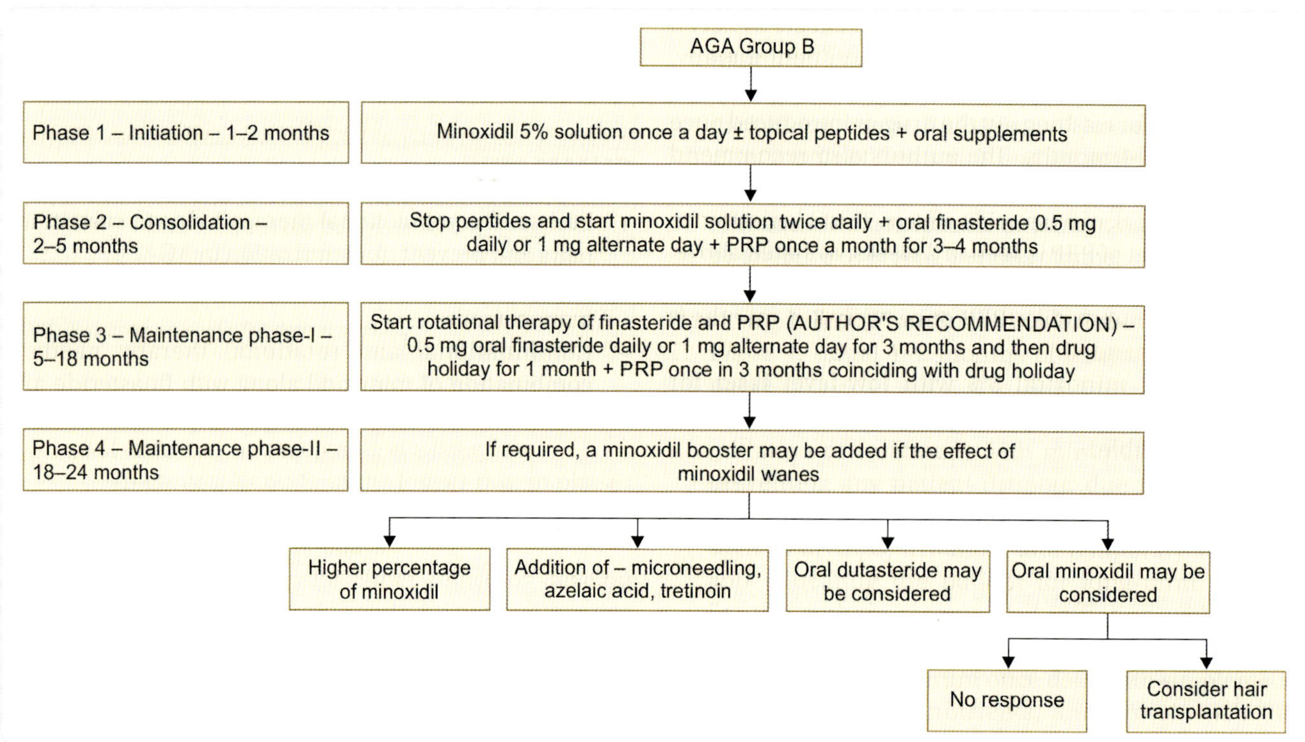

FLOWCHART 2: Algorithm for group B patients: Treatment algorithm using rotational therapy for androgenetic alopecia (AGA) group B (patients who are apprehensive about taking finasteride).
(PRP: platelet-rich plasma)

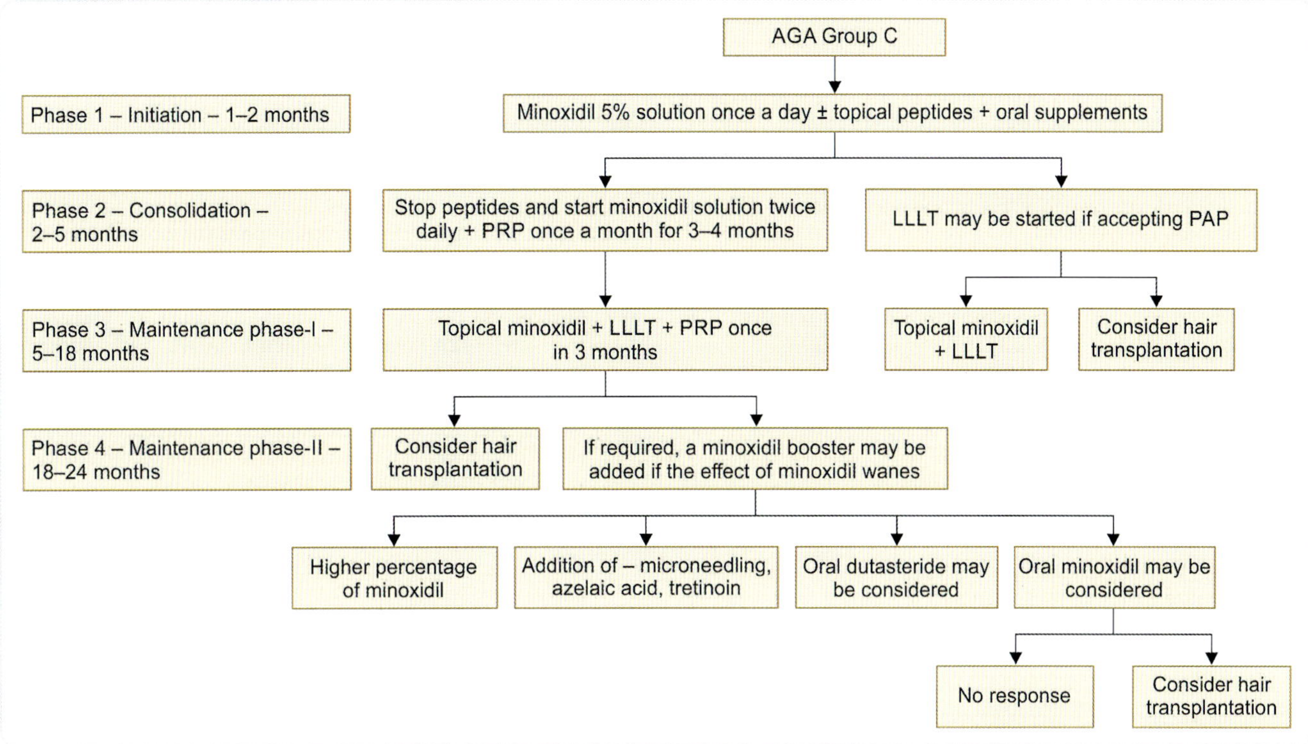

FLOWCHART 3: Treatment algorithm using rotational therapy for androgenetic alopecia (AGA) group C (patients who either refuse or develop side effects of finasteride and who need alternative treatments).
(LLLT: low-level laser therapy; PRP: platelet-rich plasma)

REFERENCES

1. Choi CW, Kim BR, Ohn J, Youn SW. The advantage of cyclosporine A and methotrexate rotational therapy in long-term systemic treatment for chronic plaque psoriasis in a real world practice. Ann Dermatol. 2017;29:55-60.
2. Weinstein GD, White GM. An approach to the treatment of moderate to severe psoriasis with rotational therapy. J Am Acad Dermatol. 1993;28:454-9.
3. Fanouriakis A, Tziolos N, Bertsias G, Boumpas DT. Update on the diagnosis and management of systemic lupus erythematosus. Ann Rheum Dis. 2021;80:14-25.
4. van de Kerkhof PC. Therapeutic strategies: rotational therapy and combinations. Clin Exp Dermatol. 2001;26:356-61.
5. Traish AM. Post-finasteride syndrome: a surmountable challenge for clinicians. Fertil Steril. 2020;113:21-50.
6. Pereira AFJR, Coelho TOA. Post-finasteride syndrome. An Bras Dermatol. 2020;95:271-7.
7. Mysore V, Kumaresan M, Dashore S, Venkatram A. Combination and rotational therapy in androgenetic alopecia. J Cutan Aesthet Surg. 2023;16:71-80.
8. Kanti V, Messenger A, Dobos G, Reygagne P, Finner A, Blumeyer A, et al. Evidence-based (S3) guideline for the treatment of androgenetic alopecia in women and in men—short version. J Eur Acad Dermatol Venereol. 2018;32:11-22.
9. Mysore V, Shashikumar BM. Guidelines on the use of finasteride in androgenetic alopecia. Indian J Dermatol Venereol Leprol. 2016;82:128-34.
10. Lee SW, Juhasz M, Mobasher P, Ekelem C, Mesinkovska NA. A systematic review of topical finasteride in the treatment of androgenetic alopecia in men and women. J Drugs Dermatol. 2018;17:457-63.
11. Sharma A, Chouhan K, Bhatia S, Dashore S. Platelet-rich plasma in androgenetic alopecia. Indian Dermatol Online J. 2021;12(Suppl. 1):S31-40.
12. Gentile P, Garcovich S. Systematic review of platelet-rich plasma use in androgenetic alopecia compared with Minoxidil®, Finasteride®, and adult stem cell-based therapy. Int J Mol Sci. 2020;21:2702.
13. Mysore V, Kumaresan M, Garg A, Dua A, Venkatram A, Dua K, et al. Hair transplant practice guidelines. J Cutan Aesthet Surg. 2021;14:265-84.
14. McClellan KJ, Markham A. Finasteride: a review of its use in male pattern hair loss. Drugs. 1999;57:111-26.
15. Kaufman KD, Rotonda J, Shah AK, Meehan AG. Long-term treatment with finasteride 1 mg decreases the likelihood of developing further visible hair loss in men with androgenetic alopecia (male pattern hair loss). Eur J Dermatol. 2008;18:400-6.
16. Rossi A, Cantisani C, Scarnò M, Trucchia A, Fortuna MC, Calvieri S. Finasteride, 1 mg daily administration on male androgenetic alopecia in different age groups: 10-year follow-up. Dermatol Ther. 2011;24:455-61.
17. Shin JW, Chung EH, Kim MB, Kim TO, Kim WI, Huh CH. Evaluation of long-term efficacy of finasteride in Korean men with

androgenetic alopecia using the basic and specific classification system. J Dermatol. 2019;46:139-43.

18. Yoshitake T, Takeda A, Ohki K, Inoue Y, Yamawaki T, Otsuka S, et al. Five-year efficacy of finasteride in 801 Japanese men with androgenetic alopecia. J Dermatol. 2015;42:735-8.
19. Drake L, Hordinsky M, Fiedler V, Swinehart J, Unger WP, Cotterill PC, et al. The effects of finasteride on scalp skin and serum androgen levels in men with androgenetic alopecia. J Am Acad Dermatol. 1999;41:550-4.
20. Gormley GJ, Stoner E, Rittmaster RS, Gregg H, Thompson DL, Lasseter KC, et al. Effects of finasteride (MK-906), a 5α-reductase inhibitor, on circulating androgens in male volunteers. J Clin Endocrinol Metab. 1990;70:1136-41.
21. Tartagni M, Schonauer MM, Cicinelli E, Petruzzelli F, De Pergola G, De Salvia MA, et al. Intermittent low-dose finasteride is as effective as daily administration for the treatment of hirsute women. Fertil Steril. 2004;82:752-5.
22. Wessells H, Roy J, Bannow J, Grayhack J, Matsumoto AM, Tenover L, et al. Incidence and severity of sexual adverse experiences in finasteride and placebo-treated men with benign prostatic hyperplasia. Urology. 2003;61:579-84.
23. Kiguradze T, Temps WH, Yarnold PR, Cashy J, Brannigan RE, Nardone B, et al. Persistent erectile dysfunction in men exposed to the 5α-reductase inhibitors, finasteride, or dutasteride. Peer J. 2017;5:e3020.
24. Irwig MS, Kolukula S. Persistent sexual side effects of finasteride for male pattern hair loss. J Sex Med. 2011;8:1747-53.
25. Irwig MS. Persistent sexual side effects of finasteride: could they be permanent? J Sex Med. 2012;9:2927-32.
26. Shin HS, Won CH, Lee SH, Kwon OS, Kim KH, Eun HC. Efficacy of 5% minoxidil versus combined 5% minoxidil and 0.01% tretinoin for male pattern hair loss: a randomized, double-blind, comparative clinical trial. Am J Clin Dermatol. 2007;8:285-90.
27. Gugle AS, Jadhav VM, Kote RP, Deshmukh MD, Dalvi AV. Comparative study of efficacy of topical minoxidil 5% and combination of topical minoxidil 5%, topical azelaic acid 1.5% and topical tretinoin 0.01% on the basis of dermoscopic analysis in androgenetic alopecia. MVP J Med Sci. 2015;2:90-9.
28. Olsen EA, Weiner MS, Amara IA, DeLong ER. Five-year follow-up of men with androgenetic alopecia treated with topical minoxidil. J Am Acad Dermatol. 1990;22:643-6.
29. Varothai S, Bergfeld WF. Androgenetic alopecia: an evidence-based treatment update. Am J Clin Dermatol. 2014;15:217-30.
30. Katz HI, Hien NT, Prawer SE, Goldman SJ. Long-term efficacy of topical minoxidil in male pattern baldness. J Am Acad Dermatol. 1987;16:711-8.
31. Price VH, Menefee E, Strauss PC. Changes in hair weight and hair count in men with androgenetic alopecia, after application of 5% and 2% topical minoxidil, placebo, or no treatment. J Am Acad Dermatol. 1999;41:717-21.
32. Olsen EA, Weiner MS. Topical minoxidil in male pattern baldness: effects of discontinuation of treatment. J Am Acad Dermatol. 1987;17:97-101.
33. Ferry JJ, Shepard JH, Szpunar GJ. Relationship between contact time of applied dose and percutaneous absorption of minoxidil from a topical solution. J Pharm Sci. 1990;79:483-6.
34. Kubba R. Topical minoxidil in androgenetic alopecia, how good is it? Indian J Dermatol Venereol Leprol. 1990;56:187-92.
35. Rossi A, Cantisani C, Melis L, Iorio A, Scali E, Calvieri S. Minoxidil use in dermatology, side effects and recent patents. Recent Pat Inflamm Allergy Drug Discov. 2012;6:130-6.
36. McCoy J, Goren A, Kovacevic M, Shapiro J. Minoxidil dose response study in female pattern hair loss patients determined to be non-responders to 5% topical minoxidil. J Biol Regul Homeost Agents. 2016;30:1153-5.
37. Suchonwanit P, Thammarucha S, Leerunyaku K. Minoxidil and its use in hair disorders: a review. Drug Des Dev Ther. 2019;13:2777-86.
38. Roberts J, Desai N, McCoy J, Goren A. Sulfotransferase activity in plucked hair follicles predicts response to topical minoxidil in the treatment of female androgenetic alopecia. Dermatol Ther. 2014;27(4):252-4.
39. Dashore S, Chouhan K, Nanda S, Sharma A. Preparation of platelet-rich plasma: National IADVL PRP Taskforce Recommendations. Indian Dermatol Online J. 2021;12(Suppl. 1):S12-23.
40. Miao Y, Sun YB, Sun XJ, Du BJ, Jiang JD, Hu ZQ. Promotional effect of platelet-rich plasma on hair follicle reconstitution in vivo. Dermatol Surg. 2013;39:1868-76.
41. Xiao SE, Miao Y, Wang J, Jiang W, Fan ZX, Liu XM, et al. As a carrier-transporter for hair follicle reconstitution, platelet-rich plasma promotes proliferation and induction of mouse dermal papilla cells. Sci Rep. 2017;7:1125.
42. Gentile P, Garcovich S, Bielli A, Scioli MG, Orlandi A, Cervelli V. The effect of platelet-rich plasma in hair regrowth: a randomized placebo-controlled trial. Stem Cells Transl Med. 2015;4:1317-23.
43. Girijala RL, Riahi RR, Cohen PR. Platelet-rich plasma for androgenic alopecia treatment: a comprehensive review. Dermatol Online J. 2018;24(7):13030/qt8s43026c.
44. Gkini MA, Kouskoukis AE, Tripsianis G, Rigopoulos D, Kouskoukis K. Study of platelet-rich plasma injections in the treatment of androgenetic alopecia through an one-year period. J Cutan Aesthet Surg. 2014;7:213-9.
45. Stevens J, Khetarpal S. Platelet-rich plasma for androgenetic alopecia: a review of the literature and proposed treatment protocol. Int J Womens Dermatol. 2018;5:46-51.
46. Alves R, Grimalt R. Randomized placebo-controlled, double-blind, half-head study to assess the efficacy of platelet-rich plasma on the treatment of androgenetic alopecia. Dermatol Surg. 2016;42:491-7.
47. Eells JT, Wong-Riley MT, VerHoeve J, Henry M, Buchman EV, Kane MP, et al. Mitochondrial signal transduction in accelerated wound and retinal healing by near-infrared light therapy. Mitochondrion. 2004;4:559-67.
48. Chung H, Dai T, Sharma SK, Huang Y-Y, Carroll JD, Hamblin MR. The nuts and bolts of low-level laser (light) therapy. Ann Biomed Eng. 2012;40:516-33.
49. Avci P, Gupta GK, Clark J, Wikonkal N, Hamblin MR. Low-level laser (light) therapy (LLLT) for treatment of hair loss. Lasers Surg Med. 2014;46:144-51.
50. Jimenez JJ, Wikramanayake TC, Bergfeld W, Hordinsky M, Hickman JG, Hamblin MR, et al. Efficacy and safety of a low-level laser device in the treatment of male and female pattern hair loss: a multicenter, randomized, sham device-controlled, double-blind study. Am J Clin Dermatol. 2014;15:115-27.
51. Leavitt M, Charles G, Heyman E, Michaels D. HairMax LaserComb® laser phototherapy device in the treatment of male androgenetic alopecia: a randomized, double-blind, sham device controlled, multicentre trial. Clin Drug Investig. 2009;29:283-92.
52. Kim H, Choi JW, Kim JY, Shin JW, Lee SJ, Huh CH. Low-level light therapy for androgenetic alopecia: a 24-week, randomized,

double-blind, sham device-controlled multicenter trial. Dermatol Surg. 2013;39:1177-83.

53. Suchonwanit P, Chalermroj N, Khunkhet S. Low-level laser therapy for the treatment of androgenetic alopecia in Thai men and women: a 24-week, randomized, double-blind, sham device-controlled trial. Lasers Med Sci. 2019;34:1107-14.
54. Lanzafame RJ, Blanche RR, Bodian AB, Chiacchierini RP, Fernandez-Obregon A, Kazmirek ER. The growth of human scalp hair mediated by visible red light laser and LED sources in males. Lasers Surg Med. 2013;45:487-95.
55. Faghihi G, Mozafarpoor S, Asilian A, Mokhtari F, Esfahani AA, Bafandeh B, et al. The effectiveness of adding low-level light therapy to minoxidil 5% solution in the treatment of patients with androgenetic alopecia. Indian J Dermatol Venereol Leprol. 2018;84:547-53.
56. Pillai JK, Mysore V. Role of low-level light therapy (LLLT) in androgenetic alopecia. J Cutan Aesthet Surg. 2021;14:385-91.
57. Higgins C, et al. Triggering human hair follicle growth. PNAS. 2013;110(49):19679-88.
58. Kemp P. The evolution of the promise of hair cloning. How hair cell cloning will fit into your practice. Hair Transplant Forum International. 2022;32:37-43.

SECTION

2

Hair Transplantation

PART A: Basic Sciences

SECTION OUTLINE

CHAPTER 36

History of Hair Transplantation

Venkataram Mysore, Aniketh Venkataram

"Those who forget history are condemned to repeat it. And history has a way of repeating itself"

—George Santayana

The above statements are very true of hair transplantation—time and again, discoveries were ignored only to be rediscovered decades later.

EARLY DAYS

The origins of hair transplantation as we know it today can be traced back to the early 20th century. The New York dermatologist *Norman Orentreich is heralded as the father of modern hair transplantation* due to his pioneering work in the 1950s. Orentreich was investigating whether common skin conditions showed donor or recipient site dominance when he discovered that grafts transplanted from occipital scalp survived on bald scalp. He coined the term *donor dominance* to explain this basic principle of hair transplantation, which is that hair transplanted to a balding area will continue to grow as if it were in its original location. He first performed hair transplant surgery in 1952 by harvesting hair in groups of 4 mm. His paper was initially rejected by a skeptical medical community but was eventually published in 1959 in the Annals of the New York Academy of Science.[1]

As we now know, several Japanese dermatologists were using small autografts for treating alopecia even before Orentreich. *The fallout of World War II prevented these works, originally written in Japanese, from reaching the Western world for several years.* These dermatologists included Sasagawa,[2] Okuda, Tamura, and Fujita. Perhaps the most famous of these is *Shoji Okuda*. He published a series of articles in the Japanese Journal of Dermatology entitled "Clinical and experimental study of living hair transplantation" in the year 1939 (nearly 20 years before Orentreich).[3] He reported nearly 200 cases, and his technique included special round saws which were very similar to Orentreich's punches. The Okuda papers contain most of the principles of modern hair transplantation but he did not mention male pattern hair loss (MPHL) as a treatable condition, which is perhaps why Orentreich is credited with being the first to use this technique for MPHL.

Orentreich's 4-mm punch grafting technique remained the basic procedure till 1975. The benefits of using smaller grafts had occurred to several practitioners but at the time, there was no satisfactory method to harvest smaller grafts. This meant that results were frequently punctuated with an unnatural doll's look. In the 1980s, smaller grafts were prepared by dissecting the punch grafts into halves or quarters. The technique evolved even further with *Carlos Uebel in Brazil*[4] and the Moser Clinic in Vienna[5] who started harvesting a donor strip that was then dissected into grafts containing three to four hairs. *This mini/micrografting ultimately signaled the end of punch grafting.*

In hindsight, it is highly regrettable that the work of *Hajime Tamura* of Japan was not known to the Western world earlier. He performed many hair transplant procedures in Tokyo. He reported good results starting from 1939.[6] What is most remarkable is how closely his procedure resembled modern hair transplantation. He harvested donor grafts with an elliptical incision, prepared the recipient site with a thick needle, stored grafts in saline, and observed postoperative shedding. Most importantly, he advocated that single hair grafts produced better results than larger grafts. Unfortunately, he seems to have lost interest in hair transplantation after becoming a professor of urology in 1944. It is indeed clear that if his work had been better known, the history of hair transplantation might have taken a different course and punch grafting might not have been the standard practice for nearly 30 years. *In the words of Sir PG Wodehouse "Half the world doesn't know how the other three quarters live!"*

EVOLUTION OF THE DONOR STRIP

A major advance occurred when the technique was taken a step further by surgeons such as William Rassman of Los Angeles with session sizes of 3,000 odd grafts.[7] For this purpose, multiblade knives of up to 10 blades were developed. Other automatic dissection devices included those of Boudjema in France (1992).[8] The problem with all these devices, however, was that they were often difficult to use, and more importantly caused injury to follicles (sometimes in the range of 25%). This led to the popularity of *microscope-aided dissection.* This was initially started by Bob Limmer of Texas in 1987[9] and popularized by others such as Seager in 1996.[10] This stereomicroscopic dissection of grafts became so ubiquitous with hair transplantation that it is now impossible to imagine the technique without a microscope.

With microscopic dissection, *the concept of "follicular unit transplantation" (FUT) was born.* This concept recognized the existence of hairs in naturally occurring groups, and the term was *coined by Bernstein et al.* in 1995.[11] Initially, FUT was met with resistance by members of the hair transplant community, as it was perceived as difficult and time-consuming. However, it gained popularity, mainly through increased patient demand, fuelled by improved results being posted on the internet. By 2000, it was regarded as the gold standard of surgical hair transplantation. The popularity of FUT ushered in the concept of the hair transplant team as it was no longer possible for one surgeon to complete the entire procedure by himself.

At the same time, the technique was also developing in Asia. The most significant of these developments was the implanter developed by Choi and Kim of South Korea, reported in 1996.[12] This was an ingenious device into which units containing one to four hairs could be loaded and implanted into the scalp with a plunger. A similar implanter was developed by Jung Chul Kim, also of South Korea. Choi and Kim also recognized the units as bundles (or units as known in the West). As hair transplantation grew in popularity, it was natural that the procedure was tried in areas of the body other than the scalp, such as the eyebrows, chest, and pubic region. This led Hwang et al. to study *the effect of the recipient site influence on hair follicles*, and they concluded that the recipient site does affect the characteristics of transplanted hair, including their growth and survival rates.[13]

It is somewhat ironic that histological evidence for the concept of the follicular unit was provided in a landmark paper published earlier, as early as 1984 by Headington, who demonstrated the units in biopsies of the scalp, which were examined after horizontal sectioning.[14] Both Rassman and Bernstein and Kim who developed the concept of FUT were unaware of this paper when they developed their technique. The history of hair transplantation is thus replete with such missed opportunities.

The focus of hair transplantation in recent years has shifted to the donor scar. Often, despite all precautions and meticulous techniques, a wide donor scar was an undesirable result. One method to offset this was the technique of trichophytic closure, described by Drs Patrick Frechet and Paul Rose, as well as Dr Mario Marzola.[15,16] In this procedure, one of the wound edges is de-epithelialized so that hair grows through the scar.

EVOLUTION OF FOLLICULAR UNIT EXCISION

However, as donor scars were still unacceptable to many, *the technique of removing follicular unit grafts individually instead of using a donor strip once again became popular.* Known as the FOX procedure, follicular unit extraction (FUE), and follicular unit separation extraction (FUSE), *this technique is credited to Rassman et al. for their paper in 2002.*[17] FUE was first attempted by Rassman in the 90s, but he was unsuccessful due to a high rate of follicular damage. It was when the work of Masumi Inaba was brought to his attention that the technique was perfected. Inaba solved the problems that Rassman was encountering by advocating that follicular damage could be reduced by cutting only partially into the dermis. However, here too there was a missed opportunity. Dr Woods from Australia was the first one to harvest single follicular units in 1995 and presented his technique to Australian Medical Association. However, he failed to produce a medically accepted paper describing his methods.[18]

This technique of FUE shows that the technique of hair transplantation has come full circle in a sense, back

Timeline of hair transplantation:

- Pre-World War II (WW2): Sasagawa,2 Okuda, Tamura, and Fujita's works
- 1950s: Orentreich's pioneering work, coined the term "donor dominance"
- 1980s: Mini/micrografting using donor strips
- Early 1990s: Microscope-aided dissection
- Late 1990s: Follicular unit transplantation
- 2000s: Follicular unit extraction
- 2010s: Robotic surgery?

to the days of individual graft harvest (albeit micrografts instead of punches). More recently, in order to address the main drawback of FUE, which is its time-consuming nature, robotic devices have been developed to harvest follicular units. One such device is the ARTAS Robotic System by Restoration Robotics Inc., San Jose, CA, which received Food and Drug Administration (FDA) approval in 2011. This system extracts FUs one at a time, using a six-axis articulated robotic arm, with stereo cameras and force sensors. While still in its infancy, this system shows promising results.[19]

This fascinating history of hair transplantation surgery highlights the need to study the techniques used in the past in order to drive the advances of the future. After all, to paraphrase Sir Isaac Newton, *"If we can see far it is because we stand on the shoulders of giants."*

REFERENCES

1. Orentreich N. Autografts in alopecias and other selected dermatological conditions. Ann N Y Acad Sci. 1959;83:463-79.
2. Sasagawa M. Hair transplantation. Jpn J Dermatol. 1923;30:493. [In Japanese]
3. Okuda S. Clinical and experimental studies on hair transplanting of living hair. Jpn J Dermatol Urol. 1939;46:537-87. [In Japanese]
4. Uebel C. 1000 grafts per session. Hair Transplant Forum. 1992;3:9-12.
5. Hugeneck J, Kokott R. Non-tufted incisional slit grafting. Hair Transplant Forum. 1992;3:6-7.
6. Tamura H. Pubic hair transplantation. Jpn J Dermatol. 1943;53:76.
7. Rassman W. Mega-transplants in transition. Hair Transplant Forum. 1993;3:11.
8. Boudjema P, Boolauch SJ. Automated hair transplant system. In: Stough DB, Haber R (Eds). Hair Replacement: Surgical and Medical. Philadelphia: Mosby; 1996. pp. 370-4.
9. Limmer R. Bob Limmer does it all one hair at a time. Hair Transplant Forum Int. 1991;2:8-9.
10. Seager D. Binocular stereoscopic dissection microscopes—should we all be using them? Hair Transplant Forum Int. 1996;6:2-5.
11. Bernstein R, Rassman WR, Szaniawski W, Halperin AJ. Follicular transplantation. Int J Aesthet Restor Surg. 1995;3:119-32.
12. Choi JC, Kim JC. The Choi hair transplanter. In: Stough DB, Haber R (Eds). Hair Replacement: Surgical and Medical. Philadelphia: Mosby; 1996. pp. 125-7.
13. Hwang S, Kim JC, Ryu HS, Cha YC, Lee SJ, Na GY, et al. Does the recipient site influence the hair growth characteristics in hair transplantation? Dermatol Surg. 2002;28:795-8.
14. Headington JT. Transverse microscopic anatomy of the human scalp. A basis for a morphometric approach to disorders of the hair follicle. Arch Dermatol. 1984;120(4):449-56.
15. Frechet P. Donor harvesting with invisible scars. Hair Transplant Forum Int. 2005;15(4):119-20.
16. Marzola, M. Trichophytic closure of the donor area. Hair Transplant Forum Int. 2005;15(4):113-6.
17. Rassman WR, Bernstein RM, McClellan R, Jones R, Worton E, Uyttendaele H. Follicular unit extraction: minimally invasive surgery for hair transplantation. Dermatol Surg. 2002;28:720-8.
18. Williams KL Jr. Current practices and controversies in cosmetic hair restoration. Dermatol Surg. 2013;39:797-801.
19. Shin JW, Kwon SH, Kim SA, Kim JY, Na JI, Park KC, et al. Characteristics of robotically harvested hair follicles in Koreans. J Am Acad Dermatol. 2015;72(1):146-50.

CHAPTER 37

Follicular Unit: Logic and Relevance

Aniketh Venkataram, Venkataram Mysore

Key Messages

- The concept of follicular unit has been the basis for several aspects of follicular unit transplantation (FUT)—both strip dissection and extraction methods.
- It has enabled accurate calculation of the number of grafts needed, through calculation of the density in donor and area of recipient, dense packing, and consistency in results.
- The term FUT means the harvesting of FUs form donor area and then transplanting them as they are, without either clubbing them or dividing them. It was originally coined when only strip dissection was the only method of harvesting donor area. Now the term includes both harvesting methods—strip dissection (FU by strip) and follicular unit extraction (FUE). It is also used when the units are harvested from other donor areas such as beard or body.

INTRODUCTION

There are three principles of hair transplantation:

1. The principle of donor dominance already discussed in earlier chapters explains that the occipital area consists of androgen-resistant hairs, and are therefore permanent. They retain this property when transplanted to other areas.
2. In addition to donor dominance, there is also the concept of recipient influence enunciated by Tommy Hwang who demonstrated that body hair when transplanted to scalp assumes the property of scalp hair and grows longer (vice versa is also true)—a property used in body hair transplantation.
3. The donor area in occipital scalp is smaller than the potential bald area; hence, a smaller area of donor hair is available to be used to cover a much larger recipient site. Therefore, what is done in any hair transplantation is to create an illusion of hair, to cover the bald area—*it is never possible to create the same original density that the patient had!* The logic behind this seemingly imbalanced equation needs to be well understood in order to understand the possibilities and limitations of this procedure. This will enable the surgeon to maximize donor usage, achieve satisfactory recipient cover as well as plan the overall treatment plan.

THE LOGIC OF HAIR DISTRIBUTION AND THE FOLLICULAR UNIT—DONOR AREA

Logic 1: Follicular unit transplantation (FUT) gives natural-looking results as the original natural architecture and distribution is preserved.

An FU consists of 1–4 terminal hairs, with their arrectors muscle, sebaceous gland, 1–3 vellus hairs, perifollicular collagen, and nerves and vessels supplying the unit. These are naturally occurring units and each person has a different proportion of these units; 1/2/3/4/5/rarely 6 hairs. These are transplanted as they are and hence lead to natural results **(Fig. 1A)**.

Logic 2: The follicular units are small, and hence it takes small holes to place them in, and hence more holes can be made in a given area; more units can be placed and denser packing is possible leading to better results.

The unit is pyramid in shape **(Fig. 1A)**, the narrowest part being at the junction of arrectors and widest at the

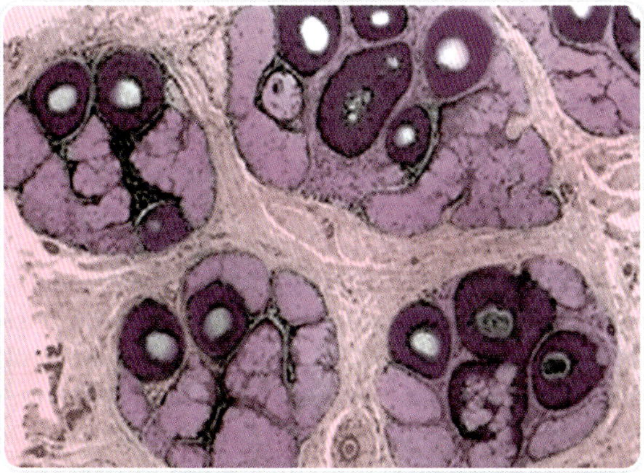

FIG. 1A: Follicular units seen by horizontal section at the level of sebaceous gland.

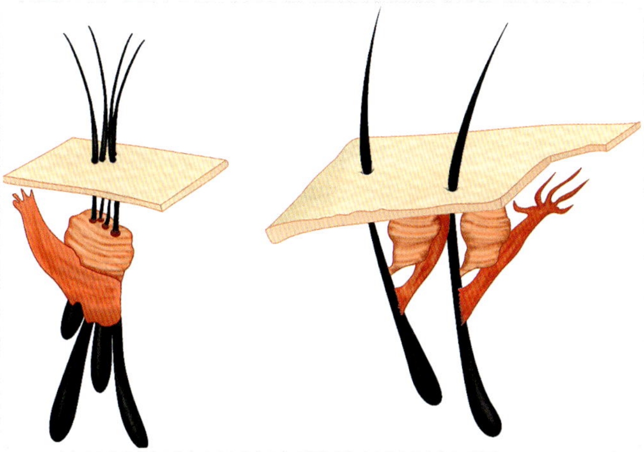

FIG. 1B: Schematic diagram of follicular unit (left) and micrograft (right)—note the larger micrograft even though it contains only two hairs.

bottom where the hairs splay. There is a small amount of dermis in between these units.

In contrast, in the previously used mini-micrografts, two neighboring follicles or FUs were clubbed together, with a lot of dermis in between as later. This means the grafts were larger and needed wider holes to place them **(Fig. 1B)**.

Logic 3: It is never possible to provide a normal density in any patient. Nor is it possible to cover entire balding scalp in stage seven baldness satisfactorily with only units from occipital scalp. What is possible to achieve is cosmetic density, to create an impression, or an illusion of density.

An average scalp is usually 500 cm^2 (50,000 mm^2) in area, with an FU distribution of 1/mm^2. Each FU (in an Indian scalp) has on an average 2-3 hairs. This leads to a total hair count of 100,000.[1] Out of the total 50,000 FUs

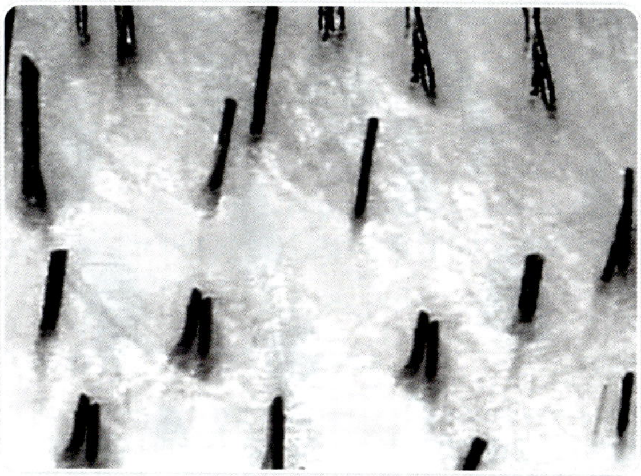

FIG. 2A: Trichoscan with low hair density—most of the units have 1–2 hairs.

on the scalp, 75%, i.e., 37,500 are on the frontal region and vertex and hence are at risk of being lost. The permanent donor area has 25%, i.e., 12,500 units. As we need 50% to appear normal, this means that a maximum of 6,250 FUs only are available for transplantation. So, in a worst case scenario, *patient would have 12.5% (6,250) follicles available to cover 75% (37,500) area achieving a density of 1/6 (18%) of normal.*[2] It, however, has to be clarified that the statistics are from Caucasian scalp and Indian data are not available.

Logic 4: A person with greater unit density will have a better result than a person with lesser unit density. A person with greater hair density (more number of larger units containing 3–4 hairs) will have a better result than a person with less hair density (more number smaller units containing 1–2 hairs).

It is important to differentiate FU density, which remains relatively constant at 1/mm^2, from hair density, which varies from 1.5 to 3/mm^2 (normal = 2/mm^2). Hence, the hair density is a function of the number of hairs per FU, rather than the total number of FUs.[2] This differentiation is important; a donor area with a lower hair density will need more number of FUs than a donor with a higher hair density to achieve the same result, as will be elucidated in the following paragraphs **(Figs. 2A to C)**.

Logic 5: Giving 40–50% of original density is sufficient to create an excellent result. This is called cosmetic density.

In the process of balding, early on, the number of FUs/mm^2 remains constant initially (though ultimately all hairs in a unit disappear); the thinning appearance is due to the reduction in the number of hairs per FU. The average person can lose up to 50% of his hair, before it is noticeably thin (i.e., a hair density of 1/mm^2).

Hence, while performing transplantation from the unaffected donor area, an FU density of 0.5/mm^2 is required in the frontal hairline to appear normal. In areas

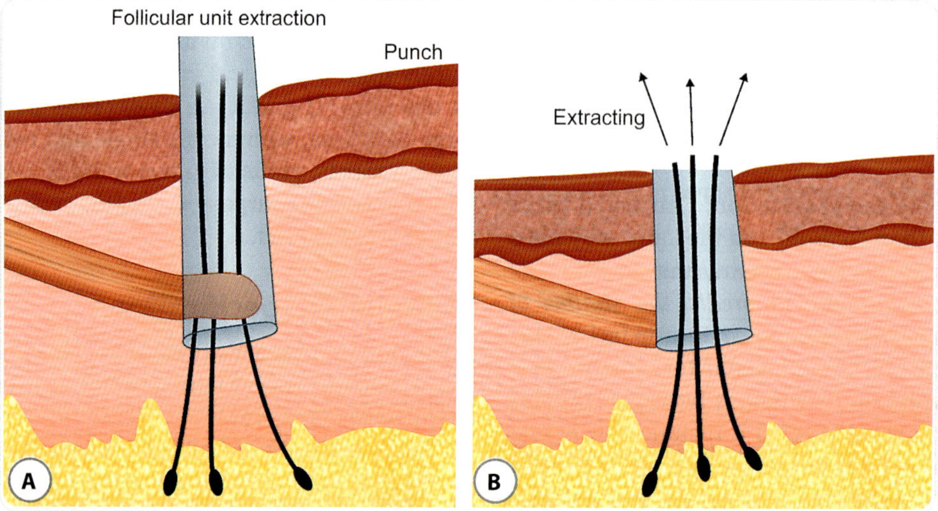

FIGS. 3A AND B: Introduction of punch and extraction of unit.

Hence, as for as possible number two neighboring units should be taken so that maximum gap between two hairs does not exceed 2 mm. This means that the total number of hairs that can be taken out safely is one in 4–6 hair units and hence does not exceed 3,000 in a person who has 12,000 units in occipital area. If more is taken out, then the ratio 1:4 is breached. If this happens, as in mega sessions (when more than 3,000 units are taken out), gaps between neighboring hair units will reach 3 mm or more, the area looks mottled, and hence patient needs longer hairs to cover the gaps, which will defeat one of the basic premises of FUE—that patient can trim and keep shorter hairs.

Logic 10: It is preferable not to extract (by FUE) more than 3,000 units from occipital scalp.

COMBINING FOLLICULAR UNIT TRANSPLANTATION AND FOLLICULAR UNIT EXTRACTION

Logic 11: FUE can be combined with strip technique to harvest larger number of grafts and cover larger areas of baldness.

The two techniques can be combined to get advantages of both:

1. FUE gives accesses to greater donor area by taking *some hairs* from everywhere in the donor-it helps us to harvest from areas where strip would never have been possible.
2. FUT by stress or follicular unit strip surgery (FUSS) allows the surgeon to take *all hairs* from one small area and retains the option of taking from the same area by including the previous scar (due to the stretchable property of skin). Hence, combining the two techniques can give larger number of hairs.

For example: A strip of 30 cm length and 1 cm wide and density of 80 units/cm^2 can give 2,400 units. FUE from above and below the strip can give another 1,600 units in the same session. Hence, 4,000 units can be obtained in one session by combining the two methods.

LOGIC OF BODY HAIR TRANSPLANTATION

The concept of recipient influence was enunciated by Tommy Hwang, who demonstrated that body hair when transplanted to scalp assumes the property of scalp hair and grows longer—a principle used in body hair transplantation.[5] This has made it possible to transplant body hair from beard, chest, and other areas when scalp hair is exhausted, and has ensured unlimited number of hairs being available. Hence, almost any area in any extent of bald scalp can now be covered. Moreover, body hair can only be extracted by FUE.

Logic 12: Body hair when transplanted to scalp grows longer and is, therefore, an alternative donor.

TWELVE COMMANDMENTS OF HAIR TRANSPLANTATION

Logic 1: FUT gives natural-looking results as the original natural architecture and distribution is preserved.

Logic 2: Since the FUs are smaller, it takes smaller holes to place them in, and hence more holes can be made; more units can be placed and denser packing is possible leading to better results.

Logic 3: It never provides a normal density in any patient nor is it possible to cover entire balding scalp in stage seven baldness satisfactorily with only units from occipital scalp. What is possible to achieve is cosmetic density, to create an impression or an illusion of density.

Logic 4: A person with greater unit density will have a better result than a person with lesser unit density. A person with more larger units containing 3–4 hairs will have a better result than a person with smaller units containing 1–2 hairs.

Logic 5: Giving 40–50% of original density is sufficient to create an excellent result. This is called cosmetic density.

Logic 6: A person with thicker hairs gets better results than thinner hairs.

Logic 7: Longer hairs create greater volume and cover greater area.

Logic 8: Hair density, not just donor density, is of importance in calculating the number of hairs that are available.

Logic 9: In frontal area, front needs to be packed densely with density decreasing as we go backward.

Logic 10: It is preferable not to extract (by FUE) more than 3,000 units from occipital scalp.

Logic 11: FUE can be combined with strip technique to harvest larger number of grafts and cover larger areas of baldness.

Logic 12: Body hair when transplanted to scalp grows longer and is, therefore, an alternative donor.

SUMMARY

Thus, understanding the logic and the mathematical principles with regards to hair loss enables the surgeon to plan and economize donor graft supple to achieve a balanced, aesthetically pleasing appearance in the long run, and avoid mistakes.

REFERENCES

1. Bernstein RM, Rassman WR. The aesthetics of follicular transplantation. Dermatol Surg. 1997;23(9):785-99.
2. Bernstein RM, Rassman WR. The logic of follicular unit transplantation. Dermatol Clin. 1999;17(2):277-95.
3. Bernstein RM, Rassman WR. Follicular transplantation. Patient evaluation and surgical planning. Dermatol Surg. 1997;23: 771-84.
4. Bernstein RM, Rassman WR. Follicular unit hair transplantation. Dermatol Surg. 1997;23:771-84.
5. Hwang ST, Kim HY, Lee SJ, Lee WJ, Kim DW, Kim JC. Recipient-site influence in hair transplantation: a confirmative study. Dermatol Surgery. 2009;35(6):1011-4.

CHAPTER

38

Surgical Anatomy of the Scalp

Sandeep Sattur, Indu S Sattur

Key Messages

- Knowledge of scalp anatomy is one of the mandatory requirements for successful hair restoration surgery. Scalp is an acronym for the layers of tissue that cover the skull, made up of five layers: Skin, connective tissue, aponeurosis, loose areolar tissue, and pericranium.
- The vascular supply, as well as the nerves, is oriented in a centripetal manner, which has significant implications in planning incisions and anesthetizing the scalp.
- The scalp laxity can be improved to some extent by scalp laxity exercises, which utilize the property of mechanical creep.

INTRODUCTION

The importance of the knowledge of scalp anatomy for a hair transplant surgeon cannot be overemphasized. A hair transplant surgeon can reap the rewards with a good understanding of the anatomy of the scalp and also pay a price for poor planning if he/she is not well versed with it.

SCALP

Scalp may be defined as the soft tissue covering of the skull, including the skin. It extends anteriorly to the region of the eyebrows up to the supraorbital margin. Posteriorly, it extends up to the external occipital protuberance and superior nuchal lines. On both sides laterally, it is limited to the superior temporal line at the level of the zygomatic arch and the external auditory meatus.

The scalp is made up of five different anatomical layers and is an acronym for the various tissues that make it up **(Fig. 1)**:

1. Skin
2. Connective tissue
3. Aponeurosis
4. Loose connective tissue
5. Pericranium

S—Skin

The skin on the scalp is one of the thickest on the body (thin epidermis, thick dermis), ranging from 3 mm (vertex) to 8 mm (occiput), and endowed with abundant pilosebaceous units. It is richly vascularized and is sensitive to touch, pain, and temperature.[1]

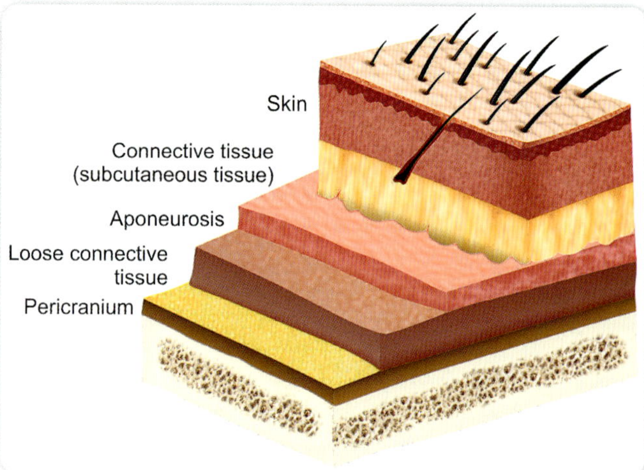

FIG. 1: Layers of the scalp.

C—Connective Tissue

The connective tissue of the scalp is made up of subcutaneous fat and is divided into multiple small compartments by tough fibrous septa which bind down the scalp skin firmly to the muscles and aponeurosis, making dissection in this plane difficult and bloody.

A—Aponeurosis

The aponeurosis, also called galea aponeurotica or epicranial aponeurosis, is the third layer of the scalp and is in conjunction with the occipitofrontalis muscle. The occipitofrontalis muscle has occipital and frontal bellies separated by the aponeurosis into which the muscle bellies are inserted. It exists as a fibrous sheet mostly over the vertex area, where it connects the occipitalis muscle posteriorly (arising from the superior nuchal line) to the frontalis muscle, which inserts into the dermis of the skin in the region of the eyebrows and bridge of the nose. Laterally, the aponeurosis blends as a thin sheet with the temporalis fascia and becomes indistinct over the zygomatic arch.

L—Loose connective tissue

The loose connective tissue is the fourth layer of the scalp and is also referred to as the subgaleal space. It is bounded by galea above and has pericranium as its floor. It is largely avascular, containing only a filmy layer of loose fibroareolar/connective tissue.

P—Pericranium (Periosteum)

The pericranium (periosteum) adheres to the suture lines of the skull, in the scalp region; these are the coronal, sagittal, temporal, and lambdoid sutures. The pericranium is a dense membranous or fibrous sheet loosely fused on its outer aspect to the galea aponeurotica, from which it is readily separable via the subgaleal space. It is usually of similar thickness to the galea and is easily bluntly dissected from the outer table of the skull as an intact sheet.[1,2]

VASCULATURE OF THE SCALP (FIG. 2)

The blood supply of the scalp is maintained by five pairs of arteries, which are branches of the external and internal carotid arteries with a small contribution from the bone perforators from meningeal vessels. The unique aspect of scalp blood supply is that all the vessels are oriented in a centripetal aspect, i.e., from the periphery to the center. The arteries of the scalp start getting smaller as they approach the midline and on the way anastomose generously with each other on the same side as well as those from the opposite side. This makes it possible for large areas of the scalp to survive the blockade of one of the feeding arteries.[1,2]

Branches of the external carotid artery:
- Occipital, whose pulse can usually be felt with careful palpation above the superior nuchal line.
- Posterior auricular
- Superficial temporal, whose pulse can be felt over the zygomatic arch immediately in front of the tragus of the ear

Branches of the internal carotid artery:
- Supraorbital artery
- Supratrochlear artery

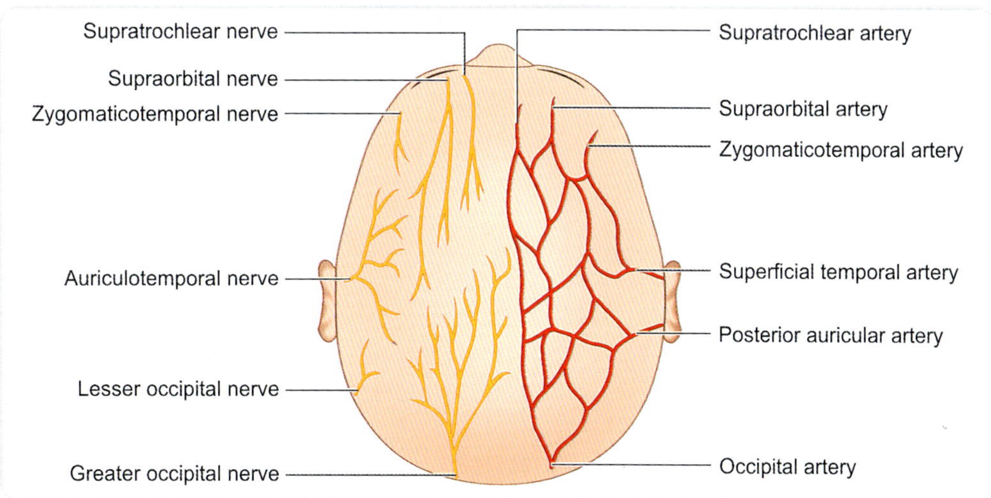

FIG. 2: Vascular and nerve supply of the scalp.

Sensory Nerve Supply of the Scalp

The sensory nerve supply of the scalp follows the vascular anatomy, is centripetal, and is located anatomically in the subcutaneous layer of the scalp. The cutaneous nerve supply of the scalp is derived from all three divisions of the trigeminal (V) nerve and from the second and third cervical nerves:[1,2]

1. From the ophthalmic division of the trigeminal nerve—the supratrochlear and supraorbital nerves
2. From the maxillary division of the trigeminal nerve—the zygomaticotemporal nerve
3. From the mandibular division of the trigeminal nerve—the auriculotemporal nerve
4. The lesser occipital nerve (C2)
5. The greater occipital nerve (C2, 3)
6. The third occipital nerve (C3)

Motor Nerve Supply of the Scalp

The motor nerves supply the various muscles adjacent to and contiguous with the galea.

- The temporal branch of the facial nerve supplies the frontalis muscle and anterior and superior auricular muscle.
- The posterior auricular branch of the facial nerve supplies the occipitalis muscle.
- The anterior and posterior deep branches of the mandibular division of the trigeminal nerve supply the temporalis muscle.
- The posterior auricular branch of the facial nerve supplies the posterior auricular muscle.

Topographical Zones of the Scalp (Fig. 3)

For the purpose of surgical planning and uniformity of descriptions, the scalp can be divided into four major surgical zones:[3] Frontal zone, midscalp zone, vertex (crown) zone, and evolving zones of hair loss.

Frontal Zone

The frontal zone extends from the front hairline back to a horizontal line drawn between the frontotemporal corners.

From a surgical perspective, when only the frontal area is transplanted, a modification of this designation termed *frontal transplant zone* is used. It is that area of the normal hair-bearing scalp that lies between the anterior hairline and a line initially drawn vertically from the left and right tragus and then gently curved so that if, for any reason, only the frontal area is transplanted but the hair loss progresses posteriorly, the appearance of the patient will be more natural looking than a noncurved one.

Midscalp Zone

The midscalp zone is the relatively horizontal part of the scalp, which is bordered anteriorly by the frontal zone, laterally by the hair-bearing parietal humps or fringes, and posteriorly by the anterior border of the vertex zone.

Vertex (crown) Zone

The vertex (crown) zone is the posterior part of the balding area often referred to as the crown. It is round or oval in

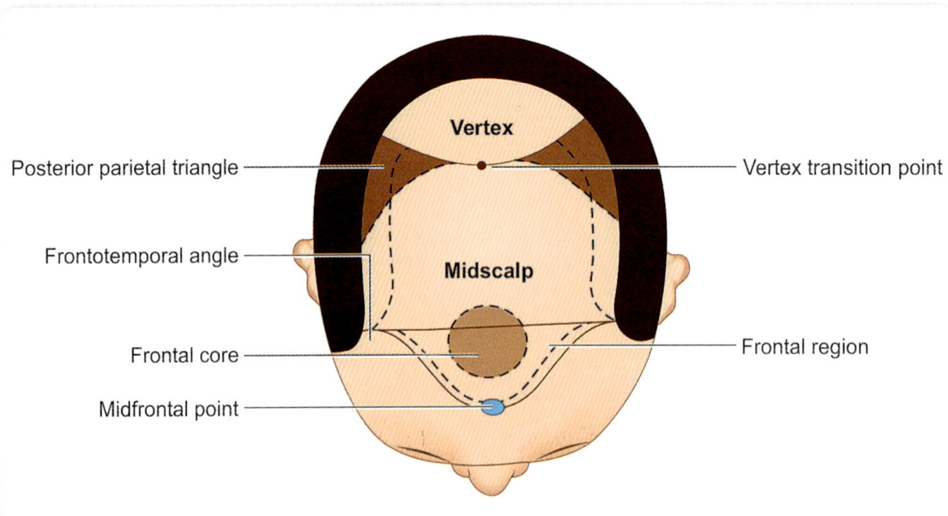

FIG. 3: Topographical zones of the scalp.

shape and is unique due to the whorl arrangement of hair. It extends from the posterior border of the midscalp to the curved parieto-occipital fringe of the hair.

Evolving Zones of Hair Loss

The evolving areas of pattern hair loss are zones that are peripheral to the frontal, midscalp, and vertex areas. These are areas in which there is persisting hair but on wetting the hair or examining under trichoscope, it is obvious that this hair will be lost eventually. The importance of these areas is including them in the surgical planning and/or approaching these areas with the use of medications such as oral finasteride (men) and topical minoxidil (men and women).

The shape of the balding area is triangular in the front, rectangular in the middle, and circular or oval in the vortex. As we go backward, the width and, hence, the area increase. Though the frontal area is the smallest, it needs more grafts per unit area to achieve a satisfactory result.

APPLIED ANATOMY OF SCALP IN HAIR TRANSPLANTATION

Bleeding during Strip Harvest

The principal blood vessels and nerves of the scalp lie in the subcutaneous layer, and when an incision is made in the scalp, the divided vessels retract between the fibrous septa and, therefore, cannot be picked up by artery forceps in the usual way. Also, any attempt to do so has the potential to damage the follicles in the wound edge. The best way to deal with this is by pressing firmly down on the underlying skull with your fingers, thus compressing the spurting vessels. Firm pressure for 5–10 minutes helps to control the bleeding. However, bleeding in the bed of the wound, which is significant, can be cauterized using bipolar cautery; this helps to limit the thermal damage.

The indiscriminate use of cautery can also damage the neurovascular structures in the bed of the donor harvest wound, and its use in the wound edges may damage follicles, leading to a wider hairless scar.

Role of Tumescence (Tumescent—Firm and Swollen)

The blood vessels lie in the lower part of the subcutaneous layer. The hair bulb is located in the subcutaneous layer; while harvesting the strip or while extracting the follicles in follicular unit extraction (FUE), the plane of dissection or intervention is, therefore, close to the level of the vessels, which can be the potential cause of bleeding during strip harvest or extraction of grafts in FUE. Also, in the absence of musculocutaneous perforators, *transection of these vessels in the periphery while harvesting the strip may compromise the blood supply to the posterior central scalp due to the centripetal nature of blood supply, leading to ischemia, postoperative pain, tissue necrosis, and scarring.*

Injecting tumescence fluid (solution containing normal saline with very dilute anesthetic and epinephrine concentration) into the subcutaneous layer of the scalp serves to:

- Increase the distance from the follicles (residing in the upper fat) to the nerves and larger blood vessels (lying deeper just above the fascia)—helps to effectively increase the distance between the vascular plane and the plane of dissection, thereby reducing the chances of injury to these structures.[4]
- Increase the rigidity of the donor area (that helps to decrease follicular transection during the harvest)
- Decrease bleeding by mechanical pressure of the injected fluid (hence, injection of substantial volume is necessary) as well as vasoconstriction of small vessels
- Produce more uniform anesthesia
- Reduce the total amount of anesthetic required
- Since larger nerve fibers are blocked, it also prolongs the duration of anesthesia.
- Subcutaneous compression and bilevel vasoconstriction in both donor and recipient sites resulted in an increased upwardly angled exit angle of the hairs to be harvested, an increased separation of individual hair shafts, and reduced bleeding.[5]
- Tumescent anesthesia is one of the most effective means of avoiding bleeding during strip harvesting.

Undermining

It is generally recommended that one should restrict the width of the strip to 1–1.2 cm in a patient with average scalp elasticity to avoid scarring—if this is done, no undermining is required to close the donor wound. However, in cases when there is suboptimal scalp laxity or the strip width is >1.2 cm, minimal undermining may help to close the wound.

According to Patrick Frechet, the galea is the main source of wound tension upon closure. So it is helpful to detach the superficial structures from the galea before closure. Undermining is usually done about a millimeter or two below the level of the bulbs of the hair follicles. Undermining should be between 5 and 10 mm throughout the length of the donor wound.[6]

It is important to know that undermining is a double-edged sword. It can free the subcutaneous layer from the galea but can also reduce blood supply to the hair follicles, especially the ones located in the wound edge (can lead to significant postoperative telogen effluvium). Also, the process of undermining can itself lead to damage to blood vessels.

Plane of Cleavage

The fourth layer of the scalp, which is composed of loose areolar tissue, behaves like a plane of cleavage, in that it readily lends itself to surgical dissection (also responsible for scalp avulsion when hair is caught in the machinery). The presence of this layer is limited to the areas where the galea exists. It extends from the superior nuchal lines (to which the occipitofrontalis muscle and galea aponeurotica attach) and proceeds anteriorly into the forehead. The lateral limit of this space ends where the galea blends with the temporalis fascia. *The surgical importance is that in the areas where this layer exists, wide excisions are possible.*

With reference to donor harvest, when a strip is harvested below the superior nuchal line, there is a restriction of the width as well as an increased chance for the scar to stretch. The vessels are also larger here and hence an increased chance of bleeding. *Therefore, it is not advisable to take a strip from below the nuchal line.* Another fact associated with this layer is that edema fluid and blood which collect in this loose connective tissue layer track freely under the scalp but cannot pass into the occipital or temporal regions because of the posterior attachment of occipitofrontalis and the lateral attachment of temporalis fascia. *It, therefore, tracks forward and accounts for the postoperative forehead swelling and bilateral periorbital ecchymosis seen after hair transplantation.*

Nerve Block

A nerve block involves the infiltration of a small volume of anesthetic around a nerve trunk. It substitutes a single injection for a large number of injections and anesthetizes a large area with a small amount of anesthetic. Blocking the nerves allows infiltration in the target area to be painless, and the dose of anesthetic required in infiltration later is much less. Knowledge of the surface anatomy of the superficial nerves of the scalp goes a long way in delivering these blocks.

Another way to achieve a similar result is to create a ring of neurological blockade, which effectively blocks the main nerves of the scalp in a circumferential manner. This aspect is dealt with in more detail in the chapter on *Anesthesia*.

Placement of Incisions

Where crease lines exist, their direction generally coincides with the lines of minimum tension.

These tend to be longitudinal in the limbs and scalp and circumferential in the neck and trunk **(Fig. 4)**. The lines of minimum tension are surgically important for two main reasons: Elliptical excisions achieve the greatest width of tissue removal when made parallel to the lines, and incisions made along or parallel to the lines heal with a minimum of scarring, while incisions made across them heal less well.

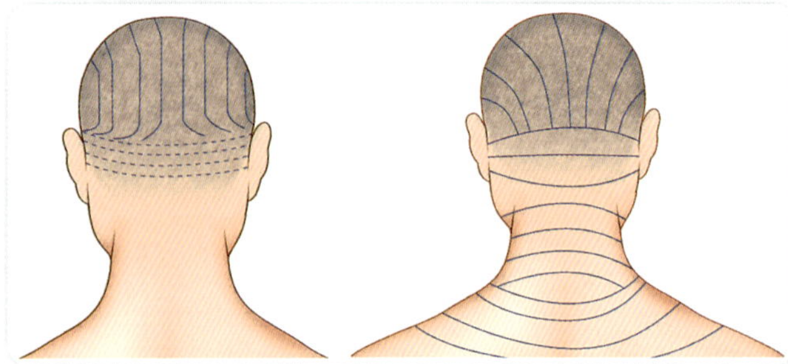

FIG. 4: Lines of tension on the scalp.

In the donor area (occipital area of the scalp), the lines of minimum tension run horizontally and hence the strip is always oriented in a horizontal manner.

Scalp Elasticity (Laxity)

Scalp elasticity or laxity is one of the limiting factors in donor strip harvest and essentially is a function of two components: (1) The ability of the scalp to glide on the pericranium (glidability) and (2) the ability to extend or stretch (stretchability or extensibility). The first component is related to undermining in the subgaleal space and is more relevant to scalp flap dissection and alopecia reductions. The second component depends on the viscoelastic properties of the scalp skin and is relevant to wound closure. Scalp laxity varies from patient to patient and should be assessed in the preoperative consultation before deciding the restoration plan. It is important in determining the amount of tissue tension during donor strip closure and ultimately the amount of donor tissue that can be safely harvested during hair transplantation. Scalp laxity is generally assessed by standing behind the seated patient and with the patient's neck flexed forward. Gross assessment can be done by checking the mobility of the scalp using both thumbs about 5–7 cm apart, placed firmly on the occipital scalp, and moving them closer to each other in both directions (mediolateral and superoinferior). This is combined with the assessment of the general glidability of the scalp over the skull. These are gross assessments, are subjective, and can be unreliable to the inexperienced surgeon.

The earliest reports of objective assessment of scalp elasticity were mentioned by Bosley in 1980. He made two marks, 10 cm apart, on the midscalp and then with maximum compression, he measured the same marks and graded the compressions to determine the amount of scalp tissue that could be harvested.[7]

Feldman described another system wherein he injected saline to determine the degree of expansion caused (in contrast to the above methods in which assessment is made by compressing the scalp).[8] Mohebi et al. devised an instrument called the laxometer to measure the scalp laxity. The instrument has three components: (1) The mobile part, (2) the tracing ring, and (3) the measuring rod. After placing the course surface of the mobile part of the laxometer, it is moved up and down. Free movement of the mobile part of the laxometer represents the mobility and laxity of the scalp in the studied areas **(Fig. 5)**.

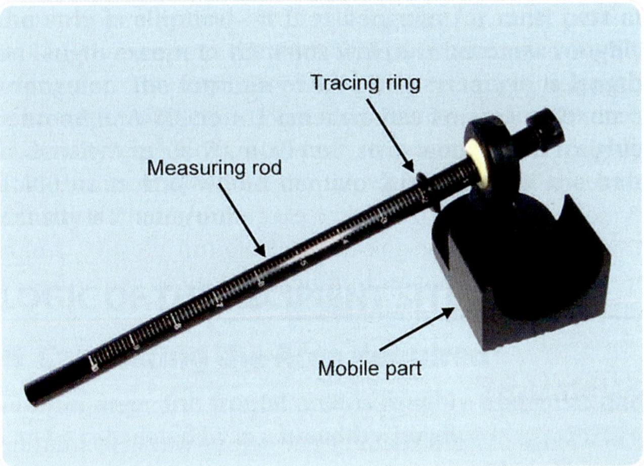

FIG. 5: Laxometer.

Scalp mobility is measured by moving the tracing ring up or down over the measuring rod to its highest and lowest positions. The final position of the tracing ring records the maximum mobility of the scalp, which represents the safe distance necessary for optimal donor closure after removal of a strip. The handheld device accurately measures scalp laxity to ensure safe and appropriate donor removal.[9]

Mayer and Pauls devised a technique to measure scalp elasticity that was reproducible, objective, and quantifiable **(Figs. 6A and B)**. They defined scalp laxity as the percentage of the original distance that the lines placed 5 cm apart on the horizontal axis move when compressed maximally by the examiner's thumbs. This is measured by a simple ruler.

They worked out a formula for the same:

$$\text{Scalp elasticity} = \frac{(50\,\text{mm} - X)(100\%)}{50\,\text{mm}}$$

where X is the measurement when the skin is compressed between the examiner's thumbs. The range of scalp elasticity is 10–45%, with 10% being a tight scalp and 45% being extremely lax.[10]

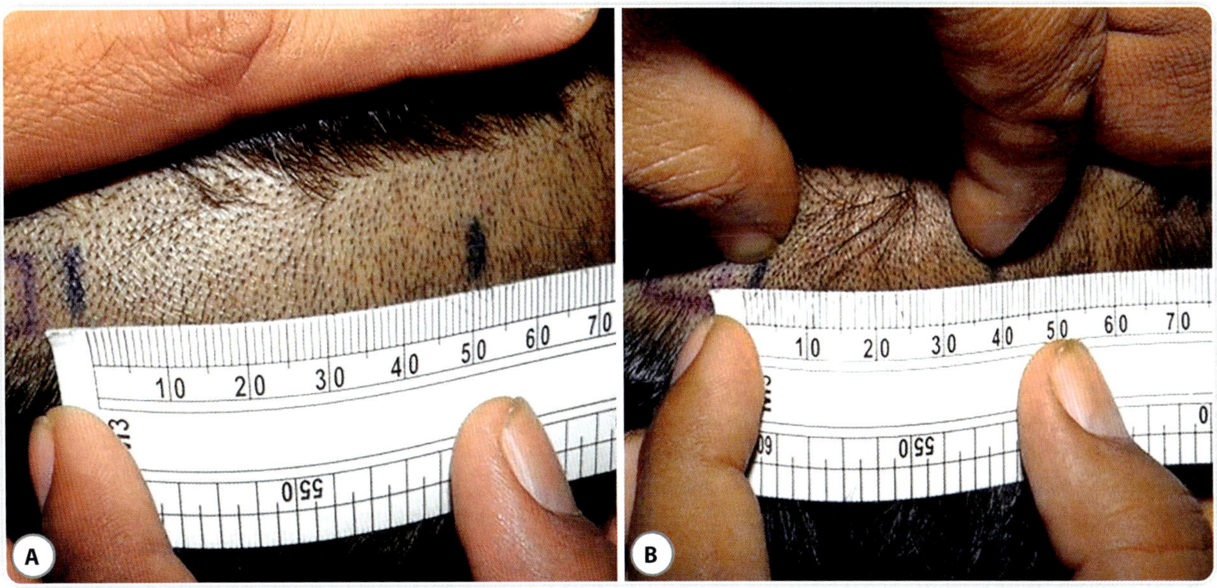

FIGS. 6A AND B: A technique to measure scalp elasticity.

Note: Quantification of Scalp Elasticity (Mayer-Pauls Scale)

$$\text{Scalp elasticity} = \frac{(50\,\text{mm} - X)\ (100\%)}{50\,\text{mm}}$$

Where 'X' is the measurement when the skin is compressed, average is 24–26%
Tight scalp is 10% → strip width not exceeding 8–10 mm
45% is extremely elastic → strip width can be between 15 and 20 mm

Extreme laxity could also pose a problem, and this was described by Bernstein as the "scalp laxity paradox."[11] In spite of the absence of tension closures, these patients heal with widened scars and could have dermal collagen abnormalities or could be subclinical variants of Ehlers–Danlos syndrome. If the laxity exceeds 30%, then it should be marked as a potential red flag.

An experienced surgeon not only evaluates scalp laxity preoperatively but also tests it during donor strip harvest. One way to be prudent is to excise a test strip of about 5 cm and determine the maximum width that can be harvested and the wound be closed without tension. Once ascertained, further strips could be harvested with the same width.

Scalp laxity is the least at the junction of parietal and occipital scalp, and this is an area where the donor scar usually stretches. Hence, strip width can be variable, minimum at places of tightness and slightly increased at places of laxity.

PROPERTIES OF MECHANICAL CREEP AND STRESS RELAXATION

Successful scalp reconstruction and donor strip harvest often require intraoperative use of the intrinsic skin viscoelastic properties, specifically stress relaxation and creep. Stress relaxation is defined as the decrease in the amount of force necessary to maintain a fixed amount of skin stretch over time. Mechanical creep is defined as the elongation of skin with a constant load over time beyond intrinsic extensibility.[12]

This property is utilized in closing wounds by presuturing (stay sutures), intraoperative tissue expansion, skin-stretching devices, and skin retraction with undermining and has been described as the vehicle harnessed for wound closure with presuturing, intraoperative tissue expansion, skin-stretching devices, and skin retraction with undermining.[13-15] The fundamental basis for these properties lies in the fact that as force is applied to a leading skin edge, tissue thickness decreases from extrusion of fluid and mucopolysaccharides, realignment of dermal collagen bundles, elastic fiber microfragmentation, and mechanical stretching of the skin. The extent to which these occur depends on the inherent properties of the tissue and the amount of force applied. When the properties of mechanical creep and stress relaxation are relevant intraoperatively, the viscoelastic attributes of the skin can greatly assist in reconstruction and allow for tension-free closure in circumstances where initial closure is difficult.

The best application of mechanical creep is the scalp laxity exercise described by Dr S Wong and Hasson. These exercises are performed by the patient in the preoperative period and have been proven to improve scalp elasticity to facilitate tension-free closure. Another application is the use of towel clips to keep the wound edges of the strip approximated till the final suturing is done. This constant force exerted by the jaws of the towel clips, in the direction of wound closure, helps in realigning collagen bundles leading to tension-free closure and better donor scars.

SUMMARY

Knowledge of scalp anatomy goes a long way in facilitating optimal and complication-free hair transplantation and scalp surgery. Hair transplant surgeons today understand scalp anatomy and its finer details, including histology, much more than their counterparts a few decades ago.

Tips and Pearls

- A strip should not be taken from below the superior nuchal line as loose connective tissue is absent below the line.
- The width of the strip should be proportionate to the scalp laxity. The need for future sessions should be factored in while deciding the strip width. The paradox of scalp laxity should be kept in mind, which may lead to stretched scars.
- Scalp laxity can be improved by scalp exercises starting 4–6 weeks prior to surgery.

REFERENCES

1. Seery GE. Surgical anatomy of the scalp. Dermatol Surg. 2002;28(7):581-7.
2. Ellis H, Vishy M. The surgical anatomy of the scalp. Surgery (Oxford). 2014;32(1):1-5.
3. Beehner M. Anatomy and landmarks. In: Haber R, Dow D (Eds). Hair Transplantation. Philadelphia: Elsevier Saunders; 2006.
4. Khan S. Nerve block and local anesthesia. In: Haber R, Dow D (Eds). Hair Transplantation. Philadelphia: Elsevier Saunders; 2006.
5. Field LM, Namias A. Bilevel tumescent anesthetic infiltration for hair transplantation. Dermatol Surg. 1997;23(4):289-90.
6. Frechet P. Donor harvesting with an invisible scar. Hair Transplant Forum Int. 2005;15:119-20.
7. Bosley L, Hope CR, Montroy RE, Straub PM. Reduction of male pattern baldness in multiple stages: a retrospective study. J Dermatol Oncol. 1980;6:498-503.
8. Feldman CS. Tissue laxity based on donor tissue ballooning. Hair Transplant Forum Int. 2001;11:119.

9. Mohebi P. Laxometer II. Instruction to use. Hair Transplant Forum Int. 2014;24(3):1-5.
10. Mayer M, Pauls T. Scalp elasticity scale. Hair Transplant Forum Int. 2005;15(4):9-10.
11. Bernstein R. Scalp laxity paradox. Hair Transplant Forum Int. 2002;12(1):9-10.
12. Wilhelmi BJ, Blackwell SJ, Mancoll JS, Phillips LG. Creep vs. stretch: a review of the viscoelastic properties of skin. Ann Plast Surg. 1998;41(2):215-9.
13. Liang MD, Briggs P, Heckler FR, Futrell JW. Presuturing—a new technique for closing large skin defects: clinical and experimental studies. Plast Reconstr Surg. 1988;81(5):694-702.
14. Frechet P. Scalp extension. J Dermatol Surg Oncol. 1993;10: 616-22.
15. Unger M. Advantages and disadvantages of the Unger pATE procedure. Am J Cosmet Surg. 1997;14(2):155-8.

implanted, remain unaffected by androgenetic factors.[5-9] Correctly evaluating safe donor area characteristics will help to define the surgical plan. It defines the limitations, cosmetic results, possible contraindications to the procedure, expected number of grafts, and possible coverages. The donor area evaluation includes calculating follicular unit density, hair shaft diameter, anagen-telogen ratio, hair and skin color, hair texture such as curl, wave or frizz, scalp thickness and laxity, and retrograde alopecia.

Donor hair follicles harvested outside the "defined safe donor area limit" **(Figs. 1A to C)** are androgen sensitive. If these are implanted, such hair follicles will likely be lost from recipient area.

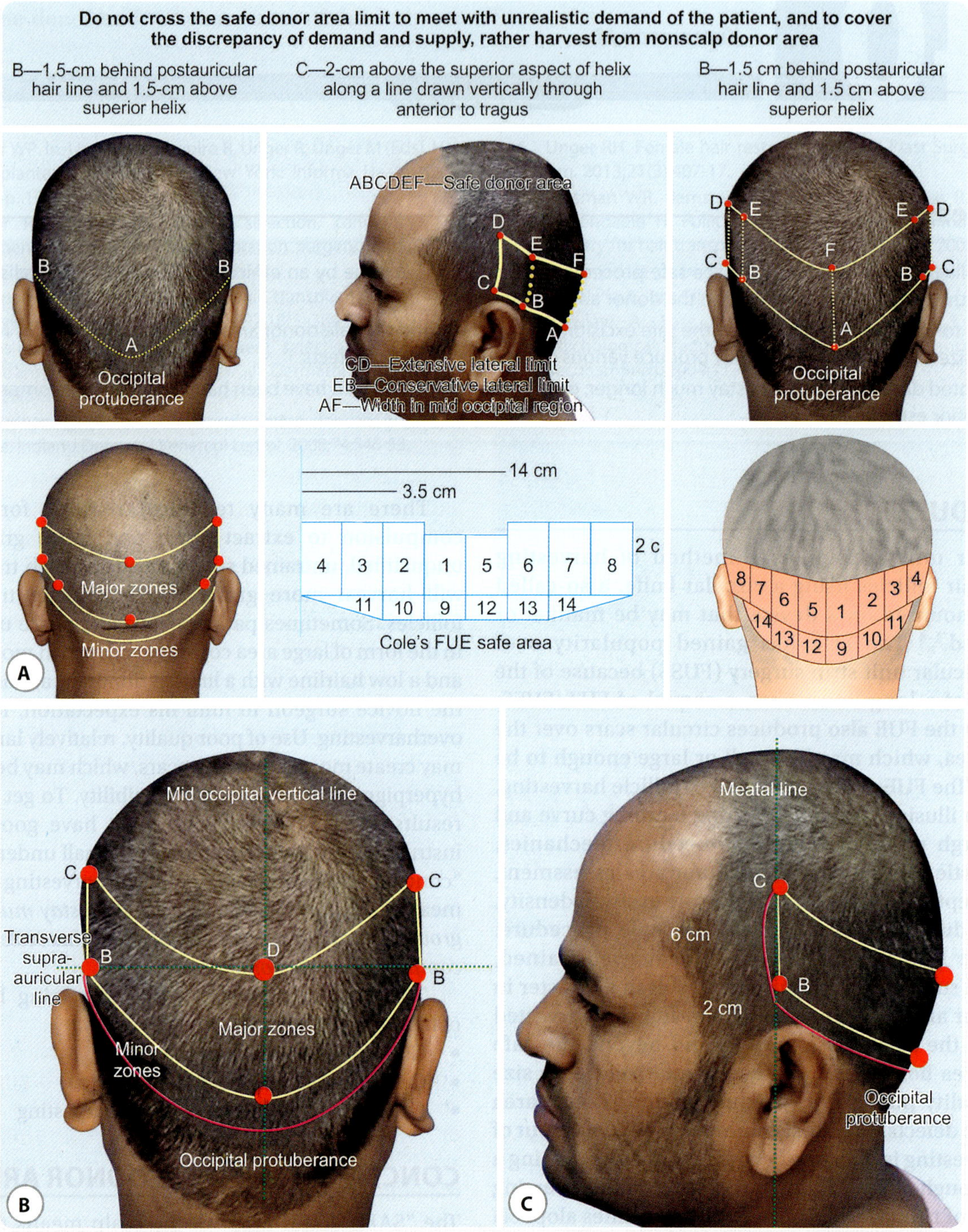

FIGS. 1A TO C: Safe donor area.

Often a surgeon crosses the safe donor area limit to harvest more donor grafts. Progressing hair loss caused by androgenetic alopecia (AGA) will expose the scars of grafts harvested from the unsafe zone.

The surgeon shall define and mark the safe donor area limit and harvest from safe donor area only. Sometimes to prevent the accidental crossing of the safe donor area limit, the surgeon can shave only the safe donor area or limit this by sticking the medical-grade sterile tape.

Note: Refer to Chapter 41 for details of Graft Harvesting From Safe Donor Area and Graft Calculation for Recipient Area: Current Concepts.

CONCEPT OF SAFE EXCISION DENSITY

Safe excision density is the number of grafts harvested without compromising the cosmetic density of the donor area.[10-13] Most FUE experts recommend 10–15 excisions/cm^2 as a safe single pass density in a person with a baseline average density of 65–75 grafts/cm^2. Dr James Harris reports a routine use of higher excision density 20–25 grafts/cm^2 without problems so as the author also does. A rough estimate of 20–25% of graft excision of existing density can be done safely. However, every donor area differs in density, thickness, color contrast, hair curl, and multifollicular units (MFUs) density. From a robust donor area, one can undoubtedly excise more grafts than a donor area that looks thin. Exceeding the safe excision limit will decrease the residual density and hair mass, causing more scarring and resulting in scalp show or poor esthetics of the donor area.

There are many compulsive reasons for overharvesting. The unqualified, untrained surgeon causing high transactions will harvest more grafts to compensate. Sometimes patient expectations are unrealistic in the form of large area coverage with much more density and a low hairline with a limited donor area; this imposes the novice surgeon to fulfil his expectation, leading to overharvesting. Use of poor quality, relatively large punch may create more prominent scars, which may be hypo- or hyperpigmented, causing scar visibility **(Figs. 2 and 3)**.

Residual Density

The residual density is the hair follicles density left over in the donor area after graft harvesting. The cosmetic density

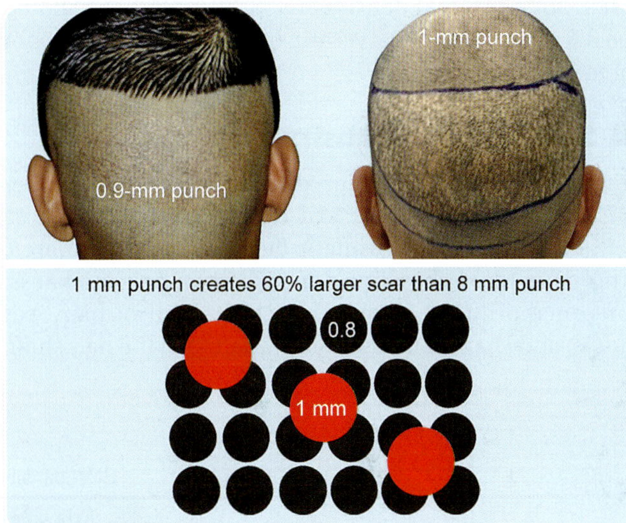

FIG. 3: Large-sized punch will create bigger visible scar.

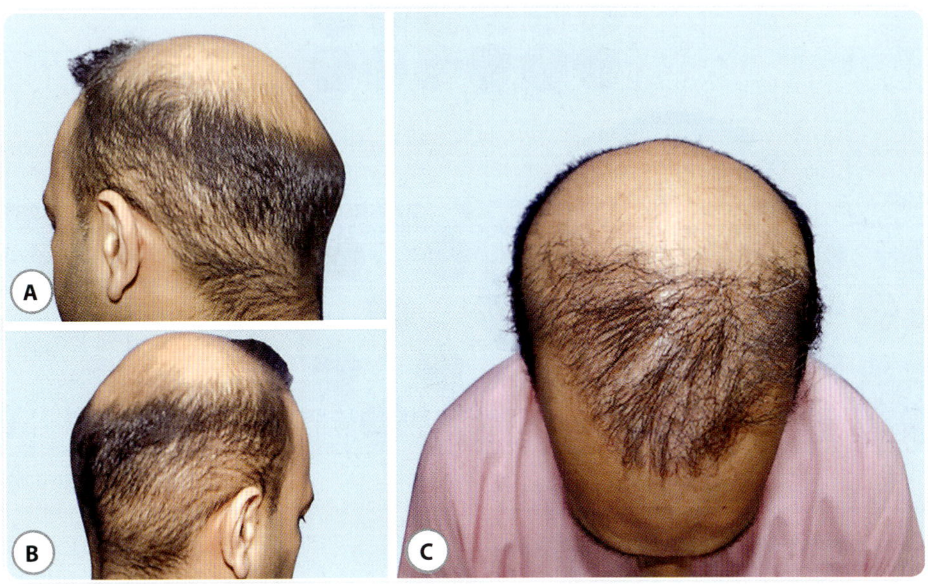

FIGS. 2A TO C: Significant donor scalp show.

of the donor area is significantly compromised if the residual density of the donor area is <35–40 grafts/cm^2. Although other than several grafts, the donor cosmetic density depends on hair thickness, MFU density, color contrast, and hair curl. Let us take an example.

Suppose a surgeon harvests grafts from a donor area having a density of 70 grafts/cm^2.

He harvests 15 grafts/cm^2 in first-pass excision. The leftover residual density will be 70–15 = 55 graft/cm^2. Then during his second pass excision, again he harvests 15 grafts/cm^2, then the residual density will be 55–15 = 40 graft/cm^2. However, suppose the surgeon continues to harvest even 10 grafts/cm^2. In that case, the final residual density will be 30 grafts/cm^2, which will cause significant scalp thinning and poor cosmetic density of the donor area. So, a residual density of >35–40 grafts/cm^2 should be left after the final harvesting of follicles over the donor area **(Fig. 4)**.

Safe Excision Density

The maximum safe excision density is the total number of grafts that can be excised from a given donor area without affecting the cosmetic density of the donor area. This depends on baseline donor density, hair thickness, presence of MFU, color contrast, the curl of hair, exit angle, and shape and thickness variation of the hair shaft. A rough estimate of 50% of existing grafts can be excised safely.

Coverage Value

The coverage value of hair on the scalp depends on the thickness of hair and hair density per square cm. This can be calculated as:

$$\text{The scalp area covered by hair mass unit} = \text{hair density} \times \text{thickness of hair}$$

Suppose the hair density = 170 hair/cm^2 and the thickness of hair is 0.05 mm

$$\text{The coverage value will be} = 170 \times 0.05 = 8.5$$

The coverage value helps in the number of hair follicles excision from a given donor area or parieto-occipital donor area zone. The coverage value of different zones of the total area can be different, because hair density and sometimes thickness may vary in different zones of the parieto-occipital donor area. It has been estimated that a minimum coverage value of five for the donor area should be left after the excision of grafts to prevent scalp show. A lower coverage value limits the safe excision density.

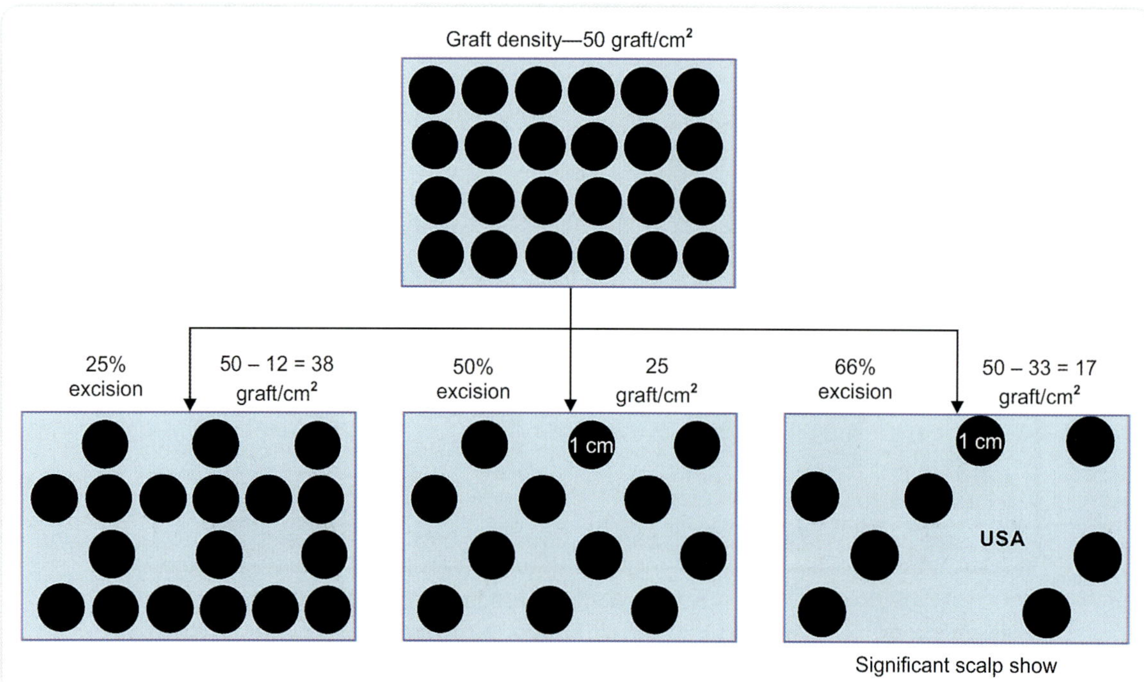

FIG. 4: Residual density.
(USA: uncovered scalp area)

Now let us calculate how many hair follicles can be extracted from a donor area having a coverage value of 8.5.

$$\text{Number of hair follicle excision} = \frac{\text{Coverage value of donor area} - 5.5}{\text{Thickness of hair}}$$

$$= \frac{8.5 - 5.5}{0.05} = 60 \text{ hair follicles/cm}^2$$

If we take as an average two hair per graft, so graft excision density = $\frac{60}{2}$ = 30 grafts/cm^2. So, a donor has a density of 170 hairs/cm^2, with a hair thickness of 0.05 mm, and safe graft excision is 30 grafts/cm^2 area.

So, coverage value of the donor area helps in the safe excision of grafts/hair.

There can be two ways of calculating coverage value. One by using a micrometer for measurement of hair thickness and a dermoscopy for donor density calculation. Another more precise way is the KE-BOT system developed by Koray Eradogan.[11]

CONCEPT OF HEALTHY HAIR FOLLICLE HARVESTING

The FUE graft harvesting is a blind procedure, and there are likely chances of injury/transection of donor grafts during excision. The transection can be complete or partial.[14] The higher transection rate will reduce the recipient area coverage. If the surgeon notices a higher transection of hair follicles, he will harvest more grafts to accomplish the required healthy donor hair follicles. The higher transections are probably the common cause of overharvesting donor hair follicles. Apart from hair follicles transection injuries, the graft may sustain various types of other injuries during harvesting, such as decapping, fracture of hair follicle shaft, desheathing, and iatrogenic splaying[15,16] **(Fig. 5)**. It is advisable to learn FUE under the supervision of a senior qualified FUE surgeon, practice it, and then perform it. In order to reduce the hair follicle transections, it is advisable to align the punch and full length of FUE handle to hair shaft angle, and engage the punch to epidermal blush of hair **(Figs. 6A to C)**.

Size of Punch

The FUE harvesting of hair follicle also leaves a tiny circular scar. The size and the quality of the FUE scar depend on the size and the quality of the punch. The size of a 1-mm punch creates a 60% larger scar than an 8-mm punch **(Fig. 3)**. Reducing the size of the punch will reduce the total scar, but at the same time, higher transection is a possibility.[1-3,17] So, the surgeon shall make a judgment of punch size, graft thickness, and total grafts to be harvested. Using a too large-sized punch may create moth-eaten deformity.[3,4] Using a large-sized punch and harvesting more MFUs (cherry-picking) will exhaust the donor and limit the extraction of grafts in successive extraction stages **(Figs. 2 and 3)**. The author believes using the same punch

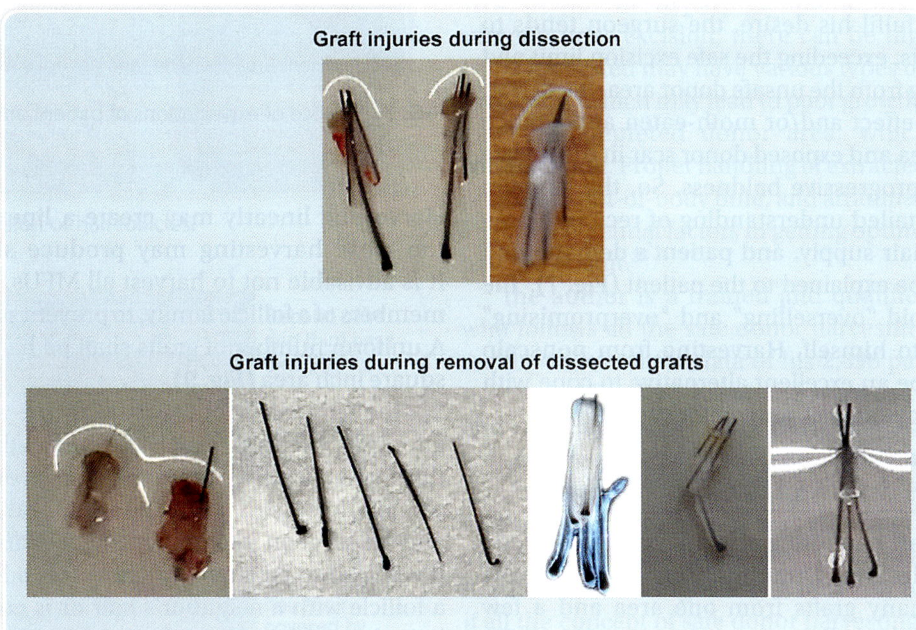

FIG. 5: Various injuries to hair follicle.

CHAPTER 41

Graft Harvesting from Safe Donor Area and Graft Calculation for Recipient Area: Current Concepts

Anil Kumar Garg, Seema Garg

Key Messages

- Occipital area represents the donor, but the entire occipital area is not the donor.
- Unger's safe donor area (SDA) definition is considered as the gold standard in SDA definition.
- A proper delineation of SDA and efficient utilization of the donor area remain the most significant factor in producing a satisfactory outcome in hair transplant (HT).
- There is no clear cut defined SDA, and it varies among races.
- Reverse pattern hair loss, diffuse androgenetic alopecia, and possibility of miniaturization in occipital scalp donor area are to be considered while delineating the donor area.

INTRODUCTION

Hair transplant surgery is based on the concept of harvesting the follicular units (FUs) from the occipital region, which is considered as relatively androgen resistant and transplanting them to the bald area.[1] A proper delineation of SDA and efficient utilization of the donor area remain the most significant factor in producing a satisfactory outcome in HT. There is no clear cut defined SDA, and it varies among races. Recently, with the advent of mega sessions of follicular unit extraction (FUE), with grafts being harvested by larger and larger parts of occipital scalp, questions have been raised as to what is SDA and whether it is wise to harvest from all areas of occipital scalp. Likewise, new concepts such as reverse pattern hair loss, diffuse androgenetic alopecia, and possibility of miniaturization in occipital scalp have also come to the fore.[2] It has long been recognized that although occipital area represents the donor, entire occipital area is not the donor. So, a number of workers have reported on the topic of "which part of occipital scalp is the safe donor." This chapter focuses on the concept of donor area in an otherwise normal patient.

UNGER'S SAFE AREA

Safe donor area was first suggested by Unger et al.,[3] in 1994, and this continues to be the global standard. They had described an SDA for over 80% of patients (under the age of 80 years). Such an area would consist of more or less a parallelogram in the parietal–occipital area, whose inferior border would be chosen by the surgeon on the basis of ≥10 hairs per 4-mm diameter circle **(Figs. 1A to D)**. This number would provide a "cushion," allowing for a subsequent decrease in density with aging to eight hairs per 4-mm diameter circle. (The number of hairs per 4-mm diameter circle could be increased if one wanted to approach the donor area in an even more conservative fashion.) The superior border of the parallelogram would be 71.7 mm superior to the inferior border. The anterior border of the parallelogram would similarly contain at least 10 hairs per 4-mm diameter circle and would angle somewhat anteriorly, parallel to the postauricular hair margin. A narrower more or less parallelogram would sit on the inferior one, with its posterior border beginning in the midparietal area. Its anterior border would be 28.6 mm anterior to a line drawn vertically from the tragus and would be parallel to the temporal hairline, unless

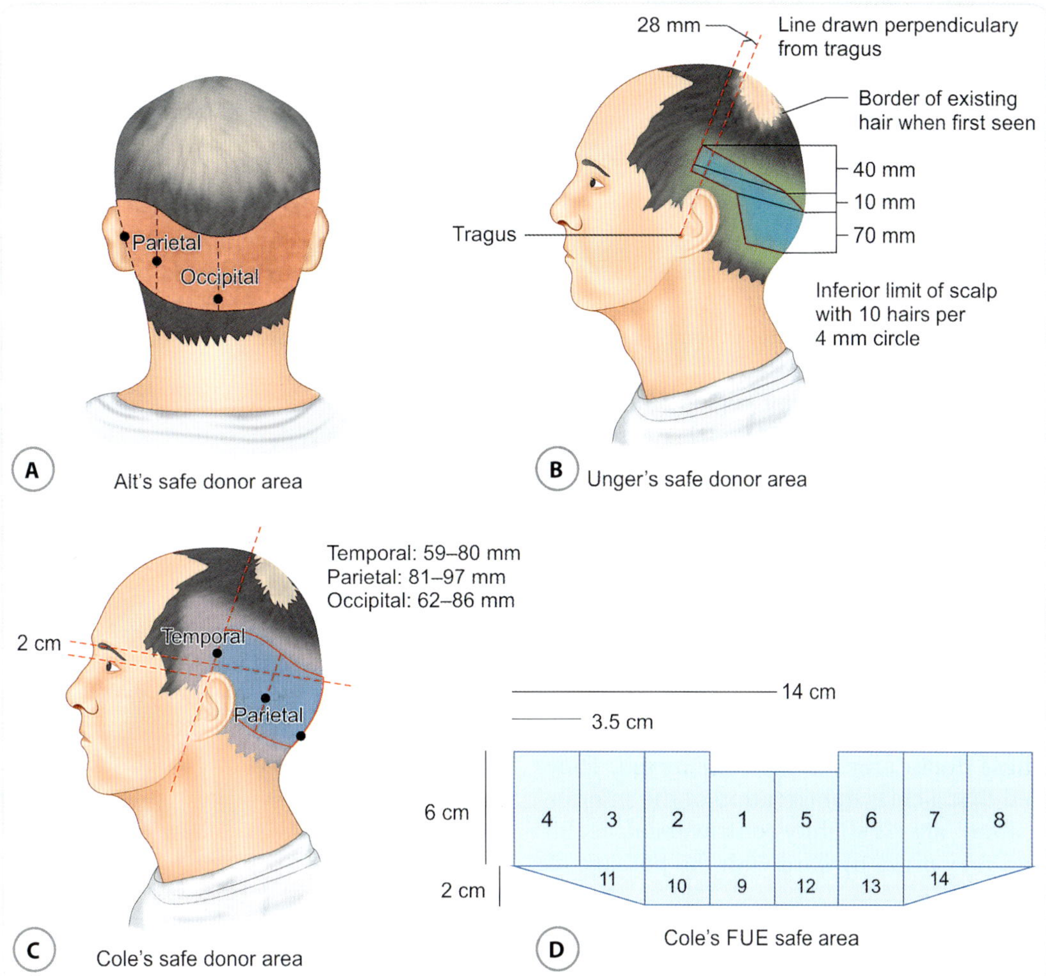

FIGS. 1A TO D: Safe donor area illustrations. (A) Alt's safe donor area; (B) Unger's safe donor area; (C) Cole's safe donor area; (D) Cole's follicular unit extraction (FUE) safe donor area.

there were good reasons to suspect the area anterior to the tragus would not remain sufficiently dense over the long term. This superior parallelogram would be 12.3 mm high (again subject to clinical findings and family history). Its superior border would drop somewhat inferiorly as it progressed posteriorly to meet the midline point of the safe occipital donor area. Lastly, in the midtemporal area, the "safe" donor area would extend 55.6 mm superior to the superior parallelogram and then descend on a line drawn to meet the SDA in the midparietal area. It is important to point out that this design incorporates permanent hair whose long-term density would be eight hairs or more per 4-mm diameter circle, but that according to this criterion less dense permanent hair would persist superior and inferior to these boundaries in virtually all patients. Some of this less dense hair in some patients could be used as additional donor material if it were necessary.[3] The aforementioned noted boundaries are not suggested as perfectly safe for all patients, but represent the implications of the only objective scientific evaluation of this area. On the basis of that investigation, they would be very safe in approximately 80% of patients under the age of 80 years. More restrictive areas can be chosen, for example, if one prefers to plan for patients who might live 80 or more years or if the patient has a father or maternal grandfather with type VII male pattern baldness.

ALT'S SAFE AREA

Alt suggested that a line drawn perpendicularly from the external auditory canal should define the anterior border of the safe area **(Figs. 1A to D)**.[4] In majority, the anterior border of this SDA was 6.5–7 cm wide and steadily narrowed posteriorly. A horizontal line drawn from a point 2 cm superior to the reflection of the skin of external ear and the scalp to the point where the line intersects the midline of occiput defines the superior border of SDA. Alt had also suggested that at least 2.5 cm of unharvested permanent hair should remain superior to the most superior donor area to provide adequate long-term camouflage of donor scars.

COLE'S SAFE AREA

Cole suggested a definition of the donor area for FUE procedure based on his study on 64 Caucasians and 30 Asians.[4] According to Cole, the total permanent donor area was 203 cm^2. He proposed a subdivision of donor area into 14 regions: 8 major regions (richer in follicles) and 6 minor regions **(Figs. 1A to D)**. The regions 1 and 5 measure 3.5 × 5 cm, regions 2, 3, 4, 6, 7, and 8 measure 3.5 × 6 cm, and the minor regions 9–14 measure 3.5 × 2 cm.

BERNSTEIN AND RASSMAN DEFINITION OF SAFE DONOR AREA

Bernstein and Rassman[5] have suggested that the SDA consists of approximately 25% of the scalp and that only half of these donor areas could be removed. They have suggested that a clear demarcation of the inferior border of the donor area is slightly controversial, as the inferior margin may move upward with the passage of time.[5]

SAFE DONOR AREA DEFINITION BASED ON PARIETAL WHORL BY PARK

Park et al.[6] defined the SDA in relation to parietal whorl (PW) involving 1,008 Korean adult males. They concluded that the progression range of vertex alopecia to the occipital side is the most critical factor in establishing the SDA. The objective and scientific prediction of the progression of vertex alopecia to the occipital side will allow the anticipation of the maximum progression range of vertex alopecia and the available SDA of each patient. According to this study, when the PW is anteriorly positioned, vertex alopecia initiates more anteriorly, and when the PW is positioned closer to the occipital side, vertex alopecia progresses posteriorly. Thus, the progression range of alopecia is verified to occur more extensively when the PW is positioned closer to the occipital side. Even though the PW may be anteriorly positioned, if the alopecia of the vertex area progressively spreads to the occipital side, the outcome becomes the same irrespective of the PW position. Hence according to Park et al.,[6] the location of the PW gives an idea to the extent of superior margin of SDA, and the authors had suggested that alopecia mostly progresses within 6 cm of the PW toward the occipital side among their study group and 97.5% of the study group had their occipital fringe 4.5 cm below the PW. This area below the occipital fringe was considered as SDA **(Fig. 2)**.[6]

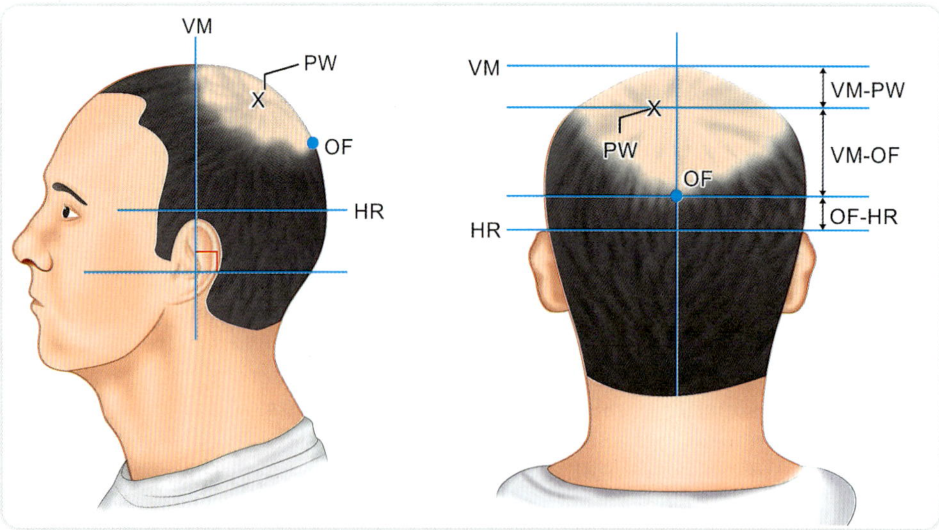

FIG. 2: Landmarks for measurement of parietal whorl position.
(VM: vertical bimeatal line; PW: parietal whorl; OF: occipital fringe; HR: horizontal plane, which connects the upper border of the helical rim)

SUMMARY

It is worth emphasizing that there can never be one valid, totally SDA for all patients. A family history, assessment of the future progression of the androgenetic alopecia, and clinical examination would be necessary to confirm the boundaries of SDA. One should always err on the side of caution.[7] There is a paucity of literature regarding the SDA in Asians and particularly Indian population. More studies are required for assessing whether the same findings reported from the studies of Caucasians are applicable to other race and ethnic groups.

Tips and Pearls

- There can never be one valid, totally SDA for all patients.
- A family history, assessment of the future progression of the androgenetic alopecia, and clinical examination would be necessary to confirm the boundaries of SDA.
- Reverse pattern hair loss, diffuse androgenetic alopecia, and possibility of miniaturization in occipital scalp donor area are to be considered while delineating the donor area.

REFERENCES

1. Yepuri V, Mysore V. Effects of hormones on hair. In: Mysore V (Ed). Hair Transplantation, 1st edition. New Delhi, India: Jaypee Brothers Medical Publishers; 2016. pp. 21-3.
2. Kumaresan M, Mysore V. Controversies in Hair Transplantation. J Cutan Aesthet Surg. 2018;11:173-81.
3. Unger W, Solish N, Giguere D. Delineating the "Safe" donor area for hair transplanting. Am J Cosmet Surg. 1994;11:239-43.
4. Devroye J. An overview of the donor area: basic principles. In: Unger WP, Shapiro R, Unger R, Unger M (Eds). Hair Transplantation, 5th edition. New York: Informa Health Care; 2011. pp. 247-62.
5. Bernstein RM, Rassman WR. Follicular transplantation. Patient evaluation and surgical planning. Dermatol Surg. 1997; 23:771.
6. Park JH, Na YC, Moh JS, Lee SY, You SH. Predicting the permanent safe donor area for hair transplantation in Koreans with male pattern baldness according to the position of the parietal whorl. Arch Plast Surg. 2014;41:277-84.
7. Kumaresan M, Deepa, MS. Occipital donor area grading and profile in Indian population. J Cut Aesthet Surg. 2023;16: 101-6.

CHAPTER 42

Antithrombotic Therapy and Hair Transplantation

Vaishalee Kirane, Aniketh Venkataram

Key Messages

- It is important to be aware of all drugs being consumed by a patient while planning surgery.
- Since hair transplantation is a cosmetic procedure, benefits and risks of the procedure and of changing the drugs should be considered carefully.
- Hair transplantation can be planned in a patient on anticoagulants safely, but with proper counseling and after physician consultation.

INTRODUCTION

As the number of patients seeking hair transplantation (HT) is rising, so is the number of patients on antithrombotic drugs for cardiac comorbidities. There is a significant area of overlap in these two groups, particularly in middle-aged males who are increasingly seeking HT. Hence, the hair transplant surgeon needs to be aware of the protocols and precautions of these patients. In simple terms, the questions to be answered are as follows:

Should antithrombotics be stopped for a hair transplant surgery?

- If *yes*:
  - What are the protocols to be followed?
  - Is the risk of thrombosis justifiable for a cosmetic procedure?
- If *no*:
  - Can HT still be performed safely and successfully?
  - What additional precautions are needed during surgery?

As a baseline recommendation, in order to decrease the risk of excessive bleeding, it would be prudent to advise avoidance or discontinuation of different agents that inhibit platelet function and clotting.[1] **Box 1** contains a list of prescription medications that can increase the risk of bleeding. This list can also be given to the patients in the preoperative instruction package. *However, the issue is more complex and needs a thorough understanding of the need for potentially lifesaving drugs and, at the same time, safe performance and fulfillment of a patient's emotional need for a cosmetic surgery.*

BOX 1 Medications that can increase bleeding.[2]

- Aceclofenac
- Acetylsalicylic acid
- Clopidogrel
- Danazol
- Diclofenac
- Dicoumarol
- Dipyridamole
- Escitalopram
- Enoxaparin
- Fluoxetine
- Ibuprofen
- Indomethacin
- Ketoprofen
- Naproxen
- Pentoxifylline
- Piroxicam
- Sertraline
- Sulindac
- Ticlopidine
- Tranexamic acid
- Warfarin

Source: World Federation of Hemophilia (drugs that can cause bleeding.)

BRIEF OVERVIEW OF ANTITHROMBOTICS

There are two main classes of drugs:

1. *Antiplatelets*:
   a. Inhibit platelet aggregation and function
   b. Affect bleeding time
   c. Used for prevention of thrombosis in patients after coronary stent implantation/stroke/myocardial infarction

   d. For example: Aspirin, ticlopidine, clopidogrel, abciximab, and eptifibatide
2. *Anticoagulants*:
   a. Inhibit the coagulation pathway
   b. Affect clotting time. Normal target international normalized ratio (INR) 2.0–3.0/2.5–3.5
   c. Used in patients with atrial fibrillation, mechanical heart valves, and venous thromboembolism
   d. For example: Warfarin, rivaroxaban, and dabigatran

Aspirin

Platelet activation and the production of platelet products are enhanced by thromboxane, the synthesis of which is inhibited by cyclooxygenase enzyme. Aspirin inhibits cyclooxygenase enzyme and thus interferes with platelet function.[3] A study by C Lawrence showed that intraoperative bleeding complications occurred only in patients receiving aspirin who had a prolonged bleeding time. Patients with a normal bleeding time can continue aspirin or nonsteroidal anti-inflammatory drugs (NSAIDs) therapy before dermatologic surgery.[3] Another study showed that the use of anticoagulants and platelet inhibitors can increase the risk of intraoperative and postoperative hemorrhagic complications in cutaneous surgery.[4] NSAIDs action of inhibiting cyclooxygenase is reversible and dependent on the presence of the circulating drug and therefore its half-life. For example, ibuprofen has a short half-life, and further, it is a nonessential drug unlike aspirin.

Warfarin

Warfarin depletes the reduced form of vitamin K and thus interferes with the production of vitamin K-dependent clotting factors II, VII, IX, and X. It is a lifesaving medication, and stoppage of the drug can lead to a serious medical episode. Its stoppage for a cosmetic procedure such as HT raises ethical questions. However, a number of practitioners have carried out hair transplants on patients who did not discontinue their warfarin and have reported acceptable levels of intraoperative and postoperative bleeding.[4] If warfarin is discontinued, then long-acting heparin is to be started 6 days prior to the date of surgery. The last dose of heparin is given on the morning of the day before surgery and restarted soon after surgery as is deemed fit by the managing physician—usually 36 hours. Warfarin is restarted at the same time as the heparin is discontinued.

Clopidogrel

Clopidogrel bisulfate is an inhibitor of adenosine diphosphate-induced platelet aggregation. It is frequently prescribed in order to reduce atherothrombotic events for patients with cardiac stents, recent myocardial infarction, or stroke as well as for those with an established peripheral arterial disease. Platelets exposed to clopidogrel are affected for the remainder of their life span (approximately 7–10 days). Thus, it will need to be stopped 7–10 days before surgery and only with the agreement of the prescribing physician.

Manchikanti and other authors showed that the recommendations derived from the comprehensive assessment of the literature and guidelines are to continue NSAIDs and low-dose aspirin during interventional techniques. However, the recommendations for discontinuation of antiplatelet therapy with platelet aggregation inhibitors such as clopidogrel and ticlopidine are variable with clinical judgment to continue or discontinue based on the patient's condition and the risk factors. Low-molecular-weight heparin (LMWH) may be discontinued 12 hours prior. Warfarin should be discontinued or INR be normalized to 1.4–2 or less based on risk factors.[5]

RECOMMENDATIONS FOR PERIOPERATIVE MANAGEMENT OF ANTITHROMBOTICS

There are two main factors which guide the perioperative management:

1. *Risk of bleeding if antithrombotics continued:* HT is classified as low risk for serious bleeding as far as morbidity/mortality is concerned. However, this bleeding might affect the cosmetic outcome even though it might not harm the patient.
2. *Risk of thrombosis if antithrombotics stopped:* Normally classified into low risk and high risk **(Box 2)**.

This risk assessment has to be taken into consideration, and a cardiologist seeing the patient should also be consulted to decide on a plan of action jointly.

BOX 2 Classifications of risk for antithrombosis.

High risk

- Any mechanical heart valve
- Atrial fibrillation with $CHADS_2$* score > 2 or history of stroke or transient ischemic attack or rheumatic valvular heart disease
- Recent venous thromboembolism (within 3 months)
- Recurrent venous thromboembolism receiving long-term anticoagulation

Low risk

- Atrial fibrillation with $CHADS_2$ score of ≤2 and no history of stroke or transient ischemic attack
- Single venous thromboembolism occurring > 3 months ago and with no other risk factors

*Score for stroke risk assessment in atrial fibrillation

Management of Anticoagulants[6,7]

- Warfarin stopped or reduced for 5 days prior to surgery
- INR lowered to 1.5, checked day before surgery
- *If high risk of thromboembolism*: Bridging anticoagulation with LMWH from 4 days prior to 3 days postsurgery
- *Low risk of thromboembolism*: No need for bridging anticoagulation
- Warfarin resumed on the evening of surgery

Management of Antiplatelets

- Aspirin is continued throughout the perioperative period. It need not be stopped.
- Clopidogrel is stopped 5–7 days prior to surgery and restarted within 24 hours of surgery.

If the patient has undergone a stent placement recently, then antiplatelet drugs are critical and cannot be stopped. Hence, the surgery should be postponed for the following durations:

- 6 weeks for bare metal stents
- 12 months for drug-eluting stent

TABLE 1: Summary of recommendations for perioperative management.

Day	Anticoagulant	Antiplatelet
–5	Stop warfarin in all	Stop clopidogrel
–4	Start LMWH in high-risk cases	Aspirin continued throughout
–3		
–2		
–1	Measure INR. Last dose of LMWH 24 hours prior to surgery	
Surgery	Restart warfarin in evening	
+1	LMWH dose 24 hours after surgery	Restart clopidogrel
+2		
+3	Last dose of LMWH	
+4	Measure INR, continue regular warfarin dose	

(INR: international normalized ratio; LMWH: low-molecular-weight heparin)

Intraoperative Precautions[6,7]

Patients on antithrombotics are at an increased risk of bleeding, both in the donor and in the recipient area. This can cause increased popping and postoperative hematoma.

Bleeding can be reduced by an adequate amount of tumescent fluid. However, this may raise the blood pressure and pulse rate and hence should be discussed with the cardiologist. Any bleeding can also be controlled with adequate and patient gauze compression.

SUMMARY

With proper knowledge and precautions, HT can be safely performed in patients on antithrombotics. The perioperative management of the commonly used antithrombotics is summed up in **Table 1**.

REFERENCES

1. Langtry JA, Maddin WS, Carruthers JA, Rivers JK. Is there a rationale for the drugs used in hair transplantation surgery? Dermatol Surg. 1998;24:967-91.
2. World Federation of Hemophilia. Drugs that can cause bleeding. [online] Available from https://wfh.org/about-bleeding-disorders/. [Last accessed October, 2023].
3. Lawrence C, Sakuntabhai A, Tiling-Grosse S. Effect of aspirin and nonsteroidal anti-inflammatory drug therapy on bleeding complications in dermatologic surgical patients. J Am Acad Dermatol. 1994;31:988-92.
4. Goldsmith SM, Leshin B, Owen J. Management of patients taking anticoagulants and platelet inhibitors prior to dermatologic surgery. J Dermatol Surg Oncol. 1993;19:578-81.
5. Manchikanti L, Falco FJ, Benyamin RM, Caraway DL, Kaye AD, Helm S 2nd, et al. Assessment of bleeding risk of interventional techniques: a best evidence synthesis of practice patterns and perioperative management of anticoagulant and antithrombotic therapy. Pain Physician. 2013;16(2):SE261-318.
6. Douketis JD, Spyropoulos AC, Spencer FA, Mayr M, Jaffer AK, Eckman MH, et al. Perioperative management of antithrombotic therapy: Antithrombotic Therapy and Prevention of Thrombosis, 9th edition: American College of Chest Physicians Evidence-based Clinical Practice Guidelines. Chest. 2012;141(2):e326S-50S.
7. Yagyu K. Guidelines for perioperative antithrombotic therapy in hair restoration surgery: management of patients with coronary heart disease, mechanical heart valve, and atrial fibrillation. Hair Transplant Forum Int. 2012;22(2):1-5.

CHAPTER 43

Emergencies and Resuscitation in Transplantation

Murali Chakravarthy

Key Messages

- Though dermatosurgeries are office procedures, surgical emergencies may occur, though they are rare.
- Dermatological surgeons should be fully aware of procedures for resuscitation in such eventualities.
- Syncope, bleeding, and issues concerning lignocaine use are the common events that might occur.
- Monitoring devices, basic resuscitation equipment, and adequately trained staff are needed to manage an emergency.
- The adage "if you are prepared for an emergency, it ceases to exist" appears to be apt under these situations.

INTRODUCTION

Office-based dermatologic procedures and cosmetic surgeries performed on a day care basis have become the trend of the day. Such procedures are supported by anesthesiologists at certain centers and by resident doctors or nurses at others. The support provided by the anesthesiologists in these situations is referred to as "monitored anesthesia care."[1] With society getting more and more litigant, it is time that dermatologists attend to quality and safety issues while dealing with these "patients," who do not usually suffer from the disease. Complications, though uncommon, have been reported in 6% of such procedures: Bleeding or hematoma in 3%, infections in 2%, and vasovagal reactions in 1%. Bleeding occurred more frequently in men or in patients taking anticoagulation, antiplatelet, or immunosuppressive agents in prolonged procedures. Vasovagal reactions were associated with patients younger than 50 years of age.[2,3]

The preparedness of dermatologists in dealing with such crises affects the outcome of the situation. The emphasis is on the patient safety and adequate infrastructure to deal with the complications that may arise during the procedure. The availability of monitoring devices, basic resuscitation equipment, adequately trained staff, and the ability to manage an emergency should always be borne in mind of the dermatologic surgeons prior to starting the scheduled procedure at the office.[4,5] It may be misconceived by a few dermatologic surgeons that complications are rare, and therefore, the therapeutic agents and knowledge to deal with the crises in their office may not be required. Providing infrastructural support to deal with crises in day care surgery not only makes day care procedures safer for the patient but also avoids potential medicolegal complications. This chapter discusses the spectrum of emergencies that are commonly encountered by the dermatosurgeon and the basic guidelines to manage these emergency situations. Dermatologic surgery is mostly cosmetic; therefore, the potential for medicolegal issues is high in the event of adverse outcome. In the author's view, the entire team in the dermatologic surgeon's procedure room should be trained to provide at least basic life support (BLS), if not advanced cardiac life support (ACLS). Dermatologic surgeons need to practice and adopt the "safe surgery saves lives" campaign as proposed by the World Health Organization.[6] A few of the points for safe surgery are mentioned in **Box 1**.

Several emergency issues may be encountered in the practice of surgical dermatology.[7] These are illustrated in **Box 2**.

BOX 1 Patient safety issues that have to be practiced in dermatosurgical patients.

- Identify all patients by name and check if the patient has consented to the procedure. All adult patients should provide consent themselves
- Ask the patient to show the site and side of the procedure
- Take history of allergies, if any
- Instruct the patient to continue all the medications that he has been prescribed
- Insert an intravenous cannula and maintain a running drip of Ringer's lactate. Other fluids, such as dextrose and saline, may be infused depending on the requirements
- In diabetic patients, check the blood sugar by "glucostrip" method
- Connect electrocardiogram and pulse oximetry in all the patients. If access to the chest is difficult to obtain, loose-fitting clothes allowing access to the chest may be worn
- Prepare the local anesthetic infiltration yourself. If you have a well-organized team, all medications should be loaded while a witness confirms the name of the medication
- It is the author's practice to load 1:200,000 adrenaline in a 20-mL syringe for all cases (it is prepared by diluting 1 mg or 1 mL of adrenaline to 10 mL; discard 9 mL of this and dilute the remaining 1–20 mL). This solution may be used to treat several problems such as hypotension, bradycardia, bronchospasm, anaphylaxis, and allergy, among others

BOX 2 Various emergency issues.

- Anaphylaxis
- Syncope
- Lignocaine-related issues
- Breathlessness
- Chest pain
- Bleeding
- Acute stroke
- Status epilepticus
- Hypotension
- Hypoxia
- Cardiac arrest

ANAPHYLAXIS

Anaphylaxis is a sudden, violent manifestation of an acute immunological reaction, which might become life threatening at times. It is produced by a complex mechanism involving the immune system. The manifestation may vary from pruritus and urticarial in milder cases, and inspiratory stridor, laryngeal edema, bronchospasm, hypotension, and cardiac arrhythmias in more severe ones. Classic anaphylaxis manifests with a massive cardiovascular collapse within minutes of exposure to the offending antigen. The outcome of such events depends mainly on the preparedness of the team. It is a good practice to start the monitoring devices prior to any interventions. It has been shown that the presence of a professional watching the patient's vitals improves the detection of anaphylaxis and its treatment.[8]

BOX 3 Management of anaphylaxis.[10]

- Place the patient supine on the examination table, preferably Trendelenburg position (head down)
- Loosen the clothing
- *Assess the vital signs*: Heart rate, blood pressure, and oxygen saturation
- Maintain the airway, breathing, and circulation
- Start oxygen by face mask
- Efforts to minimize further antigen exposure should be made. Call for help. It is prudent to have a mechanism to call for help without having to leave the patient, such as a call bell or "code blue"
- Secure an intravenous access if not already in place
- Adrenaline is the drug of choice. About 0.3–0.5 mL of adrenaline, 1:1,000 is administered intravenously, subcutaneously, or intramuscularly. Repeat the dose at 5–10-minute interval. It is the author's practice to inject 4–5 mL of 1:200,000 adrenaline intravenously when bronchospasm, severe hypotension, and bradycardia are encountered
- If the patient has severe hypotension—start intravenous fluids, preferably colloid, if not improving, start inotropes such as dopamine
- Nebulized beta-agonists, such as albuterol with or without intravenous aminophylline, may be considered in patients with severe bronchoconstriction. Simultaneously, ranitidine 1 mg/kg intravenous (IV), while a steroid may prevent a delayed reaction. Give hydrocortisone, 5 mg/kg, or approximately 250 mg intravenously (prednisone, 20 mg orally, can be given in mild cases)
- Monitor patients for 2–4 hours for a minor attack and in case of severe anaphylaxis, preferably admit the patient and monitor for 24 hours

Common causes of such anaphylaxis in a dermatologic practice are adverse reactions to intravenous antibiotic agents, local anesthetic agents, and other allergens such as latex rubber. **Box 3** shows the management of anaphylaxis. Anaphylactoid reactions are similar but are not immunologically mediated. They may be prevented by prior administration of corticosteroids and antihistaminic agents. These are common subsequent to the administration of radiological ionic dyes and a few anesthetic agents, such as atracurium and suxamethonium, which are likely to release histamine.[9] However, these are not common in dermatosurgical practice.

SYNCOPE

Syncope is a vagal-mediated unconsciousness, commonly associated with extreme bradycardia and, at times,

BOX 4 Tips for avoiding syncopal attacks.

- Explaining the patient about the procedure and allaying anxiety often helps in reducing the incidence of syncope as also performing the procedures in a supine position
- Shielding the eyes and placing a surgical sheet to block the patient's view of the operated area may help prevent the occurrence of syncope. A distracting conversation may be beneficial
- Following the procedure, the patient should slowly sit up and be observed for several minutes while postoperative instructions are being discussed. Sitting up suddenly and standing immediately after the procedure could also result in syncope after the completion of the procedure[11]

pulseless states. It is commonly encountered in anxious patients. It is often confused with anaphylaxis if it occurs after an injection. Starting of an intravenous cannulation, surgical incision in inadequately anesthetized areas, and even the sight of blood might trigger it. An early sign of syncope, prior to loss of consciousness, is profuse sweating and cold skin. Vagal-induced bradycardia in the setting of decreased systemic vascular resistance can initiate collapse. Pseudoseizure activity may occur, characterized by brief clonic activity. Blood pressure may initially decrease but is restored with supine position. The tips for avoiding syncopal attacks are mentioned in **Box 4**.

Management of Syncope

Place the patient in supine and preferably in a head down (Trendelenburg) position. Monitor vital parameters such as heart rate, blood pressure, and pulse oximetry. Reassure the patient and maintina decubitus position. Start intravenous access. Administer injection atropine 1 mg if heart rate is <40 beats/min and intravenous fluids if blood pressure continues to be low. If alone, one should call for help and step up the monitoring only after minimal monitoring has been started to begin with.

LIGNOCAINE-RELATED ISSUES

Patients with multiple allergies and atopy are more likely to develop lignocaine allergy.[12] Most of the adverse reactions that are clinically seen are, in fact, manifestations of the overdosage of the local anesthetic by inadvertent intravascular injection in extremely vascular areas such as the scalp and face. It can also occur in cases of tumescent liposuction when dosages over 55 mg/kg are used. In such cases, signs of overdosage are often delayed. A case of lignocaine overdosage leading to death late at midnight, after liposuction has recently been reported.[13] Toxic reactions to lignocaine resulting from overdosage cause central nervous system or myocardial depression or excitation, perioral numbness, nausea, seizures, or coma. Vasovagal syncope may be misdiagnosed as an allergic reaction and should be distinguished properly.

Methylparaben and propylparaben are the preservatives added to lignocaine and various cosmetics to increase their shelf life. Some of the adverse reactions seen during the administration of lignocaine may indeed be due to these preservatives.[14] Patients who are allergic to sulfa drugs may develop adverse reactions to "sulfites," which are added as preservatives to lignocaine. Anxiety regarding the use of needles and/or the effects of epinephrine in lignocaine can lead to palpitations, panic attacks, and vasovagal events that the patient may remember as an allergic reaction. Patients admitting to having had previous incorrectly allergic reactions should be properly investigated prior to submitting for dermatologic surgery. The dermatologic surgical procedure in patients with allergic manifestations may be electively performed under general anesthesia, and management of such cases in a hospital with a full backup should be planned.[15]

BREATHLESSNESS

The etiologies of breathlessness may be cardiac, respiratory, or anxiety related. Patients with asthma and obstructive airway disease should be well investigated by a pulmonologist and rendered "dry" before scheduling for dermatologic surgery. Such patients should be advised to use the routine inhalers before arriving for surgery.[16] Dermatologic surgeons should also check the preoperative "basal" values of oxygen and carbon dioxide. In the absence of this knowledge, one may find it difficult to achieve the normal values of partial pressures of oxygen and carbon dioxide. Patients with "cardiac asthma" should be well prepared with diuretic and peripheral vasodilator therapy. At times, cardiac patients manifest with dyspnea when subjected to myocardial ischemia. Even young, obese individuals might present with dyspnea of cardiac origin. Patients with respiratory compromise should not be operated without the guidance of pulse oximetry. If the oxygen saturation decreases during surgery, methods to administer the bronchodilator nebulization must be kept handy. Dyspnea, which does not abate with treatment, whether of cardiac or pulmonary origin, is a reason to stop the scheduled procedure and to reschedule at a later convenient time. Dyspnea due to anxiety will respond well to a small intravenous dose (0.5–1 mg) of anxiolytic such as midazolam. Appropriate preoperative counseling is sufficient in most patients to avoid anxiety-related problems.

CHEST PAIN

Chest pain may be a manifestation of not only coronary arterial ischemia but also anxiety. However, fear, stress of pain, and procedure can also precipitate an acute myocardial infarction in any patient prone to ischemia. Although most dermatologic surgical procedures are day care and performed in young, healthy individuals, at times, if a high-risk patient is being subjected to aesthetic surgery, thorough evaluation would be mandatory.

If a patient complains of chest pain during the procedure, place the patient supine and check the vitals. Activate physician/emergency medical services. Record an electrocardiogram, which may be compared against the basal. If you are suspecting coronary ischemia, a tablet of nitroglycerine 5 mg should be placed immediately under the tongue. One must be aware of possible headache and hypotension following this measure. An intravenous cannula should be inserted immediately (if not already done), and a patent intravenous line is important for further management. If, with these measures, the chest pain settles, and the patient is hemodynamically stable, one can proceed with the surgery. If the pain is unabated and electrocardiographic changes persist or worsen, the scheduled procedure should be deferred with. The patient may undergo the scheduled procedure after consulting with a cardiologist.

Patients at risk for myocardial ischemia should be thoroughly evaluated and medically optimized prior to the procedure. In the author's opinion, it may be wise to have "monitored anesthesia care" for all patients.

BLEEDING

A major surgical bleeder is rare in cutaneous surgeries. A patient receiving antiplatelet medications for concomitant comorbidities may pose special issues. Such patients may be better prepared by stopping the antiplatelet medication at least for 2 weeks prior to the planned procedure. Although the hemorrhage associated with cutaneous surgery may not be life threatening, its other effects, such as causing a menacing hematoma and lifting of flaps compromising their viability, may be of nuisance value.[17,18]

ACUTE STROKE

Patients on antiplatelet or antithrombotic therapy[19] and their sudden discontinuation, patients with carotid bruit, patients with prior history of stroke, and patients with cardiovascular disease are all at potential risk for stroke.[18] Preprocedural evaluation by a physician or a neurologist has to be considered in such patients. During the procedure, the dermatologist's role chiefly concerns the detection phase of a sudden neurologic deficit. This may include an alteration in consciousness (confusion, coma, and seizures), aphasia, dysarthria, facial weakness or asymmetry, extremity weakness, paralysis, sensory loss, ataxia, visual loss, or vertigo. Immediately activate the physician or emergency medical services. A definitive hospital-based intervention must occur within 3 hours of the onset of the stroke symptoms to be beneficial. Meanwhile, attend to the airway, breathing, circulation (ABC) of resuscitation and monitor vitals and manage accordingly till the physician arrives.

STATUS EPILEPTICUS

Dermatologists do encounter diseases with potential epileptic manifestations in conditions such as tuberous sclerosis and systemic lupus erythematosus **(Box 5)**. It is wise to obtain any past history of seizures and antiseizure medications.[20] If the patients are epileptic on treatment, one should advise them to continue the treatment until the day of surgery.

COLLAPSE

Most commonly, syncope, anaphylaxis, hypoglycemia, and cardiac arrest are reasons for collapse of a patient. These issues may be addressed as discussed in the chapter. However, associated with a vasomotor collapse are some of the key issues mentioned here, which need attention.

BOX 5 Management of status epilepticus.

- Stop the ongoing procedure. First priority is always the maintenance of airway. Use an oral or nasopharyngeal airway as and when required (inserting these airways are out of the routine for dermatological surgeons, so it is advisable for them to learn the insertion of these airways from their anesthesia or critical care colleagues)
- If available, oxygen can be delivered by face mask
- Monitor the vital signs
- Place the patient on a soft, flat surface away from sharp objects
- Look for and prevent tongue bite
- If seizures have stopped and the patient is breathing and has a pulse, place the patient in a recovery position (modified lateral position). It will allow the clearance of any pooled secretions
- Secure a peripheral intravenous line and send blood sample for blood glucose and serum electrolytes
- The benzodiazepine midazolam or lorazepam 1–2 mg or diazepam 5–10 mg intravenously will stop the seizures
- Call for physician and evaluate for seizures etiology and further management options

HYPOTENSION

Low blood pressure may result from bleeding, syncope, anaphylaxis, acute myocardial infarction, and secondary to medications such as sedatives/anesthetic agents. Patients may complain of giddiness (or orthostatic hypotension).

Management

Place the patient in supine position and check vital signs, such as pulse rate and blood pressure. Treat the underlying cause. Tachycardia with low blood pressure indicates blood loss; start the patient on intravenous fluid crystalloids. Ringer's lactate 5–10 mL/kg bolus over 15 minutes can be administered and the blood pressure checked. If good response continues, intravenous fluid (Ringer's lactate) at the rate of 2–4 mL/kg/h may be continued. If there is no response to the fluids, check for continued blood loss and send a sample of blood for checking the hemoglobin level. In the absence of matched donor blood, it is vital to maintain the circulating blood volume by administration of colloids such as starch solutions. More damage might be caused by allowing hypovolemia than anemia.[21,22] If hypotension persists, one should seek a physician's opinion and have a provision for starting an inotropic infusion such as injection dopamine 5 μg/kg/min should be commenced.

HYPERTENSION

Known hypertensive, elderly, female, and anxious patients are prone to increased blood pressure during the procedure. Accelerated hypertensive patients can also present with giddiness and severe headache. Optimization of blood pressure for known hypertensives, reassuring the patients, premedicant such as alprazolam, and sedatives such as midazolam and lorazepam would help in the control of blood pressure. Involvement of a physician would be helpful if basic interventions do not reduce the blood pressure.

Infections after dermatological procedures are not only rare but usually insignificant. These procedures are majorly aesthetic ones, and these "patients" do not suffer from any major systemic illnesses; the expectations about outcomes are usually high. Absence of infection after the procedure is one such expectation. The dermatologic surgeon must attend to infection control measures in providing a clean ambiance while conducting the procedure, using standard precautions, preoperative decolonization of methicillin-resistant *Staphylococcus aureus* (MRSA), and surgical prophylaxis. Post procedure, the patients may be advised about care of the wound and reporting early if signs of infection come up.

Preoperative preparation: It is common knowledge that *S. aureus* is a common cutaneous commensal; it is impossible to eradicate it. While conducting surgical operations requiring skin incision, the colony count of these organisms has to be reduced. The methods to achieve this are as follows:

- *Preoperative chlorhexidine 2% v/v wash*: The patients have to bathe twice daily for 3 preoperative days. This solution cannot be applied over the scalp and face. Those wishing to operate on the scalp and the face may use triclosan solution.
- *Intranasal mupirocin ointment*: All surgical patients must be requested to use mupirocin ointment twice daily for 5 days preoperatively. This decolonizes the nasal mucosa of MRSA.
- *Surgical preparation*: It is recommended that we must use chlorhexidine tincture 2% W/V to prepare the skin. This solution has been found to be superior to using povidone iodine; its residual action is longer than that of povidone iodine. Whether chlorhexidine or povidone iodine is used, one must wait for at least 3 minutes prior to incision. The commonly found practice of "rubbing off" excess solution using a gauze should be shunned, and instead, the solution must be allowed to dry by itself; only then the antibacterial effect is maximized.
- *Preoperative surgical prophylaxis*: It is recommended by the Center for Disease Control and Prevention that a single dose of first- or second-generation cephalosporin be administered intravenously 15–60 minutes prior to incision. Administering 1.5 g of cefuroxime suffices in most adults. If the surgery continues beyond 4 hours, a similar dose must be administered.
- *Normoglycemia and normothermia*: It has been shown that intraoperative blood sugar and temperature maintenance are absolutely essential. Cutaneous surgeries are no exception to these recommendations.

HYPOXEMIA

Patient developing desaturation during the procedure requires attention. Hypoxemia may be secondary to pain-induced hypoventilation, pulmonary embolism (during liposuction), cardiac failure, or bronchospasm due to anaphylaxis.

Management

The management steps of hypoxemia are mentioned here.

1. Stop the procedure and start oxygen by face mask, 4 L/min.
2. Talk to the patient and encourage them to breathe deeply.

3. Assess the vitals and talk to the patient. Reassure them.
4. Determine the underlying cause.
5. Notify the physician.
6. Treat the underlying cause.

CARDIAC ARREST[7,23]

The most common cause of cardiac arrest is ventricular fibrillation. Other arrhythmias such as pulseless ventricular tachycardia and pulseless electrical activity also lead to cardiac arrest.

Cardiac arrest is confirmed when the patient is not responding, pulse is not felt, and blood pressure is not recordable. Immediate measures to be taken are:

- Activate the emergency department/notify the physician or an anesthesiologist.
- Start cardiopulmonary resuscitation as per the American Heart Association (AHA) guidelines 2010.[23]
- Start chest compression at the rate of 100/min.
- Get an automated external defibrillator device. Diagnose ventricular fibrillation and defibrillate.
- Continue chest compressions.
- Begin ventilation.
- Administer oxygen.
- Obtain intravenous access.
- Administer epinephrine or vasopressin.
- Assess adequacy of clinical practice redesign efforts.
- Intubate trachea.
- Additional drug therapy.
- Post-resuscitation care and shift of the patient to a higher medical center for further management.

NERVE INJURY

Inadvertent nerve damage is one of the most dreaded complications of dermatologic surgery. Effects of local anesthesia, inadvertent pressure, or tension due to positioning are the common cause. Nerve injuries may result in transient, either reversible or permanent. Patients should always be warned of the possibility of nerve injury during the discussion of the informed consent. Patient should be frequently asked about any discomfort induced by prolonged positioning.

GENERAL RESUSCITATION PLAN AT THE DERMATOLOGIC OFFICE

Training of each and every staff member at the dermatologic office with clearly defined roles for each staff is a must in managing an emergency scenario **(Box 6)**.

BOX 6 General resuscitation plan.

- Dermatologist or a physician should play the role of the team leader
- Patient is assessed by the team leader, and they assign tasks to their team members
- Assigned staff member activates the emergency medical services or contacts a physician or an anesthesiologist
- One staff member gets the automated external defibrillator and attaches it to the patient to analyze the rhythm and shock accordingly
- One staff member plays the role of chest compressor and other staff member takes care of the airway
- Another staff member can serve as the recorder of the event times, serial vital signs measurements, securing intravenous access, administering medications, and communicating with the family members

Preferably, an anesthetist should be available on the premises, particularly when surgeries such as liposuction are being performed. In his absence, a person trained in ACLS should be available.

Various roles played by the staff members can be practiced several times so that they can act accordingly in an emergency situation. Cardiopulmonary resuscitation (CPR) training, which includes BLS and ACLS, is conducted by various health organizations in accordance with AHA. All the staff members should undergo the BLS course, whereas the dermatosurgeon/team leader or the nursing staff should undergo both BLS and ACLS courses.

LIST OF RESUSCITATION EQUIPMENT

The basic resuscitation equipment in the form of crash cart should be made available in each dermatologist's office **(Fig. 1)**.

The telephone remains the most important piece of emergency equipment in the dermatosurgeon's office; it provides the first link in the chain of initiating the emergency medical services process.

The crash cart should comprise the following:

- Portable oxygen cylinder with face mask or nasal prongs, oral or nasopharyngeal airways, intravenous cannulas, tubings, fluids, and suction apparatus.
- *Medications*: Epinephrine 1:1,000, lorazepam, diazepam, diphenhydramine, dextrose 50%, nitroglycerine tablets, baby aspirin.
- Automated external defibrillators (AED) are computerized devices consisting of adhesive electrodes that

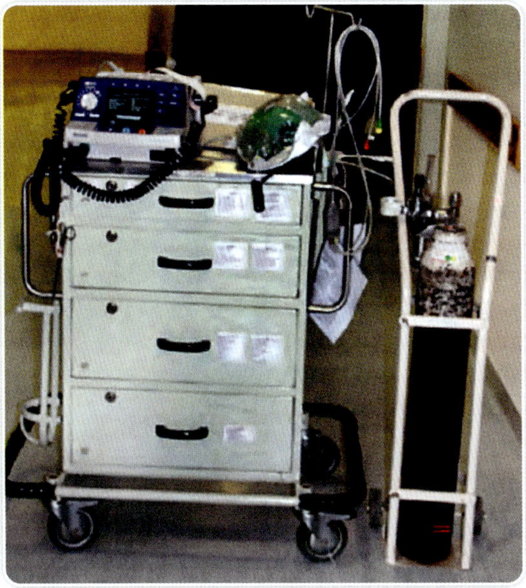

FIG. 1: Crash cart used by the author.

recognize cardiac rhythms and deliver an electrical shock across the chest wall to terminate the ventricular fibrillation. They are portable and user friendly. Adhesive electrodes are placed over the patient's cardiac apex and upper right chest to detect the cardiac rhythm. With audible and visual prompting, the device advises the operator to press the button and deliver a defibrillating shock.

- Laryngoscope, endotracheal tubes, and Ambu bag.
- The crash cart inventory should be periodically reviewed and renewed as necessary.
- CPR is a life-saving measure that supports the pumping of blood by the heart, thus allowing oxygen to reach the brain. It is more effective when done as early as possible. The conduct of CPR is guided by AHA guidelines recently updated in 2010.[23]
- CPR includes recognition of cardiac arrest, activating emergency medical services, and to get an AED, performing BLS and ACLS.
- *Components of BLS*: The primary survey includes "circulation, airway, breathing."
- *Circulation*: Chest compression keeps the blood pumping to the vital organs. It is done at the rate of 100 compressions per minute, at an adequate depth of 2–2.5 inches, and allowing complete chest recoil.
- *Airway and breathing*: Opening the patient's airway by performing the head tilt chin lift, and giving breath by mask-mouth. Chest compression to ventilation ratio is 30:2.
- *Defibrillation*: Once the AED arrives, switch on the defibrillator, and attach the adhesive electrodes to the patient's chest. Clear the patient, and once the defibrillator analyzes the rhythm, follow the defibrillator's instructions.

All the medic and paramedic staff members in the dermatology setup should be trained in performing BLS, performing chest compressions, maintaining the airway, and handling the AED.

Components of ACLS: The secondary survey

- *Circulation*: Obtain intravenous access, attach electrocardiogram leads, and monitor for arrhythmias or cardiac arrest. Use of drugs/intravenous fluids to manage rhythm and blood pressure.
- *Airway*: Maintain airway patency—use of airways, advanced airway management if needed using a laryngeal masks airway/endotracheal tube.
- *Breathing*: Give supplemental oxygen; assess the adequacy of ventilation by noting the chest rise, oxygen saturation, and capnography (expired carbon dioxide measurement).
- *Differential diagnosis*: Find and treat the reversible causes of cardiac arrest, which is easily remembered in a mnemonic form as five Hs and five Ts.
- *Hs*: *H*ypovolemia, *h*ydrogen ion (acidosis), *h*yper/*h*ypokalemia, *h*ypoglycemia, *h*ypothermia.
- *Ts*: *T*oxins, *t*amponade, *t*ension pneumothorax, *t*hrombosis (coronary and pulmonary), *t*rauma.
- General supportive care of the patient and specific pharmacologic therapy aimed at underlying event causing cardiac arrest should be initiated once the patient is successfully resuscitated.

DOCUMENTATION OF THE EVENTS

All adverse events and the measures taken are to be documented, discussed with the patient, and a discharge summary of the event to be issued to the patient. The exact time of the event may not be relevant, but the flow of events and their management may be important. Such documentations are important from the medicolegal viewpoint too.

There are certain tips given for the avoidance of complications in **Box 7**.

SUMMARY

Complications in dermatosurgery office-based procedures, although rare, do occur, and the outcomes of such

BOX 7 Tips for the avoidance of complications.

- Thorough preoperative evaluation and optimal management of coexisting medical illness[24]
- Preprocedural counseling and premedication to allay anxiety. Explanation in detail of the procedure and post-procedural care
- Basic monitoring facilities: Pulse oximetry, noninvasive blood pressure, and electrocardiogram should be made available
- Avoidance of drugs that have previously caused reactions
- Involvement of anesthesiologist (standby anesthesiologists to provide monitored anesthesia care) as and when required, at the earliest, and discussion of various anesthetic options available in the conduct of safe procedure
- Establishment of clear post-procedural instructions

events are related to the initial diagnosis and early management. Thorough preprocedural evaluation and the identification of high-risk patients,[24] optimization of coexisting medical illness with medications, will go a long way in preventing adverse events during the procedure. Good communication and patient rapport are important. High-risk cases and technologically advanced procedures should be scheduled under monitored anesthesia care and in a hospital with full-fledged emergency backup facility. A well-planned and organized office setup under the leadership of a dermatologist proves to be beneficial to the patients and reduce the medicolegal complications too.

REFERENCES

1. Bing J, McAuliffe MS, Lupton JR. Regional anesthesia with monitored anesthesia care for dermatologic laser surgery. Dermatol Clin. 2002;20;123-34.
2. Amici JM, Rogues AM, Lasheras A, Gachie JP, Guillot P, Beylot C, et al. A prospective study of the incidence of complications associated with dermatological surgery. Br J Dermatol. 2005; 153:967-71.
3. Fader DJ, Johnson TM. Medical issues and emergencies in the dermatology office. J Am Acad Dermatol. 1997;36:1-16.
4. Chan BC, Patel DC. Perioperative management and associated rate of adverse events in dermatological procedures performed by dermatologists in New Zealand. Australas J Dermatol. 2009; 50:23-8.
5. Natalie LS. Dermatologic surgical complications. Medscape; 2009.
6. World Alliance for Patient Safety. Guideline 15. WHO Guidelines for Safe Surgery. Geneva: World Health Organization; 2008.
7. Fader D. Acute emergencies in the dermatology office. In: Gloster HM (Ed). Complications in Cutaneous Surgery. United Kingdom: Springer Science Publications; 2008.
8. Tang AW. A practical guide to anaphylaxis. Am Fam Physician. 2003;68:1325-33.
9. Lieberman P. Anaphylaxis and anaphylactoid reactions. In: Middleton E (Ed). Allergy: Principles and Practice, 5th edition. St. Louis: Mosby; 1998. pp. 1079-89.
10. The diagnosis and management of anaphylaxis. Joint Task Force on Practice Parameters, American Academy of Allergy, Asthma and Immunology, American College of Allergy, Asthma and Immunology, and the Joint Council of Allergy, Asthma and Immunology. J Allergy Clin Immunol. 1998;101:S465-528.
11. Parry SW, Kenny RA. The management of vasovagal syncope: a review. Q J Med. 1999;92:697-705.
12. Gmyrek R. Local and regional anesthesia. Medscape; 2011.
13. Araujo LM, Amaral JL. Allergy to lidocaine: case report. Rev Bras Anestesiol. 2004;54:672-6.
14. Larson CE. Methylparaben–an overlooked cause of local anesthetic hypersensitivity. Anesth Prog. 1977;24:72-4.
15. Venkataram M, Nischal KC. Guidelines for administration of local anesthesia for dermatosurgery and cosmetic dermatology procedures. Ind J Dermatol Venereol Leprol. 2009;75:68-75.
16. Licker M, Schweizer A, Ellenberger C, Tschopp JM, Diaper J, Clergue F. Perioperative medical management of patients with COPD. Int J Chron Obstruct Pulmon Dis. 2007;2:493-515.
17. Alcalay J, Alkalay R. Controversies in perioperative management of blood thinners in dermatologic surgery: continue or discontinue? Dermatol Surg. 2004;30:1091-4.
18. Rausher EG. Overview preoperative evaluation and management. Medscape; 2011.
19. Kovich O, Otley CC. Thrombotic complications related to discontinuation of warfarin and aspirin therapy perioperatively for cutaneous operations. J Am Acad Dermatol. 2003;48:233-7.
20. Gloster HM. Acute emergencies in dermatology office. Complications in Cutaneous Surgery. United Kingdom: Springer Publications; 2007. p. 15.
21. Bacter CR, Canizaro PC, Carrico CJ, Shires GT. Fluid resuscitation of hemorrhagic shock. Postgrad Med. 1970;48:95-9.
22. Krausz MM. Initial resuscitation of hemorrhagic shock. World J Emerg Surg. 2006;1:14.
23. Panchal AR, Bartos JA, Cabañas JG, Donnino MW, Drennan IR, Hirsch KG, et al. Adult Basic and Advanced Life Support Writing Group. Adult Basic and Advanced Life Support: 2020 American Heart Association Guidelines for Cardiopulmonary Resuscitation and Emergency Cardiovascular Care. Circulation. 2020;142(16_suppl_2):S366-468.
24. Leshin B, McCalmont TH. Preoperative evaluation of the surgical patient. Dermatol Clin. 1990;8:787-94.

CHAPTER 44

Anesthesia for Hair Transplantation

Indu S Sattur, Sandeep Sattur

Key Messages

- Hair transplant is a surgery of fairly prolonged duration performed in a conscious patient.
- Anesthesia that is effective for that duration makes the procedure comfortable for the patient.
- Thorough knowledge of anesthetic agents and surface anatomy of sensory nerves of the scalp is mandatory for achieving the same.
- Screening of patients for red flags (medical risk stratification) should be practiced diligently.
- The ability to resuscitate the patient in an emergency is necessary for a hair transplant surgeon.
- Equipment for monitoring the patient during the hair transplant procedure and for resuscitating a patient in an emergency should be present in the hair transplant procedure room.

INTRODUCTION

One of the important concerns for a patient considering hair transplantation (HT) is the level of pain during the procedure. A frequent question from people who are considering surgical hair restoration is—how much will it hurt? In other words, will the cosmetic benefit of hair restoration be worth the discomfort of surgery? Fear of discomfort can be a potent reason to avoid elective surgery. Moreover, hair restoration may need multiple sessions for optimal coverage. It is imperative to make the experience as pleasant as possible for the patient. The fact is that hair transplant is not entirely painless, but the pain is usually at an acceptable level for most patients. Experience says that the pain perceived during HT is inversely proportional to the motivation level of the patient **(Fig. 1)**. Proper selection and administration of anesthesia is one of the key components of a successful hair transplant surgery.

What separates the anesthesia for HT from anesthesia for other skin surgeries are three basic differences:

1. Extensive area to be anesthetized
2. Maintaining the anesthesia for a prolonged period of time (6–8 hours)
3. *Conscious patient*: A highly demanding patient who may have a fear of pain

Therefore, not only does the hair transplant surgeon have to minimize discomfort through proper technique but also have to minimize toxicity through judicious use of vasoconstrictors and nerve blocks and minimize total dosage. All of these require proper monitoring throughout the procedure.

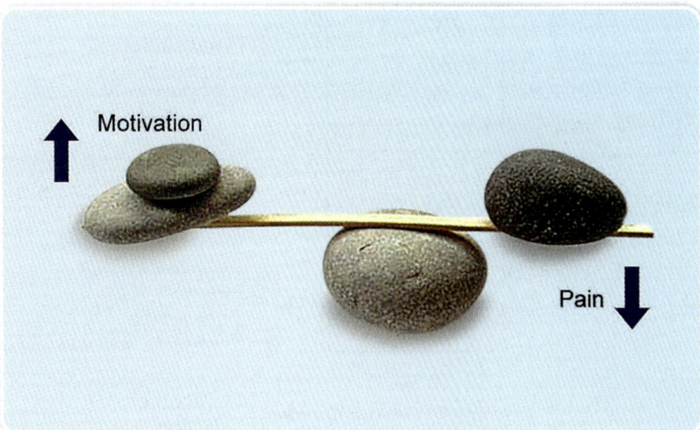

FIG. 1: Relation between motivation and pain threshold.

PHARMACOLOGY

Local anesthetics are chemicals that produce reversible loss of sensation in a portion of the body. The earliest local anesthetic drug discovered was cocaine, which was isolated in 1860 by Albert Niemann and introduced into practice by Karl Koller, a Viennese surgeon, who used it topically in ophthalmic surgery.[1]

Procaine was first synthesized in 1905 by the German chemist Alfred Einhorn who gave the chemical the trade name novocaine (from the Latin nov, meaning new, and caine, which means a common ending for alkaloids used as anesthetics). It became the first local anesthetic to gain wide acceptance.[2] However, its popularity declined after the introduction of lidocaine/lignocaine. It was the first amino amide-type local anesthetic, synthesized under the name "xylocaine" by Swedish chemist Nils Lofgren in 1943.[3] This was followed by prilocaine in 1959, bupivacaine in 1965, and ropivacaine in 1997. Most recently, purified active enantiomers, such as levobupivacaine, have also been introduced.

The pharmacological effects, including potency, onset of action, metabolism, duration of action, etc., are all linked to the chemical structure.

The local anesthetic drugs are weak bases having three basic components **(Flowchart 1)**:

1. Aromatic (lipophilic) "head"
2. Body (intermediate chain/linkage), which consists of an ester or amide bond
3. Hydrophilic "tail" (which contains a secondary or tertiary amine group)

The chemical composition decides various pharmacological benefits. The greater the lipid solubility, the greater the potency. Hence, bupivacaine is more potent than lignocaine and is, therefore, prepared as a 0.5% solution compared to 2% for lignocaine.[4] The fraction of drugs bound to protein in plasma correlates with the duration of local anesthetic activity: Bupivacaine > etidocaine > ropivacaine > mepivacaine > lidocaine > procaine and 2-chloroprocaine.

Local anesthetic drugs may be classified **(Flowchart 2)** on the basis of their central bond into *aminoamide/amides* [biotransformed in the liver (inactivated via P450)] and *aminoester/esters* (hydrolyzed by plasma esterase). The amides have a longer duration of action, are more potent, and have lower allergic potential. The two pharmacologic classes do not exhibit cross-sensitivity; hence, amide anesthetics can be administered to patients having ester anesthetic allergy.

MECHANISM OF ACTION

Local anesthetics are a group of drugs defined by their ability to prevent sodium entry into axons, thereby

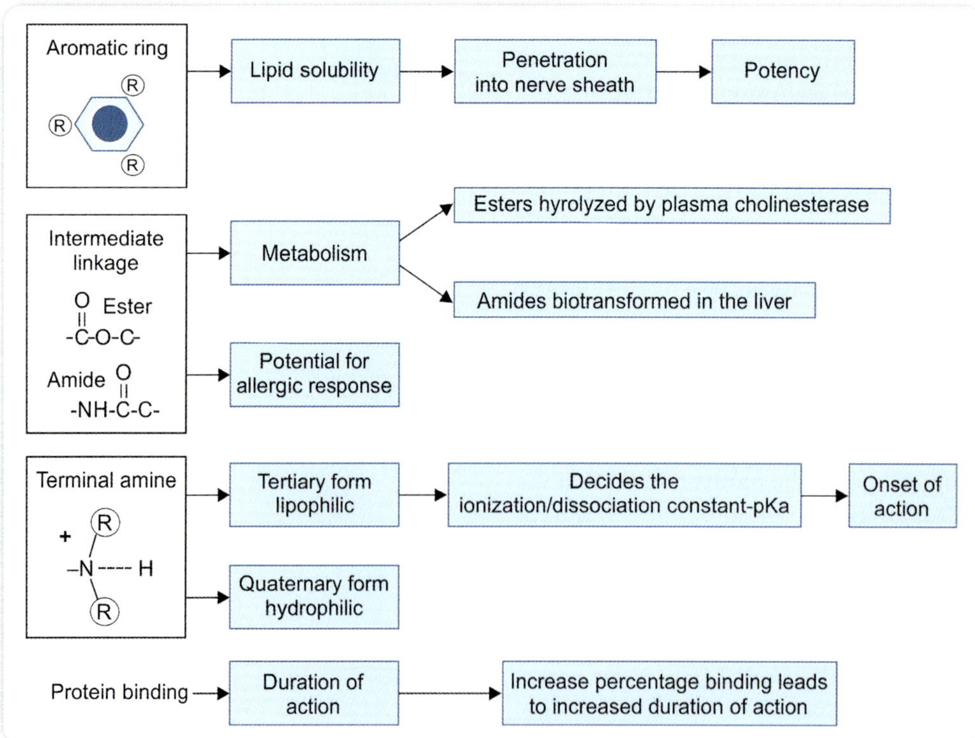

FLOWCHART 1: Impact of chemical structure on various pharmacological actions.

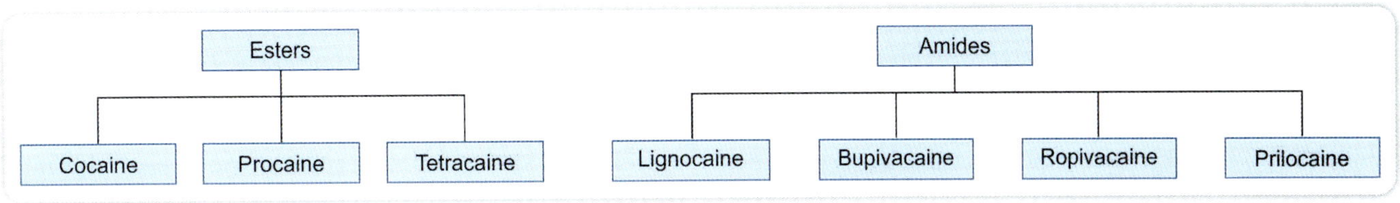

FLOWCHART 2: Classification of local anesthetics.

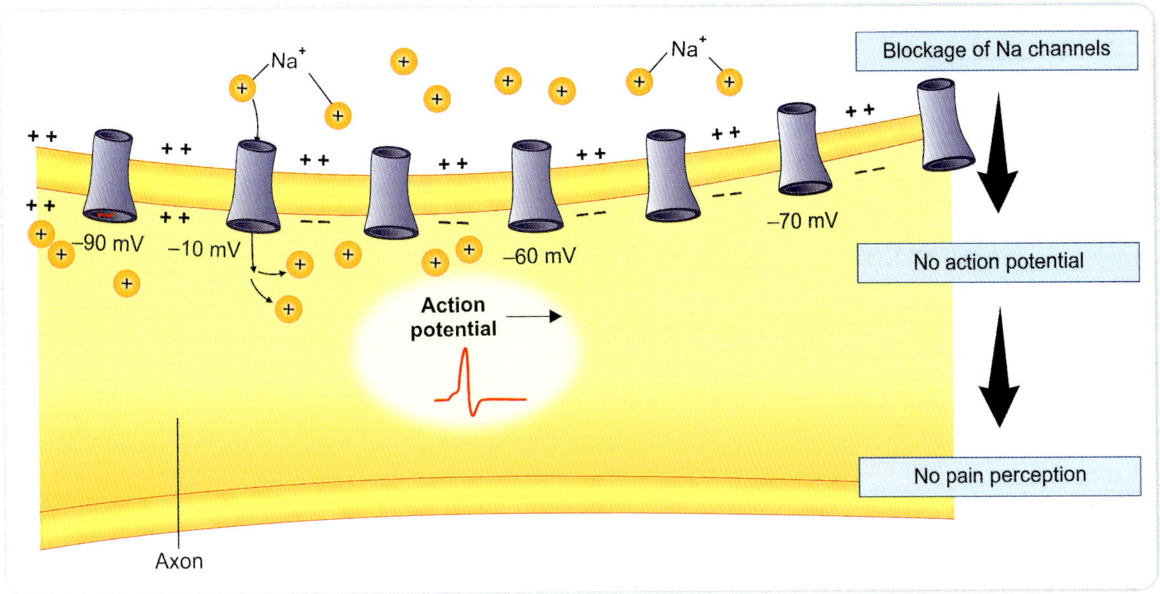

FIG. 2: Mechanism of action of local anesthetics.

preventing the generation of propagated action potentials in axons. Drugs classified as local anesthetics reversibly block action potential propagation in axons by preventing the entry of sodium that produces the potentials.[5]

All local anesthetics are membrane-stabilizing drugs **(Fig. 2)**:

- They temporarily block fast sodium channels in excitable tissues (which include nerve fibers, skeletal muscle, and cardiac muscle).
- They are also the cause of toxicity of local anesthetic drugs (which are toxic to the heart and brain, both structures being rich in fast sodium channels).
- All nerve fibers are sensitive to local anesthetics, but generally, those with a smaller diameter tend to be more sensitive than larger fibers.

Other actions of these drugs, however, such as anti-inflammatory actions by interaction with G-protein receptors, are also thought to be relevant to their use to prevent or treat pain.[6,7]

Local anesthetics used in HT are:

- Lignocaine with or without epinephrine
- Bupivacaine
- Ropivacaine
- Levobupivacaine
- Eutectic mixtures containing lignocaine
- Tetracaine or prilocaine

Lignocaine

Lignocaine is an intermediate-acting local anesthetic agent (amide type) indicated for the production of local or regional anesthesia and in the treatment of ventricular tachycardia.

Lignocaine or lidocaine is the most common local anesthetic used in HT surgery. It has a quick onset of action (within 1–5 minutes), which lasts for about 30–60 minutes when used alone and up to 2 hours when combined with epinephrine.

The maximum dose [total daily dose (TDD)] for local infiltration is 300 mg or 4.5 mg/kg of body weight. This can be increased to 500 mg or 7 mg/kg after adding epinephrine.

In the author's opinion, the actual volume/dose of lidocaine used is much less than the TDD if one can maintain the right concentration (between 0.5 and 1%)

and dosing interval. It is best to give top-ups before the onset of pain. Combining lidocaine with bupivacaine and, if required, the use of neuroprotective medications such as benzodiazepines help in keeping the dose optimum.

Additional administration of tumescence provides deeper, longer anesthesia and also helps to prolong the duration of anesthesia and minimize the total dose.

The commonly available commercial preparation is a plain 2% solution, which contains 21.3 mg of lignocaine hydrochloride with additives sodium chloride and preservative methylparaben. 1% solution contains 10.7 mg of lignocaine per milliliter. It also comes in combination with adrenaline/epinephrine, where, in addition to the lignocaine, it contains adrenaline in a concentration of 1:200,000. A preservative-free lignocaine preparation is also available, which can be used for intravenous (IV) administration in cardiac emergencies.

Bupivacaine

Bupivacaine is the most commonly used long-acting local anesthetic for HT surgery. As it has a lower dissociation constant (pKa), it has a more delayed onset of action (5–10 minutes) compared to lignocaine. But because of greater lipid solubility, it has more potency and longer duration of action, which ranges from 2 to 4 hours.

As it is more potent than lignocaine, it is available in two strengths—between 0.25 and 0.5%. The maximum daily dose is 175 mg. The use of bupivacaine is limited because of its potential cardiac toxicity. Bupivacaine produces a significantly greater depression of left ventricular (LV) pressure than ropivacaine, mepivacaine, or lidocaine. Though these effects are rare with safe dosages, nevertheless, there is potential for catastrophic events to occur.

Ropivacaine

The cardiotoxicity of bupivacaine stimulated interest in developing a less toxic, long-acting local anesthetic. The development of ropivacaine, the S-enantiomer of 1-propyl-2′,6′-pipecoloxylidide, is the result of that search. Ropivacaine is an amino-amide local anesthetic first registered for clinical use in 1996.[8]

The S-enantiomer, like most local anesthetics with a chiral center, was chosen because it has a lower toxicity than the R-enantiomer. This is presumably because of slower uptake, resulting in lower blood levels for a given dose. Ropivacaine undergoes extensive hepatic metabolism after IV administration, with only 1% of the drug eliminated unchanged in the urine. Ropivacaine is slightly less potent than bupivacaine in producing anesthesia when used in lower concentrations. However, in concentrations of 0.5% and higher, it produces dense blockade with a slightly shorter duration than that of bupivacaine. In concentrations of 0.75%, the onset of blockade is almost as fast as that of 1.5% mepivacaine or 3% 2-chloroprocaine, with reduced central nervous system (CNS) toxicity and cardiotoxic potential and a lower propensity for motor blockade than bupivacaine. For these reasons, ropivacaine has become one of the most commonly used long-acting local anesthetics in peripheral nerve blockade. Various clinical trials have evaluated the safety profile of ropivacaine and found it to be safe.[9,10]

Levobupivacaine

In recent years, levobupivacaine, the pure S (–) enantiomer of bupivacaine, emerged as a safer alternative for regional anesthesia than its racemic parent. In pharmacodynamic studies, levobupivacaine has demonstrated less affinity and depressant effects on myocardial and central nervous vital centers and a superior pharmacokinetic profile.[11] Clinically, levobupivacaine is well tolerated in a variety of regional anesthesia techniques. It is extensively metabolized with no unchanged drug detected in the urine or feces. Reports of toxicity with levobupivacaine are scarce; occasional toxic symptoms are usually reversible with minimal treatment with no fatal outcome.[11] Surgical sensory block of similar characteristics and recovery over equal dose ranges of levobupivacaine and bupivacaine has been confirmed in surgical patients.[12] The properties of levobupivacaine in peripheral nerve blockade are less well studied than those of ropivacaine; however, research results suggest that they seem to parallel those of bupivacaine. Therefore, levobupivacaine could be a more suitable and less toxic alternative to bupivacaine.[12]

ARTICAINE

Articaine is a moderately potent, short-acting amide local anesthetic with a rapid metabolism, more popular in the dental field. It has also been used for a variety of purposes such as spinal, epidural, ocular, regional, and local anesthesia. Due to its low lipid solubility, high degree of plasma binding, rapid metabolism, and quick elimination, it is a potent anesthetic with low systemic toxicity in most clinical situations. It spreads well in most tissues. However, it should not be used in patients who are known to be allergic to sulfites as sodium metabisulfite is used in articaine + epinephrine solutions as a preservative.

Toxic reactions are usually due to an inadvertent intravascular injection or use of excessive dose. To avoid overdoses, the maximum recommended dose (MRD) must not be exceeded, and aspiration test should always be performed prior to all local anesthetic injections.[13-15]

DELIVERING ANESTHESIA PREOPERATIVE PREPARATION/ SEDATION (FLOWCHART 3)

Having a relaxed and calm patient on the morning of the surgery is a step in achieving a smooth procedure.[16] In the author's experience, this is best and safely achieved by a light anxiolytic given the night before the surgery and a reassuring attitude by the surgeon and his team before and during the surgery.

Preoperative use of anxiolytics goes a long way in normalizing blood pressure (white coat hypertension). Alprazolam 0.5 mg given the previous day serves the purpose adequately.

Many hair transplant surgeons use systemic agents to sedate the patient before the procedure to reduce the pain of local anesthetic injections. Agents commonly used are benzodiazepines (diazepam, midazolam, etc.), propofol, fentanyl, opioids, ketamine, etc.[17] *All these agents should ideally be used only by or in the presence of a qualified anesthetist.*

An important point to remember is that if one is using IV sedation, then the procedure room should be equipped with monitoring equipment such as pulse oximeter and blood pressure monitor and resuscitation equipment such as laryngoscope, endotracheal tubes, oxygen cylinders, and defibrillator. An anesthetist should be available for supervision. It is also important to keep the patient nil by mouth preoperatively if IV sedation is used.

Techniques to Reduce Pain of Injection

Most of the pain associated with a hair transplant is during injection of the local anesthetic. It is also the time when there is an increased incidence of vasovagal episodes due to the pain of the injections in susceptible patients.

The pain of the injection is primarily due to increase in tissue pressure due to the increased volume of the anesthetic injected. The pain is directly proportional to the speed of injection. Rapid injection causes more pain. Contributory factors are the temperature and pH difference between the injected fluids and the local tissues. Also, the depth of injection has a bearing on the amount of pain. Pain is much less when injected into the subcutaneous tissue compared to superficial injection into the dermis.

There are many techniques to reduce the perception of this pain. They could be used singly or in combination.

Reassurance: Constant dialogue with the patient and verbally keeping him/her engaged in conversation and alleviating his/her concerns go a long way in reducing pain. A pleasant ambiance and music help minimize the apprehension.

Concomitant physical stimulation: This is based on the gate control theory of Ronald Melzack and Patrick David Wall, which states that nonpainful input closes the "gates" to painful input, thus preventing pain sensation from traveling to the CNS.[18] Stimulation of the skin using a vibrating device in the same dermatome results in reduced perception of painful stimuli.

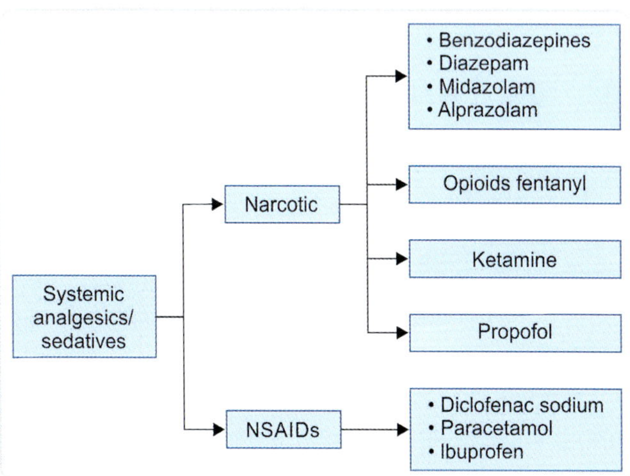

FLOWCHART 3: Systemic analgesics/sedatives.
(NSAIDs: nonsteroidal anti-inflammatory drugs)

Topical Anesthesia

Eutectic mixtures help in reducing the initial pricking pain felt on piercing the skin with a needle. These mixtures need to be applied at least an hour before the injection of anesthetic. Common mixtures used contain lignocaine with tetracaine or prilocaine.

These agents cause dermal anesthesia by migration of lidocaine and prilocaine/tetracaine into the epidermal and dermal layers of the skin, which they accumulate in the vicinity of dermal pain receptors and nerve endings. Topical anesthesia helps to blunt the initial sharp pain caused by the needle prick. It is helpful for apprehensive patients.

Carbonation and pH Adjustments

There have been different schools of thought with regards to altering the temperature and pH of the anesthetic solutions. The general practice is to use the local anesthetic solutions at room temperature. The expected benefit of doing so was to reduce the pain of injection. Many studies have concluded that warming and buffering of the local anesthetic injections prior to injecting has been shown to reduce the pain of injection.[19-21] There are some studies that have felt otherwise, i.e., there is no difference in the pain of injection with the warming of the solution.[22] There is also a view that adding sodium bicarbonate solution to raise the pH may enhance postoperative edema if administered in the frontal area.

In order to overcome the pain, attempts have been made to devise devices. A small disposable device has been launched, which numbs the injection site by simultaneously cooling the surrounding skin. It is a disposable syringe-attachable dispenser that delivers a precise stream of numbing vapocoolant to the skin just ahead of the tip of the needle just before the skin is pierced and does not leave patients with postinjection numbness.

There is very little data on this with regards to use in HT and safety and efficacy ratings.

Role of Adrenaline/Epinephrine

Adrenaline is a vasoconstrictive agent, which is added to the local anesthetic solution. Addition of adrenaline to the local anesthetic helps to prolong the duration of anesthesia, reduce the peak serum level of the local anesthetic, increase the intensity of the anesthetic blockade, and, by virtue of local vasoconstriction, help in reducing surgical bleeding.

Addition of adrenaline is routinely used in all areas of local anesthesia except where there are end arteries, such as in the fingers and toes. The usual concentration of adrenaline used in anesthetic solutions ranges from 1:200,000 to 1:400,000. More concentrated solutions are not used commonly. It is important to deliver adrenaline to the right areas, specifically the subcutaneous layer (where the larger blood vessels are present), to get optimum benefit.

In hair transplant surgery, it is used in nerve block for local infiltration, and it is a part of tumescent solution.

One must remember that using adrenaline has its advantages as well as disadvantages. It is essential for hair transplant surgery, but if not used judiciously, it can increase the risk of localized vascular compromise or the risk of systemic side effects, particularly in those with a history of cardiac problems. This needs to be kept in mind, as the amount of local anesthetic administered may be fairly large. This is also particularly important in body HT where larger areas are under anesthesia.

BLOCKS FOR HAIR TRANSPLANT PROCEDURE

A nerve block involves the infiltration of a small volume of anesthetic around a nerve trunk. The rationale of a nerve block is that it substitutes a single injection for a large number of injections and anesthetizes a large area with a small amount of anesthetic.

Blocking the nerves allows infiltration in the target area to be painless; the dose of anesthetic required in infiltration later is much less and helps in prolonging the duration of anesthesia.

The common blocks used in HT are:
- Greater occipital nerve block
- Supraorbital and supratrochlear block
- Zygomaticofrontal block
- Auriculotemporal block

With these blocks, most of the scalp can be anesthetized. The cutaneous nerve supply of the scalp is derived from all three diversions of the trigeminal (V) nerve and from the second and third cervical nerves:
- *From the ophthalmic nerve*: The supratrochlear and supraorbital nerves
- *From the maxillary nerve*: The zygomaticotemporal nerve
- *From the mandibular nerve*: The auriculotemporal nerve
- The lesser occipital nerve (C2)
- The greater occipital nerve (C2, 3)
- The third occipital nerve (C3)

A proper knowledge of surface anatomy is essential for delivering these blocks. **Figures 3 to 6** demonstrate the anatomical landmarks for these blocks.

Occipital Nerve Block

Points of Injection

- 2–3 cm lateral to the inion (external occipital protuberance)
- Placing three fingers at the level of the superior nuchal line with the middle finger on the external occipital protuberance

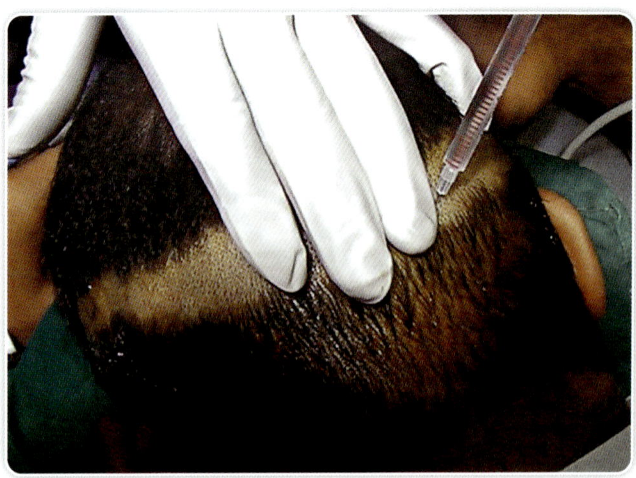

FIG. 3: Occipital nerve block.

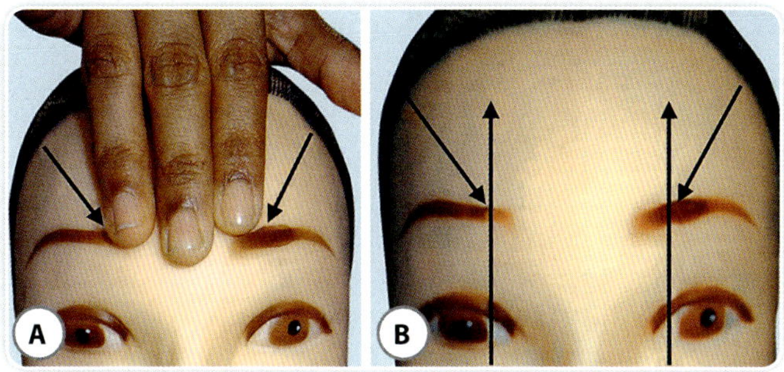

FIGS. 4A AND B: Supraorbital block.

Surface Marking of the Supraorbital Nerve

- Palpation of the supraorbital notch
- Three fingers centered vertically over glabella, major branches of supraorbital emerge just lateral to the fingers
- Medial limbus/iris line

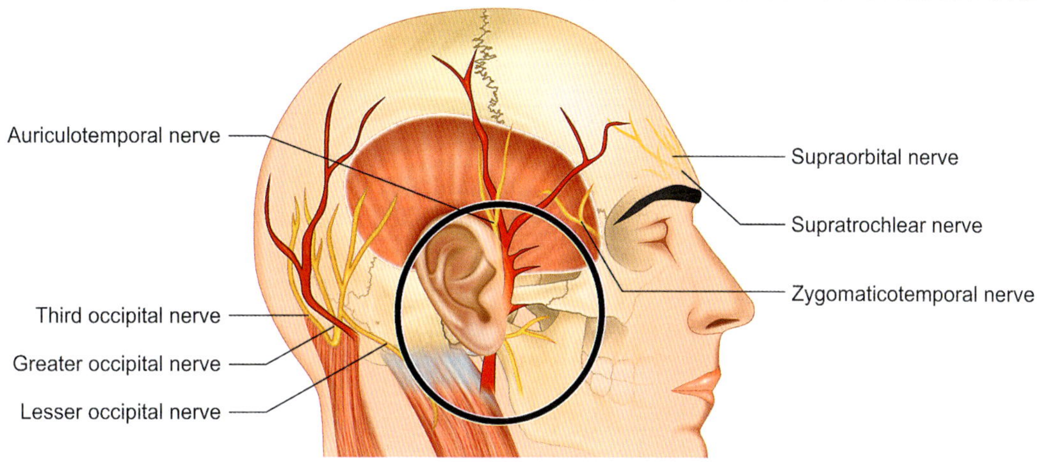

FIG. 5: Auriculotemporal block.

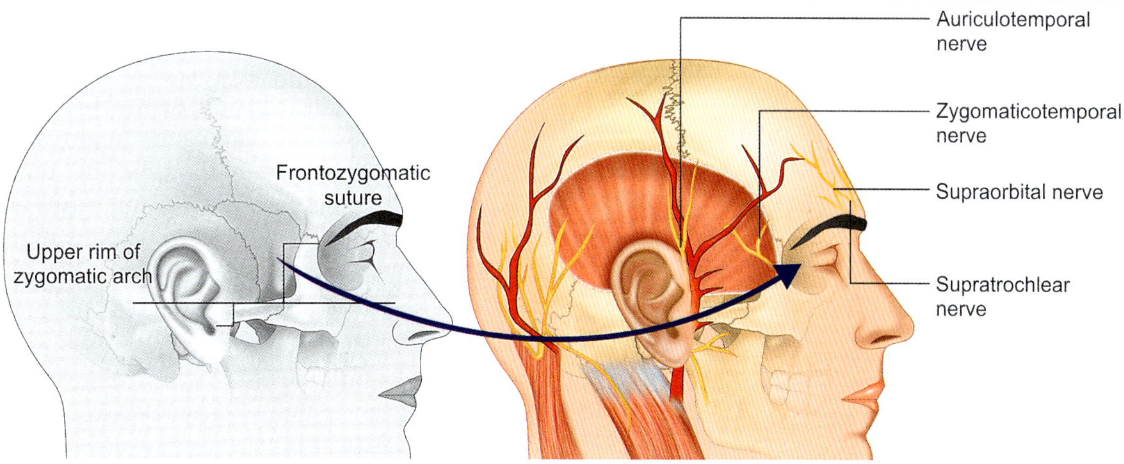

FIG. 6: Zygomaticotemporal block.

Auriculotemporal Nerve

- Auriculotemporal nerve originates from the posterior trunk of the mandibular nerve.
- It passes in front of the tragus in close proximity to the superficial temporal artery.
- It supplies part of the auricle, temporal, and temporoparietal scalp.

Surface Landmarks of Zygomaticotemporal Nerve

1.5 cm lateral to the outer canthus on the zygomatic arch.

GREATER OCCIPITAL NERVE BLOCK AND DONOR AREA ANESTHESIA

Posterior scalp is supplied by the cervical nerves and the anterior part by the branches of the trigeminal nerve. Greater occipital nerve is formed by the medial branches of the dorsal rami of cervical nerves C2. The nerve courses backward between the first and the second cervical vertebrae. After traveling through the semispinalis muscle, the nerve runs on the lateral aspect of external occipital protuberance [2–3 cm lateral to the inion (external occipital protuberance)], with the occipital artery, which usually lies just medial to this nerve.

With the patient in the prone or lateral position, the donor area is cleansed using an antiseptic solution. Placing three fingers at the level of the superior nuchal line with the middle finger on the external occipital protuberance, the point of injection is just lateral to the lateral finger on either side. About 1 cc of anesthetic solution (lignocaine 1% with adrenaline or bupivacaine 0.25%) with concurrent vibration stimuli proximal to the aesthetic area. A needle is then inserted dermally through the previously anesthetized wheal, and the anesthetic is injected slightly to the right and then left until a solid line of the anesthetic is created. Finally, the whole donor area is infiltrated at the superficial dermal level with a mixture of 0.5% lignocaine adrenaline and chilled saline, which raises the base of the follicles away from the neurovascular plane. After donor strip closure, 5 cc or 0.25% bupivacaine is injected into the suture line for prolonged aesthetic effect.

The same is also injected before the patient goes home for postoperative pain relief—the greater occipital protuberance is palpated. Placing three fingers at the level of the superior nuchal line with the middle finger on the external occipital protuberance, the point of injection is just lateral to the lateral finger on either side. It is injected on both sides, making sure that the needle is not placed intravascularly.

Supraorbital and Supratrochlear Blocks

With the patient supine, the supraorbital notch is palpated. After careful preparation of the skin, a 27-G needle is inserted just lateral to the supraorbital notch; with the needle directed medially and downward, 1 mL of anesthetic solution (lignocaine 1% with adrenaline or bupivacaine 0.25%) is injected after careful aspiration to prevent intravascular placement. To block the supratrochlear nerve, the needle is withdrawn to the skin level and directed medially toward the tip of the nose; 1 mL of anesthetic solution (lignocaine 1% with adrenaline or bupivacaine 0.25%) is injected. The block can be achieved by an inferior approach. Here, the direction after palpating the supraorbital notch is upward and lateral.

Zygomaticotemporal Block

The zygomaticotemporal nerve emerges from a small foramen in the frontal process of the zygomatic arch near the lateral orbital margin, and it innervates the temple and the hairline just superior to that. It can be located 1.5 cm lateral to the outer canthus on the zygomatic arch.

Palpate the orbital rim and the zygomatic arch. About 1–1.5 cm lateral to the lateral canthus with the needle directed medially on the zygomatic arch, about 1 cc of anesthetic solution (lignocaine 1% with adrenaline or bupivacaine 0.25%) can be injected.

Auriculotemporal Block

The auriculotemporal nerve originates from the posterior trunk of the mandibular nerve. It passes in front of the tragus in close proximity to the superficial temporal artery and supplies part of the auricle, part of the temple, and the temporoparietal scalp.

The auriculotemporal block can be achieved by passing the needle deep into the dermis, just in front of the tragus. It is important to palpate the superficial temporal artery and make sure with aspiration that the needle is not intravascular. Because in some individuals, branches of facial nerve may be close by, possibility of temporary facial nerve palsy should be kept in mind.

Advantages of the Blocks

A smaller quantity of local anesthesia is needed to anesthetize a larger area of scalp. Using blocks definitely helps to reduce the multiple needle pain of infiltration.

Disadvantages of the Blocks

Blocks are unpredictable, especially the auriculotemporal and zygomaticotemporal blocks. Experience is needed to execute these correctly. Also, normal variation in the branching of these nerves may lead to incomplete anesthesia. The blocks have to be generally combined with conventional regional infiltration. Apprehension on the part of the patient may be more as the injections for the blocks are given a little away from the area of actual surgery, particularly for supraorbital and supratrochlear blocks. Blocks also take a longer time to act than infiltration.

Infiltration anesthesia: After the nerve blocks, local infiltration is used to complete the anesthesia. In the donor area, apart from the greater occipital nerve block, it is very important to use tumescence, which has diluted concentration of lignocaine (0.5%) with adrenaline. This anesthesia is delivered in the dermis and subdermal regions. Not only it helps to create a clean field, but it also increases the distance between the follicular bulbs and the vascular zone.

Similarly, the recipient area is infiltrated using dilute lignocaine and bupivacaine with or without adrenaline, just anterior to the proposed hairline. One disadvantage of using excessive adrenaline is postoperative telogen effluvium and vascular compromise; hence, the physician should be mindful of the total dosage being administered.

TUMESCENT ANESTHESIA

Hair transplant surgery is unique in that it requires a large area of the scalp to be anesthetized and maintain the anesthesia for a prolonged period of time. This has to be achieved without causing systemic toxicity. The principle of tumescent anesthesia comes in useful to achieve this objective.

Tumescent anesthesia finds its origins in liposuction and involves the use of large volumes of dilute lignocaine and epinephrine.[23] This technique helped to achieve prolonged anesthesia and profound hemostasis. Tumescent anesthesia can have added benefits beyond the ones mentioned earlier.

Therefore, injecting tumescence fluid (solution containing normal saline with very dilute anesthetic and epinephrine concentration) into the subcutaneous layer of the scalp serves to:

- Increase the distance from the follicles (residing in the upper fat) to the nerves and larger blood vessels (lying deeper just above the fascia)—helps to effectively increase the distance between the vascular plane and the plane of dissection, thereby reducing the chances of injury to these structures[24]
- Increase the rigidity of the donor area (which helps to decrease follicular transection during the harvest)
- Decrease bleeding by mechanical pressure of the injected fluid (hence, injection of substantial volume is necessary) as well as vasoconstriction of small vessels
- Produce more uniform anesthesia
- Reduce the total amount of anesthetic required

Since larger nerve fibers are blocked, it also prolongs the duration of anesthesia.

The disadvantages of tumescent anesthesia are:

- Larger amount of adrenaline is used, which may cause tachycardia and related problems in patients with cardiac insufficiency.
- Adrenaline may cause ischemia and postpartum telogen effluvium.
- The large amount of fluid may lead to postoperative edema.

Patient Evaluation before Hair Transplant Surgery

Therefore, we owe it to our patients and ourselves to be prepared for these unlikely events (Carlos Puig).

Hair restoration surgery is one of the safest cosmetic procedures with very low risk of complications. There is no registry that tracks hair restoration surgery complication data; most surgeons describe their complication rates as being <1%. There is an even lower incidence of life-threatening emergencies during hair restoration surgery. But if such a catastrophic incidence occurs in one's clinic/office, it can be disastrous.

Hair transplant is a superficial cutaneous procedure but a surgery nevertheless. HT surgery differs from other outpatient cutaneous surgeries, mainly in the following ways:

- Duration (an average duration of 5–6 hours)
- Body surface area involved
- Amount of local anesthetic administered
- Conscious patient
- The surgery is often performed by physicians who may not have had surgical postgraduation.
- It is also performed as an outpatient surgery, usually in the clinic/office setting.
- There is a recent disconcerting trend wherein large parts of the surgery are performed by technicians without medical supervision by a physician.

There are many medical conditions that might make the procedure problematic, and these need to be checked for before the surgery. Whenever significant medical conditions are present, it is always prudent to obtain medical clearance from the patient's primary care physician or appropriate specialist.

Red Flags (Risk Stratification)

The comorbidities that may impact the procedure are hypertension, diabetes mellitus, coronary artery disease, patient on aspirin, clopidogrel or other anticoagulants, epilepsy, etc.

Prehypertensive Patients

Patients who are known hypertensives need to be well controlled before surgery. An assessment by a treating physician is indicated. If diastolic pressure remains above 100, it is better to reschedule the surgery. The patient should be told specifically not to omit the dose on the morning of the surgery.

Coronary Artery Disease

It is a good practice to perform an electrocardiogram (ECG) in all patients posted for HT surgery, even in young patients. However, a resting ECG does not rule out cardiac problems. One needs to look at potential risk factors such as hypertension, family history, and diabetes.

Patients with active disease are not candidates for HT. Stable cardiac patients can be taken up after consulting the treating cardiologist. ECG monitoring during the surgery may be helpful in such patients. ECG + two-dimensional echocardiogram (ECHO) is to be obtained in relevant cases, especially in those showing preoperative ECG changes [coronary heart disease (CHD) affects Indians with greater frequency and at a younger age than counterparts in developed countries]. If the patient complains of chest pain, nausea, weakness, or breathlessness, it is better to think about transferring the patient for further treatment to a cardiac center.

Patients on Anticoagulants

A bleeding diathesis, significant enough to impact the surgery, can generally be picked up in the patient's history; however, medications may not be always revealed and should be asked for specifically through a checklist. Patients often do not report taking aspirin and this must be asked about, as well as other nonsteroidal anti-inflammatory drugs (NSAIDs). Clopidogrel, in particular, can significantly increase bleeding during the procedure and alcohol, of course, can also increase bleeding. A proper assessment of the coagulation profile in patients who have not undergone any surgical treatment before is a good option.

Anxious Patients

White coat hypertension is a common phenomenon on the morning of surgery. There are increased chances of bleeding intraoperatively if not controlled. Use of anxiolytics will help.

Diabetes

Preoperative assessment of blood sugar, along with glycated hemoglobin, is necessary in diabetics. Hypoglycemia is seen sometimes in diabetic patients during surgery. It is a good practice to do a preoperative glucose check before beginning the surgery. Maintain the patient's glycemic levels during surgery by giving regular carbohydrate feeds.

Smokers

It is a good policy for smokers to be instructed to stop smoking 2 weeks before and for 2 weeks post- transplant. Wound healing can get significantly affected in smokers.

Screening for human immunodeficiency virus (HIV), Australia antigen, and hepatitis C virus (HCV) is important to identify a patient's immune status and liver function and to take adequate precautions for the operating personnel.

DRUG INTERACTIONS AND COEXISTING MEDICAL CONDITIONS

Prior to the hair transplant surgery, it is important for the surgeon to take a complete medical history and follow up any questions with the patient or by a consultation with the patient's physician.

Though local anesthetics are remarkably safe at therapeutic doses, the surgeon operating on patients with medical comorbidities must address two basic concerns pertinent to the use of local anesthetic agents: Existing systemic diseases that may be exacerbated by the anesthetic agent and medications that may have adverse interactions with local anesthetic agents.

Hypertension

Use of epinephrine/adrenaline in patients who are known hypertensive or suffer from ischemic heart disease is decided in consultation with the treating physician. As epinephrine/adrenaline is produced in the body, there is no real contraindication to using it.[25] If the patient's blood pressure is well controlled and the physician has approved, it is safe to proceed with the hair transplant.

Knowledge of potential adverse interactions between the vasoconstrictors in anesthetic agents and antihypertensive agents is important. The significant interaction between nonselective beta-blockers, such as propranolol, has to be kept in mind. The adrenaline in the anesthetic agent causes an unopposed alpha-receptor-mediated vasoconstriction, which can theoretically produce a hypertensive emergency and a profound vagally mediated reflexive bradycardia.[25,26] Other antihypertensive medications, such as the central sympatholytic drugs, for example clonidine and methyldopa, and the peripheral adrenergic antagonists such as reserpine, as well as the direct vasodilators, may potentiate adrenergic receptor sensitivity to sympathomimetics, resulting in a magnified systemic response to vasoconstrictor-containing anesthetics.[27]

The maximum total dose of adrenaline in a cardiac patient should not exceed 0.04 mg or 40 μg.[25]

Asthma

Well-controlled asthma should not pose a problem. However, caution has been recommended based on Food and Drug Administration warnings that drugs containing sulfites can be a cause of allergic reactions in susceptible individuals.[28] This preservative is used in some preparations of lignocaine with adrenaline. Studies suggest that sodium metabisulfite, which is used as an antioxidant agent in dental local anesthetic solutions containing vasoconstrictors to prevent the breakdown of the vasoconstrictor, may induce allergic, or extrinsic, asthma attacks.[28,29] Also, patients with controlled asthma who have not been exposed to local anesthetic, as well as patients with a history of multiple drug hypersensitivity reaction (DHR), should undergo a local anesthetic sensitivity test.[29,30]

Antipsychotic Drugs

There are no contraindications for the use of any local anesthetics, with or without vasoconstrictors, in patients taking lithium, monoamine oxidase inhibitors, fluoxetine, etc. For bipolar patients taking a phenothiazine type of drug such as chlorpromazine or risperidone, fluctuations in blood pressure are common. In fact, in Japan, adrenaline is contraindicated for use in patients receiving antipsychotic therapy because the combination of adrenaline and an antipsychotic is considered to cause severe hypotension.[31]

MONITORING DURING HAIR TRANSPLANT SURGERY

It is important to have IV access in all patients before starting the surgery. Emergency drugs needed for vasovagal syncope and allergic reactions should be kept handy.

Potential medical emergencies seen during HT are:

- Vasovagal syncope
- Allergies
- Hypertension
- Hypotension
- Hypoglycemia
- Myocardial infarction

TABLE 1: Adverse reactions to local anesthesia.

Type of reaction	Details
Localized or systemic	Allergic
Systemic	Cardiac/vascular
	Central nervous system (CNS)
Localized	Tissue toxicity

Vasovagal reactions are the most common emergency event to occur during HT. It is a reflex stimulation of the autonomous nervous system, leading to bradycardia and hypotension. The patient commonly complains of feeling faint, weak, or nauseated. This may happen at the beginning of the surgery when anesthesia is being administered or at the end of surgery when the patient gets up from a prolonged supine posture. The patient may have sweating and is pale with feeble slow pulse. If this is not picked up earlier, there may be full syncope, with or without tonic-clonic muscle contractions. These events are usually triggered by pain, sight of blood, fear, anxiety, etc. It is treated by putting the patient in a head-low position and IV atropine. Sometimes, severe cases may need IV fluids to correct the hypotension **(Table 1)**.

Allergic Responses to Local Anesthesia

True allergic reactions to local anesthetics are very rare adverse reactions when compared to myorelaxant or latex allergies. At the most, they represent <1% of all adverse local anesthetic reactions. They have mainly been described with ester-type local anesthetics. However, allergic reactions to local anesthetics have been documented even with amide-type local anesthetics. Contact dermatitis (type IV reaction) is the most often reported allergic reaction to several amide-type local anesthetics. Adverse local anesthetic-induced reactions by immunoglobulin E (IgE)-mediated allergic mechanisms (type I reaction: Anaphylactic shock or urticaria) are still debated.[32] Current available data on adverse reactions to local anesthetics has reiterated the overall safety of these agents in clinical practice. Adverse reactions to local anesthetics are more often than not secondary to other causes rather than true IgE-mediated allergy.

Role of Skin Testing

The investigation of patients with suspected allergy to local anesthetics should begin with a detailed history of previous surgery under local anesthesia, which should then help to determine whether skin testing and challenge are warranted. There are proponents of skin testing who suggest incremental challenge in patients with a history of previous allergy to local anesthetic.[33] A review by Bhole et al.[24] surmised that incremental challenge in patients with negative skin tests invariably demonstrates that the patient is tolerant of the relevant local anesthetics (incremental challenge means that the exposure to the drug is very gradual, beginning with a scratch test to a full-blown subcutaneous injection). So, they proposed that a single subcutaneous injection of the particular local anesthetics after negative skin tests is likely to be an adequate substitute for incremental challenge in this group of patients. For those patients with positive skin tests (skin prick, intradermal, or both), they suggested that skin testing and challenge with an unrelated local anesthetic be used to predict future safety.[34]

Allergic reactions are characterized by cutaneous lesions, urticaria, edema, or anaphylactoid reactions. They may occur as a result of sensitivity either to the preservative in the multiple-dose vials or to local anesthetic agents. True allergic reactions as a result of sensitivity to lidocaine are extremely rare and, if they occur, should be managed by conventional means.

Systemic Toxicity (Fig. 7)

Compared to other local anesthetics, bupivacaine is *cardiotoxic*. Adverse drug reactions (ADRs) are *rare* when it is administered correctly. Most ADRs relate to administration technique (resulting in systemic exposure) or pharmacological effects of anesthesia.

Systemic absorption of local anesthetics is determined by:

- *Site of injection*: IV > tracheal > intercostal > caudal > paracervical > epidural > brachial > sciatic > subcutaneous

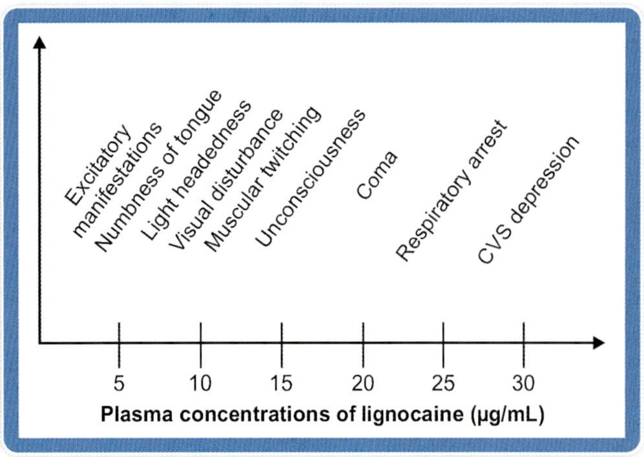

FIG. 7: Systemic toxicity linked to serum levels.

- *Dose*: Peak blood concentrations of local anesthetics correspond proportionally to the total dose administered.
- *Addition of vasoconstrictor*: Epinephrine, in concentrations of 5 μg/mL, is commonly used to decrease the absorption of local anesthetics. A 5 μg/mL (1:200,000) dose of epinephrine will significantly reduce the peak blood levels of lidocaine regardless of the site of administration.
- *Pharmacologic profiles of the local anesthetic*: In general, local anesthetics that are highly tissue-bound are absorbed at a slower rate. In addition, absorption is dependent on the individual local anesthetics' intrinsic ability to cause vasodilatation.

Toxic side effects of local anesthetic drugs occur due to elevated blood levels of the anesthetic agents. This is usually due to:

- Accidental rapid IV injection
- Rapid absorption, such as from a very vascular site
- Absolute overdose if the dose used is excessive (which may happen if track is not kept of the amount of local anesthetic used and the time in which it was used)

Managing systemic toxicity is possible if one is aware of the signs and symptoms of the same. The earlier manifestations are due to CNS excitation, with problems such as abnormal involuntary movements, confusion, and seizures. Subsequent manifestations include CNS depression with a cessation of convulsions and the onset of unconsciousness, respiratory depression, or arrest. This biphasic effect occurs because local anesthetics first block inhibitory CNS pathways (resulting in stimulation) and then eventually block both inhibitory and excitatory pathways (resulting in overall CNS inhibition). *If the patient suddenly becomes very talkative or excited, it is possibly an early sign of systemic toxicity to lignocaine.*

Higher serum concentrations of local anesthetics cause cardiovascular effects. Local anesthetics block sodium channels through a fast-in, slow-out mechanism that affects impulse conduction through the heart and nerve tissue. In the heart, this mechanism depresses V_{max} (i.e., the rate of depolarization during phase 0 of the cardiac action potential) and may lead to reentrant arrhythmias. Additionally, conduction through the sinus and atrioventricular nodes is suppressed. Acceleration of the ventricular rate has been reported in patients with atrial arrhythmias. Lidocaine may also elevate fibrillation thresholds.

Note: Often, while giving multiple injections, the surgeon may not aspirate prior to injection, leading to intravascular injection and resultant toxicity. Therefore, care has to be exercised at all stages.

Managing Complications

Remember:

- A—airway
- B—breathing
- C—circulation

Airway is the first thing to be tackled in patients with an altered level of consciousness. Open and clean the airway with suction. A simple way to open an airway is the jaw thrust. After clearing and maintaining the airway, confirm that the patient is breathing by auscultation and check the oxygen saturation with the pulse oximeter. After confirming that the patient is breathing, check the blood pressure, and if it is low, start infusion of fluids.

Although it is rare, serious emergencies can occur during a hair transplant surgery. Hence, it is very important for a hair transplant surgeon to have some training in life support, the necessary resuscitation equipment including a defibrillator, all the emergency drugs, and a plan to transfer the patient to another facility for further treatment. In the event the transplant surgeon or his staffs are not well versed with life support skills, then having a standby anesthetist is an option.

SUMMARY

The proper selection and administration of anesthesia form one of the most important tenets of successful hair transplant surgery. Ensuring patient comfort, both physically and psychologically, helps to improve the experience and facilitates a smooth surgery. Knowing the action, duration, dosage of various agents, and potential toxicity of the anesthetic agents helps to execute a safe and comfortable hair transplant procedure.

Tips and Pearls

- Administer preoperative anxiolytics such as lorazepam the night before.
- Enjoy pleasant ambience and music.
- Use concomitant stimulation of the adjacent skin with a vibrator during injection.
- Use the smallest needle possible and inject very small volumes very slowly, at each prick. Give as few pricks as possible— use a longer needle.
- Use tumescent anesthesia.
- Use blocks.
- Administer booster shot (of long-acting anesthetics such as bupivacaine/levobupivacaine/ropivacaine) at the end of surgery.
- Continuous monitoring is vital.
- Either be trained in advanced life support or have a qualified anesthetist standby for the surgery. Emergency trolley should be ready.

REFERENCES

1. Niemann A. Über eine neue organische base in den cocablättern. Arch Pharm. 1860;153:129-55.
2. Einhorn A. On the chemistry of local anesthetics. MMW Munch Med Wochenschr. 1899;46:1218-20.
3. Löfgren N, Lundqvist B. Studies on local anesthetics II. Svensk Kemisk Tidskrift. 1946;58:206-17.
4. Becker DE, Reed KL. Essentials of local anesthetic pharmacology. Anesth Prog. 2006;53(3):98-109.
5. Hille B. Ionic Channels of Excitable Membranes, 3rd edition. Sunderland, Massachusetts: Sinauer Associates Inc.; 2001.
6. Hollmann MW, Herroeder S, Kurz KS, Hoenemann CW, Struemper D, Hahnenkamp K, et al. Time-dependent inhibition of G-protein coupled receptor signaling by local anesthetics. Anesthesiology. 2004;100:852-60.
7. Wildsmith JAW. Lidocaine: a more complex story than 'simple' chemistry suggests. Proc Hist Anesth Soc. 2011;43:9-16.
8. McClure JH. Ropivacaine. Br J Anaesth. 1996;76:300-7.
9. Graf BM. The cardiotoxicity of local anesthetics: the place of ropivacaine. Curr Top Med Chem. 2001;1(3):207-14.
10. Li M, Wan L, Mei W, Tian Y. Update on the clinical utility and practical use of ropivacaine in Chinese patients. Drug Des Devel Ther. 2014;8:1269-76.
11. Burlacu CL, Buggy DJ. Update on local anesthetics: focus on levobupivacaine. Ther Clin Risk Manag. 2008;4(2):381-92.
12. Shipton EA. New formulations of local anaesthetics—part I. Anesth Res Prac. 2012;2012:546409.
13. Snoeck M. Articaine: a review of its use for local and regional anesthesia. Local Reg Anesth. 2012;5:23-33.
14. Nizharadze N, Mamaladze M, Chipashvili N, Vadachkoria D. Articaine—the best choice of local anesthetic in contemporary dentistry. Georgian Med News. 2011;190:15-23.
15. Kambalimath DH, Dolas RS, Kambalimath HV, Agrawal SM. Efficacy of 4% articaine and 2% lidocaine: a clinical study. J Maxillofac Oral Surg. 2013;12(1):3-10.
16. Nusbaum BP. Techniques to reduce pain associated with HT: optimizing anesthesia and analgesia. Am J Clin Dermatol. 2004;5(1):9-15.
17. Wolf BR. Overview of anesthesia. In: Unger W (Ed). Hair Transplantation, 5th edition. New York: Informa Health Care; 2005; pp. 227-37.
18. Melzack R, Wall PD. Pain mechanisms: a new theory. Science. 1965;150(3699):971-9.
19. Davidson JA, Boom SJ. Warming lignocaine to reduce pain associated with injection. BMJ. 1992;305:617-8.
20. Mader TJ, Playe SJ, Garb JL. Reducing the pain of local anesthetic infiltration: warming and buffering have a synergistic effect. Ann Emerg Med. 1994;23:550-4.

21. Sultan J. Effect of warming local anaesthetics on pain of infiltration. Emerg Med J. 2007;24(11):791-3.
22. Allen MJ, Bunce C, Presland AH. The effect of warming local anesthetic on the pain of injection during sub-Tenon's anesthesia for cataract surgery. Anesthesia. 2008;63:276-8.
23. Klein JA. Tumescent technique of regional anesthesia permits lidocaine doses of 35 mg/kg for liposuction. J Dermatol Oncol. 1990;16:248-63.
24. Bhole MA, Manson AL, Seneviratne SL, Misbah SA. IgE-mediated allergy to local anaesthetics—separating fact from perception: a UK perspective. Br J Anest. 2012;108(6):903-11.
25. Budenz AW. Local anesthetics and medically complex patients. J Calif Dent Assoc. 2000;28(8):611-9.
26. Becker DE, Reed KL. Local anesthetics: review of pharmacological considerations. Anesth Prog. 2012;59(2):90-103.
27. Becker DE. Drug interactions in dental practice: a summary of facts and controversies. Compendium. 1994;15:1228-44.
28. United States Department of Health and Human Services. Warning for prescription drugs containing sulfites. FDA Drug Bull. 1987;17:2-3.
29. Seng GF, Gay BJ. Dangers of sulfites in dental local anesthetic solutions: warning and recommendations. J Am Dent Assoc. 1986;113:769-70.
30. Bernstein IL, Li JT, Bernstein DI, Hamilton R, Spector SL, Tan R, et al. Allergy diagnostic testing: an updated practice parameter. Ann Allergy Asthma Immunol. 2008;100(3 Suppl. 3): S1-148.
31. Higuchi H, Yabuki A, Ishii-Maruhama M, Tomoyasu Y, Maeda S, Miyawaki T. Hemodynamic changes by drug interaction of adrenaline with chlorpromazine. Anesth Prog. 2014;61(4): 150-4.
32. Fuzier R, Lapeyre-Mestre M, Mertes PM, Nicolas JF, Benoit Y, Didier A, et al. Immediate and delayed-type allergic reactions to amide local anesthetics: clinical features and skin testing. Pharmacoepidemiol Drug Saf. 2009;18:595-601.
33. Canfield DW, Gage TW. A guideline to local anesthetic allergy testing. Anesth Prog. 1987;34:157-63.
34. Khan S. Nerve block and local anesthesia. In: Unger W (Ed). Hair Transplantation. Philadelphia: Elsevier Saunders; 2006.

PART B: Donor Area

SECTION OUTLINE

- Donor Strip Harvesting—Planning, Preoperative Assessment and Preparation
- Donor Strip Surgical Methods
- Donor Strip: Suturing Techniques
- Trichophytic Closure
- Follicular Unit Extraction: Logic, Case Selection, and Indications
- Physics of Follicular Unit Excision
- Follicular Unit Excision: Instrumentation and Technique
- Punches in Follicular Unit Extraction
- Different Machines in Follicular Unit Excision
- Comparison of Follicular Unit Excision and Follicular Unit Transplantation (Strip): A Critique
- Long Hair Follicular Unit Extraction
- Follicular Unit Extraction Mega and Giga Sessions
- Follicular Unit Excision: Do's and Don'ts

REFERENCES

1. Bernstein RM, Rassman WR. The aesthetics of follicular transplantation. Dermatol Surg. 1997;23(9):785-99.
2. Shiell RC. A review of modern surgical hair restoration techniques. J Cutan Aesthet Surg. 2008;1(1):12-16.
3. Khanna M. Hair Transplant with Strip Harvest: Indications, Contraindications, and Technique. Indian J Plast Surg. 2021; 54(4):451-5.
4. Headington JT. transverse microscopic anatomy of the human scalp. Arch Dermatol. 1984;120:449-56.
5. Mohebi P. The Laxometer: increasing the safety of hair transplants that use a large number of grafts. Hair Transplant Forum Int. 2012;22(6):226-7.
6. Dua K, Uprety S, Dua A. Donor Harvesting: Strip Dissection. J Cutan Aesthet Surg. 2018;11(4):190-4.
7. Khanna M. Hair Transplant with Strip Harvest: Indications, Contraindications, and Technique. Indian J Plast Surg. 2021; 54(4):451-5.
8. Mayer ML. Evaluation of scalp elasticity. In: Unger W, Shapiro R, Unger R, Unger M (Eds). Hair Transplantation, 5th edition. London, United Kingdom: Informa Healthcare; 2011. pp. 267-70.
9. Lam SM (Ed). Hair Transplant 360 for Physicians, Volume 1. JP Medical Ltd.; 2015.

CHAPTER

46

Donor Strip: Surgical Methods

Mayank Singh, Aparna Acharya

Key Messages

- Do not compromise on the quality of instruments, operation theater (OT) space, or magnification.
- Follicular unit transplantation (FUT) surgeries are a team work.
- Getting an aesthetically acceptable scar along with optimal yield of follicles from the safe donor zone should be the aim of every FUT surgery.

INTRODUCTION

Dissection of a strip of full-thickness skin from the safe donor zone is the first and the most crucial step of FUT procedures.

This step will determine the number of follicles that would be harvested and the quality of the resultant scar.

Since both these aspects will be the deciding factors for the success of the procedure, it is imperative that the FUT surgeon is well versed with dissection of the strip.

It requires good surgical training, technique, and knowledge to get an aesthetically acceptable scar along with sufficient harvest of good quality follicular units.

There are various ways in which the strip harvest can be done. Here, we have discussed each step of the strip harvest, variations in the techniques, and the merits and demerits of each.

After completing the initial preoperative formalities and ensuring that all the preoperative check lists are taken care of, we proceed with the actual strip harvest.

PREPARATION OF THE SURGICAL TROLLEY (FIG. 1)

The items include:

- Surgical blade no. 15 or 10
- BP handle
- Skin hooks

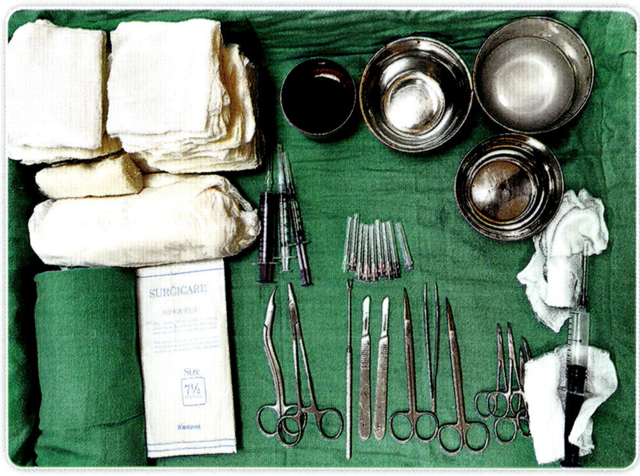

FIG. 1: Surgical trolley.

- Tooth forceps
- Artery forceps
- Fine tissue cutting scissors
- Suture cutting scissors
- Needle holder
- Curved and straight Jeweler's forceps
- Haber's spreader (if being used)
- Syringes
- Suction and cautery (if being used)
- Petri dishes
- Intumescence solution

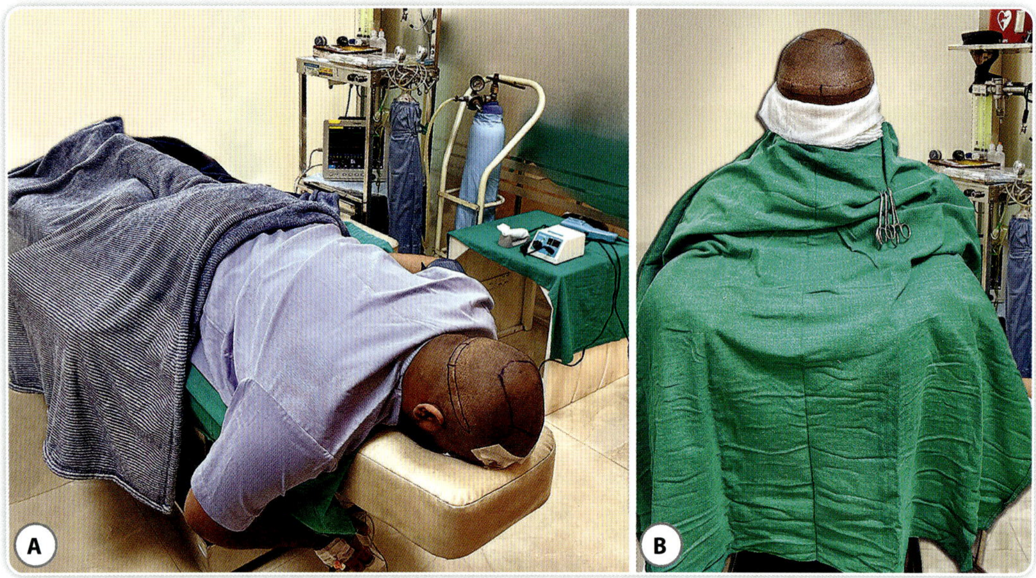

FIGS. 2A AND B: (A) Prone position of patient for anesthesia administration; (B) Sitting position of patient for follicular unit transplantation (FUT) harvestation.

- Normal saline
- Hypodermic needles/customized blades for slit making
- Surgical drapes
- Towel clips
- Gauze pieces
- Sterile bandage
- Povidone-iodine solution
- Wooden tongue depressor

STERILIZATION OF THE INSTRUMENTS

All the metallic instruments, drapes, gauze pieces, bandage, Petri dishes, tongue depressors, etc. are sterilized by autoclaving.

POSITION OF THE PATIENT (FIGS. 2A AND B)

Placing the patient in a sitting or a prone posture for the procedure is individual surgeons' choice. There are lesser chances of a vasovagal syncope in prone position as it will naturally ensure adequate circulating volume.

The sitting posture will offer certain benefits:

- It is more comfortable for the patient, especially obese ones.
- Patient can be engaged and distracted by using TV screen or mobile phone during the procedure.
- The incision angle naturally lies in the same plane as follicular exit angles offering minimal damage to the follicles during placing the incision.

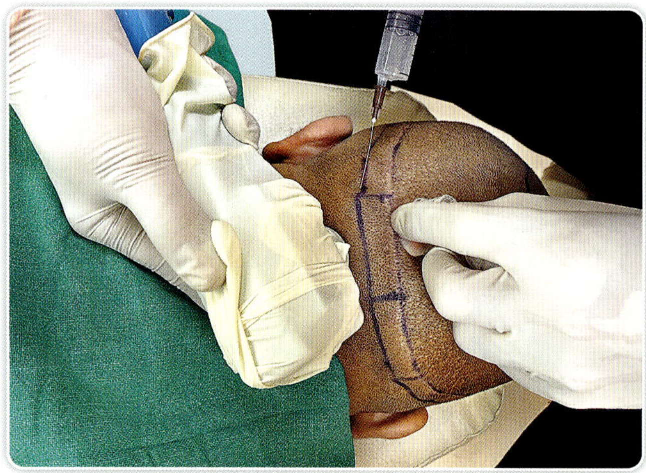

FIG. 3: Anesthesia administration with vibration.

- We prefer to do the procedure with patient in prone position for local anesthesia infiltration followed by sitting position for strip harvest so that we get advantages of both the postures.

Routine preoperative preparation of scrubbing, painting with Betadine, and draping is done.

ANESTHESIA (FIG. 3)

Intumescence anesthesia is used as a ring block. The lower border of the strip is infiltrated with diluted local anesthetic agent using a 26G needle along with continuous vibration.

Composition of intumescence fluid is 20 mL of 2% plain xylocaine, 10 mL of 0.5% L-Bupivacaine, 1 ampoule of adrenaline, 1 ampoule of hyaluronidase, 1 ampoule of 20 mg/mL triamcinolone, and 70 mL of normal saline.

Some surgeons give occipital block prior to infiltration anesthesia. Surface marking for occipital block is 1 cm below and lateral to the occipital protuberance. 1 mL of 1% lignocaine with 1:100,000 adrenaline is injected on each side.[1]

INCISIONS (FIG. 4)

After anesthesia infiltration, scoring incision is placed along the lower border of the strip. It is then deepened to the level of deep dermis.

There are different techniques for making the scoring incision.

- *Single blade*:
  - Advantage of single-blade technique is that the strip breadth can be kept variable at various places.
  - Disadvantage is, it is more time consuming as superior and inferior incisions will be done separately.
- *Double blade*:
  - Advantage of this technique is economy of the time as both the incisions are made simultaneously.[2]
  - Disadvantage is, the strip breadth is same throughout the incisions and checking for the follicular exit angles may be difficult as both the incisions are made simultaneously.
- *Multi blade*:
  - Advantage is getting thinner strips for easier dissection of slivers and follicular units.
  - Disadvantage is, if the incision is placed deeper, multiple rows of the follicles might be transected simultaneously.[3]

Also, the strip breadth would be the same throughout, which is not desirable.

The authors use single-blade technique with strip dimensions variable through its length. *The central 9–10 cm in-between mastoid areas is around 1.5–1.7 cm in scalps with average laxity. The width at mastoid area is around 1–1.3 cm. The lateral segment is again flared to 1.3–1.5 cm.*

These variations in the strip width will ensure maximum follicular yield while ensuring a tension-free closure and an aesthetic scar at the same time. This is because the skin laxity at the mastoid region is lesser than anywhere else along the strip.[4]

STRIP DISSECTION

Strip dissection can be either sharp or blunt.

Sharp Dissection

- *Fast tracking*: The strip is dissected directly downward till the level of the dermal papilla. It is important to be in the plane of exit angles of the follicles to avoid damage to the follicular units.
  This method is quick. If the surgeon is inexperienced, the dissection plane could be wrong and it will damage the entire row of follicles along the edge.[5]
- *Open technique* **(Fig. 5)**: In this technique, the entire further dissection is done under direct vision by retracting edges of the incision.

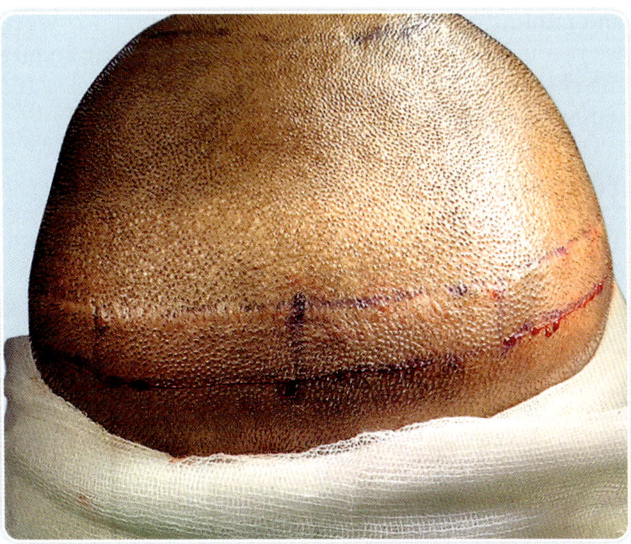

FIG. 4: Scoring incision.

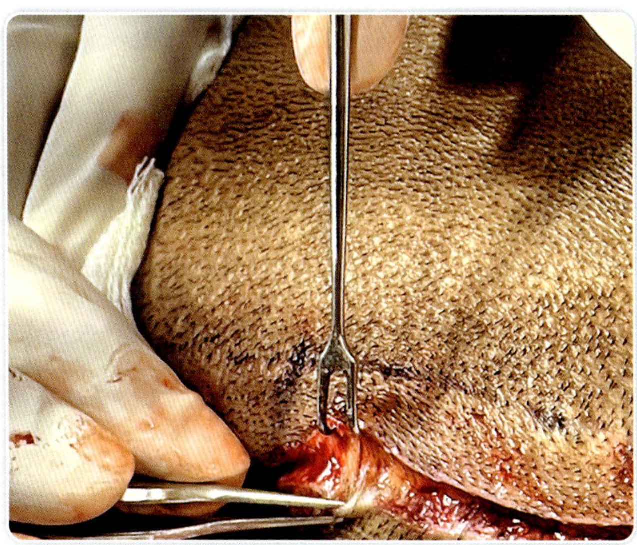

FIG. 5: Open technique.

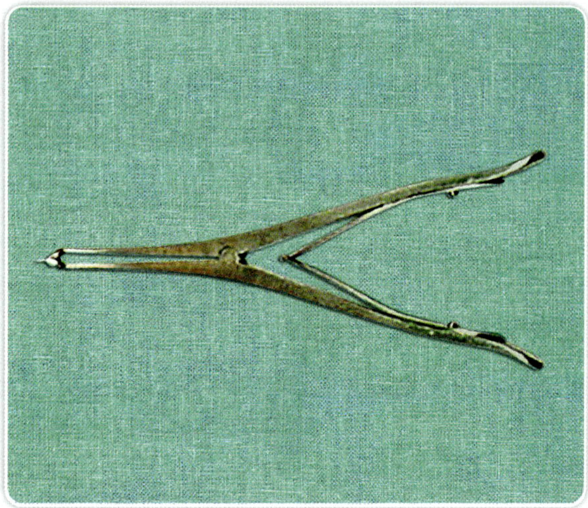

FIG. 6: Haber's spreader.

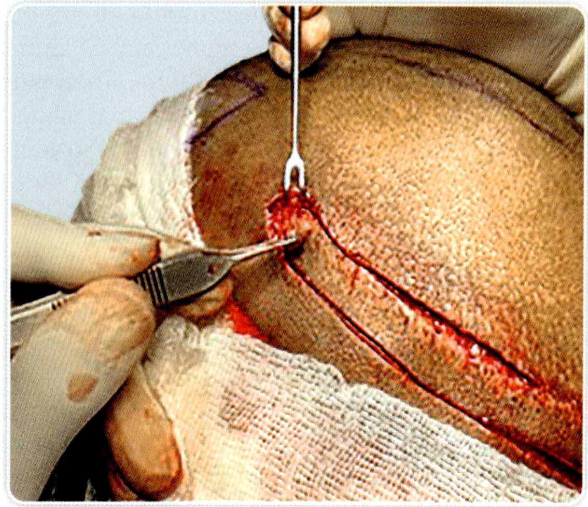

FIG. 7: Strip dissection.

A skin hook and a tooth forceps can be used for this purpose. The surgeon will hold the tooth forceps and the assistant will give continuous traction with the skin hook. By these ways the incision is deepened till the subcutaneous fat under direct vision. Only one assistant is needed for this method.

- *Double traction method*: In this method, the assistants will retract both the edges of the incision with either a single- or a double-pronged skin hook and the surgeon will deepen the incision. Depending upon the number of assistants, the number of skin hooks used can be 2, 3, or 4.[5]

Blunt Dissection (Spreader Technique) (Fig. 6)

Haber's spreader: It is an instrument which aids in the blunt dissection for deepening the incision. Prongs of the spreader are aligned within the incision and pressed to open the spreader. These prongs open up the incision till the deeper plane without the need of a sharp dissection.

Hemostat can be used in a similar manner instead of the spreader. Only disadvantage of the hemostat is that it will fatigue the surgeon more as intrinsic small muscles of the hand are used unlike the spreader. This spreader method is very useful while doing surgeries for patients with extremely curly hair as seen in African ethnicity and in patients with grey hair. In both these patients, the visibility of the follicles is low, either due to the curl or transparency. So, there are higher chances of transactions of the follicles in the sharp dissection methods.

However, this technique is not so useful in rigid and firm scalps where it can lacerate the tissues instead of spreading.

STRIP SEPARATION (FIG. 7)

Proceeding in the way described earlier, strip dissection of both the borders is done till the subcutaneous level. After this, the strip separation is started from one corner of the incision. It is vitally important to remain in the correct surgical plane while separating the strip. It is identified by a continuous traction on the strip and on the edges of the incision with skin hooks.

Sharp dissection is done keeping a thin layer of subcutaneous fat along the follicular bulbs to protect them.

Any major bleeder is ligated with Vicryl 3-0 suture in a **Figure of 8**. Continuous subcutaneous suturing obliterates the dead space and also helps control generalized oozing.

A liberal use of cautery will ensure a bloodless field and minimize the risk of hematoma formation. However, we recommend avoiding use of electrocautery to reduce the chances of effluvium of the surrounding follicles and patient discomfort.

TRICHOPHYTIC CLOSURE (FIG. 8)

Trichophytic closure is the way of ensuring hair growth through the linear scar, thus reducing the scar visibility.[6]

In trichophytic closure, the edge of the incision is deepithelized. It can be done for superior, inferior, or both the edges.

Deepithelization of the superior border may lead to hair growing in an upward direction, giving an unnatural look.

Deepithelization of both the borders may lead to hair growth in a perpendicular direction with respect to the scar, again making it look unnatural.

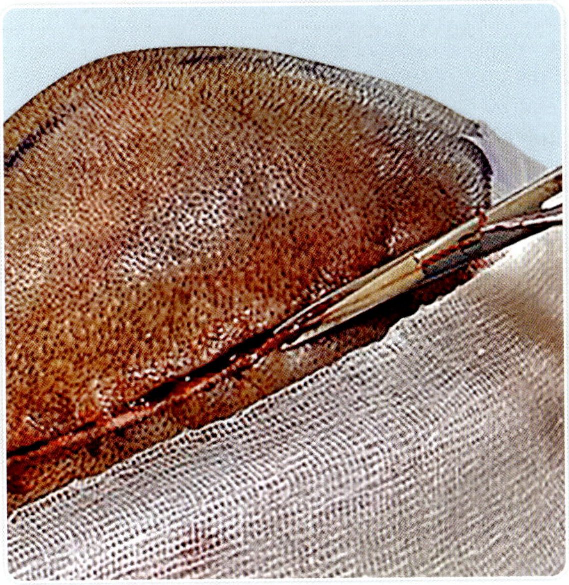

FIG. 8: Trichophytic closure dissection.

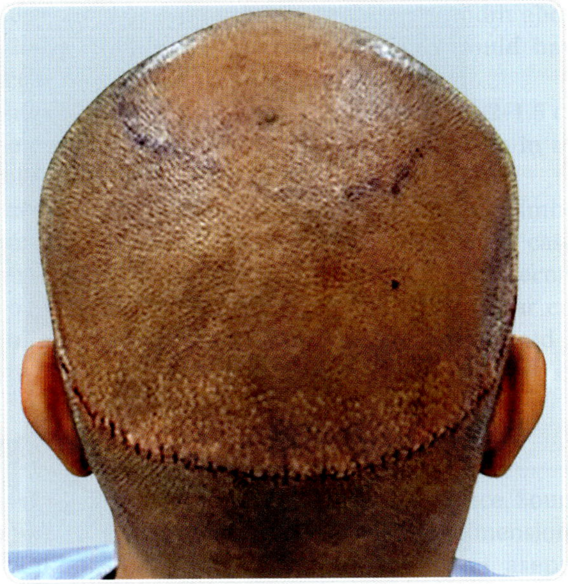

FIG. 9: Post-suture completion.

Deepithelization of the lower border ensures the hair growth in a downward and natural direction. Hence, this is the authors' preferred method.

Deepithelization is done with sharp-pointed scissors, a surgical blade or a custom-made device.[7]

Procedure

An incision is made approximately 1 mm from the edge, including a single row of follicles. The epidermis of the lower flap border is removed with fine scissors. This excised part should be very thin and translucent. The incision depth should not exceed 1 mm as it might cause damage to the sebaceous gland and bulge area, which may impact the follicular growth and can lead to cyst formation.

After removal of the trichophytic strip, the skin defect is closed.

CLOSURE TECHNIQUES (FIG. 9)

Single Layered

In cases where strip width is less than a cm a single-layered closure may be done in a continuous manner with 3-0 or 4-0 Prolene.

Double Layered

Inner layer includes subcutaneous tissue with bits of galea to prevent widening of the scar. It is done with 3-0 or 4-0 Vicryl running sutures. Continuous suturing is faster but needs adequate experience and surgical skills to get proper vertical alignment of superior and inferior rows of follicles. Outer layer is closed with Vicryl Rapide 4-0 or Prolene 4-0 in a continuous manner.

Alternatively, for the inner layer polydioxanone suture (PDS)/nonabsorbable nylon interrupted sutures can be used. Interrupted suturing is slower, but it has better chances of proper alignment even at the hands of an inexperienced surgeon.

If nonabsorbable sutures are used for skin closure, the suture removal is done on 10th postoperative day.

We use Vicryl Rapide for the skin closure as it dissolves in about 3–4 weeks and the patient does not need to come for suture removal. It has a disadvantage of getting slightly more prominent cross hatching scars.

Staple Closure

The skin approximation may be performed with staples. This technique saves labor and time and gives a better aesthetic outcome. However, it may cause more pain and discomfort.[8]

It is important that the skin edges are perfectly aligned and the cross hatching is minimal. Superior and inferior hair follicles should be aligned vertically to get a better cosmetic outcome.

Postoperative Dressing

Many surgeons dress only the donor area suture line leaving the recipient area open. We prefer an enclosed dressing for the entire scalp with paraffin gauze and Neosporin ointment. This ensures that the recipient bed

REFERENCES

1. Shiell RC. A review of modern surgical hair restoration techniques. J Cutan Aesthet Surg. 2008;1(1):12-6.
2. Khanna M. Hair Transplant with Strip Harvest: Indications, Contraindications, and Technique. Indian J Plast Surg. 2021; 54(4):451-5.
3. Stough DB. Tension donor dissection: the ultimate strip harvesting method. Hair Transplant Forum Int. 2006;17:77-8.
4. Khanna M. Hair Transplant with Strip Harvest: Indications, Contraindications, and Technique. Indian J Plast Surg. 2021; 54(4):451-5.
5. Pathomvanich D. Donor harvesting: a new approach to minimize transection of hair follicles. Dermatol Surg. 2000;26:345-8.
6. Frechet P. Minimal scars for scalp surgery. J Dermatol Surg. 2007;33(1):45-56.
7. Venkataram M. Changing trends in hair restoration surgery. Indian J Dermatol Venereol Leprol. 2006;72(2):103-11.
8. Muthuvel K, Lakshmikanthan S, Subburathinam D. Outcomes of staple closure of the donor area during hair transplant by follicular unit transfer. J Cutan Aesthet Surg. 2014;7(2):103-6.
9. Kim JC, Hwang S. The effects of dehydration, preservation, temperature and time on hair grafts. In: Unger WP, Shapiro R (Eds). Hair Transplantation, 4th edition. New York: Marcel Dekker; 2004. pp. 285-6.
10. Cole JP, Reed WM. The optimal holding solution and temperature for hair follicle grafts. Hair Transplant Forum Int. 2012;22: 17-21.
11. Dua K, Uprety S, Dua A. Donor Harvesting: Strip Dissection. J Cutan Aesthet Surg. 2018;11(4):190-4.

CHAPTER 47

Donor Strip: Suturing Techniques

Manoj Khanna

Key Messages

- Proper suturing techniques are vital to ensuring proper healing and fine scars.
- Two-layered sutures are important to decrease wound tension.
- Type of suture material is variable and depends on the preference of surgeon.
- A fine donor scar is of paramount importance. It should preferably be inconspicuous so that it is not apparent that a hair transplant procedure was performed.

INTRODUCTION

Donor strip excision has already been dealt with in detail in the earlier chapter. Suturing technique, type of suture, and the materials used are vital for ensuring a minimum scar, which are described in this chapter.

Our goal while harvesting the strip is to remove as many follicles as possible and simultaneously achieve an inconspicuous or minimally visible scar in the donor area. A good donor site scar has the following characters:

- Thin line, not more than a couple of millimeters wide
- Flush with the surface
- Hair growing through the scar
- The scar line is not easily visible unless one shaves the scalp.

This is not just a theoretical description but a realistic achievable goal. Nothing less should be expected from a good aesthetic surgeon. Satisfactory result of donor site closure comes from a meticulous technique and precise planning of the donor site, including the location and width of the strip to be removed in relation to the scalp laxity and proper harvesting technique, which preserves the hair follicles at the edge of donor wound during "trichophytic closure." It needs to be emphasized that an aesthetically acceptable donor scar is as important as getting good results in the recipient area. It determines the patient's attitude for future surgeries, if required, with respect to both the choice of the surgeon and the preference of technique.

PATIENT POSITIONING

In our attempt to harvest the perfect strip and subsequent closure of the gap, we should also appreciate the importance of time. Ideally, harvesting of the strip and closure of the donor site should not take more than 45 minutes. The patient lies prone, which is a relatively uncomfortable position. Although the scalp is numb, the rest of the body is not. We prefer to give the patient oral anxiolytic medication, such as alprazolam 0.5–1.0 mg, 45 minutes before starting the procedure. Every member of the surgical team works synchronously in perfect harmony. Speed with efficiency is nothing but economy of motion done with precision.

The surgeon usually stands on the right side of the patient, or according to his/her dominant right hand. The first assistant stands diametrically opposite to the surgeon, and the second assistant is positioned at the head of the table. The second assistant holds the head steady, guides the patient to turn the head from side to side during the procedure, and aids in hemostasis. Nothing is more unpleasant than blood spilling over the face during

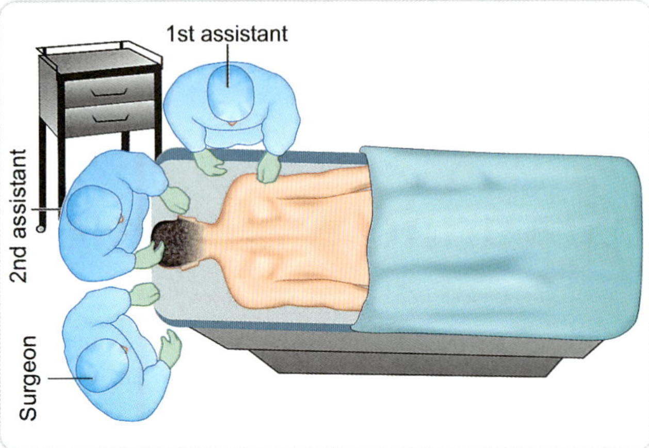

FIG. 1: Position of surgeon and assistants.

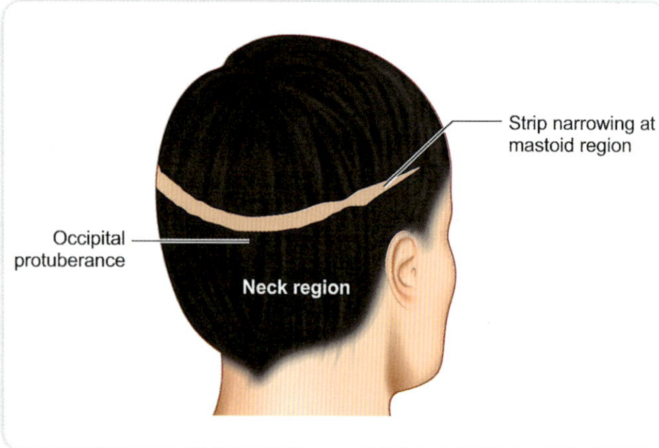

FIG. 2: Shape of the strip—schematic diagram.

surgery of an awake patient. The first assistant positions the surgical trolley between himself and the assistant at the head end of the patient **(Fig. 1)**.

Before starting the harvest, we strap the hair above the superior margin of the donor site by a skin tape (e.g., transpore, micropore) applied from forehead, circumscribing the scalp. The hair below the donor zone in male patients is usually small and directed downward, not causing much inconvenience. But, in female patients, securing the longer hair below the donor area with a paper tape may be preferable.

SUTURE MATERIALS

Suture materials used for closure may be absorbable or nonabsorbable and can be monofilament or multifilament. After using all types of sutures, we have found a two-layered closure to be most rewarding. The deeper layer is closed with a nonabsorbable monofilament 2-0 interrupted suture. The superficial layer is closed with a continuous running nonabsorbable suture such as 4-0 Prolene, which is blue-colored and easily visible during removal. An absorbable running suture of 4-0 Vicryl Rapide is used if the patient is unable to come back for suture removal. Staples have generally not found favor with surgeons because of the associated pain and discomfort while lying down in the postoperative period.

POINTS TO REMEMBER WHILE HARVESTING DONOR STRIP

All efforts are made to reduce tension of closure and preserve the much needed hair follicles at the edge of the donor site wound. Various factors have a bearing on the final donor site scar.

The site of donor strip should be appropriately chosen. The midpoint of the donor strip site should lie just above the occipital protuberance. If made any lower, it will spill over to the neck. Contraction of the neck muscles in the postoperative period can result in scar widening.

The scalp in the mastoid region has minimal mobility and is at the lateral end of the occipital ridge. It is crucial to minimize tension in this region by reducing the width of the strip here **(Fig. 2)**. It is also important to note that taking the incision too far anteriorly may result in scar visibility if the temporal fringes lose hair later.

Initial superficial scoring is done with #15 blade, taking care not to incise too deep beyond the dermis **(Fig. 3)**. We avoid using the scalpel for deeper dissection to avoid damage to the hair follicles. Two double-pronged hooks are used to separate the strip from the adjacent tissue after the epidermis and dermis have been scored. Distraction is done by the two hooks, placed on either side of the incision lines. Distraction force is applied only to the hook on the side of the strip, which is to be excised. The other hook on the incision line, away from the strip which will be excised, is merely held in position for stabilization and not for any force of distraction **(Fig. 4)**. This prevents separation of the skin flap from the galea in the floor, which makes proper closure difficult.

Leaving some amount of fatty tissue over the galea while harvesting the strip is very useful. Maintaining the plane of dissection just below the hair follicles **(Fig. 5A)** and above the level of galea gives a nice supple scar, which is not tethered to the tissue below. Efforts are taken to avoid injury to the underlying galea, which will cause scarring and adherence. Also, injury to the neurovascular bundle, which is in this plane of loose areolar fatty tissue is avoided **(Fig. 5B)**. This reduces the incidence of paresthesia and

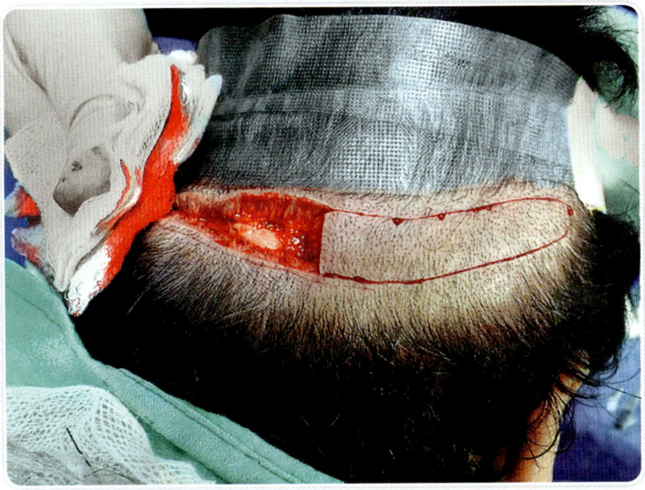

FIG. 3: Scoring strip.

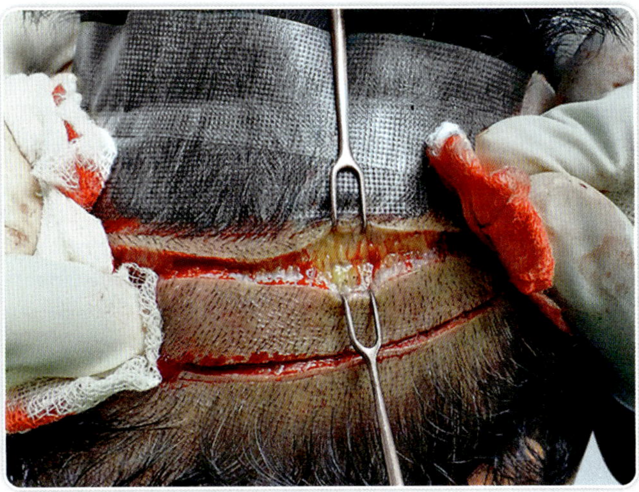

FIG. 4: Double skin hook traction.

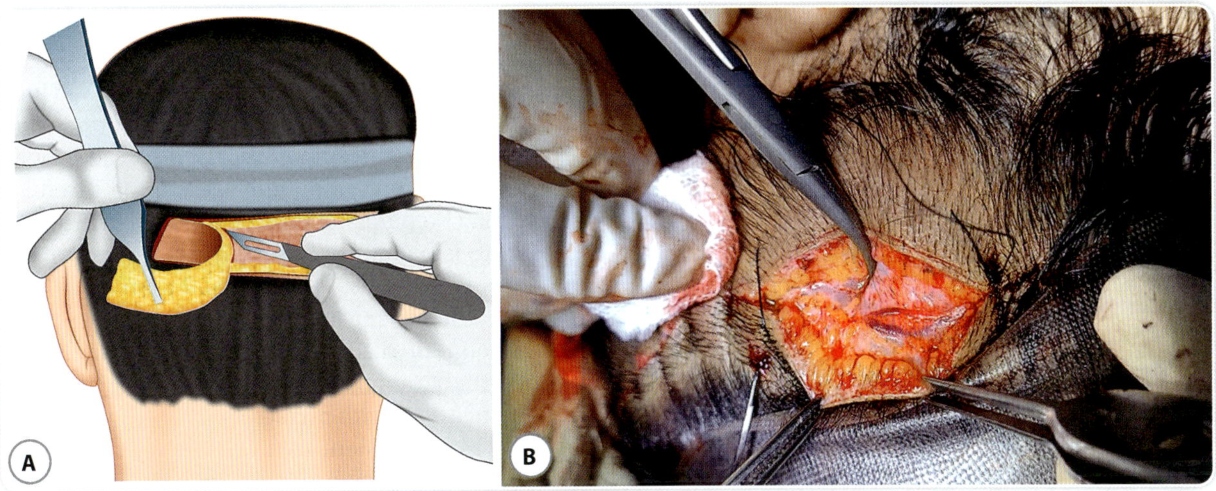

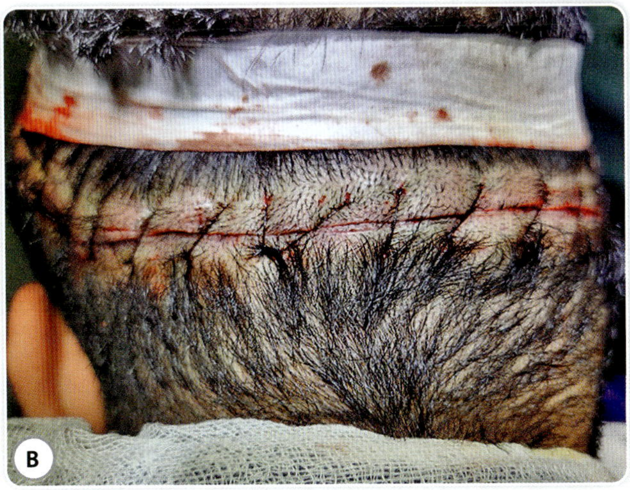

FIGS. 5A TO C: (A) Strip harvested leaving some amount of fatty tissue over galea; (B) Neurovascular bundle saved during excision of donor strip due to distraction technique; (C) Temporary closure of wound with 2-0 Nylon, causing "rapid tissue expansion" and reducing tissue edema, thereby facilitating wound closure.

anesthesia around the donor site in the postoperative period, which, though temporary, is distressing to the patient. If the strip to be harvested is long, we harvest it in segments, usually three—right, central, and left. We temporarily close the wound with running 2-0 Nylon sutures after harvesting each segment. This helps to reduce the edema sooner and also stretches the skin by "rapid tissue expansion," bringing the edges closer and thereby reducing the tension on the subsequent closure **(Fig. 5C and Fig. 6)**.

Electrocautery is carefully used to achieve hemostasis without damaging any hair follicles. Small bleeding points from the fat and deeper parts of the wound edges can be dealt with diathermy at very low settings. Any dermal edge bleeding is compressed with a gauze, and it subsequently stops, usually while skin closure is being done. Adequate hemostasis is a must as any clots below the suture line will delay wound healing and increase the risk of hematoma formation and infection.[1]

Suture Technique

During the earlier days of hair transplant (HT) surgery, the technique of donor site closure was like general surgeons. If the scalp was found to be sufficiently lax and could be closed without tension, a single-layer closure usually with a continuous 4-0 Prolene suture would be performed. If it was seen that there was significant tension, a two-layered closure would be done with an absorbable 2/0 suture for deeper layer in addition to the superficial layer.[2,3] But it was noted that these closures were ridden with recurring problem of wide scars, no matter how meticulously the suturing was done. The scar would leave a bald zone of 0.4–1 cm across the back of the head at the incision site. Sometimes, there would be hypertrophy of the same and result in a very unsightly scar. The tradeoff between a scalp full of hair while leaving behind a bad scar is disliked by the patient whose main interest is to enhance himself cosmetically in the bald area but without disfigurement of the donor area. This wide scar is a telltale sign of a HT and is the cause of unhappiness and discomfort. It was also observed that patients with very lax scalp having minimal tension during closure paradoxically developed wider scars as the loose skin continued to stretch in the postoperative period. Patients with tight scalp usually have better scars as they do not stretch easily in the postoperative period.

Our experience from the earlier days has led us to believe that in the cases of "scar widening," any scar gradually stretches up to 6–24 months after surgery. Our attempts to prevent this by using absorbable suture which lasts longer have been unsuccessful **(Table 1)**. Polydioxanone suture (PDS), which is fully absorbed in 6–7 months, loses 50% of its initial strength by 4 weeks.[2] Nonabsorbable suture, on the other hand, does not allow the scar to stretch. But as a surgeon, the apprehension of leaving behind a foreign body in the scalp is well founded. In our experience, the deeply buried nonabsorbable suture (Ethilon) poses no extra risk if placed properly. In case of a very thin scalp, one needs to be careful as the suture may be palpable if placed too superficially. But if the suture is palpable or spits, it can be removed easily under local anesthesia with a small 2-mm stab incision. We believe achieving a good cosmetic scar far outweighs this infrequent discomfort, and we have been using nonabsorbable sutures for deep buried stitches with good results since 2006 with no regrets.

A 2/0 monofilament suture (3/8 circle, 45 mm Nylon) is appropriate for the described technique. The needle is passed just below the hair follicles and above the level of galea transversely, on both edges of the wound **(Figs. 7A and B)**. We have found that this plane of suturing brings together the edges of the wound and holds them in place

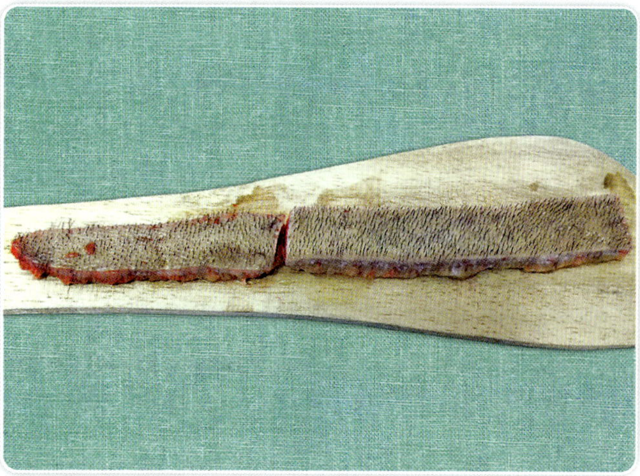

FIG. 6: Harvested strip.

TABLE 1: Number of weeks resulting in 50% loss in tensile strength of different sutures.

Number of weeks					
1	**1–2**	**2**	**2–3**	**3**	**3–4**
Plain surgical gut	Chromic gut		Dexon	Vicryl	PDS
Vicryl Rapide	Dyed Monocryl		Polysorb		Maxon
Undyed Monocryl			Biosin		

(PDS: polydioxanone suture)

with sufficient strength. Undermining of the wound edges is never done. Our objective here is to appose the edges together with minimum possible trauma to the surrounding tissue and hair roots, leaving a minimum amount of suture material behind. The surgeon begins the deep closure by passing the needle away from himself, from one side of the wound, and then brings back the needle toward himself from the other side while catching enough tissue. The knot is tied toward the surgeon's end. The surgical assistant, with the help of fine artery forceps in one hand, gently pushes down the tissue with the bulge of the underlying galea, below the suture's knot **(Fig. 7C)**. Simultaneously, the assistant, with the help of dissecting forceps in the other hand, apposes one edge of the wound toward the other side **(Fig. 7D)** while the knot is tightened. As the surgeon throws the first loop and tightens it, the underlying forceps is slid out from below the knot, achieving a tight closure. Now, the assistant prevents loosening of the first throw of the suture by holding the knot gently with mosquito forceps, and the surgeon secures a snug tight second knot. Only "reef knots" are given with three throws, as any more are not required and may make the suture palpable. The suture is cut flush on the knot by the assistant, under direct vision, by gently retracting the edge of the wound. The deeper layer of the entire wound is closed in this way, and good apposition of the edges of the incision can be achieved before trichophytic excision **(Fig. 8A)**.

In order to create a minimally visible scar, a trichophytic closure is performed in the superficial layer. This is a technique that addresses the age-old problem of a bald closure line. The aim is to get hair to grow through the scar. An epidermal strip of 1–2 mm width is removed from either edge (usually lower) of the incision line **(Figs. 8B and 9)**, leaving the intact hair roots below. The wound is sutured, approximating the edges of the donor strip wound, with the hair roots, without the epidermis, present in one margin. The incision is parallel to the hair, and thus the wound edges are beveled at both margins. Thus, after de-epithelializing the lower edge, the ledge of the superior incision conveniently advances over it. As the donor site heals, hair grows through the scar from the hair roots in the "trichophytic margin," making the stitch line inconspicuous.

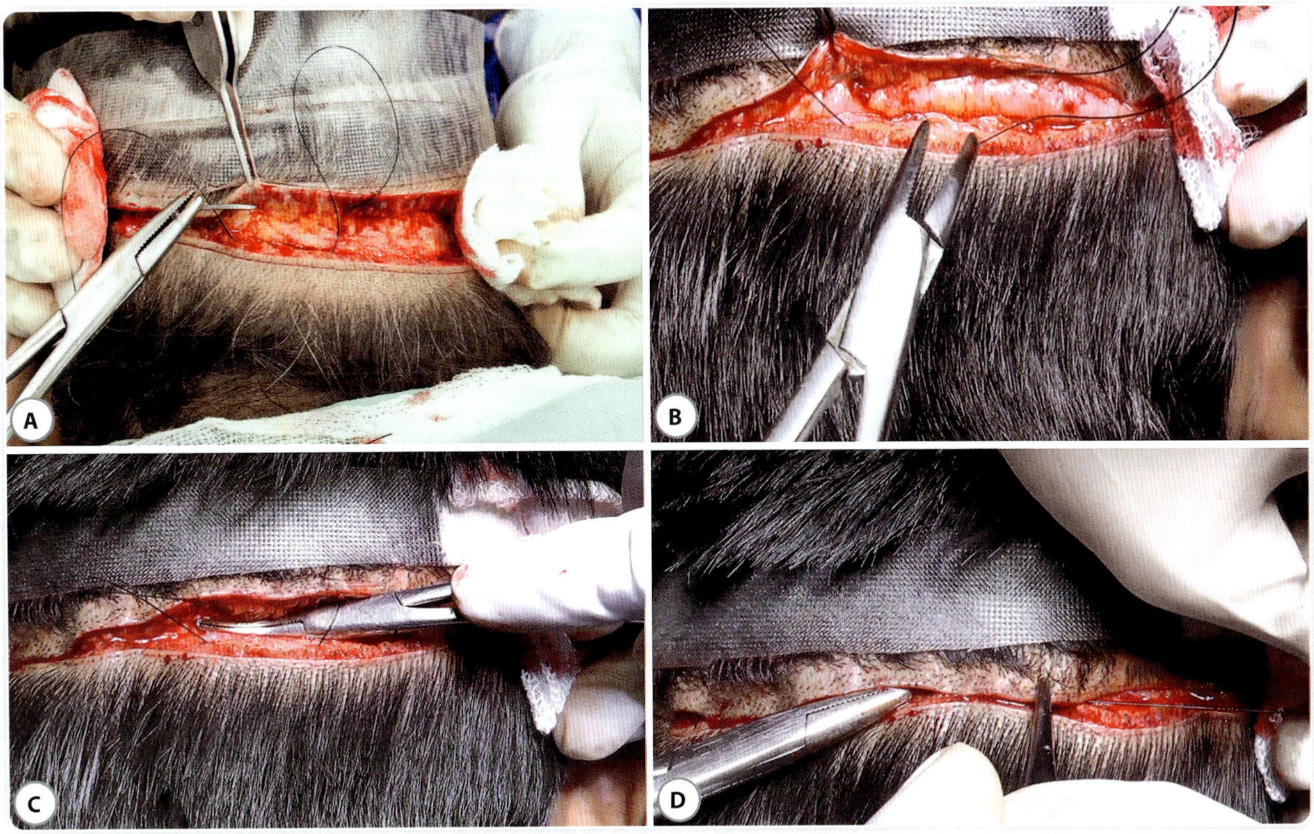

FIGS. 7A TO D: (A) Deep suturing with Ethilon. (B) Deep suturing. Note the needle bite well below the hair follicles. (C) Depressing the deep tissue before tightening the knot during deep closure. (D) Apposing the edges with toothed dissecting forceps while tightening the first knot.

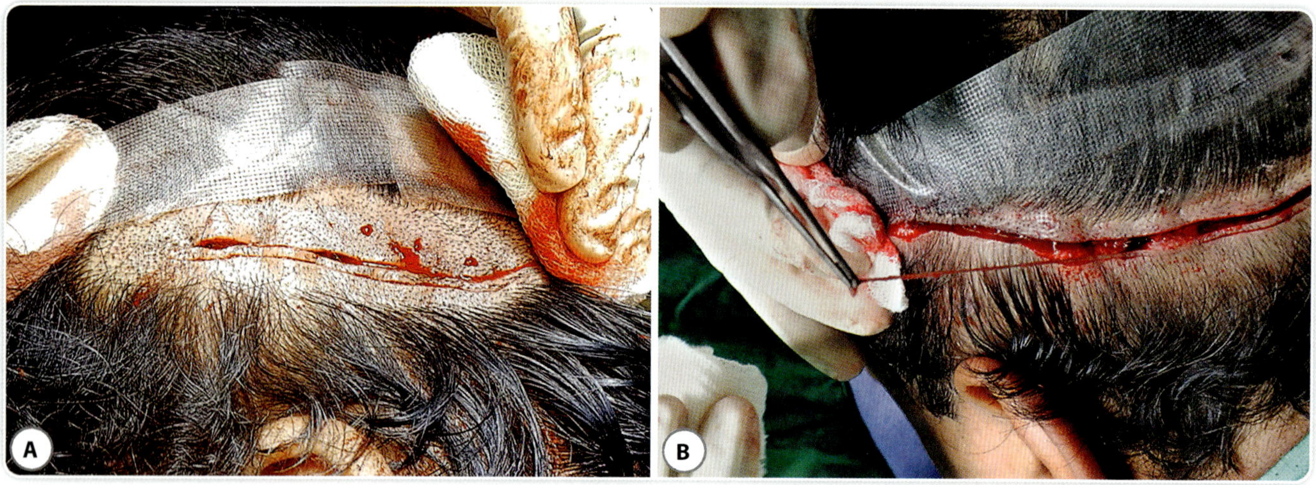

FIGS. 8A AND B: (A) Apposed skin edges after deep closure, with scored trichophytic incision; (B) Trichophytic edge excision.

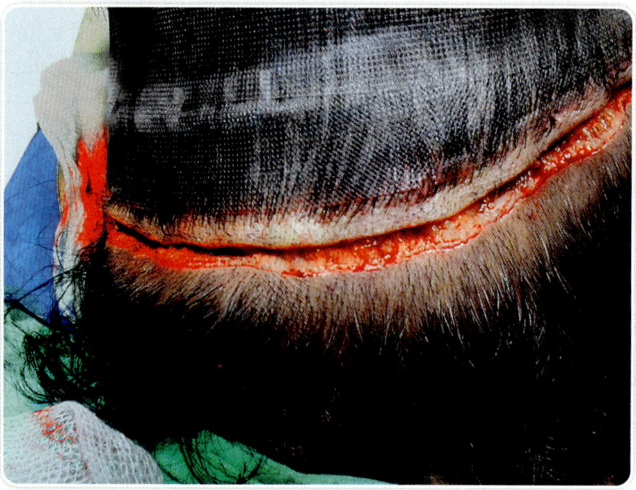

FIG. 9: After trichophytic excision.

We usually perform the superficial skin closure with nonabsorbable fine suture 4-0 Prolene, which is blue in color and can easily be identified during suture removal on the 10th to 14th postoperative day. Skin closure may also be done with short-lasting absorbable suture of 4-0 Vicryl Rapide if the patient cannot come for suture removal. It must be stated that occasionally, the absorbable suture does not fall off in 2 weeks, and this leads to increased scarring with hatch marks. It is advisable to ask the patient to send photos of the stitch line after 2 weeks of surgery if he/she is unable to come and visit any surgeon in his vicinity if the sutures have not fallen off.

Running suture is used for skin closure in either case. The surgeon begins by placing a knot 1 mm beyond the end of the incision and penetrates the skin perpendicular to the surface. A tissue purchase of 3–4 mm is sufficient. It is important that the depth of the bite should be above the underlying hair roots to prevent any injury to them. We find the 16-mm needle of the 4/0 suture to be ideal. Larger needles can penetrate deeper and may damage the hair roots. I prefer to begin by giving 20 or more loose continuous bites with the suture without tightening it, using only the proximal 15–20 cm of the suture from the needle. This shorter length of suture facilitates taking equidistant symmetrical bites along the wound. The assistant holds the hair down in place in the gap between his left four fingers and thumb across the edges of the wound while holding the extra length of the suture beyond the 20 cm firmly below his thenar eminence. After taking 20 or more bites at a time **(Figs. 10A and B)**, I tighten the continuous suture, pulling one loop after another to bring the wound edges together with equal controlled tension. A specially designed mosquito forceps with a fine curved tip is used to make this step quicker and easier **(Fig. 10C)**. The extra length of the suture is thus withdrawn, with minimum tension at the edges of the wound, avoiding squashing of tissue, and with good symmetrical closure **(Figs. 11A and B)**. All these aid in achieving a good scar. We have found this technique to be quicker and, at the same time, avoid excess tension on the wound edges. The classical technique of pulling the entire length of the suture with each throw results in unequal bites along the skin edge with extra tension which may jeopardize the fine vascularity of the edges of stitch line, resulting in delayed healing, marginal necrosis, and poorer quality of the final scar.

The use of staples has also been documented, with some surgeons preferring it because of increased speed of closure. Most published series, and our experience, however, suggest more pain and discomfort in the immediate postoperative period and more discomfort

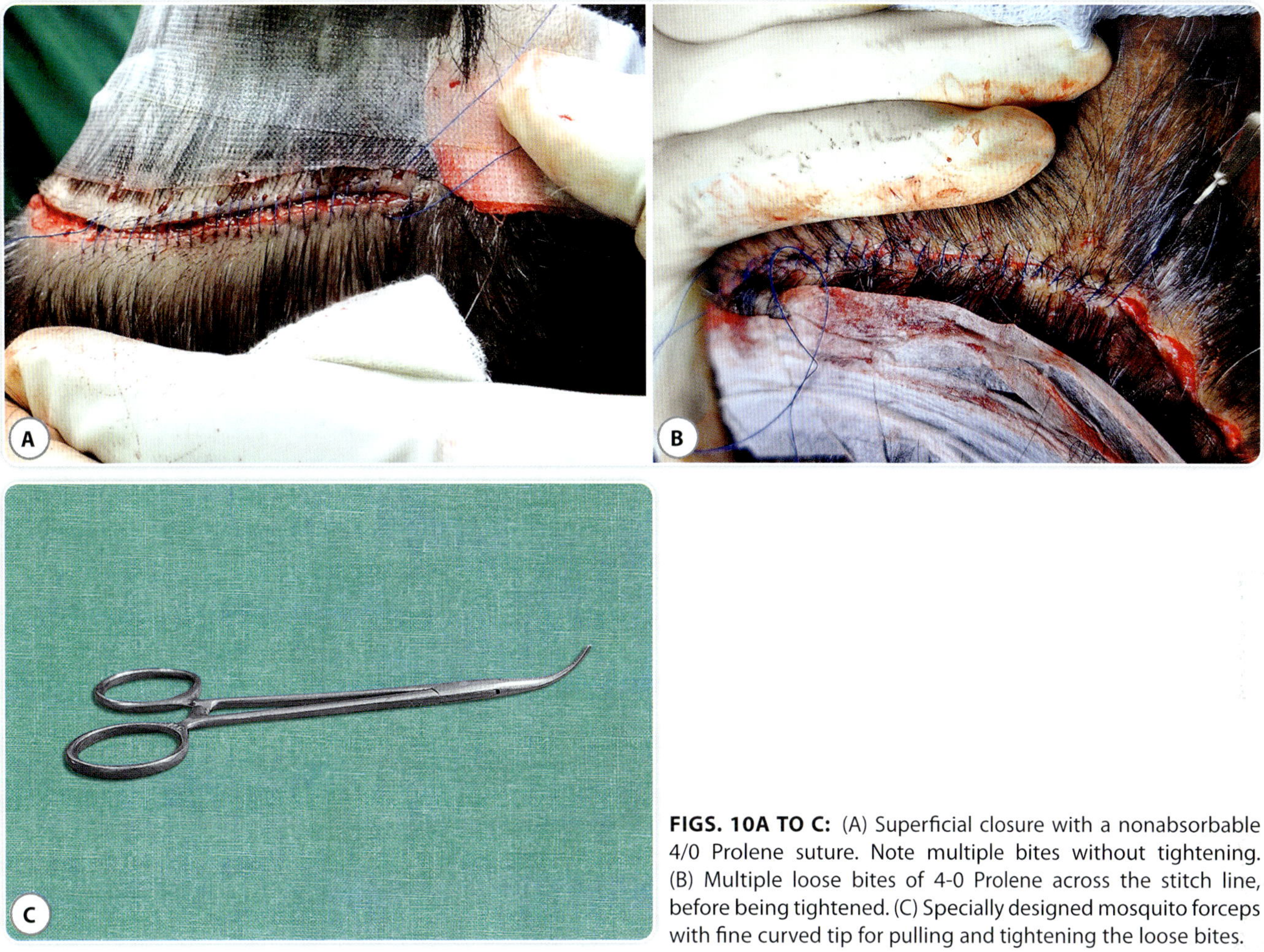

FIGS. 10A TO C: (A) Superficial closure with a nonabsorbable 4/0 Prolene suture. Note multiple bites without tightening. (B) Multiple loose bites of 4-0 Prolene across the stitch line, before being tightened. (C) Specially designed mosquito forceps with fine curved tip for pulling and tightening the loose bites.

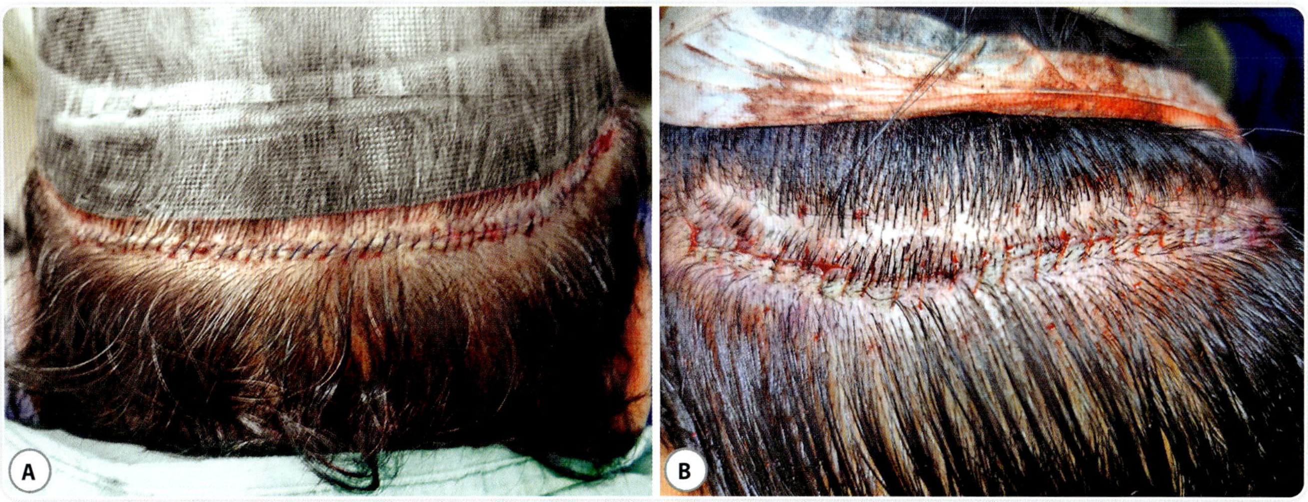

FIGS. 11A AND B: (A) After skin closure with 4-0 Prolene. Please note the symmetrical stitches. (B) Final closure with 4-0 Vicryl Rapide. Note the equidistant skin bites without tension.

at the time of staple removal as compared to the suture removal.[4]

Various techniques may be employed to facilitate closure if the scalp is not lax. A mere delay of 30–45 minutes before removal of the temporary 2-0 Nylon suture redistributes the tumescent fluid in the tissue and causes rapid tissue expansion. Some surgeons have tried to induce laxity by injecting hyaluronidase into the donor strip. Towel clips come in handy to approximate the wound edges together and provide on-table tissue relaxation. Similar effect can be achieved by using interrupted heavy temporary tension suture to bring the edges together. These are gradually removed as the suturing advances.

Postoperative Period

After suturing the donor site, the patient will be turned into the supine position and will undergo subsequent steps of the procedure. The creation of recipient site slits and then transplanting hair into them is a long process during which period the patient will lie over the stitch line. We infiltrate the donor stitch line, whenever necessary, with 10 mL of 0.25% bupivacaine to anesthetize the suture line for another 3–4 hours.

Donor site sutures are removed between the 10th and 14th postoperative day. The blue-colored Prolene is easy to identify. It is advisable to get a checkup after 14 days if absorbable sutures are used and to remove them if still present. Absorbable sutures, when present for long, have been seen to create prominent scars with crosshatching. The main objective of closure with an absorbable suture is that in the event the patient needs to get any suture removed by untrained personnel, it will be minimally present. I always give a video to the patient displaying the technique for absorbable suture removal, which can be shown for guidance, to the personnel not from the clinic, helping in removing the sutures if required.

SUMMARY

- Proper donor closure with the right suture material is very important to produce a thin scar.
- Using skin hooks during harvest is a great technique as it avoids damage to hair follicles and vessels.
- Two-layered suturing is useful for better approximation of wound edges and creating finer scars.

REFERENCES

1. Unger W. What's new in hair replacement surgery. Dermatol Clin. 1996;14:783-802.
2. Ethicon (Johnson & Johnson). Wound Closure Manual. [online] Available from https://anwresidency.com/simulation/guide/resources/Ethicon_Wound_Closure_manual.pdf [Last accessed October, 2023].
3. Bernstein RM, Rassman WR, Rashid N. A new suture for hair transplantation: poliglecaprone 25. Dermatol Surg. 2001;27:5-11.
4. Bernstein R. Staples versus monocryl. Dermatol Surg. 2001;27:5-11.

CHAPTER 48

Trichophytic Closure

Sandeep Sattur, Indu S Sattur

Key Messages

- Any incision in a hair-bearing area leaves behind a scar that is hairless.
- Trichophytic closure of donor wound helps to reduce the hairlessness of the donor scar, making it less obvious.
- If carefully performed in appropriate situations, this technique can be a useful way of leaving imperceptible donor scars after strip harvest.

INTRODUCTION

Any incision on the scalp heals with a scar that is devoid of hair. Patients undergoing hair transplantation, especially those who sport short hair, are concerned with visibility of the donor scar. The scar from strip harvest is obvious due to two reasons—the scar is linear in orientation (straight line scars always stand out) and it is hairless. This is a cause of concern to those patients who wish to wear their hair very short after the surgery. Trichophytic closure attempts to address the second reason by getting hair to grow through the scar, thereby helping to camouflage the scar.

TRICHOPHYTIC CLOSURE

Historically, the principle of trichophytic closure has been used in various aesthetic and reconstructive surgeries of the face and scalp.[1] Beveling of the incision was called the "hair camouflaging incision" by Kridel et al.[2] The purpose was to avoid visible scars and loss of hair in the temporal area in patients undergoing facelift surgery.

The credit for coining the term "trichophytic" goes to Mayer and Fleming.[1,3] This procedure was first described almost simultaneously by Marzola, Rose, and Frechet with respect to hair transplant donor area management. Paul Rose prefers to call this as "ledge closure."[3-6]

RATIONALE OF TRICHOPHYTIC CLOSURE

The basis of trichophytic closure is the presumption that superficially transected follicles in the edge of the donor wound would grow through the resultant scar. It involves a limited and controlled deepithelialization of one of the edges of the resultant donor wound, post strip harvest. It gives the benefit of camouflaging the scar by the hair growing through it. Another advantage of this is that theoretically, the growing hairs (through the scar) limit spreading of the scar.[3]

ANATOMICAL CONSIDERATIONS AND PREREQUISITES FOR TRICHOPHYTIC CLOSURE

When planning for trichophytic closure, all the principles that are followed for nontrichophytic closure should be followed. Scalp laxity should be optimal. A tight scalp or a wide strip can lead to increased tissue tension during closure, which may result in a wide or hypertrophic scar. The width of the strip is an important factor that influences the final outcome of the donor scar. Maintaining optimal width is important. Minimizing transection of follicles, during strip harvest, will ensure proper growth of these follicles at the edge of the scar. This helps to optimize the benefit accrued from the trichophytic closure. Use of magnification, clean field (use of

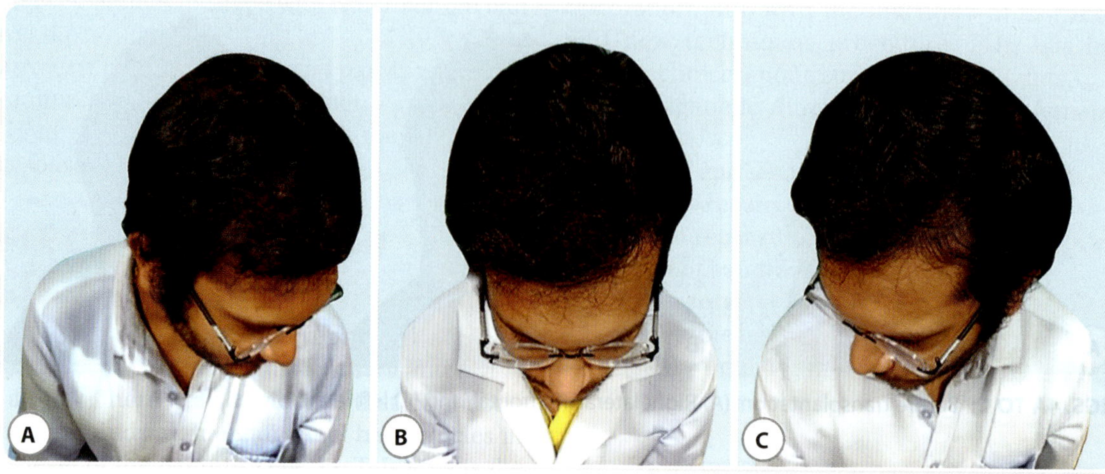

FIGS. 5A TO C: Same patient 12 months postoperation with 3,900 follicular unit grafts (FUGs) and having 10,800 hair follicles.

Such patients may need harvesting from multiple donor areas, including beard, chest, back, forearm, and other areas. In the author's opinion, 1,200–1,500 grafts from the scalp donor area are necessary for frontal hairline and frontal area to create naturalness **(Figs. 6A and B)**. In patients with advanced baldness, behind this area, nonscalp area grafts can be implanted for better coverage of balding scalp while selecting patients with advance degree of baldness and compromised scalp donor area. Hence, proper examination of the nonscalp area is equally important as many patients do not have sufficient density in beard and other nonscalp donor areas. SMP also has a role in supplementing hair transplant when the patient runs out of, or does not have enough, donor hair.[13]

Candidates of any age group with unrealistic expectation (such as coverage of entire scalp from frontal area to vertex in one sitting) should be discouraged. Candidates with body dysmorphic syndrome will never be satisfied with even good hair restoration work and hence should be avoided.

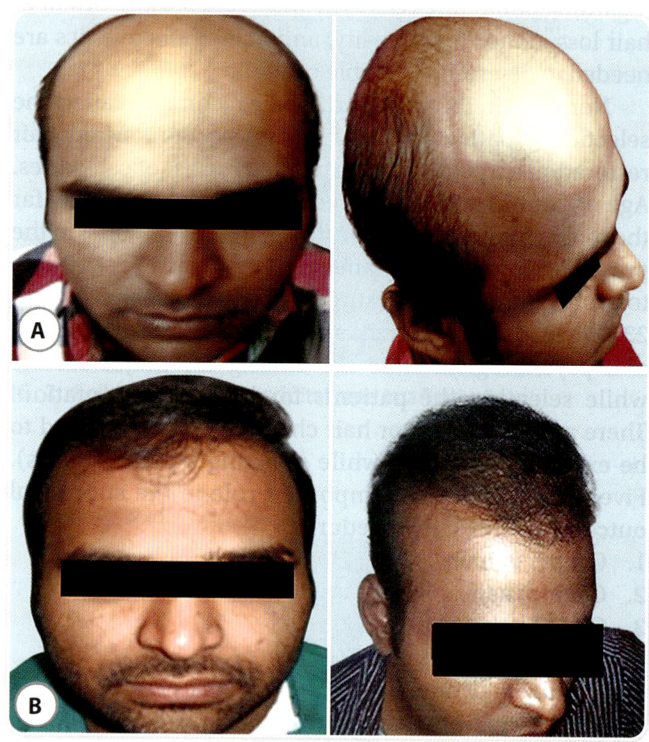

FIGS. 6A AND B: (A) A 26-year-old man with a poor scalp donor, Norwood class VII: Before pictures. (B) After 18 months and a total of 3,500 FUGs were transplanted (1,600 scalp FUGs and 1,900 beard and chest FUGs).

(FUGs: follicular unit grafts)

Selection of Female Candidates for Follicular Unit Extraction (Figs. 7 and 8)

The reader is referred to the chapter 83 Hair transplantation in female pattern hair loss for details. FUE can be performed safely in women, as trimming over donor is not an issue—hair from above covers the trimmed area easily. Ludwig grade II, pattern baldness patients are the most suitable candidates for selection.

Selection of female patients for hair restoration is always challenging, unlike male pattern hair loss (MPHL). The etiopathogenesis of female pattern hair loss (FPHL) is multifactorial, and many causes may coexist in the same patient. It is important that a woman with hair loss undergoes full history, clinical examination, and investigations prior to case selection. Women with Ludwig class II baldness are good candidates for the hair

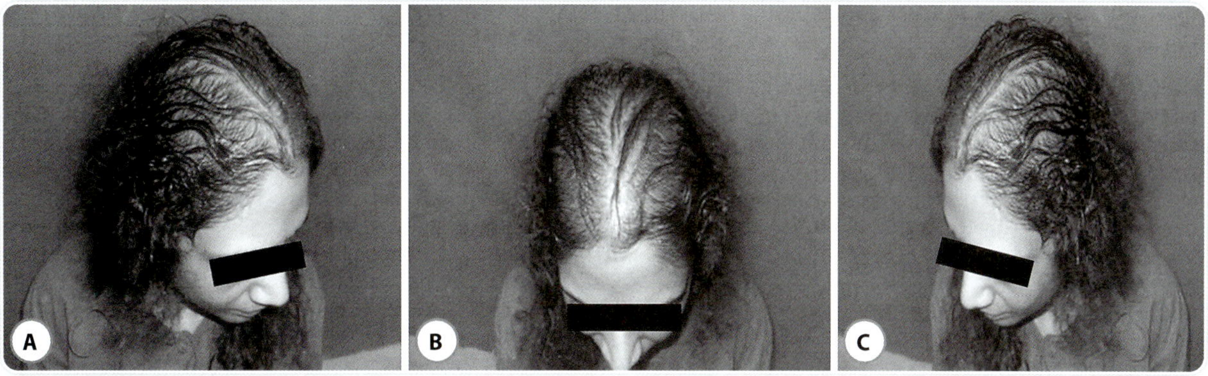

FIGS. 7A TO C: FPHL before grafting.
(FPHL: female pattern hair loss)

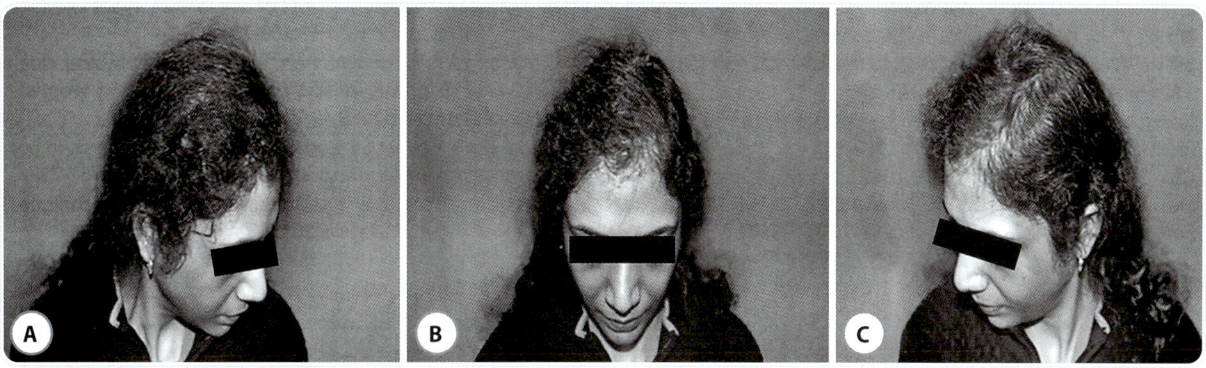

FIGS. 8A TO C: Results in FPHL after grafting 1,050 FUGs.
(FPHL: female pattern hair loss; FUGs: follicular unit grafts)

transplant.[14-16] Even 1,000–1,200 grafts are sufficient to produce satisfactory results. Women with Ludwig class III baldness are always poor candidates for the surgery because there is diffuse thinning all over the scalp, including occipital area, and the chances of getting good-quality grafts are low. With the advancement in the field of scalp micropigmentation, it is now possible to select any female candidates. Scalp micropigmentation is a cosmetic treatment where the provider deposits tiny dots of medical-grade pigment color on the scalp. These dots give you a way to make it look like you have fuller thicker hair.

INDICATIONS OTHER THAN ANDROGENETIC ALOPECIA

One of the advantages of FUE is that it can be performed for several indications as follows:

- Cicatricial alopecia
- Reconstruction of eyebrows and eyelashes
- Repair surgery
- Burn scar repair
- Vitiligo surgery

CONTRAINDICATION

In the author's opinion, there is no absolute contraindication of FUE hair transplant. However, one can avoid selecting candidates in the following situations:

- Extremely curly hairs as chances of transection of follicles are high.
- Patients with unrealistic expectations.
- Patient with large bald areas and not willing for nonscalp harvesting of the grafts or has a poor nonscalp donor.

SUMMARY

The FUE surgical procedure is an important advancement in the field of hair restoration surgery. With proper instrumentation and newer techniques, it is now possible to select almost all patients for FUE procedures. However, curly hairs of African American patients may require a patch test to confirm the patient's candidacy. In the author's opinion, success in the FUE procedure depends on customization of every candidate of baldness in different ways; in fact, even poor scalp donor candidates can be selected if their nonscalp donor area is good.[17,18]

REFERENCES

1. Harris JA. New methodology and instrumentation for follicular unit extraction: lower follicle transection rates and expanded patient candidacy. Dermatol Surg. 2006;32:56-62.
2. Onda M, Igawa HH, Inoue K, Tanino R. Novel technique of follicular unit extraction hair transplantation with a powered punching device. Dermatol Surg. 2008;34:1683-8.
3. Mayer ML, Pauls T. Scalp elasticity scale. Hair Transplant Forum Int. 2005;15:122.
4. Mohebi P, Pak J, Rassman W. How to assess scalp laxity. Hair Transplant Forum Int. 2008;18:167.
5. Rassman WR, Bernstein RM, McClellan R, Jones R, Worton E, Uyttendaele H. Follicular unit extraction: minimally invasive surgery for hair transplantation. Dermatol Surg. 2002;28:720-8.
6. Rassman W, Harris J, Bernstein R. Follicular unit extraction. In: Haber R, Stough DB (Eds). Hair Transplantation. Philadelphia: Elsevier Saunders; 2006. pp. 133-37.
7. Poblet E, Jimenez F, Ortega F. The contribution of the arrector pili muscle and sebaceous glands to the follicular unit structure. J Am Acad Dermatol. 2004;51:217-22.
8. Norwood OT. Male pattern baldness: classification and incidence. South Med J. 1975;68:1359-65.
9. Cole J. Mathematics of follicular unit transplantation. Sixth annual meeting of the International Society of Hair Restoration Surgery, Washington, DC. September 16-20, 1998.
10. Rassman WR, Pak JP, Kim J. Scalp micropigmentation: a valuable technique for use in hair loss. In: Lam SM (Ed). Hair Transplant 360 (Advances, Techniques, Business Development, and Global Perspectives). New Delhi: Jaypee Brothers Medical Publishers; 2014. p. 349.
11. Rassman W, Pak J, Kim J. Combining follicular unit extraction and scalp micropigmentation for the cosmetic treatment of alopecias. Plast Reconstr Surg Glob Open. 2017;5(11):e1420.
12. Cole J. Harvesting the fallows. ISHRS, San Diego, California; 2006.
13. Birch MP, Lalla SC, Messenger AG. Female pattern hair loss. Clin Exp Dermatol. 2002;27:383-8.
14. Ludwig E. Classification of the types of androgenetic alopecia (common baldness) occurring in the female sex. Br J Dermatol. 1977;97:247-54.
15. Hamilton JB. Patterned loss of hair in man: types and incidence. Ann NY Acad Sci. 1951;53:708-28.
16. Olsen EA. The midline part: an important physical clue to the clinical diagnosis of androgenetic alopecia in women. J Am Acad Dermatol. 1999;40:106-9.
17. Saxena K, Savant SS. Body to scalp: evolving trends in body hair transplant. Indian Dermatol Online J. 2017;8(3):167-75.
18. Saxena K. Beard over scalp matching a novel technique. ISHRS Annual Meet, Malaysia; 2013.

CHAPTER 50

Physics of Follicular Unit Excision

Aniketh Venkataram, Deeksha Rao Venkataram

Key Messages

- Knowledge of torque and rotations per minute (RPM) parameters is crucial to enable optimal harvest.
- Keep the torque settings as low as needed based on the laxity.
- Set the angular speed settings as high as tolerated based on the hair diameter.
- This combination would hit the sweet spot of having low transection while optimizing the speed of harvest.

INTRODUCTION

Follicular unit excision (FUE) is the preferred technique of hair transplantation worldwide, accounting for nearly 80% of all cases performed. The reasons for its popularity are easy to comprehend: No significant scarring, minimal pain, rapid healing, and less staff requirements.[1,2]

The technique involves the use of a hollow punch to separate the graft from its adhesions, which is then removed and grafted. Some of the criticisms of this technique include the tendency for graft transection and a longer time needed for surgery. While initially handheld nonpowered punches were used for this purpose, innovations led to the development of motorized punches. Many further innovations have been developed to minimize transection and increase speed. Some of these innovations include punch modifications and variations in motor design, for example, rotatory, oscillatory, and multiphasic.[3-6]

Surprisingly, there is a dearth of literature on the relationship between the physics of motors and FUE harvest. We believe that this is a fundamental concept of FUE harvest, and knowledge of the same can greatly benefit surgeons.

BASICS OF DRILL PHYSICS

The two most important parameters for a drill are torque and angular speed [measured in rotations per minute (RPM)].[7]

Torque is a measurement of the force with which the drill rotates. Just as force is what causes an object to have linear acceleration, torque is what causes an object to have angular acceleration. In drill terms, the more resistance to drilling, the greater the torque required. Torque is not a direct representation of speed. If a drill does not have enough torque to overcome the resistance presented, the slower it will work.

Angular speed is a simpler concept to understand. It is the number of times the drill head completes a 360° rotation in 1 minute and is measured in RPM. A drill can rotate at the same RPM with different torque settings. Intuitively, this tells us that the higher the RPM, the faster the drill will rotate, provided it has enough torque to overcome the resistance presented.

Next, we need to understand the relation between torque and angular speed, which work in tandem to produce power.

$$\begin{aligned}\text{Power of a drill (Watts)} &= \text{energy (Joules)/time (seconds)}\\ &= \text{torque (Nm)} \times \text{angular speed (RPM)} \times K\end{aligned}$$

where K is a constant and equals $2\pi/60$.

This equation tells us that power is directly proportional to both torque and angular speed. But what is more important to us in the world of hair transplantation is the transection rate of grafts and the time taken for the harvest.

The time taken is inversely proportional to the power applied, that is, inversely proportional to both torque and angular speed. If we raise either of these parameters, the time taken to perform the procedure will reduce.

Energy is directly proportional to both torque and angular speed. Raising both parameters would increase the energy delivered to the graft during harvest. It stands to reason that the higher the energy delivered to the graft, the higher the chance of transection.

Hence, the balancing act we must play is to calibrate our torque and angular speed settings so that we can reduce the time taken for the harvest while not delivering too much energy that can potentially damage the graft.

GRAFT CHARACTERISTICS

In overly simplified terms, the two components of a graft are the follicle itself and the perifollicular soft tissue. As we engage our drill on the soft tissue, the strength or weakness of this tissue represents the resistance the drill has to overcome.[8]

The follicle itself is what we are most interested in protecting. Transection of the follicle is what characterizes a failed graft harvest. Hence, the follicle strength represents the upper limit of the energy we can expend during graft harvest.[9]

$$\text{Breaking force} = \text{Breaking stress} \times \text{area of cross-section,}$$
and breaking stress is a constant for a given material.

Hence, the most important parameter indicating the strength of a follicle to be broken is its area of cross-section, for which the diameter is a proxy.

STUDY

We performed a study on the role of angular speed and torque parameters to optimize the FUE graft harvest for minimal time and number of transections. Patients undergoing FUE for the first time were selected for the study after due consent. A total of 20 patients were chosen, 10 for torque variation and 10 for RPM variation.

All patients were analyzed before the procedure for the following:

- Hair density as measured by TrichoScan over the occipital area
- Hair thickness as measured by TrichoScan over the occipital area
- Tissue laxity measured by resistance to stretching. For this, two points were marked over the occipital scalp 2 cm apart. These two points were maximally stretched with skin hooks and the new distance was noted. The change in distance was calculated as a percentage of the original reading. This essentially measures the tissue strain or laxity.

FOLLICULAR UNIT EXCISION HARVEST

We decided to analyze the effect of varying torque and angular speed independently. Based on our prior records, we saw that the most common setting we used was 11 Nm torque and 1,100 RPM angular speed. We decided to use this as the baseline and have one higher and one lower setting in this design of experiments (DOE).

Torque Variation

- The angular speed was kept constant at 1,100 RPM.
- 100 grafts were harvested at torque settings of 7, 11, and 15 Nm.
- This was done in each of the 10 patients.

Angular Speed Variation

- The torque was kept constant at 11 Nm.
- 100 grafts were harvested at RPM settings of 700, 1,100, and 1,500.
- This was done in each of the 10 patients.

OUTCOMES

The harvest was analyzed for the following:

- Time taken per 100 grafts
- Number of transections—partial and total
- Suction of follicles into the punch

RESULTS

Torque Variation

Effect on Time

On average, increasing torque led to a reduction in the time taken to harvest the grafts, although this was not uniformly reproduced in all cases **(Fig. 1)**.

Effect on Transection Rate

- At low tissue laxity, 15 Nm had the lowest transection rate.
- At intermediate laxity, 11 Nm had the lowest transection rate.
- At high laxity, 7 Nm had the lowest transection rate.

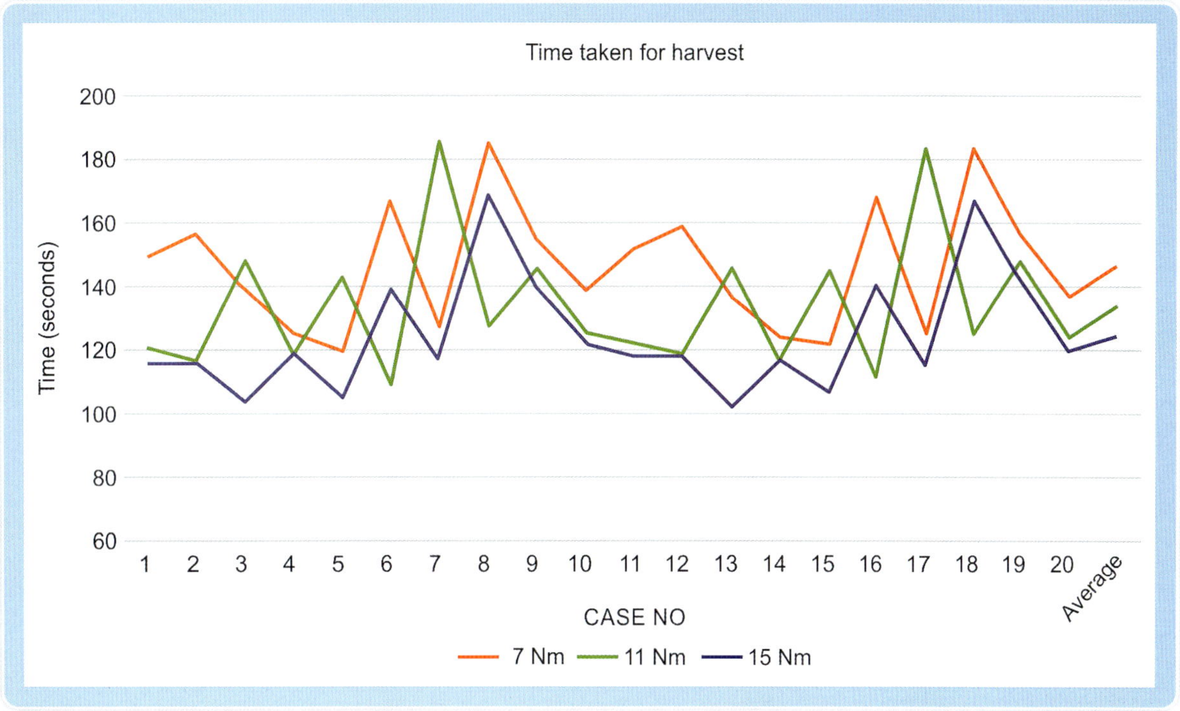

FIG. 1: Variation of time taken with torque.

This data suggests that the lower the tissue laxity, the higher the torque required **(Fig. 2)**.

Effect of Hair Diameter

No discernible pattern was found between torque and hair diameter **(Fig. 3)**.

Angular Speed Variation

With increasing angular speeds, the time taken to perform the harvest is reduced. This was seen in almost every case **(Fig. 4)**.

Effect of Angular Speed on Transection Rate

With lower hair diameter, 700 RPM speed had the lowest transection rate, while 1,100 and 1,500 RPM speeds had higher transection rates.

At intermediate diameter, 1,500 RPM had higher transection, while 700 and 1,100 RPM were comparable. At high diameter, all three speed settings had comparable transection rates.

This data shows that the higher the hair diameter, the higher the speed tolerability **(Fig. 5)**.

No discernible patterns were found between angular speed and tissue laxity **(Fig. 6)**.

OTHER FINDINGS

It was incidentally found that at higher angular speeds, there was a tendency for grafts to be sucked into the core of the punch rather than be left behind in the tissue bed. This tended to slow down the harvest as the graft stuck in the core had to be extracted before the harvest could continue.

DISCUSSION

Time Taken

We noticed that the average time taken reduced as both torque and RPM were increased. However, this correlation was more noticeable with angular speed than with torque, and this was felt clinically as well. Hence, if we had to increase one setting to reduce the time taken, we would choose to increase the angular speed.

Torque

The torque required is dependent on the amount of resistance the drill has to overcome. To measure this resistance, we used tissue laxity. The more lax and pliable the tissue, the less resistance it offers. In our study, we saw that with lower laxity, higher torque was needed to reduce

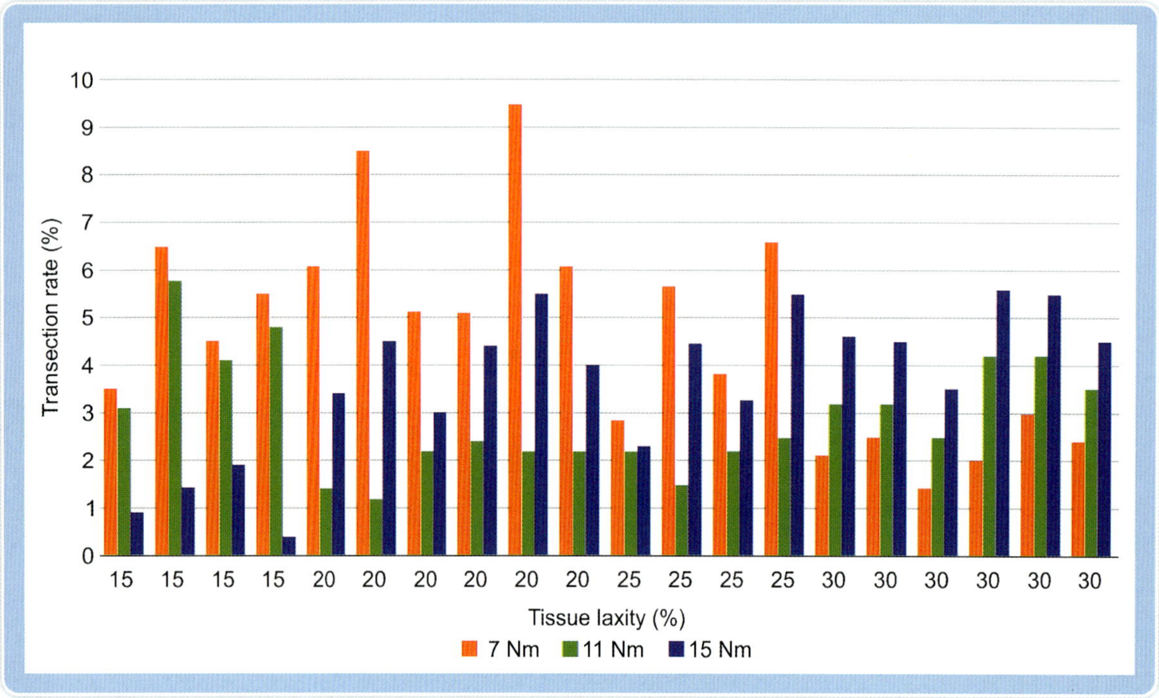

FIG. 2: Correlation between torque and tissue laxity.

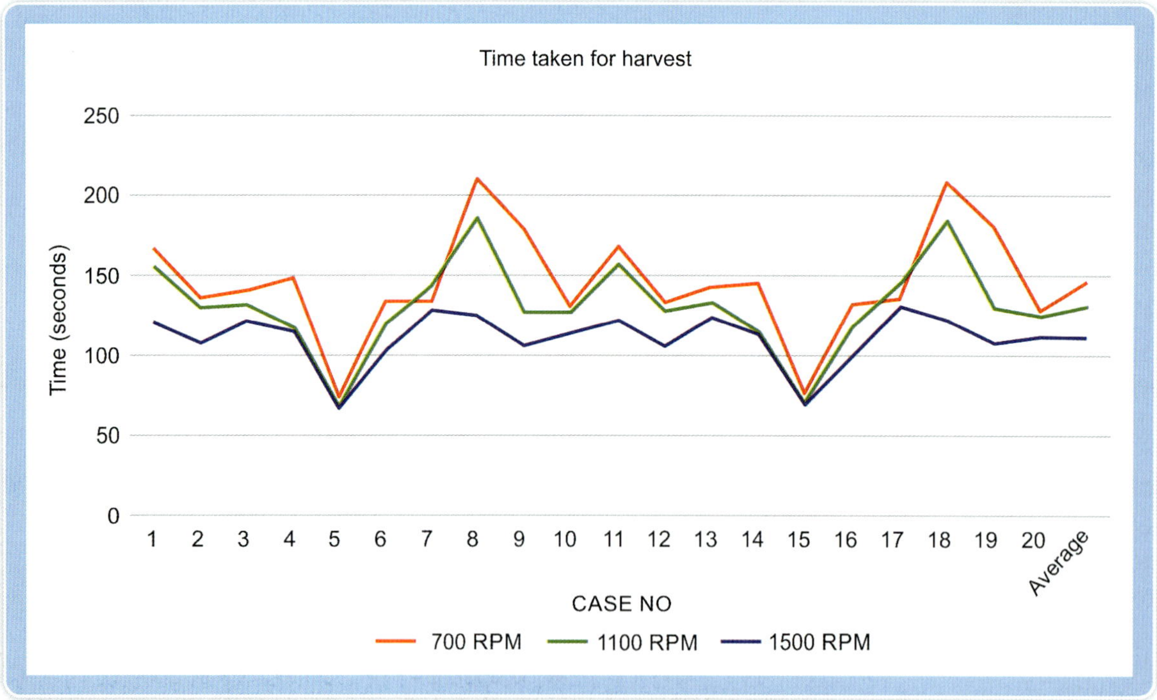

FIG. 3: Correlation between torque and hair diameter.

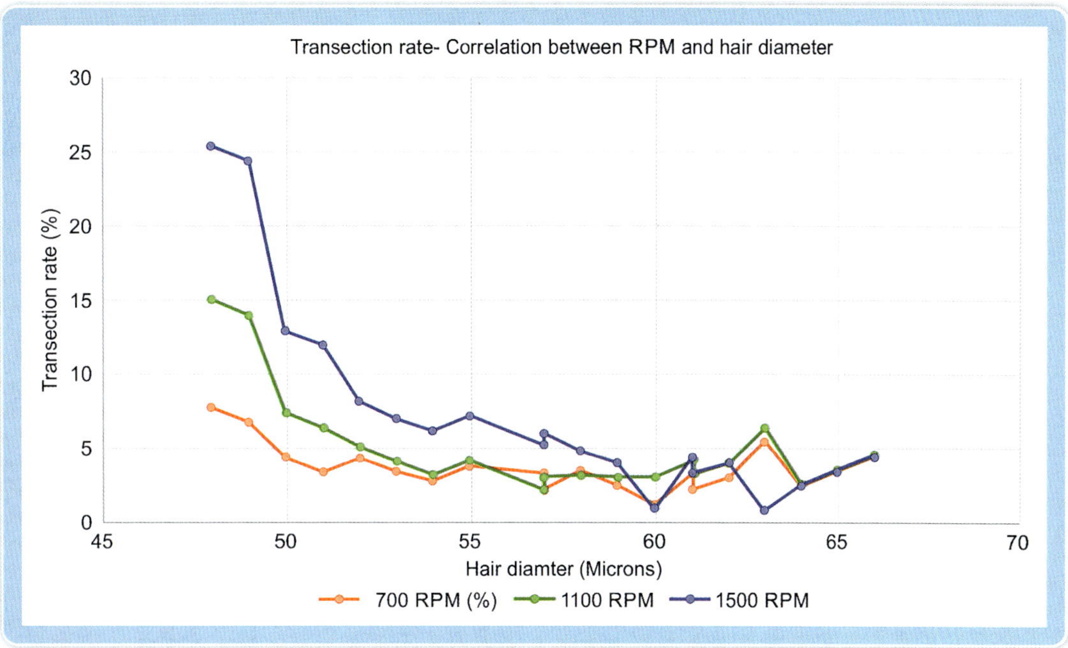

FIG. 4: Variation of time taken with change in RPM.
(RPM: rotations per minute).

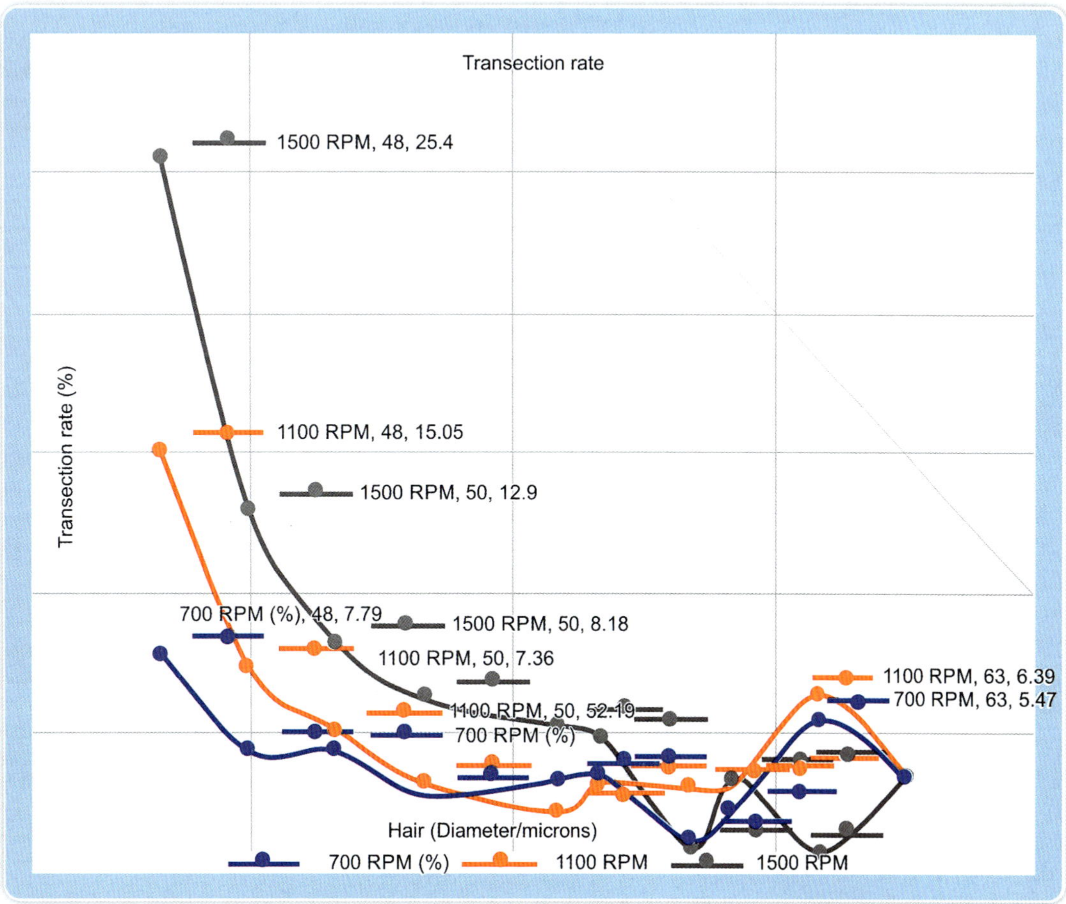

FIG. 5: Correlation between RPM and hair diameter.
(RPM: rotations per minute)

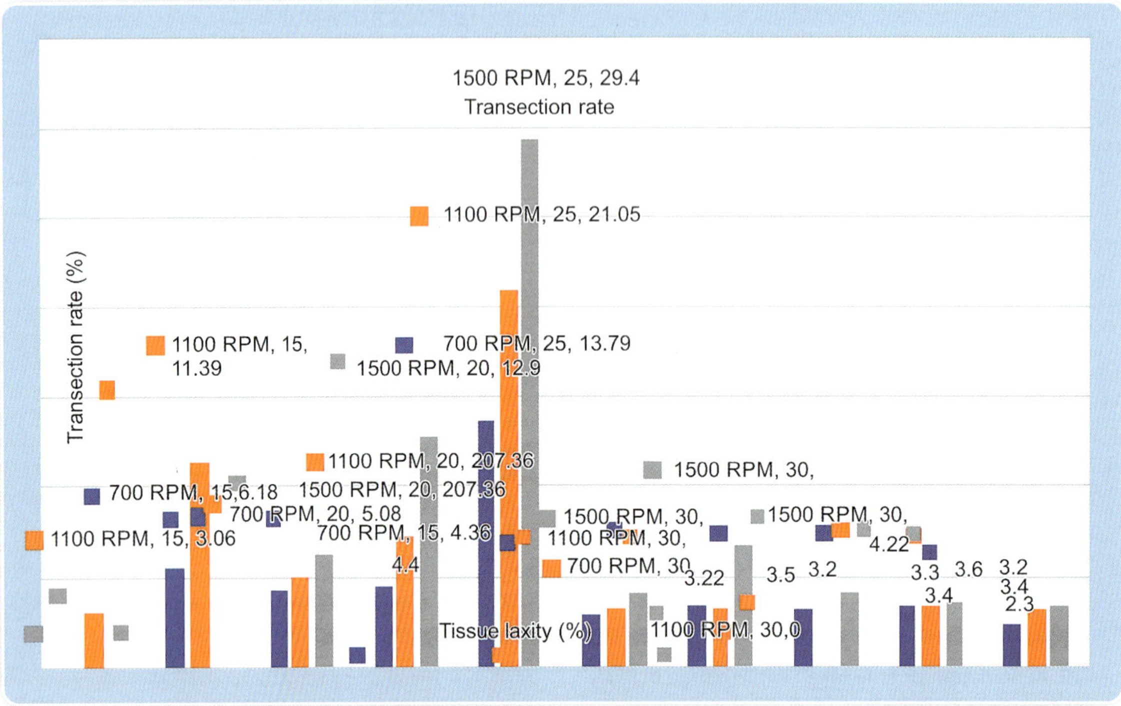

FIG. 6: Correlation between RPM and tissue laxity.
(RPM: rotations per minute)

transection rate, while low and intermediate torque settings did not fare as well. As the laxity increased, lower torque settings performed well. We could not discern any noticeable pattern with hair diameter. Hence, we believe that there is a minimum amount of torque needed for a particular skin quality in order to be able to perform the harvest.

Angular Speed

Angular speed refers to the rate at which the drill rotates. As mentioned already, it has a significant effect on the time taken for the harvest. We did not notice any pattern between angular speed and tissue laxity. At low hair diameter, the transection rate was lowest at a low RPM setting. As the hair diameter increased, higher RPM levels were tolerated. Hence, we believe that angular speed can be increased up to a certain threshold depending on the hair diameter, beyond which transection rates would be unacceptable.

At the same time, we also noticed that at higher angular speed settings, there was a tendency for grafts to be sucked into the punch and had to be extracted. This can be explained by Bernoulli's principle, which states that an increase in speed leads to a decrease in pressure. This slowed down the harvest, though the grafts were uninjured. If we found this happening, we would reduce the RPM till the suction was not seen.

TABLE 1: Adjusting torque and rotations per minute (RPM) based on tissue laxity and hair diameter.

	High laxity (low resistance)	Low laxity (high resistance)
Low hair diameter	Lower torque Lower RPM	Higher torque Lower RPM
High hair diameter	Lower torque Higher RPM	Higher torque Higher RPM

Calibrating Settings

With these findings, our process is to keep the torque settings as low as needed based on the laxity and the angular speed settings as high as tolerated based on the hair diameter. This combination would hit the sweet spot of having low transection while optimizing the speed of harvest **(Table 1)**.

APPLICATIONS

The applications of these findings are nearly universal. It is difficult to give an exact figure for torque and RPM to be used, as these would vary from person to person based on machine, punch, operator force, etc. We found that 11 Nm and 1,100 RPM were our most common settings. We would advise all practitioners to find their most common settings and then vary them as needed:

- From patient to patient—as described above
- Within the same patient, from donor area to area. For example, chest donor usually has fine hair and RPM would have to be kept low. Beard has thicker hair and RPM can be increased.
- Within the same donor area. For example, the lower occipital scalp offers more resistance and torque would have to be increased. The higher parietal scalp offers less resistance and torque can be lowered.

There is an increasing tendency for FUE instruments to get more complicated and thereby more expensive. While several of these innovations are useful and scientific, to ignore the very basics of drill physics is putting the cart before the horse. Whatever the characteristics of a given machine, they work on the principles of torque and angular speed. Understanding how to vary these can help one get consistent harvest with almost any instrument. At the same time, these are pretty basic settings in any micromotor drill and would be an inexpensive way to optimize harvesting.

The limitations of this study include the vagaries of tissue and hair quality between different individuals. We have tried to minimize this by having each patient act as its own control and perform the different settings for comparison in each patient. Operator bias was reduced by having all harvests performed by a single operator. The same punch and motor were used in all cases to reduce instrument errors.

SUMMARY

In conclusion, based on our findings, we believe that the ideal mechanism to optimize harvest is to keep the torque as low as needed and the angular speed as high as tolerated to optimize harvest. This would enable us to reduce the time taken for the harvest while also reducing the energy delivered and hence the grafts transected. We hope these findings enable hair transplant surgeons to optimize their harvest techniques.

REFERENCES

1. International Society of Hair Restoration Surgery (2015) Practice Census results. International Society of Hair Restoration Surgery, 303 West State Street, Geneva, IL 60134, USA. [online] Available from http://www.ishrs.org/statistics-research.htm. [Last accessed September, 2023].
2. Rassman WR, Bernstein RM, McClellan R, Jones R, Worton E, Uyttendaele H. Follicular unit extraction: minimally invasive surgery for hair transplantation. Dermatol Surg. 2002;28:720-8.
3. Cole JP. An analysis of follicular punches, mechanics, and dynamics in follicular unit extraction. Facial Plast Surg Clin North Am. 2013;21(3):437-47.
4. Cole JP. Follicular extraction punch and method. Patent US. 2005;2005(0203545):A1
5. Ng B, Harris JA. How I do it: powered blunt dissection with the SAFE system for FUE (part 1). Hair Transplant Forum Int. 2010;20(6):188-9.
6. Tykocinski A. Dealing with a Hybrid Trumpet punch. Hair Transplant Forum Int. 2017;27(1):14-6.
7. https://www.dewalt.ca/why-dewalt/featured-articles/what-torque-really-means#:~:text=Torque%20is%20the%20force%20the,actually%20needed%20to%20complete%20applications.
8. Dumitrescu TF, Pesce GLA, Ball RJ. Optimization of drilling resistance measurement (DRM) user-controlled variables. Mater Struct. 2017;50:243.
9. Question. [online] Available from https://www.toppr.com/ask/question/a-force-f-is-required-to-break-a-wire-of/. [Last accessed September, 2023].

CHAPTER 51

Follicular Unit Excision: Instrumentation and Technique

Kuldeep Saxena

Key Messages

- Follicular unit excision (FUE) procedures have advanced progressively from manual to powered to robotic FUE.
- Many variations have been observed in the field of FUE technique.
- Proper understanding of various techniques gives an idea to the beginners to finally decide instruments and methodology that suit them.
- Several devices have been developed by surgeons. However, punch plays a significant role in the successful outcome of the FUE procedure.

INTRODUCTION

Follicular unit excision (FUE) has brought about transformational evolution in the management of alopecia, mainly pattern baldness. When compared to the strip harvesting method, the technique of FUE involves less trauma, faster healing, and less visible scarring. These advantages have contributed to changing the image of hair restoration surgery and a greater demand for hair transplant surgeries among patients of male and female pattern baldness.

Rassman et al.[1] published the first paper on the methodology of FUE, utilizing 1-mm sharp punches manually, and called it FOX procedure.[2,3] Dr Ray Woods and Angela Campbell from Australia had earlier practiced FUE, but they never shared their technique with other physicians. While manual techniques undoubtedly benefited patients as well as surgeons, longer operating time, higher rates of transection, and tedious and laborious work limited the transplant size. The evolution of the technique in the last decade has seen the introduction of newer instrumentation and innovative techniques, which have contributed to lesser operative time, larger (mega) sessions, less fatigue, and decreased transection rate.[4-7]

Beginners entering the field of FUE hair restoration surgery should understand each and every technique and instruments used for graft harvesting and finally decide the instruments and methodology that suit them. Unlike other surgeries where rigid recommendations and specifications about technique, methods, and instruments can be provided, in FUE hair transplant surgery, innumerable differences are being observed, from surgeon to surgeon. The subject is evolving, and many of the innovations do not have the support of publications but are nevertheless significant and need consideration. The basic logic of FUE is as follows:

- Follicular unit (FU) is the best architectural unit of hairs.
- Preservation of the units and transplantation of the units in their natural pattern yield the best cosmetic results.
- The unit is pyramidal in shape with a wider bottom and a narrow top.
- The narrowest and also the tightest part is where the arrectores muscle holds the hairs together.[8]
- If the hold of arrectores is loosened, then the units become loose and come out easily.
- It is possible to loosen the hold with a small punch < 1 mm in diameter.

IMPORTANT INSTRUMENTS USED IN FOLLICULAR UNIT EXCISION

Proper selection of instruments while performing FUE is the most important factor that contributes to the successful outcome of the procedure. Handles, punches, and tensioners are important tools in the FUE procedure. Apart from these, there are various devices and systems **(Figs. 1 and 2)**.

Handle

The handle is the tool by which the punch is held, carried, and its depth controlled. There are some different handles for the manual FUE technique. The most popular are the Versi handle and the Cole isolation technique (CIT) manual punch handle. In manual handles, the punch is screwed onto the tip of the handle to fix it, and the body of the handle is held and rotated similar to skin biopsy punches to advance the punch. In motorized FUE devices, the punch is attached to the rotating tip of the handle which uses the rotational movement to advance the punch. This is held with the dominant hand just like holding a pen or whichever way is comfortable to the operating surgeon **(Fig. 3)**.

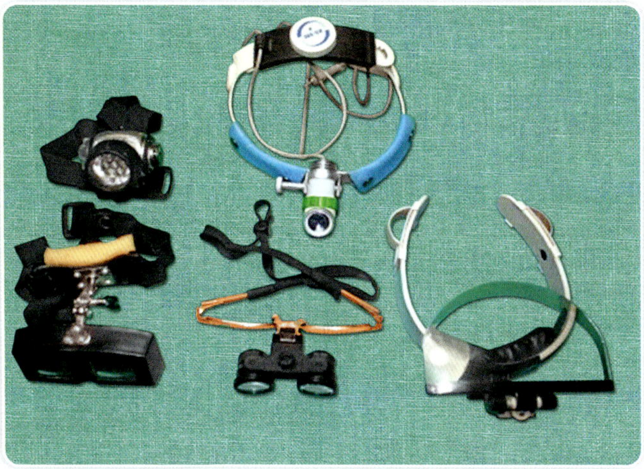

FIG. 1: Various cold light source and magnifying loupes.

Punch

Irrespective of any technique, whether it is manual, power, automated, or robotics, the punch remains the most important tool in the FUE procedure. Various punch sizes ranging from 0.75 to 1.25 mm in diameter are available for FUE. However, 0.8–0.9 mm punches are preferred for scalp FUE, and 0.7 mm is the preferred size for body and beard FUE procedures. An ideal punch should be small enough to minimize the residual scalp defect and to avoid adjacent FU damage but large enough to prevent transection of any individual follicle within the isolated FU. The decision to use a particular size of punch depends on the surgeon's experience and the average diameter of the hair follicles. Punches >1 mm in size may produce visible scarring in the donor area **(Figs. 4 to 6)**.

Types of Punches

- *Cannula punch*: This is a cylindrical punch usually made of stainless steel.
- *Titanium nitride (TiN) punch*: This is a sharp punch whose tip is coated with TiN, so that the punch has a characteristic gold-colored tip. This improves the life span of the sharp cutting edge of the punch.
- *Serrated or wave punch*: This is a punch with a serrated cutting edge that offers small points of contact with the

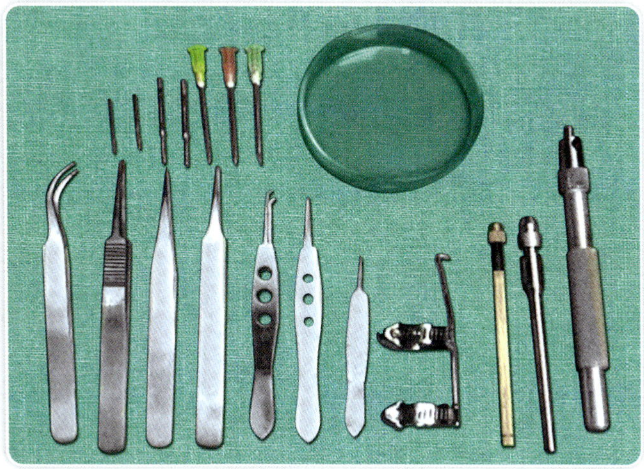

FIG. 2: Surgical instruments used during follicular unit excision (FUE) procedure.

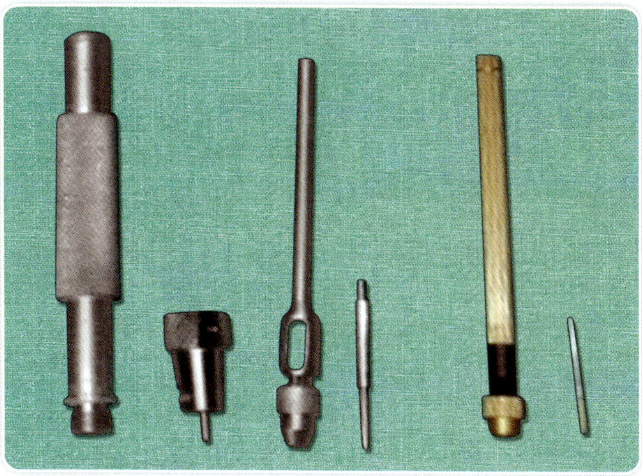

FIG. 3: Various handles used during manual follicular unit excision (FUE).

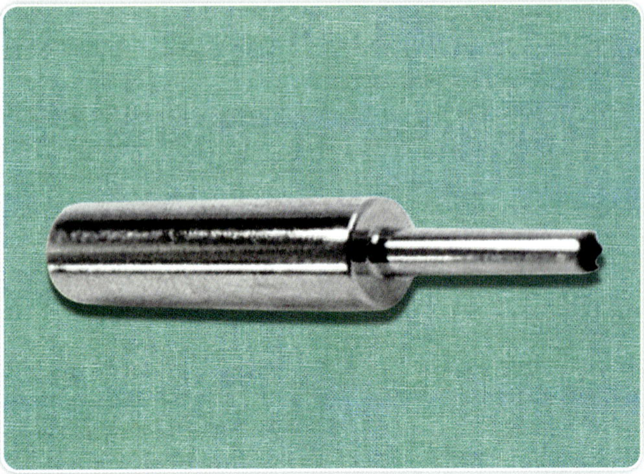

FIG. 4: Serrated punch.

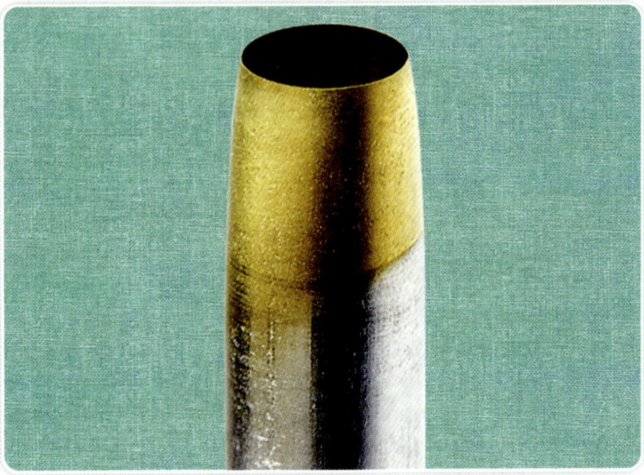

FIG. 5: Tin-coated punch.

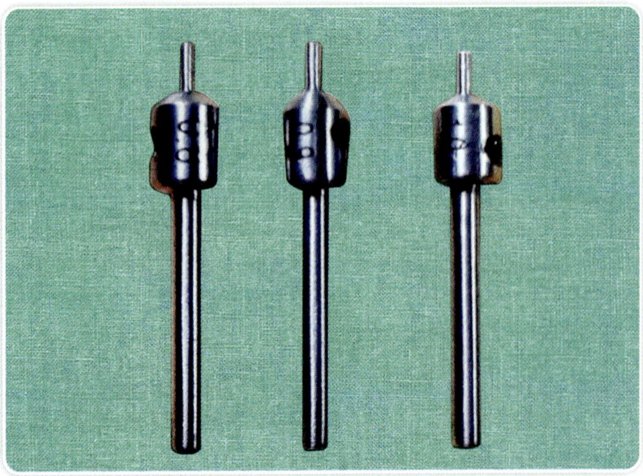

FIG. 6: Sharp punches with guard.

skin. This is also called a triple wave punch; the design reduces the surface area in contact with the skin, thus reducing friction and consequently minimizing axial forces required to cut the skin, which may help in reducing follicular transection rates during harvesting as comparatively lesser force is required.

- Hybrid punches are designed to combine the benefits of sharp and blunt punches; they have a sharp cutting edge that typically flares away **(Fig. 7)**.

Sharp edged-out punch has a cutting edge on the outer part of the bevel to protect the graft inside the punch.

The flared punch has the cutting edge facing outward to protect the graft but also creates a difference in pressure that helps the graft into the punch lumen.

Various Diameters of Punch

All punches have external, internal, and cutting-edge diameters. The cutting-edge diameter is the main measurement of the punch and should be used as the main point of reference while doing the FUE procedure. The cutting edge may be the inside bevel of the punch, outside bevel of the punch, or middle bevel of the punch (depends upon the design of the punch).

Sharpness of Punch

Follicular unit excision punches vary from having a sharpened cutting edge (sharp punch) to an edge that is

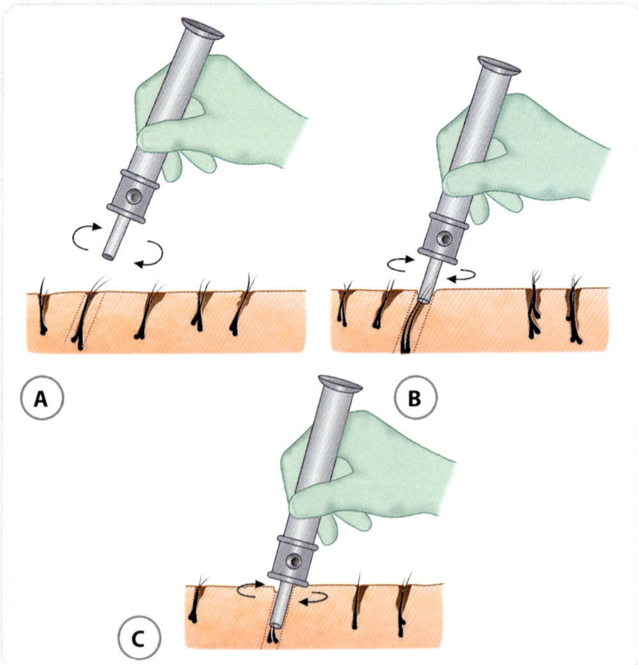

FIGS. 7A TO C: Hybrid punch.

not sharpened (dull punch). Different FUE hair transplant surgeons adopt different approaches; however, with sharp punches, one can finish the procedure in lesser time. Advantages of the sharp punch include the ability to easily penetrate through the scalp and a reduced number of rotations/oscillations required to remove the FU. Its disadvantage is that there is an increased risk of transection of the follicle due to its sharp edge. Advantages of the blunt punch include reduced transection of the FUs and reduced trauma to tissue surrounding the follicles during extraction. Its disadvantage is that an increased number of oscillations/rotations is required to penetrate the scalp and reach an appropriate depth, which creates excessive heat, tension, friction, and torsion on the grafts and the surrounding tissue. Also, more axial force is required which may cause graft displacement and transection. Hence, it is advisable for beginners to begin with blunt punches and graduate to sharp punches later to save time.

Tensioners

The ARTAS Robotic System uses external tissue tensioners to stretch the tissue for efficient superficial cutting of the epidermis and dermis. The KD spreader is a modified skin hook designed and patented by Dr Kuldeep Saxena to act as a skin tissue tensioner. It fits the index finger of the nondominant hand of the surgeon or the assistant. It can be used during graft extraction to give traction and countertraction. It is also useful for dilating the incision sites if grafts are stuck during extraction and for dilating the slits and guiding the grafts into the premade slits during implantation.

Power Devices/Systems Used in Follicular Unit Excision

- *Powered Cole Isolation Device (PCID)*: This programmable device developed by Cole allows for a more precise control of rotation, oscillation, speed, rate, and arc of oscillation.[9]
- *Harris SAFE system*: Developed by Harris, it utilizes an unsharpened, dull, or blunt punch (0.8–1.2 mm) with full rotation at variable speeds and a fixed depth of incision.[10]
- *True device*: Aseptico Porta-Tip—AEU-03SS and Osada SH28S handpiece. This is a rechargeable rotary hand engine with variable speed control and autoclavable handpiece. A silicone collar is fitted onto the punch and adjusted for precise control of incision depth.
- *Alphagraft*: This is another FUE device that uses a rotating sharp punch to harvest follicles from the donor area.
- *Devroye device*: The Devroye WAW system uses short, oscillating arcs from the epidermal to the dermal layer. The Short-Arc-Oscillation Flat Punch FUE System (SFFS) employs a quick and shaking movement that ranges between 180° and 90°. This shaking motion may increase detachment compared to a typical circular movement. The primary benefit of this approach is that it can reach a significant depth in the skin, often up to 4–5 mm, without causing harm to the follicles. The small oscillation arc prevents twisting and reduces torsional stress to the tissue, making it less damaging than rotation movement. As a result, the risk of transection and cutting damage is minimized.[11,12]
- *Mamba device*: The Mamba FUE device, created by Dr Roberto Trivellini, is a versatile programmable motor that combines several features such as in-line suction, complete rotation, oscillation, and vibration. Additionally, it utilizes a distinct "edge-out" punch design characterized by a flat shape. The Trivellini system takes advantage of suction to produce traction on the graft, stretching it and facilitating penetration of the punch. It has a touch-sensitive function called the SmartReact™ system that triggers the preprogrammed suction and rotation/oscillation/roto-oscillation/vibration features once the device makes initial contact with the skin around the FU, eliminating the need for a foot pedal. As a result, the device has been proven to enhance the quality of grafts, minimize damage, and facilitate a more gentle extraction process.[13-16]
- Dr UGraft Zeus is an all-purpose FUE device that can perform a wide range of hair extraction procedures. It is capable of extracting hair from the head, regardless of whether it is shaved or not, and is suitable for people of all ethnic backgrounds. The device can also extract hair from the beard and body, as well as harvest long-haired grafts without the need to switch punches, drivers, or acquire specialized skills. One of the main advantages of this device is that it addresses the issues that often lead to inconsistent performance in FUE devices, such as changes in skin firmness and thickness. It also overcomes the challenges associated with unpredictable hair curliness and angles by utilizing its own technology to navigate hair follicles, which is an area where FUE practitioners often face difficulties. The device includes a user-friendly dashboard with a personalized tab, allowing users to input their preferred settings, such as speed, torque, and three different movement modes. Additionally, users have the option to specify the duration of each movement mode and choose between automatic and manual retrieval of scores, which can be activated

using a foot pedal. In automatic mode, users can select intervals ranging from 0 to 4 seconds with increments of 0.25. Moreover, if the operator selects a preset, they may need to adjust any of the mentioned parameters to accommodate a specific skin phenotype.

An all-purpose punch called the Intelligent Punch—Dr UPunch i—is used, which is frustoconically shaped and has been optimized at multiple levels to incorporate solutions to several technical challenges known to contribute to FUE graft attrition (lost or nonviable grafts from transections, crush injuries, and complete desheathing), poor scarring profiles, and user experiences.[17,18]

- *KD's FUE station*: KD's FUE extractor claims a precise and fast FUE extraction process even in a beginner's hand when compared with a conventional or dental motorized tool. Decimal fraction control of repetition per minute (RPM) through microprocessor-based control of a motorized tool allows the physician to adjust RPM minutely, thus reducing transection of the grafts even in a beginner's hand. The device has a user-friendly touchscreen allowing users to minutely control the rotation and oscillation of the tool.[19]

Automated Devices/System Used in Follicular Unit Excision

Automated FUE is a term used for suction-assisted FUE where the device performs all the steps of hair transplantation from harvesting of grafts to implantation of grafts in the recipient area. Presently available Neograft and SmartGraft automated systems work on the principle of suction-assisted follicle extraction and follicle storage, follicle handling, and implantation.[20]

In the automated harvesting process, a rotating punch dissects the tissue around the hair shaft just past the follicle depth. As soon as it crosses the dermal layer and touches the loose fatty layer, the suction force is exerted. This prevents trauma while extracting FUs as the process of extraction is untouched. Punched grafts are collected in a container attached to the handpiece of the machine through special tubes.

Both Neograft and SmartGraft systems use a rotating punch for scoring the grafts and negative pneumatic pressure for suction of grafts. These devices claim precise and fast FUE compared with other motorized systems. However, a major drawback of this system is an increased transection rate of grafts because you have to advance the punch a little bit deeper to entirely cut the surrounding follicular tissues.

ARTAS robotic hair transplant system: This is a computer-assisted and physician-controlled system that combines numerous features, including image-guided robotic arm, dissection punch, and vision mapping, as well as tracking technology.[21] This device claims precise and fast FUE compared with other motorized tools, but major drawbacks of this system are as follows:

- It is prohibitively expensive.
- Extraction is possible from only the occipital zone.
- Pulling and storage of graft is still manual.

How ARTAS Works—the ARTAS Hair Studio™

Surgery is performed while the patient is in a prone position with their face down in the pillow. After infiltration of local anesthesia over the donor area, ARTAS uses an external tissue tensioner to stretch the tissue and thereby increase the distance between two FUs.

Robotic FUE involves a two-step process for graft harvesting, where a V-sharp punch first pierces the skin followed by an unsharpened rotating punch inserted deeper to release the graft. Vision mapping and tracking technology evaluates follicular density and hair exit angle based on the physician input data. Liberated grafts are finally plucked manually with forceps.

(Details of ARTAS can be referred to from the chapter 74 on Robotic Hair Transplantation).

TECHNIQUES OF FOLLICULAR UNIT EXCISION

Techniques of FUE are mainly divided into manual and power FUE.

Characteristics of the Techniques

- *Rotating extraction*: The punch is rotated a full 360° cycle in the same direction during penetration of the skin. This is usually performed by a motor. This method is more commonly used.
- *Oscillating extraction*: The punch is rotated back and forth in opposite directions through different arcs, going deeper at fixed or variable RPM during penetration. This may be performed by hand or by motor.
- *Rotating and oscillating extraction*: This is a combination where rotation is followed by an oscillation and is employed during penetration of the punch. The duration of each individual cycle can also be simultaneously controlled.

Manual Follicular Unit Excision

Sharp and dull punches (sizes 0.8–1.1 mm) or their combination can be used for graft extraction. In a one-step method, the punch is inserted to the desired depth

(3–4 mm) in a single incision, using a rotational force or oscillating force (tangential forces) and axial force (force exerted by the operator parallel to the axis of the punch) or a combination of rotational and oscillation forces. In a two-step method, a sharp punch is used initially to score the skin using a rotational or oscillating force along with axial force. Then, either another sharp or dull punch or needle is inserted through the same incision to the desired depth using a rotational or oscillating action to free the FU from the attachment of arrector pili muscles. Freed grafts can then be collected with a forceps and stored **(Figs. 8 and 9)**.

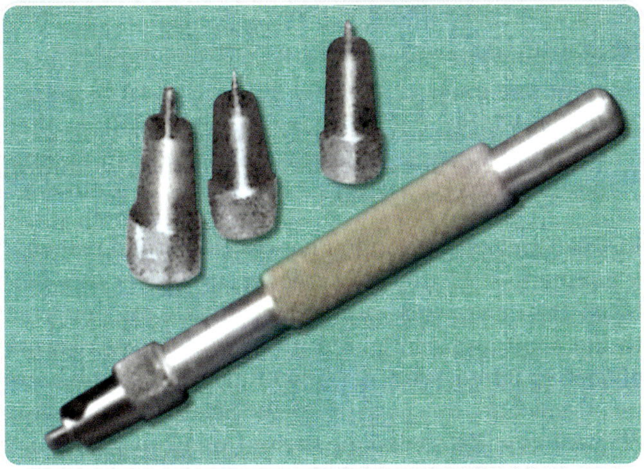

FIG. 8: Manual follicular unit excision (FUE) instrument.

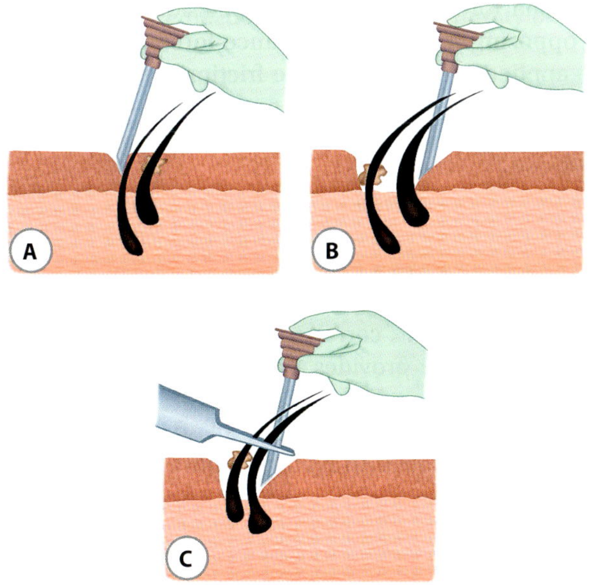

FIGS. 9A TO C: Follicular unit excision (FUE) using a manual punch.

Important Points

- *Donor tension or traction*: Tension is applied to the donor area to stabilize the hair follicles over the underlying tissue for proper extraction. It is applied by a variety of means, including tumescence, clamps, and manual or stretching forces applied by other means, such as simple manual pulling by the assistant or tensioners or stapling a latex material from one side of the scalp to the other or by using a KD spreader, an author-patented device.[22,23]
- *Scoring*: Incision of the epidermis and dermis with the punch, which produces circumferential or circular incision around a FU, to free it of the surrounding soft-tissue attachments is called scoring. Depth control is very important while scoring. Tactile feedback correlating with resistance in tissue and hair shaft provides a clue to the surgeon while scoring deeper into the skin. Resistance is felt on cutting the arrector pili muscle, and the punch may transect the roots if scoring is carried out beyond this point. An average depth of punch insertion while scoring is 2–4 mm in the scalp.
- *Pulling*: It involves giving anterior traction for the removal of the grafts, after it has been punch incised. The graft may be pulled with one hand, with a single forceps, or two hands with two forceps. The pulling forces must be parallel to the direction of hair growth and directed upward or outward from the hair follicle.

Power Follicular Unit Excision

Manual FUE methods are time consuming, and different transection rates are reported by different surgeons. Power FUE utilizing motor-driven punches allows for more precise control of rotation, oscillation, arc of oscillation, and speed with lesser rates of transection **(Figs. 10 and 11)**.

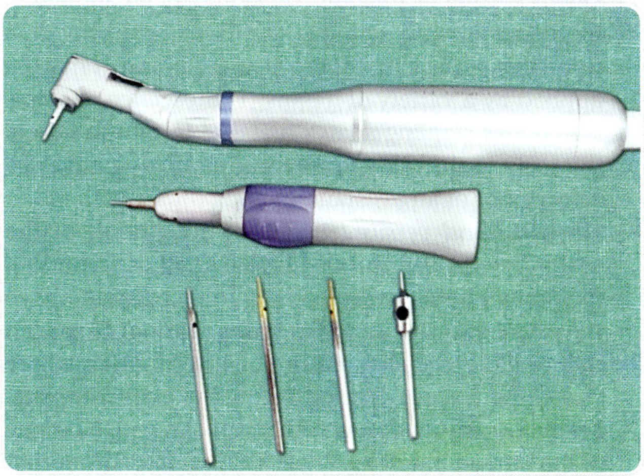

FIG. 10: Straight and contra-angle handpiece of follicular unit excision (FUE) device.

Tips and Pearls

Finally, the most important aspect of FUE is transection—every effort needs to be made to avoid transection, and the following steps are offered as tips:

- Depth control when punch produces incision.
- Proper position of the operating surgeon and patients.
- Prone position for occipital area FUE and lateral decubitus position for temporoparietal area.
- Traction and countertraction over the donor area.
- Use of tensioners or spreaders, especially on tight scalp.
- Adequate lighting and proper magnification are essential.
- Insertion of punch at the proper angle during FUE.
- Repeated checking of grafts during the procedure.
- Anterior or lateral traction over the donor area while collecting punched grafts.

SUMMARY

The FUE technique is an important advancement in the field of hair restoration surgery. The minimally invasive nature of the surgery not only caught the attention of a patient but was also accepted among physicians.

Regular innovation in this field improved the technique and instrumentation, thus minimizing the higher transection rate and reducing the operative timings. The author firmly believes there is no single device which is perfect for all patients. A hair transplant surgeon should understand various available options for FUE and their advantages and limitations. This makes the procedure better and brings good clinical outcomes.

REFERENCES

1. Rassman W, Haris J, Berstein R. Follicular unit extraction. In: Haber RS, Stough DB (Eds). Hair Transplantation. Philadelphia: Elsevier Saunders; 2006. pp.133-42.
2. Bernstein RM, Rassman WR, Szaniawski W, Halperin A. Follicular transplantation. Int J Aesthet Restor Surg. 1995;3:119-32.
3. Bernstein RM, Rassman WR. Follicular transplantation. Patient evaluation and surgical planning. Dermatol Surg. 1997;23:771-84.
4. Tykocinski A. Hybrid trumpet punch for FUE harvesting. Hair Transplant Forum Int. 2017.
5. Trivellini R. Trivellini hair transplant technology. Hair Transplant Forum Int. 2018.
6. Umar S, U Graft Power FUE Device, FUE Asia Delhi 2023.
7. Saxena K. Micro rpm adjustment vs. conventional dental motors for FUE extraction. FUE Asia, Delhi; 2023.
8. Poblet E, Ortega F, Jiménez F. The arrector pili muscle and the follicular unit of the scalp: a microscopic anatomy study. Dermatol Surg. 2002;28:800-3.
9. Cole J. Harvesting the fallows. ISHRS, San Diego, California; 2006.
10. Harris JA. Follicular unit extraction: the SAFE System. Hair Transplant Forum Int. 2004;14(157):163-4.
11. Devroye J. Powered FU extraction with the Short-Arc-Oscillation Flat Punch FUE System (SFFS). Hair Transplant Forum Int. 2016;26(4):129-136.
12. Devroye J. Available from www.devroyeinstruments.com. [Last accessed October, 2023].
13. Trivellini R. An innovation in suction assisted FUE. Hair Transplant Forum Int. 2016;26(2):58-9.
14. Trivellini R. The Trivellini system and technique. Hair Transplant Forum Int. 2018;28(5):188-90.
15. Gupta AK, Love RP, Mohebi P, Trivellini R. Advances in hair transplantation technology: multiphasic device for follicular unit Excision. Skinmed. 2019;17(4):241-6.
16. Trivellini RL. Trivellini Flared. [online] Available from https://www.trivellinitech.com/product/trivellini-flared. [Last accessed October, 2023].
17. Chauhan K. Zeus Follicular Unit Excision Machine. AHRS Annual Meeting Indore 2023.
18. Umar S, Lohlun B, Ogozuglu T,Carter MJ. A novel follicular unit excision device for all-purpose hair graft harvesting. Clin Cosmet Investig Dermatol. 2021;14:1657-74.
19. Saxena K. Dental motor vs. micro adjustment motor for FUE. AHRS Annual Meeting, FUE Asia, Delhi; 2023.
20. Saxena K. Human hands vs automated implanters. AHRS Annual Meeting, Mumbai, India; 2011.
21. Wasserbauer SM. Robotic-assisted harvest of follicular units. The ISHRS 19th Annual Scientific Meeting, Anchorage; 2011.
22. Saxena K. KD spreader: a slit dilating device in hair transplantation. ISHRS 24th World Congress, Las Vegas, USA; 2016.
23. Saxena K. Safe and easy hair transplantation utilizing KD spreader. Plast Aesthet Res. 2018;5:5.

CHAPTER 52

Punches in Follicular Unit Extraction

Sukhbir Singh

Key Messages

- Extraction or excision of hair follicles is an important step of hair transplant.
- An appropriate punch is the best friend of hair transplant surgeon.
- A variety of punches are available for use like sharp, dull, and hybrid.
- Every surgeon uses his/her punch depending on thickness, hair curl, and ethnicity.
- Various factors determine which punch to use as detailed in the chapter.

INTRODUCTION

Follicular unit extraction (FUE)/excision has gained popularity over the years. This has indeed become one of the most common procedures done worldwide. One of the most important steps in hair transplant surgery is extraction or excision of hair follicles. This should be performed with utmost care to minimize the transection rate of the follicles from the permanent zone (back of scalp). So, an appropriate punch is like a "Best Friend" for the hair transplant surgeon. Each surgeon has his or her own preference, but basic principle of usage remains the same and aim is always to keep the transection rate to the lowest.

DYNAMICS OF FOLLICULAR UNIT EXTRACTION

- Follicular extraction or excision requires two forces:[1]
  i. Axial *(penetrating force)*[1]
  ii. Tangential force (rotation or oscillation)[1]
- *Torque*: It is the force applied through an angle and involves rotational movement.

These dynamics are important to understand since, depending on the forces and torque, one decides what type of punch is suitable to a surgeon. There are various other variables which decide which punch to use or not.

HISTORICAL PERSPECTIVE

First hair transplant in history[2] was performed by a Japanese doctor, Dr Shoji Okuda (1886–1962) in 1937. He used a crude punch made up of metallic tube with two ends and called it a round saw.[3] The punch diameter was 1–5 mm. The grafts extracted using this crude punch was called micro round skin flaps,[3] which consisted of skin and the hair follicles, which were then transferred to the recipient site.

PUNCH METALLURGY[1]

A good punch has a sharper edge (can be dull too), wall which is thin, and should have high precision. Punches which are used nowadays consist of variety of elements including Fe, C, Cr, etc.[1] The addition of chromium to these elements makes the punch resistant[1] to corrosion.

PUNCH VARIABLES

An appropriate punch would be the one which not only minimizes transection rate, but also improves the speed of extraction/excision. This will lead to less surgeon fatigue and better results. There are various factors based on which we decide what punch to use. There are various variables listed as under:

- Punch diameter[1]
- Cutting edge location[1]
- Punch wall thickness[1]
- Punch edge sharpness[1]
- Punch edge shape[1] (smooth vs. contoured)
- Punch tip length
- Special punch types

Human scalp hairs exit at various angulations mostly acute. This is very important to identify during extraction, so that the surgeon can adjust the inferior edge of the punch accordingly since it makes contact with the skin first. When the punch makes contact with the inferior edge first, the force is applied in direction of the rotation and the tissue applies resistance in the opposite direction.

Punch Diameter[1]

Punches vary in diameter from 0.6 to 1.5 mm. Punch diameter should be chosen wisely as too small a punch creates higher follicular transection and too big a punch creates a larger circular defect, which leads to more scarring and visibility. One important factor for choosing the right diameter is ethnicity of an individual. Like in Indian scalp using punch diameter <0.8 mm will lead to more transections. As African hairs are more curled they need not only slightly higher punch diameter but also different punch design to minimize transection. It is advisable not to use >1 mm punch as it will decrease interfollicular epidermis and it is likely to heal with hypopigmented scars. Cole defined three diameters, i.e., (i) internal diameter, (ii) external diameter, and (iii) diameter of cutting edge. It is very important to check from the manufacturer the correct internal diameter of the punch.

Cutting Edge Location[1]

Cole further defined the cutting edge location and the bevel according to each as shown in **Figure 1**. They are:

- Cutting edge on the inside with a bevel which is outside (type 5 punch)[1]
- Cutting edge in the middle and bevel also in the middle (type 4 punch)[1]
- Cutting edge on the outer side with bevel toward inside (type 3 punch)[1]—this type creates least follicular damage and gives good quality extractions.

Punch Wall Thickness[1]

Thin wall punches are usually preferred. The presence of thin wall helps to reduce the resistance as the punch makes contact with the skin. This leads to better quality grafts and decreased transection rates.

Punch Edge Sharpness[1]

There are either sharp or dull punches. In a sharp punch the contact area is small. When the surgeon uses the sharp motorized punch, the resistance of tissue is exceeded much more quickly leading to easy extraction. This leads to lesser force meaning a lower torque. This is in contrast to the dull punch in which the contact area is larger and a higher force (higher torque) is needed to exceed the tissue resistance. An individual surgeon has their own choice, but I prefer a sharp punch which increases my speed of extraction and leads to less fatigue as the force applied is quite minimal.

Blunt FUE punches were invented by Dr James Harris.[4,5] He used a blunt cutting tip for extraction/excision. He invented the "Safe System", which involves manual extraction using two different steps. The first step involves scoring to a depth of 0.3–0.5 mm. This is followed by using a blunt punch to remove the graft from the skin. Harris used the dull Hex punch with the

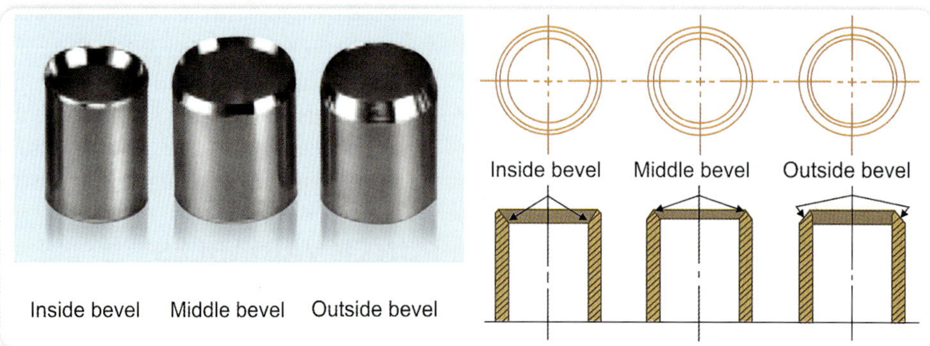

FIG. 1: Bevels.

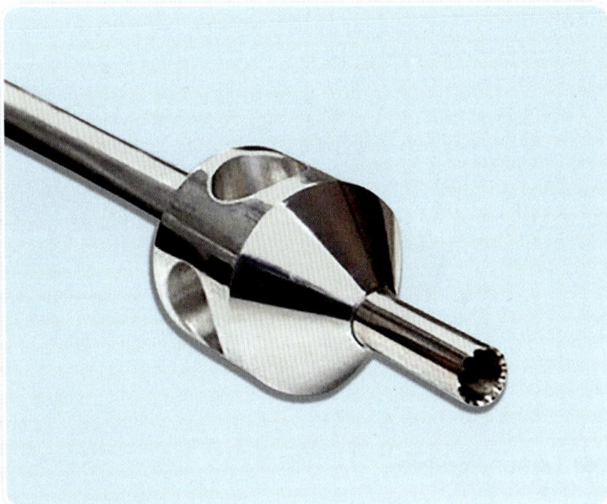

FIG. 2: Serrated Ertip punch.

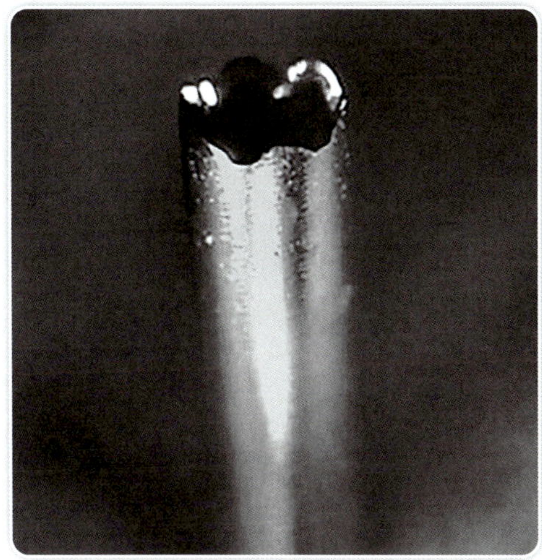

FIG. 3: Surrounded Cole punch.

motorized extraction. This helped to improve the speed as compared to manual extraction and also decreased the transaction. Dull punch has its own set of problems including slower extraction speed as compared to sharp punch[2] and higher incidence of buried grafts.

Punch Edge Shape[1]

The blunt punch surface can be either:

- *Rounded*: Where the cutting tip surface touching the skin is convex.
- *Flat*: Where the cutting tip surface touching the skin is flat. The advantage with flat punch is that it can penetrate deeper into the skin without damaging the hair follicle.[2]

Sharp punches have lot of varieties. They are:

- *Serrated Ertip punch as shown in **Figure 2***: This punch has sharp and serrated edges, which help in smoother extraction with less force. The wall of this punch is thin. All these factors help in easier extraction due to reduced friction and lesser transection rates.
- *Triple wave punch*: This punch consists of stainless steel (grade 303) and a coating of titanium nitride. The design mimics the wave pattern, which helps to reduce friction during extraction by decreasing the total surface area of the punch.
- *Surrounded Cole punch*:[1] This punch **(Fig. 3)** has multiple cutting edges, has a thin wall, and is more sharper than triple wave punch. This decreases the force required to overcome skin resistance and helps in decreasing the follicle transection rates.

Punch Tip Length

Punch length usually varies from 3 and 5 mm. Typically I use 0.9 mm, 4 mm tip length for graft extraction, but

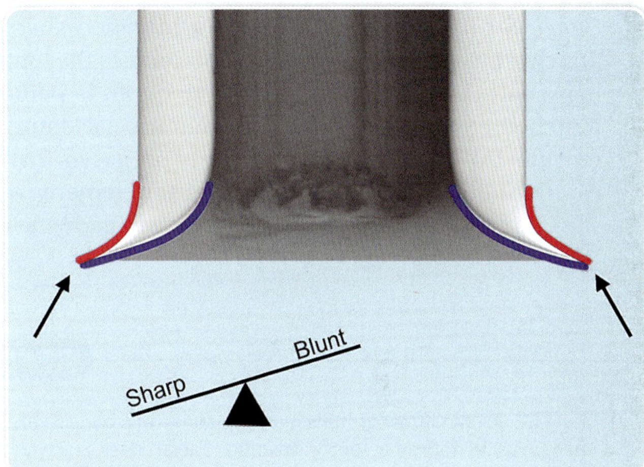

FIG. 4: Hybrid punch.

sometimes we require 5 mm also depending on graft length. It is always advisable to do some test grafts so that exact length of punch can be used to prevent high transection rates.

Special Punch Types

- *Hybrid FUE punch*: This was invented by Dr Sanusi Umar **(Fig. 4)**. In this punch, the cutting tip is *flared away* from the central axis of the punch cylinder and the follicles. The follicles abuts the blunter portion of the punch while the sharp cutting tip faces and cuts away the surrounding tissue, thereby decreasing the transection rates.
- *Trivellini's flared rim punch (Trumpet)*: This punch **(Fig. 5)** has been designed with a sharp cutting edge of 40° and has a 30° angulation from the front plane

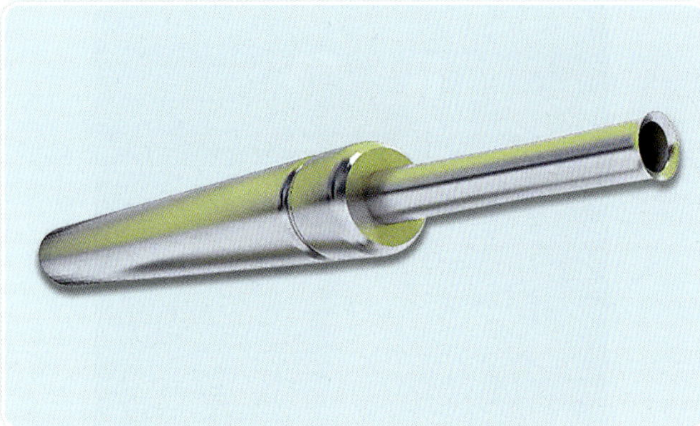

FIG. 5: Trumpet punch.

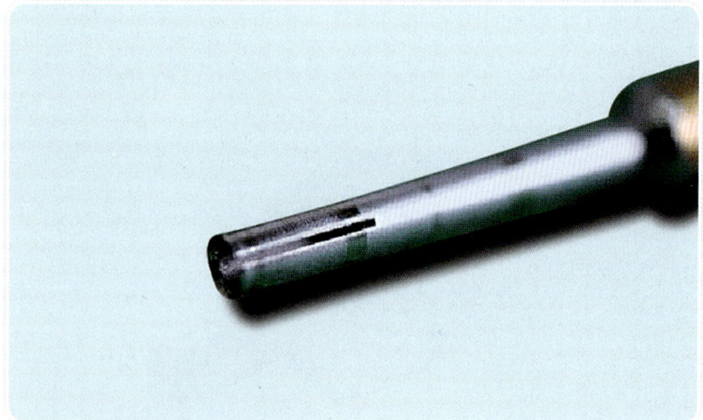

FIG. 6: Long hair punch.

to the side of the edge. The sharp cutting and robust edges help in easy and quick extraction with minimal transections.

- *Punch for long hair FUE*: This is a modified sharp punch with a slit **(Fig. 6)** that accommodates the long hair shaft inside the punch while the graft is being punched either by motorized or manual oscillatory movement. Oscillatory movement is preferred than rotational movement to avoid entanglement of surrounding hairs. Various surgeons have made their own punch for long hair FUE, the most common being Trivellini's punch for long hair FUE in an unshaven scalp.

Tips and Pearls

There are a variety of punches available for usage by the competent surgeon. Depending on the hair follicle length, ethnicity, and surgeon's personal choice, one can choose which punch best suits his/her patient with minimal transection rate and extraction of good quality grafts.

REFERENCES

1. Cole J. An analysis of follicular punches, mechanics, and dynamics in follicular unit extraction. Facial Plast Surg Clin North Am. 2013;21(3):437-47.
2. Garg A, Garg S. Donor donor harvesting: follicular unit excision. J Cutan Aesthet Surg. 2018;11(4):195-201.
3. Inui S, Itami S. Dr Shoji Okuda (1886–1962): the great pioneer of punch graft hair transplantation. J Dermatol. 2009;36:561-2.
4. Harris JA. Conventional FUE. In: Unger (Ed). Hair Transplantation, 5th edition. London, UK: Informa Health Care; 2011. pp. 291-2.
5. Harris JA. The SAFE System: new instrumentation and methodology to improve follicular unit extraction (FUE). Hair Transplant Forum Int. 2004;14:163-4.

CHAPTER 53

Different Machines in Follicular Unit Excision

Kavish Chouhan, Megha Tandon

Key Messages

- Follicular unit excision (FUE) has established it's reputation as a safe and minimally invasive technique of hair restoration.
- The advancements in techniques, punch shapes, and motorized devices have significantly reduced the rate of follicle damage and improved the speed of FUE.
- It is crucial for hair restoration surgeons to have knowledge about the various devices accessible, as well as comprehend how these tools can be tailored to the specific hair and skin characteristics of each patient.
- The inclusion of the robotic hair restoration system is a significant enhancement to the methodologies employed in hair restoration surgery.

INTRODUCTION

Hair transplantation has made significant progress over the years, starting from the time when Dr Orentreich introduced the punch hair transplant technique in the 1950s. Since then, the field has evolved to include more approaches such as follicular unit transplantation (FUT) in the 1990s and the latest method called follicular unit excision (FUE).[1,2] FUE, also referred to as the FOX procedure,[3] follicular unit separation extraction (FUSE) method,[4] Wood's technique,[5] and follicular unit (FU) isolation method,[6] is a minimally invasive hair restoration surgery that offers several suggested benefits for patients, including reduced discomfort after the surgery, quicker recovery time, the option to utilize body hair as a potential donor area, a potential increase in the availability of scalp donor hair (due to reduced scalp laxity restrictions), and less noticeable scarring.

In all techniques of extracting hair follicles, a punch is used to cut the tissue, and a punch driver is used to move the cutting tip of the punch. The punch driver can be operated manually by the practitioner, who rotates a handheld punch in a manner similar to a skin biopsy. The challenges faced with the utilization of manual punches to extract grafts were its slow process, with only a limited number of grafts obtained during a single session due to time constraints. Alternatively, it can be mechanical, with the punch mounted on an electromechanical drill device, which is often borrowed from dental drill systems. As FUE progressed, the instruments used to extract FUs also progressed to more advanced mechanically or electronically assisted devices, eventually leading to the latest advancement in a robotic FUE device.

EVOLUTION OF MOTORIZED DEVICES

The advancements in techniques, punch shapes, and motorized devices have significantly reduced the rate of follicle damage and improved the procedure's speed. These advancements include the utilization of sharp punches with depth control, blunt rotating punches, and different punch shapes such as flared, hybrid, and edge-out. These modifications aim to prevent the inadvertent cutting of follicles beneath the skin, ensuring better preservation during the transplantation process. Moreover, the introduction of motorized devices incorporating rotation, roto-oscillation, oscillation, vibration, suction, and hydration has further contributed to the successful extraction of grafts.

Different surgeons have created multiple FUE systems, each with its own advantages and disadvantages.

Suction-assisted Motorized Device

Boudjema created the first motorized instrument in the 1990s, which was later named Calvitron and was the first device of its kind.[7] In Asia, it was initially referred to as Omnigraft, but it is now recognized as NeoGraft.[8,9] NeoGraft and SmartGraft are two commercially available hair transplantation machines that employ a handheld surgical device that uses rotating sharp punches for scoring the grafts and negative pneumatic pressure for the suction of grafts. These devices utilize pneumatic pressure to insert the grafts into premade slits with another handpiece **(Fig. 1)**. They boast about their accuracy and speed in performing FUE compared to other motorized systems. Nevertheless, a significant drawback of this system is the higher rate of graft damage as the punch needs to penetrate deeper to fully sever the surrounding follicular tissues.[10,11]

Cole Isolation Device

In 2004, the programmable Power Cole Isolation Device (PCID) was introduced, which involved the use of a sharp punch with a thin wall and depth control.[12-14] The depth of the incision could be customized to suit the specific scalp characteristics and FU variation of each patient **(Fig. 2)**. The successful extraction of the FU graft can be achieved by making a precise cut beneath the arrector pili muscle. Furthermore, the size of the punch and the angle of the incision can be modified to match the specific characteristics of the patient's individual FUs more effectively. The Mini-Powered Cole Isolation Device (mPCID) functions similar to the PCID but in a smaller size.

Harris SAFE System

Dr James Harris, an American physician, introduced the Surgically Advanced Follicular Extraction (SAFE) system for hair extraction in 2004 that involves a two-step process **(Fig. 3)**. The first step entails using a sharp punch (measuring 1 mm in diameter) to score the skin at

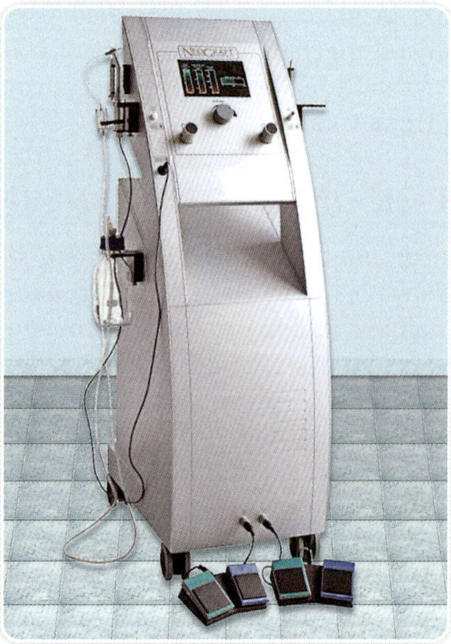

FIG. 1: Neograft[9].

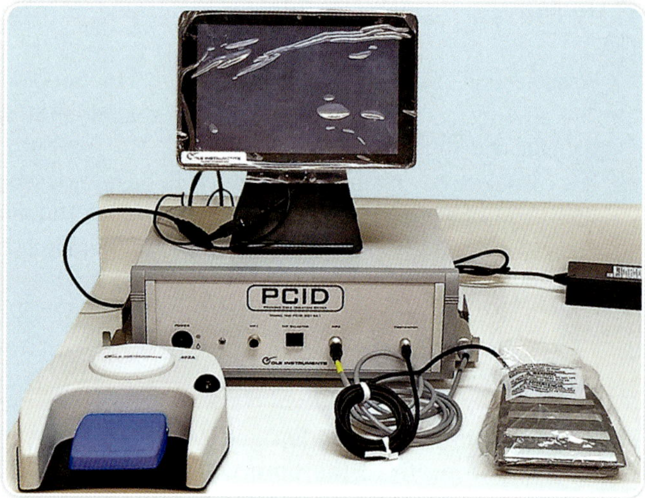

FIG. 2: Programmable Power Cole Isolation Device (PCID).
Courtesy: With permission from Cole Instruments Inc., Alpharetta, GA

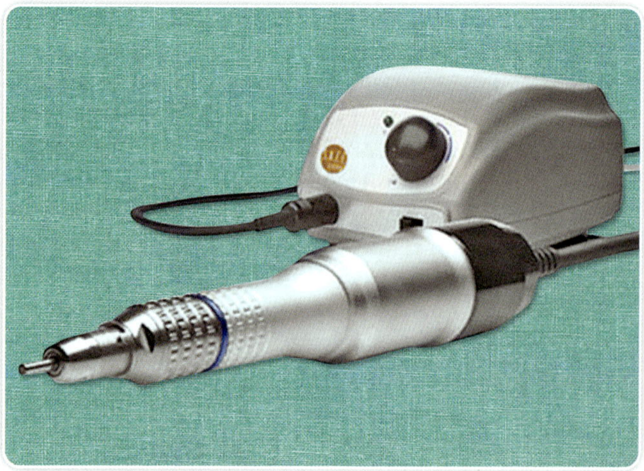

FIG. 3: Harris SAFE system[9].

a depth of 0.3–1.5 mm, just below the epidermis. During the second phase, a blunt punch is employed to carefully cut deeper into the dermis surrounding the FU, typically measuring between 4 and 6 mm. It is crucial to ensure that the follicles remain protected and are not exposed to any sharp edges. Over time, the blunt dissecting punch was combined with rotation, which eliminated the need for the sharp punch as the rotation permitted the initial incision to be made by the blunt punch. This improvement made it possible to harvest the graft in a single step, known as the Powered SAFE Scribe.[15-18]

True Device

True modified the Aseptico Porta-Tip-AEU-03SS machine and the Osada SH28S handpiece to create a precise punch tool that uses rotation at different speeds.[9] The tool uses Cole Serrounded Punches with sizes ranging from 0.8 to 1.25 mm and is equipped with a silicone collar to ensure consistent and accurate depth of incision **(Fig. 4)**.

Alphagraft

Alphagraft is an alternative device that employs a rotating sharp tool to extract follicles from the donor area **(Fig. 5)**.

KD's Follicular Unit Excision Station

This device incorporates both electropneumatic and physician control systems, combining a wide range of features. It covers every aspect of the FUE process, starting from painless anesthesia to the harvesting of FUs, graft hydration, creation of recipient sites, and implantation of grafts **(Fig. 6)**.[19,20] The FUE extractor developed by KD offers a precise and fast extraction process, even for beginners, surpassing the performance of traditional or motorized dental tools.[21] The motorized tool's rotations per minute (RPM) can be finely adjusted through a microprocessor-based control system, allowing physicians to minimize graft damage, even in the hands of beginners. Additionally, this device holds three internationally recognized patents for its automated graft hydration system. It also incorporates human-assisted automated incisions and automated forceps expansion during graft implantation.

Devroye Device

The Devroye WAW system uses short, oscillating arcs from the epidermal to the dermal layer. The Short-Arc-

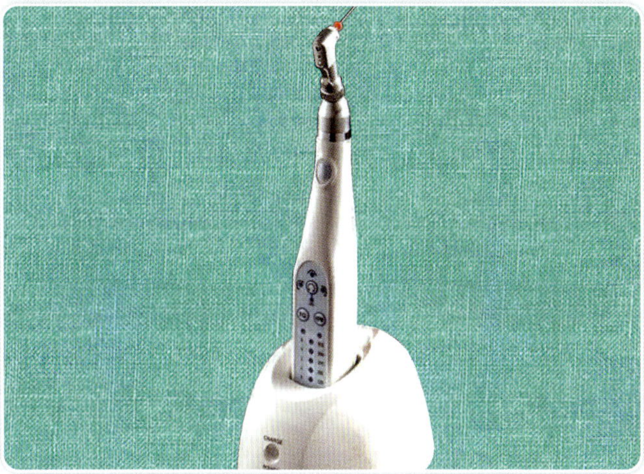

FIG. 5: Alphagraft[9].

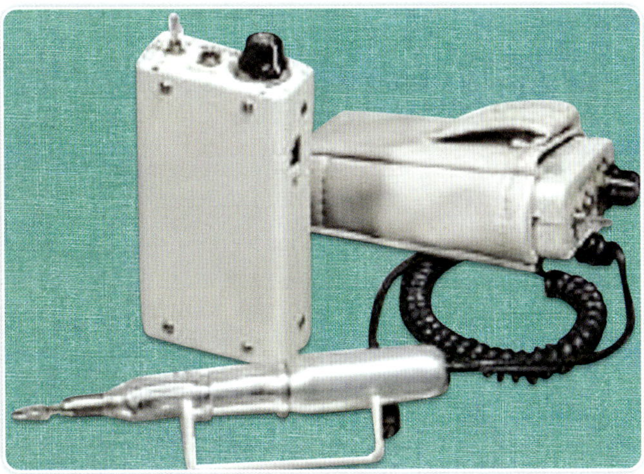

FIG. 4: True device[9].

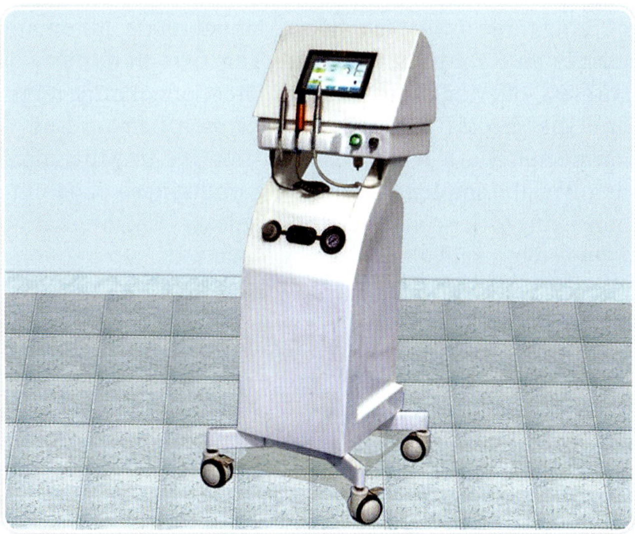

FIG. 6: KD's follicular unit excision station.

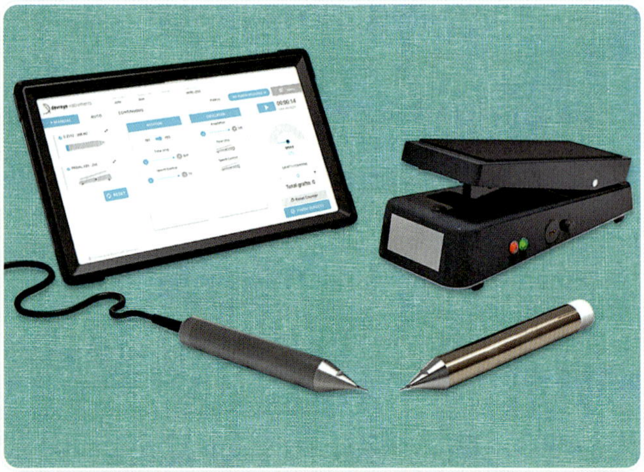

FIG. 7: WAW DUO follicular unit excision System.
Courtesy: With permission from Devroye Instruments, Brussels.

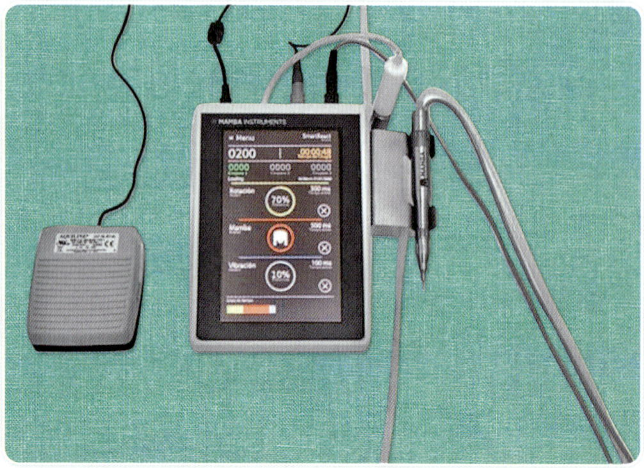

FIG. 8: Trivellini device[9].

Oscillation Flat Punch FUE System (SFFS) employs a quick and shaking movement that ranges between 180° and 90°. The primary benefit of this approach is that it can reach a significant depth in the skin, often up to 4–5 mm, without causing harm to the follicles. The small oscillation arc prevents twisting and reduces torsional stress to the tissue, making it less damaging than rotation movement. As a result, the risk of transection and cutting damage is minimized.[22,23] The original WAW FUE system was initially designed using a wired handpiece and operated solely with oscillatory movement, allowing for adjustment of the oscillation angle.

The new iteration, known as the WAW DUO FUE system, was introduced in 2022 and incorporates various advancements compared to the classic system **(Fig. 7)**. It comprises four main components: Two handpieces, a pedal, and a tablet equipped with a dedicated application offering three available modes: Manual mode, automatic mode, and continuous mode. The first handpiece is wireless, offering users significant freedom of movement, and the second handpiece serves as a backup and is connected via a wire. The next notable improvement involves the implementation of a multiphase capability consisting of two consecutive movements: A slight rotation followed by oscillation.

Mamba Device

The Mamba FUE device, created by Dr Roberto Trivellini, is a versatile programmable motor that combines several features such as in-line suction, complete rotation, oscillation, and vibration **(Fig. 8)**. Additionally, it utilizes a distinct "Edge-Out" punch design characterized by a flat shape. The Trivellini System takes advantage of suction to produce traction on the graft, stretching it and facilitating penetration of the punch.[24] It has a touch-sensitive function called Smart React that triggers the preprogrammed suction and rotation/oscillation/roto-oscillation/vibration features once the device makes initial contact with the skin around the FU, eliminating the need for a foot pedal. As a result, the device has been proven to enhance the quality of grafts, minimize damage, and facilitate a more gentle extraction process.[25-27]

Shiao 4-D Device

Created by Dr TK Shiao, similar to the Mamba, this device integrates customizable multifunction controls. The movement of the punch is initiated by touch (similar to the Mamba device). Sharp punches are utilized in the system. The handpiece is disposable and can be easily produced at a low cost using a 3D printer **(Fig. 9)**.[9,28]

There are various motorized movements incorporated alone or in combination in the machines used for FU harvesting:

- *Rotation*: Blunt punches need more force compared to sharp punches to make the first cut. This force is due to an increase in axial force, but using more axial force can cause the targeted FU to become misaligned and result in the cutting of the follicle. By rotating the punch, a rotational force or torque is generated, which reduces the amount of axial force required to penetrate the tough epidermis.[12] This is particularly beneficial for blunt punches that have a thick wall. Rotating the punch is useful when removing grafts at an angle where only a small part of the punch makes the initial incision on the skin.[29]

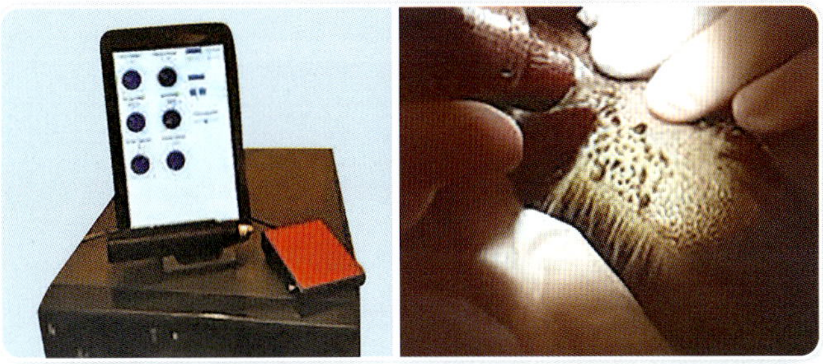

FIG. 9: Shiao 4-D device[9].

- *Oscillation*: This action involves repetitive arcs that alternate between clockwise and counterclockwise directions. The length of these arcs can be either short or wide, depending on the operator, and some machines have the ability to adjust the speed of these arcs. This movement is most effective when the punch is deep within the dermal layer, and the majority of the FU graft is located inside the punch.[22-24]
- *Roto-oscillation*: This movement is a blend of rotational and oscillatory actions, where rotation is typically performed initially, followed by oscillation.[13,26,27]
- *Vibration*: When the edge of the punch is situated deeply in the dermal layer, and the excised graft is primarily located inside the punch lumen, vibrating the punch can be beneficial. In contrast to rotation, this particular motion does not cause significant torsional strain or only produces minimal amounts of it when oscillating. It aids in gently loosening the graft within the punch and separating the perifollicular tissue from the walls of the punch. This motion is typically used together with the Harris hexagonal-shaped punch,[15-18] the Trivellini Edge Out™ punch, and flared tip punches.[24,26,27] Additionally, Umar has described the utilization of ultrasonic frequencies to vibrate the Dr.UPunch Curl™, which is known as Dr UGraft Sonic FUE™, and this technique makes it easier to extract grafts from thick skin.[30]
- *Multiphasic*: Certain motorized FUE devices are capable of executing the previously mentioned movements in a specific order.

TOWARD THE NEWER AVENUES

Dr UGraft Zeus

Dr UGraft Zeus is an all-purpose FUE device that is capable of extracting hair from the head, regardless of whether it is shaved or not, and is suitable for people of all ethnic backgrounds.[31] An all-purpose punch called the Intelligent punch—Dr U Punch i (Dr U Devices Inc, Manhattan Beach, CA) is used, which is frustoconically shaped and has been optimized at multiple levels to incorporate solutions to several technical challenges known to contribute to FUE graft attrition (lost or nonviable grafts from transections, crush injuries, and complete desheathing), poor scarring profiles, and user experiences.[32] Other advantages of this system are as follows:

- It is capable of extracting hair from the beard and body, as well as harvesting long-haired grafts without the need to switch punches or drivers or acquire specialized skills.
- It addresses the issues that often lead to inconsistent performance in FUE devices, such as changes in skin firmness and thickness.
- It overcomes the challenges associated with unpredictable hair curliness and angles by utilizing its own technology to navigate hair follicles, which is an area where FUE practitioners often face difficulties.
- The machine incorporates torque in a manner that allows the punch to stop once it has separated the graft from its lateral attachments. Consequently, instead of relying on the practitioner's experience or using mechanical guards, automatic depth control with a timeout mechanism, the all-purpose FUE device primarily relies on the tissue's resistance to determine the optimal depth.

The device includes a user-friendly dashboard with a personalized tab, allowing users to input their preferred settings, such as speed, torque, and three different movement modes. **Figures 10A and B** illustrate this feature. Additionally, the new driver system design incorporates an optional fluid flush system.[32]

Image-guided Robotic Device

In 2006, a biotechnology and engineering company from the United States unveiled an automated FUE extraction device with the aim of reducing the impact of variations in skill and experience among practitioners. The ARTAS robotic system is a combination of physician-controlled and computer-assisted technologies, incorporating various features such as an exclusive imaging technology, a computer interface terminal, several video cameras, a video display, a robotic arm device, a suction system for lifting harvested grafts, and a comfortable chair that positions the patient correctly for the robot **(Fig. 11)**.

How ARTAS works: The robot scans and converts the visual characteristics of the donor area into digital format, analyzing each FU. Using a customizable mathematical algorithm, the machine randomly extracts FUs.[33-35] The

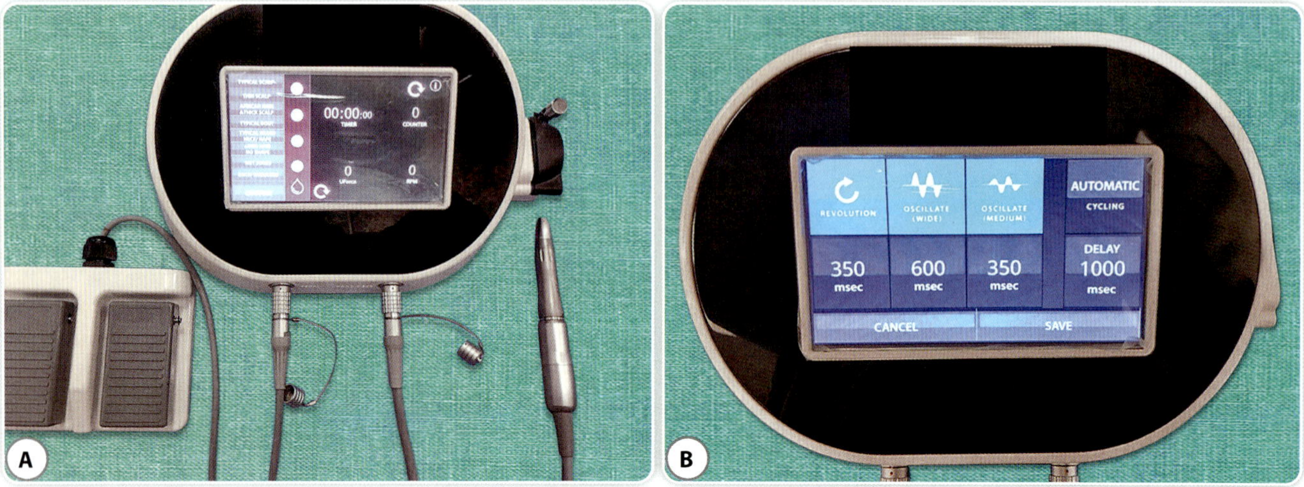

FIGS. 10A AND B: Dr UGraft Zeus. (A) The system, consisting of the console, handpiece, foot pedal, and optional fluid integration. The dashboard shows six presets, custom mode, torque control, speed, timers, and reset features. (B) The dashboard displays three movement modes, adjustable movement duration, score intervals, and automatic/manual modes.

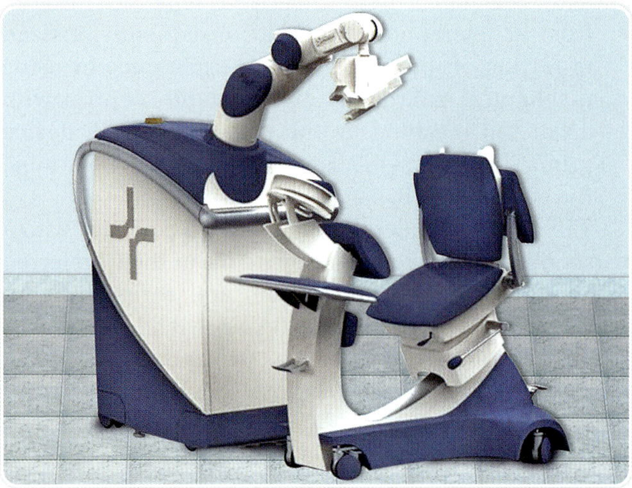

FIG. 11: ARTAS[9].

spacing between harvested grafts is carefully chosen to minimize the visibility of graft sites when the patient's hair is cut very short. Additionally, the computer program calculates the density of FUs and the angle of hair growth.

Equipped with a dual-bore needle apparatus, the robotic arm consists of a sharp needle tip for skin penetration and a surrounding coring blunt needle for deeper tissue insertion. This design reduces the risk of hair transection and facilitates the removal of selected FUs. The sharp needle includes markings to determine penetration depth, while pressure sensors in the robotic system assess the forces required to penetrate the tissue. If the force threshold is exceeded, the system automatically stops and requires parameter adjustments. Both the physician and the assistant are equipped with emergency stop buttons to halt the operation of the machine. The emergency stop button is located on the handheld "pendant" device, which the physician utilizes to control the different functional aspects of the device.

The ARTAS Hair Studio™ is a cutting-edge software bundle that accompanies the ARTAS robotic system for FUE. This software offers significant advantages for both patients and doctors by enhancing the consultation and design phase of the hair restoration procedure, resulting in an improved overall experience.

SUMMARY

The perfect FUE procedure necessitates meeting two conflicting demands: Acquiring a large quantity of hair-rich grafts with minimal transection and utilizing small-sized punches while keeping the extraction costs low.

Hair restoration surgeons frequently use FUE as a technique, and thus it is crucial for them to have knowledge about the various devices accessible as well as comprehend how these tools can be tailored to the specific hair and skin characteristics of each patient, in order to attain the most favorable graft harvesting results **(Table 1)**.

TABLE 1: Summary of different machines in follicular unit excision (FUE) and their features.

Device	Motions	Punch shape	Punch tip	Depth control	Suction	Hydration	Long hair extraction (using same punch)	Approximate price (USD)
NeoGraft/Omnigraft	Rotation	Cylindrical/round	Sharp	No	Yes	Yes	No	$5,465.00
Programmable Power Cole Isolation Device	Rotation Oscillation Roto-oscillation	Cylindrical/round Window	Sharp	Yes	No	No	No	$ 17,500
Harris Powered Safe Scribe	Rotation	Cylindrical/round	Blunt	Yes	No	No	No	$320.00
True Device: Aseptico Porta-Tip-AEU-03SS Osada SH28S handpiece	Rotation	Cole Serrounded™ Punch	Sharp	Yes	No	No	No	$695.00
KD's FUE station	Rotation	Cylindrical/round	Sharp	No	No	No	No	$4,270.00
Shiao 4-D device	Rotation	Cylindrical/round	Sharp	Yes	No	No	No	$9,700.00
Devroye WAW system	Oscillation	Hybrid Tornado	Flat Serrated	No	No	No	No	$10,944.50
Devroye WAW DUO FUE system	Rotation Oscillation	Hybrid Tornado	Flat Serrated	No	No	No	No	$16,368.00
Trivellini system	Rotation Oscillation Roto-oscillation Vibration	Edge out Flared	Sharp	No	Yes	No	No	$9,990.00
Dr UGraft Zeus™	Rotation Oscillation	Flared (textured)	Sharp	Innate (no physical depth stop)	No	Yes	Yes	$15,000.00
ARTAS	Rotation	1st cylindrical/round 2nd cylindrical/round	Semi-sharp, inner bevel, 2- or 4-pronged Dull	Yes	No	No	No	$76,517.00

REFERENCES

1. Orentreich N. Autografts in alopecias and other selected dermatological conditions. Ann N Y Acad Sci. 1959;83:463-79.
2. Bernstein RM, Rassman WR, Szaniawski W, Halperin A. Follicular transplantation. Int J Aesthetic Restorative Surg. 1995;3:119-32.
3. Rassman WR, Bernstein RM, McClellan R, Jones R, Worton E, Uyttendaele H. Follicular unit extraction: minimally invasive surgery for hair transplantation. Dermatol Surg. 2002;28:720-7.
4. Poswal A. Donor sealing: a novel method in hair transplant surgery. Indian J Dermatol. 2006;51:55.
5. Woods R, Campbell AW. Chest hair micrografts display extended growth in scalp tissue: a case report. Br J Plast Surg. 2004;57:789-91.
6. Kingsley S. Sharing experiences of follicular isolation technique? Follicular unit extraction. Hair Transplant Forum Int. 2004;14:15-6.
7. Boudjema PJ. Device for transplanting small diameter hair grafts. Patent US5827297A; 1998.
8. Harris JA. History of FUE: a retrospective. In: Lam SM, Williams KL (Eds). Hair Transplantation 360: Follicular Unit Extraction (FUE), Volume 4. New Delhi, India: Jaypee Brothers Medical Publishers; 2016. p. 7.
9. True RH. A 2019 guide to currently accepted FUE and implanter terminology. Hair Transpl Forum Int. 2019;29(3):98-106.

10. Saxena K. Automated FUE: FUE hair restoration major procedures minor Incisions 1st eds, India 2007:79-82.
11. Saxena K. Human hands vs automated implanters, AHRS Annual Meeting, Mumbai, India; 2011.
12. Cole JP. An analysis of follicular punches, mechanics, and dynamics in follicular unit extraction. Facial Plast Surg Clin North Am. 2013;21(3):437-47.
13. Cole Instruments. [online] Available from www.coleinstruments.com. [Last accessed September, 2023].
14. Cole JP. Follicular extraction punch and method. Patent US 2005/0203545 A1; 2005.
15. Harris JA. New methodology and instrumentation for follicular unit extraction: lower follicle transection rates and expanded patient candidacy. Dermatol Surg. 2006;32(1):56-61.
16. Harris JA. Follicular extraction method and device. Patent US 2005/0267506 A1.
17. Ng B, Harris JA. How I do it: powered blunt dissection with the SAFE system for FUE (Part I). Hair Transpl Forum Int. 2010;20(6):188-9.
18. Ng B, Harris JA. How I do it: Powered blunt dissection with the SAFE system for FUE Part II: the extraction phase. Hair Transpl Forum Int. 2011; 21(1):16-7.
19. Kavya, Saxena D, Saxena K. Indian Patent Journal. IN number 202321007369 in 2023.
20. Saxena K. Automated forceps expansion technique (AFET). A teaching tool for FUE graft implantation. ISHRS Prague World Congress, Czech Republic; 2017.
21. Saxena K. Automated incision technique. FUE Europe Manchester Annual Meeting; 2019.
22. Devroye J. Powered FU extraction with the short-arc-oscillation flat punch FUE system (SFFS). Hair Transpl Forum Int. 2016; 26(4):129-6.
23. Devroye J. www.devroyeinstruments.com Accessed May 9, 2020.
24. Trivellini R. An innovation in suction assisted FUE. Hair Transpl Forum Int. 2016;26(2):58-9.
25. Trivellini R. The Trivellini system and technique. Hair Transpl Forum Int. 2018;28(5):188-90.
26. Gupta AK, Love RP, Mohebi P, Trivellini R. Advances in hair transplantation technology: multiphasic device for follicular unit excision. Skinmed. 2019;17(4):241-6.
27. Trivellini RL. Trivellini flared. [online] Available from https://www.trivellinitech.com/product/trivellini-flared/. [Last accessed September, 2023].
28. Shiao T-K. Mechanized punch for cylindrical excision of hair follicles. US Patent 2016/0166272 A1; 2016.
29. Rassman W, Pak J, Kim J. Follicular unit extraction: evolution of a technology. J Transplant Technol Res. 2016;6(2):1-14.
30. Umar S. Coming soon – Dr.UGraftÔ sonic FUE. [online] Available from https://ugraft.com/news/coming-soon-dr-ugraft-sonic-fue/. [Last accessed October, 2023].
31. Umar S. What Is The Dr.UGraft™ Hair Transplant System? https://ugraft.com/what-is-dr-ugraft-hair-transplant-system/. Accessed March 30, 2020.
32. Umar S, Lohlun B, Ogozuglu T, Carter MJ. A novel follicular unit excision device for all-purpose hair graft harvesting. Clin Cosmet Investig Dermatol. 2021;14:1657-74.
33. Canales M. Robotic hair transplantation: experience and results of first human clinical testing. Presentation at the ISHRS Annual Meeting, Las Vegas (NV), September 26–30, 2007.
34. Rose PT. The latest innovations in hair transplantation. Facial Plast Surg. 2011;27(4):366-77.
35. Harris JA. Robotic-assisted follicular unit extraction for hair restoration: case reports. Cosmet Dermatol. 2012;25(6):284-7.

CHAPTER 54

Comparison of Follicular Unit Excision and Follicular Unit Transplantation (Strip): A Critique

Kumaresan M

Key Messages

- There are two different techniques in hair transplant (HT)—follicular unit transfer (FUT) and follicular unit excision (FUE), both have their advantages and disadvantages.
- Both FUE and FUT are equally effective in generating high-quality grafts.
- Follicular unit transplantation results in a linear scar, whereas FUE produces punctate scars that are easily concealed.
- Distinct subgroups of HT patients are eligible for FUE, FUT, or both procedures.
- FUE has a short learning curve and limited infrastructure in terms of man power and machinery.
- Any HT surgeon should master both the techniques and should have both the facilities to provide optimum care to the patient

INTRODUCTION

Hair transplant (HT) surgery is performed by two different techniques of harvesting the donor follicular unit (FU) grafts from the safe donor area (SDA). Strip or follicular unit transfer (FUT) employs excision of an ellipse of scalp tissue and is subjected to further dissection to isolate the FU and results in a linear scar over the donor area. Follicular unit excision (FUE) employs punches to isolate and excise the FU one by one from the donor area and avoids the linear scar but results in several punctate scars over the donor region. FUE has definitely contributed to the enhancement of donor area to other body parts and enhanced patient comfort. It has removed the fear of surgery and led to greater acceptance of HT among public. However, FUE has also led to "minimalization" or even trivialization of the surgery, leading to all and sundry claiming to be experts and to several ethical issues.[1] The FUT linear scar and FUE transection rates are frequent topics of debate. This chapter analyzes the pros and cons of these two different techniques.

DONOR REGION SCARRING

The linear scar of the strip surgery is a significant concern for patients who wish to wear their hair very short **(Fig. 1)**. Although the thin linear scar is easily concealed by the hair

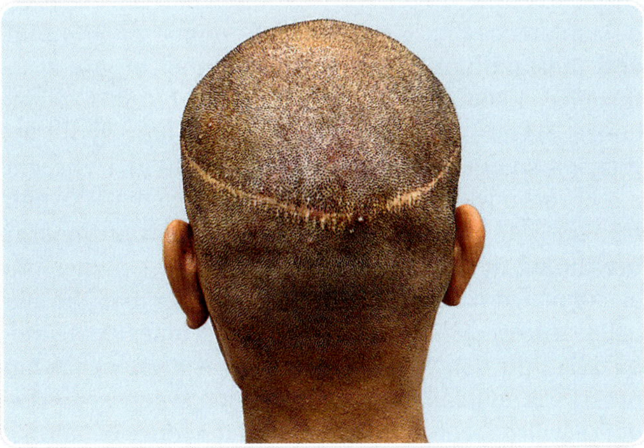

FIG. 1: Linear scar post follicular unit transfer (FUT).

above the scar, there are patients who have scars that have widened, and there are also patients who have several scars from multiple procedures. The healing tendency of the patients has variability leading to highly unpredictable scarring.[1] Strip excision is a surgical technique that needs expertise and adherence to proper closure techniques. Of late, there has been an influx of doctors of all specialties into this field, who may not have the necessary surgical skill. Aggressive harvesting to obtain large number of grafts, over 3,000–3,500 from strips over 2 cm wide, leads to wide scars.

Several techniques have been introduced to minimize the width of the strip scar:

- Limiting the width of the donor strip to <1.5 cm
- Minimizing the tension while closing the wound
- Double-layered closure
- Undermining the edges
- Careful dissection along the line of incision to avoid damage to the follicles
- Including the previous strip scar
- Trichophytic closure
- Insertion of few grafts into suture at the end of the surgery[2-6]

Proper planning and execution greatly reduce the problems associated with scar formation in strip surgery. In spite of such meticulous procedure, some individuals end up with a bad scar.[7]

Follicular unit excision was propagated with the claims of scarless surgery since it does not involve excision of a large portion of the scalp and even claimed to be a nonsurgical method. Although a linear scar is not created with FUE, circular scars are created **(Figs. 2A and B)**, and hence, it is not proper to use the terms scarless or no scar.

The total area of excision is greater with FUE than with strip harvesting. This is apparent when one calculates the circumference of a 1-mm punch (1 mm × π = 3.14 mm) and then multiplies this by the number of grafts, for instance, 1,000 grafts (1,000 × 3.14 = 3,140 mm, which equals 314 cm). In comparison, in a strip harvest of 1,000 grafts, assuming an average density of 80 FUs/cm^2 and a 1-cm strip width, the length of the scar created would be 12.5–37.5 cm (12.5 cm per 1 mm width of the scar, presuming the scar width ranges 1–3 mm). Hence, the accumulated scarring area of FUE is greater than the area of linear scarring in FUT.[8] If a patient becomes extensively bald (i.e., the donor fringe becomes very narrow), the line of FUT will generally still remain hidden, whereas the dots of FUE will be seen above (or below) the fringe of hair.[1]

With each subsequent session, the scarring in FUE is additive. For example, if the first FUE session is 2,000 grafts, there will be 2,000 tiny round scars **(Fig. 3)**. With a second session of 2,000 grafts, there will be a total of 4,000 scars. In contrast, with FUT, the first scar is completely removed in the next procedure. Even though the scar may be longer in the next session, with FUT, regardless of the number of procedures, the patient is left with only one scar. The scarring and distortion of the donor scalp from FUE make subsequent FUE sessions more difficult **(Fig. 4)**.[6]

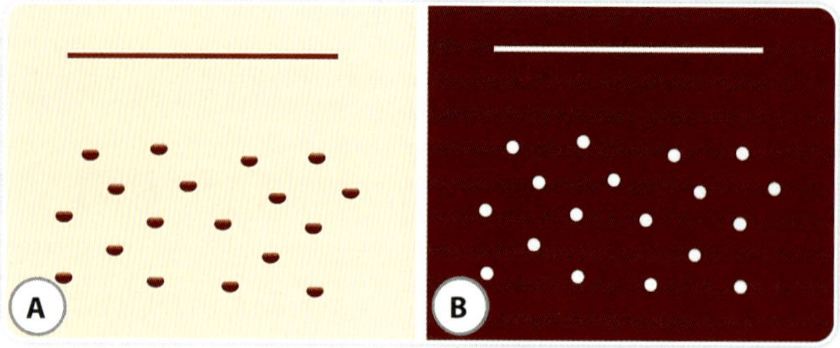

FIGS. 2A AND B: (A) Linear versus dot-like scars in fair skin; (B) Linear versus dot-like scars in dark skin.

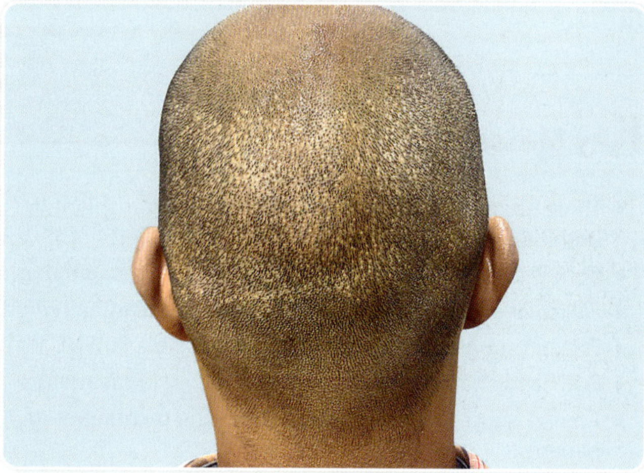

FIG. 3: Hypopigmented scars post follicular unit excision (FUE).

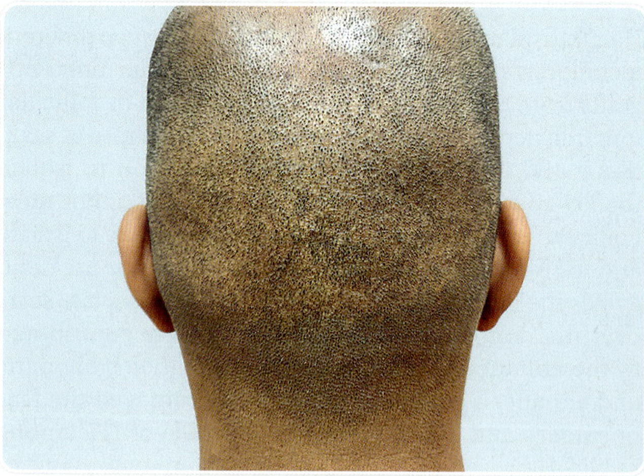

FIG. 4: Scarring and distortion of follicular unit (FU) post follicular unit excision (FUE).

QUALITY OF GRAFTS

Quality of FU grafts harvested determines the survival and longevity of the implanted FU. High-quality grafts are ones that are obtained from the most permanent part of the donor area, undamaged, and contain a protective layer of tissue around the follicles. The protective dermis reduces mechanical injury during insertion and from drying when the grafts are outside the body. FUT typically yields high-quality grafts, especially when clinical assistants are extensively trained in stereomicroscopic dissection.1

In FUE, the grafts quality were not up to the mark during the initial phase, but with the technological advancements in the punches and the FUE machines, the quality of grafts improved so much that these can be compared to as good as a properly dissected FU grafts from FUT. Smaller punches used in FUE yield grafts that have very little tissue surrounding the follicles and are more prone to dehydration and damage because of manipulation during insertion of grafts, which might lead to reduced survival of the grafts in FUE.[8] The lack of perifollicular tissue is often a result of "pulling" on the graft to remove it in FUE. No adequate studies are available to compare survival rates of grafts between FUT and FUE.

TRANSECTION RATES

Follicle transection rates reflect the quality of harvesting, where a lower transection rate indicates a higher quality procedure.[9-11] The transection rate is defined as the ratio of transected follicles to the number of total follicles excised (intact plus transected) and is given as percentage.[12]

Follicular unit excision is a blind procedure in contrast to FUT. Strip, which is an open procedure with dissection, is performed under stereomicroscopic dissection. FUE involves releasing the hold of arrectores; however, the level of attachment of arrectores cannot be visualized. It is this fact, coupled with the pyramidal shape of the unit (with splaying of hairs at lower end) that results in transection. Transection occurs because of anatomical characteristics of hair follicles (HFs) varying between regions of the scalp and between patients.[12] Partial transection decreases the total number of hairs in the graft and thus reduces the overall yield. Completely transected hairs do not grow. Hence, there is a need to reduce the transection rate in FUE to as minimum as possible. In those individuals who had underwent mega sessions of FUE earlier, the transection rate is greater in subsequent sessions because of angulation and scarring created during the previous surgery.[6]

However, it is also true that FUE techniques and instrumentation have improved over the years; transection rates have fallen from a high of around 10–20% few years back to 2–5% now. The time for extraction has also come down with better instrumentation, and it is now possible to complete a 3,000-graft session in approximately 8 hours in 1 day.[1] All these have resulted in increased popularity of the technique.

GRAFT YIELD

In FUT, the donor strip is removed from the midportion of the permanent zone and the entire FU within the strip can be harvested, but there is a limitation to the width that can be safely harvested. The number of grafts per harvest for FUT depends on the area size, hair density of the donor strip, and whether FUs or individual HFs are dissected as grafts.[13] In FUE, the surgeon is only able to harvest about one of every five follicles in a given area or 20% (this compares with 100% using FUT/strip).[8,14] Combining FUE and strip harvest improves the graft yield, particularly in grade 6–7 Norwood scale, whereby the entire SDA in mid occiput is harvested by strip, and the FUE is employed to harvest the grafts from those SDA regions inaccessible to strip excision.

However, in contrast to the above facts, there is one aspect where FUE is superior—FUE is the only method to extract body hair. This offsets the above limitation for the number of grafts from scalp.[1]

TECHNICAL EXPERTISE

Follicular unit transfer needs greater surgical skill for proper closure and microscopic dissection. The surgical skill required to master FUE is different from FUT. In FUE, which is a blind procedure, surgeon should be able to align the punch to the angle of the follicles, presume the depth of the incision, and avoid transection.[15] Patients with curly or very wavy hair may be difficult to treat when FUE is used. The recent innovations in FUE machinery have enabled the harvesting of curly hair with ease. In comparison, strip harvesting is suitable for all types of hair. FUE can be a tedious process, and both patient and physician may experience fatigue. This can limit the amount of grafts that can be harvested in a single session.[15] The physician may need to use high power loupes 4×–6×. Working at a shorter focal distance can be tiresome and lead to neck problems.[13,15]

COMPLICATIONS

Follicular unit transfer is associated with significant postoperative pain, hypertrophic scars, folliculitis, cyst formation, wound dehiscence, and restriction of postoperative mobility. In contrast, FUE has lesser postoperative downtime, faster healing of the donor area, and rapid recovery. Chances of hypertrophic scarring and keloids are rare in FUE. However, some complications, though minor, can occur in FUE such as burying of grafts, pinpoint white scars in donor area, and moth-eaten appearance in donor area because of overharvesting, epithelial cysts, donor site infection, and necrosis of donor area.[16]

TEAM AND SETUP

Strip harvesting requires a larger staff, larger theater, stereomicroscopes, and larger space than FUE, and the technicians have to be taught how to dissect under microscope, which can be time-consuming. For novice surgeons, this is a major disadvantage. For FUE, the surgeon can organize the surgery with just one or two assistants, also needs less stringent theater requirements.[17]

SUMMARY

Strip harvesting and FUE are both acceptable techniques for harvesting donor grafts. Each technique has advantages and disadvantages. **Table 1** summarizes the comparison of the two techniques. Combining FUT and FUE improves the graft outcome and the yield. FUT scores higher when multiple sessions of HT are required for a candidate and to have maximum optimization of the grafts from SDA. FUE is well suited for patients who insist on not having a linear scar. It may be an excellent choice for young patients seeking small procedures. FUE is the only choice for harvesting trunk, leg, and arm hair, and it is an excellent way to camouflage strip scars. However, the simplicity of the technique has also meant that unqualified people (technicians) have started performing this procedure independently, without supervision of surgeons. Surgeons should learn all types of surgery and use the technique for each patient as per their requirements.

TABLE 1: Comparison of the two techniques.[1]

Features	FUT	FUE
Scar	Single linear	Multiple round
Donor healing	Long time required	Short time
Limitation in exercise after surgery	Yes	No
Postoperative discomfort	Yes	Minimal
Applicability in people with greater scarring tendency	No	Yes
Body hair harvesting	No	Yes
Risk of harvesting beyond SDA	No	Yes
Graft quality	Good	Good to less than good
FU yield	Good	Good, but can be low sometimes
Scarring is additive	No	Yes
Graft survival	Good	Good but variable
Time taken to complete	Shorter	Longer
Damage to grafts	Less	Higher
All types of hair can be harvested	Yes	No (tough for curly hairs)
Surgical setup	Advanced setup required	Basic setup is sufficient
Surgical team	A big team is required	Small team can manage the surgery
Grafts outside the body tissue	Shorter time	Longer time—not if you alternate between extraction and insertion. Shorter than FUT in cases of direct hair implantation
Narrowing donor area in future can expose scar	No (FUT scar remains hidden within the narrow fringe of occipital hair even in advanced grade of AGA)	Yes
Microscopic dissection in addition to extraction	Yes	No
Buried grafts and capping	No	Yes
Size of single session limited by time	No	Yes

(AGA: androgenetic alopecia; FU: follicular unit; FUE: follicular unit excision; FUT: follicular unit transfer; SDA: safe donor area)

Tips and Pearls

- The healing tendency of the patients has variability leading to highly unpredictable scarring.
- Strip excision is a surgical technique that needs expertise and adherence to proper closure techniques.
- Although a linear scar is not created with FUE, circular scars are created.
- The total area of excision is greater with FUE than with strip harvesting.
- With each subsequent session, the scarring in FUE is additive.
- FUE techniques and instrumentation have improved over the years; transection rates have fallen from a high of around 10–20% few years back to 2–5% now.
- FUE is the only method to extract body hair.

REFERENCES

1. Kumaresan M, Mysore V. Controversies in hair transplantation. J Cutan Aesthet Surg. 2018;11:173-81.
2. Khanna M, Purohit V. Donor strip: Suturing techniques. In: Mysore V, Sattur S, Garg AK, Dua K, Patwardhan N (Ed). Hair Transplantation. New Delhi, India: Jaypee Brothers Medical Publishers; 2016. pp. 172-7.
3. Garg AK, Garg S. Donor strip harvesting: Surgical methods. In: Mysore V, Sattur S, Garg AK, Dua K, Patwardhan N (Ed). Hair Transplantation. New Delhi, India: Jaypee Brothers Medical Publishers; 2016. pp. 164-71.
4. Sattur S. Trichophytic closure. In: Mysore V, Sattur S, Garg AK, Dua K, Patwardhan N (Ed). Hair Transplantation. New Delhi, India: Jaypee Brothers Medical Publishers; 2016. pp. 178-81.
5. Garg AK, Garg S. Donor area complications of strip harvesting. In: Mysore V, Sattur S, Garg AK, Dua K, Patwardhan N (Ed). Hair Transplantation. New Delhi, India: Jaypee Brothers Medical Publishers; 2016. pp. 282-7.
6. Dua K, Dua A, Chahar M. Repeat hair transplant. In: Mysore V, Sattur S, Garg AK, Dua K, Patwardhan N (Ed). Hair Transplantation. New Delhi, India: Jaypee Brothers Medical Publishers; 2016. pp. 293-304.
7. Bernstein RM. Commentary on association between scalp laxity, elasticity, and glidability and donor strip scar width in hair transplantation and a new elasticity measuring method. Dermatol Surg. 2017;43:582.
8. Mahadevia B. Comparison of follicular unit transplantation and follicular unit extraction: a critique. In: Mysore V, Sattur S, Garg AK, Dua K, Patwardhan N (Ed). Hair Transplantation. New Delhi, India: Jaypee Brothers Medical Publishers; 2016. pp. 199-204.
9. Park JH, You SH. Various types of minor trauma to hair follicles during follicular unit extraction for hair transplantation. Plast Reconstr Surg Glob Open. 2017;5:e1260.
10. Lam SL (Ed). Hair Transplant 360 (Vol. 1). New Delhi, India: Jaypee Brothers Medical Publishers; 2011.
11. Karamanovski E. Problematic graft quality and handling. In: Unger WP, Shapiro R, Unger R, Unger M (Eds). Hair Transplantation, 5th edition. London, UK: Informa Healthcare; 2011. pp. 408-13.
12. Lorenzo J, Devroye JM, True R, Cole JP. Standardization of the terminology used in FUE: part III. Hair Transplant Forum Int. 2014;24:93-4.
13. Gupta AK, Love RP, Harris JA. Old friend or new ally: A comparison of follicular unit transplantation and follicular unit excision methods in hair transplantation. Dermatol Surg. 2020;46(8):1078-83.
14. Dua K, Dua A, Chahar M. Dos and don'ts of follicular unit extraction. In: Mysore V, Sattur S, Garg AK, Dua K, Patwardhan N (Ed). Hair Transplantation. New Delhi, India: Jaypee Brothers Medical Publishers; 2016. pp. 205-12.
15. Saxena K. Follicular unit extraction: technique and instrumentation. In: Mysore V, Sattur S, Garg AK, Dua K, Patwardhan N (Ed). Hair Transplantation. New Delhi, India: Jaypee Brothers Medical Publishers; 2016. pp. 190-8.
16. Dua K, Dua A, Chahar M. Complications of follicular unit extraction. In: Mysore V, Sattur S, Garg AK, Dua K, Patwardhan N (Ed). Hair Transplantation. New Delhi, India: Jaypee Brothers Medical Publishers; 2016. pp. 288-92.
17. Mysore V, Omprakash HM. Setting up a hair transplantation theater unit. In: Mysore V, Sattur S, Garg AK, Dua K, Patwardhan N (Ed). Hair Transplantation. New Delhi, India: Jaypee Brothers Medical Publishers; 2016. pp. 378-89.

CHAPTER 55

Long Hair Follicular Unit Extraction

Kavish Chouhan, Sayyad Ajara T Hamid

Key Messages

- Long hair follicular unit extraction (FUE) is one in a series of advances that have made FUE increasingly popular.
- Long hair FUE involves use of specialized punches and motor based on the principles of oscillation, vibration, and rotation.
- It seeks to overcome an important disadvantage of FUE—trimming of hair.

INTRODUCTION

The science behind hair transplant has evolved from an amateur plug procedure to strip surgery to the follicular unit extraction (FUE) procedure.[1] Evolution of the surgical technique has always taken inspiration from changing and evolving demands from patients. Pain, long wide scar of strip, and prolonged healing time associated with strip surgery encouraged hair restoration surgeons to focus on developing a technique such as FUE with minimum pain and scarring and shorter healing time. Present-day needs of hair transplant patients demand discretion and freedom from shaving their entire head. Long hair FUE, which is also called nonshaven FUE (NS-FUE), is the result of this exact patient demand.

ADVANTAGES OF LONG HAIR FOLLICULAR UNIT EXTRACTION OVER CONVENTIONAL FOLLICULAR UNIT EXTRACTION

- *Privacy and discretion:* When it comes to hair transplantation, long hair FUE provides a good option for patients who value privacy and discretion. Despite the growing acceptance of hair transplants in society, some individuals, including celebrities, politicians, and those who have to make public appearances, prefer to remain discreet about their procedures. In order to meet the needs of these patients, long hair FUE enables them to undergo a hair transplant with minimal visible effects immediately following the procedure, providing an inconspicuous result.
- *Natural camouflage for crusting:* A common concern expressed by patients considering shaved FUE hair transplants is visible crusting and healing after the procedure. Fortunately, long hair FUE addresses this concern by providing a natural camouflage in both recipient and donor areas, enabling a seamless and natural appearance.
- *Donor and recipient area preview:* Long hair FUE proves advantageous for patients with limited graft supply. It allows surgeons to visualize donor area during procedures, helping to optimize graft usage when grafts are scarce. Additionally, long hair FUE is an excellent choice for procedures requiring precise curvature control, such as eyebrow and eyelash transplants.

HISTORY OF LONG HAIR FOLLICULAR UNIT EXTRACTION

Hair restoration using long hair FUE is a groundbreaking technique. Modern FUE and follicular unit transplantation (FUT) techniques have been greatly influenced by the contributions of Uebel, Limmer and Bernstein, and Rassman in the 1990s.[2]

In 2006, Pitchon introduced the concept of "preview long hair transplantation," which allowed patients to have a preview of their final hair transplant result immediately postoperatively. The technique utilized by Pitchon was long hair FUT technique, in which a strip was harvested without shaving head and implanting hair in a routine way.[3]

Follicular unit extraction, pioneered by Okuda in Japan before World War II, was first described as a surgical technique in the medical literature by Rassman and Bernstein in 2002.[2] There is no linear scar associated with FUE, there is less postoperative pain, and body and beard hair can be transplanted to the scalp.

Long hair FUE was introduced in 2016 with the advantage of previewing the donor area before the procedure. NS-FUE can be divided into three types: Pretrimming (PT), direct method (DM), and long hair FUE.[2-5] In PT, the target follicles are trimmed to a length of about 1 mm before being located and removed. DM, however, involves dissecting grafts one by one with a punch tip. Both the pretrimmed and direct FUE methods are not long hair FUE in reality, since they require trimming of the follicles to be implanted. Only long hair FUE with extraction of follicular units with the entire shaft without shaving both donor and recipient areas is long hair FUE in actual sense.

In 2016, Otavio Boaventura described open punch as a new tool enabling long hair follicular units extraction by FUE method.[4]

In 2019, Erdogan proposed a design of sharp punch with a slit along the length to accommodate the shaft.[6]

In 2020, Sanusi Umar developed a bipronged punch and subsequently hybrid punch for enabling long hair FUE, which revolutionized the long hair FUE with minimum graft and shaft transection.[7]

In 2020, another punch designed by Roberto Trivellini enabled long hair FUE extraction utilizing oscillatory movement and octagonal ring punch.[8]

CHALLENGES IN LONG HAIR FOLLICULAR UNIT EXTRACTION

Despite its advantages, long hair FUE presents several unique challenges that are specific to this technique.

- *Transection of grafts and shaft:* One of the primary challenges in long hair FUE is the transection of grafts. The extraction process requires a high level of precision and expertise. The risk of transecting the follicles is supposed to be higher in long hair FUE compared to traditional FUE. This is due to the length of the hair, which can obstruct the view of the surgeon and make the extraction process more difficult. Graft extraction in the conventional FUE procedure involves anticipation of the root of the follicle by viewing the angle of emergence of shaft and aligning the punch in a way to accommodate the follicle to decrease transection rate. In long hair FUE, the presence of shaft makes it difficult to anticipate the hair direction, thus increasing the chances of transection.

  Another problem encountered in long hair FUE is breakage of the shaft of the hair follicle with or without transection of the hair follicle unit. Capping is seen when the force used for extraction is distributed unequally around the hair follicle, resulting in separation of epidermis with the shaft of the follicle from the rest of the follicular unit. Capping was more commonly encountered in case of open punch. Newer devices for long hair FUE extraction have developed more advanced ways to minimize capping and allow better graft separation.[4]
- *Slow extraction process:* Another significant challenge is the slow extraction process. Long hair FUE is a time-consuming procedure, primarily due to the complexity of extracting long hair follicles. The need to carefully extract each follicle without causing damage can significantly slow down the extraction process, making long hair FUE a more lengthy procedure compared to traditional FUE.

  Presence of hair shafts makes visualization of donor area difficult compared to shaven FUE. Moping the blood oozing from previously extracted sites in the presence of long hair and avoiding entanglement of the surrounding hair follicles pose another challenge.
- *Long learning curve:* Specialization in long hair FUE requires a significant amount of training. This technique requires a high level of skill and expertise, and surgeons need to undergo a relatively long training period to specialize in it. This can be a barrier for many surgeons who wish to offer long hair FUE as a service.
- *Postoperative effluvium:* Patients need to be made aware that transplanted follicles will undergo a period of effluvium as a part of the normal process of healing. Patients may panic seeing the shedding of transplanted follicles; they need to be reassured about the regrowth.[9]
- *Cost of devices:* Last but not least, the cost of devices used in long hair FUE is a significant challenge. Specialized tools and devices, such as the open punch, the Trivellini device, and the Zeus hybrid punch, are costly. This can increase the overall cost of the procedure, making it less accessible to many patients.

PHYSICS OF LONG HAIR FOLLICULAR UNIT EXTRACTION

In routine FUE procedures, a micromotor is commonly used with a sharp punch to cut through the epidermis and extract follicular units. The rotation mode of the micromotor facilitates the movement of the punch, allowing for the extraction of individual hair follicles. However, in long hair FUE harvesting, specialized devices are utilized, which employ a combination of oscillation, rotation, and vibration in different combinations and for varying time periods.

This combination of oscillation, rotation, and vibration serves several purposes in long hair FUE harvesting.[10] Firstly, it aids in cutting through the epidermis without transecting the hair shaft. The oscillation and vibration motions help to minimize the risk of damage to the hair shaft during the extraction process.

The hybrid punch utilized for harvesting long hair follicular units has outer cutting edge and inner blunt edge. This design, in combination with short arc oscillatory movements, allows the punch to cut through the epidermis and dermis while the inner expanded portion of the punch provides enough space for follicular tissue to glide inside the punch along with the shaft of the follicle. This allows harvesting follicles without transecting the shaft of the follicle. Once the punch has crossed dense dermal tissue, the machine automatically shifts to the next cycle of wide arc oscillations, allowing the peri-follicular tissue to separate from graft, in contrast to conventional sharp punch with rotatory movement which cuts the tissue.[10]

The oscillatory movement also reduces the chances of transection and follicle damage. The rotation mode assists in the actual extraction of the follicular unit, while the vibration motion can further aid in dislodging the follicular unit from the surrounding tissue in case of fibrosis. The textured inner region of the punch allows the graft to slide up inside the punch **(Figs. 1 and 2)**.

By incorporating these different motions in different permutations and combinations, long hair FUE devices aim to improve the efficiency and success rate of the

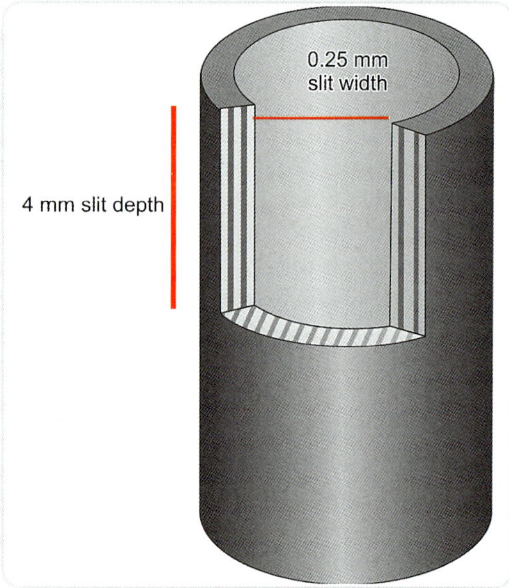

FIG. 1: Design of open punch.[4]

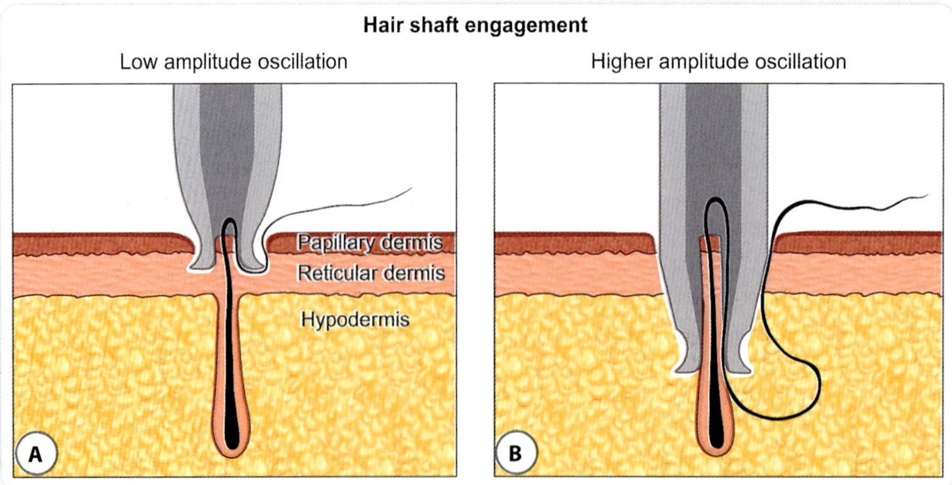

FIGS. 2A AND B: Utilization of low amplitude oscillations as they cut the epidermis without cutting the hair shaft.[10]

extraction process while minimizing the risk of transection and follicle damage. The specific combinations and durations of these motions may vary depending on the device and the surgeon's technique.

Relative placement of punch and hair shaft also seem to play a role in preventing shaft transection. Some devices recommend a 12 o'clock position; in the author's experience, the recommended placement is anywhere in between 3 and 6 o'clock.[11] The exact mechanism behind this is not elucidated. Hair shaft tissue is said to have less density and is able to withstand higher tissue pressure up to 270 MPa; hence, this process does not transect the hair shaft.[12]

It is important to note that the physics behind long hair FUE harvesting is a complex and evolving field. Ongoing research and advancements in technology continue to enhance the understanding and optimization of the physics principles involved in the technique, ultimately leading to improved outcomes in long hair FUE procedures.

DEVICES AVAILABLE FOR LONG HAIR FOLLICULAR UNIT EXTRACTION

Open Punch (Figs. 3A to C)

There are two versions of open punch, one given by Otavio Boaventura in 2016[6] and the other given by Erdogan in 2019.[6]

Entangling of long hair makes it impossible to use open punch in rotational mode for long hair FUE extraction. The punch designed by Otavio can be used for manual extraction as well as for motorized extraction using oscillation mode. The most common problem encountered with open punch is capping of tissue around the graft. A combination of the manual FUE device and open punch usually left some uncut skin around hair shafts, resulting in capping and difficult harvesting. There is also an incomplete cut of the epidermis around the graft, leading to improper extraction in this case. After some adjustments, Otavio settled on a 0.125 mm slit width and a 4.5 mm slit depth, with 1 and 0.9 mm punch diameters to minimize capping. It was harder to insert hair into the punch, but the capping issue was eliminated, manual extraction became feasible, and motorized extraction with oscillation arcs of 270–360° worked well.[4]

Zeus—UGraft System

The UGraft® Zeus™ system has revolutionized long hair FUE. It is unique due to its ability to perform long hair FUE without a groove or slot, which has not been seen in previous technologies.

Intelligent Punch™, also known as Dr. UPunchi™, is one of the key components of this system. This design is purposed to extract any type of hair follicle. As a result of the punch's spinning motion, the long hair is pulled inside by the vortex effect. This device has three stages

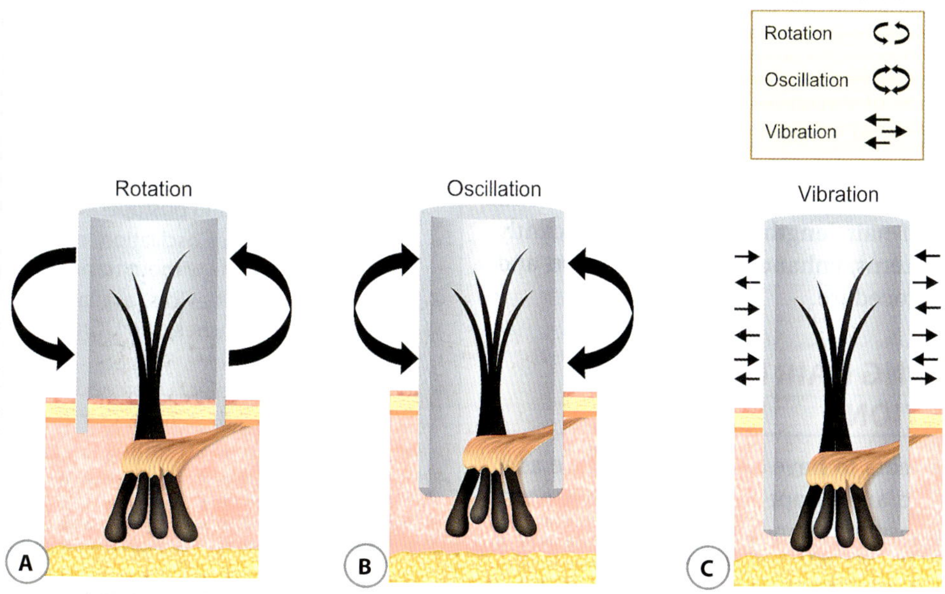

FIGS. 3A TO C: Combination of movements used in long hair FUE: (A) Rotation is used to penetrate the epidermis; (B) Oscillation is used in dermis; (C) Vibration is used to separate the perifollicular tissue.[13]

REFERENCES

1. Dua A, Dua K. Follicular unit extraction hair transplant. J Cutan Aesthet Surg. 2010;3(2):76.
2. Memon R, Avram M. The pros and cons of follicular unit extraction (FUE) versus elliptical donor harvesting (FUT). J Cosmet Laser Ther. 2022;24(6-8):63-5.
3. Mayer M. Hair transplantation in Asian and Black patients. In: Unger W, Shapiro R, Unger R, Unger M (Eds). Hair Transplantation, 5th edition. New York: Informa Healthcare; 2011. p. 431.
4. Pathomvanich D, Imagawa K. Asian hair: knowing the differences. In: Pathomvanich D, Imagawa K (Eds). Hair Restoration Surgery in Asians. New York: Springer; 2010. pp. 17-9.
5. Donor area harvesting. In: Unger W, Shapiro R (Eds). Hair Transplantation, 5th edition. New York: Informa Healthcare; 2011. p. 292.
6. Mohebi P, Cole J, Devroye J, Lorenzo J, True R. Standardization of the terminology used in FUE: part II. Hair Transplant Forum Int. 2013;23(6):210-2.
7. Mohebi P, Lorenzo J, Devroye J, True R, Cole J. Standardization of the terminology used in FUE: part I. Hair Transplant Forum Int. 2013;23(5):166-8.
8. Garg AK, Garg S. Donor harvesting: follicular unit excision. J Cutan Aesthet Surg. 2018;11(4):195.
9. Chouhan K, Kota RS, Kumar A, Gupta J. Assessment of safe donor zone of scalp and beard for follicular unit extraction in Indian men: a study of 580 cases. J Cutan Aesthet Surg. 2019;12(1):31.

PART C: Graft Handling

SECTION OUTLINE

- ❑ Graft Dissection: Techniques
- ❑ Magnification in Hair Restoration
- ❑ Graft Preservation

CHAPTER 58

Graft Dissection: Techniques

Anil Kumar Garg, Seema Garg

Key Messages

- Graft production after strip harvesting is a vital component of hair transplantation.
- It is a microsurgery and needs good hand–eye coordination, patience, and training.
- It consists of two components: Slivering and follicular unit production.
- Magnification is absolutely essential during the entire process of graft production.
- The hair follicles are very delicate and sensitive to microtrauma and desiccation.

INTRODUCTION

Graft dissection is a vital part of transplantation. To achieve healthy hair growth, we need to have healthy grafts. Magnification, proper training, good hand-eye coordination, patience, commitment, and dedication are all mandatory.

GRAFT PRODUCTION

The entire process of graft production is no less than a microsurgery, and it requires all important prerequisites of microsurgery to be followed. The surgeon's position with comfortable sitting, appropriate instrumentation, good light with magnification **(Figs. 1A to D)**, and a wet atmosphere for grafts are vital to ensuring success. A surgeon working with poor-quality instruments under inadequate light and uncomfortable position gets early fatigue, resulting in errors in dissection. Graft production in the strip method involves multiple steps with the involvement of multiple people—surgeon and technicians—it is a supply chain. Every step in the supply chain needs to be precise, steady, and quick—to deliver the ultimate end product, i.e., a healthy graft. These steps are strip harvesting (dealt with in earlier chapter), slivering, and graft dissection. Graft dissection [slivering and follicular unit (FU) separation] is discussed in this chapter.

Slivering

The first step in graft harvesting after strip dissection is slivering.

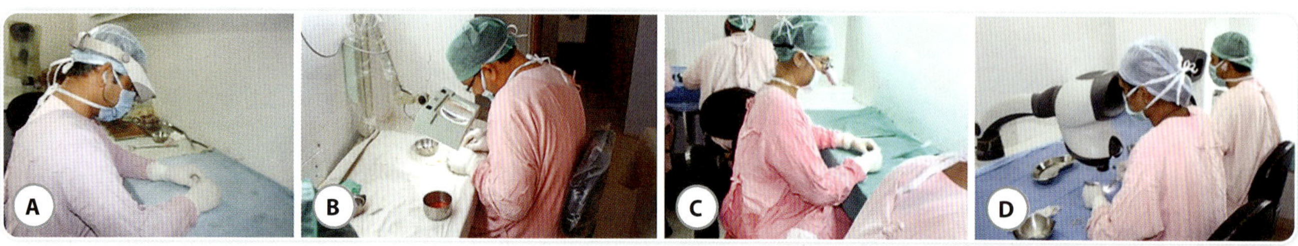

FIGS. 1A TO D: Magnification: (A) Optivisor; (B) Magnifying lens; (C) Magnifying loupe; (D) Stereomicroscope.

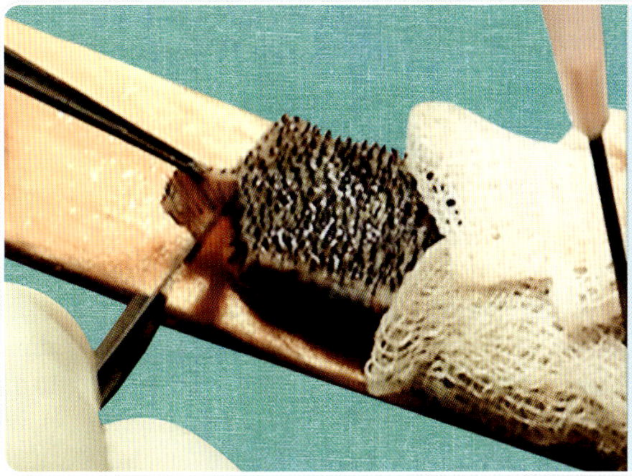

Things to remember

- Proper fixation of sliver
- Keeping sliver moist
- Use tip of scalpel while cutting
- Direction of movement of scalpel parallel to follicle direction
- Forceps holds epidermis and dermis only and traction outward and slightly upward
- Extra fat excision leaving minimal fat below bulb

FIG. 2: Process of slivering (with things to remember).

A sliver is a piece of skin with a single row of FUs derived from the skin strip—it is usually 1-1.5 cm long (depending on the width of the strip) and 2 mm wide. Dissecting a sliver from a strip needs magnification and the use of a loupe/microscope with magnification 3× is good enough to have a good visualization of follicles. A range of 2.5-6× is commonly used for slivering.[1]

Steps of Slivering (Figs. 2 to 4)

1. The skin strip is fixed on a wooden spatula using a size #25 needle at one end **(Fig. 2)**. Alternate methods of fixing include using a rubber band to stretch the strip, which is then tied onto a needle.
2. The strip is kept moist during the entire process of slivering. The skin strip can be kept moist by wrapping a moist gauze piece around it. Alternately, saline can be sprayed on the strip frequently.
3. Slivering is usually performed across the width of the strip to produce slivers that are 1-1.5 cm long **(Fig. 2)**. Some surgeons perform across the length of the strip to produce slivers 15-20 cm long **(Fig. 3)**. The latter technique is more difficult and needs experience. Slivering should be done under magnification only.[2]
4. Injection of saline into the strip can cause separation of units and aids dissection.
5. The upper edge of the strip is held by fine tooth forceps. A slight lateral traction is applied over the edge of the skin strip, and using the tip of a scalpel, the skin in between two rows of follicles is cut **(Fig. 2)**. Dissection has to be gentle. An ideal sliver should be single FU wide. Extra fat tissue below the bulb of follicles is excised, leaving a thin rim of fat below. This thin rim of fat prevents drying of the graft as well as protects it during implantation.

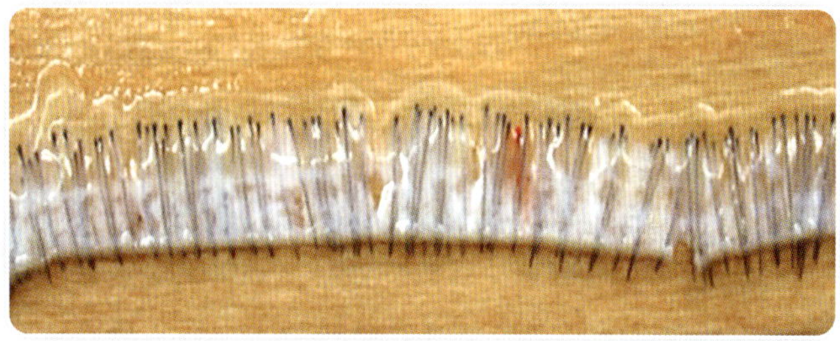

FIG. 3: Long sliver dissected across the length of the strip.

Graft Dissection

Individual grafts are dissected from slivers. Grafts contain individual FUs, which may contain one to four hairs. Occasionally, a surgeon may choose to create multi-follicular units (MFUs) that contain more than one unit. Proper magnification, good cold light, and a sharp scalpel are necessary for proper dissection.

High-quality graft refers to a consistent size and shape with intact arrectores, sebaceous glands, dermal papilla, a thin layer of surrounding dermis, and a small quantity of underlying adipose tissue. If the surrounding tissue is not sufficiently trimmed, the graft becomes too thick, i.e., "chubby," which is difficult to insert **(Fig. 5)**. In an attempt to insert a chubby graft, multiple efforts with more force cause damage to the follicle. On the other hand, if too much surrounding tissue is removed, grafts become "skinny." A skinny graft loses vital structures for growth and is prone to drying and poor growth. How chubby and how skinny a graft should be has been a matter of debate. Most surgeons agree that some tissue around the growth is preferable.

Slivers are put over a cutting surface with good illumination. An ideal cutting surface platform should be translucent, nonslippery, and sterile and should preserve

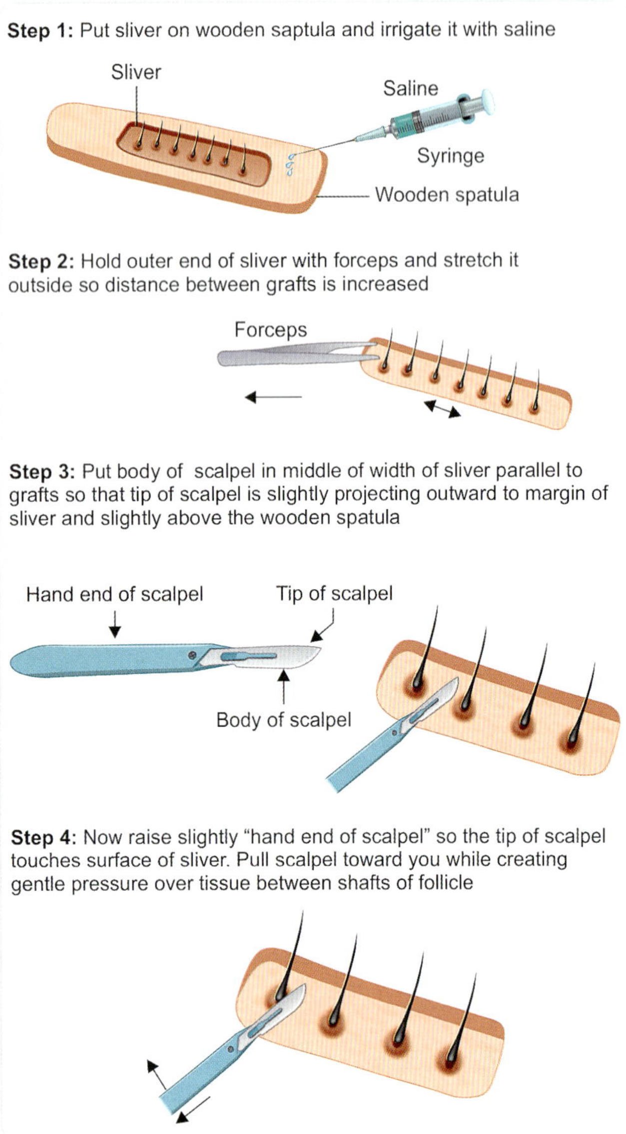

FIG. 4: Different steps of slivering and graft dissection.

the cutting edge of the scalpel. It should be hard enough so that small particles will not be scraped off and act as foreign bodies.

The yellow, rough, polyethylene surface is a good surface preferred by the author that completes all the requirements of an ideal cut surface. Many surgeons use a spatula as a dissection surface.

The author uses a stereomicroscope for follicle dissection with 6× magnification.[3] The magnification under the stereomicroscope gives good depth perception and virtual colors. This produces high-quality grafts, improves graft yield, and better visualization of nonpigmented hairs. However, there are surgeons who feel that in the case of Asian hairs, loupe dissection is adequate as hairs are pigmented and more visible as compared to Caucasian hair.

Steps for Dissection of Individual Units

1. A sliver is placed over a cutting board (polyurethane or wooden spatula) and irrigated with saline.
2. One edge (left edge for all right handers—as the scalpel is held in the right hand) of the sliver is grasped with jeweler's forceps to stretch the sliver **(Fig. 6)** the sliver is cut longitudinally with a scalpel from the epidermal end to the subcutaneous end. Cut inbetween the two follicles **(Fig. 7)**.
3. Extra epidermis is then removed **(Fig. 8)**.
4. Extra fat is removed by dissection at the lower end of the graft **(Fig. 9)**.

An ideal graft is a pear or teardrop shape with a sufficient amount of protective dermis and subcutaneous fat around the dermal papilla, intact sebaceous gland, little or no surplus epidermis, and a tiny shaft of hair left over.

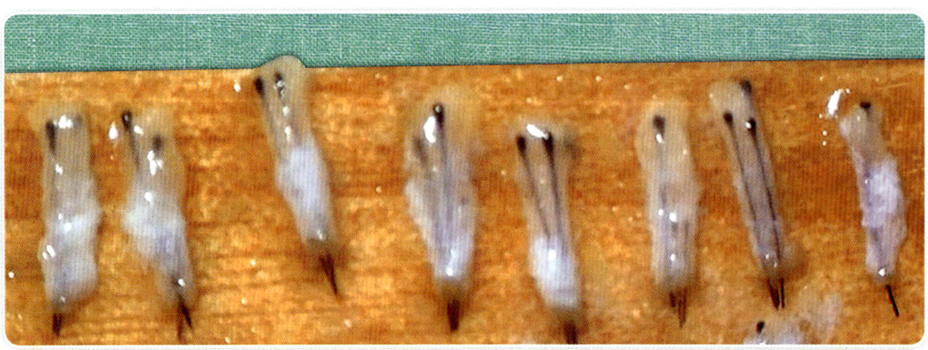

FIG. 5: Chubby grafts.

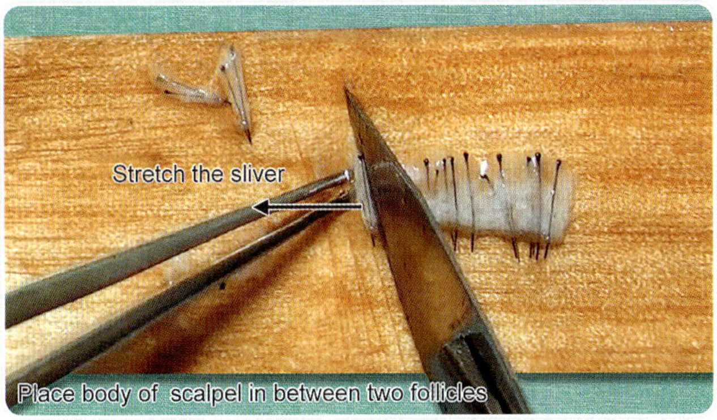

FIG. 6: Stretch the sliver by holding one end out side as shown by arrow.

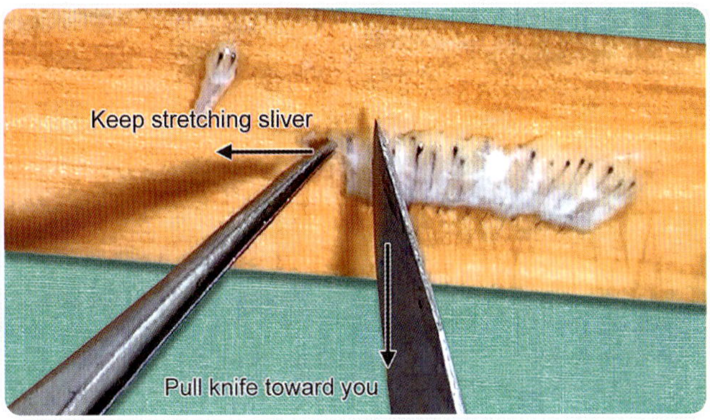

FIG. 7: Step 3—cut sliver in between two follicles.

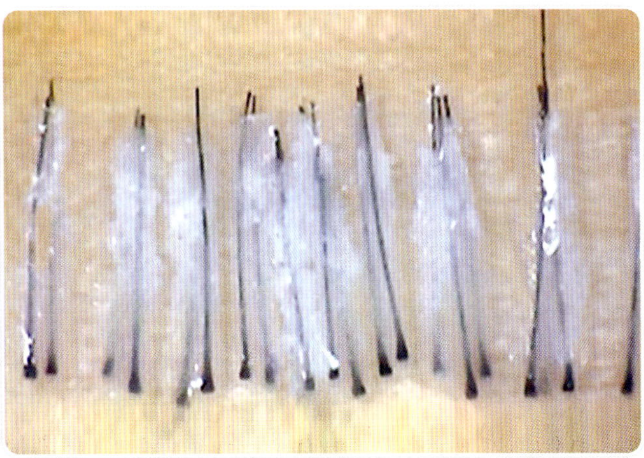

FIG. 8: De-epithelializing grafts with intact sebaceous glands.

At all steps, gentle handling of grafts is important. Grafts handling by nacked eye will create microtrauma to delicate follicles as blind man holds the hand of his friend to tight **(Figs. 10A to C)**.

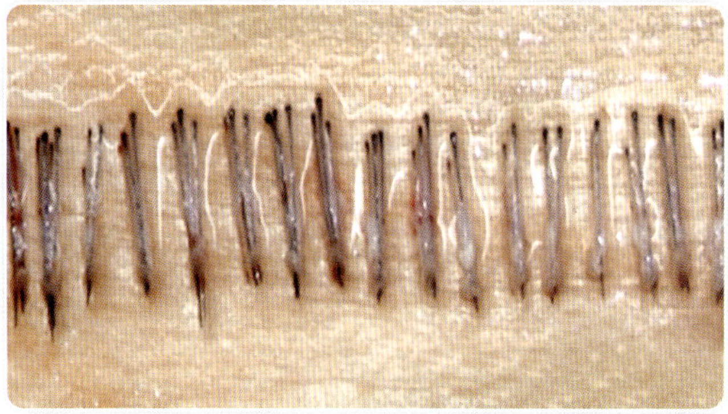

FIG. 9: Grafts after dissection.

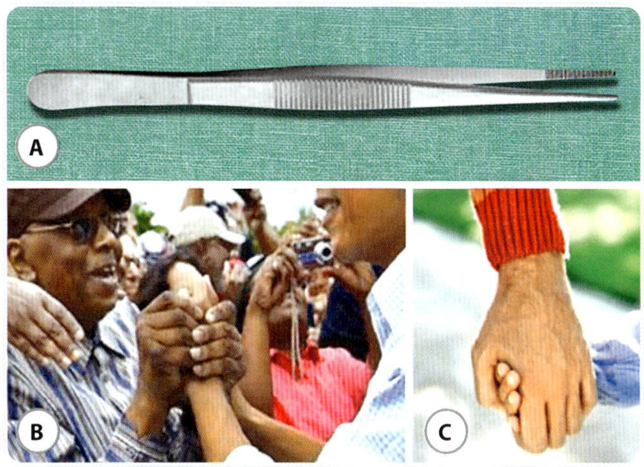

FIGS. 10A TO C: (A) Forceps; (B) Blind person holds hand tightly; (C) Gentle holding of hand.

Things to Remember during Follicle Dissection

- Keep all grafts and slivers moist.
- Hold the perifollicle tissue of the graft.
- Hold the outermost end of the sliver and slightly stretch it outward to increase the distance between grafts.
- Minimal cuts and minimal handling of graft
- Trimming if necessary
- Grafts neither skinny nor chubby
- If de-epithelialization, preserve sebaceous glands

SUMMARY

Graft dissection under proper magnification and with careful handling is the key to a successful hair transplantation. This needs training and practice. The grafts should have some dermal tissue around for survival. Gentle handling at all states is vital. Readers can practice on the training module developed by the author.[4]

Common mistakes made by beginners:

- Trying to do too fast dissection
- Getting frustrated at the slow pace
- Not removing the epidermis properly
- Not clearing the wastage from the central area of dissection
- Getting fatigued or bored
- Not sitting in the right body position

REFERENCES

1. Bernstein RM, Rassman WR. Dissecting microscope versus magnifying loupes with transillumination in the preparation of follicular unit grafts. A bilateral controlled study. Dermatol Surg. 1998;24(8):875-80.
2. Limmer B. Donor strip slivering and microscopic dissection. In: Haber RS, Stough DB (Eds). Procedures in Dermatology—Hair Transplantation. Philadelphia: Elsevier; 2006. p. 87.
3. Sandoval CA, Sandoval H. Classic microscopic dissection of follicular units. In: Unger W, Shapiro R (Eds). Hair Transplantation, 5th edition. New York: Informa Healthcare; 2011. p. 313.
4. Garg AK, Garg S. A learning module in hair restoration surgery: a simple and economic method to learn all steps of strip method of hair follicles harvesting and implantation. Indian J Plast Surg. 2017;50:230-5.

CHAPTER 59

Magnification in Hair Restoration

Amit Kerure, Komal Ahuja

Key Messages

- Magnification is an important tool to decrease damage to the hair follicle while performing various steps of hair transplant.
- Magnification devices involve using high-powered microscopes or loupes.
- Loupes are simple and easy to use, while microscopes offer higher magnification but have long learning curve.

INTRODUCTION

Hair restoration is one of the most exciting and innovative surgical fields in aesthetic surgery today. Hair transplantation is a surgical procedure that involves removing hair follicles from a donor area and transplanting them to a recipient area where hair growth is desired. The success of the procedure depends upon various factors, including the quality of hair follicles, the expertise of the surgeon, the density of the recipient area, and damage to hair follicle. However, one factor that is often overlooked but crucial in hair transplantation is magnification.

Magnification in hair transplant surgery involves using a high-powered microscope or loupes to closely examine and separate hair follicles under optimal conditions. This technology allows surgeons to precisely extract the hair follicles from the donor area with minimal damage and to transplant them into the recipient area with maximum accuracy.

HISTORY

The practice of hair transplantation for balding patients was first introduced in the 1950s in Japan. Since then, the history of magnification has been a crucial aspect that has made the procedure more advanced and effective in hair restoration. With the introduction of magnification devices, the success rate of hair transplant procedures has increased by providing a better view and more precise work. The first magnifying device used was the conventional microscopes. In the 1990s, with the introduction of operating microscopes, the field of hair transplantation was revolutionized. In recent years, the use of advanced magnification tools such as the loupes has gained popularity. However, with the advent of follicular unit extraction (FUE), the dependence on microscopic dissection has reduced.

TYPES OF MAGNIFICATION

There are various types of magnifying devices that are being used in hair transplant surgery. The most common types are mentioned in the following text.

Loupes

Magnification: 2.5–4.5×

Loupe is a miniature hand-held device that the surgeon can place directly over their eyes. It is simple, cheap, and effective for all steps of hair transplantation and is most commonly used. Compared to other magnification devices, it can be customized and offer better resolution with quality magnification.

Mechanics: It contains fundamentally two monocular microscopes with side-by-side lenses, angled to focus on an object. The magnified image that is formed has

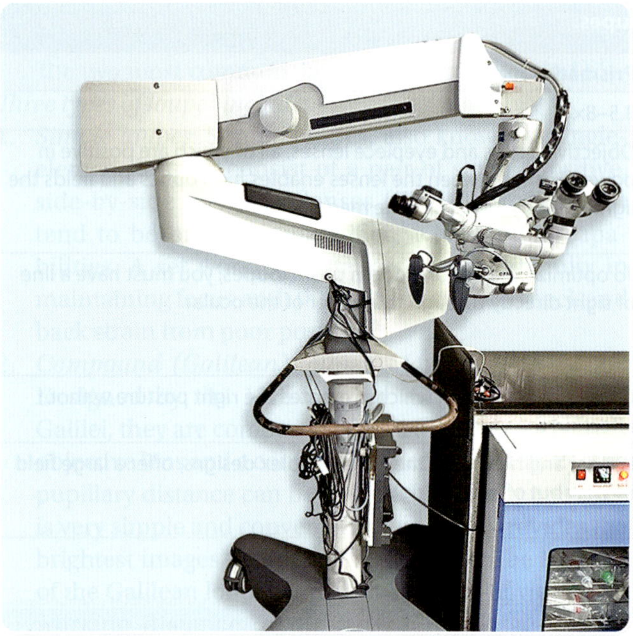

FIG. 6: Operating microscope.

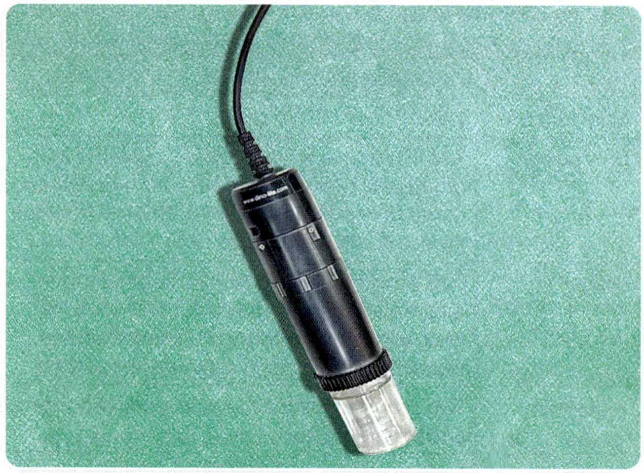

FIG. 7: Video microscope.

binocular protects against eye strain and fatigue. It incorporates fully coated optics and achromatic lenses with high-resolution and high-contrast stereoscopic vision.

Microscopes offer the ability to utilize different magnifications with the same instrument and can provide higher levels of magnification. Generally, the traits associated with the use of surgical stereomicroscopes are three-fold: Illumination, magnification, and increased precision in surgical skill delivery. Illumination and magnification delivered by an external stereomicroscope offer the advantage that it allows significantly greater magnification when compared to loupes and the ability to deliver illumination directly to the surgical field.

In hair transplant surgery, it is used to dissect hair follicles making small incision and to implant hair follicles into the recipient area.[5,6]

Video Microscope

Magnification: Up to 50× Video microscopes are computerized tools that provide real-time imaging of hair follicles on a monitor screen **(Fig. 7)**. They have the highest magnification but are expensive, have long learning curve, and are used only in some centers.

Polarized Light-emitting Diode

Magnification: Up to 2× Polarized light-emitting diode provides magnification for optimal recipient site creation during hair transplant. It has no perceived advantage in creating grafts or placing grafts compared to other magnification devices. There was less eye strain and greater ease in creating recipient sites using polarized magnification.[7]

The advantages and disadvantages of various magnifying devices are given in **Table 3**.

TABLE 3: Advantages and disadvantages of various magnifying devices.

Types	Advantages	Disadvantages
Loupes	Magnification: 2–8× Simple, cheap, easy to use, can be customized with good resolution	Lower magnification, eye strain
Magnifying glasses	Lightweight, easy to wear, eye protection	Minimal magnification
Magnifier with frame/ headband[1]	Magnification: 1.5–3.5×, lightweight, pivots out of viewing angle	Small field of view, difficult positioning for optimum viewing angle
Magnification stand[1]	Need not to be worn	Not easily portable, cumbersome to use
Operating microscope	Magnification: 10–50×	Not easily portable, extra space required, can cause strain on neck, used only in slivering and cutting steps of hair transplant
Video microscope	Magnification: Up to 50× Provide high-definition visuals for better identification and dissection of hair grafts	Expensive, requires specialized training
Polarized light-emitting diode (LED)	Magnification: Up to 2× Less eye strain, reduces unwanted reflection or glare	Less magnification

USE OF MAGNIFICATION IN DIFFERENT STAGES OF HAIR TRANSPLANT

A hair graft is a microscopic structure of 3–5 mm in length. So, if it is magnified up to 10×, 30×, or 50×, the chances of damage will decrease at each step and ultimate yield of surgery will increase.

- Magnification is used in the initial assessment of donor and recipient sites in determining the quality and quantity of hair follicles and inspection of hair shaft, bulb, and root, ensuring that the follicles are healthy and viable for transplant. Additionally, magnification is used to assess the recipient site to determine the density and pattern of existing hair follicles.[6]
- Magnification allows for precise identification and dissection of individual hair follicles, which are then extracted using either FUE or follicular unit transplantation (FUT).[6] It is also used to differentiate between different types of hair grafts, such as single-hair, double-hair, and triple-hair grafts, which are then used to ensure a natural-looking hairline.
- Magnification aids in ensuring the precise placement of hair follicles in the recipient site,[6] considering the angle, direction, and pattern of hair growth. It allows the surgeon to place hair grafts without injuring the surrounding hair follicles and hence less collateral damage, ensuring a successful and aesthetically pleasing outcome.

Magnification required in different steps of hair transplant **(Table 4)**.[8,9]

BENEFITS OF USING MAGNIFICATION

- *Better visibility*: Magnification provides a better view of the scalp and hair follicles, which makes it easier to identify and extract healthy hair follicles without damaging them.
- Reduced trauma and reduced healing time

TABLE 4: Magnification required in different steps.

Follicular unit transplantation	Follicular unit extraction
Strip harvesting: 2.5–5×	Extraction: 2.5–5×
Slivering and dissection: Ideally stereomicroscope used with magnification of 10×	
Slitting: 4×	Slitting: 4×
Implantation: 2.5–5×	Implantation: 2.5–5×

- *Improved result*: With greater precision and accuracy, surgeons can ensure that each hair follicle is placed in the correct location, resulting in a more natural-looking hairline.

FEATURES OF AN IDEAL MAGNIFICATION DEVICE

- Ideal magnification devices should provide magnification of 2.5–50×.
- They should have a good light source.
- They can be used for slivering, dissection, harvesting, and implantation of hair follicle.
- They should be affordable and maintenance free.
- They should be capable of changing angle, direction, and orientation of all three working axes.

CHOICE OF A MAGNIFICATION DEVICE

Overall, the types of magnification used depend on the surgeon's preferences and specific needs of the hair transplant procedure.

Important criteria to look for while choosing magnification devices are magnification required (2.5–4×), light source, field of vision (7–9 cm), space available, budget, and easy to use.

Tips and Pearls

- A binocular loupe with magnification of 2.5–5× appears to be the most useful magnifying device.
- As magnification increases, the field of view decreases and the amount of light coming through the lens also decreases, making the field of view darker.
- Adjustment period for wearing loupes is usually 2–3 weeks.
- Starting with a low magnification and gradually increasing it make it easy to adapt to a higher magnification.
- While loupes improve visual acuity, this improvement is significant when combined with illumination.

SUMMARY

- Magnification in hair transplant surgery is mandatory at each step to avoid transection during the process of harvesting, slivering, and dissection of follicular units. The use of magnification results in better outcomes and superior aesthetic results.
- When used properly, magnification devices can be beneficial to the surgeon by promoting better posture, preventing eye strain, and providing enhanced visualization of operating field and instruments.[1]

REFERENCES

1. Chodkiewicz HM, Joseph AK. Magnification for the dermatologic surgeon. Cutis. 2017;99:413-7.
2. Liang CA, Levine VJ, Dusza SW, Hale EK, Nehal KS. Musculoskeletal disorders and ergonomics in dermatologic surgery: a survey of Mohs surgeons in 2010. Dermatol Surg. 2012;38:240-8.
3. Sethu M. A simple and innovative technique to offload the microsurgical loupe. Int Microsurg J. 2022;6(1):3.
4. Stanbury SJ, Elfar J. The use of surgical loupes in microsurgery. J Hand Surg Am. 2011;36(1):154-6.
5. Bernstein RM, Rassman WR. Dissecting microscope versus magnifying loupes with transillumination in the preparation of follicular unit grafts. A bilateral controlled study. Dermatol Surg. 1998;24(8):875-80.
6. Cooley JE, Vogel JE. Follicle trauma and the role of the dissecting microscope in hair transplantation. A multicentric study. Dermatol Clin. 1999;17(2):307-12.
7. Avram MR. Polarized light-emitting diode magnification for optimal recipient site creation during hair transplant. Dermatol Surg. 2005;31(9 Pt. 1):1124-7.
8. J Cutan Aesthet Surg. 2010;3(2):76-81.
9. Indian J Plast Surg. 2008;41(Suppl):S56-S63.

CHAPTER 60

Graft Preservation

Nirmal B

Key Messages

- Grafts in hair transplantation surgery are subjected to various stresses right from extraction till implantation.
- Graft storage solutions help in graft survival and optimal growth.
- Solutions are classified as extracellular fluid (ECF)-like and intracellular fluid (ICF)-like solutions.
- ECF-like solutions are cheaper and easily available.
- ICF-like solutions are expensive and are optimally chilled.

INTRODUCTION

The number of grafts transplanted has increased as the field of hair transplantation surgery has progressed over the years. With an increase in the number of grafts harvested and mega sessions, there is a corresponding lengthening of the time of grafts spent outside the body. This has meant that grafts are exposed to various stresses from the extracted time till they obtain revascularization in the recipient area. Appropriate biopreservation of hair follicle grafts when they are out of the body in the absence of nutrients is hence an important factor in the survival of grafts. This has become even more relevant with the advent of the follicular unit extraction (FUE) method of extraction and harvesting of nonscalp hair as donor hair, which are slower processes and involve greater handling of grafts by the surgeon.

POSSIBLE STRESSES ENCOUNTERED BY GRAFTS

The potential sources of injury for graft during transplantation are:

- Mechanical injury during harvesting
- Injury sustained during transit time from donor to recipient
- Injury during implantation
- Injury in the postoperative period

Some of these processes cause mechanical trauma, while others cause chemical alterations. It is, therefore, important to understand the molecular process in a graft after its extraction and till it gets its own blood supply from the recipient area. Mechanical injuries to the graft that occurs during dissection, extraction, and implantation are all dealt with in different chapters, and this chapter focuses on tissue injury during the transfer of the graft and various graft-holding solutions.

Cellular and Molecular Considerations

Cells receive energy in the form of adenosine triphosphate (ATP) through glycolysis, Krebs cycle, and electron transport chain. Glycolysis converts glucose into pyruvate, and in aerobic conditions, pyruvate is oxidized to form ATP through the Krebs cycle and electron transport chain. In the absence of oxygen, pyruvate is converted into lactic acid.

Cessation of circulation once the grafts have been extracted leads to shift from aerobic to anaerobic metabolism, resulting in the production of lactic acid. Short interruptions in the supply of oxygen and glucose can be made up with energy from the lactic acid cycle;

however, this is self-limiting as H^+ ions have negative feedback on the anaerobic production of ATP and, hence, can be detrimental with the passage of time.[1]

Adenosine triphosphate-driven pumps maintain osmotic balance, free radical generation, membrane phase changes, organelle instability, and water flux. These cell membrane pumps control the movement of various ions, including sodium, potassium, magnesium, calcium, and chloride and counter-balance the osmotic gradient on either side of the cell membrane.

Graft-holding Temperature

The temperature of the graft-holding solution should be maintained at a steady level that is specific to the solution throughout the transplantation process. Lowering the temperature reduces cell metabolism. The Q10 equation principle states that for every 10°C drop in temperature, cell metabolism lowers by 50%.[2] This reduction in cellular metabolism and nutrition demand because of hypothermia is, therefore, advantageous. Several devices have been devised to provide cooling of the grafts, most of which include a container to hold ice and above which a petri dish is placed to keep the grafts.

Though this reduction in cellular metabolism and nutrition demand because of hypothermia is advantageous up to a point, on the flip side, it can also result in cell destruction due to the following causes.

Decreased activity of ATP-dependent sodium-potassium pump in hypothermia: Proper functioning of the pump is necessary to keep sodium outside and potassium inside the cell. Malfunction results in increased sodium within cells, subsequently causing increased chloride inside the cell to balance the charges and increased osmotic pressure inside the cell **(Fig. 1)**. This shifts water from extracellular fluid (ECF) into the cell, resulting in cellular swelling and lysis.[3-5] Grafts become bloated and may be misinterpreted as chubby, well hydrated, healthy grafts.[6]

- Glucose serves as energy during cold storage. However, excessive glucose results in the production of lactic acid, causing more cellular acidosis. Hence, glucose should be present in very low levels to prevent acidosis.[7]
- Cells outside the natural environment require an effective buffer at low oxygen concentrations. Bicarbonate is not an effective buffer in lower temperatures.[8]
- The lipid bilayer membrane may change phase to a gel phase at a lower temperature from a more physiological fluid state at a higher temperature.
- Cooling also results in decrease in natural defense mechanisms to free radicals, resulting in apoptosis.[9]

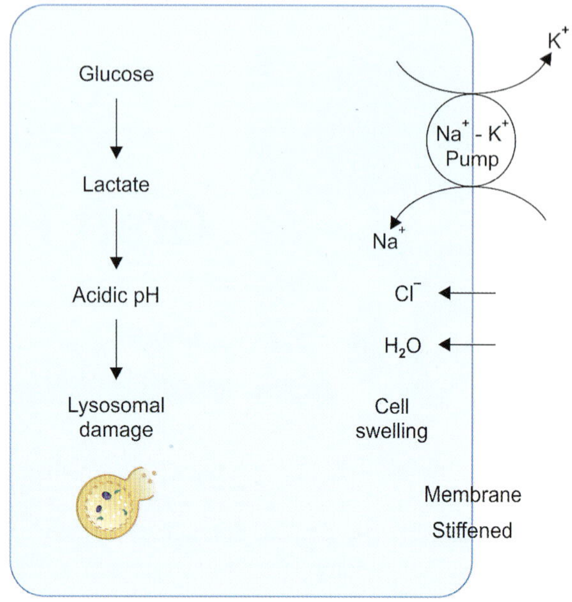

FIG. 1: Cold injury.

Reperfusion Injury

The graft is dependent on the passive perfusion of oxygen and glucose from the host dermis up to 48 hours. The graft develops its own blood supply within 3–5 days, and hence, it is thought that the first 5 days after implantation are crucial for survival. Any factor that affects the graft during this period, such as dislodgement, poor vascular supply, or postoperative bleeding, can adversely affect graft survival. Thereafter, proper reperfusion sets in.

Reperfusion is a stage when a graft, under ischemia, transplanted in the recipient area is exposed again to blood circulation, receiving a blast of oxygen **(Fig. 2)**. However, it brings its own set of problems from graft-reperfusion injury. Reperfusion injury is marked when compared to ischemia and hypoxia. The causes of reperfusion injury include production of free radicals, rise in intracellular calcium, and loss of membrane phospholipids.[10] Ischemia causes accumulation of hypoxanthine, which, when reperfused with oxygenated blood, leads to the formation of free radicals that damage cell membranes and deoxyribonucleic acid (DNA).[6] Reperfusion injury is one of the causes of poor results following hair transplant surgery and can be reduced with the inclusion of scavengers of free radicals in the graft-holding solution.[11]

Effect of Drying

Drying of grafts has been held to be one of the main causes of tissue injury. Survival rates of grafts decreased from 94

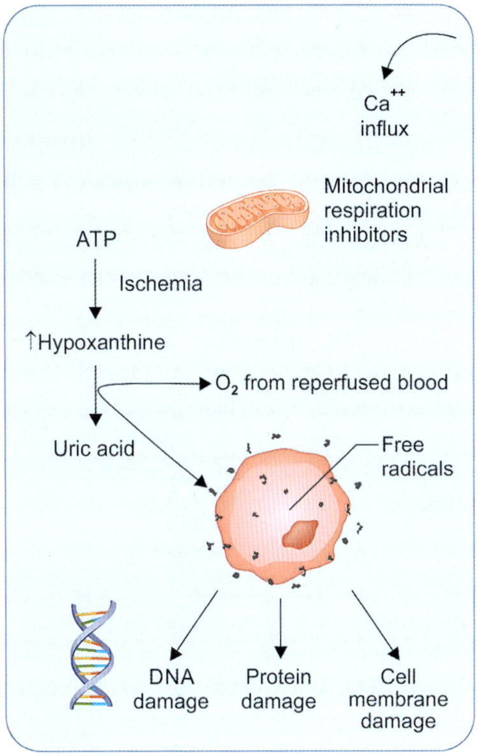

FIG. 2: Ischemia–reperfusion injury.
(ATP: adenosine triphosphate; DNA: deoxyribonucleic acid)

to 68% when grafts were allowed to dry on gauze for 5 and 30 minutes, respectively. Hair regrowth was affected even when grafts were kept on surgical gloves for 3 minutes.[12] It is, therefore, recommended that during implantation, more than 20 grafts should not be kept on the surgeon's hand, and regular spraying needs to be performed. A cup-like device that holds the grafts in a holding solution has been devised to overcome the problem of drying.

It is, therefore, important to maintain the graft in a moist environment. Repeated spraying with fluids is important during transfer, soon after implantation, and also in the postoperative period.

GRAFT-HOLDING SOLUTIONS

Graft-holding or storage solutions play an important part in hair transplant surgery as graft dehydration has detrimental effect on the survival of grafts. Several studies have sought to determine graft survival and the time the grafts spend outside the body. Limmer performed an in vivo study using chilled normal saline (NS) with follicular unit grafts. The results of graft survival were 95% in 2 hours, 90% in 4 hours, 86% in 6 hours, 88% in 8 hours, 79% in 24 hours, and 54% in 48 hours.[13] Limmer related a good "rule of thumb," stating that the loss was roughly 1% for every hour. Other studies endorsed these findings and stressed the need for completing the transplantation quickly.[14,15] There is no doubt that the duration that the graft spends outside the body needs to be as short as possible. The fact that there is little graft loss in the first 4 hours leaves a window of opportunity for the dissecting team. However, in larger sessions and for beginners who need longer time to complete the dissection, this is a disadvantage. Hence, the search is for a solution that can enhance this graft survival.

TABLE 1: Characteristics of holding solutions.[12]

Holding solution	pH	Buffer
Normal saline	5.0	None
Ringer's lactate	6.5	Lactate
PlasmaLyte A	7.4	Acetate
HypoThermosol	7.6	Hydroxyethylpiperazine ethane sulfonic acid

Ideal Graft-holding Solution

The essential characteristics of an ideal graft-holding solution are as follows:

- Maintain ionic balance across the cell membrane
- Should have the same osmolality as the grafts
- Minimize cellular swelling
- Prevent intracellular acidosis
- Prevent free radicals' formation and their elimination
- Provide high-energy substrates such as ATP
- Quicken recovery on reperfusion and rewarming
- Should be easily available
- Should be inexpensive

It is, of course, true that such an ideal solution is yet to be found. Several solutions have been used and are discussed below.

Storage solutions can be broadly classified into solutions that resemble ECF in composition (ECF-like) and those that resemble intracellular fluid (ICF-like) solutions. **Table 1** shows the characteristics of some of the holding solutions.

Extracellular Fluid-like Storage Solutions

Extracellular fluid-like solutions are similar to the normal extracellular environment of cells. They are suitable for the preservation of grafts in normothermic conditions. However, they are not suited for hypothermic conditions as they do not balance ions across membranes in hypothermia, resulting in osmotic imbalance, cellular swelling, and lysis. Hypothermia also results in decreased glycolysis and increased lactic acid production, leading to intracellular acidosis, causing lysosomal instability and apoptosis. Examples of ECF-like solutions include NS, Ringer's lactate, and tissue culture media.[1]

Normal saline, the most commonly used solution, has the advantages that it is readily available, is cheap, and has been time tested. It has an acidic pH that can impair graft survival, especially when grafts have to be placed in it for prolonged duration with longer extraction sessions. Some surgeons prefer Ringer's lactate as it has more potassium and a relatively more physiological pH. PlasmaLyte A is saline with optimized pH. It is reasonably fair to use NS for shorter surgeries while choosing optimized storage solutions for longer surgeries.[6]

Intracellular Fluid-like Storage Solutions

Intracellular fluid-like solutions are hypertonic solutions comprising higher potassium and lower sodium ions similar to the intracellular compartment. They have a larger anion concentration which does not move across the cell membrane, hence providing osmotic balance. These solutions have a higher osmotic pressure, which prevents the passive influx of water across the membranes and hence reduces cell swelling. These solutions are more expensive, and though there is a theoretical basis that they improve graft survival, there is still paucity of large clinical studies proving their superiority. Examples of ICF-like storage solutions include HypoThermosol, Viaspan (University of Wisconsin Solution), Collins, Euro Collins, CryoStor, Celsior, and Unisol.[16] Several cell culture media, such as Dulbeco's Modified Eagle's Medium (DMEM), also used in vitiligo surgery by cell suspension method, are also examples of ICF-like solutions.

HypoThermosol

HypoThermosol is an optimized hypothermic graft-holding solution. The constituents of the solution include glutathione, hydroxyethylpiperazine ethane sulfonic acid (HEPES), dextran-40, mannitol, lactobionate, and adenosine **(Table 2)**. Glutathione and a synthetic analog

TABLE 2: Constituents of HypoThermosol.

Constituents	Properties
Glutathione	Antioxidant
Hydroxyethylpiperazine ethane sulfonic acid	Buffer at low temperature
Dextran-40	Oncotic support
Mannitol	Osmotic agent
Lactobionate	Calcium chelator
Adenosine	Adenosine triphosphate regeneration

of vitamin E are potent antioxidants that act as free radical scavengers, acting as a buffer, and provide osmotic balance at low temperatures. Anions in the solution include gluconate, citrate, glycerophosphate, and anionic forms of aminosulfonic acids, such as HEPES. HEPES is an excellent buffer at low temperatures. A colloid like dextran-40 is also included for providing oncotic support. Mannitol is an osmotic agent and also acts as a free radical scavenger. It also causes vasodilatation mediated by prostaglandin.

Calcium is an important factor in apoptosis. Lactobionate is a chelator of calcium and thus minimizes cell injury due to the influx of calcium. Glucose is included at smaller concentration as higher concentrations can result in anaerobic lactic acid production under hypothermia.[17]

Liposomal Adenosine Triphosphate

Adenosine triphosphate is extremely unstable, and not all forms of ATP are efficacious. Liposomal ATP (ATP packed within liposomes) fuses with the cell membrane and delivers ATP into the cell. Liposomal ATP (VitaSol) must be diluted in the ratio of 1:10 in HypoThermosol NS. Grafts are to be stored at 14–20°C for the optimal uptake of ATP by cells.[18]

PLATELET-RICH PLASMA

Platelet-rich plasma (PRP) has been found to be useful in wound healing, orthopedics, and dentistry for a number of indications. The procedure involves the concentration of a patient's own platelets to four to seven times above baseline.[19] Alpha granules of platelets, when activated, release platelet-derived growth factor, transforming growth factor beta, epidermal growth factor, and vascular endothelial growth factor. PRP has been shown to improve graft survival, earlier hair growth, and faster healing in few studies on hair transplantation.

Platelet-rich plasma therapy makes the recipient area more fertile and receptive for transplanted hair by cell growth and differentiation, antiapoptotic activity, and neovascularization. PRP provides a favorable environment for dormant hair, leading to new hairs in shorter time.[20] Though the mechanism of action of PRP is not fully understood, results achieved clinically are promising.

Autologous plasma is easily available, is isotonic, and contains numerous growth factors and fibrin. Fibrin around the grafts not only acts as a barrier of protection but also provides a biologically active scaffold that maintains the optimal integrity of transplanted hair, preventing the graft from dehydration. Follicular units pretreated with platelet plasma growth factors before implantation resulted in significant improvement in hair growth and hair density.[21]

Advantages of autologous plasma as graft-holding solution:
- Easily available
- Relatively inexpensive
- Provides a biological scaffold for the graft
- Prevents graft from drying and desiccation
- Contains growth factors resulting in better results
- Prevents effluvium and faster regrowth

HISTIDINE-TRYPTOPHAN-KETOGLUTARATE SOLUTION

Histidine-tryptophan-ketoglutarate (HTK) solution is the gold standard for the preservation of solid organs. A low potassium-sodium ratio decreases the chances of cellular edema and damage due to ischemia-reperfusion. Deferoxamine (DFO) is an iron chelator used in organ transplantation to alleviate lipid peroxidation injury due to cold storage. HTK solution also contains strong buffer (histidine), osmotic substance (mannitol), and low-permeability amino acids (alpha-ketoglutaric acid and tryptophan) to mitigate ischemia-hypoxia injury.[22]

SUMMARY

Graft-holding solutions are essential in the transport and storage of grafts from the donor area till they are transplanted in the recipient area. An ideal holding solution lowers free radical production and maintains osmotic balance across the cell membranes, thus reducing apoptosis and cell swelling. Choosing the ideal temperature for the type of graft-holding solution is also important. However, there are no large randomized controlled trials to guide the selection of ideal holding solution in hair transplant surgeries, and current evidence is largely based on graft preservation in transplantation medicine. Knowledge about the various solutions and cellular mechanisms of various stresses in transit is quintessential to increase the yield of hair transplantation.

Tips and Pearls

- Hair follicle grafts are subjected to various stressors in transit from the donor area to the recipient site.
- An optimal graft-holding solution would reduce the trauma to grafts from reperfusion injury, free radical formation, and osmotic imbalance across cell membranes.
- Graft storage solutions are classified as ECF-like and ICF-like solutions.
- ECF-like solutions should preferably not be chilled as hypothermia leads to increased cellular osmolality and cell swelling.
- Use of cooled ECF-like solutions may cause cold injury to cells.
- ICF-like solutions are ideal for graft holding in hair transplant surgeries; however, their superiority over cheaper solutions is yet to be established.
- ICF-like solutions should be cooled to <8°C for graft holding.

REFERENCES

1. Mathew AJ. A review of cellular biopreservation considerations during hair transplantation. Hair Transplant Forum Int. 2013;23:7-11.
2. Reyes AB, Pendergast JS, Yamazaki S. Mammalian peripheral circadian oscillators are temperature compensated. J Biol Rhythms. 2008;23:95-8.
3. Mathew AJ, Baust JG, Van Buskirk RG. Improved hypothermic preservation of human renal cells through suppression of both apoptosis and necrosis. Cell Preserv Technol. 2003;1:239-54.
4. Baust JM. Advances in media for cryopreservation and storage. BioProcess Intl. 2005;3:46-56.
5. Mathew AJ. I'm losing cell viability and function at different points in my process, and I don't know why! BioProcess Intl. 2010;8:54-7.
6. Cooley JE. Holding solutions. In: Unger W, Shapiro R (Eds). Hair Transplantation, 4th edition. New York: Marcel Dekker; 2004. pp. 321-4.
7. Anderson RV, Siegman MG, Balaban RS. Hyperglycemia increases cerebral intracellular acidosis during circulatory arrest. Ann Thorac Surg. 1992;54:1126-30.
8. Taylor MJ, Pignat Y. Practical acid dissociation constants, temperature coefficients and buffer capacities for some biological buffers in solutions containing dimethyl sulfoxide between 25 and –12°C. Cryobiology. 1982;19:99-109.
9. Taylor TJ. Effect of hypothermia on the generation of free radicals. In: Baust JG, Baust JM (Eds). Advances in Biopreservation. Boca Raton: Taylor & Francis Group; 2007. pp. 39-40.
10. Cooley J. Ischemia-reperfusion injury and graft storage solutions. Hair Transpl Forum Int. 2004;13:127-30.
11. Krugluger W, Moser K, Moser C, Laciak K, Hugeneck J. Enhancement of in vitro hair shaft elongation in follicles stored in buffers that prevent follicle cell apoptosis. Dermatol Surg. 2004;30:1-5.
12. Unger W. Graft survival and growth studies. In: Unger W, Shapiro R (Eds). Hair Transplantation, 4th edition. New York: Marcel Dekker; 2004. pp. 330-2.
13. Limmer R. Micrograft survival. In: Stough D, Haber R (Eds). Hair Replacement. St. Louis: Mosby; 1996. pp. 147-9.
14. Hwang SJ, Lee JJ, Oh BM, Kim DW, Kim JC, Kim MK. The effects of dehydration, preservation temperature and time on the hair grafts. Ann Dermatol. 2002;14:149-52.
15. Gandelman M, Mota A, Arahamsohn P, De Oliveira SF. Light and electron microscopic analysis of controlled injury to follicular unit grafts. Dermatol Surg. 2000;26:25-31.

16. Bessems M, Doorschodt BM, van Vliet AK, van Gulik TM. Preservation of rat livers by cold storage: a comparison between the University of Wisconsin solution and HypoThermosol. Ann Transplant. 2004;9:35-7.
17. Mathew AJ, Baust JM, Van Buskirk RG, Baust JG. Cell preservation in reparative and regenerative medicine: evolution of individualized solution composition. Tissue Eng. 2004;10:1662-70.
18. Beehner ML. 96-hour study of FU graft "out-of-body" survival comparing saline to HypoThermosol/ATP solution. Hair Transplant Forum Intl. 2011;21:37.
19. Parsley WM, Perez-Meza D. Review of factors affecting the growth and survival of follicular grafts. J Cutan Aesthet Surg. 2010;3:69-75.
20. Garg AK, Garg S. A histological and clinical evaluation of plasma as a graft-holding solution and its efficacy in terms of hair growth and graft survival. J Cutan Aesthet Surg. 2020;13:50-6.
21. Abdelkader R, Abdalbary S, Naguib I, Makarem K. Effect of platelet rich plasma versus saline solution as a preservation solution for hair transplantation. Plast Reconstr Surg Glob Open. 2020;8:e2875.
22. Zhou Y, Zhang J, Fan Z, Hu Z, Miao Y. Evaluation of a novel graft-holding solution in hair transplantation: a randomized controlled clinical study. Dermatol Surg. 2023;49:675-81.

PART D: Recipient Area

SECTION OUTLINE

ANGLE OF SLIT (FIG. 3)

The next factor in slit making is the angle at which the slit is made. As the angle of entry becomes more acute, the depth of penetration for the same length of slit made reduces as explained below.

We know that sinθ = opposite side/hypotenuse. In our situation, sin(angle of entry) = depth/length of slit. Using this formula, the depths of penetration for a slit of 5 mm length at various angles are shown in **Table 1**.

This equation shows that the lower the entry angle, the lesser the depth of penetration and less chance of deep vascular injury. Hence, we should not use a vertical angle and make our angle acute as far as possible, mimicking the natural exit of hairs, which varies from 15° to 60°.

Inference: The more acute the angle, the less the depth of penetration

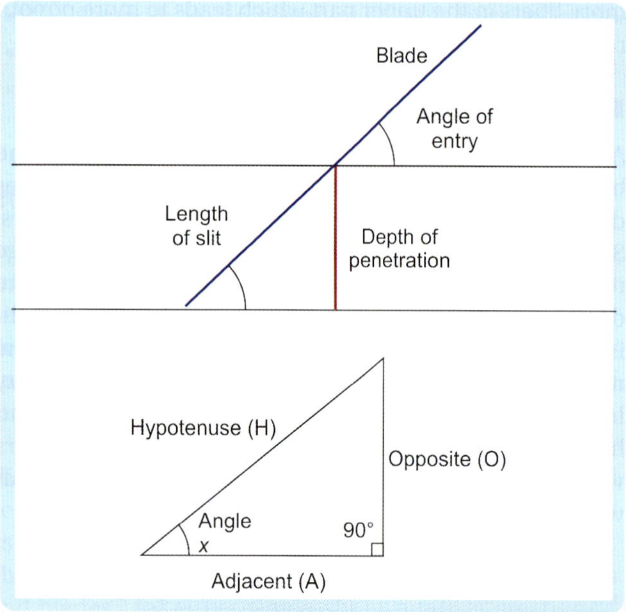

FIG. 3: Relation between angle of entry and depth of penetration.

TABLE 1: Variation between angle of entry and depth of penetration.

Angle (°)	Depth (mm)	Depth reduction (%)
90	5	0
75	4.8	4
60	4.3	14
45	3.5	30
30	2.5	50
15	1.3	74

SLIT ORIENTATION—CORONAL VERSUS SAGITTAL

The next factor to consider in slit making is the surface orientation of the slit, whether coronal or sagittal. Coronal versus sagittal is an old debate. Coronal slit making was recommended as a better way to provide better orientation of grafted hairs with respect to light reflectance and hence create a better visual impact. However, a sagittal slit was preferred by many as the more natural orientation and less likely to interfere with vasculature.

We would like to consider a different factor—the surface incision and whether it is the same as the width of the instrument **(Fig. 4)**.

In sagittal slits, the width of the blade is on the same axis as the angle of the slit. Hence, the length of the surface incision varies with the angle of the slit, similar to the above equation. **Table 2** shows the variation of surface incision for a blade of 1 mm width with angle.

As we can see, at more acute angles, the surface incision increases in length significantly. This increases the trauma to the superficial plexus, thereby offsetting the benefits of lower depth of penetration achieved at more acute angles. Also, the wider surface incision would decrease the density of packing.

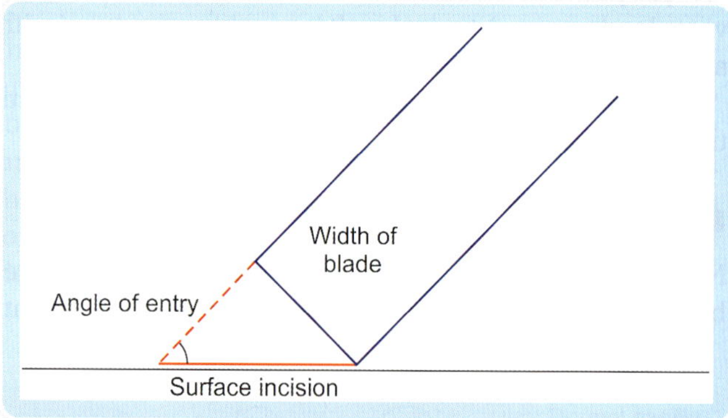

FIG. 4: Relation between angle of slit and length of surface incision for sagittal slits.

TABLE 2: Variation between angle of entry and surface incision.

Angle (°)	Surface incision (mm)	Increase (%)
90	1	0
75	1.035	3.5
60	1.155	16
45	1.415	41
30	2	100
15	3.85	285

In coronal slits, the width of the blade is perpendicular to the axis of the angle of the slit. Hence, the length of the surface incision does not change and is always the same as the width of the slit. This reduces the trauma to the superficial plexus while also preserving the deep plexus as the angle becomes more acute. Hence, the coronal slit would have the advantage of remaining the same width even after angulation.

Inference: Coronal slits do not increase the length of the surface incision, whereas sagittal slits increase the surface incision as the angle reduces.

RECOMMENDATIONS

The ideal slit is one that allows easy implantation at an optimum depth without much popout, with minimal vascular damage at optimal density.

Hence, to sum up, the slit technique that causes minimal vascular damage includes the following:

- Use of rectangular blades will reduce the damage to the dermis and vascular plexus as compared to rectangular blades and needles as the depth of penetration required is lower.
- Use of acute angle will reduce the depth of penetration for the same length of slit and reduce damage to deep plexus.
- Coronal slits will have lesser vascular damage than that of sagittal slits, whether using a single knife or multiple knives.

We believe that these recommendations provide the optimum volume slits while causing minimal vascular damage.

REFERENCES

1. Rose PT. Advances in hair restoration. Dermatol Clin. 2018;36(1): 57-62.
2. Garg AK, Garg S. Donor harvesting: follicular unit excision. J Cutan Aesthet Surg. 2018;11(4):195-201.
3. Sharma R, Ranjan A. Follicular unit extraction (FUE) hair transplant: curves ahead. J Maxillofac Oral Surg. 2019;18(4): 509-17.
4. Marwah MK, Mysore V. Recipient area. J Cutan Aesthet Surg. 2018;11:202-10.
5. Wells A. Use of blades of 0.7 to 1 mm in diameter and coronal incisions in hair transplantation: surgical approach to improve density and natural results. Rev Bras Cir Plast. 2013;28(4):593-8.
6. Atodaria PR. An innovative instrument for reducing the surgeon's time in making recipient sites. Hair Transplant Forum Int. 2014;24(4):131-2.
7. Atodaria PR, Atodaria KP. Modifications of multi slit knife for enhanced versatility in balding and vertex area hair transplant. J Cutan Aesthet Surg. 2020;13(3):247-50.
8. Atodaria PR, Atodaria KP. Reducing surgical time: an innovative and versatile instrument for creating multiple brick-pattern sagittal recipient sites in a single stroke. Hair Transplant Forum Int. 2020;30(5):180-1.
9. Ginzburg A, Agrawal S. Alternate coronal and sagittal slits in recipient area of hair transplantation to ensure the correct graft implantation by assisting surgeon. J Am Acad Dermatol. 2020;83(3):e189-90.
10. Nakatsui T, Wong J, Groot D. Survival of densely packed follicular unit grafts using the lateral slit technique. Dermatol Surg. 2008;34(8):1016-22.
11. Cormia FE. Vasculature of the normal scalp. Arch Dermatol. 1963;88:692-701.

CHAPTER 62

Recipient Area: Male and Female Hairline Design

Shalini Malhotra, Anchal Shah, Diwaker Sharma

Key Messages

- Know the anatomical landmarks of the hairline.
- Key considerations before designing a hairline.
- Balancing patient's expectations and surgeon's planning.
- How to proceed step by step to design a hairline that looks natural.
- Mistakes made and lessons learned.

INTRODUCTION

Hairline is a surgeon's signature. If you get the front hairline right, you get the whole thing right. Establishing the hairline is a crucial part of any hair transplant (HT) procedure. At times, even the most skilled surgeon may go awry in designing the hairline. Although there are no specific rules on hairline placement, different factors play an important role. The crucial component of HT procedure is not just the technique but also planning and expectation management.

ANATOMICAL LANDMARKS (FIGS. 1 TO 5)

Midfrontal Point

The midfrontal point (MFP)[1,2] is the most anterior midpoint of the frontal hairline. The MFP should be positioned 7–10 cm from the glabella on a vertical line drawn from the glabella to the trichion. Factors to consider while deciding the position of MFP are the age of the patient, grade of androgenetic alopecia (AGA), and facial contour.

Midpupillary Point

The midpupillary point (MPP) is the second point to be marked laterally to the MFP on a line drawn vertically upward from the pupil. The hairline curves posteriorly upward from here.

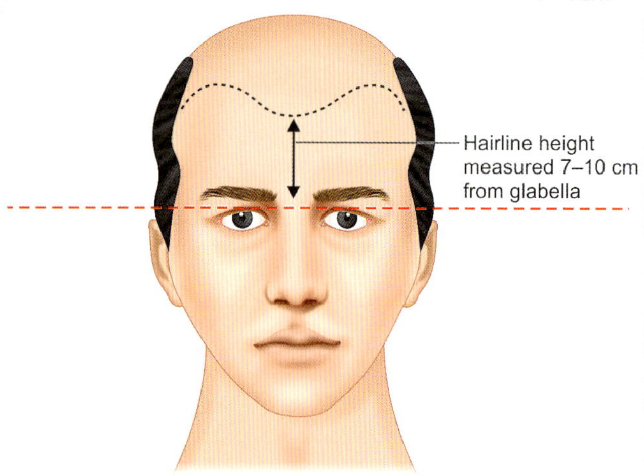

FIG. 1: The midfrontal point (MFP) lies 7–10 cm above the glabella.

Frontotemporal Angle

The frontotemporal angle (FTA)[2,3] is the meeting junction of the frontal and temporal hairline. The hairline should be directed upward on the side view. To locate the FTA, a line should be drawn vertically upward from the lateral epicanthus. *Red flag*: If the hairline looks straight or slopes downward on the side view, it will look artificial.

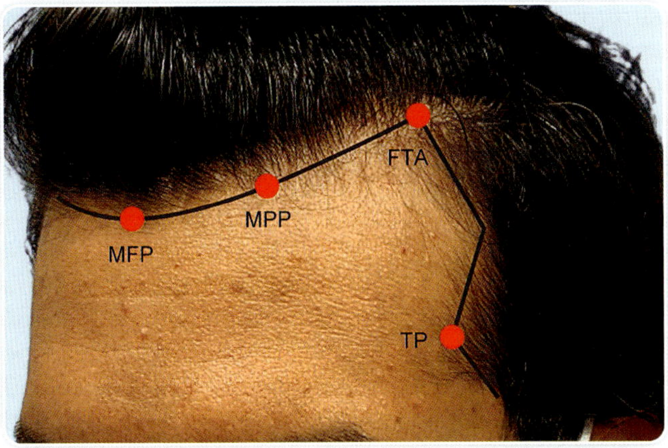

FIG. 2: Marking the hairline.
(FTA: frontotemporal angle; MFP: midfrontal point; MPP: midpupillary point; TP: temporal point)

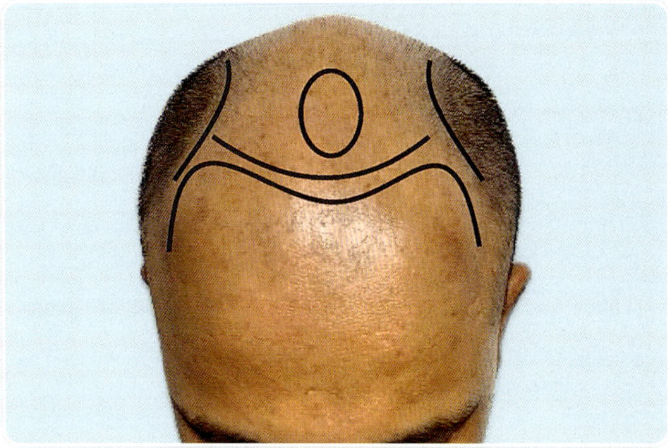

FIG. 5: Hairline pattern in Indian males.
Note: The shape of the frontal hairline, frontal tuft area, and parietal humps.

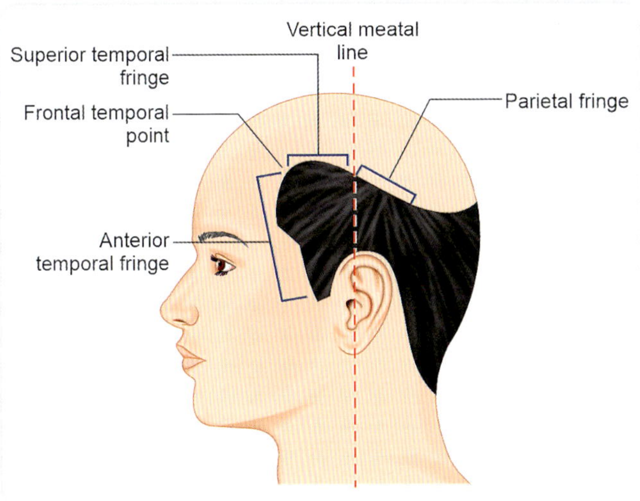

FIG. 3: Anatomical landmarks on the lateral view of the hairline.

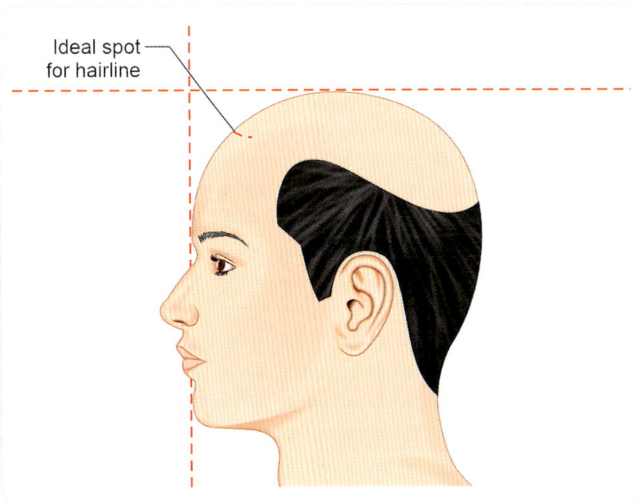

FIG. 4: Marking the midfrontal point.

Temporal Point

The temporal point (TP) is the anterior protrusion located on the lower aspect of the temporal hairline.

Vertex Transition Point

Parietal Hump

The parietal hump[3,4] is important for locating FTA in severe hair loss (grades 6–8 AGA). Its anterior border is the temporal hairline. In grades 6–8 AGA, restoration of lateral hump (LH) should be considered. We need to be careful about implantation direction; as in the upper part of the LH, the direction of hair is forward, and as we move in the lower half, hair is directed downward at an acute angle of 10–15°.

HAIRLINE ZONES (FIGS. 6 AND 7)

Pearl tip: Micro- and macroirregularities are created.[4,5]

Transition Zone

The anterior 0.5–1 cm area of the hairline is defined as the transition zone (TZ). It is irregular and ill-defined with sparse density. Grafts with 1 follicular unit (FU) should be used in TZ to give a natural and soft look to the hairline. Grafts with 2 FUs should be implanted behind the TZ.

Defined Zone

The defined zone (DZ) area lies behind the TZ. It is preferred to implant grafts with 2 and 3 FUs in this zone. The direction of implantation should be downward and forward. We can create a converging effect for a better density illusion.

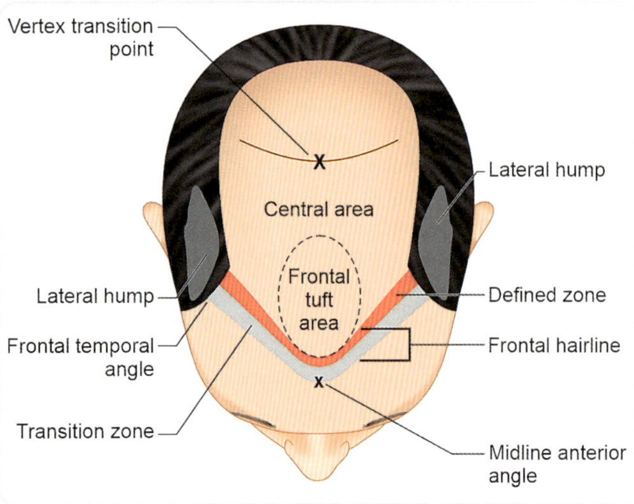

FIG. 6: Zones and markings on the scalp.

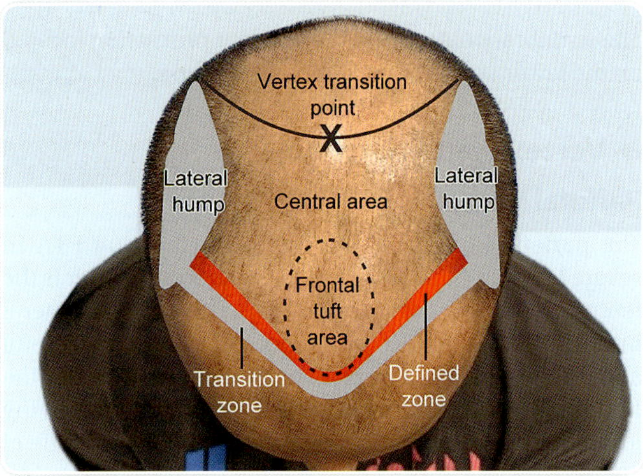

FIG. 7: Zones and markings on the scalp.

Frontal Tuft

The frontal tuft (FT) is also called the central tuft; this oval area overlies the central portion of the DZ directly behind the TZ in the midline.

PATIENT FACTORS FOR DECIDING HAIRLINE POSITION[5,6]

Age

The hairline should be conservatively designed anticipating future hair loss.

Sex

Men have temporal triangular recession that should be preserved to some extent in recreated hairlines. Women's hairline usually curves into the temples without any recession.

Ethnicity

Hispanics, Asians, and Blacks have flatter hairlines than Caucasians.

Patient Expectations

The surgeon should be careful of patients with body dysmorphic disorder who have higher and unrealistic expectations from any cosmetic surgery. The surgeon and the patient should always agree with an appropriate and achievable outcome.

Available Donor Area

Advanced balding will reduce donor availability.

Hair Characteristics

The number of hair per FU, shaft diameter, curl, and color of hair all affect the placement of the TZ and TPs.

Facial Features

The hairline must match the facial contour. The hairline on a narrow head has a less flaring design, while a rounded head favors a rounded, flared design.

Styling Patterns

The hairline level should be adjusted as per styling direction and length of hair the patient wishes to keep.

Points to remember:

- Explain *aging* and future hair loss.
    - What is the *worst-case scenario* for future hair loss?
    - Is it even possible to be *aggressive* in the placement of a hairline at a lower level and be able to implant all the areas behind it?
    - Importance of *medical therapy* to maintain existing hair
- What is the patient's *facial structure*? Wide, vertical, rounded? Forehead long or short? Facial features change with aging.
- What is the patient's *styling* pattern?
- What is the *direction* of existing hair?
- What are the patient's *preferences*?

YOUNG PATIENTS WITH EXPECTATIONS OF A LOW HAIRLINE

Hair loss can be chronic, progressive, and unpredictable. Norwood's study showed that 10% of men in their 60s will have stage VII hair loss, and Unger found that 20% of men in their late 60s will become stage VII. Explain donor area depletion in young patients with high expectations for future transplants.

Practical Tips Based on Experience

- Many young men in their early 20s are very distraught about their maturing hairlines and temporal recession, and they can be extremely insistent on addressing these concerns with HT procedures
- For such cases, I insist on the following:
  - Assess the risk of advanced hair loss
  - Convince them for a long-term medical therapy
  - Always plan for a conservative hairline design

Warning Signs in Young

- Well-defined area of baldness at a very early age in life
- "Whisker hair" (curled, "oily" appearing hairs around the ears and lower neck)
- A wide area of miniaturization on top
- An indistinct fringe border
- Family history of males with Norwood stage VII or advanced stage VI

TOOLS REQUIRED TO DESIGN A HAIRLINE

- Skin marking scale
- Skin marker
- Laser hairline device
- Mirror

Step-by-Step Approach[7]

1. *Marking the MFP:* Mark the MFP 7–10 cm above the glabella.
2. *Marking the MPP*: Mark the MPP from a line drawn upward from the pupil.
3. *Locate the* frontotemporal angle-refer to **Flowchart 1**.
4. Draw a gentle curve connecting the MFP to MPP to FTA. This makes your anterior hairline.
5. *Approaches to temporal peak designing (if required)*:
   - Blunting of FTA
   - TP restoration
   - Curved anterior temporal contour
6. *Evaluating the drawn hairline*:
   - Look straight at the patient at the level of his/her eyes.
   - Look for equal weightage on both sides.
   - The patient himself may have asymmetry in frontotemporal recession, hair pattern, and bony prominences.
   - The overall alignment appears horizontal to the MFP.
   - When viewed from the sides, the hairline should curve upward and backward.
7. *Show the patient his drawn hairline in a mirror.*
   - Explain the natural curve of the hairline drawn.
   - Explain regarding future recession and thinning patterns.

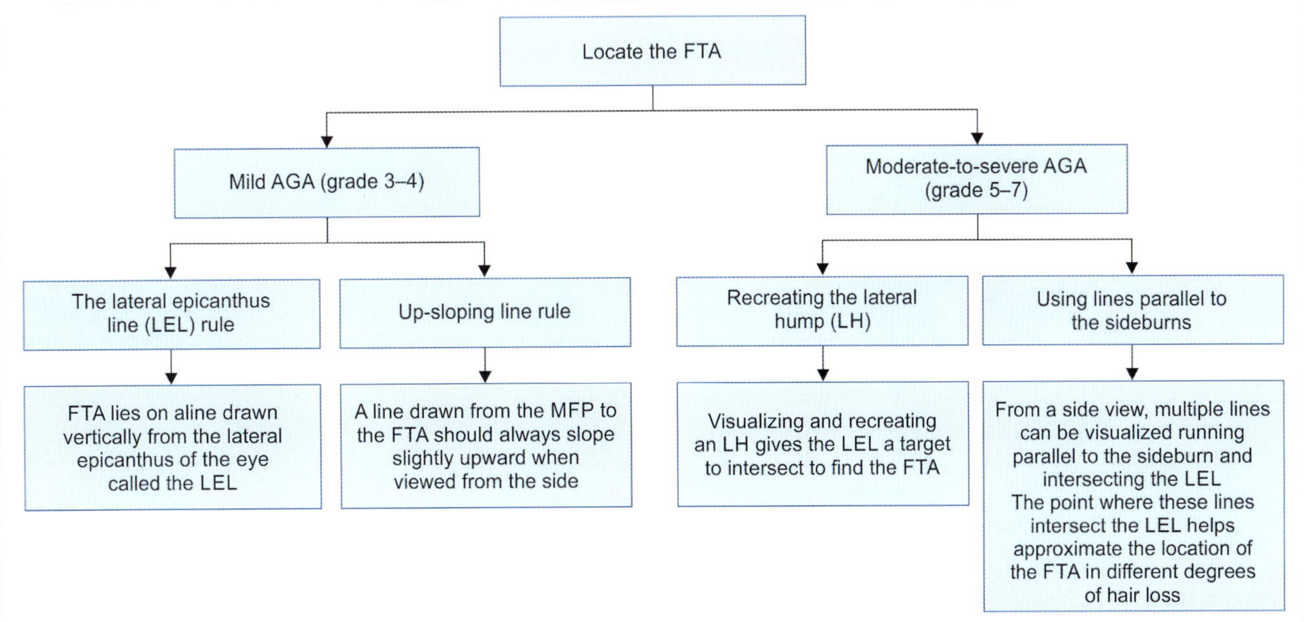

FLOWCHART 1: Locating the frontotemporal angle.
(AGA: androgenetic alopecia; FTA: frontotemporal angle; MFP: midfrontal point)

- Balance and adjust according to the patient's expectations and feasibility.

Points to Remember

- Most of the cases that we see in clinical practice have asymmetry in the location of FTA and TPs. So while designing a hairline, carefully look for asymmetry. While counseling patients regarding the hairline position, this should be informed and documented
- An illusion of a lower hairline can be created by a widow's peak
- There is recession of temporal hairline and lateral fringe in cases of severe hair loss. The lateral epicanthal line (LEL) cannot intersect here. Hence, recreation of these areas is recommended
- The MFP and TPs show recession in proportion to each other. Hence during reconstruction, this proportion needs to be maintained
- Always design the hairline in such a way that it merges with the future hair loss pattern

TEMPORAL AREA

Pattern of hair loss in the temporal area—*Meyer's classification* **(Fig. 8)**:

N—no thinning and/or recession of TP

T—mild thinning of the temporal area with thinning and/ or recession of TP

P—the recession of the temporal area and the TP is in line with the sideburn.

R—further recession of TP and area creating a reverse (concave) pattern

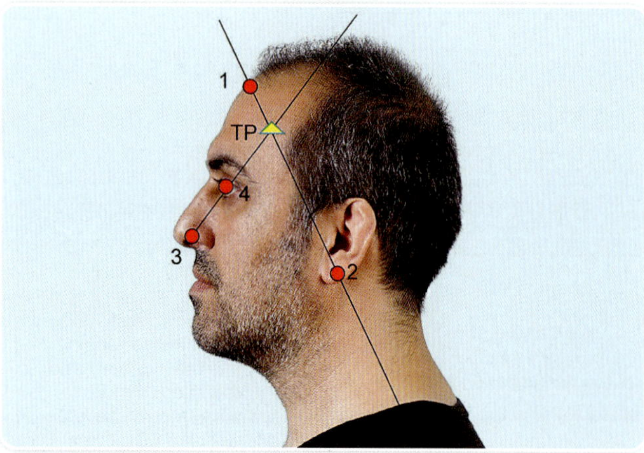

FIG. 8: Meyer's method for locating temporal point (TP). 1: midfrontal point (MFP); 2: ear lobule tip; 3: base of the nose; 4: mid pupillary point (MPP). The TP is at the intersection of these two lines.

- The *TP* is created at a point of intersection of two imaginary lines drawn as follows:
  - *Line one* is from the tip of the earlobe to the midfrontal point.
  - *Line two* is from the base of the nose to the center of the pupil.
- It is always a challenge to recreate the temporal area. It is very difficult to match the direction, texture, and caliber of hair in this area.

Should a Temporal Hump be Created in a Young Patient? (Figs. 9 to 11)

Young patients usually have No (N) or Mild Thinning (T) in the temporal area. They should be prescribed oral and

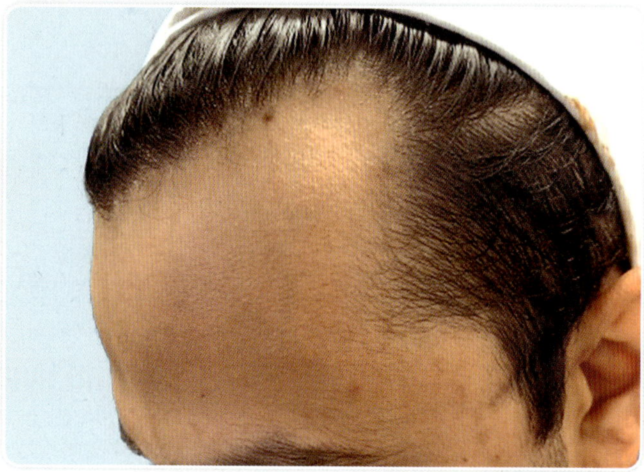

FIG. 9: Young male with grade 3 androgenetic alopecia (AGA) with thinning (T) of temples.

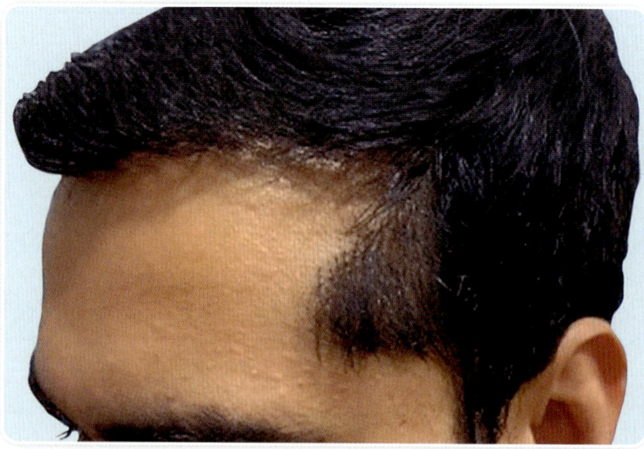

FIG. 10: Overzealous reconstruction of anterior temporal area (ATA) giving it a bushy look.

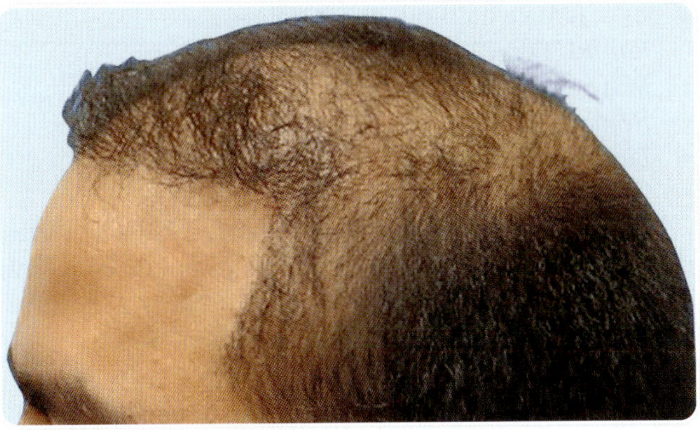

FIG. 11: Inappropriate anterior temporal area (ATA) advancement and shape distortion.

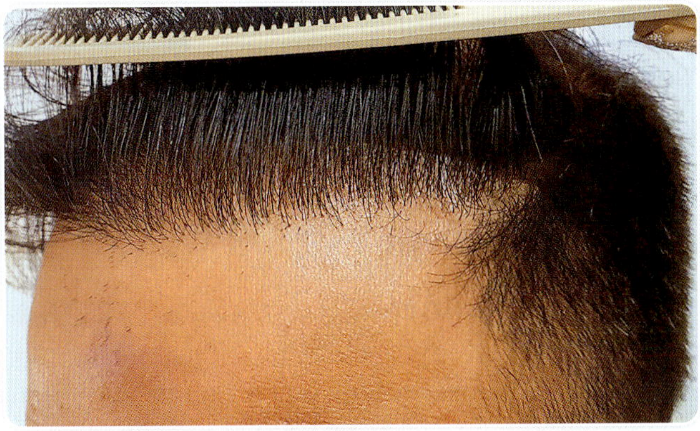

FIG. 12: Macro- and microirregularities make the hairline look natural.

topical medicines to maintain this hair. If at all required, it is better to augment the temporal hump with fine hair instead of bringing it anteriorly.

How to Get that Acute Angle During Slit Creation?

To make the slits for anterior areas, the bevel of the blade should be directed parallel to the epidermis and incisions should be made perpendicular to the hair direction. The angle of hair is directed posteriorly and inferiorly in this area.

How to Select the Hair for the Anterior Temporal Area?

Fine hairs can be selected from the supra-auricular, supra-postauricular area, or the nape of the neck to match with the finer hair of the anterior temporal area (ATA).

MAKING THE HAIRLINE LOOK NATURAL (FIG. 12)

Microirregularity[8]

The hairline should look like a beach shore viewed from the cliff, i.e., irregularly irregular. This should not be defined, which means clusters should have five to eight grafts at unequal intervals. In total, roughly 200 grafts are needed to create microirregularity. Few sentinel hairs should be scattered in the TZ.

Macroirregularity

The hairline when looked at from the frontal view should look curved with the slope upward on the sides. It is also called *snail tracking/mounds/protrusions*. The angle of the grafts in the first two rows should be acute (10–15°).

USAGE OF SHARP IMPLANTERS FOR HAIRLINE RECONSTRUCTION

- Using implanters in a one-step stick-and-place method without creating any reception holes is my preferred method to implant grafts
- This method gives practically a bloodless field, and since implanters are lightweight and easy to maneuver, it becomes very easy to implant grafts at an acute angle of 10–15° at the hairline
- We must always tense the skin to ease the insertion and diminish popping
- Always ensure an avascular plane of entry and implantation
- Use implanter needles with a smaller diameter (0.8–0.9 mm) to implant the front two rows of the hairline with grafts having single roots
- Ensure correct depth of insertion
- The implanter gives us the technical possibility to recreate an illusion of normal density.
- Achieving appropriate density and correct angle is a matter of practice

IMPLANTATION TIPS AND TRICKS

- Existing miniaturized hair gives clues about the angle and direction to be considered for implantation
- It is preferred to have more density in the hairline and central forelock to give a fuller look
- Make sure you do not end up in vascular compromise or necrosis while creating a higher density
- Always follow the standard implantation density and take into consideration the patient's age and desired area of coverage
- The transition from density to softness is a matter of the surgeon's expertise

V-SHAPED HAIRLINE RECONSTRUCTION

V-shaped hairline reconstruction has been shown in **Figures 13 and 14**.

ROUND-SHAPED HAIRLINE RECONSTRUCTION (FIGS. 15 AND 16)

Female Hairline

Most females already possess an intact, natural hairline. In such cases, we usually implant the hair behind this to give a natural dense look to the hairline.

Types of female hairlines are as follows:
- *Round* **(Fig. 17)**
- *M type* **(Fig. 18)**
- *Rectangular* **(Fig. 19)**
- *Bell-shaped* **(Fig. 20)**
- *Triangular* **(Fig. 21)**

Some females have naturally occurring high hairlines, traction alopecia, or those who have cosmetic concerns; in such cases, hairline lowering is required.

Marking the Female Hairline

- *MFP*: It is usually set 6–7 cm above the glabella (bit lower than in males).

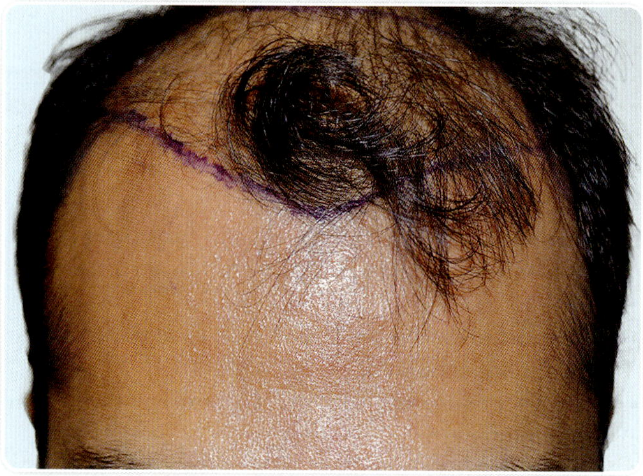

FIG. 13: Planning the V-shaped hairline.

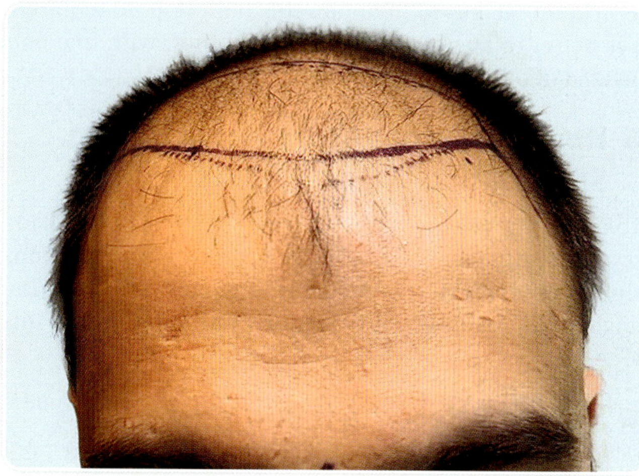

FIG. 15: Planning the rounded hairline.

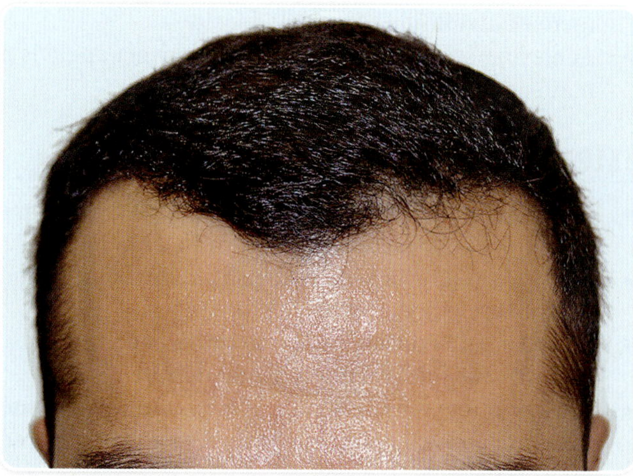

FIG. 14: Reconstructed V-shaped hairline.

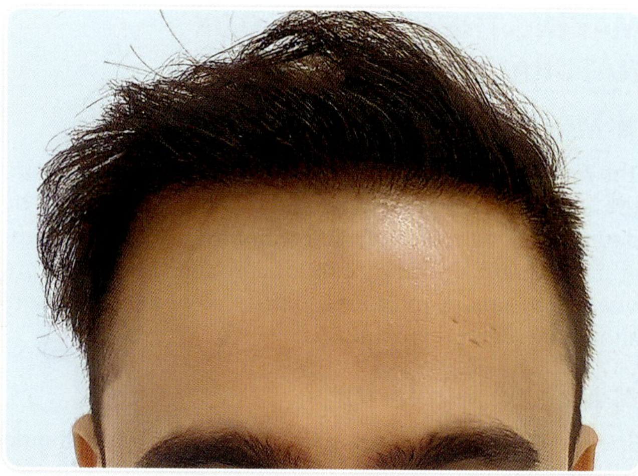

FIG. 16: Reconstructed rounded hairline.

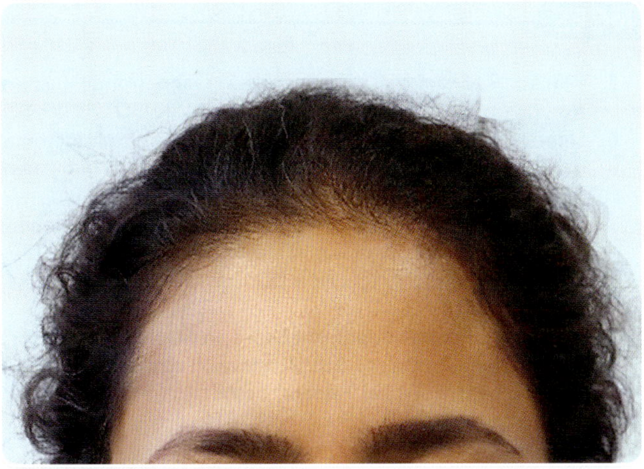

FIG. 17: Rounded female hairline.

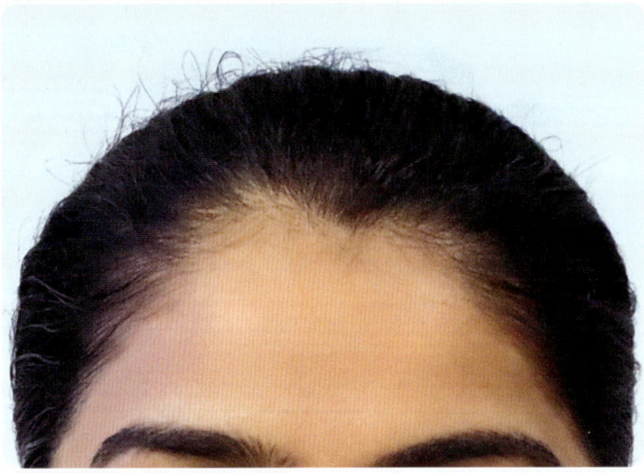

FIG. 18: M-shaped female hairline.

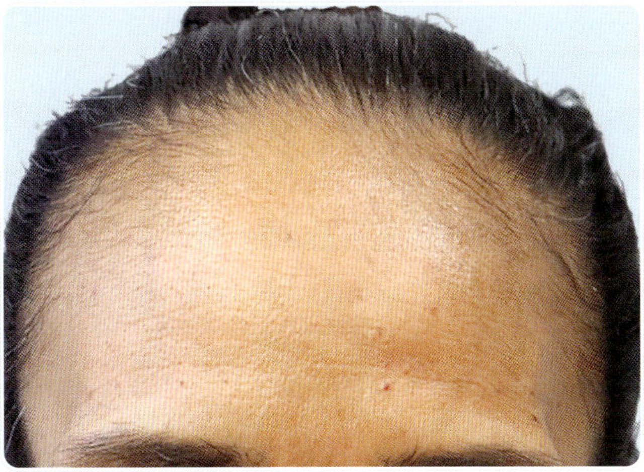

FIG. 19: Rectangular female hairline.

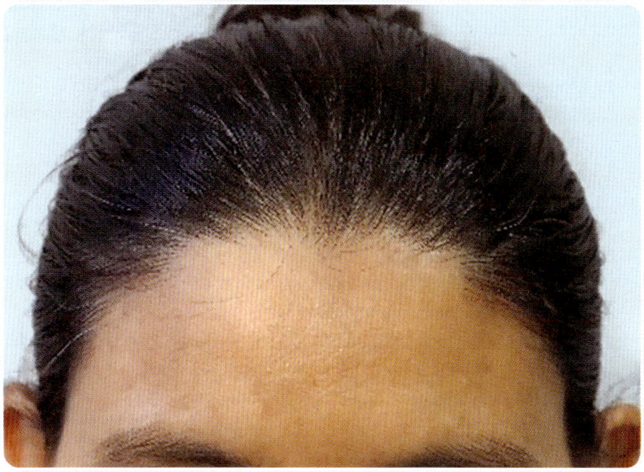

FIG. 20: Bell-shaped female hairline.

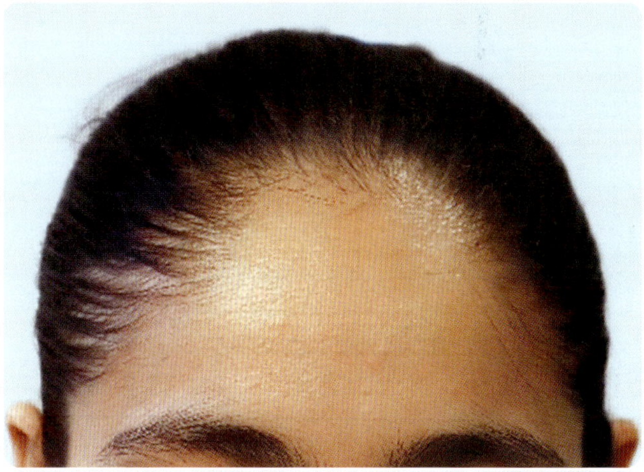

FIG. 21: Triangular female hairline.

- Draw a horizontal line through the MFP.
- Mark points on each side on the epicanthal line positioned 1–1.5 cm posterior to this horizontal line.
- Mark points on each side just anterior to anterior temporal fringe, 0.5–1.5 cm anterior to the above-marked points.
- Connect these points using a curved line.

Tips and Pearls

- The marking of the anterior hairline is one of the most important and permanent factors that stay with the patient for the rest of his/her life.
- Too low or too straight, or an imbalanced hairline does not reflect well.

REFERENCES

1. Unger W. Hairline zone and "egg." In: Unger W, Shapiro R (Eds). Hair Transplantation, 5th edition. London, United Kingdom: Informa; 2011. pp. 372-4.
2. Beehner M. Hairline design in hair replacement surgery. Facial Plast Surg. 2008;24(4):389-403.
3. Garg A. Men—crucial aspects of hair transplant design. In: True R, Garg A, Garg S (Eds). Practical Guide to Hair Transplantation: Interactive Study for the Beginning Practitioner. New York, NY: Thieme Medical Publishers; 2021.
4. Garg AK, Garg S. Decoding facial esthetics to recreate an esthetic hairline: a method which includes forehead curvature. J Cutan Aesthet Surg. 2017;10(4):195-9.
5. Shapiro R, Shapiro P. Hairline design and frontal hairline restoration. Facial Plast Surg Clin North Am. 2013;21(3):351-62.
6. Sirinturk S, Bagheri H, Govsa F, Pinar Y, Ozer MA. Study of frontal hairline patterns for natural design and restoration. Surg Radiol Anat. 2017;39(6):679-84.
7. Sethi P, Sanke S, Bansal A, Kumar A. Designing the anterior hairline. In: Sethi P, Bansal A, Kumar A, Sanke S (Eds). Step by Step Hair Transplantation. New Delhi: Jaypee Brothers Medical Publishers; 2019.
8. Knudsen R. Hairline design strategies and techniques. In: Lam SM (Ed). Hair Transplant 360 (Advances, Techniques, Business Development & Global Perspectives), Volume 3. New Delhi: Jaypee Brothers Medical Publishers; 2014.

CHAPTER 63

Temporal Triangle and Parietal Hump

Anil Kumar Garg, Seema Garg

Key Messages

- In advanced stages of hair loss where the temporal peak point and frontal temporal fringe have receded significantly, there is a need to restore the side framing of the face.
- Mayer's guidelines help in the placement of the temporal points.
- Parietal eminences or posterior parietal triangle is an important area to maintain the contour of scalp and needs attention to restore with mid-scalp in advancing grade of baldness.
- In advanced grades of baldness, where the parietal hump has receded downward, there is a need to reconstruct the parietal hump.
- It is preferable to avoid coverage of vertex in younger individuals <30 years old.
- Medical management is the preferred treatment modality for vertex hair loss in younger individuals <30 years old.

INTRODUCTION

Androgenetic alopecia[1] is one of the common causes of hair loss in men. The usual presentation is receding of anterior hairline (AHL) with loss in the frontotemporal area of the scalp.[2] When hair loss further progresses, it leads to hair loss in the parietal and occipital areas leading to a drop-down of the parietal hump.[3] The usual priority of reconstruction is the frontal area, followed by mid-scalp and crown.[4] Because of the limitation of donor hair follicle supply, the temporoparietal region remains uncovered or minimally covered.[4]

In this chapter, we cover the temporal triangle and mid-scalp including parietal hump and parietal eminence.

TEMPORAL FRINGE (TRIANGLE)

A hair transplant aims to restore the framing of the face. The anterior hair and temporal fringe recede because of androgenic alopecia, compromising the facial aesthetic. Receding of AHL leads to the widening of the forehead in the vertical direction, while receding of temporal fringe leads to an increase in the width of the forehead. A prominent forehead significantly affects the aesthetic appearance of the face. Until around 2000, there was a reluctance to perform reconstruction of the temporal lines and temporal points because of the poor technique of hair angle implantation, giving unnatural results, a shortage of grafts, and future loss in the temporal area. Now, reconstruction of the temporal line and the point has become necessary because of the critical contribution of the temporal area to facial aesthetics.[4] This also resolves the problem of lowering the hairline.

Pattern of Hair Loss in the Temporal Area—"Mayer Classification"[5]

Hair loss in the temporal area may range from thinning to significant receding of the temporal fringe. Based on the pattern of hair loss in the temporal region, Mayer has classified hair loss pattern into four ways **(Figs. 1A to D)**:

1. *Class N*—no thinning or recession of temporal point in this category
2. *Class T*—mild thinning of the temporal area with thinning and recession of the temporal point

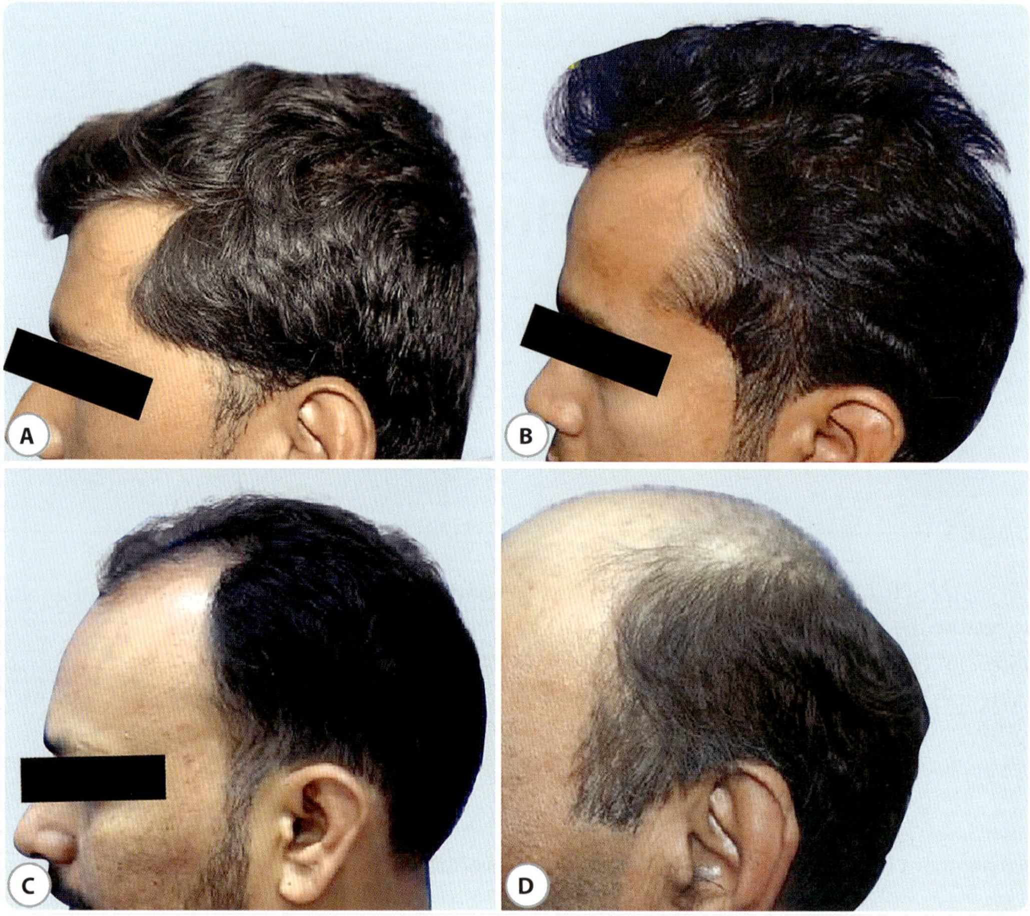

FIGS. 1A TO D: Mayer's classification of pattern of hair loss in temporal fringe: (A) Class N; (B) Class T; (C) Class P; (D) Class R.

3. *Class P*—recession of the temporal area and the temporal point aligns with the sideburn
4. *Class R*—significant recession of temporal fringe leading to a reverse pattern of normal (the normal pattern is convex, but, in this pattern, it becomes concave).

Mayer's Guideline for Placement of Temporal Points

Mayer has given a guideline for reconstructing the temporal peak point and fringe. As per Mayer's guideline,[5] the temporal point is a point of intersection of two imaginary lines drawn as follows:

1. Line one is from the tip of the earlobe to the mid-frontal point (MFP).
2. Line two is from the base of the nose to the center of the pupil.

The temporal peak/point is the intersection of these two imaginary lines **(Figs. 2A and B)**. The temporal point is placed on the lateral and above the lateral end of the eyebrow over the forehead. The angle of hair in this area should be kept as flat as possible. The existing hair helps to determine the direction of graft implantation. The direction of hair in the temporal area changes gradually. In the upper area, hair faces forward and downward, gradually sweeping downward and backward facing to the ear.

There can be some variation in the direction of hair. The angle of insertion is 0–5° **(Figs. 3A to C)**. Single- or two-hair follicular unit (FU) grafts are used to graft the temporal area. The usual density is approximately 20–25 grafts/cm^2.

The distance between mid-frontal and temporal peak points in the lateral profile shall be <3 cm. The recession of mid-frontal and temporal peak points is also in proportion, so to maintain the aesthetics of the face, the proportion between the temporal peak and the mid-frontal point shall be maintained **(Fig. 4)**.

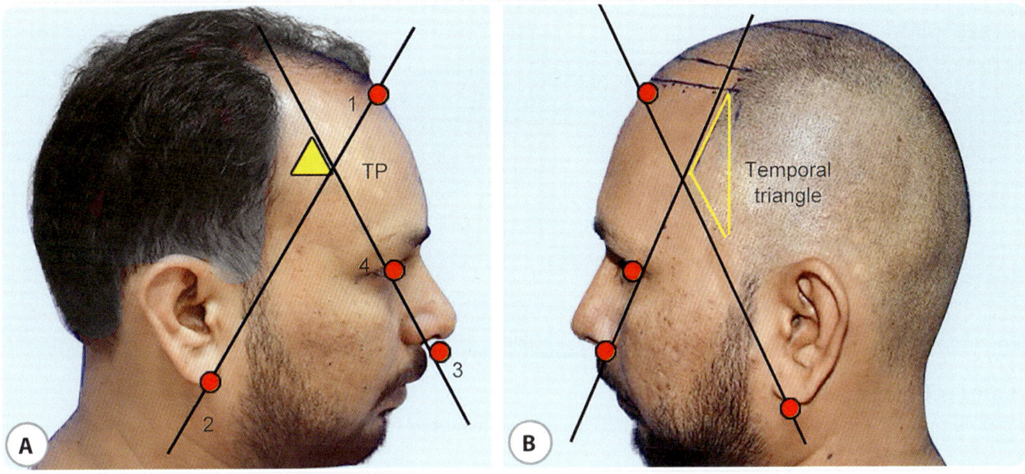

FIGS. 2A AND B: Mayer's guideline for placement of temporal points (TP).

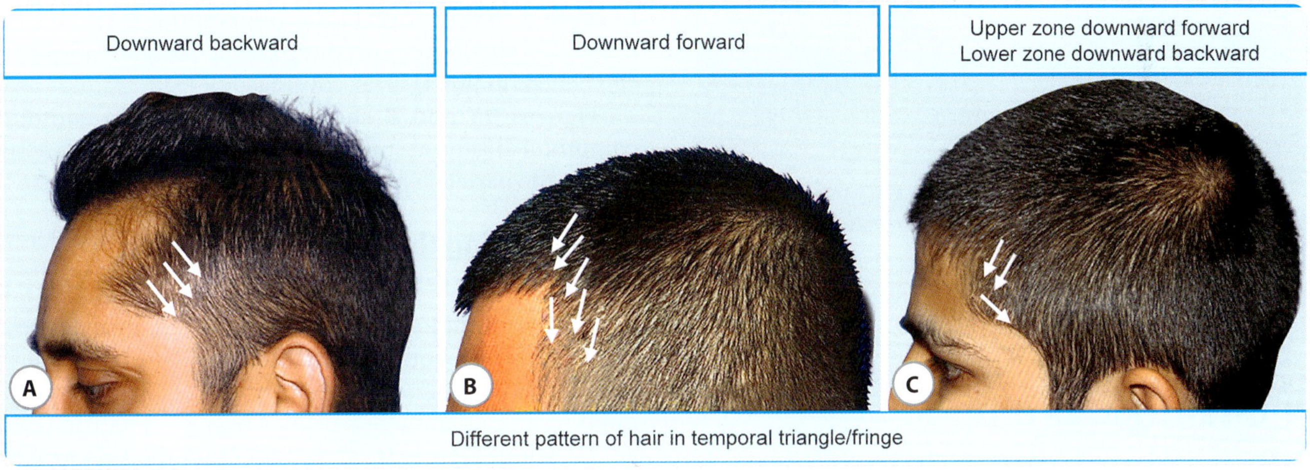

FIGS. 3A TO C: Variations in the direction of hairs in temporal fringe.

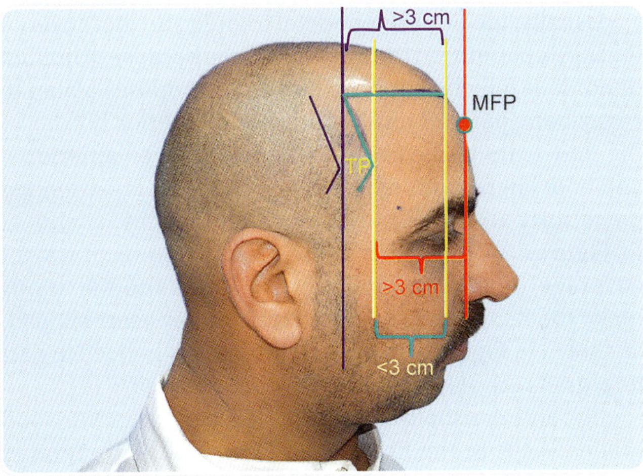

FIG. 4: Relation of temporal peak point and mid-frontal point.
Note: The distance between TP and MFP shall be <3 cm.
(MFP: mid-frontal point; TP: temporal point)

CASE STUDIES

Case 1 (Figs. 5A to C)

In this case, the temporal peak point was not receded, but the anterior border of the temporal fringe was concave. This triangular area of the temporal fringe was reconstructed without a change in the location of the temporal point.

Case 2 (Figs. 6A and B)

Receded temporal fringe in a 36-year-old man with limited supply of donor follicles, so conservative reconstruction of temporal fringe was done as shown in **Figures 6A and B**.

Case 3 (Figs. 7A to D)

Reconstruction of temporal fringe in class P temporal fringe hair loss, done using 300 single FU grafts harvested from the postauricular scalp donor area.

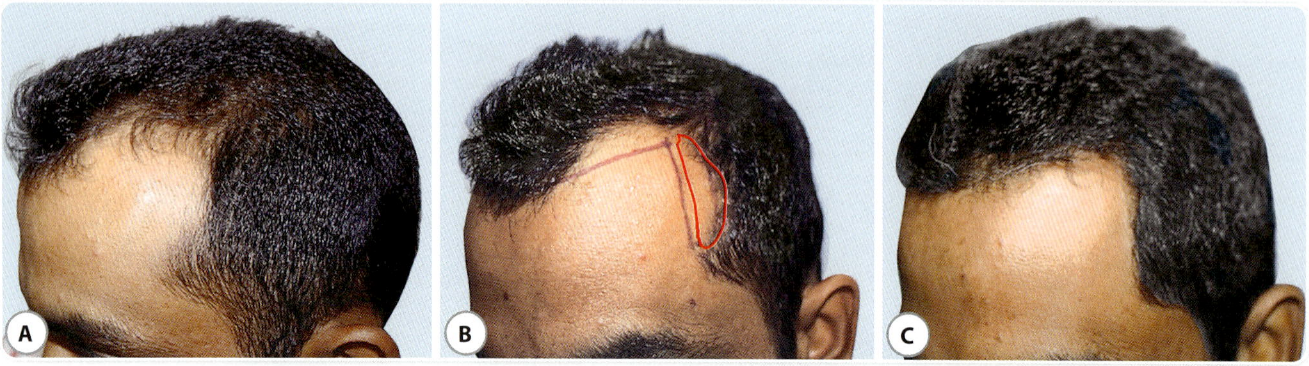

FIGS. 5A TO C: Case I—Reconstruction of temporal fringe.

Note: Temporal point at normal position but the temporal fringe was concave. The temporal triangle was marked and the concave fringe was covered using hair follicles.

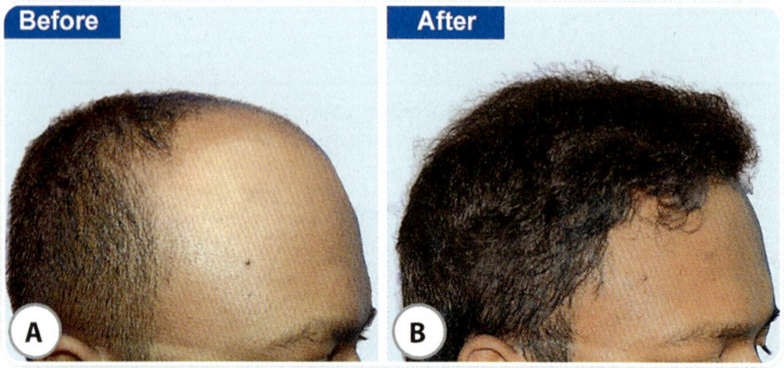

FIGS. 6A AND B: Advance grade of baldness with limited supply of donor follicles, so conservative reconstruction of temporal triangle done.

Case 4 (Figs. 8A to D)

Advance grade of baldness in a man of 60 years. The temporal fringe was reconstructed using 360 grafts.

MID-SCALP

The mid-scalp is a horizontal, slightly curved area of the scalp. Hair faces forward in the central region and turns laterally toward the side. If existing hair is present, follow the angle and direction. The hair angle is 25–35°. Usually, the recommended density is 20–30 grafts/cm^2, depending on the available donor area. Multi FU grafts should be used for grafting in the mid-scalp area **(Figs. 15A to C)**.

Parietal Eminence (Posterior Parietal Triangle)[6]

The parietal eminence is one of the essential islands of the scalp, and there is a need to transplant the parietal eminence. It is advisable to include parietal eminence as an extension of the mid-scalp area, especially in cases where there is a possibility of going in a higher grade of baldness and/or area showing thinning.

The parietal eminence maintains the balance in the frontal and lateral profiles and restores the skull's contours. In limited donor availability, preferential attention to parietal eminence or posterior parietal triangle transplant can benefit indirect vertex coverage.

Figures 9A and B show the loss of scalp contour compromising the aesthetics of the face, and also in lateral profile, the parietal eminence thinning looks prominent.

Transplanting the Parietal Eminence (Posterior Parietal Triangle)

Anteriorly, the mid-scalp area is bounded by an imaginary line connecting both the tragi, laterally on both sides' parietal humps, and posteriorly by vertex transition point.[7] Parietal eminence or posterior parietal triangles are shown in **Figure 10**. If we look from the side profile of a face, the posterior parietal triangle/parietal eminence area shadows the central vertex area, and the central vertex area is visible only in the posterior profile of the scalp.

Usually, the posterior parietal triangles are not covered during implanting in the mid-scalp area because of limited donor hair follicles supply. The author proposes a plan to cover both parietal eminences. The posterior border of the mid-scalp in the central area is advanced anteriorly, and both lateral ends of the posterior border are extended posteriorly to cover the parietal eminences as shown in **Figures 3A to C**. This is the graft economical way of coverage of parietal eminences. These modifications make the recipient area's posterior border heart-shaped, as shown in **Figures 11A to C**. If thinning is noticed in part line, grafts are also implanted in part line area.

The author usually does 4,500–5,000 grafts in Norwood grades V–VII in the first stage of hair transplantation.[2,8] Day 1, 2,500–3,000 grafts are harvested from the scalp using follicular unit extraction (FUE), and around 2,000 grafts from the beard are extracted.[8] On the first day, all scalp hair follicles are implanted all over the planned

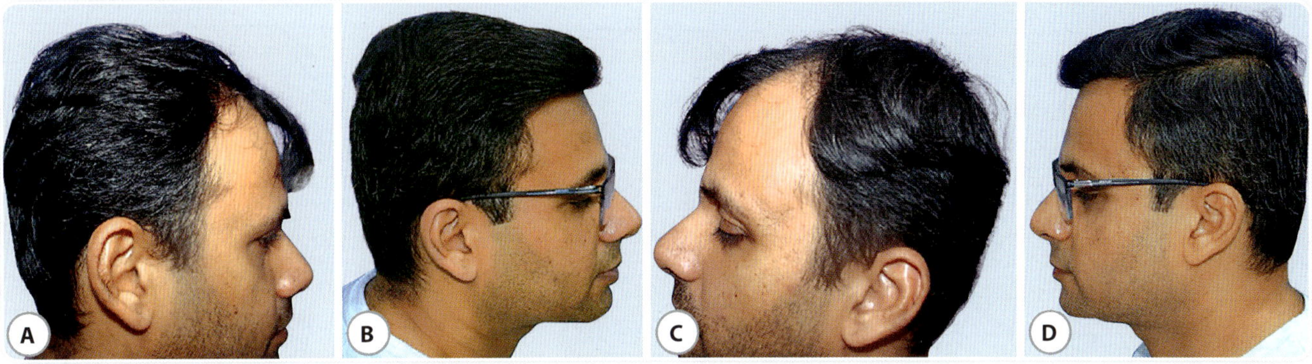

FIGS. 7A TO D: Reconstruction of P-class hair loss of temporal fringe. Class P temporal fringe/triangle reconstructed in Norwood grade (NG) VI. 300 grafts implanted in each temporal area.

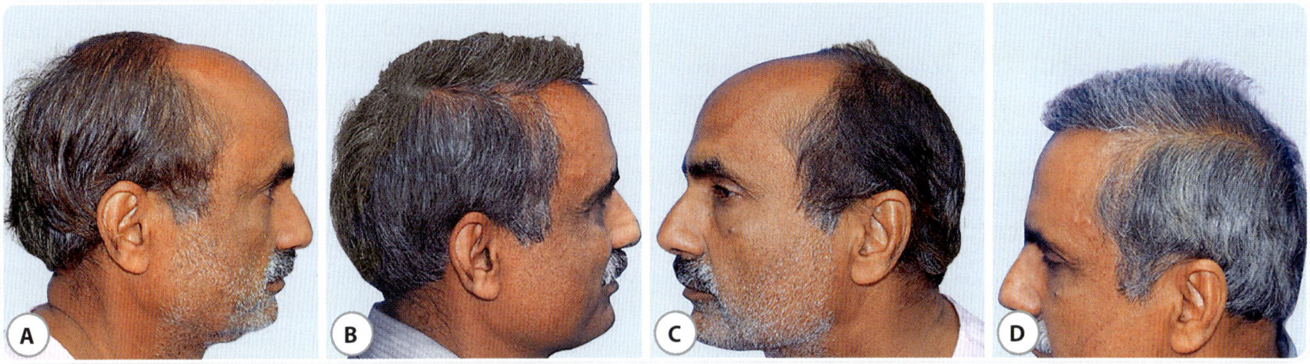

FIGS. 8A TO D: Reconstruction of R pattern hair loss of temporal fringe. Class R temporal fringe/triangle reconstructed in Norwood grade (NG) VI. 360 grafts implanted in each temporal area.

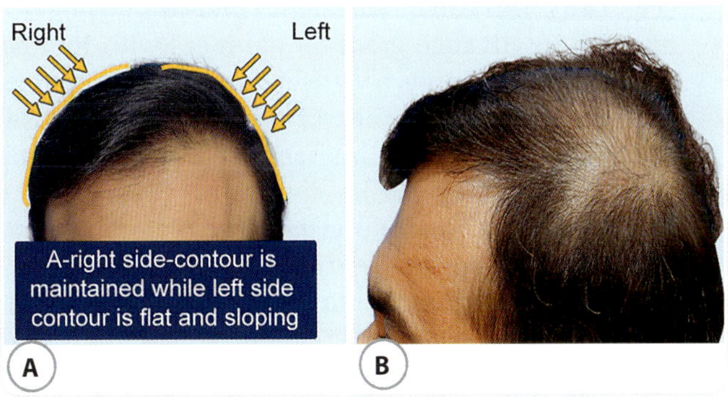

FIGS. 9A AND B: Results after 11 months of hair transplant, whose front and mid-scalp were transplanted. Even after hair transplant patient is showing loss of contour on his left side (A) and thinning in the parietal area (posterior parietal triangle) and part line.

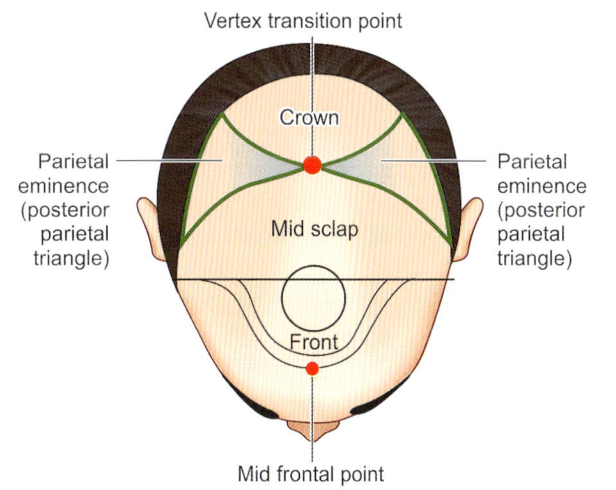

FIG. 10: Scalp major zones and posterior parietal triangles or parietal eminence areas.

area, leaving gaps in between for beard grafts. On the second day, donor hair follicles are harvested from the beard. The beard follicles are implanted between the scalp hair follicles that were implanted a day before, using the combination grafting technique of scalp and body hair.[9] The author uses autologous plasma as graft holding solution.[10] The areas transplanted are frontal, mid-scalp, and parietal eminence areas (posterior parietal triangle) as per the plan shown in **Figures 11A to C**. They cover the frontal and mid-scalp areas with extension to parietal eminence on both the sides.

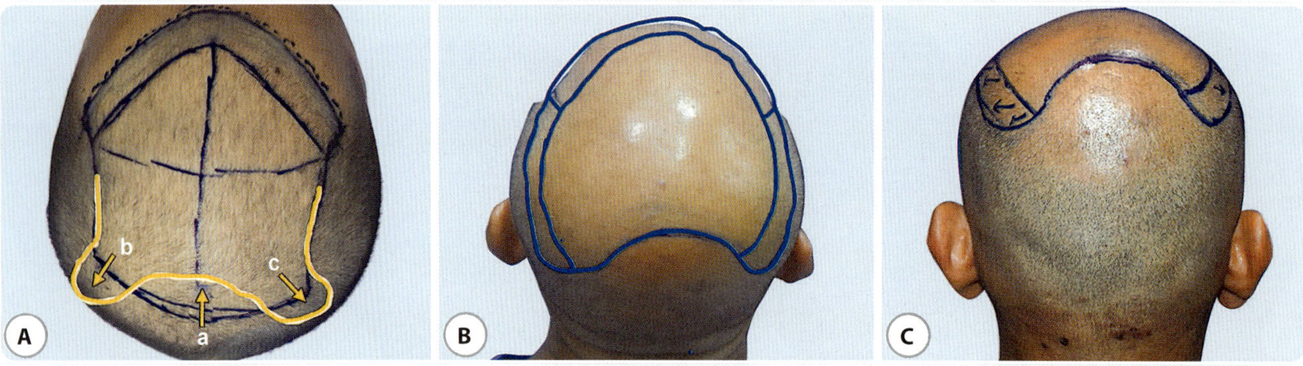

FIGS. 11A TO C: Modification to cover posterior parietal area by extending posteriorly laterally in areas "b" and "c." The final area looks like a heart shape.

Results

Case 1 **(Figs. 12A and B)**—This young man had hair loss and thinning in the front, mid-scalp, and crown. A total of 5,256 grafts were implanted in 2 days. On day 1, 3,030 grafts were harvested from the scalp and on day 2, 2,226 grafts were harvested from the beard. Front and mid-scalp, including parietal eminence (posterior parietal triangle), were transplanted. After 8 months of hair transplant, the results showed good coverage over parietal eminence.

Creation of Parietal Hump or Fringe

Recreation of AHL needs two important landmarks: The MFP and the frontotemporal point (FTP).[3] A few guidelines must be followed to achieve an aesthetically pleasing result.

Firstly, the FTPs should be located on the lateral canthal line, and the FTP should be at the same level as or above the MFP. If the FTP is relocated lower than the MFP, the frontotemporal angle will appear too broad and unnatural.

In cases where there is advanced baldness, the lateral fringe (parietal hump) has dropped to a point where the lateral end of the frontal hairline is disconnected. In such a condition, if the FTP is relocated at the drooped parietal hump, this can result in the FTP being lower than the MFP, which would create an obtuse frontotemporal angle **(Figs. 13A and B)**. To avoid this, the receded parietal hump must be uplifted or restored so that the reconstructed hump is at the same level of MFP **(Figs. 13A and B)**.

The direction of hair changes in the lateral fringe area **(Fig. 14)**. In the upper area, the hairs face forward and then turn inferiorly as we move lower. The anterior portion of the parietal hump blends into the upper temporal line. The existing hair always helps in deciding the angle of implantation of the follicle. **Figures 15A to C** show a case of hair loss in the mid-scalp zone, with a lowering of the lateral hump and receding of the temporal area. All three areas were reconstructed.

Steps to recreate parietal hump (temporal-parietal hump) **(Figs. 16A to F)**:[7]

- *Step I*: The height of the parietal hump will depend on the position of the FTP. To position or relocate FTP, we need three planes or lines. The intersections of these three lines will relocate the FTP as shown in **Figure 16A.**
- *Step II*: As the FTP shall be at the level or just above the MFP, a horizontal line is drawn at the level of the MFP **(Fig. 16B)**. This can be called the "mid-frontal line."
- *Step III*: In advance grade of baldness with limited donor follicles supply, a vertical line is passed in front of tragus. This vertical line will intersect the previously drawn horizontal line. This can be called the "tragus temporal line" **(Fig. 16C)**.
- *Step IV*: The FTP should be on the vertical lateral canthal line. So, a line is passed upward and then backward to intersect the previous two-line intersection **(Fig. 16D)**. This line can be called the "lateral canthal line." That is how these three planes or line intersections will relocate the new FTP.
- *Step V*: A curved superior parietal fringe border is drawn as shown in **Figure 16E**. This is the parietal hump or temporo-parietal fringe that will give a base to FTP, and the AHL will connect the MFP and newly relocated FTP.

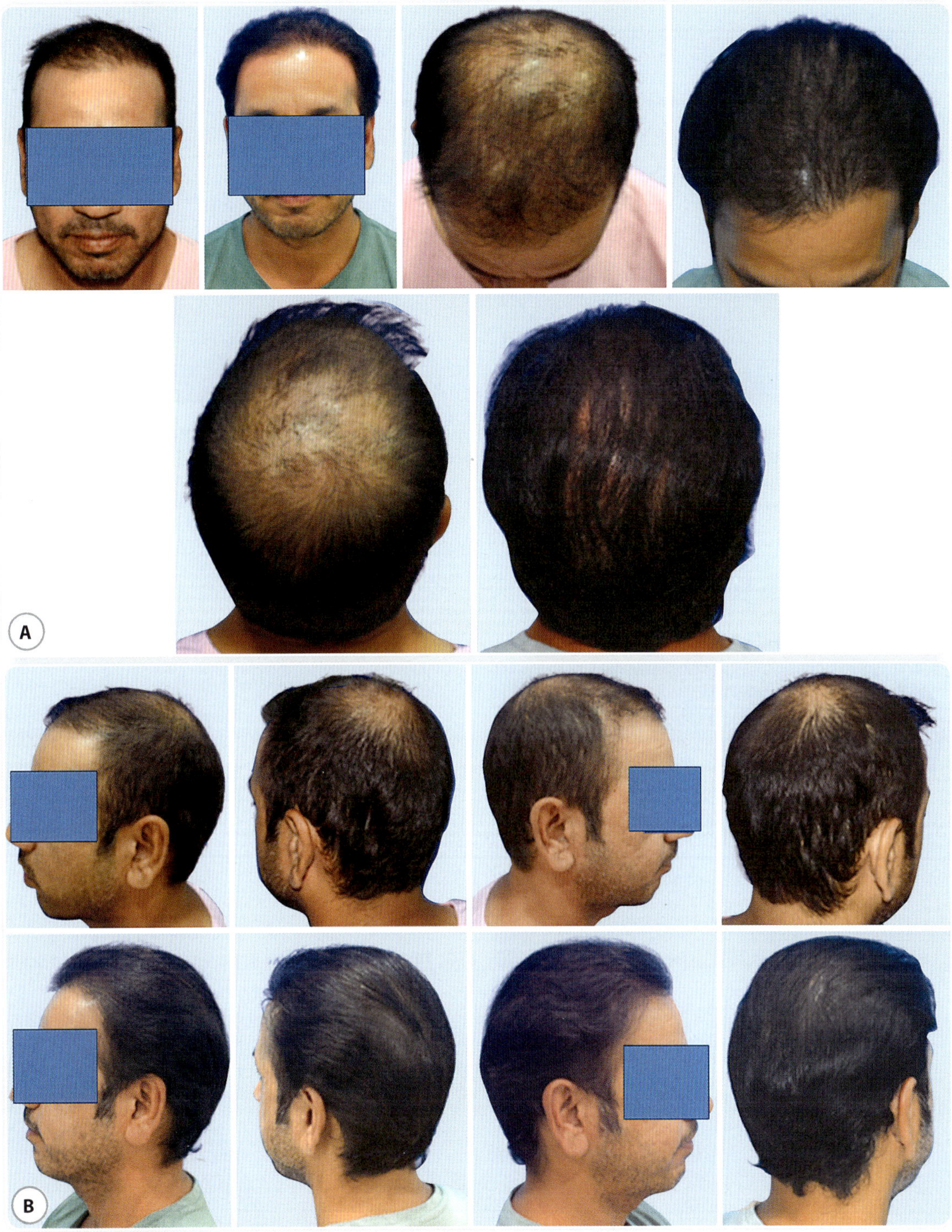

FIGS. 12A AND B: Eight months postoperative results. Hair transplant using 5,256 grafts in frontal, mid-scalp area, including parietal eminence, was done.

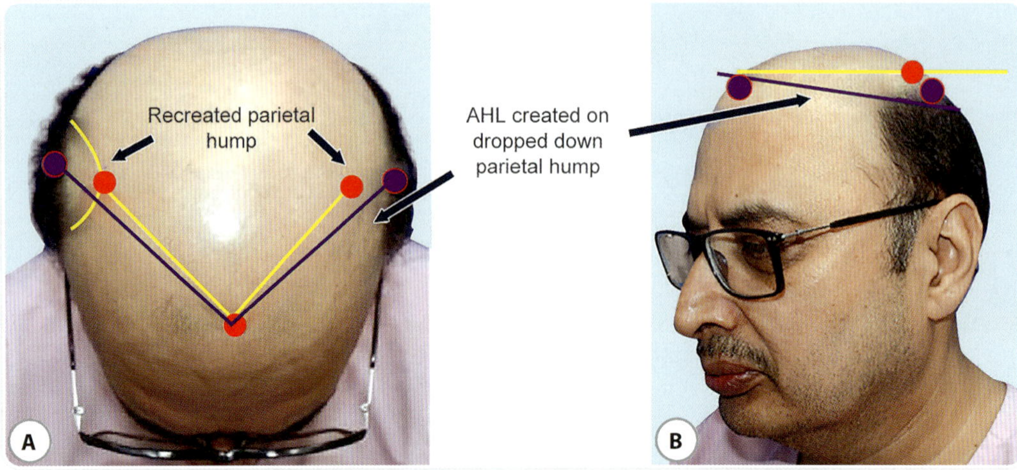

FIGS. 13A AND B: Logic of creating the parietal hump. (A) *Parietal hump* is needed to relocate frontotemporal point so that a natural AHL can be reconstructed; (B) If we mark FTP as over receded/dropped down parietal hump, then the FIP will be at lower level to MFP, which will make an unnatural AHL.

(FTP: frontotemporal point; AHL: anterior hairline)

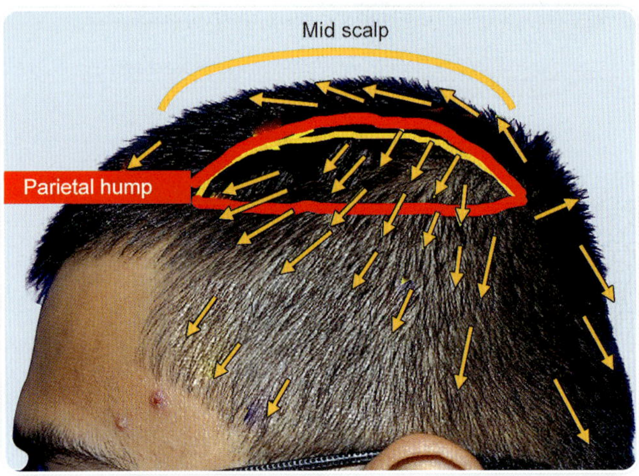

FIG. 14: Direction of hair in parietal hump and mid-scalp.

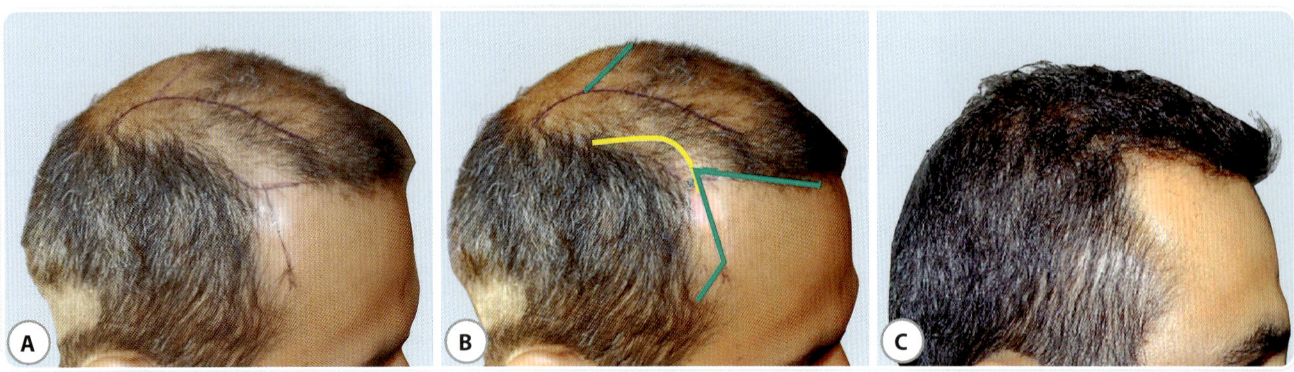

FIGS. 15A TO C: Loss of hair in temporal fringe, mid-scalp, vertex, and lowering of the parietal hump. Reconstruction of temporal fringe, mid-scalp, and parietal hump. Vertex was not covered. Restoral of parietal hump, temporal triangle, and mid-scalp, without crown coverage.

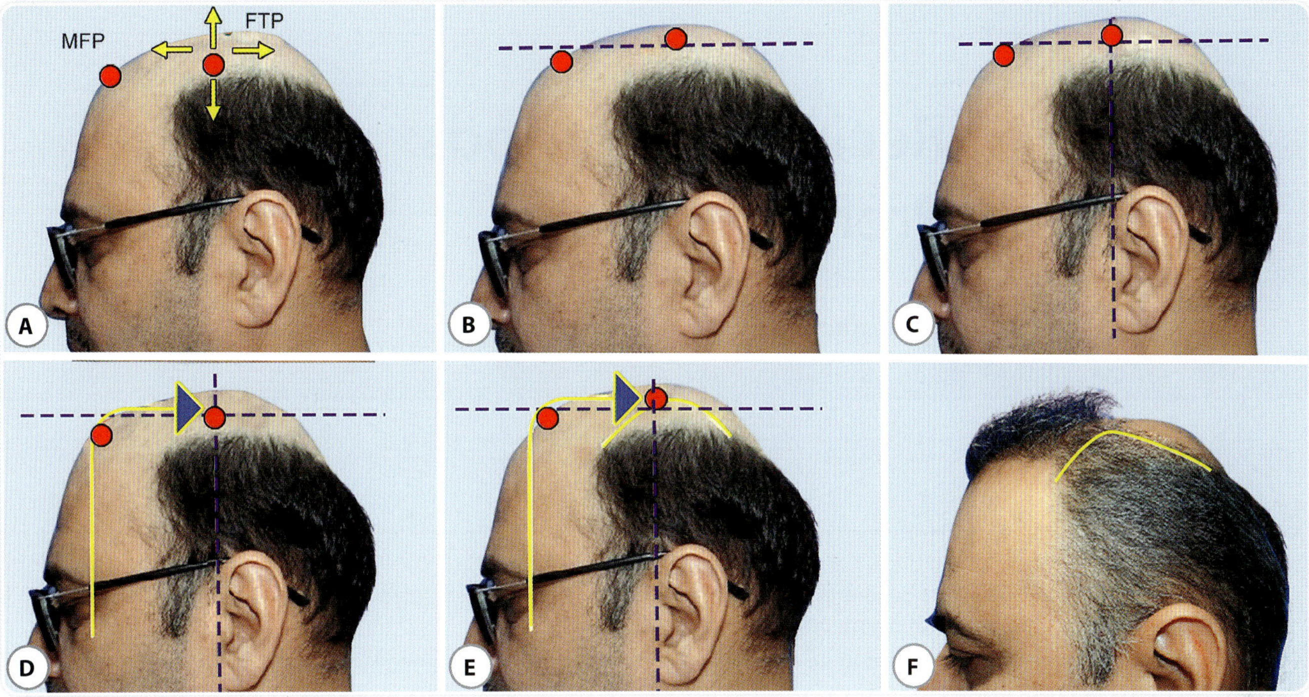

FIGS. 16A TO F: Steps to recreate parietal hump (temporal–parietal hump): (A) Step 1—to relocate a point (FTP), we need three lines/planes' intersection. (B) Step II—first line/plane FTP shall be at the level or just above MFP. (C) Step III—second line/plane. Vertical line passes anterior to tragus. (D) Step IV—third line. The FTP shall be a vertical line of lateral canthus. (E) Step V—the parietal hump height is the level of FTP as placed. (F) Reconstructed AHL and parietal hump.

(AHL: anterior hairline; FTP: frontotemporal point; MFP: mid-frontal point)

SUMMARY

Receding of the temporal fringe leads to an increase in the width of the forehead. A prominent forehead significantly affects the aesthetic appearance of the face. To restore esthetics, it is advisable to recreate a temporal fringe depending on the availability of donor hair follicles.

Recreating the parietal hump in cases of advanced-grade baldness is essential for aesthetic relocation of the FTP. Transplanting bilateral parietal eminence is an indirect way of covering the vertex in a graft-economical way.

REFERENCES

1. Rathnayake D, Sinclair R. Male androgenetic alopecia. Expert Opin Pharmacother. 2010;11(8):1295-304.
2. Gupta M, Mysore V. Classifications of patterned hair loss: a review. J Cutan Aesthet Surg. 2016;9(1):3.
3. Tamashunas NL, Bergfeld WF. Male and female pattern hair loss: treatable and worth treating. Cleve Clin J Med. 2021;88(3):173-82.
4. Jimenez F, Ruifernández JM. Distribution of human hair in follicular units. A mathematical model for estimating the donor size in follicular unit transplantation. Dermatol Surg. 1999;25(4):294-8.
5. Mayer ML, Perez-Meza D. Temporal points: classification and surgical techniques for aesthetic results. Hair Transplant Forum Int. 2002;12(4):147-58.
6. Garg AK, Garg S. Aesthetic importance of the parietal eminence area (posterior parietal triangle), an essential island of scalp requiring hair restoration. Hair Transplant Forum International. 2022;32(3):87-9.
7. Bernstein RM, Rassman WR. Follicular transplantation. Patient evaluation and surgical planning. Dermatol Surg. 1997;23(9):771-84.
8. Garg AK, Garg S. Donor harvesting: follicular unit excision. J Cutan Aesthet Surg. 2018;11(4):195.
9. Garg AK, Garg S. "Combination grafting" of scalp and body hair to enhance the visual density of hair transplant and coverage of higher grade of baldness. J Cutan Aesthet Surg. 2020;13(2):163.
10. Garg AK, Garg S. A histological and clinical evaluation of plasma as a graft holding solution and its efficacy in terms of hair growth and graft survival. Indian J Plast Surg. 2019;52(2):209.

CHAPTER 64

Recipient Methods: Preformed Slits

Manoj Khanna

Key Messages

- The premade slits method offers several advantages: It is quick, allows overall planning, permits increased density if required, and allows freedom for the surgeon to perform other tasks.
- However, it needs expertise for implantation, especially in between existing hairs, needs an experienced team to execute, and is assistant-dependent.
- The density of hair at various zones should be natural in relation to each other. Density is visually appreciated rather than counted in numbers.
- Graft survival needs to be cared for, especially in megasessions.

INTRODUCTION

The final goal of a hair transplant surgery is to match the patient's expectation of naturalness and density. A mere mathematical approach does neither. Hair transplant is a blend of science and art. Simply harvesting hairs from the permanent zone and transplanting them to bald areas is not the end of the story. The hair transplant should be aesthetically pleasing and natural not only for today but in future times to come. Naturalness, if absent, draws the attention of the eye; it mandates the surgeon to evaluate both at an individual graft level, where the single graft should have a natural direction, and as a whole where the pattern of placement throughout the bald region as well as the hairline should be appropriate. Also, as the balding progresses with age, the blending between areas of transplanted and preexisting hair zones should be without any abrupt gaps. We have evolved from using large minigrafts to follicular unit (FU) grafts, yet the most important quest remains, i.e., to ascertain a technique that creates the best balance between naturalness and density.

Recipient area planning and graft placement techniques form vital parts of the hair transplantation process. Hairline design has been dealt with in the earlier chapter. This chapter deals with recipient area planning, graft placement, and graft density, with particular reference to the preformed slit technique.

RECIPIENT AREA PLANNING

The recipient scalp is divided into different zones **(Fig. 1)**. The reader is also referred to the previous chapter 62 on Recipient area: Male and Female Hairline design and also the chapter 81 on Designing the Vertex for more details.

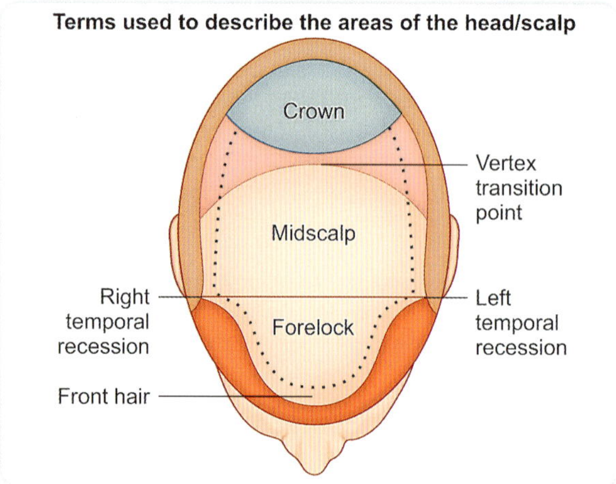

FIG. 1: Different zones on the bald area of the scalp.

Different Zones on the Bald Area of the Scalp

- Most anteriorly lies the hairline. It is broader at the lateral sides than at the center. It is 1.5–2 cm in width. The hairline gradually diminishes in density from behind to front in the hairline, to blend with the forehead anteriorly. Hairs in this zone are directed anteriorly and leave the scalp at an acute angle of 10–20°.
- Behind the hairline is the frontal region, which is supported by the temporal fringe of hair laterally. The hairs are still directed anteriorly, but the angle at which they leave the scalp is about 20–35°. For convenience, we may say that it is the area anterior to a line joining the apices of the two laterally lying frontotemporal points. While transplanting the scalp in a frontal-type pattern, we tend to include, along with the frontal region, an area lying backward intruding the midscalp region at its lateral borders because this part lies in a more vertical plane than the rest of the midscalp region and is appreciable when the patient is seen from the side.
- The point where the temporal fringe meets the frontal hair is the frontotemporal point and the anterior-most point of this lateral fringe is the temporal point. These are important landmarks, and their correct position and restoration are very important aesthetic goals. Receding temporal points make the forehead look wider. The entire midscalp region is supported by the temporal and the parietal fringe of hair at its lateral border.
- There is a transition zone between these two where the hairs change direction ever so gradually from anterior to anterolateral. This transition zone is called the lateral crease. Those people who part their hair do it at this level; hence, it is very important to give good density in the lateral crease zone.
- Posteriorly, the scalp transitions from a horizontal to a vertical plane, and this point is called the vertex transition point.
- Below this is the vertex or the crown zone. The vertex is peculiar in its hair distribution. The hair in the vertex area is arranged in a whorl pattern, and it requires a significant amount of hair follicles to recreate what was lost and maintain aesthetic pleasantness.
- Below the crown lies the occipital fringe of permanent hair.

A beginner is advised to have a close look at the hair of people around him, study their natural direction and angle at which they leave the scalp, analyze the gradual changes that occur in the transition zones, and envision a three-dimensional (3D) image in one's mind to apply during hair transplants.

BASIC PRINCIPLES OF DENSITY

Illusion of Density

Density is more a perception than an absolute mathematical figure, although arithmetic helps. A key point to understand is that we are limited by the total number of FUs available for transfer. The donor area or the zone of permanent hair is only 25% of a normal scalp. An appearance of fullness will be perceived when approximately 50% of the original hair volume is present. As more and more hairs are lost, a decrease in density is visible. The optical principle being when light falls on an object, it gets reflected to the observer's eye—this is how we see the world around us. The more the light is reflected from the hair rather than the scalp, the more is the illusion of a greater density. All those factors that increase the light reflected from the scalp rather than the hair will increase the perception of baldness. Any factor that helps in more light appearing to be reflected from the hair will aid to give an illusion of more density. These factors are mentioned below:

- The intensity of light falling on the scalp is one of the factors responsible for thinning being noticed—often people first realize that they have lost a significant amount of hair when someone points that out at a party under a bright focused light.
- The color contrast between hair and scalp plays a crucial role as dark-haired individuals with light scalps realize hair loss much earlier.
- Hair curl increases the draping of the scalp by the hair, giving a fuller appearance with a relatively lesser number of hairs.
- The diameter of hair is another important factor. A 0.01-mm increase in the caliber of the hair increases the density by 36%;[1] hence, apart from focusing on hair transplant, we should also take care of measures to enhance the thickness of hair.
- The angle of the hair leaving the scalp, orientation of hair, distribution or spacing between grafts, and type of graft, i.e., single FU or multiple FUs, are some of the other factors that affect the apparent density. Hair sticking out at right angles will cover less of the scalp than hair leaving at a natural acute angle. We generally tend to mimic the natural angle at which hair leaves the scalp, and this gives the most pleasing result. This is of utmost importance to prevent grafts from looking artificial.

A normal scalp contains approximately 100,000 follicles, with an average hair density of 80–100 follicles/cm^2. Appearance of fullness is maintained with up to 50% of density. Thus, technically speaking, 40–50 follicles/cm^2 would be required to cover the bald zone.

Still, this is more than one may be able to harvest in a single session. Keeping in mind the previously discussed factors, zones of importance are implanted with greater density than the less important and transition zones.

Distribution of Density

- From the front view, we first see the hairline and frontal tuft zone; thus, they require denser placement of hair follicles, i.e., 25–40/cm^2. The hairline gradually thins from behind forward, and follicular distribution becomes sparser as we approach the plain hairless forehead. The hairline zone merges with the frontal tuft region behind.
- The 1.5-cm anteriormost area is the hairline zone. In the initial 1 cm, the density is kept a little more than the frontal region, and thereafter, it is gradually reduced in each row. The final 2 mm of the transition zone is made with a thinner needle (19 or 20G) in sparsely arranged irregular mounds. A straight line with densely packed follicles gives an abrupt and unnatural hairline.
- The next region of importance is the lateral crease region, which is a thin strip extending from the frontotemporal point in front to the vertex transition zone. It is necessary to give good density to this region for two reasons. Firstly, most people part their hair along this line, and hence the zone should have good hair density to drape the scalp well in this region. Secondly, if the hairs are parted, the hair growing in this region will overlap the midscalp region. We can thereby reduce the number of required hair follicles in the midscalp region due to this overlap. The posterior band of the lateral crease region is somewhat visible from the lateral profile also. The left-side lateral crease or right-side lateral crease will depend on the patient—whether he parts from left to right or vice versa; usually, right-handed patients part from left to right. These regions must be grafted with the maximum density possible without rationing. If the number of follicles available for transplant is low, these areas are to be transplanted first, and usually, it is better to give good density here, rather than trying to compromise with follicles for the frontal or midscalp region.
- The next zone of importance is the frontal tuft region followed by the midscalp. One can gradually decrease the density of follicles as one progresses backward. Very often, we leave the midscalp region and find later that the patient is happy and does not want any further hair to be put in the midscalp region as it is the least noticeable and partly gets covered by the lateral crease hair.

Vertex zone transplantation is a different entity altogether. We transplant it separately because the follicular requirement here far exceeds what is anticipated. This region stands vertically like a billboard, and even a slight fault in either density or direction is immediately noticeable. A bald or thinning vertex is much more normal-looking than a poorly transplanted one. This aspect is dealt with in a separate chapter 80 on Vertex Transplantation.

Rather than absolute numbers, the required follicular density is better explained in relative terms; the highest density is required in the most important zones and the lesser density should be placed in subsequent regions to maintain naturalness and give an equilibrium.

Megasessions

Since the advent, development, and improvisation of follicular unit transplantation (FUT), the usual session of placing a few hundred minigrafts has now become a task of placing several hundreds or thousands of grafts comprising single and multiple FUs.[1] There is no definition as such of a megasession, but arbitrarily, one may say any session >2,500 grafts would be termed a megasession. It is the result of the natural evolution of the technique. Subtle changes in the preexisting technique have culminated to form a megasession. To understand this point better, we must see the process of hair transplantation as a whole and come to a realization that the only limiting factor to perform a megasession is time. We organize the surgical team and the operating setup, fine-tuning every step with one goal in mind; to save time in each step and ensure the maximal survival of transplanted hair. Performing a megasession is not a casual jog in the park—it is more like running a marathon that requires much more preparation and attention to detail. It is tiring for both the team and the patient. Thus, we need a well-lubricated system that conveniently sees through the procedure and lets us get prepared for the next-day surgery session at the same time.

The rationales behind performing a large session, which is both time consuming and labor intensive, are many. Besides obvious aesthetic reasons for obtaining complete coverage in one session, there are a few technical aspects as well: The donor site is limited in the number of hairs, and multiple incisions of multiple procedures reduce their availability as more hair follicles get trapped in the scar tissue of each session and may not be easily dissected out for transplantation.

- Multiple sessions mean that the modern busy patient has to come for surgery multiple times and spend more time.
- Apart from the type of hair loss, the pattern of placement of graft is very much influenced by the number of follicles available to provide the most

optimal result. It is like trying to paint a masterpiece with a limited quantity of paint. Even if a small session is performed, the surgeon has to make it look presentable, and not just do one half, mathematically. Logically speaking, the more the number of available follicles, the better they are suited to produce a desired effect. This is a good example where the whole is much more than the sum of its parts.

The technique of FUT has helped the surgeon to extrapolate and calculate the required number of recipient sites. Since 1996, we have been doing FUT almost exclusively. We find that this produces the best and most natural results. Separating follicles into "predetermined number of hairs" grafts strips away the finer resting hairs, which are not so clearly visualized. Maintaining the FU structure prevents that as well as preserves the microvascular plexus present in the FU. It is also easy for the surgical assistants to dissect out FUs that naturally lie separated from each other. FUs of different numbers of hair can be easily densely packed and have excellent survival rates, and avoid the pluggy appearance of previously used larger grafts.

However, megasession needs experience and attention to detail—in particular factors affecting the graft and causing injury.[2,3] These have been dealt with in a separate chapter 60 on Graft Preservation.

GRAFT PLACEMENT

There can be three approaches to creating the recipient area sites and placing the grafts:

1. One technique is to "stick and place," where the surgeon makes a recipient site and then immediately places the graft. This is a time-tested technique, but it is slow and good for a much smaller session requiring a lower number of hair grafts.
2. The second method is to make preformed slits.
3. The third method is by using implanters. We discuss here the preformed slits technique, and the other two techniques are discussed in separate chapters.

Preformed Slits

We use preformed slits and have found several advantages of using this technique. The surgeon begins the recipient site creation by initially visualizing it in his mind. *Using the preformed slit technique allows him to paint his canvas efficiently in a flow.* As the design begins to form, any required adjustments are easily made. We also find a much better control of bleeding with this technique; the assistant presses down on the areas where slits have been made, and a few minutes of gentle compression achieves hemostasis. Surgical sessions take a long time, and in a high-volume center catering to two to three patients every day, the surgeons also need time for consultations and reviewing previously transplanted patients. Once the recipient sites have been made, the team of surgical assistants can implant the FU grafts. This allows the surgeon to perform other important tasks such as consultations, follow-up, supervision, or planning for the next case.

Sagittal versus Coronal Slits

A slit may be viewed as a small line that may be oriented coronally (i.e., perpendicular to the anteroposterior plane) or sagittally (which is parallel to this plane) **(Figs. 2A to C)**. While sagittal slits are generally preferred, coronal slits have been claimed to create a better illusion of density. Visually, FU grafts placed coronally would provide maximal apparent density like a couple of cards placed to create a wall preventing any light to escape from the scalp. But this has its disadvantages too; it may have a profound effect on the way the hair will fall after full growth as well as a theoretical risk of jeopardizing the radially arranged blood supply of the scalp if the slits are placed very close. Such orientation is good for people who back brush their hair and in the temporal region. Recreating the temporal hairline requires very acute angled slits and fine single follicular grafts—sagittal slits are preferred. If the slits are placed coronally in the temporal region, the graft can move sideways inside the slit and change lateral orientation, but in a sagittally placed slit, the graft may move in the vertical plane, and the angle at which the hair leaves the skin may increase. We have been creating slits in the sagittal plane since the beginning and have found no specific advantage of one technique over the other. It is preferable that the surgeon follows whatever he is comfortable with. Often, the two types are used in combination too, in different areas.

Slits versus Holes

In the earlier days of hair transplant when punch grafts and then the minigrafts were used, the recipient sites were cored out using round or rectangular punches, creating round or rectangular slots. Both followed a similar principle; such punches were hollow and would cut out a core of tissue. This central core was pulled out using jeweler's forceps and left behind small round or eye-shaped slots. Round slots could be made by 0.75–3-mm-sized punches; similarly available sizes for the rectangular punch were between 1.6 and 4 mm. Precut grafts were required for these slots. In the quest for achieving natural-looking results, newer techniques evolved, and the use of FU grafts became the dictum, and these older techniques went out of favor.

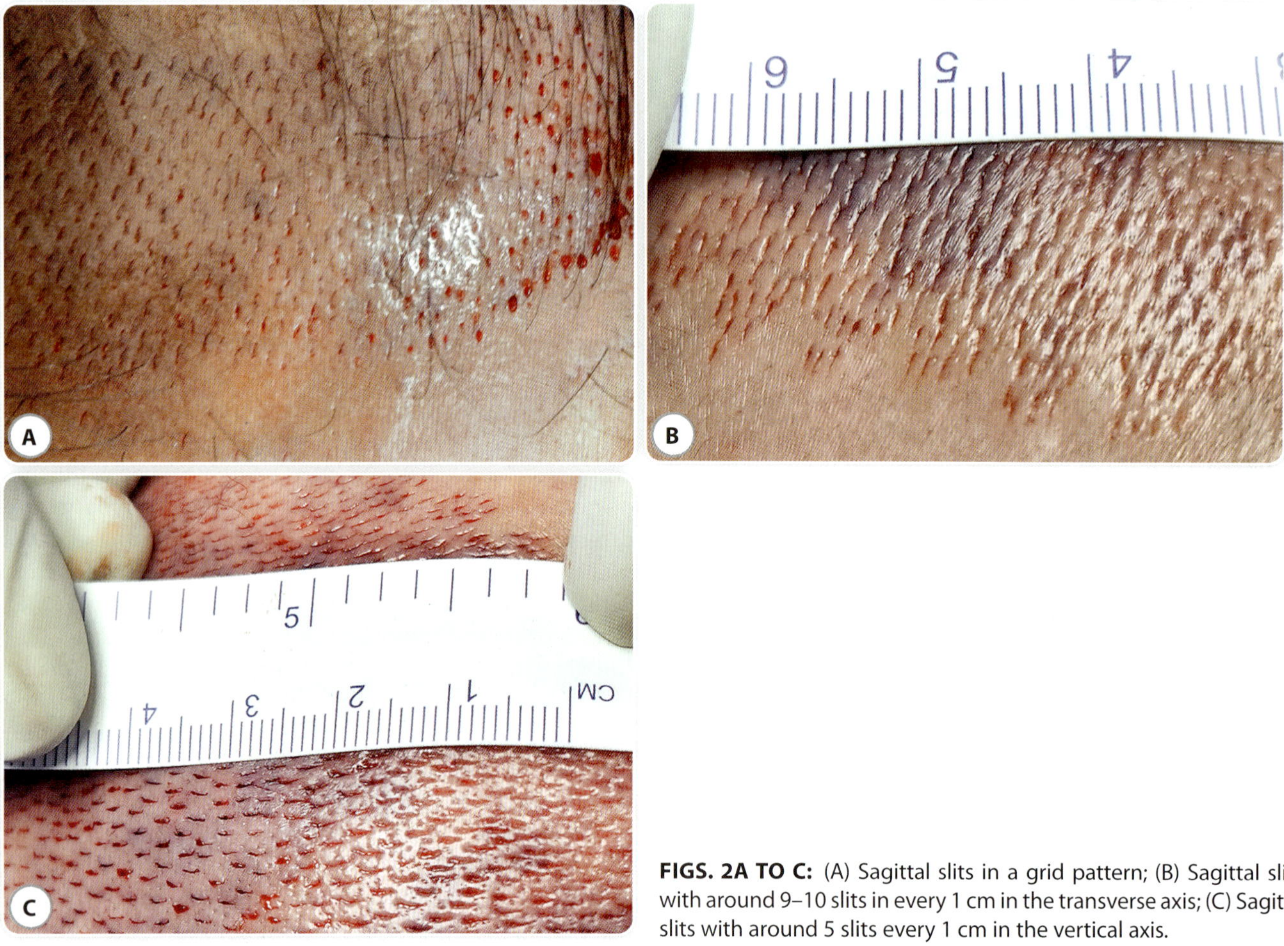

FIGS. 2A TO C: (A) Sagittal slits in a grid pattern; (B) Sagittal slits, with around 9–10 slits in every 1 cm in the transverse axis; (C) Sagittal slits with around 5 slits every 1 cm in the vertical axis.

The advantage of creating a punch was that it would remove the extra skin from the recipient site. If this was not punched out, the gap between the grafts would increase resulting in pluginess. Round holes would also cause more bleeding or popping and were also more time-consuming as each central core needed to be removed in a separate movement. Nowadays, when the small follicular graft is being prepared with little epidermis and dermis around it, the need for a round hole and the need to punch out tissue have disappeared. Hence, a simple needle or thin blade slits are sufficient to hold the graft. These sites can be made in a single stroke, are small, allow close and dense packing, and lead to pleasing aesthetic results.

INSTRUMENTS TO MAKE SLITS

No. 18, 19, and 20G needles, depending on the diameter of the harvested hair, are preferred by the author for making slits. Designer blades of different sizes are available. Several surgeons custom-make the blades by cutting an ordinary safety razor blade with a blade cutter. Each has its advantage, and a surgeon may choose any instrument or a combination of any of these tools.

Procedure

The patient lies supine on the comfortable operating table. The controls for changing the height of the table and the head end should be within the easy reach of the surgeon to make adjustments as and when required. The surgeon sits at the head end on a comfortable chair, whose height is adjustable and under proper illumination from above. We prefer using optivisor loupes with 2–3× magnification. Among the numerous available loupes, these are more efficient, and it is very easy to swipe the loupe upward to see the progress of the design created from time to time with the naked eye. The surgical assistant stands to the left of the surgeon but keeps the trolley of instruments in a position that allows the surgeon ample space to move around comfortably **(Figs. 3A and B)**.

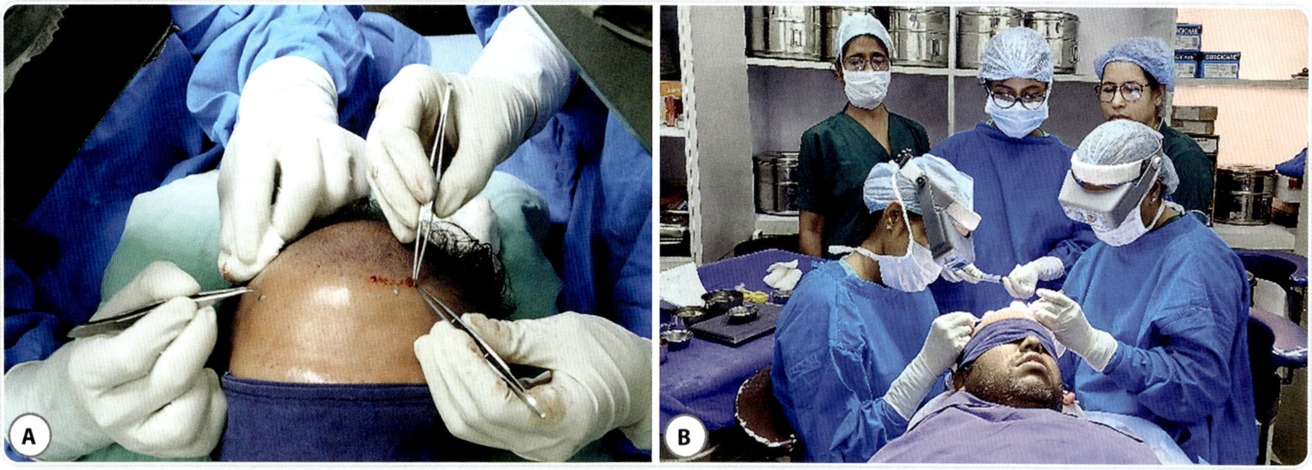

FIGS. 3A AND B: (A) Two assistants implanting; (B) Two transplanters and one assistant working together.

The hand of the surgeon must be in the most ergonomically efficient position to create correctly angled recipient slits. The slits are made with 18, 19, or 20G hypodermic needles, depending on the caliber of the hair. The needle is attached to a Luer-lock syringe, which serves as the handle **(Figs. 4 and 5)**. The 18G needle slits are used to place two- and three-hair FUs, while the 19/20G needle slits are used to place single-hair FUs. For areas of the scalp where extremely acute angles are required, such as the temple and frontotemporal regions, the needle is double bent at 90° **(Fig. 4)**. The area is tumesced with normal saline as the surgeon progresses from one region to another. Saline is infiltrated in the superficial layer with a 26G needle **(Fig. 6)**. The surgeon holds the mounted needle in his hand between the first three fingers in a tripod grip and stabilizes it by resting his hand on the scalp. The assistant uses one hand to stretch the scalp and the other to aid in hemostasis and keeping the field of surgery clean. While slits are being created for the hairline, the assistant gives gentle tug over the forehead making the skin taut for easy penetration. A sharp needle must be used, and as soon as it becomes blunt, it is replaced. Blunt needles make shallow slits and can result in popping while transplanting the hair follicles. *Depth control is important—too deep a slit leads to bleeding and a buried graft. Too superficial a slit leads to popping.*

The slits are made in rows, but two adjacent rows do not have slits exactly one behind the other or else the transplant will look very unnatural. Also, grafts placed one behind another will make the final density appear much less. Neither are the slits made at random in a haphazard manner. The best way is to make an interlocking grid pattern, which reduces the see-through effect as shown in **Figures 2A to C**. This allows placing the grafts very close to each other and gives good apparent density.

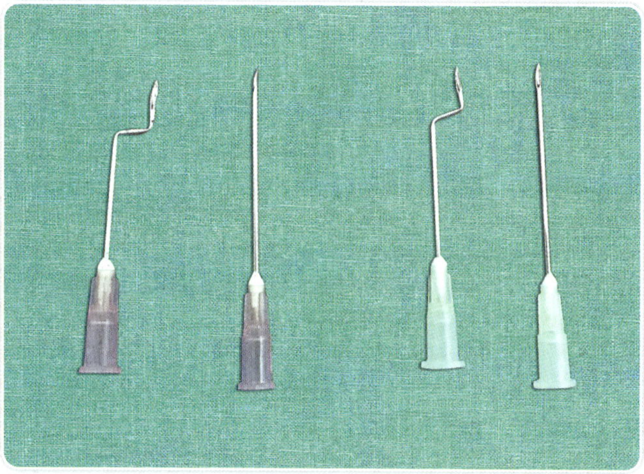

FIG. 4: Different types of needles—bent and straight.

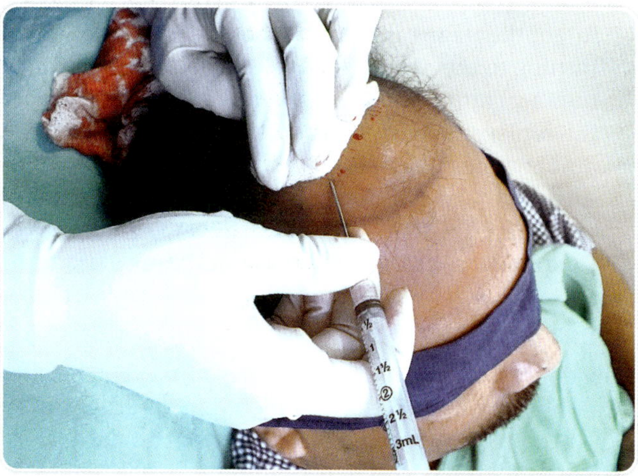

FIG. 5: 18G needle attached to a syringe for making slits.

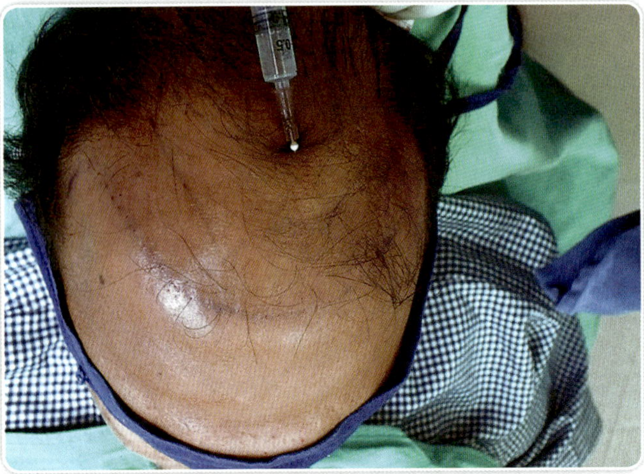

FIG. 6: Administration of saline for tumescence.

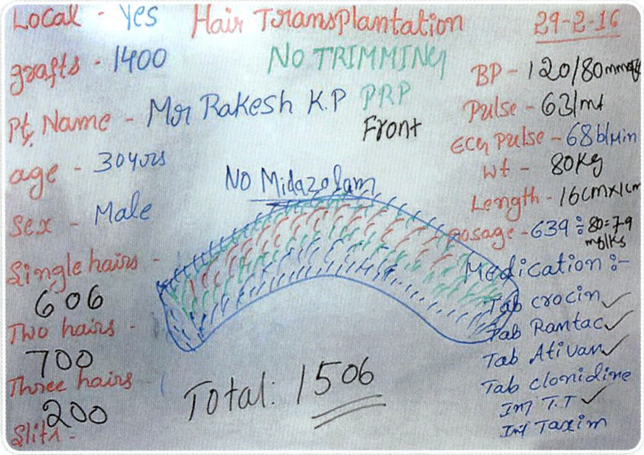

FIG. 7: Documentation of counted grafts with a map on a board.
Courtesy: Dr Venkataram Mysore.

Counting

Counting is important in this technique as the number of slits must match the number of grafts dissected. Making hundreds of slits may at times becomes monotonous, and the surgeon may lose count of the slits. It is preferable that a precise method of counting be adopted by the surgeon. Different methods can be used for this purpose:

- Both the surgeon and the assistant keep an individual count independent of each other and collaborate after a few slits. The instruments on our trolley serve as a precise counter. Four empty needle caps are placed to the left of a central towel clip, and after the count of every hundred, one of them is shifted to the right. So, the surgeon just has to count up to 100 at a time. At the fifth count of 100, one separate towel clip is placed aside to denote 500, and the caps shift back to the left of the central towel clip. Number counts have a tendency to slip away from the short-term memory with the slightest distraction, just as we forget the page number in a book immediately after turning to the next page. All our staff members know how to count, and in case one has to be relieved, the replacement staff can resume counting from the point where it was left.
- Alternately, an assistant can write the counted number on a board **(Fig. 7)**.
- Counting machines are available and can be used.

Dense Packing

How dense is dense? What is the maximum safe density? While the required density is mentioned earlier, there have been claims, by surgeons, that they can pack 50–70 FU/cm^2. There has also been an opinion that too much packing would affect dermal vascularity and create an environment of ischemia leading to less graft survival.[4-7] The available occipital donor area determines the upper limit of the number of grafts that can be harvested. So, the more that are packed in one zone, the less would be available for other areas. The availability of body hair has increased the availability of donor hair. Nevertheless, the general principle to give optimum density remains as discussed earlier. Greater density in specific instances such as actors, if requested, may be given in a second session, rather than too much packing in the first.

Humorously, "dense packing" conveys a meaning of stuffing grafts into a very small space. The author is often asked by many students about the mathematics of the number of slits to be made per square centimeter. There is no precise and fixed answer. Patients do not count the density but appreciate it visually. It takes experience to analyze all the factors, including the thickness of the hair, the number of available follicles, the color, direction, and frizziness, etc., to find an appropriate number of slits to be made in a given area for a good result. During the crucial early period of training, I often inquire from students about the required density to be placed in different parts of the scalp before beginning slit creation in each area. How close can two grafts be placed and whether they will survive or not are again frequently asked questions. No definite answer can be given here as well. Few tips I would like to give: Keep the angle and tilt similar in nearby slits, and do not slit into the adjacent slit, which then becomes one big slit instead of two.

Graft Placement and Insertion

The surgical assistant gives gentle pressure for a few minutes over the area after slitting is complete to achieve hemostasis. Waiting for some time is very beneficial. Then, we gently wash the scalp with Betadine surgical scrub to remove any clots lying superficially.

Transplanting the dissected hairs takes time and expertise. The patient must be comfortable on the operating chair, just as earlier when the slits were being made. By the time all the slits have been made, most of the follicular dissection would have been completed. We try and utilize all available hands on the deck. We prefer the technique of two assistants implanting together as this speeds up the process. We have observed that the grafts are most prone to injury during the implantation phase. It is important that the team should not get tired. The mental pressure of speeding the process in cases of a large number of grafts can take its toll on accuracy. Grafts get continuously shifted across hands and Petri dishes and have a lot of time and opportunity for desiccation injury in between.[2,3] Implantation should be performed by trained assistants who know how to sustain the effort over long periods of time. Implantation is done under magnification, and the assistants wear loupes. The two assistants sit at the head end of the patient, one to the right and one to the left. One or two assistants can stand by the trolley to arrange the direction of the grafts, which they arrange in bunches of 25 of 1, 2, 3, or 4 FU in the tray on a stockinet immersed in saline. The aim is to make the implanting assistant free from all trivial hassles and to let him focus completely on the accurate implantation of the graft without having to look around.

Hence, proper arrangement and alignment of grafts is important to facilitate efficient placement. The grafts can be placed either on the implanter's left hand, either on the dorsum or index finger, or on the forehead of the patient. Other devices for carrying grafts have been devised, such as plastic cups or metal cups, that can be fixed on the finger of the implanter or assistant. The grafts are handed over to the implanting assistants in a manner that it does not interfere with their work. The grafts are given in groups of 5–10 at a time and aligned such that the direction need not be adjusted before insertion. It is time-consuming to reorient the grafts with every insertion.

The way one holds the graft during implantation is also important; it should be held gently just above the bulb. For follicular unit excision (FUE) grafts, which are thinner and more fragile, the graft should be held by the shaft of the hair to avoid injury to the hair follicle.

Introduction of the graft into the slit can be made by different methods:

- Introduce the tip of the forceps into the slit keeping an eye on the tip, not on the bulb of the graft. Move the graft gently in the direction of the slit without scraping or grazing the lateral walls; the bulb will automatically follow wherever the tip of the forceps goes—let go of the forceps and gently slide it out. This should be a very smooth swift action, all in one motion.
- Another way is to open the slit first with another forceps held in the nondominant hand and then use the dominant hand to push the graft inside.
- A third way is to open the slit first with a needle in the nondominant hand and then use the dominant hand to push the graft inside.
- Lastly, some centers practice the "buddy" method—here, one assistant opens the site, and the other assistant introduces the graft. This is particularly useful in the final stages of insertion, amid grafts in a densely packed area. It is also useful in areas such as eyebrows or mustache.

The direction of the slits is such that a right-handed person sitting on the left is at a disadvantage because the slits open to the left away from him. The technique of implantation on the left side differs from the right and requires much more practice. On the right side, the forceps held in the right hand place the graft into the slit, which is oriented toward the right. But on the left side, the slit is oriented toward the left, and the graft is ideally placed into the slit using the left hand to slide in the graft. It is, therefore, beneficial for a left hand-dominant person to sit on the left side for implantation.

Identification of Sites

Proper magnification is required so that the grafts are placed in a nontraumatic fashion and no slits are missed out. One technique is to use forceps (or a needle) to recognize the next slit. While implanting the hair FU, the tip of the forceps (or the needle) is inserted gently into the next slit.

Staining the Slits

Using a dye to stain the edges of the slit helps in easier identification during implantation, especially in dark-skinned patients. After the creation of slits, a few drops of methylene blue or gentian violet **(Fig. 8)** are smeared over the recipient area and kept for a few minutes, and then the scalp is cleaned with normal saline. The dye stains the slits and thus prevents missing any slit during implantation.

PROBLEMS ENCOUNTERED IN PRESLITS METHOD

- *Skipped area for slits:* Sometimes, certain areas may have denser packing, and here some areas may be skipped during slit making. It is, therefore, important for the surgeon to inspect the area after making all the slits, look for skip areas, and make more slits as required.

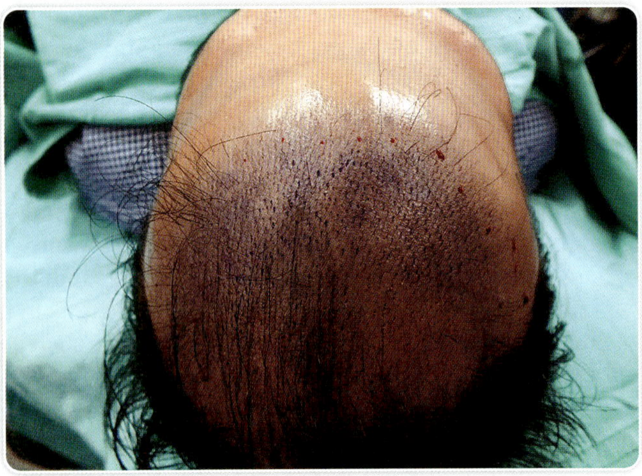

FIG. 8: Staining the slits with gentian violet.

- As slits are made, two slits may coalesce and form a larger slit. Care is needed to prevent this while making the slits.
- *Depth control*: Any surgeon who is a beginner may often make slits with variable inappropriate depth leading to problems as pointed out earlier.
- Some slits, which are smaller, may close after some time.
- *Direction*: It must be maintained and needs to be uniform and should not vary—it will lead to inappropriate hair direction later if done incorrectly.
- Identification of the slits may be a problem for beginners (described earlier).
- The technique needs proper coordination between the dissecting team and the surgeon; the number of grafts dissected and the number of sites made should be the same. The number of sites for each type of unit: 1/2/3/4 hair units need to correlate with the precise number of grafts of each type. This needs experience and competence. An inexperienced team may end up dissecting fewer grafts than slits; the team may also end up dissecting units of grafts of sizes different from the sizes of sites made by the surgeon.
- Likewise, the implanting team needs to have the experience and competence to implant the right graft into the right site in the right direction within the right time. An inexperienced team may either implant smaller units into larger sites (as it is easier), may implant in the wrong direction, or may take too much time to implant.
- Popping may be a problem

For all these reasons, this technique is suited more for a team that is experienced. A beginner can choose the "slit and place" or "implanter" technique, and then as they gain experience, adopt the preformed slit technique. In the beginning, they can create 50–100 slits and implant, and then another 50–100 slits and progress thereon.

Popping

The term "popping" refers to previously planted grafts popping out of the skin while inserting an adjacent graft. This frustrating event unnecessarily prolongs the duration of surgery and leads to additional handling and possible damage to grafts. Popping may occur for the following reasons:

- If the graft is too big in girth (chubby graft) for the recipient size
- If the incision is too shallow
- Tough, thick scalp or areas of scar tissue transmit displacing forces easily and result in more popping
- Excessive bleeding also increases popping; therefore, gentle handling while inserting the graft is important. Any rough handling increases local trauma and bleeding, resulting in more popping.
- Density of slits is also an important factor; the greater the density, the more the popping, particularly for beginners. However, it is not correct to decrease the density and compromise on the result. Rather, the technique should be improved to match the requirement.
- Improper technique—this is a common reason. A beginner fails to identify the right direction, the right-sized hole, and the right force of implantation.

Tips to Avoid Popping

The most important tool to avoid popping is proper technique, practice, and experience; to identify the right direction, the right-sized slit, the right-sized graft, and the right force of implantation, any of these, if incorrect, may result in popping.

- While inserting the new graft, the compressive forces from the lateral and inferior directions tend to displace the graft outward when a new graft is placed behind it. When the forceps with the bulb end of the graft is pushed down to the depth of the slit, while releasing the forceps, the forces from below can displace the adjacent graft upward, and it may slip back out just behind the forceps. So, the direction of the implanting force needs to be parallel to the existing slit. The graft needs to go in smoothly and gently along the direction of the slit. While pushing in the graft, stop the forceps about halfway into the slit and slip the remaining graft gently in. This coordination during the insertion is very important and needs practice and experience.
- Bleeding increases popping. The deeper the forceps goes while implanting, the more the chances of

bleeding, which results in popping. If this happens, just press for a few minutes and then reinsert the graft. Bleeding is more if tumescence is improper or if the patient is hypertensive, smokes, or has been on antiplatelet drugs. These have been dealt with in earlier chapters.

- To reduce popping, one can trim the graft a little more and make it fit for the recipient site.
- It is a good practice to make a few slits initially, and check by placing grafts into them, and the depth of the slits can be adjusted likewise.
- Another useful technique is to begin planting from anterior to posterior. The same forces which tend to pop out the graft when being placed from back to front now push the graft against the back wall of the slit when a new graft is placed **(Fig. 9)**.
- Proper tumescence and anesthesia prevent bleeding.
- It is important to complete the process as quickly as possible. With prolonged surgical time, the effect of adrenaline wears off leading to rebound vasodilatation and bleeding. Injection of additional tumescence itself can cause popping. The team also starts getting tired, and efficiency drops. The patient also gets fatigued and may become fidgety.

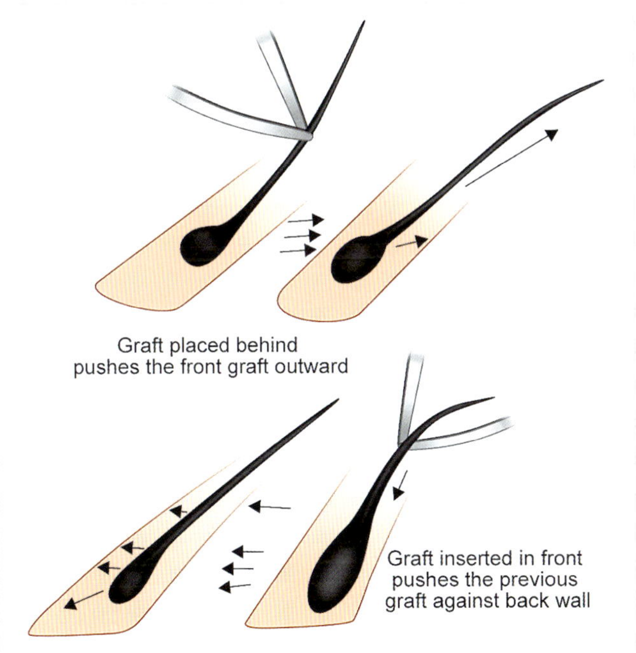

FIG. 9: Schematic diagrams showing how the graft placed behind pushes the graft in front outward; the graft placed in front pushes the graft behind backward.

POSTIMPLANTATION CARE

Once all the grafts are placed, the scalp is made wet with copious saline. Gentle dabbing with saline-soaked gauze is done to remove any clots. A stick swab or an earbud soaked with saline can be used for this purpose. The graft adheres to the walls of the slit immediately by fibrin adhesion and stops any bleeding in the process. Even scalps that bleed profusely during the implantation go completely quiet once all the grafts are in place. Any undue bleeding from any of the slits signifies that the graft has been displaced. At this point, we infiltrate the donor region with 7–10 mL of 0.5% bupivacaine to provide prolonged analgesia.

Postoperative Period

A strip of gauze is applied over the donor site for soakage and a sports headband is applied across the scalp, covering the donor site behind and across to below the transplanted zone in the forehead in the front. The recipient site is left open. The headband is not tight enough to hamper the venous drainage of the scalp but prevents edema from the scalp sliding down to the face. The reader is referred to the chapter 68 on Immediate Postoperative Care for details.

The grafted area is kept moist with a few drops of normal saline every 30–60 minutes for the first 24 hours after the transplant. The patient is given all the postoperative instructions in detail, and all his queries are answered. Special emphasis is given to explain him the importance of avoiding any trauma to the transplanted hair for the first 3 weeks. The patient is advised to sleep at night with the head elevated by one or two soft pillows below the head.

SUMMARY

A preformed slit is a very useful technique with several advantages, including complete control, attaining good density, and completing the procedure faster. However, it needs proper technique and experience, for both the surgeon and the team. A surgeon needs to be proficient with all techniques and should adopt the technique to the needs of the patient.

Tips and Pearls

- The recipient area needs careful planning.
- A hair transplant surgeon should be familiar with all techniques of graft insertion.
- A proper technique is vital to prevent popping.

REFERENCES

1. Cole J. Mathematics of follicular unit transplantation. Sixth Annual Meeting of the International Society of Hair Restoration Surgery, Washington, DC, September 16–20, 1998.
2. Gandelman M, Mota AL, Abrahamsohn PA, De Oliveira SF. Light and electron microscopic analysis of controlled injury to follicular unit grafts. Dermatol Surg. 2000;26(1):25-31.
3. Limmer BL. Micrograft survival. In: Stough DB (Ed). Hair Replacement: Surgical and Medical. St. Louis, Missouri: Mosby; 1996. pp. 147-9.
4. Farjo B, Farjo N. Dense packing: surgical indications and technical considerations. Facial Plast Surg Clin North Am. 2013;21(3):431-6.
5. Nakatsui T, Wong J, Groot D. Survival of densely packed follicular unit grafts using the lateral slit technique. Dermatol Surg. 2008;34(8):1016-22.
6. Alhaddab M, Kohn T, Sidloi M. Effect of graft size, angle, and intergraft distance on dense packing in hair transplant. Dermatol Surg. 2005;31(6):650-3.
7. Limmer BL. The density issue in hair transplantation. Dermatol Surg. 1997;23(9):747-50.

CHAPTER 65

Recipient Methods: Stick-and-Place

Sandeep Sattur, Indu S Sattur

Key Messages

- Correct and atraumatic graft placement is the key to a successful outcome in hair transplantation.
- Grafts can be inserted using premade incisions or with stick-and-place (S&P) technique or using mechanical devices called implanters.
- The S&P technique is a technique where the surgeon makes an incision and immediately inserts the graft.
- This technique has the advantages of accuracy, total surgeon control, and suitability for hairy areas.

INTRODUCTION

After the grafts have been harvested, the next critical step in hair transplantation is graft insertion, also called placement or implantation. There is more than one way to do so, and the technique one employs depends upon the preference, expertise, and aptitude of the person implanting.

GRAFT PLACEMENT TECHNIQUES

Graft placement techniques can be divided into three basic categories:

1. *Incision first or premade incisions*: All incisions are made in one go followed by implantation.
2. *Simultaneous site creation and immediate implantation* [stick-and-place (S&P)]: Incision is made, and this is followed immediately with graft placement.
3. *Graft insertion using implanters* (GII): The incision is made and the graft is placed almost simultaneously with the use of a special mechanical device, the implanter. It could be considered as a subtype of S&P in the true sense.

Each method has its own advantages and disadvantages and will be considered in different chapters. This chapter discusses the "S&P technique."

Stick-and-Place Technique

The S&P technique of graft insertion involves creating the recipient site and simultaneously inserting the graft. This is done either by a single person or by two people where one creates the slit and the other inserts the graft. Graft insertion by S&P requires well-trimmed grafts and good coordination between the hands as the process involves creating the site with a sharp instrument with one hand and withdrawing that to allow the graft to be inserted by the other hand. *It can be likened to putting your foot into the shoe using a shoe horn.*

Instrumentation for Stick-and-Place

The following instrumentation is used by the author. However, one can use other devices to create the recipient sites:

- Hypodermic needles (19G, 20G, 21G: 1.5 inch long) or chisel blades which could be customized or Minde's knife

- Angular implanting forceps, fine tipped
- Magnification in the form of loupes/magnifying visors (good quality with at least 3× magnification)

Prerequisites for Stick-and-Place

- Proper body and hand positioning of the surgeon/assistant (adjust the patient's head and chair height)
- Good illumination

Technique of Stick-and-Place

The technique of S&P can be split up into the following steps:

1. *Creating incision*:
   i. The choice of needle size depends on the size of grafts, commonly used needles are 21G, 20G, and 19G hypodermic needles **(Fig. 1)** with 1.5-inch length.
   ii. Insert the needle only up to the bevel.
   iii. Withdraw the needle slightly to hold the site open.
2. *Grasping the graft*:
   i. Grasp the graft at the subcutaneous tissue below the bulb or just lateral to it **(Fig. 2)**, or just above it gently (without crushing); do not hold either over the bulb or higher up where the bulge area resides. Some surgeons hold the graft below the bulb, over the fat.
   ii. Grasping it higher can cause the follicle to bend over itself (J-phenomenon).
3. *Insertion of graft*:
   i. Withdraw the needle slightly.
   ii. Slide the graft along the bevel into the recipient site (just like a foot being inserted into a shoe using a shoe horn).
   iii. When the graft is three-fourths inside, withdraw the needle completely and simultaneously push the graft.
   iv. It requires coordination of both hands.
4. *Adjusting the position of the graft*:
   i. Push the graft inside the recipient site gently.
   ii. Make sure it is flush with the skin or slightly above it.
5. *Improving efficiency in S&P*: It is important to understand that S&P is based on the "work as you go" principle and allows for a lot of customization. But if one has to improve the efficiency of the technique there are a few points to be kept in mind:
   i. Choose the size of the needle for creating the recipient site as per the size of the graft being implanted.
   ii. Make sure the grafts are well trimmed and do not have frills.
   iii. Density in S&P is achieved through multiple passes as it may not be able to achieve full density in the first pass. The first pass should aim to create 50–60% density while the second pass will increase density. It is always ideal to use a fresh needle when going for the second pass. Depending upon the individual properties of the skin, one needle usually lasts for 20–30 slits.
   iv. A common problem that can arise is placing the incisions in a line, which not only reduces the illusion of density but also makes it look artificial.
   v. Organize the grafts and keep them in the field of view of the surgeon so that efficiency and speed may be increased. The grafts can be placed on a spatula, on a thick sterile cloth on the forehead, or

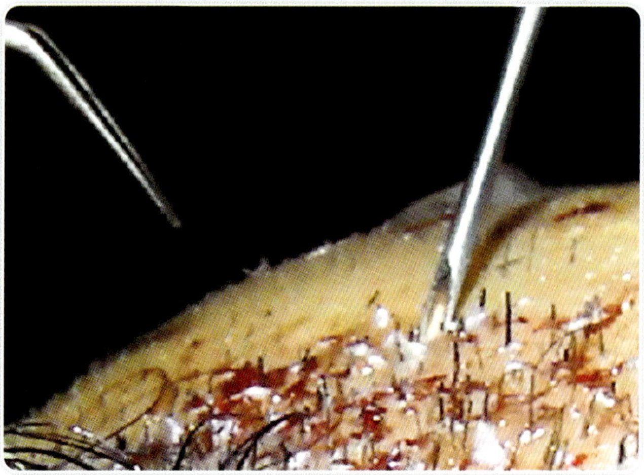

FIG. 1: Hypodermic needle used to create a recipient site. The direction of the needle has to be parallel to the surrounding hair or as standard direction and angulation for the given recipient area.

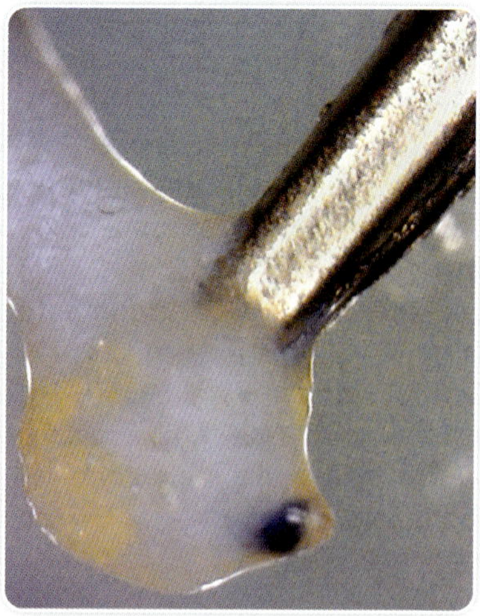

FIG. 2: The graft has to be grasped just lateral to the bulb or below it.

on the surgeon's index or middle finger or dorsum of the hand. Special containers (finger cups) which can be hooked onto the finger have also been devised.

vi. *Word of caution:* Avoid desiccation of grafts by keeping only a small number of grafts and also irrigate the grafts constantly with saline.

6. *Modifications*:
   i. The method can be combined with premade slits. One of the disadvantages of preformed slits is that there may be gaps between slits or some slits may be missed. S&P is an excellent technique to fill such areas.
   ii. Usually, for the left side, the needle is held in the left hand and the graft in the right hand. While working on the right side, the graft is in the left hand with a forceps and a needle in the right hand to make a slit. This needs practice.

The Pros and Cons of Stick-and-Place

Pros

- Less bleeding
- Ability to work in areas of thinning amid hairs
- Adaptability to special areas (eyebrows, mustache, beard, etc.) and size of grafts
- Ability to control depth, angle, and direction depending on the recipient areas (the needle can be bent at right angles as shown in **Figure 3**, which acts not only as a depth guard but also helps to keep the angulation consistent)
- No missed sites or piggybacking
- Can be used in combination with preformed slit method when slits are missed
- With experience, high density can be achieved **(Figs. 4A and B)**.

Cons

- Long learning curve
- More surgeon dependent, more effort and time commitments on the part of the surgeon
- Possibility of differences in density and angle of implantation if two people are implanting simultaneously.

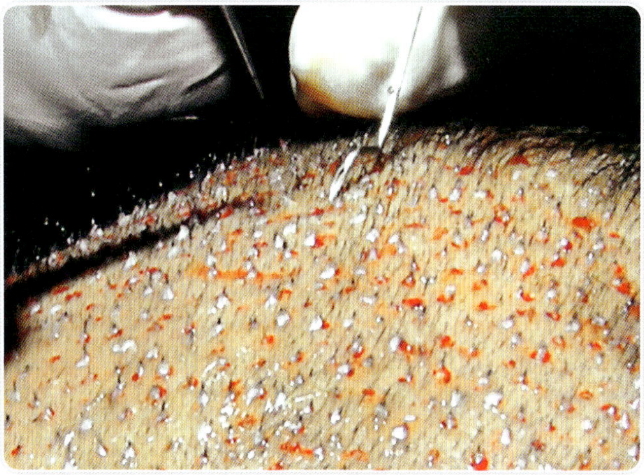

FIG. 3: Modifying the needle tip to act as a guard against the depth as well as keeping a uniform angulation.

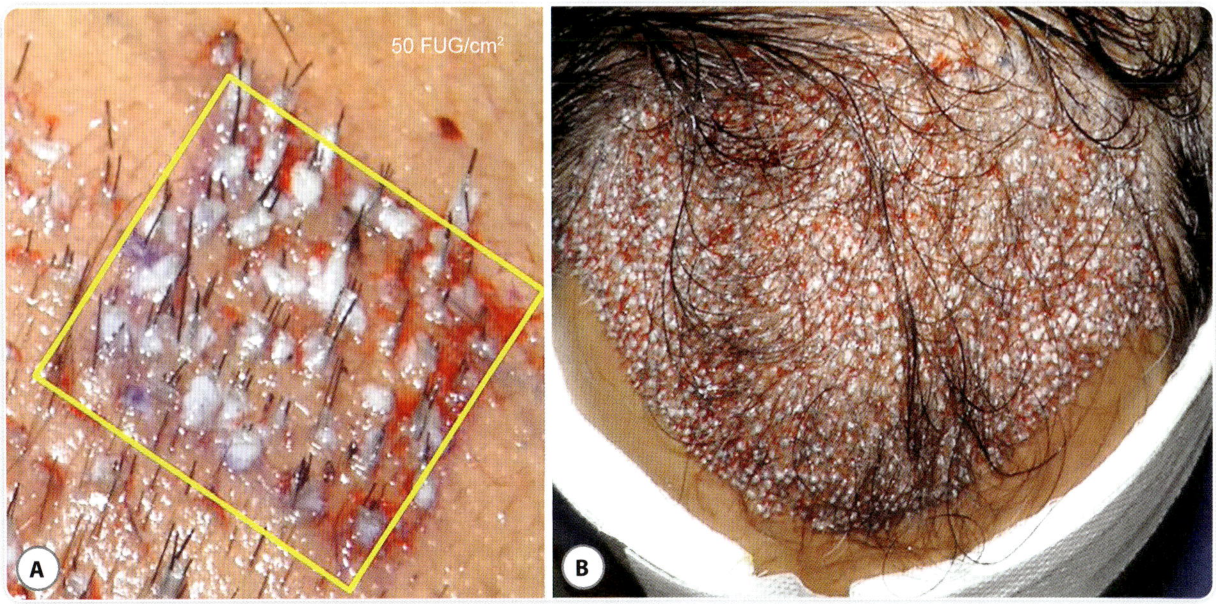

FIGS. 4A AND B: The density achieved by the stick-and-place (S&P) technique.

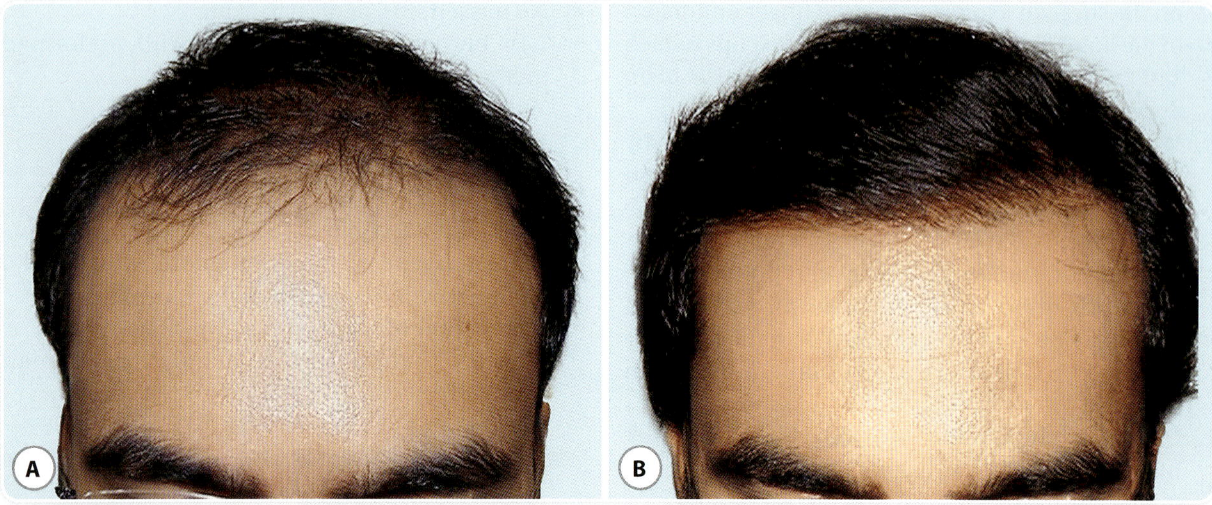

FIGS. 5A AND B: Results after implantation with the stick-and-place (S&P) technique.

- It is somewhat slower than other methods, though experienced surgeons can perform this technique very quickly **(Figs. 5A and B)**.

SUMMARY

With regard to the popularity of techniques, premade incisions and implantation are the most popular. But many centers/surgeons use a combination of techniques, especially when dealing with implantation in areas of thinning. Moreover, the author always uses S&P for final touches to the hairline and to increase densities with the help of additional passes. In summary, it is best to use the technique that one is comfortable with and one that the team is fluent in.

CHAPTER 66

Implanters

Syed Mubashir

Key Messages

- Implanters represent an attempt at automation of recipient implantation.
- The advantages include quick implantation and use in hairy areas.
- Both steps, site creation and implantation, are completed in one step.
- The disadvantage includes the cost of the devices.

INTRODUCTION

Description of implanters: Implanters have the following characteristics:

- Needle
- External diameter where follicular units can be placed
- *Channel*: It should allow the graft to move easily and does not cause any decapitation or trauma; the minimum ratio of external diameter to channel should be 10:8.
- *Bevel*: A large bevel with a fine wall facilitates the loading of hair grafts.
- *Tip*: The tip can be either sharp or blunt; blunt ones increase popping.
- *Surgical steel*: Good steel needles having high tensile strength can last longer as compared to bad steel with low tensile strength as it gets bent.

IMPLANTER BODY

- As far as length and width are concerned, they are the same in all brands of implanters; their size does not vary much.
- Body shape varies in brands, and it facilitates its use depending upon the surgeon's comfort.

There are three basic steps of hair transplantation:

1. Harvesting
2. Graft preparation
3. Plantation

Each step is of vital importance and should function smoothly to ensure a satisfactory outcome. It is like establishing a supply chain.

Implantation consists of two steps:

1. Site creation
2. Insertion of graft in the created site using implanter will help in improved results because of minimal graft handling, more graft placement in less time, and thereby reducing body out of time.[1] In follicular unit excision (FUE), however, there is a greater chance of trauma and consequent poor growth with forceps because the follicles themselves are touched.[2] Implanters answer this problem.

IMPLANTERS

Implanters were devised in an attempt to automate and quicken the process of implantation.

Criteria for an Ideal Transplanter

An implanter should be the following:

- Small
- Lightweight
- Convenient length
- Minimum joints
- Disposable
- No or easy learning curve
- Economically viable

- Work without electricity, suction, or spring device
- Available in various sizes for different size of units
- With good quality steel having high tensile strength
- Cause no damage to the graft
- Can be easily handled and maneuvered in the surgeon's hand
- Popping should be less
- Easy sterilization
- Able to create suitable opening size and depth of the cavity
- Should have depth control

Popular Implanters Used in Hair Transplantation

- OKT implanters (Optimally Kept Transplanter), Choi implanter
- Lion implanter
- KEEP (Koray Erdogan Embedding Placer) implanter
- Mohebi inserter
- Rainbow implanter
- SAVA implanter
- KNU (Kyungpook National University) implanter

Choi Implanter

The Choi implanter **(Fig. 1)** consists of a needle with a bevel where the graft is placed, a body that holds the needle, and a plunger or a pusher with a spring to push the graft into the site **(Fig. 2)**.

Method of Use

As shown in **Figures 3A to C**, the hair unit is loaded into the bevel of the implanter of the right size. The implanter is then placed on the recipient area, and the plunger is pushed (like in a ball pen), which makes a slit and places the graft at the same time.

ADVANTAGE

The advantage of this implanter is quick and easy implantation.

Disadvantages

- It has too many parts.
- Frequent change of the needle
- Implantation process is blind **(Fig. 2)**.
- Learning curve
- It is more suitable for straight hair but not for curved hair.

The implanter should be held with the second, third, and back part of the fourth finger from the upper middle and lower part equidistant, and the thumb positioned in the middle front opposing other fingers to hold it. Traction can be given anteriorly with two fingers of nondominating hand on the forehead and in case of posterior area with two fingers of nondominating hand posterior and downward. In this position, we perform a forward movement, and with a little pressure, the bevel slips easily into the dermis. As needle has penetrated the required depth, the second finger changes the position to the upper part of the plunger and depresses it, and at the same time, we remove the needle from the scalp.

If the length of needle is too long, it can cause burying of grafts leading to folliculitis, and if the length of needle is short, it can cause pop out of grafts.

- 0.8–0.9 mm—single root graft
- 0.9–1.0 mm—double root graft
- 1.0–1.2 mm—triple root graft

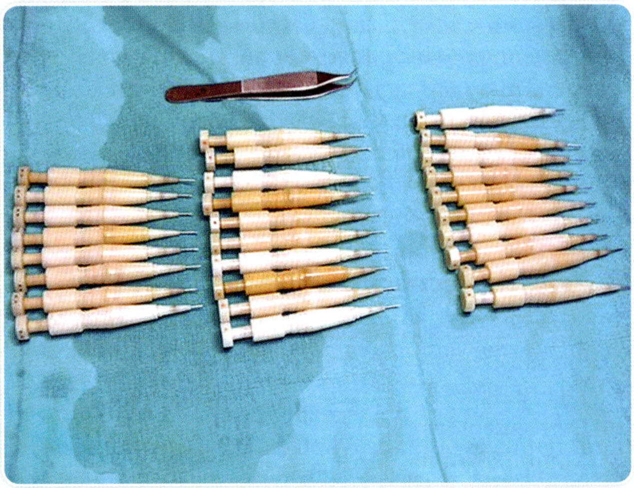

FIG. 1: Choi implanter [later modified as KNU (Kyungpook National University) implanter].

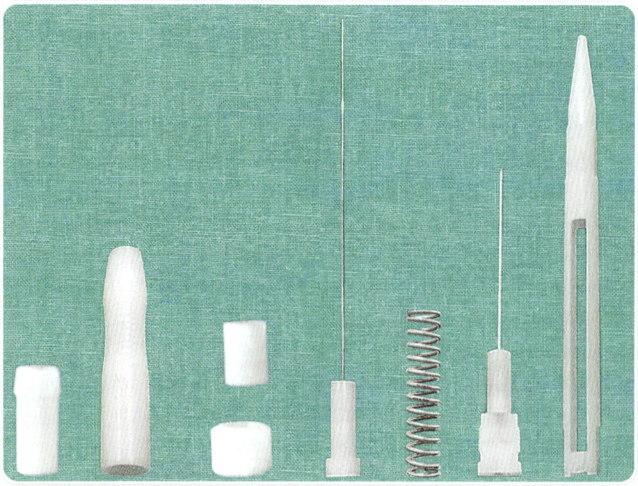

FIG. 2: Parts of a Choi implanter.

SAVA Transplanter (Figs. 4A and B)

SAVA transplanter performs the following functions:

- Creates the site
- Has depth control
- Makes a spiral cavity
- Keeps the mouth of cavity open
- Stretches the cavity walls apart
- Acts as a slide during plantation

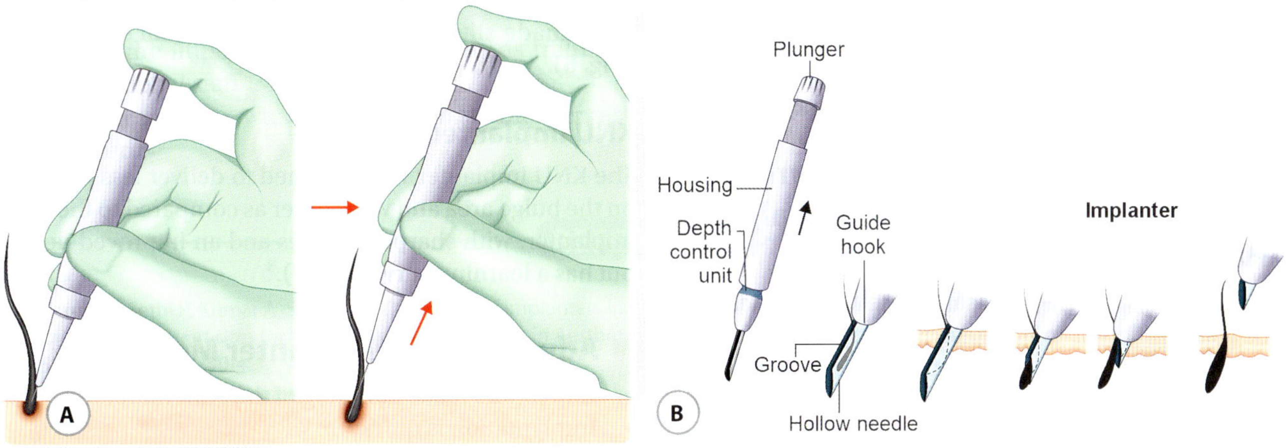

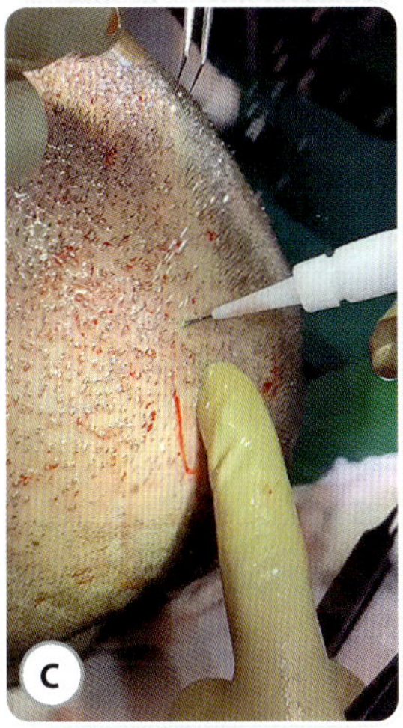

FIGS. 3A TO C: Use of a Choi implanter.

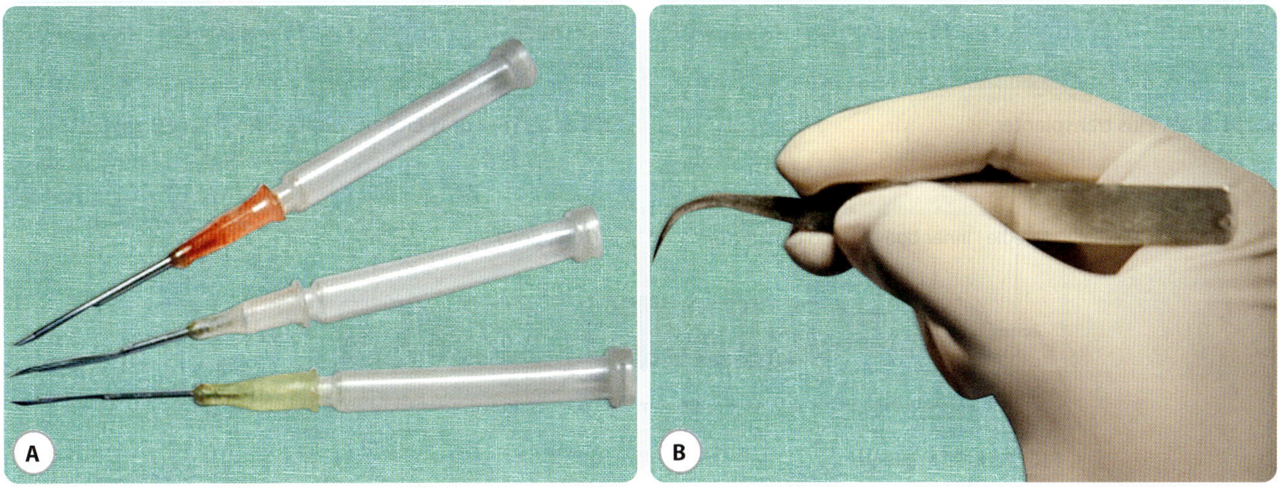

FIGS. 4A AND B: (A) SAVA transplanter and (B) SAVA introducer.

CHAPTER 67

Overview of Different Methods of Recipient Site Implantation

Venkataram Mysore

Key Messages

- Different methods of recipient insertion include premade slits, slit and place, and implanters.
- The preslit method is quick, allows proper planning, and allows free time for the surgeon.
- The slit and place technique is accurate, is fully under the surgeon's control, and is useful in hairy areas.
- The implanter method is quick and allows plantation in hairy areas.
- Each method has its advantages and disadvantages, and the surgeon needs to be aware of all methods so that he can use the right method for the right situation.

INTRODUCTION

The previous chapters have discussed different methods of implantation. Each method has its own advantages and disadvantages. A surgeon needs to be proficient in all methods so that different methods can be used for the benefit of the patient in a given situation. This chapter summarizes the different approaches and presents an overview.[1] The advantages and disadvantages of different methods are summarized in **Table 1**.

METHOD 1: PREFORMED SLITS AND PLACE

This method is popular with many surgeons as it has the advantages of speed and lesser surgeon's involvement time. It allows overall planning and control for the surgeon as he can plan the entire recipient session in one step. It also gives time for the surgeon to perform other tasks (as his task of making the slits gets over quickly) and perform other procedures. However, the following challenges are faced:

- It needs greater coordination between the surgeon and the dissecting team. As the dissection of grafts lags behind the process of making slits (which is faster), there can be a disparity in the number of slits made and the final outcome of the number of grafts dissected.
- If the number of sites is less, the surgeon has to spend more time making new ones. If sites are created more than required, then slits will remain unused or fresh harvesting has to be done. Likewise, it is a challenge to precisely make an estimate of the specific number of slits for one hair, two hair, and three hair grafts beforehand. Therefore, this method needs an experienced surgeon and an experienced team for proper execution.
- Bleeding from created sites may continue throughout the procedure, which makes sites messy, wet, and slippery. Hence, the method needs proper tumescent anesthesia.
- With time, identification of sites may become difficult, small slits may close, and hence some slits may be missed during implantation, especially in dark-skinned people.
- A large amount of local anesthetic may leak out with the fluid from these sites, making the pain-relieving effect unpredictable.
- Making uniform distribution of slits needs experience; skip areas may occur. These may need a visit by the surgeon to make more slits in that area.

TABLE 1: Summary of features of different methods.

Features	Preformed slit and graft placement	Slit and place	Implanters
Description	All slits are performed in one go and grafts are placed by assistants, one by one after all slits are made	Each slit is performed followed by immediate placement of each graft	Hairs are placed into implanters (sharp or dull) and then implanted
Handling grafts	Grafts may get crushed in inexperienced hands	Grafts may get crushed in inexperienced hands	Minimum handling of grafts
Speed	Quick	Slower	Quick
Instruments	Forceps, needles	Forceps, needles	Dull implanters—place grafts in premade slits Sharp implanters—single step
Surgeon's dependency	Surgeon can make the slits and then assistants can place grafts, less surgeon time	Surgeon dependent	Surgeon dependent in sharp implanters
Accuracy	Calculations of number of slits needs to be accurate, needs experience	Accurate	Accurate
Placement	Some slits may be missed, some slits may close	Accurate	Accurate
Bleeding	Bleeding may occur during initial placement	Bleeding while making slits making graft placement difficult	Bleeding may push the graft out in sharp implanters
Identification of slits	Maybe difficult with time	Not a problem	Problem with dull but not sharp implanters
Grafting in between existing hairs	Difficult	Easy	Very easy
Angulation, precision of placement	Since done by assistants, may vary	Accurate	Accurate
Skill needed	Needs skill and experience	Needs skill and experience	Easier
Cost	Cheap	Cheap	Cost of devices

- Popping may occur if the slits are placed too close to each other.
- It is more difficult to adopt, when implantation is required between existing and previously planted hair.
- Once slits are all made, then the job is entirely left to the assistants to implant the grafts. This can lead to lack of control, poor handling of grafts, and poor communication with patients.

However, it is important to note that an experienced surgeon and a team can overcome these challenges.

METHOD 2: IMPLANTATION BY STICK AND PLACE

This method has some advantages: Graft placement is immediate, causing less bleeding; it is easier to implant between hairs, and variations are possible as the process progresses gradually. There is also total surgeon control as he is present throughout the surgery. It is particularly useful for beginners. It is particularly useful for areas such as eyebrows and the temporal angle where frequent changes in direction are needed. It is also useful at the end of a preformed slit insertion process for skip areas.

However, this method has the following disadvantages:

- *During creating sites*:
  - Lack of depth control for a beginner; it depends on the feel of surgeon.
  - If the site created is deep, there may be bleeding. Hence, immediate placement may be difficult. This is common with beginners.
  - Creating sites in close proximity may lead to popping; hence, dense packing may be difficult.
  - Since each graft needs a different-sized hole, frequent change of needles is necessary.

- *During placement*:
  - During placement, grafts may be crushed, squeezed, bend, destroyed, or pushed too deep to produce pitting, particularly in the hands of a beginner.
  - Overall, this procedure is slower and time consuming.
  - A surgeon's involvement is more as he has to be present throughout surgery.

Again, it has to be pointed that all the challenges apply to beginners only.

IMPLANTERS

Implanters have had a checkered history. Sharp implanters were first introduced in the 1990s in Korea but did not achieve much popularity in other parts of the world because of the time of involvement of surgeon and the cost of implanters. However, with the advent of follicular unit extraction (FUE), they made a reentry in the last decade in the form of dull implanters. The FUE grafts were thought to be more fragile, and hence needed minimum handling. Sharp implanters were used to make slits (hence surgeons' involvement) and place grafts in one step. The disadvantage of extensive surgeon involvement was removed by the introduction of dull implanters, which were used to only hold and place the grafts into premade slits.

Advantages

Implanters have some advantages:

- Implanters make handling of the graft minimal.
- Implantation is quick.
- It is easy to use in between existing hairs.
- Implantation in different angles is possible.
- Depth control is possible.

Disadvantages

Implanters have the following disadvantages:

- Additional cost as they are disposable
- Dissection needs to be precise as the graft needs to be loaded into the slit on the needle of the implanter. Since FUE grafts come out ready for implantation, this is not an issue for FUE grafts.
- Loading the implanter with the graft needs training and additional staff. This is made easier in newer implanters with slits that allow grafts to be rolled into the slits.
- Popping can occur, in which case a graft has to be placed by the above other method.

DIRECT HAIR TRANSPLANTATION[2,3]

Follicular unit extraction and introduction of implanters also made possible a new method of recipient process called direct hair transplantation (DHT) or direct hair implantation. Implantation of FUE grafts immediately after extraction into premade slits is referred to as direct hair transplantation and has become popular. In this method, first described by Pradeep Sethi and Arika Bansal, there is an important reversal of steps. Traditionally, donor excision was first performed, and then recipient sites were created followed by implantation. However, in DHT, the process is reversed. Recipient slits are created first. This is followed by extraction of grafts by FUE with the patient usually sitting on an FUE chair. As soon as they are extracted, the recipient team implants the grafts through implanters into the premade slits.

This method has the advantage *that out-of-body time is minimized* as grafts immediately go into the recipient sites. FUE grafts being ready for implantation without any need for dissection are well suited for direct implantation. Implantation can be done either by traditional forceps and needle or through implanters. This has also brought down the duration of hair transplantation (HT) using FUE and made the process faster. It is particularly useful while extracting from beard and body.

The disadvantages of the method are that two teams are needed to work simultaneously, thereby increasing manpower. The method is tedious to perform as the field available is narrow and angulation of grafts may be difficult in some areas.

The method signifies an important advance in HT by FUE. It removed one main disadvantage of FUE: Longer duration and also had one advantage: decreased out of body time—leading to better survival of grafts. A modification called immediate HT has been used by the author, where extraction is done in batches of 500–700 grafts, and these are implanted either immediately (directly as mentioned above) where feasible or in batches after extraction where it is tedious due to lack of field of operation. Since it is possible to extract 500–700 in about 20–30 minutes, out-of-body time is reduced to maximum of 30 minutes. It also makes implantation more comfortable for the surgeon.

Tips and Pearls

- The greatest advantage of premade slit and place is that a surgeon's involvement is least and takes least total surgical time. It allows a surgeon to perform other tasks or even start another case. Its biggest disadvantages are that there could be miscalculations in the number and errors in orientation as it is assistant dependent. So, it is a method for teams led by an experienced surgeon and an experienced team. It still needs additional implantation by slit and place at the end for any skip areas.
- The greatest advantages of stick and place are its control and accuracy due to its near total surgeon involvement. It is also suitable for hairy areas. However, it gives little time for the surgeon to do other tasks. It is also time consuming. It is a method of choice for beginners.
- The greatest advantages of the implanter method are its speed, accuracy, and near total surgeon control and utility in hairy areas. The disadvantages are expense of devices, need for more precise dissection for placement in the implanter, and need for additional staff to load implanters.
- A surgeon should be proficient in all methods so that he can use the right method for the right patient in the right situation.

REFERENCES

1. Marwah MK, Mysore V. Recipient area. J Cutan Aesthet Surg. 2018;11(4):202-10.
2. Sethi P, Bansal A. Direct hair transplantation: a modified follicular unit extraction technique. J Cutan Aesthet Surg. 2013;6(2):100-5.
3. Mysore V. Direct hair transplantation (DHT): an innovative follicular unit extraction (FUE) technique of hair transplantation. J Cutan Aesthet Surg. 2013;6(2):106.

PART E: Postoperative Care and Complications

SECTION OUTLINE

CHAPTER 68

Immediate Postoperative Care

Venkataram Mysore

Key Messages

- Proper care of the donor area and transplanted grafts is important in the immediate postoperative period to ensure smooth recovery.
- Avoiding dryness and heat is of importance.
- Postoperative pain, edema, and crusting need to be managed properly.

INTRODUCTION

Postoperative care after hair transplant surgery is important, both from the view of the current surgery and from the view of possible future surgeries. Postoperative pain, edema, healing, etc., all affect patient comfort, particularly in the strip technique. Proper physician understanding and patient education are, therefore, particularly important.[1,2]

NATURAL COURSE OF EVENTS

Donor Area

In the donor area, after the strip technique, some postoperative pain is anticipated. A feeling of tension, heaviness, and numbness is all common. Occasionally, oozing of red-tinged fluid can also occur, with staining of the pillow cover, leading to anxiety. Sutures disappear between 10 and 14 days depending on the suture used, and if they do not, it is preferable to remove them. The scar appears initially erythematous, and this is often a concern to the patient.

Follicular unit extraction (FUE), on the other hand, is associated with very little postoperative issues. The sites heal dramatically within 1 day.

Recipient Area

The grafts, when transplanted, undergo a shift from the anagen phase to the telogen phase. Hence, there is a natural loss of hairs in the second week about which the patient needs to be forewarned. The growth then occurs after a lag phase of about 3 months. The hairs then grow 1–1.25 cm a month, which is the natural pattern of scalp hair. However, since each hair has its own cycle, it is not necessary that all hairs fall. Early use of minoxidil may decrease this hair fall. It is also important to differentiate this hair fall from shock loss, which denotes the loss of existing hairs after surgery and is particularly common over the donor area adjacent to the suture area and also over the recipient area when grafting is done amid preexisting hairs.

The objectives of postoperative care are as follows:

- Patient comfort, including management of postoperative pain
- Postoperative wound care to reduce crusting and ensure optimum healing
- Counseling on return to activities
- Prevention of complications

General care of the patient in the immediate postoperative period: While generally, in most patients, the

POSTOPERATIVE EDEMA[5-7]

Postoperative edema can be a major concern for patients, particularly those who need to travel or return to work early. It is, therefore, important to factor in the possibility of forehead and eyelid edema occurring on day 4 or 5 and often persisting for 3–5 days. In the author's experience, this edema is more common in elderly patients, perhaps due to the lax skin. Several measures, such as the use of a headband, injection of steroid triamcinolone into the frontal scalp, oral steroids for 3–5 days, mixing steroids into a tumescent solution (Abbassi solution), and lying down for prolonged periods to avoid the effect of gravity, have all been advocated. Once it occurs, it persists for 3–5 days, and in the author's experience, masterly inactivity, frequent counseling, and watchful expectancy are all that are needed. Cold compresses are usually advised, and while their efficacy is doubtful, they at least help in keeping the patient engaged and focused.

Measures to avoid postoperative edema:
- Headband
- Injection of steroid triamcinolone into the frontal scalp
- Oral steroids for 3–5 days
- Mixing steroids into a tumescent solution (Abbassi solution)
- Lying down for prolonged periods to avoid the effect of gravity

Exercise

Follicular unit extraction patients can start all exercises and yoga after one week. Strip technique, on the other hand, imposes certain restrictions, and mild exercise can be started from day 2. Jogging and swimming can be done once the donor area is healed. Neck stretching exercises are preferably avoided for 6–8 weeks to prevent tension on the donor area and a possible wider scar in strip technique.

Minoxidil Use[8,9]

Early minoxidil is advocated as it may prevent postoperative telogen effluvium and promote growth. However, evidence for this is debatable. Minoxidil frequently causes itching and hence may lead to the dislodgment of grafts. It is, therefore, the author's practice to start the application after 7 days.

Use of Hair Pieces and Wigs

There is a concern that early use of these may lead to infection and folliculitis. This is particularly true in the hot Indian environment. Also, the clips and sticking tapes used to fix them may have an impact on the grafts. Hence, it is preferable to avoid using hairpieces for about 10 days. If used, it should be limited to a few hours per day depending on the weather.

Graft Dislodgment

Patients view this very seriously and often with panic. Education, therefore, that all grafts may fall after 5 days is absolutely essential. Early dislodgment with mild bleeding also needs prior counseling with instruction to apply firm pressure on the bleeding area for a minute. Patients may demand that the dislodged graft be reimplanted, but there is little sense in reimplanting them as they quickly die due to dryness.

SUMMARY

The summary of postoperative care is shown in **Box 1**. The details are mentioned in the **Annexure**.

BOX 1 Summary of postoperative care.

- Patients should be prescribed post-transplant analgesics with nonsteroidal anti-inflammatory drugs, particularly in follicular unit transplantation (FUT)
- Massage, cold compresses with ice, and oral steroids are needed to avoid or improve frontal swelling during the first week after transplant
- Post-transplant prophylaxis with oral antibiotics is usually needed[10]
- Patients need to continue their treatment, such as anticoagulants, antiaggregant therapy, antihypertensive and antidiabetic therapies, and vitamin supplements, as per the advice of the concerned treating physician, 24–48 hours after hair transplant
- Nonabsorbable stitches should be removed between 10 and 14 days after FUT
- The recipient area needs to be kept and maintained moist by spraying the area with water or normal saline every 2–3 hours during the first 3–5 days after transplant. Patients may start washing their hair gently, without rubbing the scalp
- Rubbing should be avoided and grafts should not be disturbed during the first week
- Rubbing the scalp to eliminate the crusts is allowed 5–7 days after transplant
- A mild shampoo is allowed with a neutral shampoo during the first week after transplant
- Brushing is allowed after 2 weeks. Cutting hair is allowed after a month
- A cap or hat may be worn immediately after surgery
- Direct sunlight and heat should be avoided for at least 2 weeks
- While walking is allowed immediately, sports or physical activity and swimming should be avoided during the first week after hair transplant
- Minoxidil can be started after 1 week

ANNEXURE 1

Postoperative Instructions

After going back: Please note that hair transplantation is a very predictable surgery; all postoperative events are already informed to you, so there are no surprises and hence there is no need for any anxiety. Do not be worried about pain as it is not much.

On the day of surgery

- Have light food, your usual food, rice, *dal*, chapatti, *rasam*, or any nonspicy food.
- Do not smoke and do not drink alcohol.
- Take medicines as per the prescription. All capsules to be taken after food or with a glass of milk but not on an empty stomach. Remember that tramadol capsule is for pain. It acts for about 4–6 hours, so you may need one more capsule at night. Do not hesitate to take one if needed, but take it after milk/food.
- Be your usual self; bedrest is not needed. You may watch TV, listen to music, read, and work on computer.
- Avoid exertion
- Avoid jerky movements of the head. Avoid pressure on the head.
- Go to bed early.
- Use soft, thin pillows. You may lay on the back of the head. You may turn sideways, but do not sleep with the hand under the head.
- If you feel pain at any time, take one additional cap of tramadol but with a glass of milk. If there is any urgent problem beyond what is already mentioned, you may contact us at _______.

Next day

- You need to come back for removal of the bandage. You cannot remove this yourself. Time for this will be informed to you.
- Before coming, you can take a bath for the body but not for the head.
- You can have breakfast as usual. Take capsules after breakfast.
- When you come to the clinic, our nurse will remove the bandage and show how to clean and how to shampoo. Always feel free to ask any doubts.
- You may go to the office if you feel like, by wearing a cap (any type of cap, which is not tight). You can drive. Avoid exertion.
- You need to massage the forehead (as shown in the clinic) 3 times a day to prevent swelling of the forehead.

Cleaning of grafts

- *After removal of the bandage*: Note that moisture is very important for grafts. So, wet the hairs in both the donor and recipient (grafts) areas either by spray or by a wet pad; do not be hesitant to put water; water should be clean; use mineral water or boiled cooled water; you may add a small amount of Johnson's baby shampoo to the water. Do wetting as often as you can (2–6 times) for the first 4 days.
- *First week*: Do not disturb the grafts by rubbing/combing. Rest of the scalp may be cleaned by baby shampoo if you wish; otherwise, water is enough.
- *Second week*: Mild rubbing is allowed; you may apply oil if you want. You may start using minoxidil lotion twice daily. Grafts fall off at this stage; do not panic. They will come back by 3–4 months.

Donor area

- It also needs cleaning, with spray just as grafts. After cleaning, put mupirocin ointment twice daily. After 1 week, gently rub the stitch area so that stitch becomes gradually loose. After 2 weeks, use Hexilak cream.

Exercise

- Walking is allowed. Neck stretching can put tension on the donor suture area; hence, neck-stretching exercises are to be avoided for up to 2 months. Swimming is allowed after 2 weeks.

Postoperative swelling

- This may appear in 5% of patients only, on the forehead which may come down to eyelids on day 4/5. If so, do not worry, it will disappear in 2–3 days. Apply ice cubes as follows:
    - Take ice cubes.
    - Keep them in a piece of cloth. If you do not have ice, take a wet cloth in cold water.
    - Keep the ice pack on the swollen area for 2–3 minutes for 4–5 times for 2 days.

Sutures

- Sutures can be removed anytime after 10 days by our nurse; this is a simple, painless procedure taking about 10 minutes.
- For those who are from outside Bengaluru, absorbable sutures are put, and these will be absorbed by 2 weeks.
- Hair may start falling by 2 weeks. Do not panic; the roots are firmly in place. Sometimes, you may see whitish material sticking onto roots; do not worry about it. They will start growing by 3–4 months; you will see full results in 9 months.

Apply minoxidil lotion twice a day (1 mL) and take tablet finasteride after 1 week. Minoxidil may cause some dryness/dandruff; Some patients may develop a few boils on the grafts area after 4–6 weeks. These are temporary; do not worry.

Note: Some patients are too anxious to clean grafts; so they may see grafts with greenish-brown materials sticking to the skin; this only needs proper cleaning. Note that after 7 days, rubbing is allowed. Anytime you have doubts, contact us by e-mail or telephone if urgent. Feel free to contact us at any time. Our staff will contact you for feedback after 1 month and after 6 months.

REFERENCES

1. Vañó-Galván S, Bisanga CN, Bouhanna P, Farjo B, Gambino V, Meyer-González T, et al. An international expert consensus statement focusing on pre and post hair transplantation care. J Dermatol Treat. 2023;34(1):1-8.
2. Mysore V, Kumaresan M, Garg A, Dua A, Venkatram A, Dua K, et al. Hair transplant practice guidelines. J Cutan Aesthet Surg. 2021;14(3):265-84.
3. Perez-Meza D, Leavitt ML, Trachy RE. Clinical evaluation of GraftCyte moist dressings on hair graft viability and quality of healing. Int J Cosm Surg. 1998;6(1):80-4.
4. Hitzig GS. Enhanced healing and growth in hair transplantation using copper peptides. Cosm Dermatol. 2000;13:18-22.
5. Hwang S. Gravity position to prevent facial edema in hair transplantation. Hair Transplant Forum Int. 2009;19(3):77-80.
6. Abbasi G. Hair transplantation without postoperative edema. Hair Transplant Forum Int. 2005;15(5):157.
7. Nordstrom RE, Nordstrom RM. The effect of corticosteroids on postoperative edema. In: Unger W, Nordstrom R (Eds). Hair Transplantation. New York: Marcel Dekker; 1988. pp. 391-4.
8. Kassimir JJ. Use of topical minoxidil as a possible adjunct to hair transplant surgery. A pilot study. J Am Acad Dermatol. 1987;16(3 Pt 2):685-7.
9. Bouhanna P. Topical minoxidil used before and after hair transplantation. J Dermatol Surg Oncol. 1989;15(1):50-3.
10. Tsilosani A, Gugava M. Is there a rationale for use of antibiotics in hair transplantation surgery? Georgian Med News. 2005;122:7-10.

CHAPTER 69

Complications of Hair Transplantation: An Overview

Narendra Patwardhan, Vaishalee Kirane, Venkataram Mysore

Key Messages

- Complications in hair transplantation (HT) can result from general or specific causes.
- Most complications are infrequent and minor and can be avoided by detailed history-taking, thorough examination, and evaluation to rule out cutaneous and systemic problems.
- The most common donor site surgical complication is donor scarring.
- The most common recipient site complication is postoperative edema.
- Most complications can be avoided or managed by a proper surgical technique.

INTRODUCTION

Hair restoration surgery (HRS) is usually a safe procedure and is associated with very few complications. However, as in all surgeries, the risk of complications cannot be discounted. They can be classified as follows:

- Complications that are common to all surgeries such as lignocaine reactions, pain, infection, bleeding, and keloids.
- Others that are specific for hair transplantation (HT)[1-5]
- Complications during anesthesia
- Complications in the donor area—intraoperative and postoperative
- Complications in the recipient area—intraoperative and postoperative
- Complications in special areas and situations
- Complications of special techniques such as follicular unit extraction (FUE)
- Poor and unsatisfactory results

The factors that may be responsible for these complications include the following:

- Unsuitable candidate selection, improper preoperative counseling, errors in preoperative assessment, and inappropriate surgical planning
- Poor technique during donor area harvesting
- Errors during the storage of the grafts
- Poor technique during recipient area implantation

These complications are dealt with in three chapters, with this chapter focusing on a general overview. Complications of the strip technique and FUE are dealt with in subsequent chapters.

GENERAL COMPLICATIONS

- *Adverse reactions to drugs*
  - Local anesthetic agents can give rise to adverse systemic reactions falling into four categories: (i) Toxic, (ii) psychogenic, (iii) idiosyncratic, or (iv) allergic. The overwhelming majority are psychogenic in nature and related to fear.
    - True immunologic reaction to a local anesthetic is rare.
    - All patients should be asked if they have received local anesthesia earlier. Those who have not should be tested with a test dose prior to surgery.
  - Analgesics and antibiotics prescribed during HT surgery can cause gastritis, which can be prevented by the administration of antacids and H2 blockers.
    - These drugs even carry the risk of serious cutaneous hypersensitivity reactions such as erythema multiforme, Stevens-Johnson

syndrome (SJS), toxic epidermal necrolysis (TEN), or erythroderma, which will need to be managed accordingly. Proper history-taking about any prior known drug allergies will surely help in their prevention.

- *General intraoperative complications*
  - Tachycardia can occur when tumescent fluid containing adrenaline is given. This is usually transient. However, in a cardiac-compromised patient, this may pose a risk. Hence, in all patients, particularly those who are above 40 years of age, an electrocardiogram (ECG) and physician assessment are indicated.
  - Syncope can be a complication, particularly if it is a long surgery. This may be due to pain, postural hypotension, lignocaine toxicity, poor hydration, hypoglycemia, etc.

Preventive Steps for Complications

- Proper anesthesia and analgesia
- Making the patient sit first for a short time before standing upright
- Minimizing total lidocaine usage by reducing the total surgery time
- Maintaining proper water, electrolyte, and nutrition balance
- Administering clonidine 0.5 mg preoperatively to help prevent syncope due to its anticholinergic and analgesic activity (personal study)

Pain Management during and after Surgery

- Pain during surgery or postoperatively is a common complication that can be managed with proper surgical technique and the use of analgesics.
- Factors contributing to pain include a wide strip, bleeding, wound tension, and large sessions with inadequate anesthesia.
- Adequate analgesia can be achieved with medications such as paracetamol, codeine, and similar analgesics.
- Postoperative administration of prednisolone can help reduce wound edema, inflammation, and pain.

Postoperative Hiccups

- Postoperative hiccups are a rare but distressing complication that can last up to 2–3 days.
- The exact cause is not known, but it may be due to stimulation of the sensory divisions of C2, C3, and C4 nerves, which also innervate the diaphragm through the phrenic nerve.[6]

DONOR SITE COMPLICATIONS IN STRIP HARVESTING

- *Bleeding*: The scalp is highly vascular, and bleeding is expected. Patients on anticoagulant drugs such as warfarin or antiplatelet drugs need to discontinue them at least 1 week before surgery. Strategies to prevent bleeding include tumescence, anxiety reduction, and proper surgical technique.[7]
- *Folliculitis*: Inflammation and/or infection of hair follicles can occur in the donor area. This may happen when hair gets stuck in the suture line during suturing. Folliculitis decalvans, a recurring and persistent condition, has also been reported **(Fig. 1)**.[8]
- *Infection*: Scalp surgery infections are not common due to the high vascularity of the scalp. Prophylactic antibiotics are often administered. Infection-prevention measures include aseptic surgical practices, maintaining patient resistance, and treating nasal colonization of *Staphylococcus aureus* with mupirocin ointment and preoperative scalp hair shampooing with chlorhexidine gluconate medicated soap.[9-12]

Wound Dehiscence or Necrosis

Wound dehiscence or necrosis[13] of the donor wound site is a very unusual complication and is mostly due to the excessive removal of tissue of width > 1.5 cm and wound closure under extreme tension.

Numbness

Numbness, usually transient, can occur because of the transection of superficial sensory branches during donor strip excision.

Postoperative Pain

Pain can result, especially if the donor wound is closed under extreme tension or due to damage to the underlying

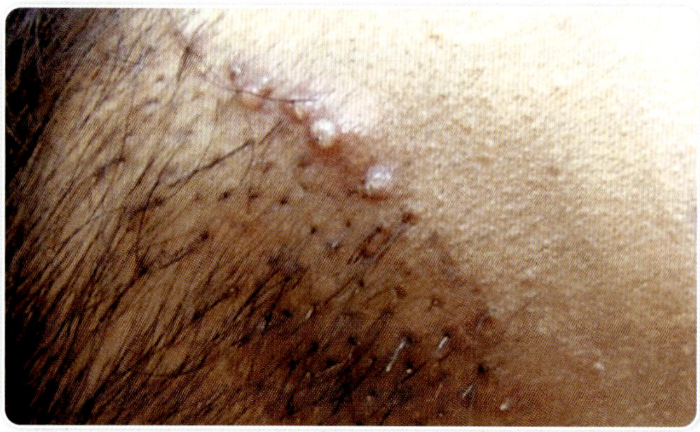

FIG. 1: Folliculitis.
Courtesy: Dr Narendra Patwardhan.

neurovascular supply. This is prevented by injecting a sufficient tumescent solution of saline to raise the donor tissues and enable cutting above the plane of the deeper neurovascular structures, also containing 0.5% lidocaine/bupivacaine and 1:50,000 epinephrine for their anesthetic and vasoconstrictive properties, respectively.[14]

Persistent Pain

Though rare, some patients complain of persistent pain and hyperesthesia[14] for several weeks, possibly due to the development of neuropraxia and neuromas. Gabapentin and intralesional steroid injections are helpful in such cases.

Suture Extrusion

Suture extrusion can occur rarely.

Keloids

Keloids are rare on the scalp. However, hypertrophic scarring can occur.

Donor Hair Effluvium

Donor hair effluvium or donor hair shock loss may occur, particularly in the postauricular area, and more so after tight wound closure. It usually recovers in a few weeks but may cause great anxiety to the patient.

Donor Site Scars

Various preventive and corrective steps have been described to avoid a wide unsightly donor scar, for example, scalp laxity exercises done for about 4 weeks prior to HT.[15,16]

COMPLICATIONS OF FOLLICULAR UNIT EXTRACTION

Complications of FUE are discussed in a separate chapter. Other complications include the following:

- Lichen planopilaris has been reported—possibly due to precipitation of an autoimmune reaction by the transected hairs.[17,18]
- Alopecia areata is another rare complication.[19]
- Trichorrhexis nodosa has also been reported.[20]

RECIPIENT AREA COMPLICATIONS

Poor Hairline

A proper hairline in HRS is very important to give a natural frame to the face as onlookers visualize a person mainly

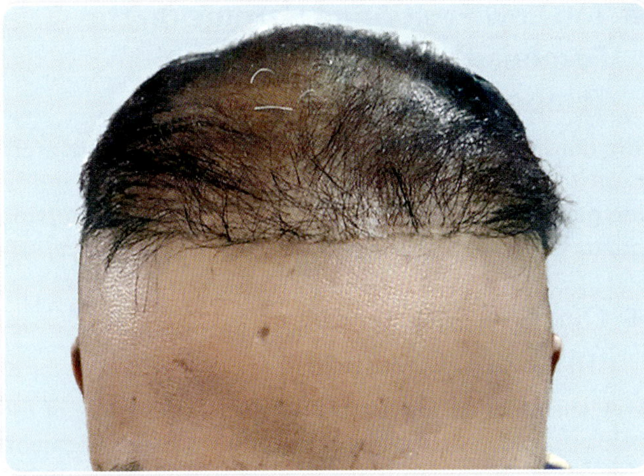

FIG. 2: A patient who came for revision shows several problems—hairline is straight, density is poor, there is poor angulation, improper direction, and the patient has lost hair behind the grafted area.

from the front. The midscalp and the vertex play the next important role. Shapiro felt that proper selection and implantation of follicular units (FUs) using skill as well as art enable surgeons to create a more natural-appearing, soft hairline while establishing the illusion of density. Several problems can occur due to an improper frontal hairline **(Fig. 2)**.

Asymmetry

If the frontal hairline given is a straight line with poor temporal angles, it will look very unnatural and nonaesthetic and eflects a poor technique. It is essential to design a natural, age-related proper hairline, making efforts to avoid asymmetry. This can be done two-dimensionally with the help of a mirror and three-dimensionally when the hairline is examined straight on. A ruler and a laser guiding system additionally can be used to help plan an appropriate frontal hairline by an inexperienced surgeon who has not developed an eye for symmetry. Hairlines differ based on gender, with female hairlines appearing more rounded, without the bitemporal recession occurring in males.[21]

Cornrow Plugs

Cornrow plugs resulted from the old punch grafting technique and are unacceptable in the modern FU hair transplant era. They especially are exposed as the residual hair recedes and then necessitate correction. They can still occur if large-size FUs are used for the front hairline.

Too Low Positioned Hairline on the Forehead and Blunting of the Temporal Angles

The hairline should never be placed below a point 6 cm from the glabella. This can result in dissatisfaction of the patient over time, especially in the case of evolving progressive hair loss behind the transplanted hairline.

Low Cosmetic Density and Unnatural Coverage

Low cosmetic density and an unnatural coverage of the bald area reflect errors in surgical and aesthetic judgment. These include performing a procedure on an unsuitable patient candidate, surgical distribution of grafts that failed to consider the possibility of future progressive hair loss in any young patient of genetic pattern hair loss, and improper counseling of having realistic expectations. The surgeon needs to consider whether there would be sufficient projected donor hair to cover any future hair loss. A corrective hair transplant procedure involves removal of the plugs, leaving behind a few hairs that will look soft and natural, combining with scalp reduction surgery as needed, and then transplanting additional FUs to give further density, using the FUE method, either from the scalp occiput or from body hairs.[22,23]

Recipient Area Edema

Recipient area edema is common on the third to fifth day after surgery, starting on the forehead and gradually spreading onto the eyelids and nose. The precise incidence varies, but it may occur in 3–8% of patients. The exact reason is not known, but several factors are thought to be responsible:

- Trauma of the surgery
- A large quantity of the tumescent solution injected into the recipient area
- Intraoperative bleeding
- Gravity which pulls the fluid down
- Lymphatic drainage of the frontal scalp
- Loose donor skin; elderly patients are more likely to experience it.
- Large sessions

A prophylactic measure includes the use of a short course of postoperative steroids. Injecting dilute steroids into the anterior scalp below the hairline can help minimize the extent of postoperative edema. An Elastoplast bandage stuck on the forehead at the end of surgery and kept in place for the next 3–5 days may also help. Abbassi injected a solution consisting of 100 cc of normal saline, 1 cc of epinephrine 1/1,000, with triamcinolone acetate 40 mg, into the recipient area and suggested that it could help to prevent the edema. A reclining position for 24 hours post surgery, though impractical, may help. Once the edema develops, applying ice packs frequently and manual massage to push fluids to the sides are also useful **(Fig. 3)**.[24]

Postoperative Pustules (Fig. 4)

Postoperative pustules occur 1–3 months after surgery and represent a foreign body reaction. They are related to improper dissection of grafts and reflect a poor dissection technique. They are sterile and, when small, heal by themselves. When large and persistent, they may need puncture and drainage of pus.

Central Scalp Necrosis (Figs. 5A to C)

Central scalp necrosis can occur after large sessions, particularly in the elderly with vascular compromise.

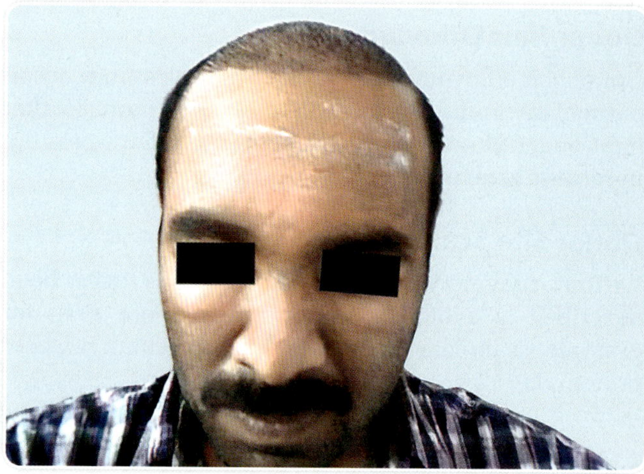

FIG. 3: Postoperative edema.

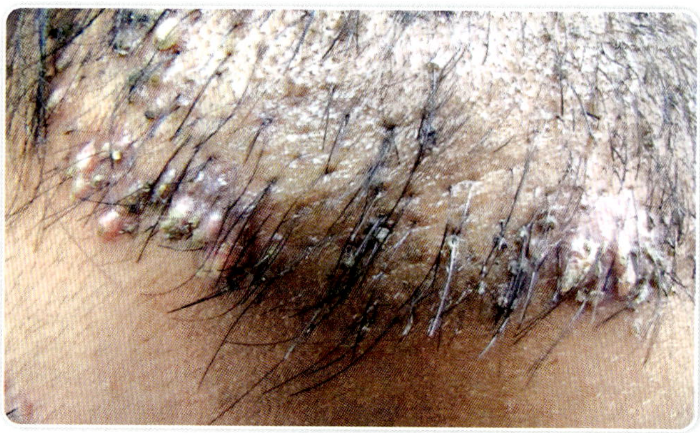

FIG. 4: Folliculitis in the recipient area.

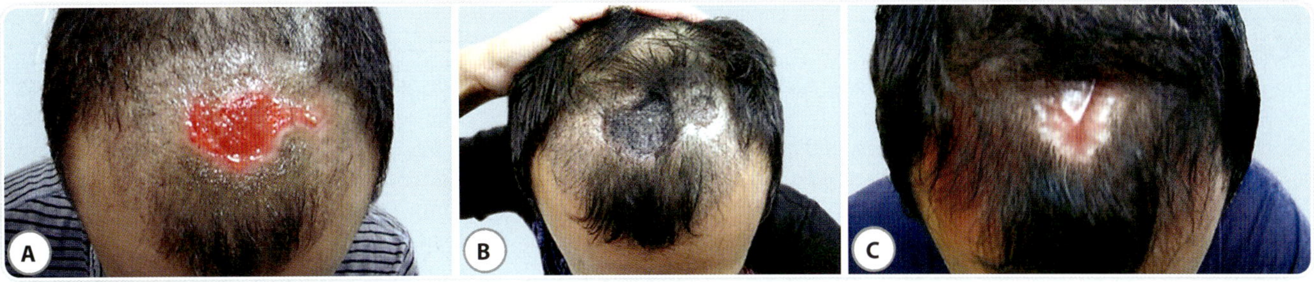

FIGS. 5A TO C: (A) Necrosis in the recipient area. (B) Eschar formed after necrosis. (C) Scar resulting from the necrotic area.

It is characterized by a dusky red discoloration of the scalp followed by extensive crusting. It heals with a central scar. While the exact cause is not known, it is postulated to be due to the fact that the central scalp receives comparatively less blood supply. Smoking, diabetes, and actinic damage may predispose to the condition.[25]

Cobblestoning

Cobblestoning occurs from elevations and indentations of the scar tissue around the hair graft resulting in an unsightly, uneven surface in the recipient area. This is when FU grafts are implanted into too small a hole or at an incorrect depth. To avoid this, grafts should be placed only 1–2 mm above the surrounding surface. Cobblestoning mostly improves with time or else the scars may need to be excised. Fractional erbium-YAG or CO_2 laser has been used to correct and resurface the cobblestoning (Venkataram Mysore, personal communication). Postoperative pitting can also occur in the recipient area **(Fig. 6)**.

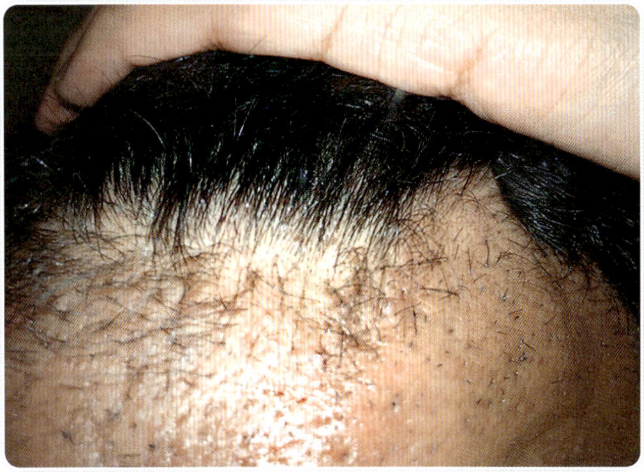

FIG. 6: Postoperative pits.

Cysts

Cysts appear as small skin-colored swellings around the transplanted hair follicles, which can become erythematous and painful. These result due to small grafts slipping under the skin or from piggybacking one graft on top of the other. Treatment consists of incising the cysts and expressing out the contents, warm compresses, or sometimes antibiotics in case of an infection.

Poor Hair Growth

Poor hair growth can occur when there is traumatic dissection of the hair grafts from the harvested strip or traumatic placement or desiccation of the grafts. It can also be a result of poor-quality donor hair, which should be identified before surgery, and thus, such patients are not selected for surgery. Decreased growth can also be due to factors such as heavy smoking, diabetes, and excessive sun damage to the scalp's skin. In some cases, a definite cause cannot be identified for poor growth, suggesting that there are yet unidentified causes for poor hair growth after transplantation.

Temporary Hair Loss

Temporary hair loss, called shock loss, is a type of telogen effluvium of the surrounding hairs occurring due to the trauma of the surgery in 10–15% of males and more in females. The patient should be forewarned about its possibility to alleviate anxiety or alarm. The use of topical minoxidil prior to surgery can help to minimize this hair loss.

Arteriovenous Fistula

An arteriovenous fistula can occur but is extremely rare.[26]

Tips and Pearls

- Thorough preoperative counseling regarding the benefits, limitations, and risks of HRS and recording in the medical chart go a long way in preventing some complications.
- Selection of a suitable candidate for surgery and proper evaluation and surgical planning of the recipient area are very important.
- Good design using sound surgical skills and techniques combined with artistry is essential for hairline reconstruction and for high perceived midscalp or vertex cosmetic density and is also important to record the same.
- Avoid complications by meticulous preoperative assessment and good postoperative management.
- Quality control for every step of the surgery should be on a continuous basis, improving whenever and wherever possible.

REFERENCES

1. Loganathan E, Sarvajnamurthy S, Gorur D, Suresh DH, Siddaraju MN, Narasimhan RT. Complications of hair restoration surgery: a retrospective analysis. Int J Trichology. 2014;6(4):168-72.
2. Salanitri S, Gonçalves AJ, Helene Jr A, Lopes FH. Surgical complications in hair transplantation: a series of 533 procedures. Aesthet Surg J. 2009;29(1):72-6.
3. Konior RJ. Complications in hair restoration surgery. Facial Plast Surg Clin North Am. 2013;21(3):505-20.
4. Perez-Meza D, Niedbalski R. Complications in hair restoration surgery. Oral Maxillofac Surg Clin North Am. 2009;21(1):119-48.
5. Lam SM. Complications in hair restoration. Plast Surg Clin North Am. 2013;21:675-80.
6. Arnold J. In: Stough DB, Haber RS (Eds). Hair Replacement. St. Louis: Mosby; 1996.
7. Otley CC, Fewkes JL, Frank W, Olbricht SM. Complications of cutaneous surgery in patients who are taking warfarin, aspirin, or nonsteroidal anti-inflammatory drugs. Arch Dermatol. 1996;132:161-6.
8. Otberg N, Wu WY, Kang H, Martinka M, Alzolibani AA, Restrepo I, et al. Folliculitis decalvans developing 20 years after hair restoration surgery in punch grafts: case report. Dermatol Surg. 2009;35(11):1852-6.
9. Kaiser AB. Antimicrobial prophylaxis in surgery. N Engl J Med. 1986;315(18):1129-38.
10. Zoumalan RA, Rosenberg DB. Methicillin-resistant Staphylococcus aureus—positive surgical site infections in face-lift surgery. Arch Facial Plast Surg. 2008;10(2):116-23.
11. van Rijen MM, Bode LG, Baak DA, Kluytmans JA, Vos MC. Reduced costs for *Staphylococcus aureus* carriers treated prophylactically with mupirocin and chlorhexidine in cardiothoracic and orthopaedic surgery. PLoS One. 2012;7(8):e43065.
12. Farjo N. Infection control and policy development in hair restoration. Hair Transplant Forum Int. 2008;18:141-4.
13. Karaçal N, Uraloğlu M, Dindar T, Livaoğlu M. Necrosis of the donor site after hair restoration with follicular unit extraction (FUE): a case report. J Plast Reconstr Aesthet Surg. 2012;65(4):e87-9.
14. Wesley CK, Unger RH, Rosenberg M, Unger MA, Unger WP. Factors influencing postoperative hyperesthesia in hair restoration surgery. J Cosmet Dermatol. 2011;10(4):301-6.
15. Unger WP. Correction of cosmetic problems secondary to hair transplantation. In: Unger WP, Shapiro R (Eds). Hair Transplantation, 4th edition. New York: Marcel Dekker, 2004. pp. 372-9.
16. Mayer M, Pauls T. Scalp elasticity scale. Hair Transplant Forum Int. 2005;15:122-3.
17. Donovan J. Lichen planopilaris after hair transplantation: report of 17 cases. Dermatol Surg. 2012;38(12):1998-2004.
18. Chiang YZ, Tosti A, Chaudhry IH, Lyne L, Farjo B, Farjo N, et al. Lichen planopilaris following hair transplantation and face-lift surgery. Br J Dermatol. 2012;166(3):666-370.
19. Rodrigues Barata AR, Camacho-Martínez F. Alopecia areata as a complication of hair restoration surgery. Eur J Dermatol. 2012;22(6):813-4.
20. Hwang ST, Park BC. Trichorrhexis nodosa after hair transplantation: dermoscopic, pathologic and electron microscopy analyses. Dermatol Surg. 2013;39(11):1721-4.
21. Shapiro R. Principles and techniques used to create a natural hairline in surgical hair restoration. Facial Plast Surg Clin North Am. 2004;12(2):201-17.
22. Bernstein RM, Rassman WR, Rashid N, Shiell RC. The art of repair in surgical hair restoration part I: basic repair strategies. Dermatol Surg. 2002;28(9):783-94.
23. Vogel JE. Correcting problems in hair restoration surgery: an update. Facial Plast Surg Clin North Am. 2004;12(2):263-78.
24. Gholamali A, Sepideh P, Susan E. Hair transplantation: preventing post-operative oedema. J Cutan Aesthet Surg. 2010;3(2):87-9.
25. Yildiz H, Ercan E, Alhan D, Sezgin M. Recipient site necrosis after tumescent infiltration with adrenaline in hair transplantation. Acta Dermatovenerol Croat. 2015;23(3):233-4.
26. Unger W. Re: Arteriovenous fistula following hair transplantation. Dermatol Surg. 2011;37(12):1816-7.

CHAPTER 70

Donor Area Complications

Mayank Singh, Aparna Acharya

Key Messages

- Preoperative assessment of scalp laxity is important.
- Good surgical technique is essential for an aesthetic scar.
- Intraoperative sterile precautions are vital.

INTRODUCTION

Strip harvest and closure of the defect are important steps in follicular unit transplantation (FUT) surgeries. Patients are almost always bothered about the aesthetics of the scar. Getting a less visible and acceptable scar demands good surgical skill and adequate experience in suturing techniques.

Most of the complications of donor strip harvesting are avoidable. In this chapter, we discuss about various possible complications, how to deal with them, and, more importantly, how to avoid them.

INTRAOPERATIVE COMPLICATIONS

- Vasovagal syncope
- Damage to the follicles
- Bleeding
- Problems in closure

IMMEDIATE POSTOPERATIVE COMPLICATIONS

- Persistent pain
- Hiccups
- Bleeding
- Edema
- Hematoma
- Wound infection
- Gaping
- Necrosis

LATE POSTOPERATIVE COMPLICATIONS

- Scar dehiscence
- Numbness
- Hypertrophic scar
- Donor area effluvium
- Neuralgia
- Hypoesthesia
- Folliculitis

DELAYED COMPLICATIONS

- Keloid
- Stretched scar
- Arteriovenous (AV) fistula

PREVENTION AND MANAGEMENT OF COMPLICATIONS

Vasovagal Syncope

Vasovagal syncope is syncope resulting from a failure in autoregulation of blood pressure and, ultimately, in cerebral perfusion pressure, resulting in transient loss of consciousness. Vasovagal reaction is an exaggeration

CHAPTER 72

Repeat Hair Transplantation

Kapil Dua, Bhawna Bhardwaj, Aman Dua

Key Messages

- Repeated hair transplants are primarily done for recipient area issues by the patients, but the donor area can be a major challenge for the surgeons.
- In patients who had undergone punch hair grafting, the donor area is badly affected, leading to a lesser number of grafts in both follicular unit extraction (FUE) and follicular unit transplantation (FUT).
- In patients with previous FUT surgery, the placement and the width of the scalp play a role in deciding whether to proceed with FUE or FUT.
- In patients who had undergone poor and overharvested FUE for the first time, revision FUE is very difficult because of the diffuse scarring throughout the donor area, and FUT in them also does not yield a good number of grafts.
- With the rise in ghost surgeries, we are encountering more patients with overharvested donor areas, including donor areas from the body. In such cases, other treatment modalities need to be considered to correct the hairline or density of the recipient area.

INTRODUCTION

Every surgeon wants the best possible results for his/her patients. Most of the times, the yield of a hair transplant is good, and the patient is satisfied. But sometimes in spite of the good growth of the transplanted hairs in terms of the number of grafts taken up by the body, the patient might still be unhappy because of the lack of cosmetic outcome as per his expectations. At other times, the hairs do not grow at all. Both these conditions are labeled as failed hair transplants, one subjective (the former) and the other objective (the latter). An unfavorable result from a hair transplant can also occur from the judgmental errors in the planning stage, which is mostly due to ignoring the fact that hair loss is progressive. All these conditions constitute the indications for repeat hair transplant, and we will deal with the causes resulting in this situation and how to deal with the same in this chapter.

INDICATIONS

The subjective causes of dissatisfaction of postoperative patients are mainly from the errors in the planning stage, whereas the objective ones are due to faults in the actual procedure, which are discussed here in detail.[1]

- *Abnormal hairline*: The hairline should be created considering the patient's age, degree of baldness, and further progression of androgenetic alopecia (AGA). Normally, it should be irregular, feathered, and in an asymmetric pattern. A misplaced hairline (either too high or low) or a straight hairline without frontotemporal angles (FTAs) or a bushy appearance can cause aesthetic problems due to which the patient wants to correct the hairline **(Fig. 1A)**.
- *Angulation of grafts*: Misdirected grafts, especially in the hairline zone, can result in an unnatural appearance, causing the hair to fall in abnormal directions instead of following the natural course.

Hence, it is pivotal to follow the natural pattern of hair of the patient during slit making **(Fig. 1B)**.

- *Unnatural appearance of grafts*: A revision surgery is also considered for patients who have undergone the old technique of punch grafting. This technique causes plugging and doll-like appearance of grafts, for which revision is attempted **(Fig. 2)**.
- *Complications due to the previous transplant*: Necrosis of the scalp can occur due to excessive use of anesthetic agents and adrenaline or higher density in the recipient area **(Fig. 3)**. Other complications such as scarring of donor and recipient areas and depleted donor area due to overharvesting also constitute the indications for revision hair transplant **(Fig. 4)**.
- *Poor growth of grafts*: This can arise due to various causes, which may include poor quality of grafts, longer outside body, time of grafts, poor graft handling, or storage injury resulting in below-par growth of grafts **(Figs. 5A and B)**.

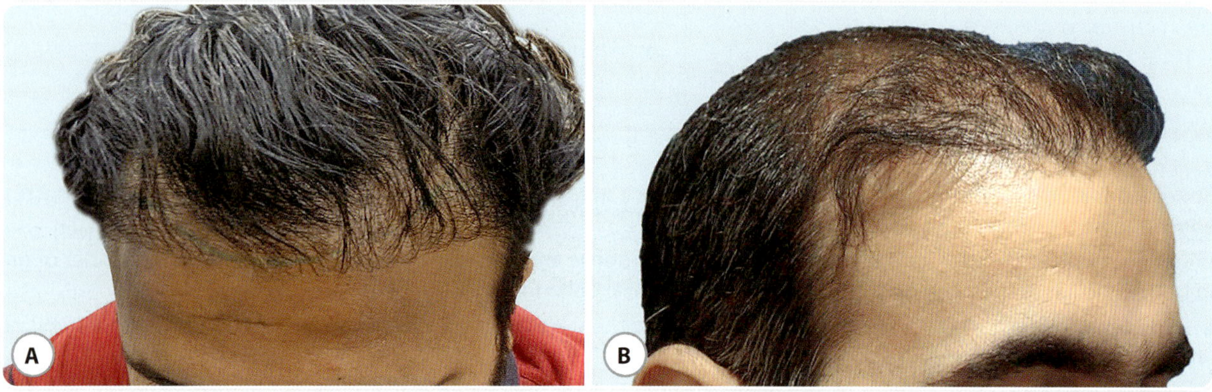

FIGS. 1A AND B: (A) A very low hairline with low FTAs. The grafts placed exhibit a higher angulation due to which the see-through appearance is seen with suboptimal density. (B) A 27-year-old patient got operated 4 years back from outside by technician. He presented to us with improper angulation and direction of grafts with low FTAs in the hairline and further progression of AGA. In spite of an unnatural-looking hairline, he did not agree to remove the wrongly implanted grafts and wanted to enhance the density in the frontal hairline and full coverage of scalp.

(AGA: androgenetic alopecia; FTAs: frontotemporal angles)

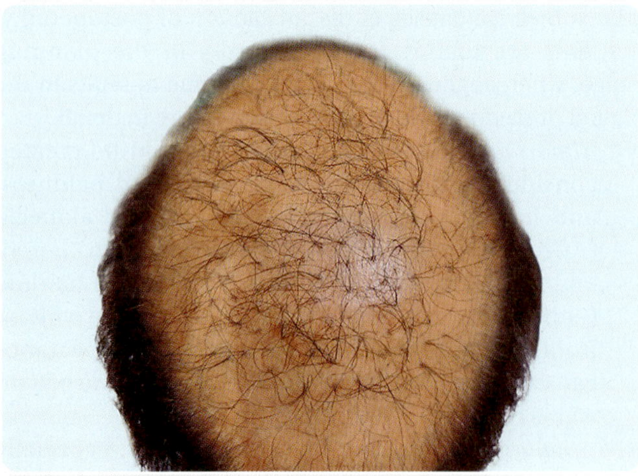

FIG. 2: Doll-like appearance of grafts.

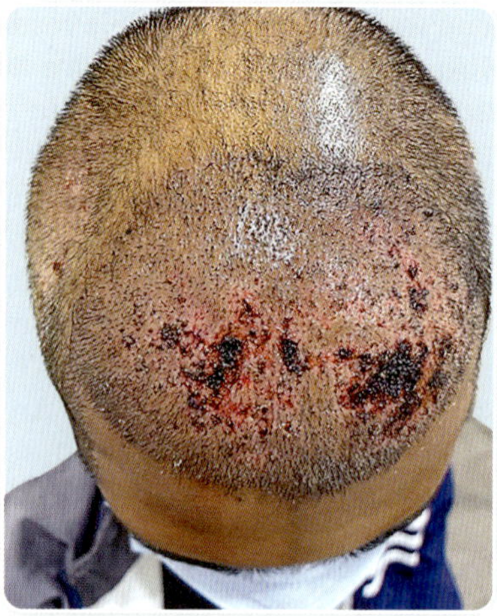

FIG. 3: Necrosis of recipient area: The patient presented to our clinic 4 days after undergoing follicular unit extraction (FUE) from outside with necrosis on the recipient area.

SEQUELAE OF PRIMARY SURGERY

When a hair transplant surgery is done, the scalp undergoes changes at the physiological level in both donor and recipient areas. There is perifollicular fibrosis, changes in graft angulation, decreased density, and reduced vascularity in the operated scalp.[2,3] This leads to a decrease in the number of grafts accessible from the donor area. Also, there is a limitation of the donor area due to overharvesting in the initial surgery/surgeries. In the recipient area too, there may be underlying fibrosis and alteration in blood supply.

All these changes contribute to increased transection of grafts and greater chances of difficulties in harvesting, overharvesting in donor area leading to visible thinning and a comparatively longer duration of the procedure. A repeat surgery is, therefore, more challenging and needs experience and expertise in management.

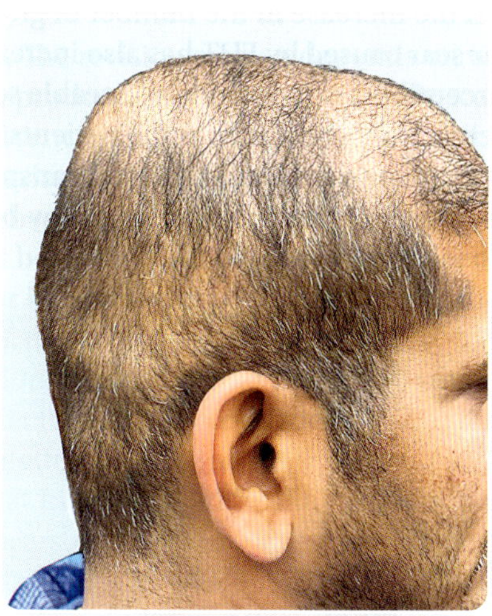

FIG. 4: Depletion of donor area.

Preoperative Assessment

Before undertaking the patients for repeat surgeries, the surgeons should evaluate the patients in detail, taking into consideration their age, family history, and patterns of baldness, reserve of donor hair, the problems faced by the patient due to the current hair pattern just like any primary surgery, and the details of the previous surgery (the type of surgery, the number of grafts extracted, the area of the scalp covered, etc.). A judicious use of the available grafts is warranted in revision surgeries to reduce long-term problems.

Repeat Surgeries

The initial hair transplantation surgery could have been done by any of the following—punch grafting, strip surgery, or follicular unit extraction (FUE). A repeat surgery can produce good results only if the primary surgery was done in an appropriate manner to facilitate the repeat procedure, which can be done by either of the techniques—strip surgery or FUE.

DONOR AREA ISSUES

Primary Surgery: Punch Hair Grafting

Around two to three decades back, punch grafting was the order of the day. Nowadays also, sometimes the authors come across patients who had undergone punch grafting previously, though such surgeries are rare now.

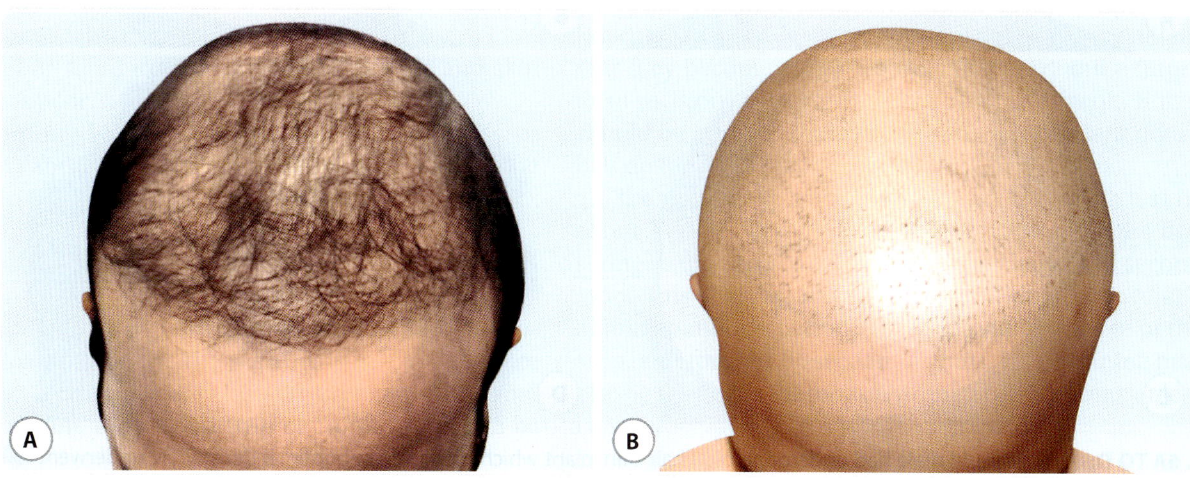

FIGS. 5A AND B: Poor growth of the transplanted grafts after follicular unit transplantation (FUT): (A) Hairline without trimming; (B) Hairline after trimming of the whole area.

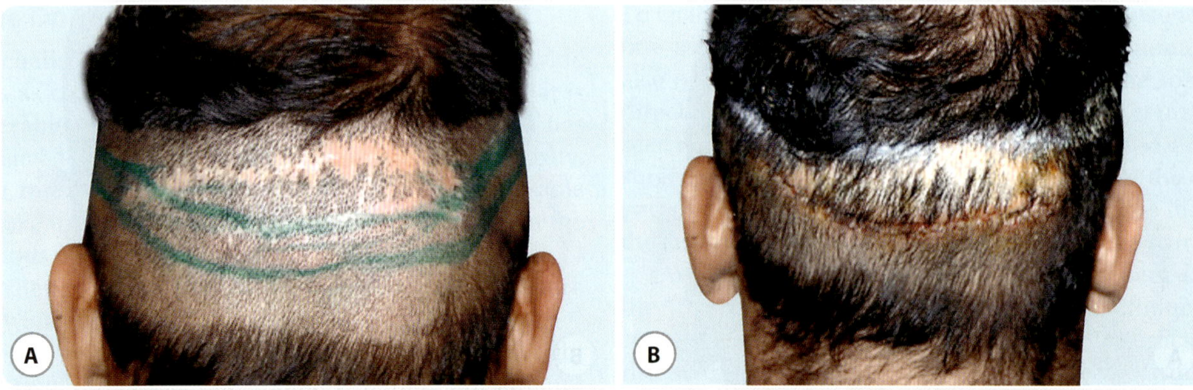

FIGS. 13A AND B: The patient had undergone two strip surgeries outside. There were two scars, one on the top which was curving down on the left side and a small one in the middle. The patient wanted another strip surgery. The authors removed another strip from the middle of the permanent zone by including the small scar in the middle of the initial surgery and removing the curved scar on the left side as well. (A) Marking of strip before the third strip surgery; (B) 10 days after the suture removal.

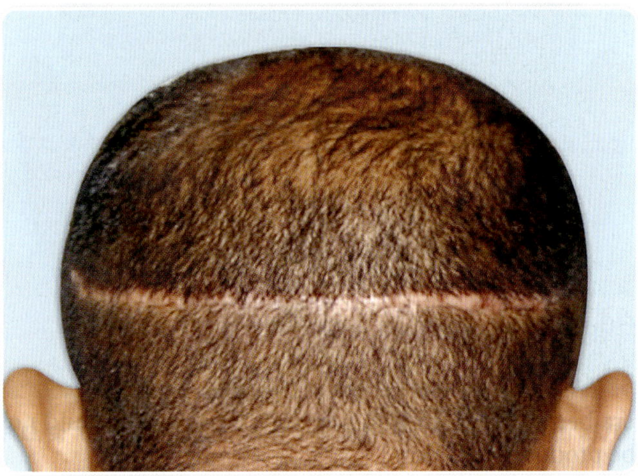

FIG. 14: Hypertrophic scar which was treated with intralesional triamcinolone injections.

Performing Follicular Unit Extraction after Follicular Unit Transplantation

Patients who have undergone strip surgery for their first session frequently ask for FUE for their second session.

In many cases, a second strip surgery may not be possible because of a wide scar, which is unresectable as mentioned earlier. FUE is also needed in patients who ask for camouflaging the donor scar. The advantage of doing FUE in such a case is that since the original scarring is only along the suture line, rest of the donor area behaves as a virgin area **(Figs. 15A to D)**. In the author's experience, the FTR in such cases is less as compared to cases needing FUE after FUE as the first surgery. The following points need to be considered:

- The surgeon has to avoid going too near to the suture line—both upper and lower margins of the suture line—as the angulation of grafts is distorted along this line. This can lead to increased transection.
- If a large number of grafts are taken out from above the strip area, it may lead to the exposure of the suture line as shown in **Figures 13A to D**. Hence, surgeon needs to be conservative in approach.
- Another point to be kept in mind is that there is sometimes a difference in the quality and density of the grafts above and below the suture line. This occurs because the best grafts are removed during the first strip surgery as a result of which the weaker or the poor-quality grafts are pulled up from below and come to lie in the middle part of the available donor area. The density of these hairs is less, and they are also thinner as compared to those above the suture line. The total number of grafts, which can be extracted in these patients, can be around 1,000–1,500 only.

Primary Surgery of Follicular Unit Extraction

With increasing popularity of FUE, FUE after FUE is becoming common. This category of patients can be further subdivided into those who had earlier undergone single session and those with multiple sittings of FUE.

- *FUE after previous single session of FUE:* If the first FUE session was a small session of 1,000–1,500 grafts, performing a second FUE is relatively easy as there is adequate unexploited donor area. This situation is similar to a first session of FUE; hence, it is not dealt with in detail.

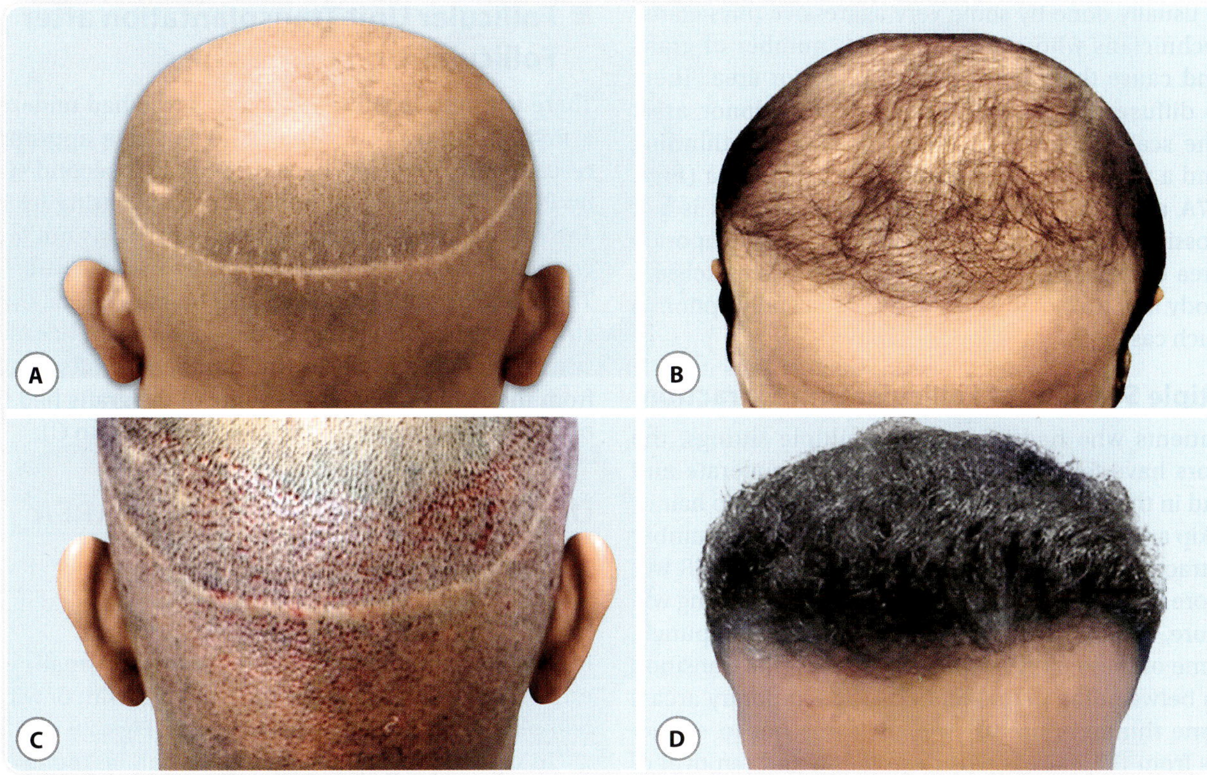

FIGS. 15A TO D: A 29-year-old male had undergone strip surgery outside, which did not yield proper results. So, the patient became wary of the strip surgery and underwent follicular unit extraction (FUE) from the scalp, beard, and body (3,000 grafts—1,750 from scalp, 630 from beard, 620 from chest).

- *Primary mega-session:* In the patients who had undergone mega-session of FUE earlier, there would be microscarring present throughout the donor area. There is a change in angulation of grafts, leading to difficulty in alignment with the exit angle of the hair, which results in higher transection rates as compared to the first-time surgery. The FTR in second surgery is more if the primary surgery was FUE (FTR in primary FUE surgery ranges from 5 to 17.5%)[13] as compared to FUT as postinflammatory changes affect whole of the donor area. There is also a risk of overharvesting associated with a repeat FUE, resulting in patchy skip areas of hair loss in the donor region, which should be avoided. The incidence of burying of grafts and thus postoperative folliculitis may also be more because of the increased fibrosis in the donor area **(Fig. 16)**.

  Subject to the above limitations, if the number of grafts extracted by the first FUE surgery is around 2,000–2,500, then the surgeon may be able to extract up to 70–75% of the number of grafts extracted in the first sitting.

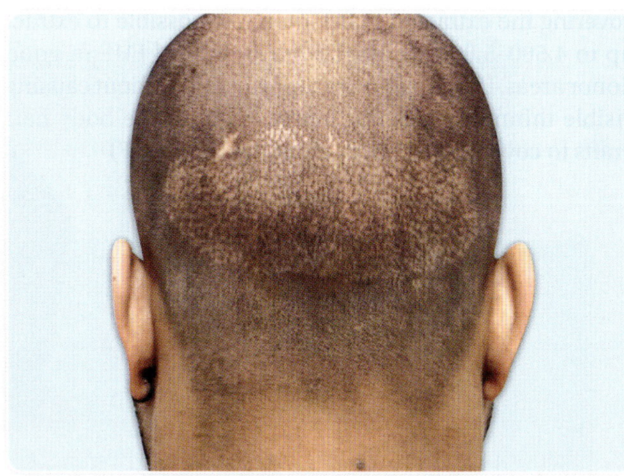

FIG. 16: A 23-year-old male with traction alopecia underwent follicular unit extraction (FUE). He got 1,200 grafts. Then he came again after 1 year to have 600 grafts to increase the density (this picture is before the second surgery).

- *Primary giga session:* The authors sometimes come across patients who had undergone an extraction of >5,000 grafts from the scalp in one sitting only. This

Continued

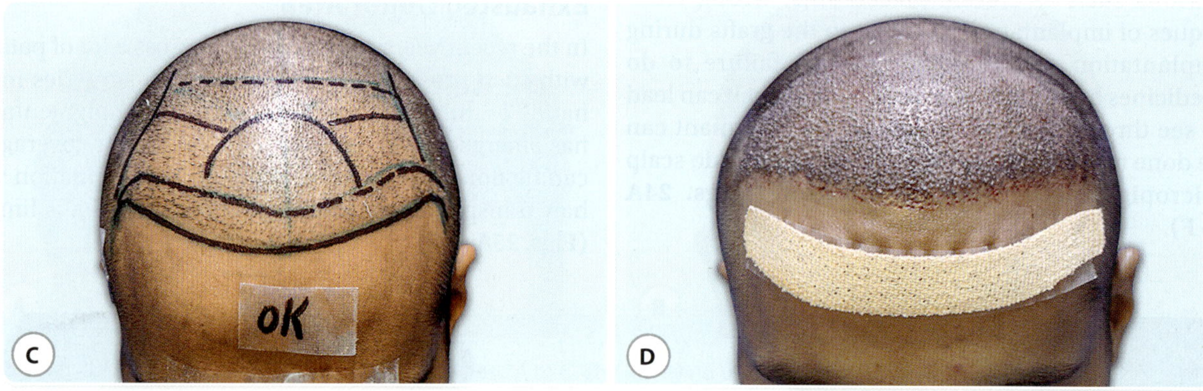

FIGS. 23A TO D: (A and B) A 32-year-old patient came with suboptimal results from previous transplant and wanted to enhance the density of anterior hairline. (C) On trimming, grafts were seen to be placed in a straight line (railroad sign) and were also regularly placed. (D) The plan was to retain the same hairline and plan to recreate transition zone. Grafts were excised from the hairline to recreate macro- and micro-irregularities, and single follicle grafts (FUGs) were placed in triangles formed to enhance the density.

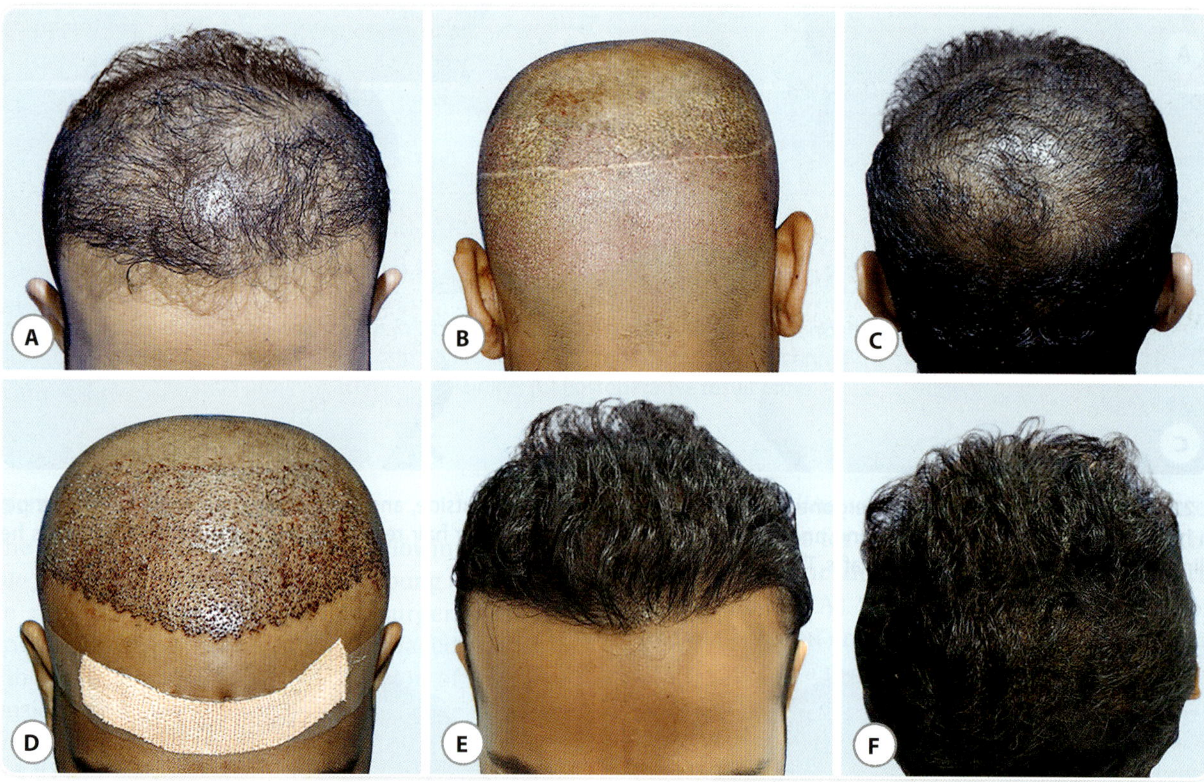

FIGS. 24A TO F: (A) A 30-year-old patient who had undergone a combination of FUT and FUE from outside. He was not satisfied with the results after a year. The hairline and crown area had suboptimal density (C). As the excision was not uniformly distributed, there was pinpoint scarring and coalescing of scars had occurred (B). The hairline was made dense using scalp hair (2,300 grafts—1,300 from scalp and 1,000 grafts from beard) (D). The mid-scalp and crown were dealt with medication, platelet-rich plasma, and SMP to camouflage the contrast (F). The results after 1 year show less visibility all over scalp (E and F).

(FUE: follicular unit extraction; FUT: follicular unit transplantation; SMP: scalp micropigmentation)

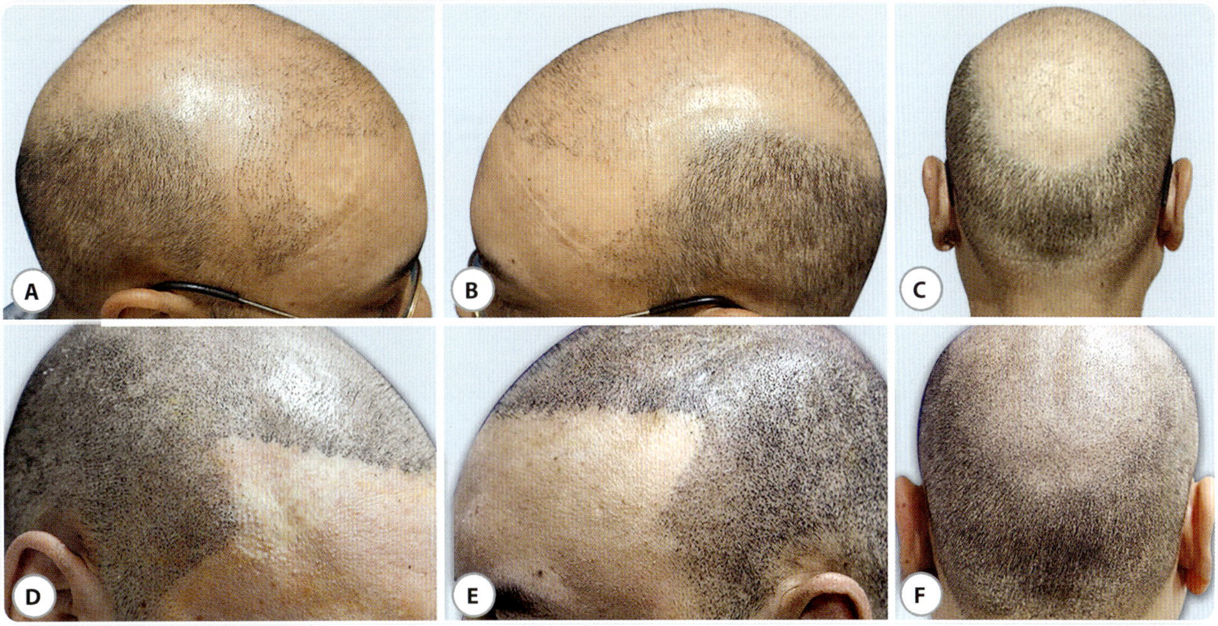

FIGS. 25A TO F: A 32-year-old patient who has undergone follicular unit extraction (FUE) from outside complained of suboptimal growth and wrong angulation presented to us with an exhausted donor area even body (A to C). He was advised scalp micropigmentation (SMP) for camouflaging. His results after three sessions of SMP (D to F).

SUMMARY

In corrective repair surgery, the judicious use of the available grafts is of utmost importance. In repair work, the distribution of grafts and the density to be achieved should be decided carefully.

REFERENCES

1. Fisher J. Revision of the unfavorable result in hair transplantation. Semin Plast Surg. 2005;19(2):167-78.
2. Bernstein RM, Rassman WR, Rashid N, Shiell RC. The art of repair in surgical hair restoration part I: basic repair strategies. Dermatol Surg. 2002;28(9):783-94.
3. Nirmal B, Somiah S, Sacchidanand SA, Biligi DS, Palo S. Evaluation of perifollicular inflammation of donor area during hair transplantation in androgenetic alopecia and its comparison with controls. Int J Trichol. 2013;5:73-6.
4. Bernstein RM, Rassman WR, Rashid N, Shiell RC. The art of repair in surgical hair restoration—part II: the tactics of repair. Dermatol Surg. 2002;28(10):873-93.
5. Limmer BL. Follicular holocaust. Hair Transplant Forum Int. 1998;8(5):11.
6. Bernstein RM, Rassman WR. The scalp laxity paradox. Hair Transplant Forum Int. 2002;12(1):9-10.
7. Smith JB, Fenske NA. Cutaneous manifestations and consequences of smoking. J Am Acad Dermatol. 1996;34:717-32.
8. Bernstein RM, Rassman WR, Szaniawski W, Halperin A. Follicular transplantation. Int J Aesthetic Restor Surg. 1995;3:119-32.
9. Bernstein RM, Rassman WR. Follicular transplantation: patient evaluation and surgical planning. Dermatol Surg. 1997;23:771-84.
10. Seery GE. Improved scalp surgery results by controlling tension vector forces in the tissues by galea to pericranium fixation sutures. Dermatol Surg. 2001;27:569-74.
11. Seery GE. Hair transplantation: management of donor area. Dermatol Surg. 2002;28:136-42.
12. Shiell RC. A review of modern surgical hair restoration techniques. J Cutan Aesthet Surg. 2008;1:12-6.
13. Kim JC, Choi YC. Regrowth of grafted human scalp hair after removal of the bulb. Dermatol Surg. 4:312-3.

CHAPTER 73

Automation in Follicular Unit Excision

Kuldeep Saxena

Key Messages

- In the last two decades, the follicular unit excision (FUE) procedure advanced progressively from manual to powered to robotic FUE.
- Automation in FUE gives enough space to beginners to flaunt skills and deliver the best results.
- Mechanical devices operated electronically, reducing human intervention to a minimum, can have significant consequences on the final results.

INTRODUCTION

Necessity is the mother of invention. Even a small change in a technique can have significant consequences on the final results. It has been certainly so with the automation techniques in follicular unit excision (FUE). Automation is defined as the technique, method, or system of automatic means, as by electronic devices, reducing human intervention to a minimum. For example, a mechanical device operated electronically that functions automatically without continuous input from an operator.

Automation has provided solutions to many of the problems in the field of hair restoration surgeries. In 2002, Rassman and Bernstein presented the first ever paper on the FUE technique, where they have done extraction of the follicles by using a manual method.[1]

Manual FUE methods are time-consuming and tiring, and different transection rates are reported by different surgeons. In order to overcome these issues, surgeons have taken the help of automation in the form of power devices from 2005 to 2023.[2,3] The FUE procedure has been refined with the help of power motors where precise control of rotation and oscillation can be performed.

AUTOMATION IN FOLLICULAR UNIT HARVESTING

The first attempt at automation in FUE is the use of DC motors that rotate the punches so that the procedure can be finished quickly. In 2009, Allen Feller introduced a motorized FUE device. After that, Cole's device and Harris (SAFE) system came into the market.[4,5] Other advancements included:

- Devroye's WAW system
- Trivellini wireless device
- Sanusi Umar device for combining oscillation and rotation
- KD's microadjustment of rpm device

All these devices solved some existing problems and helped surgeons to minimize graft transection.[6-9]

(Readers can refer to the chapter 51 on Follicular Unit Excision: Instrumentation and Technique)

ROLE OF AUTOMATION DURING LOCAL ANESTHESIA

Joanne Kieffer Helfer described and published the skin tap technique to reduce the pain of intramuscular injection.[10] This approach was developed by applying clinical experience, integrating the theories of gate control, relaxation, and distraction.[11,12]

Helfer skin tap technique is again a manual technique that has been refined by the use of a vibrator, where the use of a DC micromotor produces strong and coarse vibration over the surface of the skin.[13-15] This technique is undoubtedly a very good technique, but precision in integrating the theories of gate control, relaxation of muscles, and distraction is better achieved by automation (by using a vibrator).

The author has developed and applied for an international patent for a unique device EPIWAND™ for painless anesthesia that uses a combination of vibration and cold to reduce the pain sensation during hair transplant surgery **(Figs. 1 and 2)**.

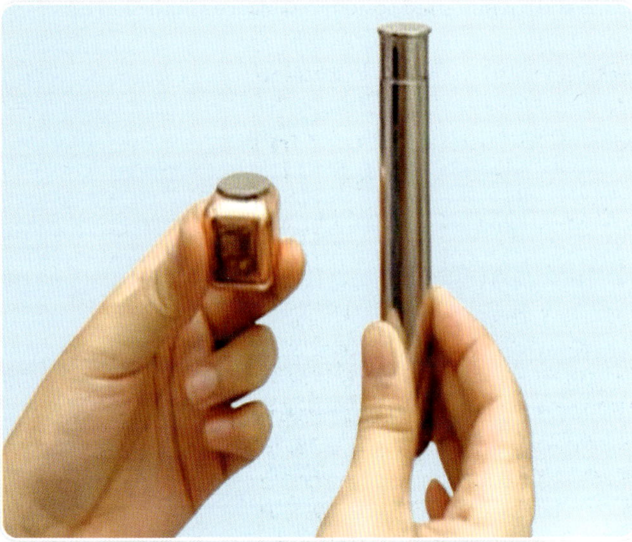

FIG. 1: Copper-coated stainless steel cube is precooled (–18°C) inside the freezer and vibrator having DC micromotor.

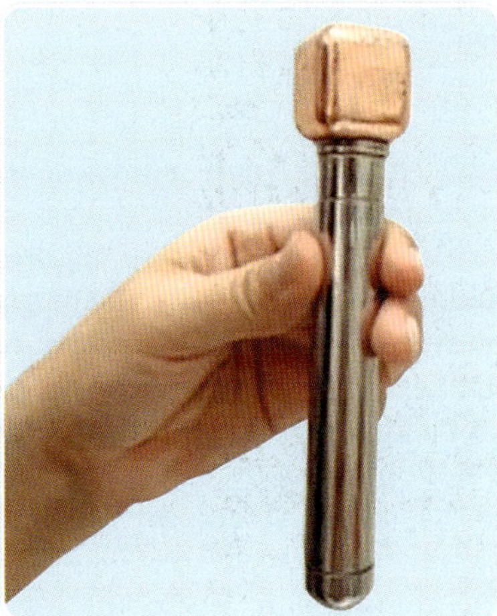

FIG. 2: During the procedure, a cooling device is attached to the vibrating device and used as a handheld device.

It is a handheld device that uses a combination of vibration and cold to reduce the pain sensation of multiple local anesthesia injections during FUE surgery. When apply over the operative side, skin surface receive two stimuli. The cooling device utilize simultaneous vibration and cold application to synergistically lessen the pain sensations.

Suction-assisted Automation in FUE

Neograft and SmartGraft are two commercially available hair transplantation machines that use a rotating punch for scoring the grafts and negative pneumatic pressure for the suction of grafts. These devices also use positive pneumatic pressure for pushing the grafts into premade slits.[16,17] These devices claim precise and fast FUE compared with other motorized systems. However, the major drawback of this system is an increased transection rate of grafts. This occurs because you have to advance the punch a little bit deeper to entirely cut the surrounding follicular tissues.

ROLE OF AUTOMATION IN GRAFT HYDRATION

Follicular unit excision grafts are devoid of fat, which can lead to desiccation.[18] It is recommended that grafts should remain hydrated throughout the procedure from harvesting to insertion. Implantation is a technician-dependent work, and many times, they forget to spray saline over the recipient area. Just to solve this issue, the author has developed an automated hydration arm in which an electronic valve facilitates opening and closing the flow of liquid through a tube without any contact between the liquid and the valve itself.[19] A sensor is also attached to the terminal end of the device that automatically lets out water after detecting movement. The tube is pinched between a fixed and a moving bar, when sensor detects movement it automatically opens valve thus opens lumen of pinched tube which in turn lets out water through lumen of the tube **(Figs. 3 and 4)**.

ROLE OF AUTOMATION DURING SLIT CREATION

Over the past, in the field of automation and robotics, more emphasis was given to harvesting of FUE grafts than to incision. However, slit creation through power devices is an equally important issue. Surgeon fatigue and imperfect hand movements are two issues that can be solved with the help of automation. An automated handheld hair transplant incision device is an exciting

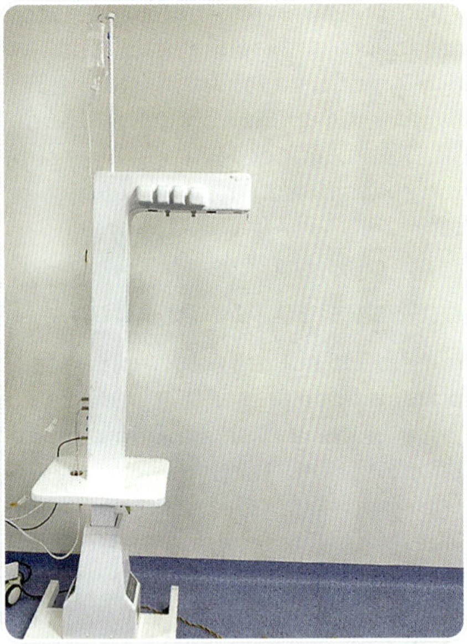

FIG. 3: Sensor-operated automated hydration system.

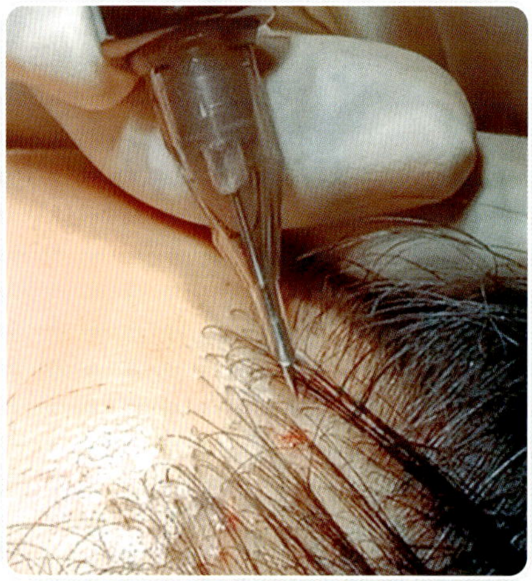

FIG. 5: Human hand-guided automated incision creation device. 1, 1.2, and 1.3 mm sized customized blades attached to it.

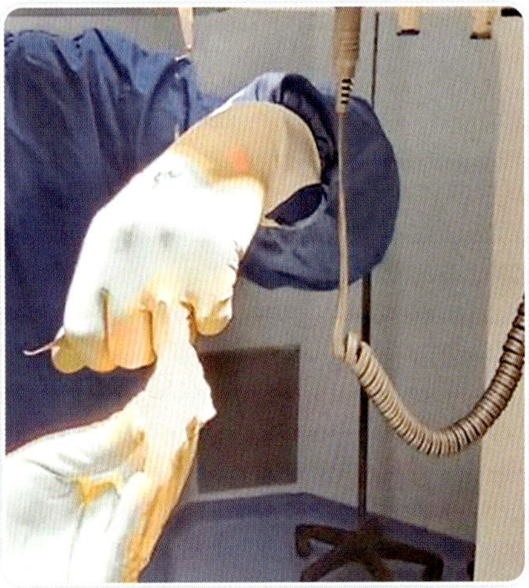

FIG. 4: Automated hydration device where you can keep hand in proximity to sensor and get saline drops over the grafts.

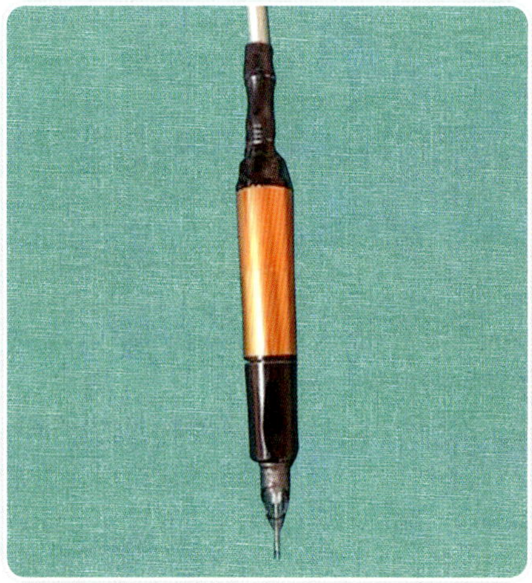

FIG. 6: Automated incision device where you can control the depth of incision.

tool for senior surgeons, in whom fatigue is always an issue. It also gives them an opportunity to enjoy fatigue-free speedy slit creation **(Figs. 5 and 6)**.

In 2015, the author developed an automated incision device working on the principle of the electropneumatic system where positive pneumatic pressure pushes the blade in a linear motion to create a slit in the recipient area, and through elastic recoil, it regains its normal position when pneumatic pressure is released.[20] This device solves the issue of surgeon fatigue but suffers from low speed.

In 2018, the author converted this device into a power incision device where the knife moves in a linear motion through electric power. Depth adjustment and speed adjustment are possible with this device. Since it is a handheld device, angles from 20° to 45° are possible as well as incision orientation like coronal or sagittal, which is not possible even with the ARTAS incision-creating arm.

In 2017, Dr Levent Acar invented a wireless handheld automated incision device with the name Robopen **(Fig. 7)**. The Robopen is fully adjustable via the in-built liquid-crystal display (LCD) screen, which also displays the incision count.[21]

The ARTAS robotic hair transplant system also has a feature of incision creation through an image-guided robotic arm.

ROLE OF AUTOMATION IN IMPLANTATION

Over the last 10 years, techniques and innovations have made it easy for beginners to implant FUE grafts.

We have observed numerous innovations in implanters. However, forceps still remain the gold standard instrument for implantation.

Though it looks very easy to insert grafts in preformed slit, there is a definite learning curve in implantation using forceps. Hand and eye coordination and fine motor skills for gentle insertion of the grafts differ from one person to another. Several attempts for inserting a graft into a tiny slit frustrate many beginners.

Keeping these factors in mind, the author has developed and patented an automated device that can solve the learning curve of the beginner and give an opportunity to the hair transplant surgeon to perform efficient and faster graft placement.

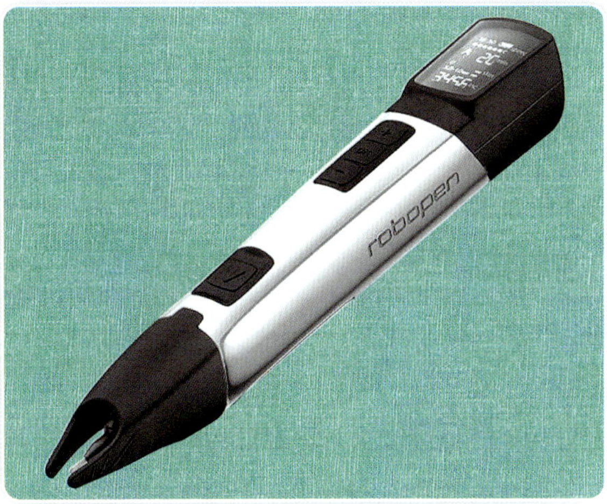

FIG. 7: Wireless handheld automated incision device—Robopen.

HOW DOES AUTOMATED ARM WORKS?

The automated forceps expansion arm works on electro-pneumatic principle where positive pneumatic pressure allows expansion of the terminal end of the forceps while the property of elastic recoil allows the terminal end of the forceps to regain its resting position. Pressing the pedal switch releases the air inside the rubber tube, thus creating positive pneumatic pressure which pushes the plunger that produces compression of spring and forward movement of forceps.[22] Forward movement of forceps releases forceps tightly holds arms thus produce expansion at its distal end.

Parts of an automated forceps expansion arm are:
- Hand piece
- Pneumatic tubing
- Compressor
- Pneumatic foot pedals

Hand Piece (Fig. 8)

- *Terminal end*: It comprises a 0.6-mm stainless wire split longitudinally to function as slit spreader forceps.
- *Body*: It has a plunger that glides within the tubular stainless steel wire and spring.
- *Tail*: It is attached to the pneumatic tubings and compressor unit with a pressure-regulating valve specially designed for air generation without producing noise.

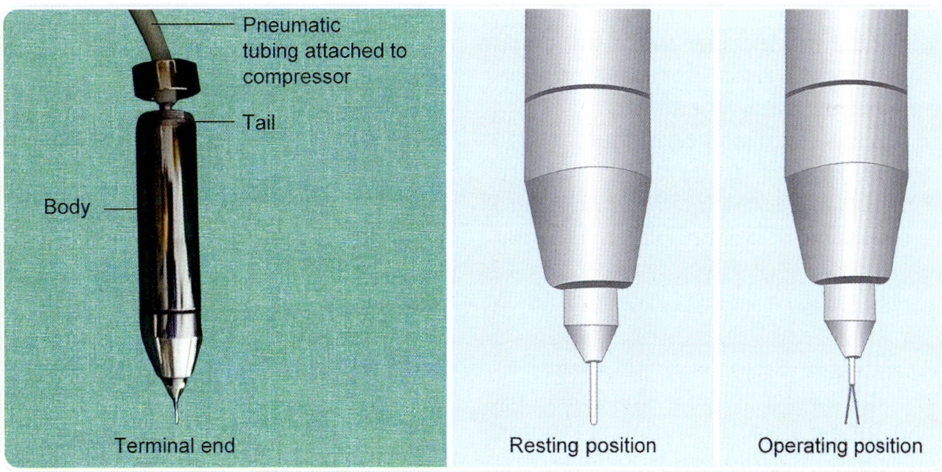

FIG. 8: Hand piece.

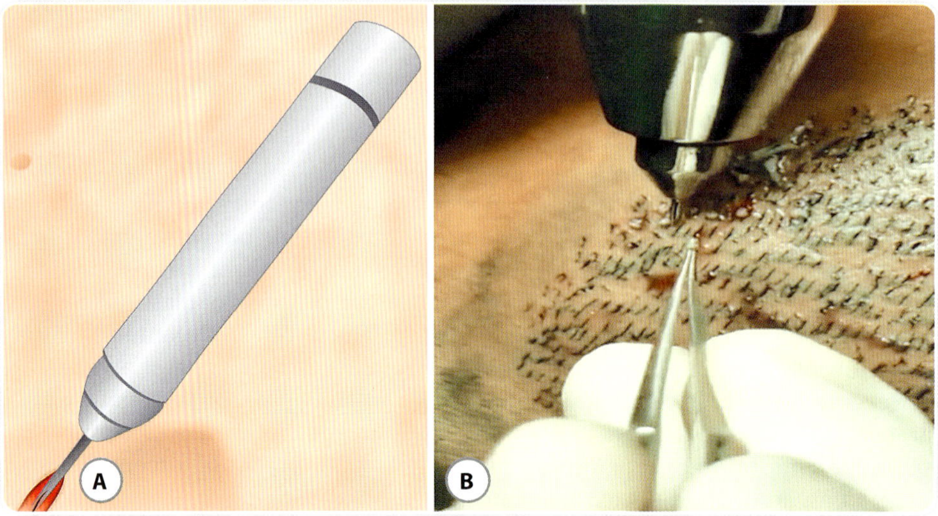

FIGS. 9A AND B: Position of the terminal end of the forceps in premade slits.

OPERATING STEPS

- *Engagement of the automated forceps*: It refers to the step when the tip of the terminal part of the automated arm is slightly inserted inside the premade slit **(Figs. 9A and B)**.
- *Expansion of the automated forceps*: After inserting the terminal portion of the arm into the premade slit, the operator presses the pedal switch that produces forward movement of the stainless steel wire. Forward movement of the wire releases wires that tightly hold arms to produce expansion at its distal end, thus causing dilatation of the sagittal slit **(Figs. 10A and B)**.
- *Implantation of the graft*: The operating surgeon holds the grafts with jeweler's forceps using another hand. The graft gently slides inside the slit while the slit is adequately dilated by automated forceps expansion **(Figs. 11A and B)**.
- *Resting position of the forceps*: Release of the pedal switch allows the forceps to retain its resting position because of the decompression of the spring.

The automated forceps expansion technique (AFET) can be used as a teaching tool to develop hand-eye coordination and motor skills. Pneumatic tubings and pedal switches are two issues that many surgeons do not prefer.

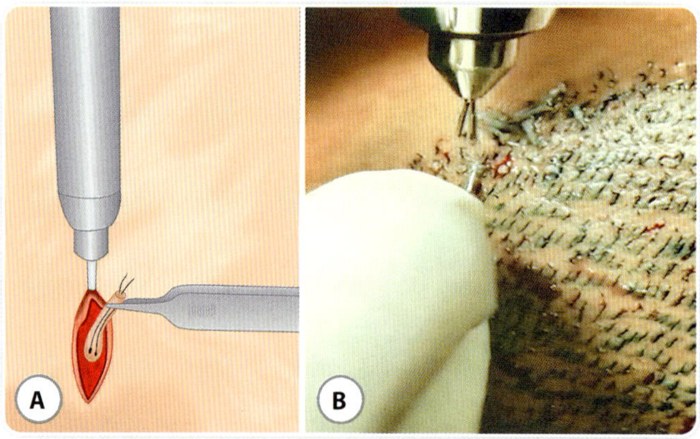

FIGS. 10A AND B: Dilatation of the slit by opening of the terminal end of forceps because of positive pneumatic pressure.

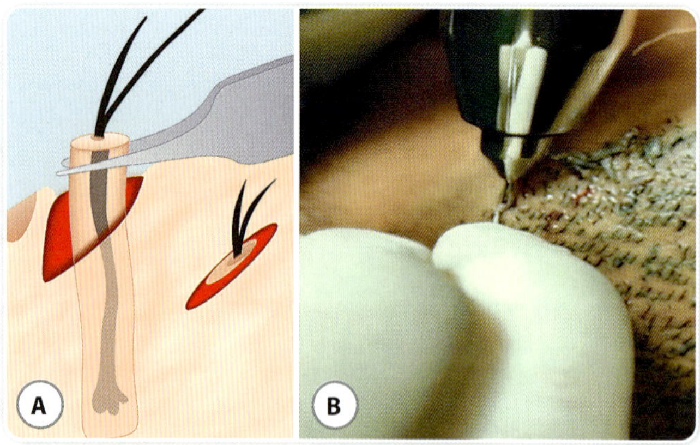

FIGS. 11A AND B: Graft gently slides inside the dilated slit using another forceps.

SUMMARY

The role of automation is to identify tasks that machines can do better than us, to help in removing human error and allowing scalability. The author believes that automation does not mean losing the human side; it means empowering the human hand to focus on more impactful work.

REFERENCES

1. Rassman WR, Berbstein RM, McClellan R, Jones R, Worton E, Uyttendaele H. Follicular unit extraction: minimally invasive surgery for hair transplantation. Dermatol Surg. 2002;28:720-8.
2. Harris JA. New methodology and instrumentation for follicular unit extraction: lower follicle transection rates and expanded patient candidacy. Dermatol Surg. 2006;32:56-61.
3. Onda M, Igawa HH, Inoue K, Tanino R. Novel technique of follicular unit extraction hair transplantation with a powered punching device. Dermatol Surg. 2008;34:1683-8.
4. Cole J. Harvesting the Fallows. ISHRS Meeting, San Diego, California; 2006.
5. Harris JA. Follicular unit extraction: the SAFE system. Hair Transplant Forum Int. 2004;14(157):163-4.
6. Tykocinski A. Hybrid Trumpet Punch for FUE harvesting. Hair Transplant Forum Int. 2017;27(1):14-6.
7. Trivellini R. Trivellini Hair Transplant Technology. Hair Transplant Forum Int. 2018;28(5):188-90.
8. Umar S, Lohlun B, Ogozuglu T, Carter MJ. A novel follicular unit excision device for all-purpose hair graft harvesting. Clin Cosmet Investig Dermatol. 2021;14:1657-74.
9. Saxena K. Micro rpm adjustment vs. conventional dental motors for FUE extraction. FUE Asia, Delhi; 2023.
10. Helfer JK. Clinical issue painless injections Helfer skin tap technique. Nurse Educ. 2000;25:272-3.
11. Melzack R, Wall PD. Pain mechanisms: a new theory. Science. 1965;150(699):971-9.
12. Melzack R. From the gate to the neuromatrix. Pain. 1999;Suppl 6:S121-6.
13. Vibration therapy for pain. Lancet. 1992;339(8808):1513-4.
14. Smith KC, Comite SL, Balasubramanian S, Carver A, Liu JF. Vibration anesthesia: a noninvasive method of reducing discomfort prior to dermatologic procedures. Dermatol Online J. 2004;10(2):1.
15. Physical methods for treatment of pain. In: Auerbach PS (Ed). Wilderness Medicine, 5th edition. Maryland, MI: Mosby; 2007.
16. Saxena K. Automated FUE. In: Saxena K, Saxena D (Eds). FUE Hair Restoration Major Procedures Minor Incisions, 1st edition. Mumbai; Cosmazone Pvt Ltd; 2007. pp. 79-82.
17. Saxena K. Human hands vs automated implanters. AHRS Annual Meeting, Mumbai, India; 2011.
18. Beler F, Southhand J. Principles of solid-organ preservation by cold storage. Transplantation. 1988;45(4):673-6.
19. Saxena K. Automation in FUE hair transplant. Annual Meeting of FUE, Europe; 2019.
20. Saxena K. Automated incision technique. FUE Europe Manchester Annual Conference; 2022.
21. Acar L. Robotic incision creating device. FUE Europe Annual Meeting, Istanbul; 2021.
22. Saxena K. Automated forceps expansion technique (AFET): a teaching tool for FUE graft implantation. ISHRS World Congress, Prague, Czech Republic; 2017.

CHAPTER 74

Robotic Hair Transplantation

Sanjay Parashar

Key Messages

- Follicular unit extraction (FUE), being a repetitive process, is amenable for automation.
- ARTAS is a robot that has evolved over the past few years, and robotic hair transplantation (HT) is a reality.
- Several challenges in robotic HT need to be addressed.

INTRODUCTION

Traditional hair transplantation (HT) techniques have some limitations and disadvantages:

- Manual follicular unit extraction (FUE) techniques rely on the skill and experience of the surgeon and assistants in extracting individual hair follicles. This can lead to variations in graft quality, transection rates, and survival rates upon transplantation.
- *Subjectivity in hairline design*: Traditional techniques often rely on the surgeon's subjective judgment and artistic skills in designing the hairline. However, subjectivity can introduce variations in hairline placement and design, potentially leading to suboptimal results or patient dissatisfaction.
- *Time-consuming procedure*: Manual extraction and transplantation is labor intensive and can be a time-consuming process. This can be challenging for both patients and surgeons.
- *Increased risk of human error*: Human error can occur during the extraction or transplantation process, leading to lower graft survival rates, graft damage, or improper placement and inconsistencies in final results.

These limitations along with the repetitive nature of the FUE process, which renders it suitable for automation, have led to the development of a robot for FUE.

INTRODUCING THE ARTAS ROBOTIC SYSTEM

ARTAS Robotic HT represents a significant advancement in the field of hair restoration **(Box 1)**. It combines cutting-edge technology, precision robotics, and artificial intelligence (AI) to revolutionize the way HT procedures are performed.[2]

The ARTAS Robotic System (ARS) incorporates AI algorithms and a robotic arm to automate and streamline the FUE process. One of the key advantages of ARTAS Robotic HT is its ability to precisely identify and extract individual hair follicles. The system utilizes advanced imaging to scan the donor area, creating a detailed three-dimensional (3D) map of the patient's scalp. This allows the robotic arm to identify and select the most suitable hair follicles for extraction based on specific criteria, such as size, orientation, and quality. The robotic arm then precisely removes the hair follicles using a minimally invasive technique, minimizing trauma to the surrounding scalp and ensuring high graft survival rates.

It also offers improved patient comfort and experience. The minimally invasive nature of the procedure results in reduced postoperative discomfort, swelling, and scarring compared to traditional techniques. Additionally, the robotic arm's speed and efficiency enable shorter procedure times, reducing the overall time patients spend in the clinic.

BOX 1 Evolution of the ARTAS Robotic System timeline.

- 2002: Restoration Robotics, the company behind the development of the ARTAS Robotic System, was founded in San Jose, California
- 2006: Restoration Robotics introduced the first prototype of the ARTAS Robotic System, which combines robotics, imaging technology, and artificial intelligence for hair restoration procedures
- 2007: United States Food and Drug Administration (USFDA) approved it for use in hair transplantation procedures
- 2011: The commercial version is launched as the first robotic hair transplantation system available for clinical use
- 2013: The ARTAS 9x system, an upgraded version of the ARTAS System, was launched. It features improved imaging capabilities and enhanced robotic arm movements[1]
- 2017: Restoration Robotics is acquired by Venus Concept, a global medical technology company focused on aesthetic medicine
- 2018: Venous Concept introduces the ARTAS iX system, an advanced iteration of the system that incorporated artificial intelligence, improved imaging technology, and a more user-friendly interface
- 2020: Venus Concept partners with allergan aesthetics to promote and distribute the system globally

Note: The ARTAS iX system continues to undergo advancements and refinements, with ongoing research, clinical studies, and software updates to further improve its performance and outcomes.

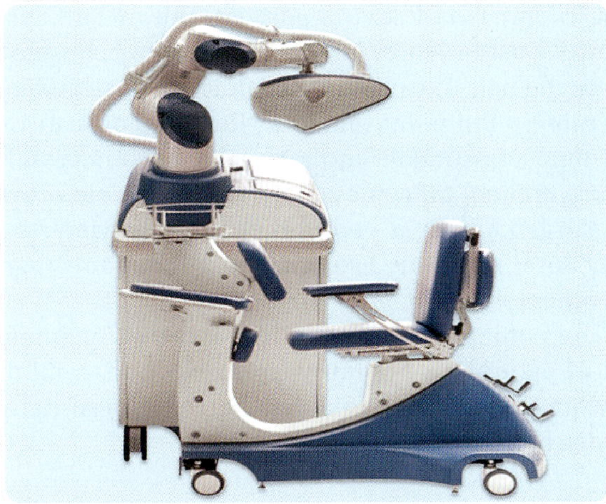

FIG. 1: ARTAS Robotic System with robotic head and arm, main console, and ergonomically designed chair.

BOX 2 Key features of ARTAS.

- High-resolution three-dimensional (3D) imaging
- Real-time analysis
- Robotic arm with precision controls, minimizing the risk of human error
- Minimally invasive extraction with utmost accuracy, ensuring minimal trauma to the surrounding scalp tissues and reducing postoperative discomfort and scarring
- Consistent graft quality, ensuring that each hair follicle is extracted intact, with minimal damage

Furthermore, the system allows for more accurate and natural-looking hairline design. The robotic arm's precision ensures precise placement of each graft, resulting in a hairline that seamlessly blends with the existing hair and facial features. This customization and attention to detail contribute to a more aesthetically pleasing and satisfying outcome for patients.

UNDERSTANDING ARTAS ROBOTIC HAIR TRANSPLANTATION

Overview of the ARTAS Robotic System Components and Functionality (Fig. 1 and Box 2)

Robotic arm: At the heart of the ARTAS System is a robotic arm that performs the critical tasks of identifying, extracting, and implanting hair follicles. The robotic arm is equipped with precision controls and computer-guided movements, allowing it to perform these tasks with exceptional accuracy and consistency.

Digital imaging system: The ARS incorporates a high-definition, 3D imaging system that captures detailed images of the patient's scalp. This imaging technology creates a comprehensive map of the donor area, identifying the density, angle, and direction of existing hair follicles. The digital imaging system provides critical data to guide the robotic arm during the extraction and implantation process.

Artificial intelligence algorithms: The ARS utilizes AI algorithms to analyze the captured images in real time. These algorithms assess and identify the optimal hair follicles for extraction based on specific criteria, such as size, quality, and suitability for transplantation. The AI algorithms also aid in precise hairline design and determine the most natural distribution of the transplanted hair follicles.

Dissection tool: The ARTAS System includes a small, rotating tool that assists in the precise dissection of follicular units. This tool helps to carefully separate and extract individual hair follicles from the surrounding tissue without causing damage or transection.

Sterile chamber and storage: The ARTAS System incorporates a sterile chamber where extracted hair follicles are collected and stored during the procedure.

User interface and control console: The ARTAS System features a user-friendly interface and control console that allows the hair transplant surgeon to monitor and guide the robotic arm's movements. The surgeon can make real-time adjustments and intervene when necessary to ensure optimal outcomes. The control console provides the surgeon with a comprehensive overview of the procedure, including live imaging, extraction progress, and other relevant data.

The combination of robotics, imaging technology, and AI algorithms optimizes graft selection, minimizes transection rates, and enables the creation of natural-looking hairlines.

Integration of Artificial Intelligence Algorithms and Human Expertise

Surgeon Expertise and Decision-making

- *Surgical planning and oversight*: While the AI algorithms provide valuable insights, the expertise of the hair transplant surgeon remains essential. The surgeon evaluates the data and recommendations provided by the system and makes informed decisions based on their professional judgment and experience.
- *Real-time adjustments*: The surgeon has the ability to make real-time adjustments during the procedure. They can intervene and modify the robotic arm's actions, ensuring the desired outcomes align with the patient's specific needs and expectations.
- *Efficiency and streamlined workflow*: The combination of AI automation and human oversight optimizes the HT process, reducing procedural time and improving overall efficiency. The system assists the surgeon in performing tasks more efficiently, freeing up their focus for critical decision-making and customization.

ARTAS Robotic Hair Transplantation Procedure

Initial Consultation Process and Patient Candidacy Evaluation

The initial consultation process and patient candidacy evaluation can be enhanced using the ARTAS studio tool using a 3D image model **(Fig. 2)**.

The consultation process and patient evaluation remain the same as the conventional FUE procedure, with additional information on the technology with its pros and cons explained to the patient.

Assessment of patient characteristics:

- *Scalp analysis*: The ARTAS System's advanced imaging technology captures high-resolution 3D images of the patient's scalp that provide detailed information about hair density, quality, and the pattern of hair loss.

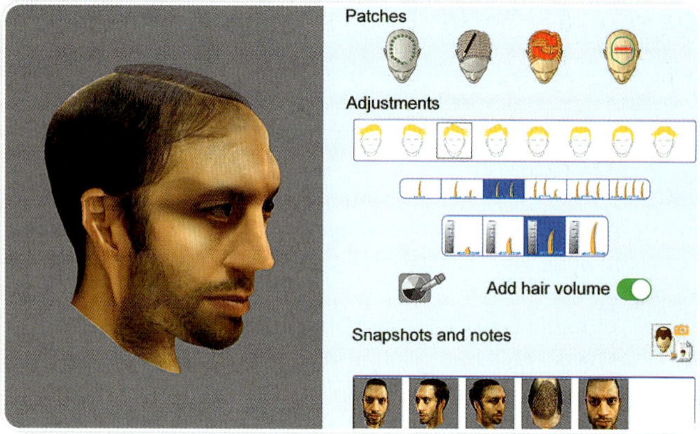

FIG. 2: ARTAS studio toolusing a 3D image model.

- *Donor area evaluation*: It assesses the donor area's density, quality, suitability, and scalp laxity.
- *Facial features and aesthetic goals*: The ARTAS System takes into account the patient's facial features, including the shape of the face, hairline position, and existing hair pattern. These factors are considered when designing a personalized treatment plan to ensure a natural-looking and aesthetically pleasing outcome.
- *Interactive patient involvement*: The ARTAS System allows for interactive patient involvement in the hairline design process.
- *Treatment plan visualization*: The ARTAS System utilizes 3D simulation technology to provide a visual representation of the proposed treatment plan, allowing the patient to visualize the potential results and make informed decisions.

Robotic-assisted Follicular Unit Extraction (RAFUE)—Step-by-Step Procedure of ARTAS Robotic Follicular Unit Extraction

Robotic chair: The patient is seated on a specially designed ergonomic chair with his/her head down on a cushion. The patient's scalp is numbed using local anesthesia. In robotic hair extraction, there is no need to use tumescent infiltration, unlike in conventional FUE. This possibly has a low risk of follicle shock.

*Robotic follicular unit extraction **(Fig. 3)***: A proprietary skin tensioner (10 × 10 cm) is applied to the scalp to stretch out the scalp. There are fiduciary markings that allow the robotic head to scan and adjust its area of work. Then the surgeon uses a remote switch to play mode. The robotic arm then moves randomly in a controlled fashion to dissect the hair follicles. A large TV screen displays a magnified view of the process with a detailed view of actual live punch action, sites selected, grafts dissected, etc. This allows the surgeon to modify any parameter they may deem necessary **(Fig. 4)**.

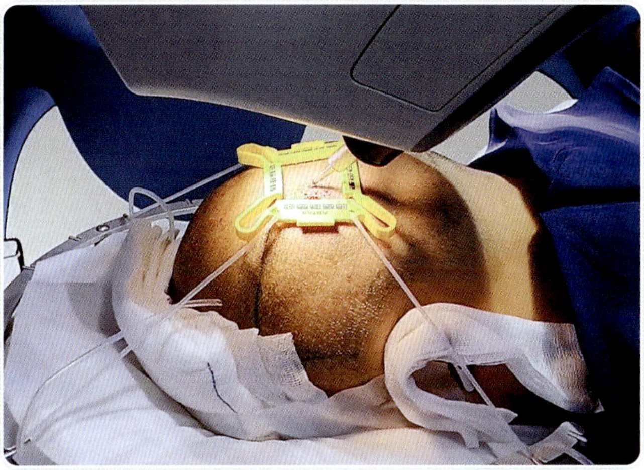

FIG. 3: Robotic follicular unit extraction after applying skin tensioner.
Courtesy: Restoration Robotics, Inc., San Jose, California, USA.

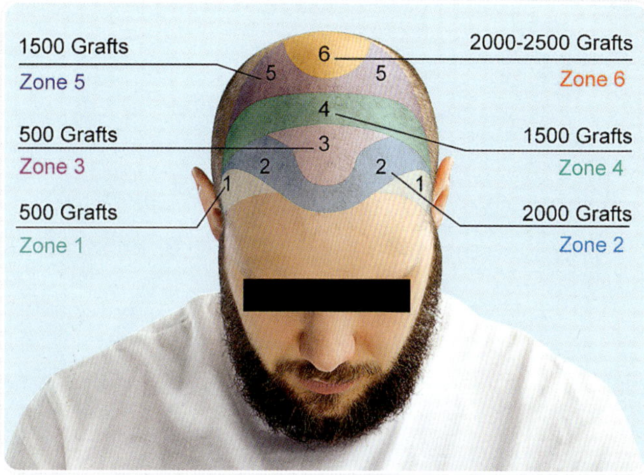

FIG. 5: Preoperative 3D plan for site making that is loaded in the system.

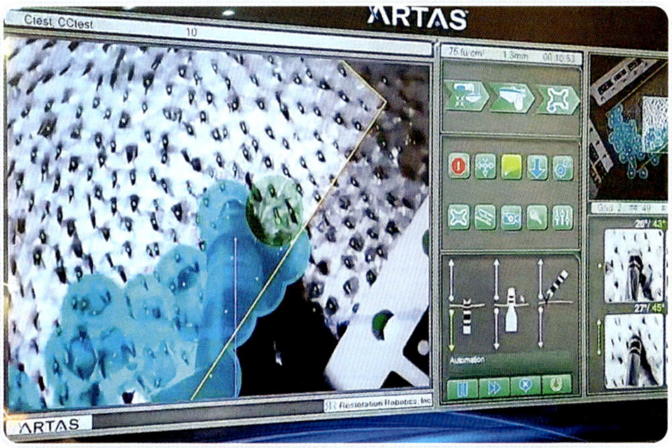

FIG. 4: TV screen displaying magnified view of the hair follicles and control parameters.

Punch selection: The ARTAS System utilizes a small dual-bore punch tool, typically ranging in size from 0.8 to 1.0 mm, to extract individual follicular units. The inner punch is sharp for epidermal incision and the outer punch is blunt for atraumatic tissue dissection. The system controls the depth of the punch tool to ensure that only the upper part of the follicle, containing the hair bulb and necessary supporting structures, is extracted. This controlled depth minimizes the risk of transection or damage to the follicles. There is an attached suction mechanism that elevates the graft, making it easy to collect. After quality check of few grafts, the robot is placed in auto mode, and it extracts about 90–100 grafts from within the skin tensioner. The grafts are then collected by an assistant, and the tensioner position is changed to the next area. The machine harvests at a speed of 600–700 grafts/h. In our experience, the graft harvest speed is not directly related to the time it takes to complete the procedure. Additional time is added to manually collect the graft (that can be done simultaneously as the robot is harvesting) and reposition the tensioner (speed improves with experience).

Dissection of follicular units: The extracted follicular units can be 1, 2, or 3 follicular groups and are carefully dissected from the surrounding tissue manually, ensuring the preservation of their integrity and viability.[3]

Sorting and storage: The individual follicular units are sorted based on their size, quality, and the number of hairs contained within each unit and stored in a suitable solution.

Recipient site creation: The 3D plan **(Fig. 5)** that is created using ARTAS Studio preoperatively is loaded in the system. A separate incision kit of size 18 or 19 G is connected to the ARTAS console. The position of the chair is changed to 180°, and the patient lies down with his/her head down. Local anesthesia is used to give a ring block in the recipient site.

The ARTAS remote is used to play the system and the robotic head adjusts its position to create tiny incisions at an angle that is predecided by the surgeon **(Fig. 6)**. It takes 20–30 minutes to prepare 1,500–2,000 incision sites.

The challenge at the moment in my practice is inadequate depth for graft insertion in some incisions that require additional manual work to dilate the incisions.

Precision in incision placement:

- *Accurate angle and direction*: The ARTAS Robot, guided by advanced imaging and robotic technology, ensures that each incision is placed at the appropriate angle and direction.

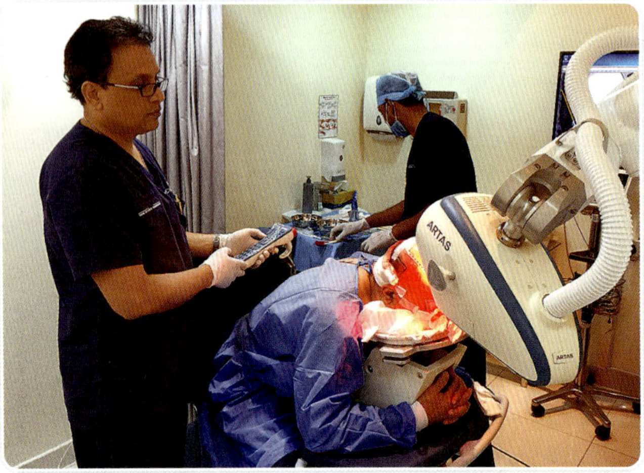

FIG. 6: Using Remote Control to adjust the depth and angle of recipient site.

- *Consistent spacing*: The robotic system maintains consistent spacing between the transplanted grafts, preventing a clustered or unnatural appearance.

Graft Placement Using Cartridge

The ARS utilizes an implantation cartridge as part of the HT process. The implantation cartridge is designed to facilitate the precise placement of harvested hair follicles into the recipient area of the scalp.

Here is how the implantation cartridge works:

- *Loading of hair follicles*: The follicles are loaded into the implantation cartridge, which is a specialized device designed to securely hold and protect the grafts during the transplantation process.
- *Calibration and positioning*: The ARS calibrates and positions the implantation cartridge for accurate and controlled graft placement. It is aligned properly to facilitate precise positioning of the follicles in the recipient area.
- *Controlled implantation*: The ARS uses its robotic arm and advanced imaging to guide the implantation cartridge to the target area on the recipient scalp. It inserts the cartridge into the scalp, and the individual grafts are placed at predetermined angles and depths.
- *Graft release*: It gently releases the individual grafts into the recipient sites. The release mechanism within the cartridge ensures that each graft is accurately placed without causing trauma to the surrounding tissues.
- *Surgeon's control and adjustment*: While the ARS assists with the initial placement of grafts, the surgeon closely monitors the implantation and manually adjusts the position of grafts.

BOX 3 Advantages and disadvantages of ARTAS.

Advantages of ARTAS:
- Less use of infiltration anesthesia, thus possibly less risk of follicular shock loss
- Less postoperative swelling and discomfort
- Less bleeding and early wound healing
- In secondary cases, graft selection is better with the ARTAS System
- Younger patients with longer heads are ideal candidates as more follicular units can be harvested

Disadvantages of ARTAS:
- If the patient is moving to a great extent, the robotic system will have difficulty aligning with the donor area
- Curvilinear areas have challenges due to the extreme angle of the follicles
- If the scalp is soft, e.g., in the nape area, it is difficult to harvest
- It is difficult to harvest curly hair
- The incision making part and implantation are still very challenging and require manual override

Personal Experience (Box 3)

We have been using ARS since 2016 at our center. Installation of the machine was challenging as we had to break a wall and use a crane to install it on the first floor of our center.

The reasons for us to enter into the field of ARTAS Robotic Hair Restoration were because of the following reasons:

- Lack of manpower due to governmental regulation issues
- I personally found it less tiring to do robotic HT, and it allowed me to carry on with my other plastic surgery-related work.
- It was easy for me to teach our junior doctors, and the learning curve was shorter than the conventional FUE technique.
- It was also possible to do more than one HT procedure in a day despite limited personnel.
- It gave us a significant marketing advantage and helped us to lead the hair restoration work in the region.
- It opened our practice for the affluents who wanted technology and surgeons to have more control than other personnel.

However, there are several challenges we must deal with using ARS. The biggest, of course, is the investment, recurring cost of consumables, and maintenance of the equipment.

REVIEW OF LITERATURE

Shin et al. conducted a study on 22 patients who underwent robotic-assisted hair restoration surgery from September 2012 to March 2013 at Seoul National University Bundang Hospital. In this study, they collected hair follicles from three grids (upper central, lower center, left lateral) to avoid variations between subjects and analyzed the technique. The harvested follicles were analyzed under a microscope by two independent nurses. According to the study, the average yield was 95.1% and the transection rate was 4.91%. They concluded that it efficiently harvests not only single hairs but multiple hairs as well.[4]

SUMMARY

The ARTAS Robot is a tool and an option to extract follicles that reduces manual fatigue and possibly improves the overall experience of the patient. The site making still has many challenges that require surgeon override. I have not experienced the implantation cartridge that appears promising, but it is too early to know its true value. There are not many comparative studies between the ARTAS robotic technique and the motorized technique to draw a conclusion at this stage. We hope to update our experience in future.

REFERENCES

1. Bernstein RM, Wolfeld MB. Robotic follicular unit graft selection. Dermatol Surg. 2016;42(6):710-4.
2. Rose PT, Nusbaum B. Robotic hair restoration. Dermatol Clin. 2014;32(1):97-107.
3. Rashid RM. Follicular unit extraction with the Artas robotic hair transplant system system: an evaluation of FUE yield. Dermatol Online J. 2014;20(4):22341.
4. Shin JW, Kwon SH, Kim SA, Kim JY, Na JI, Park KC, et al. Characteristics of robotically harvested hair follicles in Koreans. J Am Acad Dermatol. 2014;72:146-50.

CHAPTER 75

Body Hair as a Donor

Aman Dua, Bishan Mahadevia

Key Messages

- Introduction of follicular unit extraction (FUE) and concept of recipient influence led to the use of hair from donor areas other than the scalp for transplantation.
- This has been an important advance in hair restoration, as it has created a vastly greater donor area.
- However, nonscalp donor areas are used only in those with poor scalp hair and not as the first choice.
- Technique is difficult, needs patience, and is time-consuming.

INTRODUCTION

Scalp hair transplant could bring a natural and permanent solution to the hair loss patients. However, limited number of available scalp donor hairs did not always satisfy balding men, who had the need and greed for more hair. This made the surgeons look for the body hair (BH) as a source of donor hair. Driven by demand, some adventurous surgeons entered the unchartered territory of harvesting and transplanting BH. This chapter discusses different aspects of body hair transplantation (BHT).

It is important to note that BHT is a new technique, though it is being practiced increasingly, and there are very few publications on the subject. Hence, a lot of materials quoted are through the personal experience of authors or other experts.

HISTORY

In 1988, Masumi Inaba from Japan introduced the use of a 1-mm punch for extracting individual follicular units.[1] In 2002, Rassman refined the procedure and named it follicular unit extraction (FUE).[1] The first recorded case of successful BHT was in 2001 by Hirai et al.,[2] and Ray Woods of Australia first tested BHT and found it effective in 1998.[3] He documented that although the BH would typically only grow up to 4 cm, when transplanted to the scalp, it could grow up to 15 cm. However, he published his study much later, only in 2004. The evidence that there is a recipient influence, the influence of scalp dermis on the transplanted hair, was demonstrated by Tommy Hwang, which gave scientific legitimacy to the technique.[4]

BODY HAIR CHARACTERISTICS

The human body is said to have 5 million hairs. Except for scalp hair, most other BH is vellus to begin with, but a proportion of these hairs have androgen sensitivity, and they become terminal hair (androgenic hair) around puberty in areas such as the axilla and pubis of the sexes, face, chest, and back of males.[5] The majority, though, remain vellus hair throughout life. Due to a normally higher level of androgen, men tend to have more androgenic hair than women. So, BHT is practically exclusive to men. As far as the distribution and number of BH is concerned, there is a racial distribution—Ainu race in Japan is the hairiest race. Whites and South Asians have more BH than Africans, American Indians, and Orientals in general.

Body hair differs from scalp hair in several ways:

- *Hair cycle*: One important difference between scalp and most BH, of practical importance for hair surgeons, is that of the hair cycle. In the case of scalp/

TABLE 1: Hair growth rate in various regions of the body.

Region	Anagen (%)	Telogen (%)	Depth of follicle (mm)
Scalp	85	15	3–5
Eyebrow	10	90	2–2.5
Cheek	60	40	2–4
Beard	60	40	2–4
Moustache	55	45	1–2.5
Axilla	30	70	3.5–4.5
Pubis	30	70	2–4.5
Arms	20	80	2.5–4
Leg and thigh	20	80	2.5–4

Source: Modified from Richards–Meharg table.[8]

facial hair, nearly 85% of the hair is in the anagen phase, and the duration is long: 250–350 weeks. The hair cycle for BH (other than facial hair) is much shorter, and a larger number, close to 60% of BH, is in the nongrowing phase of telogen.[6] BH also has a longer telogen phase (10–24 weeks) and a shorter anagen phase (13–16 weeks), and therefore, BH grows shorter compared to scalp hair **(Table 1)**.

- *Ability to grow*: BH grows slower. Whereas scalp hair grows at 0.37–0.44 mm/day, BH grows at 0.27 mm/day. Compared to scalp hair, most BH is thinner in diameter, grows shorter, and slower. The only exception is facial hair, which grows thicker and faster than even scalp hair. Beard hair is usually the thickest hair in the body. So, they are good for producing volume when transplanted to the scalp. But, due to their thickness, they are not suitable for the hairline as they stand out and look abnormal.
- Tommy Hwang demonstrated the concept of recipient influence, where he showed that after transplantation, BH tends to acquire the growth characteristics of scalp hair (vice versa is also true—scalp hair, when transplanted to the body, tends to grow less and slowly) and tends to grow longer.[4] This finding formed the basis of BHT.
- *Type of units*: Unlike scalp hair, BH has mostly follicular units with one hair (hair-to-graft ratio: Low with mostly single hair grafts) and very few units of two or three hairs.[7] The two to three hair units may be found in the chin or sideburn areas of the beard and some chest hair or hair from the back.
- *Tendency for gray hairs*: BH is slow to gray compared to scalp hair, and this characteristic can be of use while restoring the hairline and eyebrows.
- *Curly hair*: Many patients have curly BH; even in otherwise straight-haired person, BH often looks curled, even if they are not curled. This may be because BH is usually not groomed, is sparse and thin, and curls outside the body to gain support.
- *Patterns*: BH often grows in variable directions in the same area and occasionally forms whirls. There are 15 patterns of chest hairs described in the literature **(Figs. 1 to 3)**.[9-13] This variable direction requires repeated adjustment of the punch direction and may even require frequent changes in the surgeon's position, thus making the extraction process tedious and difficult.
- *Angle of emergence*: BH exits from the skin at more acute angle than scalp hair **(Figs. 4A and B)**.
- *Location*: BH lies superficially in the upper dermis, which has dense collagen. Certain areas of the body,

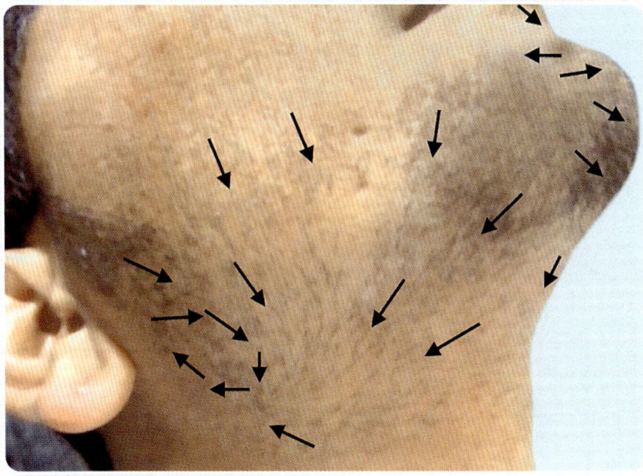

FIG. 1: Distribution of beard hair.

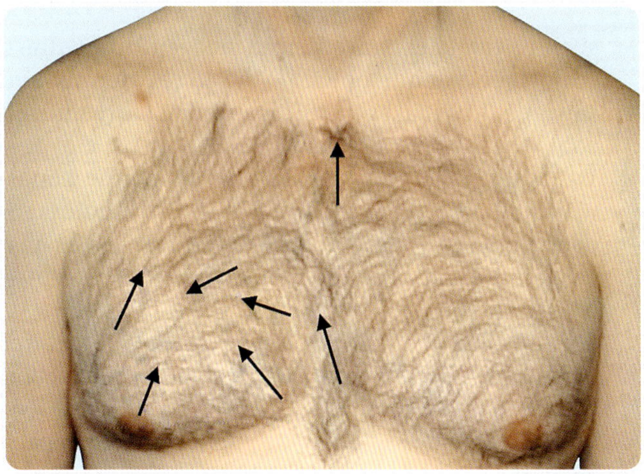

FIG. 2: Pattern of chest hair.

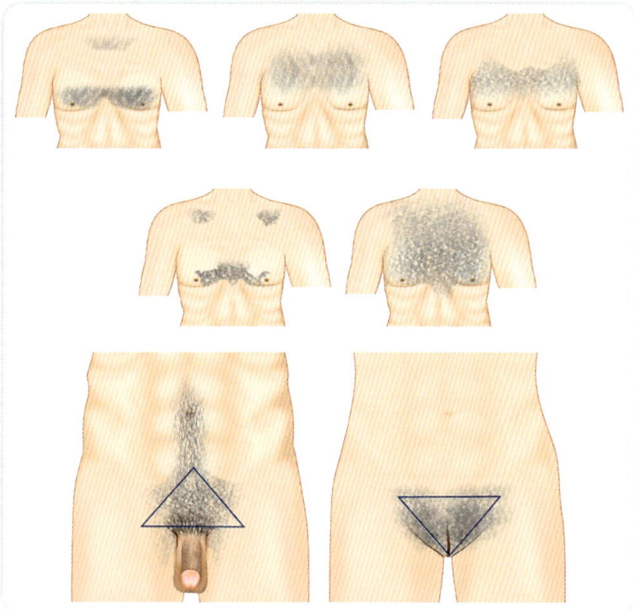

FIG. 3: Pattern of chest and pubic hair.

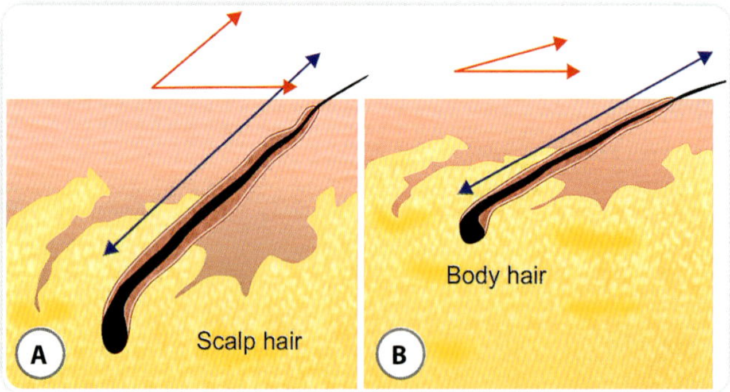

FIGS. 4A AND B: Angle of emergence of body hair.

such as the back, have dense collagen. In contrast, scalp hair extends down to the lower dermis and subcutis. This makes the BH harvesting more difficult compared to the scalp hair.

- *Wet zones*: Axilla and pubic hair have apocrine glands, which release secretions that have an unpleasant odor. Some surgeons have, therefore, advised against using these hair as donor, though this is not accepted by others.
- *Leg hair*: Shin area may take longer to heal due to lower blood supply and can have higher chances of infection of the extraction sites.
- *Yield*: Chest hair seems to give a better yield than back and arms.[7]

INDICATIONS FOR BODY HAIR TRANSPLANTATION

- Poor scalp donor area conditions, such as:
  - Deficient scalp donor area
  - Exhausted scalp donor area
  - Unhealthy scalp donor area of diffuse unpatterned alopecia (DUPA)
  - High miniaturization in the scalp donor area (>10%)
- For the camouflage of strip, punch, burns, or other injury scar in the donor area
- Recharging (also called sealing or farming) of donor area: In already depleted donor area where more scalp hair is to be used, scalp hair can be replaced by BH to show reduced thinning of donor area.
- For segmental vitiligo
- Finer BH can be used for hairline feathering. BH can be useful especially for temple point or eyebrow creation when scalp hair is very thick. BH is slow to gray, and therefore, its use in hairline can be fruitful.
- If the donor area has very curly hair, some BH (e.g., legs) can be useful if they are straight when used for eyebrow restoration.
- BH can also be used to camouflage donor strip scar.
- BH can also be implanted into the suture at the end of the strip surgery to enhance the appearance of a scar.

Who is Not a Candidate for Body Hair Transplantation?

Not everyone is a candidate for BH transplant, as some simply do not have BH, while others have a few poor-quality BH. Those with good growth of thick hair on the chest, who are well motivated and are willing for multiple sessions, form the best candidates.

How to Select Body Hair Transplantation Feasibility?

Robert True has described the torso donor index (TDI). The TDI takes into account chest hair characteristics, such as density, texture, percentage of two- and three-hair follicular units, surface area, and hair length [presented at the International Society of Hair Restoration Surgery (ISHRS) 14th Annual Scientific Meeting in Coronado, CA, in October 2006]. A composite score that can distinguish excellent and marginal candidates and noncandidates for torso-to-scalp hair transplantation is given in **Table 2.** Robert True chooses only people with index > 7 as good candidates. He also recommended doing a test transplant of 200–300 hairs first before doing more. Patients with TDI scores of 4 or less are not candidates. Patients with TDI scores of 5–7 have limited supplementary resources that may allow for focused touch-up work. Patients with TDI scores of 8 and above may have a donor resource that exceeds their scalp donor resource **(Figs. 5A and B)**.

PREOPERATIVE PREPARATION IN BODY HAIR TRANSPLANTATION

- Preshaving to the skin level of the body donor area using a razor is undertaken 2–5 days (depending upon the speed of hair growth) prior to extraction.

TABLE 2: Robert True torso donor index.

	0	1	2	Score
Density	≤20 FU/cm²	20–40 FU/cm²	≥40 FU/cm²	
Texture	Very different	Somewhat similar	Very similar	
2–3 hair FU	≤20%	20–30%	≥30%	
Surface area	≤50 cm²	50–200 cm²	≥200 cm²	
Hair length	≤2 cm	2–5 cm	≥5 cm	
Total				

Note: There are many factors that affect individual hair growth. This growth table should only be used as a generalized guide.

It avoids telogen hair and selectively shows the anagen hair.[14]

- Minoxidil application to donor sites a few weeks before surgery may shorten the telogen, convert some telogen hair into anagen hair, and may also prolong the anagen phase.
- Patients should be prepared for frequent changes in position and the need for multiple injections for anesthesia.
- Persons with keloidal tendencies and bleeding tendencies should be excluded.

DIHYDROTESTOSTERONE INHIBITORS AND BODY HAIR TRANSPLANTATION

The role of dihydrotestosterone (DHT) inhibitors such as finasteride or dutasteride in BH growth is still debated. Both increase and decrease in BH growth following DHT inhibitors have been reported in the literature.[15] Some surgeons routinely advise to stop the use of DHT inhibitor a few months before and even after BHT.

SURGICAL PEARLS

- Harvest time for BH is longer than that of scalp hair. This may be attributed to:
  - Acute exit angle
  - More superficially sitting follicles in collagenous dermis unlike scalp hair, which float in fat

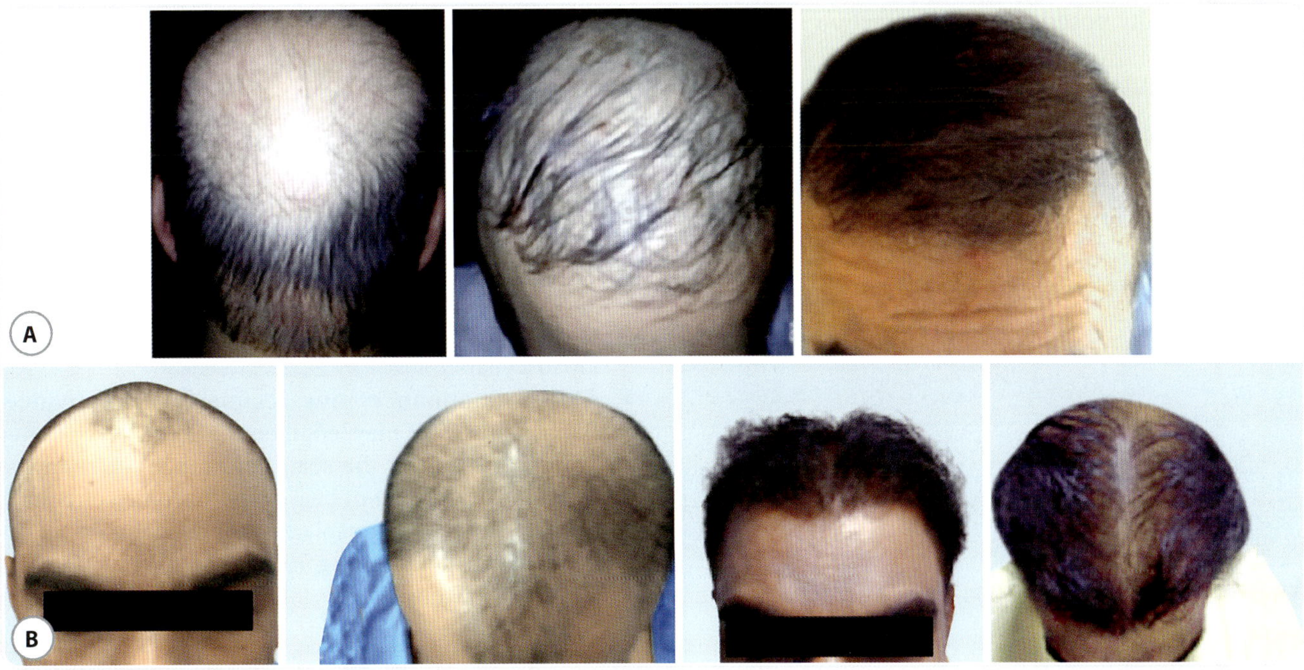

FIGS: 5A AND B: Result of body hair transplantation.

  - Absent bony support and bulky soft tissue in many situations, such as the abdomen, pubic, back, thigh, and axilla
  - Some BH are thin; hence, they do not have a strong shaft to facilitate easy extraction.
  - Awkward position for the surgeon, especially in the armpit and pubic area
  - Greatly variable direction and pattern of BH
- Traction of the skin or tumescence can help.
- BH is thinner and shorter in length; hence, good skills are required for extraction. Transection rates are also higher for BH; however, this is of less significance unlike transection of scalp hair.
- Chest and beard hairs are of better quality compared to hair from other body areas for transplanting to the scalp due to their thickness and length.
- In dark-skinned patients, harvesting is preferred from upper sideburns and under the chin area only, and the other areas are avoided to prevent visible scarring.
- Blunt punch may not be as useful as sharp punch.
- Sternal region is avoided for harvesting due to the possible risk of hypertrophic scar and keloid formation **(Fig. 6)**.
- The thicker caliber beard hair should not be transplanted in the hairline and the temples, as these areas typically have finer caliber hair. The ideal hair combination in these areas would be a mix of the scalp and finer caliber BH.[16]
- The use of the needle tip as a cutting instrument in the expanding needle concept is especially beneficial in the more difficult body donor areas, as it has reduced the difficulty posed by larger extraction sites and, at the same time, lowered the transection rates of the body donor hair.[17]
- Due care needs to be devoted to use a mix of the various donor hair in any bald area of the scalp.[16] BH is generally mixed with scalp hair and implanted on the midscalp and vertex region for better blending.

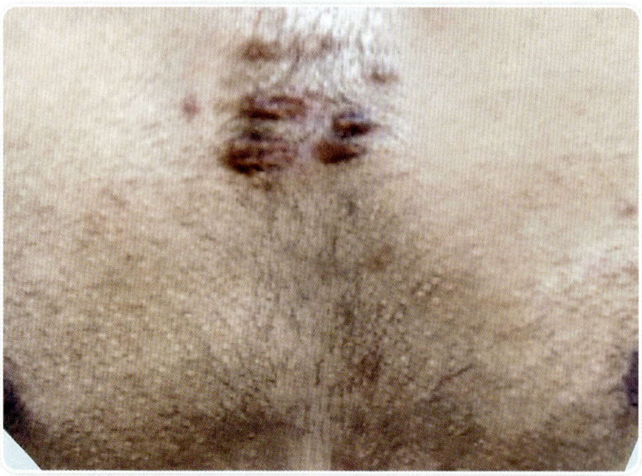

FIG. 6: Chest keloid following body hair transplantation.

Anesthesia

Anesthesia may be painful as multiple entry points are needed, and blocks are not useful. The area near the nipples is very sensitive. Maximum dose of anesthetic can limit the extraction in a day. Ring block is normally not effective. Tumescent anesthesia is preferred to cover a larger area and to use a large volume of anesthetics.[7] Using vibration, icepack or ethyl chloride spray, and thinnest possible bore needle, injecting very slowly helps reduce pain during anesthesia. Avoiding multiple punctures by the use of a long lumbar puncture (LP) needle is also useful in infiltration. It is a good idea to use diluted lidocaine so that a larger area can be harvested within the permissible dose.

Complication

- Hypopigmented/hyperpigmented pinpoint scars are common.
- Presternal or shoulders are vulnerable areas for keloids. Few test punches can be done to see for keloid tendency.
- Ingrowing hair and folliculitis due to buried grafts can happen.

POSTOPERATIVE PHASE

- Mupirocin skin ointment is applied for a week; bandaging is not required.
- Scab takes 10–15 days to go, but hyperemic pink-purple spots are visible for as long as 2 months, particularly in exposed areas.
- *Slow growth*: It usually takes 4–6 months for initial growth after transplant, and the best effect may take up to 2 years.
- Donor dominance plus recipient codominance: Transplanted BH may lengthen the growth cycles after transplantation in the scalp and may grow to more length. Coarser hair of beard may become softer over few years of being transplanted to the scalp.
- Asymmetrical harvesting of BH should be avoided for aesthetic reasons.

LIMITATIONS

Body hair has several limitations and hence needs to be used with caution and in selected cases:

- Except for facial hair, most BH has a lesser diameter than that of scalp hair, and therefore, BH generates less volume and requires more grafts for a similar volume compared to scalp hair.
- BH mostly has single hair grafts, hence, the need for more grafts for density, volume, and coverage.
- BH takes longer time to grow.
- BH is known to have less final yield, 60–80%, and sometimes has unpredictable growth.
- Long-term behavior of BH is still not known as the technique is relatively new and practiced only occasionally.
- Possibility of synchronous cycling is there although not seen usually.

Since the procedure is more time-consuming and technically difficult, the cost is likely to be higher.

SUMMARY

Donor other than scalp is a useful adjunct in modern hair surgery. Doctors need to be equipped with adequate knowledge about BH behavior, and patients need to be appropriately educated and communicated about the pros and cons. When done in the right framework, results are satisfying. However, the technique is still in its infancy, and, hence, needs further evaluation before it can be recommended as a routine method.

Treatment Pearl

- BH is a valuable source of hair in advanced baldness.
- It has limited value in enhancing volume, and hence, proper counseling is needed.
- It is time-consuming and needs experience to perform efficiently.

REFERENCES

1. Bertram N. Follicular unit extraction in the Asian population. In: Pathomvanich D, Imagawa K (Eds). Hair Restoration Surgery in Asians, 1st edition. Japan: Springer; 2010. pp. 133-40.
2. Hirai T, Inoue N, Nagamoto K. Potential use of beards for single-follicle micrografts: convenient follicle-harvesting technique using an injection needle. Ann Plast Surg. 2001;47:37-40.
3. Woods R, Campbell AW. Chest hair micrografts display extended growth in scalp tissue: a case report. Br J Plast Surg. 2004;57:789-91.
4. Hwang S, Kim JC, Ryu HS, Cha YC, Lee SJ, Na GY, et al. Does the recipient site influence the hair growth characteristics in hair transplantation? Dermatol Surg. 2002;28:795-8; discussion 798-9.
5. Bleyl SB, Braver PR, Francis-West PH. Development of skin and its derivatives. In: Schoenwolf GC (Ed). Larsen's Textbook of Embryology, 4th edition. Philadelphia: Churchill Livingstone, Elsevier; 2009. pp. 202-5.
6. Schneider MR, Schmidt-Ullrich R, Paus R. The hair follicle as a dynamic miniorgan. Curr Biol. 2009;10:R132-42.
7. Richards RN, Uy M, Meharg G. Temporary hair removal in patients with hirsutism: A clinical study. Cutis. 1990;45:199-202.
8. Mysore V. Body hair transplantation: case report of successful outcome. J Cutan Aesthet Surg. 2013;6:113-6.
9. Poswal A. Expanding needle concept for better extraction of body hair grafts. Indian J Dermatol. 2013;58:240.
10. Setty LR. The sterno-infraclavicular chest hair pattern. J Natl Med Assoc. 1962;54:486-7.
11. Setty LR. The circumareolo-pectoral series of chest hair patterns. J Natl Med Assoc. 1963;55:233-4.
12. Setty LR. Variations of the hair patterns of the chest of white males. J Natl Med Assoc. 1965;57:211-4.
13. Setty LR. The distribution of chest hair in Caucasoid males. Am J Phys Anthropol. 1961;19:285-7.
14. Setty LR. The bipartite pattern of pubic hair. J Natl Med Assoc. 1964;56:261-2.
15. Poswal A. The preshaving protocol in body hair-to-scalp transplant to identify hair in anagen phase. Indian J Dermatol. 2010;55:50-2.
16. Inadomi T. Efficacy of finasteride for treating patients with androgenetic alopecia who are pileous in other areas: a pilot study in Japan. Indian J Dermatol. 2014;59:163-5.
17. Poswal A. Use of body and beard donor hair in surgical treatment of androgenic alopecia. Indian J Plast Surg. 2013;46:117-20.

APPLICATIONS OF BEARD HAIR TRANSPLANTATION

Scalp Hair Restoration for Advanced Grade Baldness

The careful use of beard hair in scalp hair restoration is crucial to ensure patient satisfaction. The natural curl of the hair plays a significant role in how well the beard/body hair is accepted by the patient, especially if their own scalp hair is straight. To achieve the highest level of patient acceptance, it is advisable to combine scalp donor hair with beard donor hair. This holds true even if the beard hair is thick and wavy, while the patient's scalp hair is fine and straight. Therefore, a thoughtful blend of different donor hair sources is essential when addressing bald areas on the scalp.

The strategic placement of beard hair on the scalp is vital for achieving the best results. The rear frontal zone, midscalp, and vertex are the most suitable areas to utilize beard hair **(Fig. 6)**. On the other hand, the hairline and temples, which naturally consist of finer hair, should not receive transplants of thicker beard hair to maintain a natural appearance.[10]

Beard hair becomes especially valuable in patients with resource versus recipient mismatch, such as those with low donor reserve. These cases may involve issues like low-donor density, a narrow-donor fringe, retrograde alopecia, miniaturization in the superior fringe region, diffuse thinning, and fine and straight hair. In such instances, beard hair can be effectively used to augment the hair restoration process.

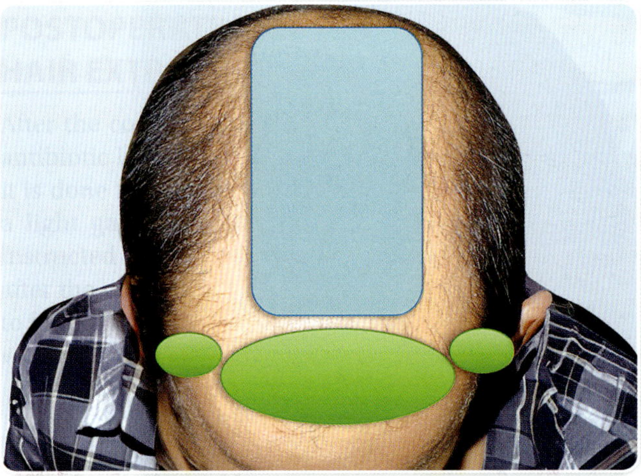

FIG. 6: The rear frontal zone, midscalp, and vertex (blue rectangle) are the most suitable areas to utilize beard hair. Frontal hairline and temporal triangles (green circles) should not receive beard hair transplantation.

Another specific indication for utilizing beard hair in scalp hair restoration is for patients who have previously undergone traditional hair restoration procedures or those with unnatural-looking transplanted hair, and no more scalp donor supply is available. The use of beard hair can offer a cosmetic repair solution in such cases.

It is prudent to use beard hair in the first session of hair transplant, particularly in younger patients. This approach helps preserve the scalp donor area for potential future sessions.

Facial Hair Restoration

Beard hair transplantation offers a transformative solution for individuals with patchy or thin beards. When considering transplanting hair from a nonscalp body area, it is best to use hair from the same area if it is available in sufficient quantity. For instance, beard hair from below the jawline can be selectively transplanted to the cheek beard, creating a fuller and more symmetrical beard. The coarser texture and natural curl of beard hair contribute to a more realistic and natural appearance.

This procedure is especially beneficial for individuals with facial scarring, a genetic predisposition for sparse facial hair, or those who have undergone medical treatments that affected beard growth. By strategically transplanting beard hair follicles to the desired areas of the face, a significant improvement in beard density and overall facial appearance can be achieved.

Scar Camouflage

Beard hair transplantation provides an effective solution for camouflaging scars resulting from previous surgeries, trauma, or burns on the face or scalp. By transplanting beard hair follicles into the scar tissue, they seamlessly blend with the surrounding hair, significantly reducing the visibility of the scar. This technique not only restores self-confidence but also enhances the overall aesthetic appearance by concealing unsightly scars.

Compared to thin-caliber body hair, the thicker consistency of beard hair offers superior cosmetic coverage in scar tissue. However, caution is necessary when dealing with cases where the scalp and beard donor hair significantly differ in caliber and color. Transplanting the thicker beard hair at a high density all along the scar may result in a linear zone of hair with a different texture and color, standing out from the rest of the hair. To avoid this, it is best to transplant beard hair at a lower density, around 20 grafts/cm^2, and combine it with donor hair follicles taken from the scalp and other suitable body areas.

Eyebrow Restoration

The eyebrows hold significant importance in framing the face and accentuating facial expressions. Unfortunately, some individuals may experience eyebrow loss due to various factors such as medical conditions, excessive plucking, or scarring. In such cases, beard hair transplantation can be an effective solution for restoring natural-looking eyebrows.

While beard hair has a coarser texture compared to eyebrow hair, its natural curl and length closely resemble that of eyebrows. This similarity makes beard hair an excellent choice for recreating realistic and aesthetically pleasing eyebrow hair. By carefully selecting and transplanting beard hair follicles into the eyebrow area, hair transplant surgeons can achieve a seamless and natural appearance.

LIMITATIONS OF USING BEARD HAIR AS A DONOR SITE

While beard hair transplantation can be a valuable resource in hair restoration, it does come with some inherent limitations that need to be carefully considered. The characteristics of beard hair, such as thickness, length, and hair cycle, may not perfectly match those of scalp hair. Studies conducted by Hwang et al. have shown that when body hair, including beard hair, is transplanted to the scalp, the thickness remains relatively unchanged, but the length and growth rate may undergo alterations.[11] The transplanted hairs tend to become longer, and their growth rate increases compared to standard scalp hair.

The process of harvesting beard hair as a donor site is more time-consuming and demands a higher level of expertise compared to traditional scalp FUE techniques. Beginners, in particular, may encounter higher transection rates during beard hair extraction. However, with the use of proper equipment and techniques, such as sharp or hybrid punches of the correct size and design, inserted at the appropriate angle and depth, and rotating or oscillating with the right speed and force, transection rates can be minimized.

It is crucial to acknowledge that the suitability of beard and body hair donor sites may be limited, especially in individuals with minimal natural body hair. For patients with sparse body hair, the availability of adequate donor follicles may be insufficient to achieve the desired hair restoration goals.

Additionally, the aesthetics of utilizing beard hair as a donor source can vary based on the patient's unique characteristics. For instance, if the patient's scalp hair is straight while the beard hair is thick and curly, achieving a natural blend may be more challenging.

Despite these limitations, beard hair transplantation remains a valuable option in specific cases, offering an additional source of donor hair for individuals with hair loss concerns. It is essential for hair transplant surgeons to thoroughly assess each patient's individual characteristics and needs, considering the potential challenges and advantages of using beard hair as a donor site to provide the most appropriate and satisfactory results.

SUMMARY

In conclusion, the utilization of beard hair as an additional donor resource has proven to be a valuable and versatile technique in the field of hair restoration for AGA. It is important to note that the color, curl, and shaft diameter of beard hairs remain consistent, necessitating careful planning when combining various donor hair types for transplantation. Besides AGA, beard hair serves as a valuable resource for individuals seeking to improve their facial aesthetics, whether it involves restoring facial hair, concealing scars, or reconstructing eyebrows.

As technology continues to advance, we can anticipate further advancements in beard hair transplantation techniques, leading to even more natural and aesthetically pleasing results for patients desiring a fuller and more vibrant appearance. However, further research is needed to better understand the potential impact of transplanting beard hair to the scalp on factors such as anagen-telogen ratios, anagen-telogen durations, growth rates, and lengths of the transplanted hair.

Fortunately, beard hair harvesting has become a well-established component of hair restoration surgery, boasting high success rates when performed with proper technique. As the field of hair transplantation continues to evolve, beard hair will undoubtedly continue to play a significant role in meeting the diverse needs and desires of patients seeking effective and lasting solutions for their hair loss concerns.

REFERENCES

1. Saxena K, Savant SS. Body to Scalp: Evolving Trends in Body Hair Transplantation. Indian Dermatol Online J. 2017;8(3):167-75.
2. True RH. Using Nonscalp Hair in Scalp Hair Restoration-Theory and Execution. Indian J Plast Surg. 2021;54(4):463-70.
3. Jimenez F, Ruifernáández JM. Distribution of human hair in follicular units: A mathematical model for estimating the donor size in follicular unit transplantation. Dermatol Surg. 1999;25:294-8.
4. Poswal A. The preshaving protocol in body hair-to-scalp transplant to identify hair in the anagen phase. Indian J Dermatol. 2010;55(01):50-2.
5. Umar S, Lohlun B, Ogozuglu T, Carter MJ. A Novel Follicular Unit Excision Device for All-Purpose Hair Graft Harvesting. Clin Cosmet Investig Dermatol. 2021;14:1657-74.
6. Garg AK, Garg S. "Combination Grafting" of Scalp and Body Hair to Enhance the Visual Density of Hair Transplant and Coverage of Higher Grade of Baldness. J Cutan Aesthet Surg. 2020;13(2):163-9.
7. Umar S. Hair transplantation in patients with inadequate head donor supply using nonhead hair: report of 3 cases. Ann Plast Surg. 2011;67:332-5.
8. Gupta J, Chouhan K, Kumar A, Chandrasegaran A. A Comparative Study on the Rate of Anagen Effluvium and Survival Rates of Scalp, Beard, and Chest Hair in Hair Restoration Procedure of Scalp. J Cutan Aesthet Surg. 2019;12(2):118-23.
9. Poswal A. Use of body and beard donor hair in surgical treatment of androgenic alopecia. Indian J Plast Surg. 2013;46(1): 117-20.
10. Gupta B, Banerjee P, Priyadarshini Y, Rathi P. BEARD-A Potential Donor Site in Grade 6 and Grade 7 Alopecia: A Case Series. J Maxillofac Oral Surg. 2021;20(4):545-50.
11. Hwang ST, Kim HY, Lee SJ, Lee WJ, Kim DW, Kim JC. Recipient-site influence in hair transplantation: a confirmative study. Dermatol Surg. 2009;35:1011-4.

CHAPTER 77

Facial Hair Transplantation

Kapil Dua, Navjot Kaur, Aman Dua

Key Messages

- In facial hair transplantation, it is imperative to understand the direction of hair in important zones of the recipient area to give it a natural look.
- Facial hair transplantation yields good results because of the increased blood supply to the recipient area.

INTRODUCTION

Facial hair transplantation includes restoration of eyebrows, eyelashes, beard, and mustache. The number of patients opting for facial hair restoration has increased over time with increasing awareness. As per the latest International Society of Hair Restoration Surgery (ISHRS), USA survey released in 2015, the number of patients undergoing facial hair transplant (face/mustache/beard) has increased from 1.50% in 2013 to 3.7%, eyebrows from 4.5 to 5.5%, and eyelashes from 0.50 to 0.6% to take the total nonscalp procedures to 10.9% compared to 7.1% earlier.[1]

Eyebrow and eyelash transplantation has been described in other chapters, and this chapter deals with beard and mustache transplantation.

BEARD AND MUSTACHE TRANSPLANTATION

Indications

The common indications are as follows:
- Scars due to trauma, burns, or surgery
- Traction alopecia (especially in the Indian Sikh population; **Fig. 1**)
- Congenital hypotrichia/atrichia **(Fig. 2)**
- Postfolliculitis scarring
- Long-standing alopecia areata
- Correction of previous transplantation surgery

Apart from these indications, many men simply want to improve the density in certain areas of their beard or mustache, depending on certain styles they would like.

Anatomy

Beard growth starts during puberty, under the influence of androgens, and increases in density till the mid-30s. For the purpose of facial reconstruction, the face can be divided into lateral and frontal aspects with different zones **(Fig. 3)**. The lateral aspect includes the sideburns, the cheek beard, the jawline beard, and the submandibular

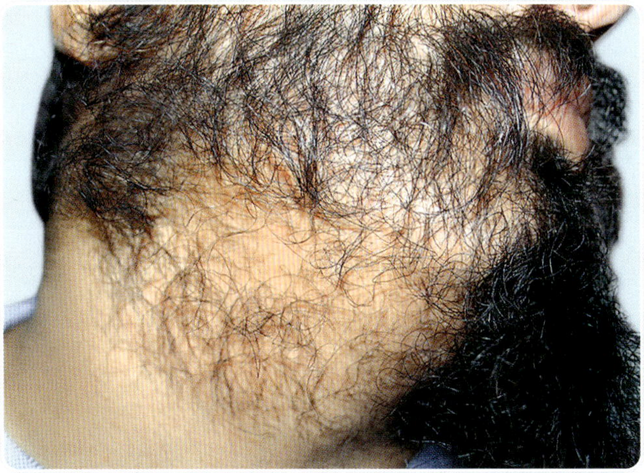

FIG. 1: Traction alopecia.

beard area. Out of these four areas, the cheek beard is cosmetically the most important. In the frontal aspect, the mustache and the goatee are the prominent features and higher densities are present in these areas. The hair below the chin and jawline that extends onto the neck is also usually considered to be part of the beard. The follicular units in the beard and mustache are usually single-haired. The caliber of beard hair is more compared to that of scalp hair. Beard hair is also typically triangular in shape compared to scalp hair.[2] The hair density in the beard is also different among various ethnic groups. Indian and Middle-Eastern men have relatively higher density.[3]

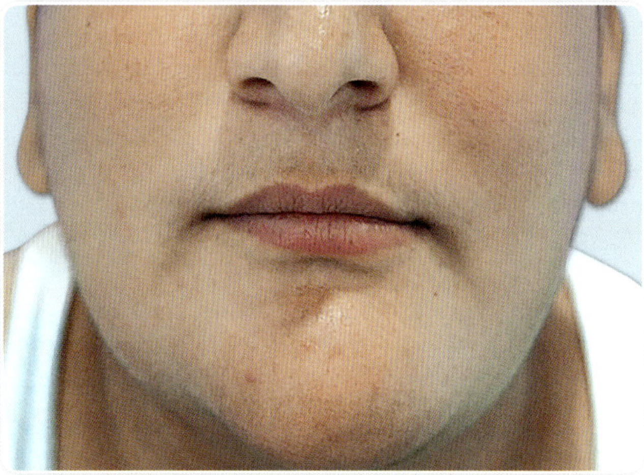

FIG. 2: Congenital hypotrichia.

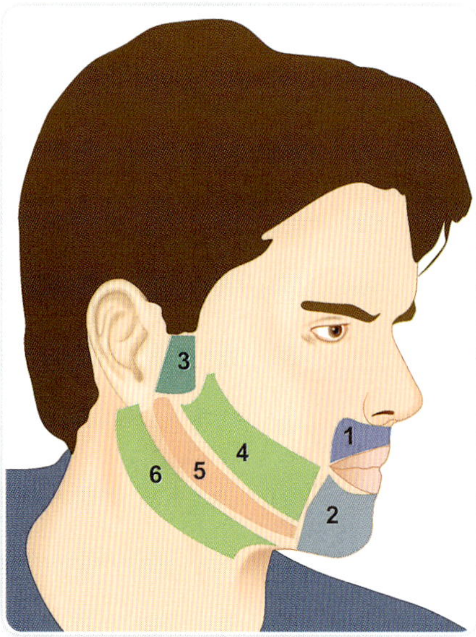

FIG. 3: Zones of beard area for planning of facial hair transplantation: (1) Mustache; (2) Goatee; (3) Sideburn; (4) Cheek beard; (5) Jaw beard; (6) Submandibular beard.

The basic principles of hair transplantation are the same, but it needs to be planned in a different way. A detailed examination of the face is required to determine the number of grafts required for the entire area that needs reconstruction. The most common indication that is encountered for facial hair reconstruction is congenital hypotrichia or atrichia. Such patients often need as many as 2,000–2,500 grafts to recreate the entire beard and mustache. The grafts are removed from the donor area in the same way as in routine follicular unit extraction (FUE) or follicular unit transplant (FUT). The midoccipital area is preferred because of the similarity in texture to beard/mustache hair.[4] However, the main difference lies in the distribution of grafts and recipient site creation.

Local Anesthesia

Local anesthesia is very painful in the facial area. Therefore, nerve blocks are preferred.

- *Auriculotemporal nerve*: This is blocked as it ascends in front of the auricle over the posterior root of zygoma, behind the superficial temporal artery. The needle is inserted about 1.5 cm anterior to the ear, at the level of tragus behind the superficial temporal artery pulsations, and around 1 mL of 2% lignocaine with 1:200,000 adrenaline is injected.[5] This nerve supplies the skin over the parotid gland and the external ear **(Fig. 4)**.
- *Infraorbital nerve*: This is blocked by giving 1 mL of 2% lignocaine with 1:200,000 adrenaline through the intraoral route by inserting the needle vertically upward with the tip pointing toward the foramen in the gingivolabial sulcus between the canine and the first premolar. This anesthetizes the infraorbital area, upper lip, and mustache area **(Fig. 5)**.

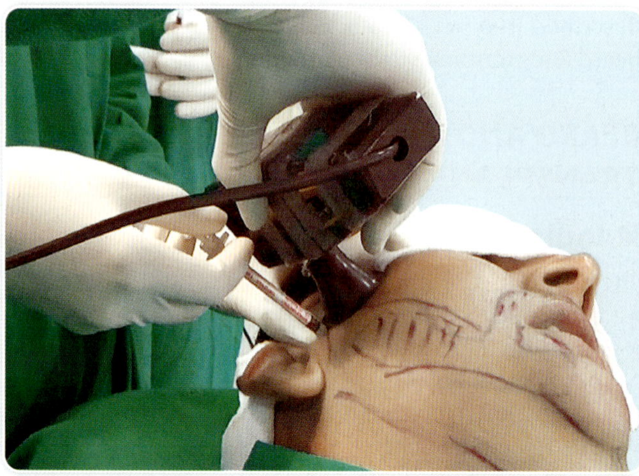

FIG. 4: Local anesthesia to the auriculotemporal nerve.

- *Mental nerve*: The nerve is blocked as it emerges from the mental foramen, which is located at the gingivolabial sulcus between the two lower premolars (1 mL of 2% lignocaine with 1:200,000 adrenaline). This helps to numb the lower lip and chin area **(Fig. 6)**.
- *Long buccal nerve*: This is blocked by injecting 2–3 cm laterally and superiorly to the angle of the mouth with the needle pointing toward the mouth and in a fanning manner. This nerve supplies the cheek area.[6]

After the nerve blocks, field anesthesia is given starting from in front of the ear advancing downward to the lower border of the beard, then across the lower border, and then over the upper border.

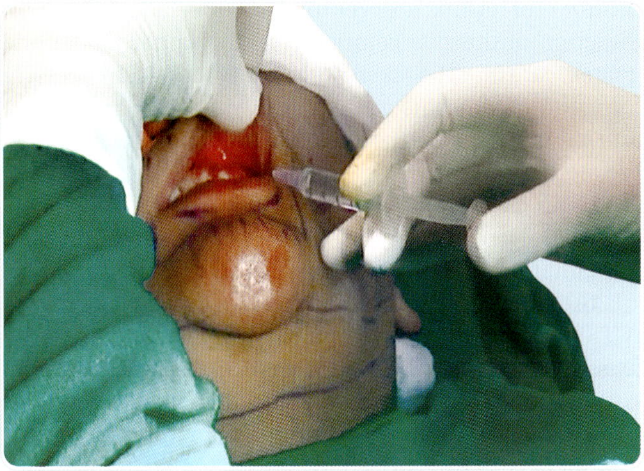

FIG. 5: Local anesthesia to the infraorbital nerve.

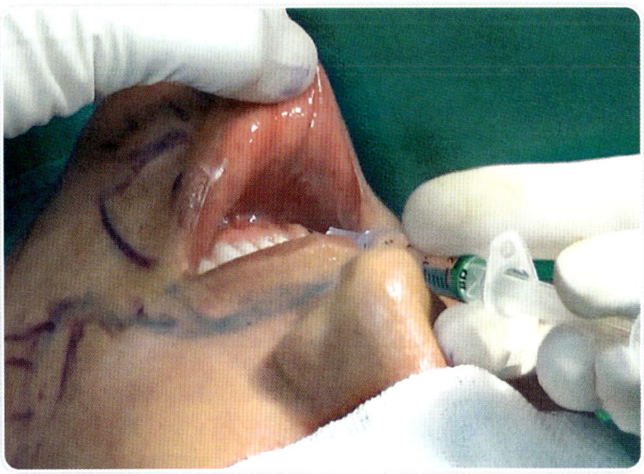

FIG. 6: Local anesthesia to the mental nerve.

Donor Area

Site and Technique

The scalp is preferred as the donor area for the beard. Beard-to-beard transplantation is done for small scar reconstruction requiring less than 100–150 grafts, for mustache reconstruction, and if the patient is willing to take grafts from the area under the chin. The grafts are usually taken out from the midoccipital area by FUE or FUT, and mostly single- or double-haired grafts are extracted **(Fig. 7)**. The total number of grafts required for mustache and beard reconstruction is usually around 1,000–1,100; the precise number, however, depends on the area.

Recipient Area

Creation of Site

Out of the six zones of the beard, the sideburns and the cheek area are the most important parts in the lateral profile. The authors prefer coronal slits because they help to assure alignment of the hair acute to and parallel to the skin. Density is kept more in the upper part of the sideburn as those hairs will grow in a downward direction, providing better coverage inferiorly due to the overlapping effect from above. The total number of grafts usually implanted in this area is around 200 per side.

On the area of the cheek, the slits are directed in a skewed pattern as they turn laterally and downward. But this is quite a big zone, and it is further divided into two parts: The border and the body. In the cheek border, less

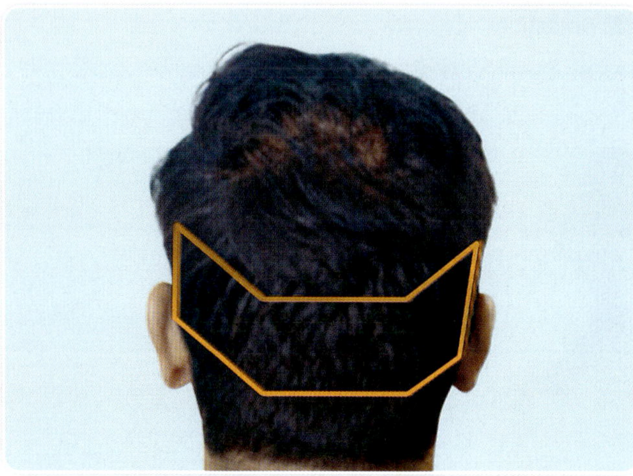

FIG. 7: Midoccipital area from where the grafts are extracted.

density is given, and single hair grafts are preferred to give it the look of the feathering zone. The cheek body is an area where a relatively higher density is given so that the maximum effect of a full beard can be achieved. Usually, two or three hair grafts of scalp hair are placed in this area. The density is kept less in the lowermost part of the cheek beard along the jawline. Usually, 500–600 grafts are required for the cheek beard on each side **(Figs. 8 and 9)**.

The jawline beard is an area where less grafts are required as a result of the overlapping effect achieved due to the hairs layering from above. The grafts are usually not implanted in the undersurface of the beard in the first sitting as it is a shadow (or less cosmetically important) area. And the authors want to implant a higher number of grafts in the more visible areas. The only exception is the traction alopecia seen in the Sikhs like the one shown in **Figure 2**, in which the undersurface of the beard also needs reconstruction.

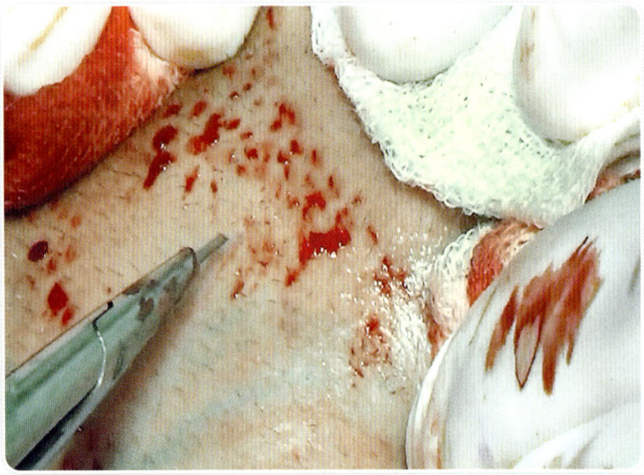

FIG. 8: Creation of site for the cheek beard (right).

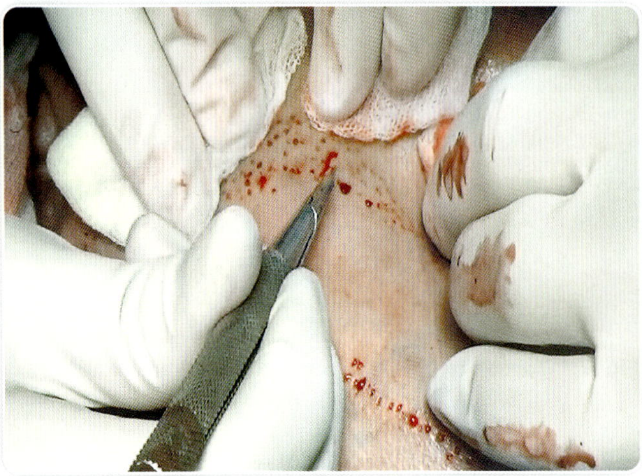

FIG. 9: Creation of site for the cheek beard (left).

The frontal aspect is cosmetically more important than the lateral aspect and requires a higher number of grafts relatively. As mentioned earlier, around 1,000–1,100 grafts are required for mustache and beard reconstruction.

The mustache usually needs around 400–500 grafts. The density is relatively higher (around 35–40 FU/cm^2) in this area and the hairs are directed downward. Usually, sagittal slits are given in this area in caudal to cephalic direction making sure that the angle of the slit is as parallel to the skin as possible. More grafts are placed in the upper part as compared to the lower part of the mustache as the layering of the hair compensates for the lesser number of grafts in the bottom part. The single-hair grafts are placed in the topmost row to give it a natural look.

The goatee is another area where a relatively higher number of grafts are required (600–700). The main direction of the slits is inferior. In the upper part of the goatee, care must be taken not to apply too much excessive force for making slits as the underlying layer has less fat and it may get cut across the inner labial surface and touch the teeth as well.

Superficial tumescence and adequate stretching of the lax facial skin are essential during the creation of slits and implantation.

The authors prefer to make the slits first with cut-to-size (CTS) blades (~0.8 to ~0.9 mm in size). But sometimes the slits close before graft placement. If so, the application of countertraction to stretch the skin will reopen the sites for placement. The difficulty encountered in this technique is that there may be more chances of bleeding. Sometimes, the stick and place method is used, in which this problem of site closure does not happen.

Implantation

Implantation may be difficult in the beard area due to muscularity and increased risk of bleeding. Adequate stretching by the assistant may be needed for implantation. During implantation, single-haired grafts are placed over the superior outline similar to the scalp hairline, and single- or two-haired grafts are placed over the other areas. Two-haired or paired grafts can be used to increase the thickness. Implantation takes a longer time compared to the scalp **(Fig. 10)**.

The beard area presents some challenges during implantation. Being a muscular area, the tissue needs to be firmed up by an assistant. Bleeding may also be more. Superficial nerves may get injured during the process, with transient paresis of facial muscles.

Postoperative Precautions

Some drooling may occur initially during the postoperative period due to the local anesthesia. Therefore, semisolid food is advised on the day of surgery after discharge. Hair growth begins after around 3 months and improves over the next year. Superficial tumescence given during surgery can also cause postoperative edema and ecchymosis, which disappear over a couple of days.

Special features: Since it is a mobile area, some restricted mobility is advised. Soft food and liquid diet are preferred. Some swelling of the area is expected postoperatively. A short course of oral steroids postoperatively reduces the edema.

Results

Results of beard and mustache transplant are shown in **Figures 11 and 12**.

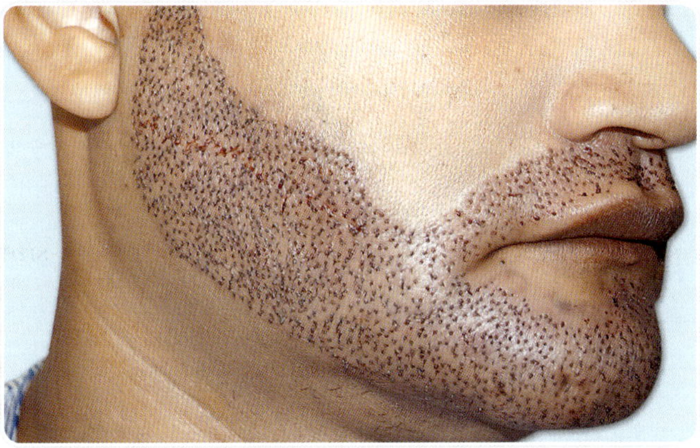

FIG. 10: Beard implantation.

EYEBROW TRANSPLANTATION

Indications

The following are the indications commonly encountered for eyebrow restoration:
- Voluntary plucking
- Trichotillomania
- Alopecia areata
- Genetic
- Traumatic
- Hypothyroidism

Anatomy

The average length of an eyebrow hair follicle is around 4.5–5 cm. The shape of the eyebrow is more arched in females and the peak of the arch lies along a vertical line between lateral limbus and lateral canthus. The shape is almost flat (nonarched) in men **(Figs. 13 and 14)**.[7]

Eyebrow Designing

The eyebrow can be divided into three sections: Head (medial, one-fifth), tail (outer, one-third), and body (between the head and tail). The head part is the most critical section and is around 5–10 mm in length. It has a square to rounded medial border and starts just medial to a vertical line drawn from the medial canthus **(Fig. 15)**.[7]

The body of the eyebrow **(Fig. 16)** is around 25–30 mm in length and is the densest, widest, and most prominent portion. Its lower border starts in a flat/horizontal direction from the head; it then slightly arches along the

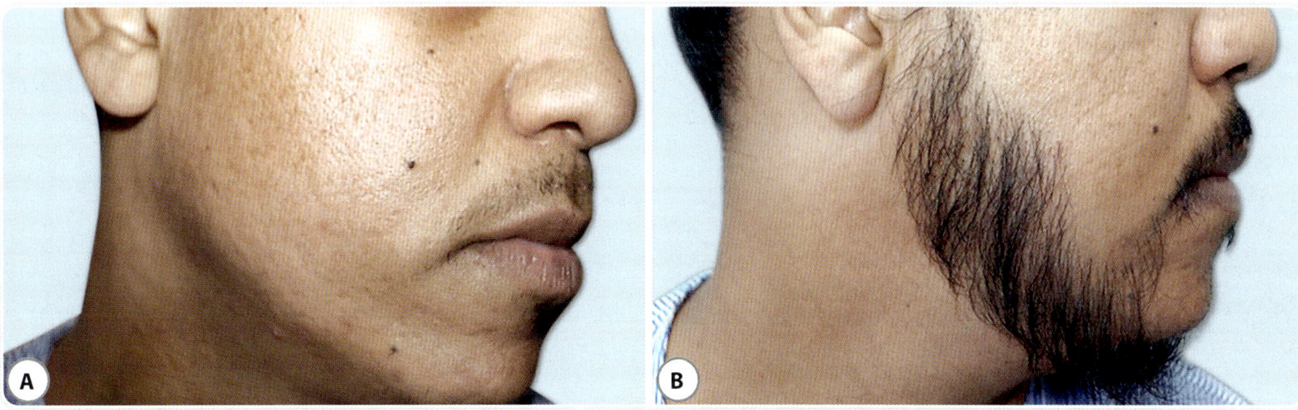

FIGS. 11A AND B: Results of beard and mustache transplant (case 1). (A) Before; (B) After 1 year.

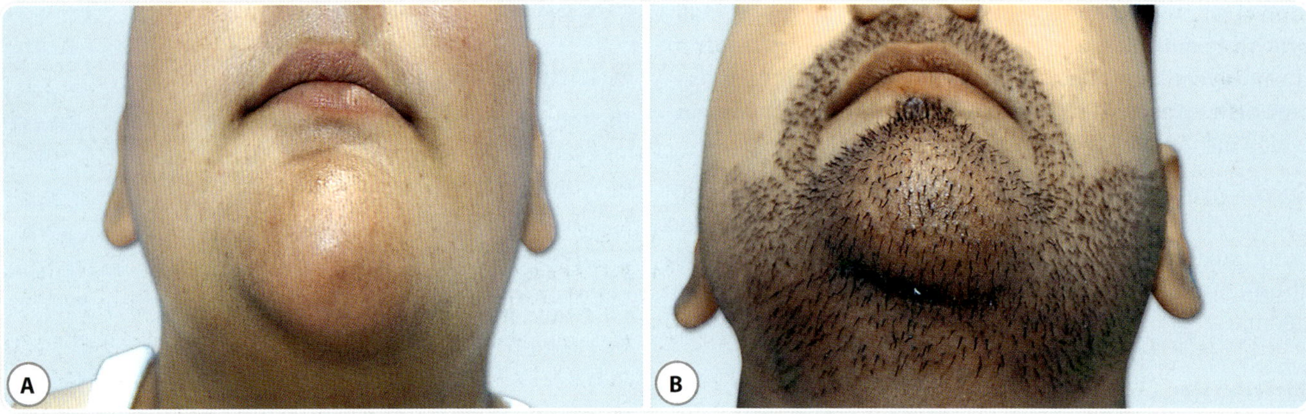

FIGS. 12A AND B: Results of beard and mustache transplant (case 2). (A) Before; (B) After 1 week.

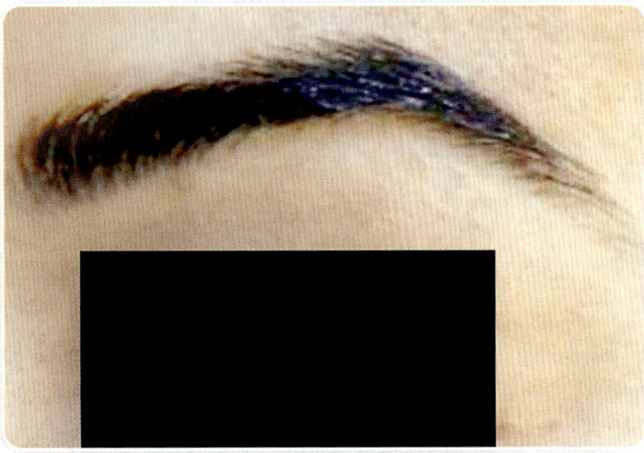

FIG. 13: Shape of eyebrow in women.

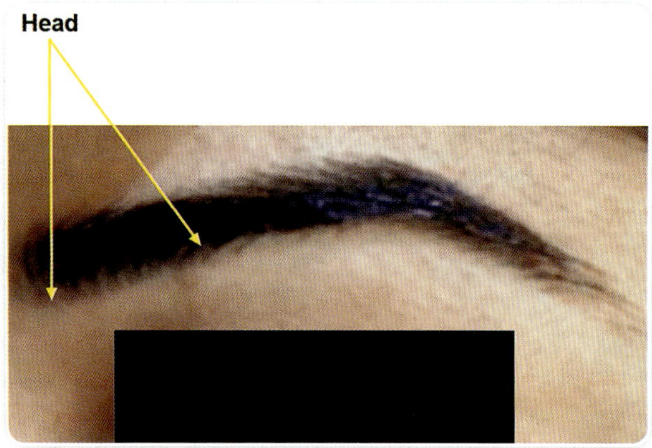

FIG. 15: Head of the eyebrow.

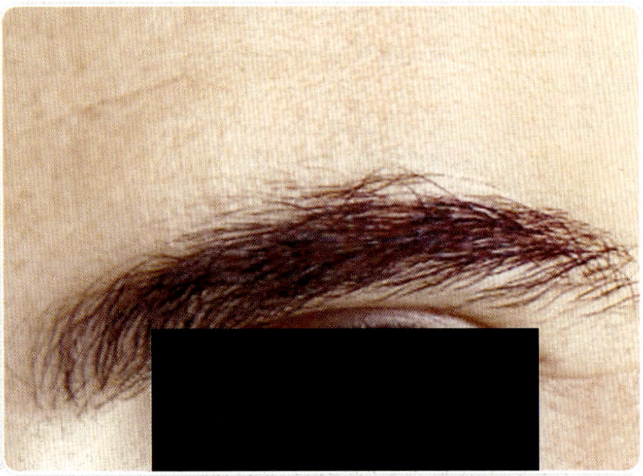

FIG. 14: Shape of eyebrow in men.

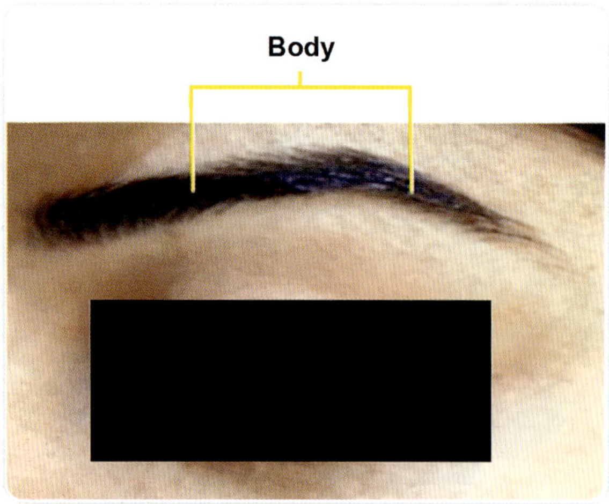

FIG. 16: Body of the eyebrow.

medial half of the body creating a subtle narrowing of the width of the outer half of the body in females.[7] In males, there is no narrowing of the lateral half of the body, and it may be kept as the widest portion to create a more masculine appearance.

The tail of the eyebrow **(Fig. 17)** averages around 10 mm in length. It is the narrowest portion and has the least density. It laterally descends from the peak of the arch in a subtle downward direction and flares horizontally.[7]

Creation of the Recipient Site

In the medial most part of the head, the direction of hair is vertical, and the grafts are placed sparsely to give a feathering appearance. At the transition of the head area into the body, there is a change of direction from vertical to horizontal. In the area of the body, the slits given on the upper border should have a slight caudal angle, while slits on the lower border should have a slight cephalic angle, resulting in cross-hatching **(Fig. 18)**. In the tail region, the slits are placed horizontally, in a slightly downward direction. In the lateral most part of the tail, sparse concentration is kept with fine one-hair grafts as it is a feathering zone. The angle should be very shallow, almost parallel to the skin, to prevent the hairs from sticking out.

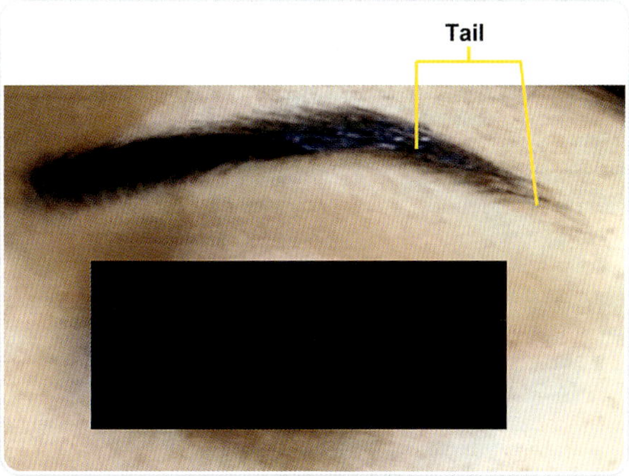

FIG. 17: Tail of the eyebrow.

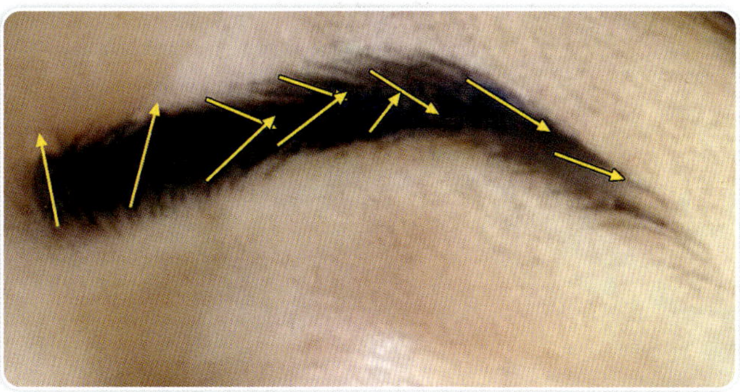

FIG. 18: Direction of hair with cross-hatching.

Donor Area

The best donor site is the midoccipital area of the scalp as the hairs have the best texture and curl and are least likely to turn gray. The other donor area that can be used is the legs. Either the strip technique or FUE can be used for graft harvesting. The donor strip of 6 × 1 cm provides around 400–450 grafts.

Implantation

Fine one-hair grafts are placed at "feathering zones" and at periphery. Two-hair grafts are placed in central areas. Grafts should be placed and rotated so that the direction of the curl complements the direction of the recipient site. After implantation, they should be evaluated again with the patient for any adjustments to be made in symmetry and overall appearance **(Figs. 19 and 20)**.

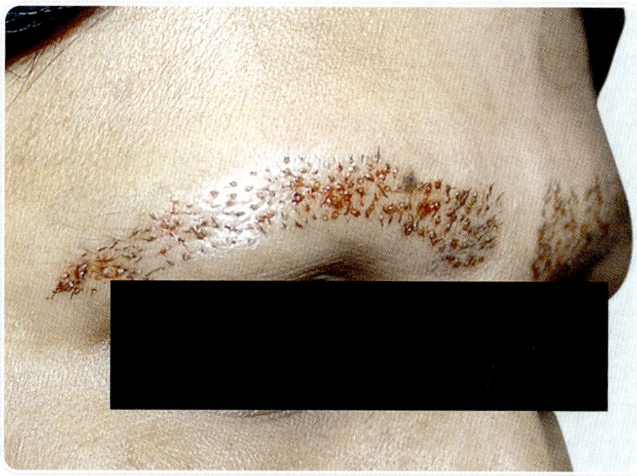

FIG. 19: Picture taken after implantation.

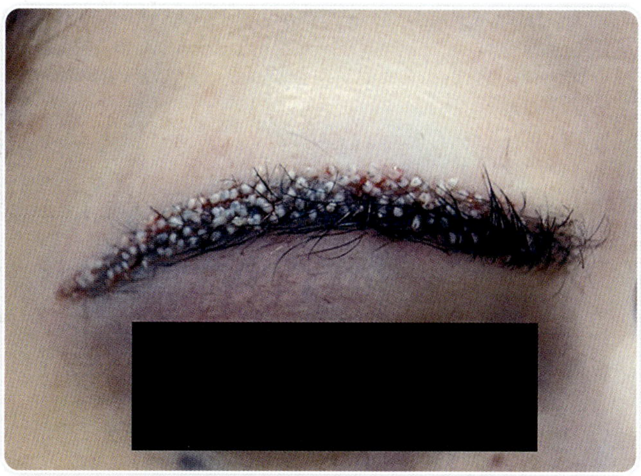

FIG. 20: Few weeks after implantation.

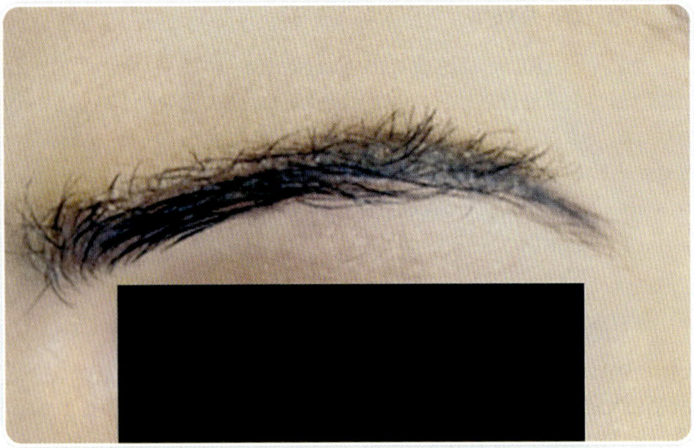

FIG. 21: Before surgery.

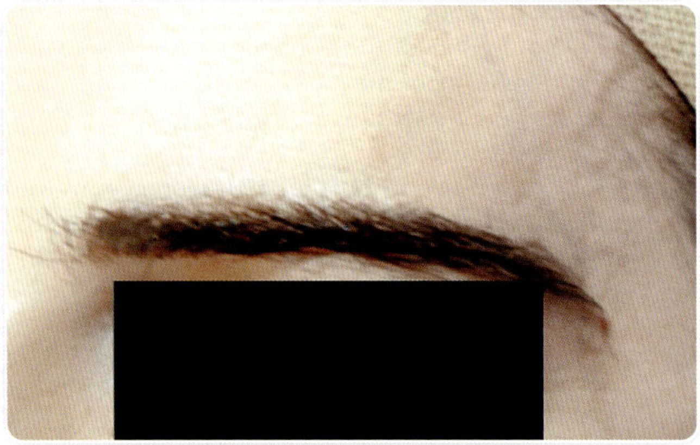

FIG. 22: After 4 months.

Postoperative Care

The eyebrows should be kept dry for 5 days. The implanted hairs will fall out in 2–3 weeks and the regrowth starts in about 3 months. Due to contracture of the skin, 10–15% may grow in an aberrant direction. These rogue hairs can be plucked or cut short or trained with gel for a more aesthetic look. If the scalp is used as a donor area, biweekly trimming is required. Around 10–15% of the patients want a revision of the eyebrow transplant surgery as they might be unhappy because of the misaligned direction.

Figures 21 and 22 show the results of eyebrow transplantation in a patient who had undergone a previous eyebrow transplantation.

SUMMARY

Facial hair transplantation needs special technique and experience.

Proper direction and placement of grafts are important to ensure a satisfactory outcome.

REFERENCES

1. International Society of Hair Restoration Surgery (ISHRS). (2015). Survey finds non-scalp hair transplants surge in popularity. [online] Available from http://www.ishrs.org/press-release/survey-finds-non-scalp-hair-transplants- surge-popularity. [Last accessed September, 2023].
2. Vogt A, McElwee KJ, Blume-Peytavi U. Biology of the hair follicle. In: Whiting DA, Blume-Peytavi U, Tosti A, Trüeb RM (Eds). Hair Growth and Disorders. 1.8.6 Duration of the Hair Cycle, Table 1.5. Berlin: Springer; 2008. p. 13.
3. Gandelman M, Epstein JS. Reconstruction of the sideburn, moustache, and beard. Facial Plast Surg Clin North Am. 2004;12:253-61.
4. Pathomva D, Imagawa K. Special procedures in hair restoration surgery: sideburn transplant and moustache transplant. In: Pathomvanich D, Imagawa K (Eds). Hair Restoration Surgery in Asians. Berlin: Springer; 2010. pp. 227-35.
5. Bebawy JF, Bilotta F, Koht A. A modified technique for auriculotemporal nerve blockade when performing selective scalp nerve block for craniotomy. J Neurosurg Anesthesiol. 2014;26(3):271-2.
6. Sanchez JP, Balingit JS, McCutcheon R. Local and Regional Anaesthetic Blocks Made Simple. Philippines: Nazarene Printers; 2002.
7. Epstein JS. Eyebrow transplantation. In: Unger W, Shapiro R (Eds). Hair Transplantation, 5th edition. New York: Informa; 2011. p. 465.

CHAPTER 78

Eyebrows Transplantation

Rajesh Rajput

Key Messages

- Eyebrows and eyelashes form important aesthetic landmarks on the face.
- Restoration of eyebrows and eyelashes needs a proper understanding of anatomy, natural design, and proper technique.
- The use of single hairs, premarking the slits flush to the surface, proper angulation and direction, and good density are all important to ensure a good outcome.

INTRODUCTION

Eyebrows add considerably to a person's beauty. Madarosis is the loss of eyebrows, and milphosis is the loss of eyelashes. The term madarosis has originated from "madao" in Greek, which means falling off.[1] Lack of eyebrows creates a distinct change in facial appearance, an attribute of the leonine facies, affecting beauty. Three important muscles of facial expression, orbicularis oculi, corrugators, and occipitofrontalis, are inserted into the dermis under the eyebrows, contributing to animation of the face with every expression. Eyebrows prevent sweat from trickling over the eyes. Eyebrow transplants were done by Okuda in Japan as early as 1939. Transplants planned just for thinning may have a risk of mismatch. It is worth mentioning that thinning eyebrows often respond to low-dose oral minoxidil (LDOM) 2.5–5 mg/day, though this is an off-label use.

INDICATIONS FOR EYEBROW TRANSPLANTATION

Common indications for surgical restoration of eyebrows are burns, trauma, Hansen's disease, stable alopecia areata, frontal fibrosing alopecia, or scarring alopecias, after expert opinion or biopsy to rule out active disease. Rarely, eyebrow transplant may be required for hypothyroidism, trichotillomania, or congenital absence of eyebrows.[2,3] Post-burns and post-traumatic eyebrow restoration is planned only after all other functional deformities are corrected, and no more procedures are required for the face.[4] Any other procedure for scar revision, flaps, skin grafts, and tissue expanders can shift the level of the reconstructed eyebrow to appear misaligned or asymmetrical.

With the present prevalence of skills and knowledge, eyebrow restoration is best done with follicular unit transplantation (FUT).[5] Previously, eyebrow reconstruction was attempted with the use of strip grafts and temporal artery-based flaps. These resulted in fibrosis, changes in the direction of hair growth, scarred borders, too thin or too bushy hair, and unnatural appearance. Eyebrows require the selective use of single hairs dissected out of a scalp strip or extracted individually as single hair units.[6] A good eyebrow should recreate a natural curve with a distinct pattern.[7]

CHARACTERISTICS OF A NATURAL EYEBROW

The eyebrows are arched rows of hairs growing in the facial skin along the upper borders of the orbit. The hairs of the eyebrows are short, thick, stiff, and nonpliable, displaying a slight curve along the body and tapering toward the end. Asians' eyebrow hairs are thinner than scalp hair, while

Caucasians' eyebrows are thicker compared to their scalp hair.[8,9]

Structure and Layout of the Eyebrow[8,10-12]

The eyebrow can be roughly divided into three parts from medial to lateral: Head, body, and tail. The medial third constitutes 10–15% of the eyebrow. It lies below the orbital margin with few staggered hairs oriented vertically. Often, you may not want to restore this area. The middle third, the body, constitutes 60% of the brow. It gradually arches upward and lies along the orbital margin. Hairs in the upper borders are directed downward and outward. Hairs in the mid-rows are directed horizontally, while rows along the lower border placed crisscross to the upper rows create a good aesthetic definition with hair overlapping along the curved longitudinal axis of the brow. The tail is the lateral part that constitutes 20–25% of the eyebrow, with hair directed horizontally. Eyebrows are less dense laterally than medially; thus, hair loss is more obvious in the lateral part.

There are two types of eyebrow patterns:

1. *Triple pattern brow*: Two rows of few medial hairs are angled slightly medially and vertically, gradually tilting outward toward the hair in the middle third growing vertically upward and outward, while the lateral third hair grows downward and outward **(Fig. 1)**. The brow is thickest medially and becomes challenging to match.
2. *Double row crisscross brow*: Hair in the upper and lower halves grow crisscross toward each other **(Fig. 2)**.

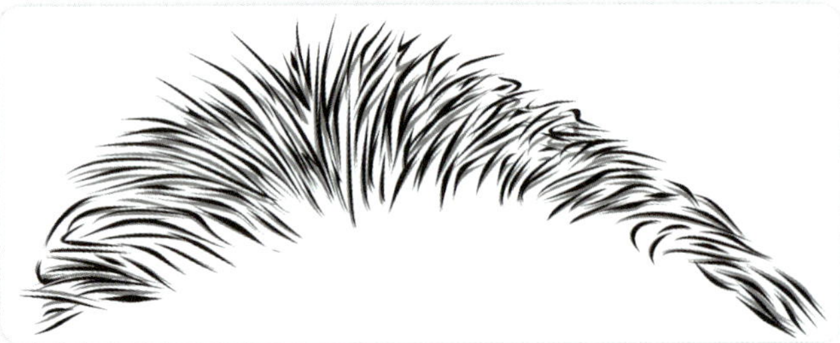

FIG. 1: Triple pattern brow.

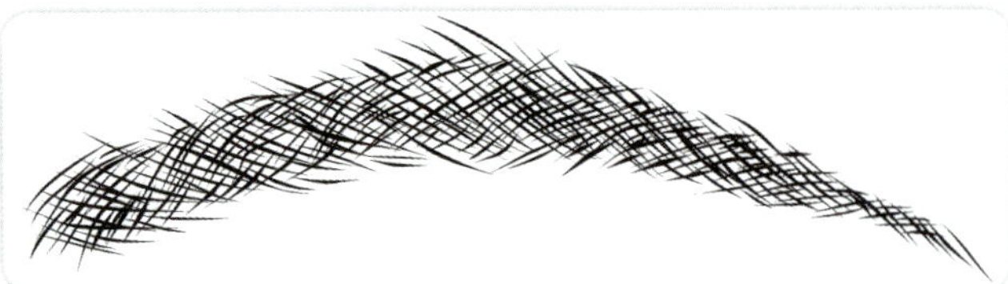

FIG. 2: Double-row crisscross brow.

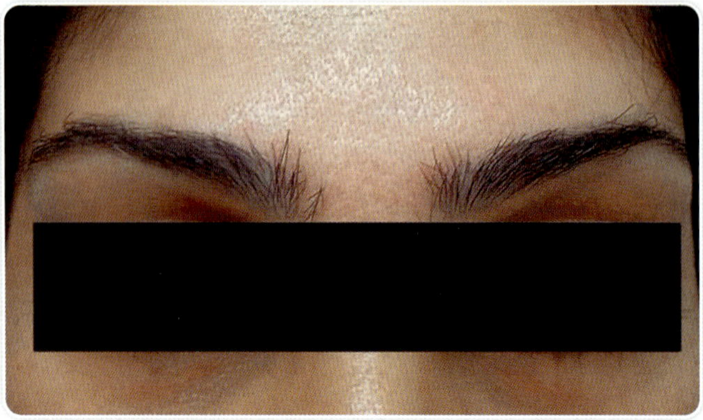

FIG. 3: Natural layout and eyebrow pattern.

The pattern and shape of the opposite brow or old photograph are a guide. A single eyebrow may require 70–130 single hair grafts placed in three to five rows. Brow slanting downward gives an elderly look. Brow placed higher gives a surprised look. An eyebrow placed low medially and raised laterally gives an angry look. The lateral end should be at the same horizontal level as the medial end or marginally higher. A horizontal brow divides a long face and makes it look rounded or shorter, while a curved brow can make a round face look longer. Female brows should be created thinner; the patients may like to draw the eyebrow for you. The female eyebrow begins slightly away from the medial canthus, is thinner, and more "C"-shaped, with maximum curvature at the lateral border of the limbus. The natural pattern of eyebrow is shown in **Figure 3**. In females, remember that the transplanted brow has thicker follicles, which are difficult to reshape with threading or plucking.

TECHNIQUE OF EYEBROW RESTORATION

Natural eyebrows are made of single hair. Thin, slow-growing hairs for eyebrow and eyelash restoration are selected from the lower neckline, below the nuchal ridge, or the lower part of the parietal scalp. Donor hairs can be harvested by either FUT or follicular unit extraction (FUE),[13] but the method of choice is FUE, which allows selectively harvesting single hair grafts and reduces donor area scarring. Single hair follicles are extracted with a 0.8-mm manual or motorized punch and implanted as micrografts. Use of an 18 G needle for harvesting single hair grafts has also been described, though this, nowadays, is not required with easy availability of punches.[14-16]

The other technique, less often used, is FUT. In FUT, an elliptical strip of scalp skin is excised 1 × 4–5 cm. The depth of the strip is restricted to the subdermal level. Restricting the thickness of the strip to the subdermal level preserves lymphatics, veins, and nerve endings, avoids neuromas and numbness, and ensures faster healing. Two-layered closure ensures a thin cosmetic scar. The scalp defect is closed in two layers. The excised strip is dissected or slivered along the width, under magnification, preferably under a stereomicroscope, creating single follicle rows of 8–12 follicles each, called slivers. Natural follicular units, having one, two, or three hairs, are dissected out from the slivers and further divided into single hair grafts for eyebrow restoration. The single hair grafts are implanted to match the required pattern, layout, and angle to create the new eyebrow.[17]

Medial eyebrow hairs are implanted pointing upward, gradually tilting outward, becoming parallel to the axis of the eyebrow in the middle third, and then sloping downward in the lateral third. Two or three rows placed in this pattern along the upper border will define the curve of the eyebrow. Then, two middle rows are placed parallel to the axis of the eyebrow, giving good body to the brow, and finally, in order to define the lower border, two rows of grafts from the lower border are placed at right angles across the grafts along the upper border. The lateral third of the brow gradually tapers into a tail having sparse spacing and thinner hair grafts. About 150 hairs are required for a thick, full eyebrow restoration. Retain 5–7 mm hair length in the grafts to identify the natural curve, guiding to match the direction and layout during implantation.[12,15]

Method of Placement of Grafts[18,19]

It is essential to place the grafts flush to the skin. Eyebrows placed at the slightest elevated angle grow out like canopies and look unacceptable. The grafts can be implanted in three ways:

1. Use of implanter device
2. Premade slits
3. Stick and place

For using an implanter, the hair grafts are loaded into the needle tip of an implanter. The implanter needle is pricked into the skin at the right angle and right depth, and a plunger is pushed to place the graft. The use of implanters can help overcome the lack of skill for graft placement. In premade slits, the slits are premade with a special 1-mm chisel blade **(Fig. 4)**, and the grafts are placed into these slits. Slits can also be made with a 19 G or 20 G hypodermic needle or a 0.9-mm blade. In the third method of stick and place, hypodermic needle punctures are made with left hand and grafts are placed immediately in the needle tracks with a forceps in the right hand. An assistant should stretch and stabilize the skin during the creation of the premade slits and during implantation

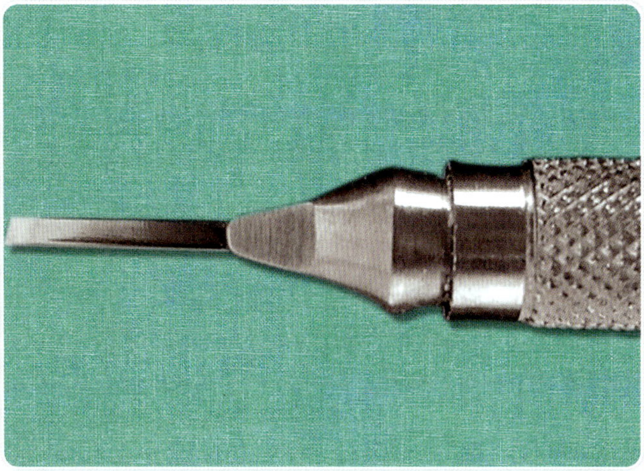

FIG. 4: Special chisel blade for making slits.

for easy placement of the grafts. The author prefers stick and place, using 20 G and 19 G hypodermic needles with minimum injury to the recipient skin **(Fig. 5A)**. The angle of the needle controls the direction, depth, and layout of the grafts. In scarring alopecias, the premade slit or the needle track must reach the avascular layer and shows punctuate bleeding through the site. The slight ooze indicates that we have reached a level of adequate blood perfusion available to the graft, suggesting better survival. Natural skin elasticity holds the grafts in place. Thick scars with no elasticity can be cored out with an FUE punch to create a track that can easily accommodate the graft without pressure. Scar areas often require a second sitting.

Spacing between the Grafts

For eyebrow restoration, the hairs are placed 1–1.5 mm apart in a staggered or brick wall partial overlap pattern. While transplanting into scars, it is best to wait for the scar to be mature, soft, supple, and not stuck to the underlying bone. In the scar, the grafts are spaced further apart at 2–4 mm to ensure good graft survival; density can be added later in a second sitting. In scars, the first sitting is best to be treated as a trial grafting.

Postoperative care: Patients are prescribed antibiotics and analgesics for 2 days. There is no dressing over the recipient areas. A thin layer of Neosporin ointment or Betadine ointment is applied to prevent drying on the grafts. The donor area is covered with Betadine ointment and pad for 2 days. A saline spray every 3 hours keeps the grafts moist and prevents dehydration. Patients are instructed not to touch the grafts for the next 2 days. Cold compresses in the periorbital area are advised three times a day to prevent swelling. The patient is allowed a head bath and removal of the donor dressing on the third postoperative day. During the bath, there should be no rubbing or friction over the grafts. A double-folded soft towel can be used to dab the areas or pat them dry. From the third day, gentle application of Neosporin ointment or Betadine with earbuds is advised twice a day. Patients are allowed or encouraged to gently rub the grafts during bathing after 10 days to facilitate removal of the crusts. Some hair will be shed along with the crusts due to anagen effluvium. Complete regrowth of the grafts takes 6–8 months. A second sitting should be planned only after 9–10 months.

RESULTS

The hair growth from grafts implanted in scar areas and alopecia areas is delayed. The grafts commence growth at 6 months instead of the usual 4 months and display good growth by 8 months. The reconstructed eyebrow not only creates an aesthetic landmark but also covers an uneven scar, with double benefit. However, density can be an issue and may need a second session **(Fig. 5B)**.[18] Patients are usually counseled for two to three sittings. In our review of eyebrow and eyelash restoration, only 9% of patients could be corrected in one sitting, 77% required two sittings, and 14% required three sittings. Scalp hair grafts grow faster than facial hair and need to be trimmed regularly.[19] Distorted growth can result from excessive handling, tight squeezing of grafts during implantation, or within an unyielding scar; there could be poor circulation from the scar bed. Injured or scarred surrounding tissue may compress the graft, leading to distortion of the angle and wavy growth. The distortion will be less pronounced in the subsequent hair cycles, and the hair will set better gradually in the next 8–10 months.[4,9] Coconut oil or Vaseline can be used to groom the hair and press it down to grow along the required direction.

Poor Growth and Failure of Graft Growth

Failure of 5–7% growth of grafts can be attributed to poor blood perfusion, compression of the grafts in the scar tissue, deep dermal scarring, too much handling, repetitive attempts of graft insertion, and implantation in the nonelastic scarred skin. This can be countered by premaking the slits or needle tracks or by extracting scar tissue with an FUE punch to facilitate graft placement. The loss of grafts and failure to grow improve with experience. The technique demands good surgical skills. The job is repetitive, time-consuming, and laborious, but the results are rewarding.

SUMMARY

- Eyebrow restoration is planned last, after completing all other surgical corrections on the face.
- Thin single hair should be selected for eyebrow restoration.
- Ensure placement of grafts extremely flush to the skin with premade tracks, slits, or implanters.
- Mimic the pattern of the opposite brow. In bilateral restoration, a crisscross pattern is of choice.
- Wait till the scar is mature, mobile, supple, and blanching.
- Reach the plane of punctate oozing in scar tissue.
- Wait 8–10 months for results in scar tissue.
- Always counsel the patient for two sittings.

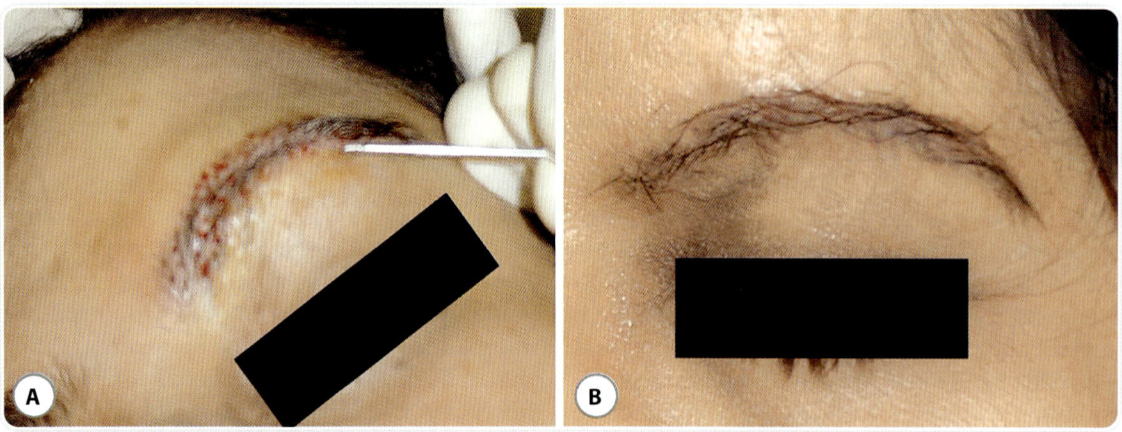

FIGS. 5A AND B: (A) Placement of grafts; (B) "C"-shaped eyebrow after construction.

REFERENCES

1. Kumar A, Karthikeyan K. Madarosis: a marker of many maladies. Int J Trichology. 2012;4(1):3-18.
2. Gandelman IM. Patient selection in hair transplantation. Annals of Brazilian Symposium on Facial Contour, Sao Paulo, Brazil; 1983.
3. Van Loey NE, Van Son MJ. Psychopathology and psychological problems in patients with burn scars: epidemiology and management. Am J Clin Dermatol. 2003;4(4):245-72.
4. Motamed S, Davami B. Eyebrow reconstruction following burn injury. Burns. 2005;31(4):495-9.
5. Avram M. Follicular unit transplantation for male and female pattern hair loss and restoring eyebrows. Ophthalmol Clin North Am. 2005;18(2):319-23.
6. Ergün SS, Sahinoğlu K. Eyebrow transplantation. Ann Plast Surg. 2003;51(6):584-6.
7. Mysore V. Controversy: synthetic hairs and their role in hair restoration? Int J Trichology. 2010;2(1):42-4.
8. Standring S. Face and scalp. In: Standring S (Ed). Gray's Anatomy: The Anatomical Basis of Clinical Practice, 40th edition. London: Elsevier; 2008. pp. 467-98.
9. Pathomvanich D. Anatomical restoration surgery of the eyebrow in Asian. Thai J Surg. 2004;25:47-52.
10. Dawber RP, Messenger AG. Hair follicle structure, keratinization and the physical properties of hair. In: Dawber R (Ed). Diseases of the Hair and Scalp, 3rd edition. London: Blackwell Scientific; 1997. p. 44.
11. Robbins CR. Chemical and Physical Behavior of Human Hair, 4th edition. New York: Springer-Verlag; 2002. p. 8.
12. Laorwang K, Pathomvanich D, Bunagan K. Eyebrow transplantation in Asians. Dermatol Surg. 2009;35(3):496-503.
13. Gandelman M. A technique for reconstruction of eyebrows and eyelashes. Semin Plast Surg. 2005;19:153-8.
14. Rassman WR, Bernstien RM, McClellan R, Jones R, Worton E, Uyttendaele H. Follicular unit extraction: minimally invasive surgery for hair transplant. Dermatol Surg. 2002;28(28):720-8.
15. Gandelman M. Eyebrow and eyelash transplantation. In: Unger WP (Ed). Hair Transplantation. New York: Marcel Deker; 1995. p. 294.
16. Bernstein RM, Rassman WR. Follicular unit transplantation: 2005. Dermatol Clin. 2005;23(3):393-414.
17. Limmer BL. Elliptical donor stereoscopically assisted micrografting as an approach to further refinement in hair transplantation. J Dermatol Surg Oncol. 1994;20(12):789-93.
18. Toscani M, Fioramonti P, Ciotti M, Scuderi N. Single follicular unit hair transplantation to restore eyebrows. Dermatol Surg. 2011;37(8):1153-8.
19. Kasai K. Eyelash reconstruction with strip composite eyebrow graft. Ann Plast Surg. 2008;60(6):649-51.

CHAPTER 79

Eyelash Transplantation

Sukhbir Singh

Key Messages

- Eyelashes add to the beauty and attractiveness of a person.
- Eyelash transplant is an uncommon but technically demanding procedure.
- Complex eyelid anatomy should be kept in mind for the same.
- There are various indications for the same most common being trauma and for beauty enhancement.

INTRODUCTION

It is a common saying that "Beauty Lies in the Eye of Beholder." Eyelashes not only add to one's beauty but also attractiveness and self-confidence. Eyelashes lost due to any reason can lead to loss of self-confidence. Though it is a delicate area, advancements in field of hair transplant have made eyelash transplant a reality as of today.

HISTORICAL BACKGROUND OF THE PROCEDURE

In 1917, Knapp[1] transplanted free graft strips from the eyebrow to the eyelid border. In 1980, Marritt[2] used a solid needle to insert hair follicles harvested from the periphery of 4-mm punch grafts into the eyelid border. Thus, various options have been used for eyelash restoration such as strip grafts from eyebrows; pedicled flaps from eyebrows; or single follicular units harvested and inserted with automated needles.[3]

EYELASH ANATOMY AND COMPARISON WITH SCALP HAIR

Eyelashes on the upper eyelid are much longer than those of the lower eyelid. Eyelash hair and scalp hair share some similar features[4] like hair shaft (the visible part), root under the skin and a bulb, which is the enlarged terminal portion as seen in **Figure 1**. The lash is made up of three structures:[5] *Medulla*—the innermost layer consisting of loose cells; *thicker cortex* surrounding the medulla to give strength and stability; and the *outermost cuticle*. The upper eyelid has more eyelashes, around 70–150 lashes and tend to curve upward with average

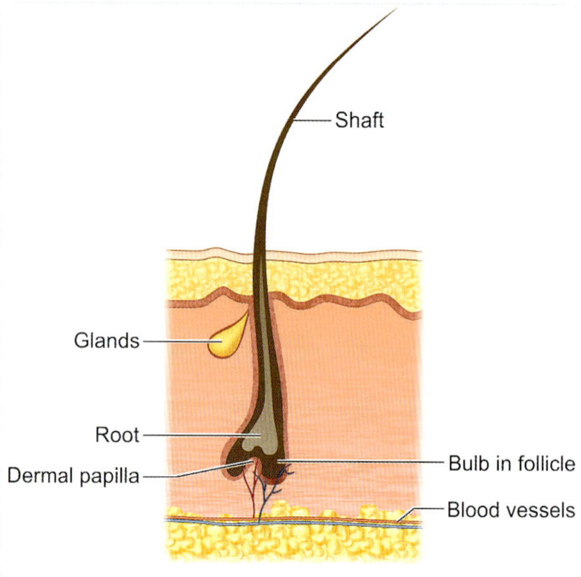

FIG. 1: Anatomy of the eyelash hair follicle.

TABLE 1: Differences between eyelash hair and scalp hair.

Eyelash hair	Scalp hair
Shorter than scalp hair	Longer than lash hair
No arrector pili muscle	Arrector pili muscle is present
Anagen phase is shorter: 4–10 weeks	Anagen phase is longer: 2–6 years
Growth rate is shorter: 0.12–0.14 mm/day	Growth rate is more: 0.3–0.4 mm/day

length of 8 mm. Lower eyelid has generally a row of 60–80 eyelashes, much smaller with a downward curve.

There are few notable differences between eyelash hair and scalp hair, which are listed in **Table 1**.[4,6-9]

Nesher et al. demonstrated that the prostaglandin analog F2α receptors were expressed in several layers of the lash follicle during its anagen phase.[10] There are two types of secretory glands in the lash follicles—Zeiss and Moll. The Zeiss glands produce sebum[10] through a holocrine mechanism, which has antimicrobial and lubrication properties and the Moll glands are apocrine glands[11] and their secretions contain variety of sugar components, which help in defense against microorganisms.[11]

ETIOLOGY OF EYELASH LOSS

Milphosis, or loss of eyelashes can occur due to various reasons:

- Congenital causes like congenital aplasia[12]
- Acquired causes like trauma (avulsion injury), burns, and tumor excision
- Iatrogenic causes like tattooing, wrong implantation methods leading to injury of healthy eyelashes
- Psychological disease such as trichotillomania
- Endocrinopathy such as thyroid disease
- Ophthalmic[13] causes like lid infestation (*Staphylococcus species*, *Demodex folliculorum*, trachoma) and/or lid inflammation (posterior blepharitis, ocular rosacea, and seborrheic blepharitis)
- Associated with eyebrow madarosis:[14] Dermatological diseases like alopecia aereata,[12] leukotrichia, and vitiligo.

PATIENT EXPECTATIONS AND EXAMINATION

Patient may seek treatment for actual eyelash loss or only aesthetic needs. Eyelash loss can involve upper eyelash (partial or complete) or both upper and lower eyelash. Eyelash examination should include detailed history along with assessment of surrounding structures like eyebrow, scalp, and beard hair. Exact reason of eyelash loss must be found out including previous localized infection or trauma, leading to scarring with eventual loss of the eyelash.

EYELASH TRANSPLANT

Donor area: The donor area is typically finer hairs from temporal area,[15] nape of neck, or postauricular scalp region. The donor area harvesting is done under local anesthesia under loupe magnification. It can be either a strip harvest or follicular unit excision (FUE), depending upon individual surgeon's expertise. Usually, single root hair follicles are used; if roots are multiple, slivering is done under loupe magnification, and single hair roots are isolated and used for implantation.

Eyelash Transplant—Steps of Technique

- *Donor area harvesting*: FUE from the postauricular scalp region and nape of the neck.
- *Local anesthesia*: Along the eyelid border. Since the amount of local anesthesia is quite less, we inject 2% lidocaine with adrenaline (1:200,000 concentration) along the eyelid border. No tumescence is used for the procedure.
- Placing of wet cotton layer covering the cornea (corneal shield can be used alternatively).
- Double twisting the 20G straight needle to make a small curve (French eye needle[15] can also be used).
- Curved needle is placed on the syringe holder.
- Passed from the upper eyelid skin side (taking care to stay above the tarsal plate) and come out at the eyelid margin (exit of eyelashes).
- The assistant then feeds the single follicular unit at the needle exit.
- The needle is pulled retrogradely.
- The follicle is placed in the desired position.
- Care is also taken to maintain the curl and proper direction of the eyelashes to prevent trichiasis and any damage to the neighboring healthy follicles.
- Few authors have described other ways for eyelash transplantation:
  - Using implanters such as Choi or Kyungpook National University (KNU) implanter, which allow the hair to be implanted at the desired angle.[16]
  - Gandelman[17] used a sewing needle. A long donor hair is harvested and is sewn into the eye of the curved needle. The root being larger than the shaft stays outside the eye. The needle is passed from the conjunctival side of the eyelid margin (6 mm from the margin) to emerge through the lid margin and pulled out. The needle is then slid down the shaft.

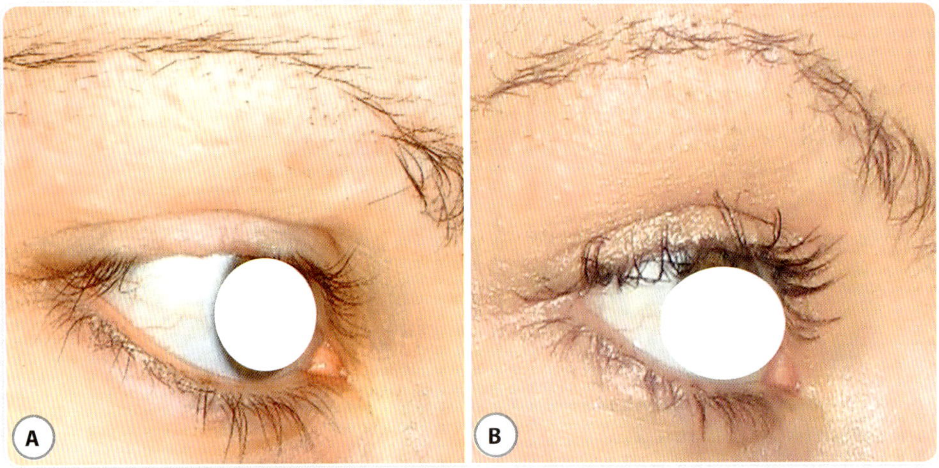

FIGS. 2A AND B: Postoperative figure of the patient post eyelash transplant 1 year.

The curve of the needle ensures the curvature of the grafted hair. Videos 1 and 2 show anaesthesia and implantation techniques for eyelash transplant.

Postoperatively

- Immediate postsurgery icing is done to prevent the swelling.
- Antibiotic cream is applied.
- No other dressing is done.
- Patient is asked to wear protective glasses.[12]

Complications

Eyelash transplant procedure requires extreme care during transplant since we are operating very close to the eye, especially the cornea which needs to be protected to avoid injury. Complications are rare if proper precautions are taken; however, the documented ones are as follows:

- Folliculitis
- Bleeding
- Scarring
- Eyelid ptosis
- Trichiasis[18]

Trichiasis[18] needs special mention as it means misdirection of the eyelashes, which can irritate the cornea, and hence it requires urgent reintervention and removal of the transplanted follicle.

Tips and Pearls

Eyelash transplant is in high demand because of the natural results and improvement in facial aesthetics it can produce if done properly as seen in **Figures 2A and B**. Vice-versa if not done well it can damage the cornea and may be the eye permanently. So, only doctors trained in these kinds of procedures should venture to do the same since it is a matter of someone's eyes and face.

POINTS

1. Leukotrichia and vitiligo can be added under indications
2. Can mention other techniques for eyelash transplantation
3. Can mention other donor areas

REFERENCES

1. Knapp P. Klin Monatsbl Augenheilkd. 1917;59:447.
2. Marritt E. Transplantation of single hairs from the scalp as eyelashes. Review of the literature and a case report. J Dermatol Surg Oncol. 1980;6:271-3.
3. Choi Y-C, Kim J-C. Eyebrow, eyelash, moustache and pubic area hair transplantation. In: Unger WP, Shapiro R (Eds). Hair Transplantation. New York: Marcel Dekker, Inc; 2004. pp. 579-84.
4. Marieb E. Le Système Tégumentaire. In: ERPi (Ed). Anatomie Et Physiologie Humaines, 3rd edition. 2005. pp. 156-208.
5. Liotet S, Riera M, Nguyen H. Les cils. Physiologie, structure, pathologie. Arch Ophtalmol (Paris). 1977;37:697-708.
6. Montagna W, Ford DM. Histology and cytochemistry of human skin. 3. The eyelid. Arch Dermatol. 1969;100(3):328-35.
7. Na JI, Kwon OS, Kim BJ, Park WS, Oh JK, Kim KH, et al. Ethnic characteristics of eyelashes: A comparative analysis in Asian and Caucasian females. Br J Dermatol. 2006;155(6):1170-6.
8. Thibaut S, De Becker E, Caisey L, Baras D, Karatas S, Jammayrac O, et al. Human eyelash characterization. Br J Dermatol. 2010;162(2):304-10.

9. Paus R, Burgoa I, Platt CI, Griffiths T, Poblet E, Izeta A. Biology of the eyelash hair follicle: an enigma in plain sight. Br J Dermatol. 2016;174:741-52.
10. Nesher R, Mimouni M, Elnaddaf H, Nemet A, Kidron D. Characterization of prostaglandin F2 alpha receptors in human eyelids. Eur J Ophthalmol. 2015;25:81-4.
11. Stoeckelhuber M, Stoeckelhuber BM, Welsch U. Human glands of Moll: histochemical and ultrastructural characterization of the glands of Moll in the human eyelid. J Invest Dermatol. 2003;121(1):28-36.
12. Gandelman M. A Technique for Reconstruction of Eyebrows and Eyelashes. Seminars in Plastic Surg. 2005;19(2):153-8.
13. Vij A, Bergfeld WF. Madarosis, milphosis, eyelash trichomegaly and dermatochalasis. Clinic Dermatol. 2015;33:217-26.
14. Kumar A, Karthikeyan K. Madarosis: a marker of many maladies. Int J Trichol. 2012;4:3-18.
15. Gandelman M. French needle technique. In: Barrera A (Ed). Hair Transplantation. St Louis, MO: Quality Medical Publishing; 2002. pp. 178-80.
16. Caputy GG, Flowers RS. The "pluck and sew" technique of individual hair follicle placement. Plast Reconstr Surg. 1994;93(3): 615-20.
17. Kasai K. Eyelash reconstruction with strip composite eyebrow graft. Ann Plast Surg. 2008;60(6):649-51.
18. Murchison AP, Wojno TH. Trichiasis after eyelash augmentation with hair follicle transplantation. Ophthal Plastic Reconstr Surg. 2007;23(4):323-4.

CHAPTER 80

Vertex Transplantation

Suneet Soni

Key Messages

- Anatomically, vertex is a challenge because of its circular shape, radiating direction of hair, presence of whorls, and possibility of expansion of baldness in a circumferential pattern.
- Vertex baldness is viewed in its entirety by a viewer and hence is noticed easily, causing much emotional distress to the patient.
- Age is an important consideration for treatment in view of possible future hair loss.
- A holistic treatment plan, which includes both medical and surgical management, needs to be discussed for vertex baldness.

INTRODUCTION

The vertex, often referred to as the crown, is the most posterior area of Norwood types III and IV or greater male pattern baldness. The most anterior border of vertex area is often shaped as a "mirror image" of its posterior border, thus creating a circular or oval form. Vertex is a round, contoured part of head that looks balder because of natural contours and whirling pattern. In Norwood type IV or V, male pattern baldness, the anterior outline of vertex area usually ends at the posterior border of mid-parietal bridge.[1] This chapter also needs to be read along with chapters on Scalp Anatomy, Hairline Design, and Recipient Methods, as they contain additional relevant information.

ANATOMY

Vertex (Crown)

The "vertex" (or the more vernacular term, "crown") is the most posterior area of male pattern baldness, which is characterized by a "whorl" arrangement of hair direction and which can range from the small, early thinning vertex in its minimal degree of baldness up to the large vertical wall of baldness seen in an advanced Norwood class VI or VII male, and includes all the variations between these two **(Figs. 1 to 3)**.

Vertex Transition Point

This is the midline point on the posterior half of the scalp, near the rear of the midscalp, where the horizontal plane starts to become vertical **(Fig. 4)**. It generally lies just

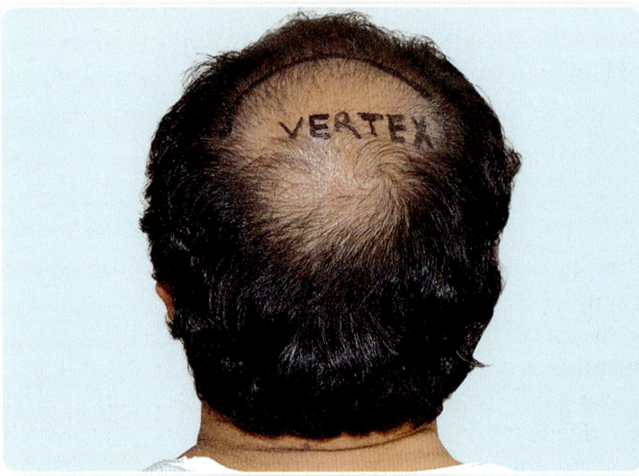

FIG. 1: Posterior view of patient showing vertex.

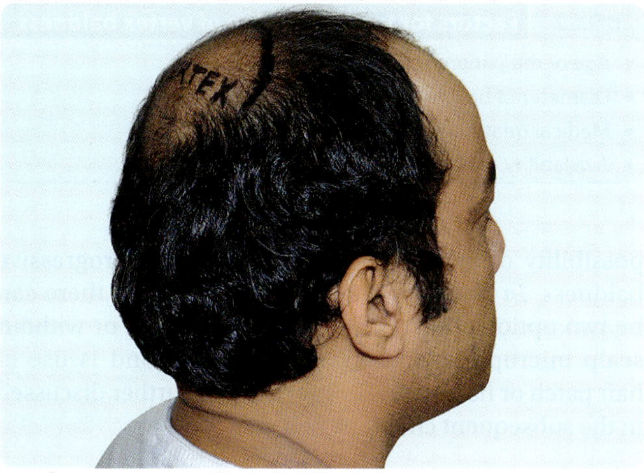

FIG. 2: Posterolateral view of patient showing vertex.

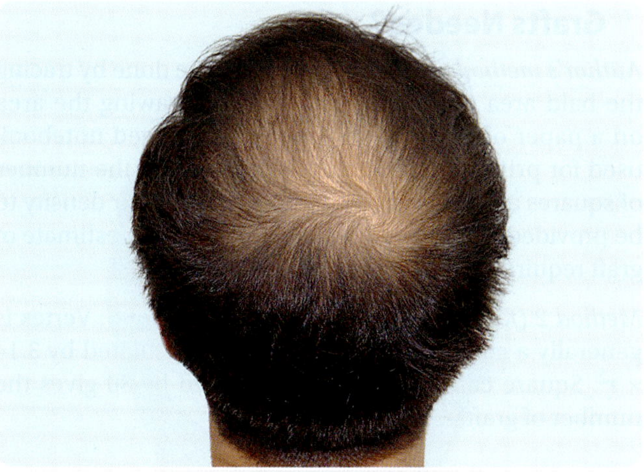

FIG. 3: Lateral view of patient showing vertex.

behind the highest part of the skull and lies approximately where the hair changes from a generally anterior direction to that of a whorl arrangement. This aspect is designed in greater detail in Chapter 81 on Designing the Vertex.

COUNSELING CHALLENGES IN VERTEX BALDNESS

The most important factor in vertex hair transplant is counseling of patient **(Box 1)**. As in all cases of hair transplantation, but even more so in vertex baldness, a young patient, particularly below 25 years of age, is not a good candidate for surgery and is better treated medically with minoxidil and finasteride. This is due to the possibility of hair loss and, more significantly, the circumferential progression of baldness in all directions. The young patient (25–30 years of age) needs to be

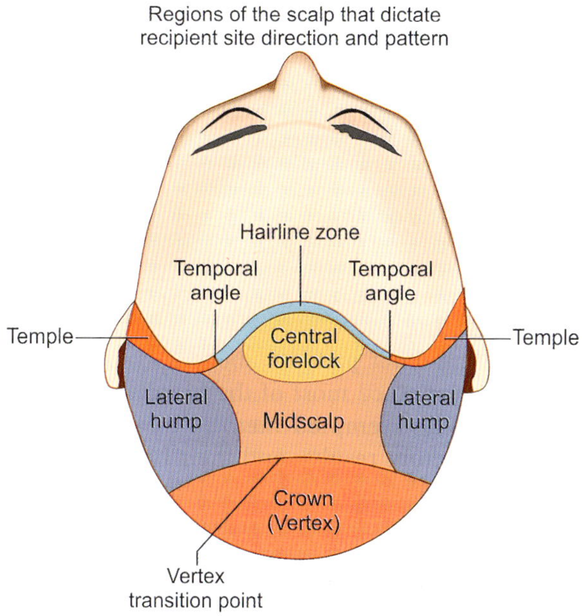

FIG. 4: Vertex transition point.

BOX 1 Treatment plan for vertex baldness.

- Always treat early cases medically
- Delay the transplant in a young patient
- Counsel him in detail with photographic evidence
- Follow-up with the patient to understand his psyche before performing the surgery
- Always consider requirement for a second or third session while planning

warned about the possibility, in the future, of evolving areas of male pattern baldness. Regular progression of vertex baldness should be monitored. By doing this, a physician is in close follow-up and gets to know the progress of baldness.[2-4] This will enable the surgeon to take appropriate decision for hair transplant at the right time. Vertex baldness affects the patient severely, as he himself cannot see it but invites comments from others; further, vertex is easily visible and is seen in its entirety-like a billboard. Photographic documentation is, therefore, particularly important in counseling.

It is the general principle to delay the vertex transplantation as much as possible, at least 35 years of age. However, surgical treatment in a young patient can be considered if:

- Vertex baldness has stabilized for >2 years
- Medical treatment has been tried but has not yielded results, resulting in frustration to patient, but after appropriate counseling

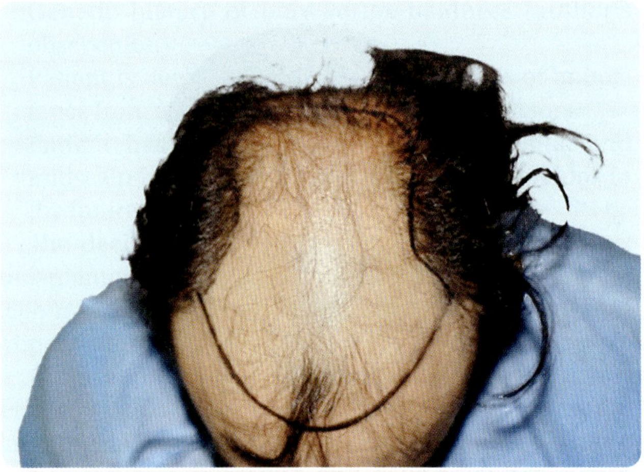

FIG. 10: Patient with higher grade baldness (top view).

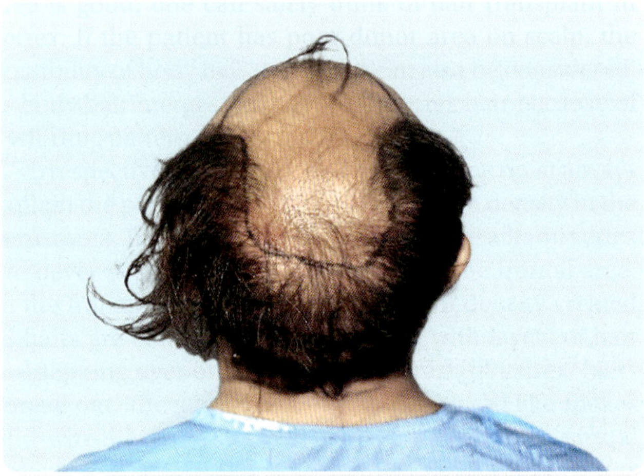

FIG. 11: Patient with higher grade baldness (back scalp view).

For example, a 35-year-old patient with higher grade baldness (grade 6) **(Figs. 10 and 11)** underwent a hair transplant procedure using 4,900 grafts **(Fig. 12)**. Among these grafts, 3,200 were obtained from FUT, 900 from FUE **(Fig. 13)**, and 800 from BHT (beard hair FUE extraction) **(Fig. 14)**.

After 1-year post operation, the patient was satisfied with a natural hairline design and good frontal area density **(Fig. 15)**. The midscalp area showed mild density coverage, and the vertex area showed low density coverage with a natural whorl design **(Fig. 16)**.

Anesthesia

Generally, donor anesthesia is adequate for lower part of vertex. Only the front part needs to be anesthetized, and hence the amount of lignocaine needed is less. Adequate tumescence is necessary as in all cases of hair transplantation.

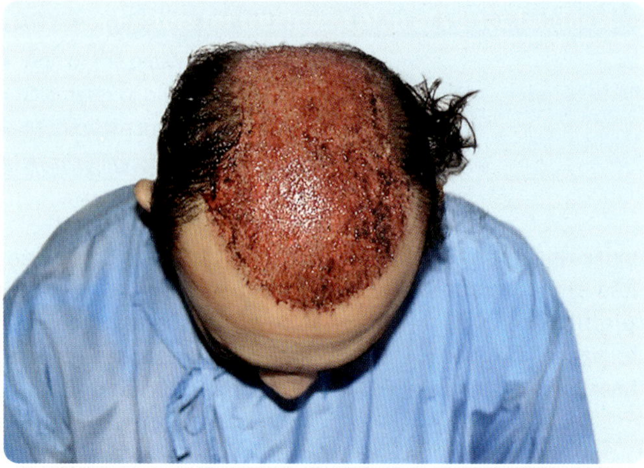

FIG. 12: Triple combination (FUT, FUE, and BHT)—4,900 grafts' implantation.

(BHT: body hair transplant; FUE: follicular unit extraction; FUT: follicular unit transplant)

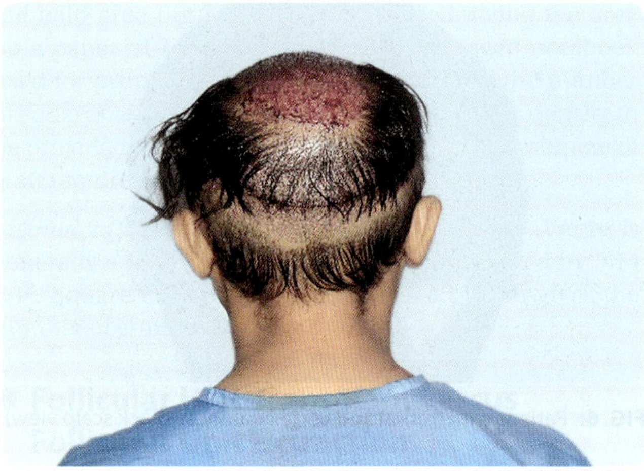

FIG. 13: Extracted 3,200 FUT grafts and 900 FUE graft (combination of FUT + FUE).

(FUE: follicular unit extraction; FUT: follicular unit transplant)

Creating Whorl Pattern

If residual vertex hairs or even vellus hairs are present, then it is best to adopt a patient's natural whorl center point as epicenter **(Fig. 17)**. Sometimes, there are two separate whorls, in which case the author likes to select only one whorl and transplant hair to spin off from it. In cases of total vertex baldness where hardly any hairs are left, it is essential to create a new whorl **(Fig. 18)**. How to select the correct location of a whorl is a tough task. The author likes to place a whorl at the right side or just inferior point of epicenter to get the maximum benefit of overlapping. In a higher grade of baldness (grade VI), the whorl center can be slightly right of midline but superior

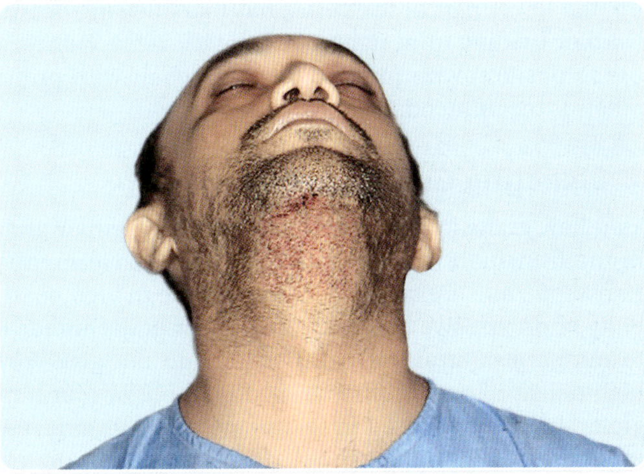

FIG. 14: 800 graft extraction from BHT (beard hair FUE extraction). (BHT: body hair transplant; FUE: follicular unit extraction)

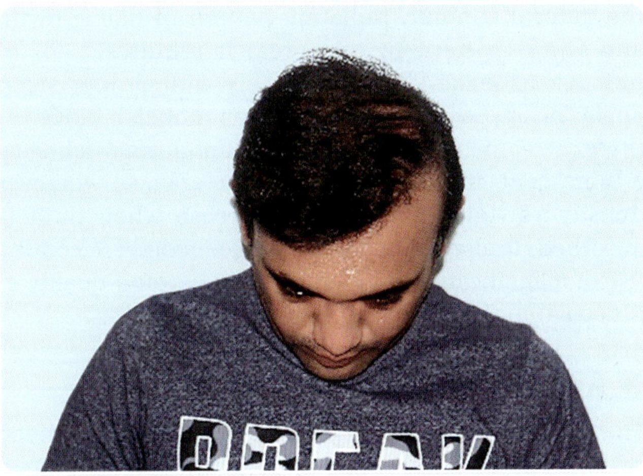

FIG. 15: After 1-year post operation (top view).

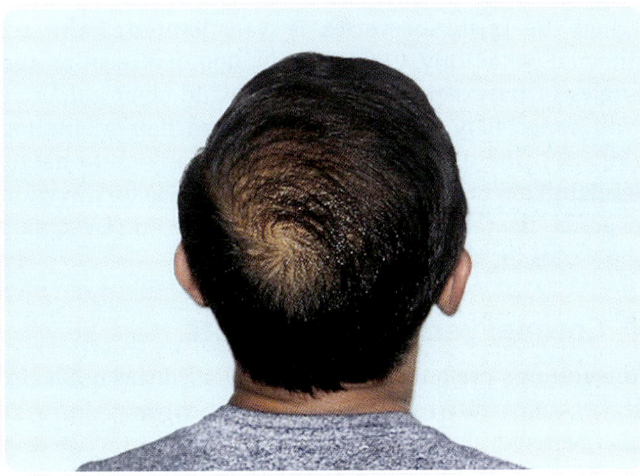

FIG. 16: After 1-year post operation—vertex area.

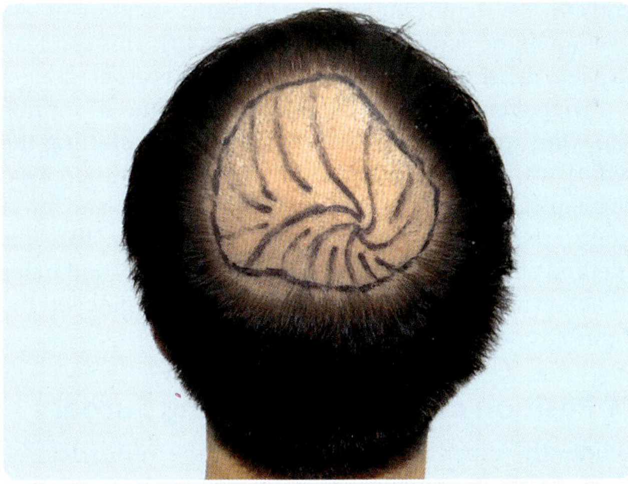

FIG. 17: Marking for vertex whorl with the aid of existing hair. Marking should be done before trimming the hair.

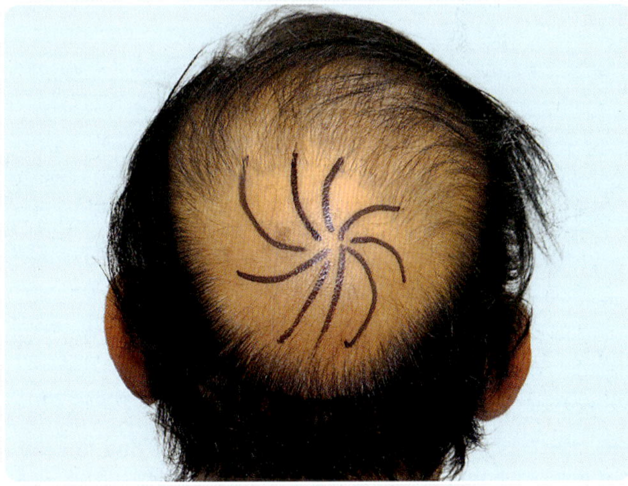

FIG. 18: Marking for vertex whorl when there are no hairs at all.

to or as midpoint of vertical height of vertex (i.e., at halfway point of a vertical line drawn from midline occipital fringe to the midline point of the anterior border of the vertex or the vertex transition point).

Whorl creation can be difficult and also consume a large number of grafts. In such cases, particularly for beginners, it is recommended that instead of a whorl, a fall can be given wherein below a particular level (lower one third), all the hairs can be planted as to flow downward. This is easier and is also effective (personal communication by Dr Rajesh Rajput).

Shifting the Whorl Posteriorly

In cases where a large area of the vertex needs to be covered with the central whorl pattern, creating the central whorl consumes a significant number of grafts, resulting in less overlap in the central vertex zone **(Fig. 19)**. This can lead to a less dense appearance in the central vertex area.

To overcome this situation, the technique of shifting the whorl posteriorly can be employed. By shifting the whorl toward the posterior region, there is increased overlap of hair in the central zone of the vertex, and fewer grafts are required to achieve a fuller look **(Fig. 20)**. This method allows for a more efficient use of grafts and helps in achieving a denser and more fuller appearance in the central vertex area.

Position of the Patient during Surgery

While the upper part (front part) of the vertex can be grafted with the patient reclining comfortably, with face up, the lower part of the vertex has hairs flowing downward or twirling from right to left or vice versa. Hence, a prone position with prone pillow or a chair with prone pillow is recommended.

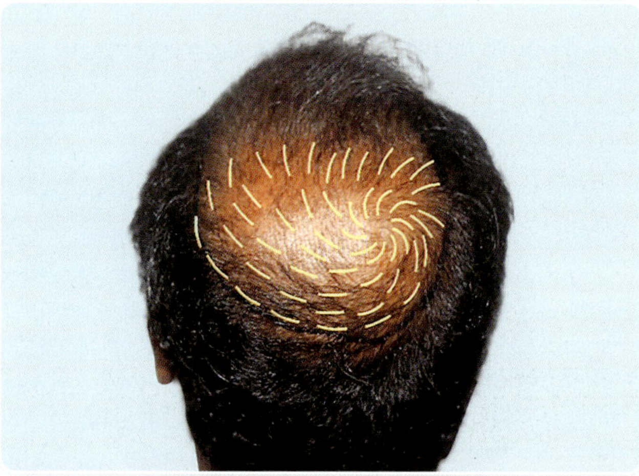

FIG. 19: Less overlap in the central vertex zone due to central position of whorl.

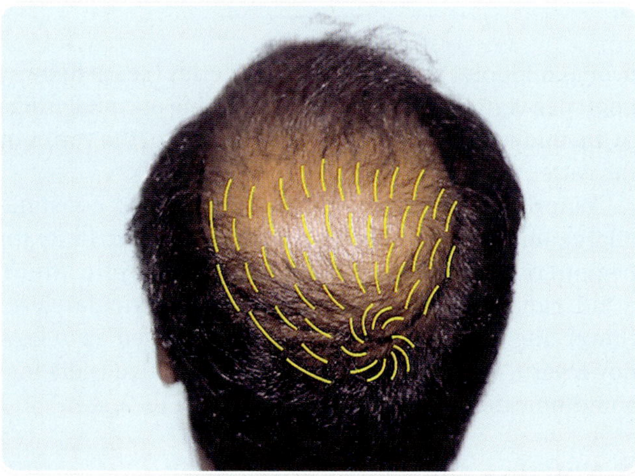

FIG. 20: Shifting whorl posterior to increasing overlap at central vertex.

Selecting Graft Sizes

Two hair grafts in the central zone and single hair graft in the transition zone are recommended. Covering the transition zone is extremely important due to high possibility of progressive baldness. Single-hair grafts are ideal to mimic a natural pattern, but they do not give very high density. In the authors' opinion, three or four hair grafts should be avoided in central areas as it gives a very unnatural pluggy appearance.[6] However, this is a matter of opinion, and many surgeons use three to four hair grafts in the totally bald part of the scalp, particularly upper vertex.

Giving density in vertex can be very tricky owing to the natural contour, radiating pattern of hair growth, and whorl pattern in that area. It requires a lot of practice to make slits very closely with proper steep angle (prior practice can be done on models); however, there are some tips. Firstly, use a lot of normal saline as a tumescent. It increases the surface area, so whatever density you give will further increase when fluid is absorbed. It also helps in reducing bleeding. Secondly, use of magnification is essential, such as good-quality 4′ binocular magnification.

Angle and Direction of Graft

The angle of recipient sites in vertex will affect aesthetic results significantly. Hair should always be placed at a more acute angle, most often 20°–45° and never approaching 90°. In the anterior and superior region of vertex, the hair will generally be directed inferiorly or angled to right or left to reflect the normal whorl pattern. When the posterior vertex is transplanted, hairs are directed posteriorly. Close examination of directions and angles of preexisting hairs will provide clear guidance with respect to proper recipient area graft/hair orientation **(Fig. 21)**. The direction changes frequently and existing miniaturized hairs should be used as a guide for direction of grafts. The reader is referred to chapter 81 on Designing the Vertex for more details.

Coronal versus Sagittal Slits

The author's preference is to do sagittal slits as it has the least trauma rate to existing hair, but coronal slits may also be used, depending on the surgeon's practice and ease.

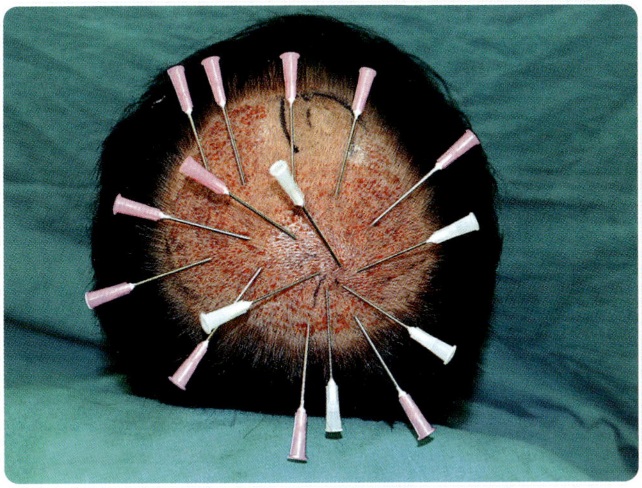

FIG. 21: Direction and angles of implantation of hair graft in vertex baldness.

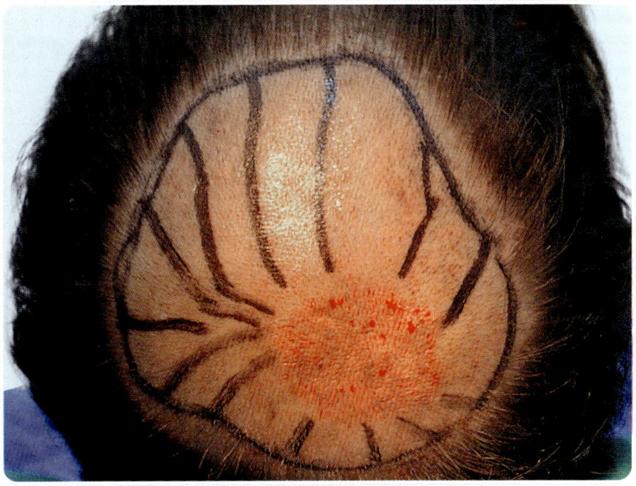

FIG. 22: Punching the slits in the vertex region is done from the center to periphery. Implantation of hair proceeds in the same way. It is important to provide hair even in the transition zone between the bald vertex and the area of thick hair in the periphery.

Method of Implantation

The author uses a preslit method. However, other methods such as slit and place, and implanters can also be used, and this is a matter of individual preference and often a combination of different techniques is needed.

Needles versus Blades

This is a matter of preference, and both needles and blades can be used. Author prefers to use 18 G and 19 G needles over blades. Needles are disposable, sharp, easily available, presterilized, and cost effective.

How to Progress to Create Whorl?

After marking the area and hairline pattern with a marker, the hairs are trimmed, and adequate tumescence with normal saline till skin blanches and becomes tense is achieved. Then slits are made first anteriorly in supine position, then in the sides in lateral position, and finally posteriorly in prone position. The creation of the slits proceeds from the center to the periphery, at each of the sites **(Fig. 22)**. After making central most part of 3–5 cm radius, the remaining anterior part in supine position is covered. Implantation proceeds in a similar fashion.

POSTOPERATIVE INSTRUCTIONS AND PROTOCOL

The patient is advised to avoid sleeping on back for the first couple of days. He should sleep on side or forehead to avoid rubbing on vertex area. The patient is also instructed to start washing his hair daily with mild shampoo after 24 hours. Detailed information is available in the Chapter 68 on Immediate Postoperative Care. The vertex is more difficult to clean by the patient himself and hence may need assistance and proper demonstration.

COMPLICATIONS

The most important complication is a dissatisfied patient because of less density than he had expected. The need of a second sitting should always be forewarned. Emptiness in the central-most part, even in high density transplant, may occur, and this possibility should also be forewarned to the patient. Photographic documentation is, therefore, of utmost importance. There could be a problem in architecture, design, and angulations which may make the result aesthetically unappealing. These are avoided by proper technique. Progression of the male pattern baldness may lead to a peripheral halo in long-term follow-up in some patients, if they do not take medical treatment properly. These patients may need further procedures **(Figs. 23A to C)**.

Results of vertex transplantation are shown in **Figures 24 and 25**.

SUMMARY

There is no debate that vertex is the most difficult region of the scalp to transplant. Theoretically, all men with male pattern baldness in the vertex can undergo hair transplant; in practice, however, certain precautions have to be taken. There are a few important factors which

REFERENCES

1. Ziering C, Krenitsky G. The Ziering whorl classification of scalp hair. Dermatol Surg. 2003;29(8):817-21.
2. Haber RS. Pathogenesis and medical therapy of male and female pattern hair loss. In: Haber RS, Stough D (Eds). Hair Transplantation (Vol. 4). China: Elsevier Health Sciences; 2006. pp. 154-47.
3. Kaufman KD, Olsen EA, Whiting D, Savin R, DeVillez R, Bergfeld W, et al. Finasteride in the treatment of men with androgenetic alopecia. J Am Acad Dermatol. 1998;39(4 Pt 1): 578-89.
4. Olsen EA, Weiner MS, Delong ER, Pinnell SR. Topical minoxidil in early male pattern baldness. J Am Acad Dermatol. 1985;13(2 Pt 1): 185-92.
5. Shaprio R. Placing grafts: an overview of basic principles and current controversies. In: Unger WP, Shaprio R (Eds). Hair Transplantation, 4th edition. New York: Marcel Dekker; 2004. pp. 533-9.
6. Barrera A, Uebel C. Hair Transplantation: The Art of Micrografting and Minigrafting, 2nd edition. St. Louis, Missouri: Quality Medical Publishing; 2014. p. 291.

CHAPTER 81

Designing the Vertex

Anil Kumar Garg, Seema Garg

Key Messages

- At a younger age, the vertex can best be treated by medication and topical solution.
- The hair restoration of the scalp is incomplete by not restoring the vertex.
- A detailed discussion with the patient is necessary before transplanting the vertex.
- Usually, transplanting the vertex is considered after the restoration of frontal and mid-scalp transplantation.

INTRODUCTION

The vertex is a posterior zone that lies between the mid-scalp and the permanent occipital zone. Hair loss in the vertex has less impact on the appearance of a person but has impact on his feeling. As it is said, "hair loss in the front hurts one's appearance, while hair loss in the vertex hurts one's feeling".

Vertex is the single most risky region of the scalp in hair transplant (HT). It is always a debate whether to transplant the vertex, considering progressive hair loss with limited donor hair availability. Pattern of hair loss, age, family history, and donor availability significantly affect the restoration of this area. So generally, it is said that "vertex is like a black hole" where hundreds of hair follicles are utilized, resulting in minimal cosmetic effect. There is always a preference to restore the facial frame first by transplanting the front area of the scalp, especially in young individuals. At a younger age, the vertex can best be treated by medication and topical solution. Transplanting the vertex can be taken after the completion of the restoration of the facial framework and at a later age. Today, techniques of harvesting and implantation have improved, and it is possible to use nonscalp donor areas to provide extra hair follicles, which improve our ability to cover the vertex. The scalp show of the vertex can be reduced by doing scalp micropigmentation.

The reader is referred to the chapter 80 Vertex Transplantation for details.

If a patient has a limited donor area and still wants an HT, the following options can be considered **(Box 1)**:

- The first option is to restore the upper area of the crown so that the individual can camouflage the remaining part of the vertex by combing hair in a posterior direction.
- The second option is to perform peripheral vertex transplant to reduce the bald area.
- The third option is to cover the entire vertex, including the anticipated future area of hair loss, with a lower-than-average density of hair.
- The fourth option is if mid-scalp hair has been lost and we are not planning to transplant the vertex, then, an anterolateral border must be created at the junction of the mid-scalp and vertex.

Detailed discussion with the patient is necessary before opting for any of these options because none of the above options cover the entire bald area of the vertex.

BOX 1 Vertex transplant.

Options for vertex transplant are as follows:

- Do not transplant the entire vertex with uniform density
- Transplant the entire vertex with graded density, less in the center and more at the periphery
- Transplant only at the periphery
- Transplant in the uppermost zone of vertex, hair in downward direction
- Create an anterolateral border of the vertex only

It is very important to visualize future hair loss in the vertex before undertaking HT. The easy way to assess this is to wet the patient's hair. This simple procedure will give useful information of future hair loss, which needs prior planning to cover this area. Blending grafts into this area of hair thinning will limit the chance of showing an unnatural balding halo as a result of progressive hair loss.

HAIR ARRANGEMENT IN VERTEX

Hair distribution and pattern in the vertex are unique and complex. Restoring normalcy means maintaining a normal existing hair pattern. It requires careful observation of existing patterns and loss with anticipated patterns of hair loss. There are different patterns of hair arrangement in the vertex (Ziering study).[1] There can be a so-called S pattern **(Fig. 1A)**, which describes a clockwise whorl; "Z" pattern which describes an anticlockwise whorl; a combination of S and Z patterns with adjacent whorls, namely an "SS" **(Fig. 1B)** or an "SZ" **(Fig. 1C)**, and there can be diffuse patterns.

Challenges in Vertex Transplantation

Limited donor hair follicle supply to cover advanced grade of baldness is one of the major limiting factors for vertex coverage. The vertex transplantation is the last priority in the aesthetic restoration sequence of the scalp. The vertex is convex in shape, having bony prominences. A convex surface has a larger surface area in comparison to a flatter surface. The hair distribution pattern in the vertex is complex, and recreation of such a pattern with limited donor follicle supply is difficult **(Figs. 2A to C)**. The whorl pattern of hair in the vertex reduces the illusion effect, which means cosmetic efficacy requiring more number of hair follicles.

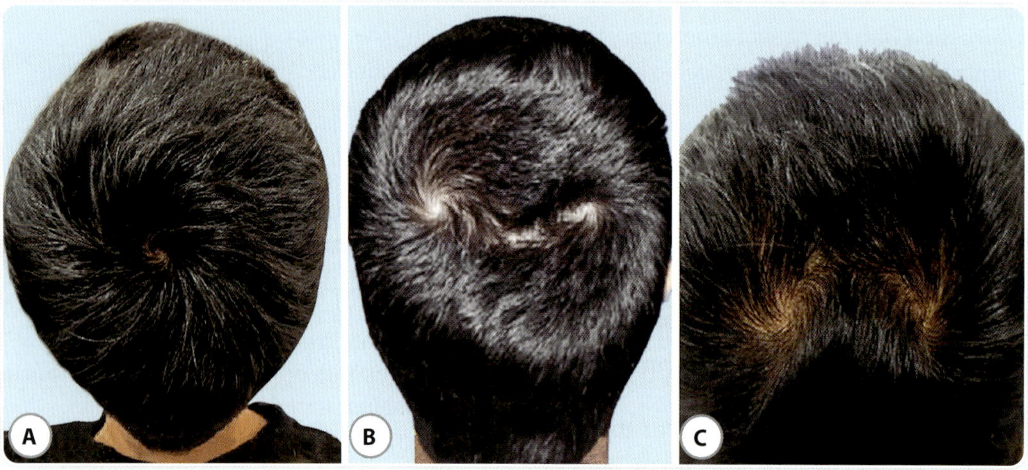

FIGS. 1A TO C: Various whorl patterns in vertex: (A) Single "S" whorl; (B) Double "S" whorl; (C) Double "S" "Z" whorl.

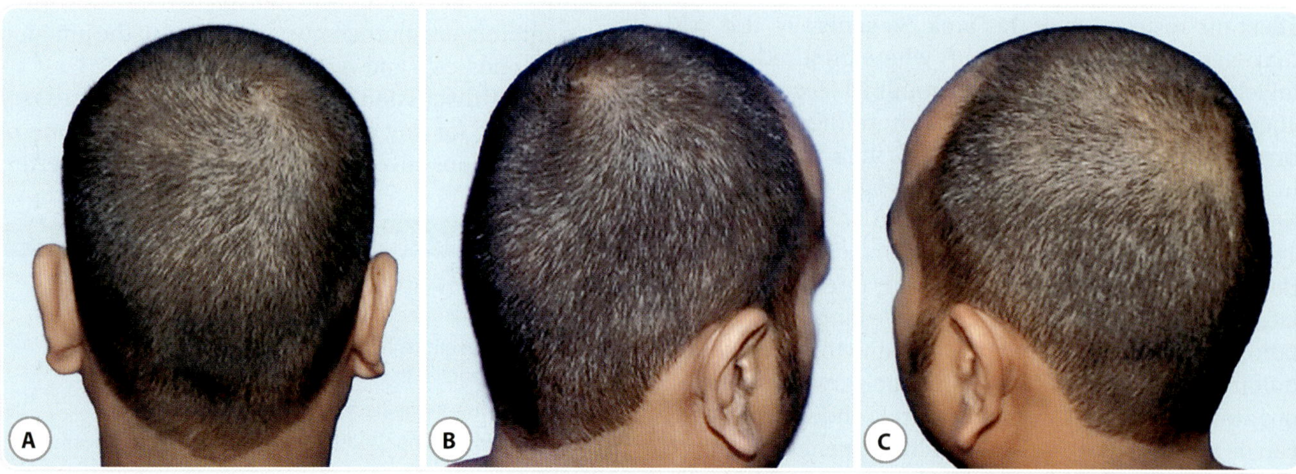

FIGS. 2A TO C: Complex hair arrangement in vertex.

Evaluating Patients for Existing Hair Pattern

The best guide is existing vellus hair in the vertex. If a patient does not have any whorl left, it is better to place a single whorl in the center, precisely on the side of the part. If the patient parts his hair from left to right, the whorl should be designed clockwise on the left side of the head so that the upper limb of the vertex arc matches the hair part and the follicles' part. Also, matching the same direction of the hair part facilitates hair styling.

Patient Position and Implantation in Vertex

Slit creation and implantation are better done in the prone position or in sitting position with the patient reclined approximately 45º and the surgeon standing. Thai massage chair is a good option for creating sites/slits as well as simultaneous extraction of follicles and implantation. We may need to put the patient in lateral position while creating slit and implanting on both lateral sides of the whorl. Planning the vertex can be divided into four parts **(Box 2)**:

1. Center of whorl
2. Upper arc
3. Lower arc
4. Vertex transition point **(Figs. 1A to C)**

Planning the Vertex Transplant

The best guide is the existing vellus ("ghost" hair).[2] Most of the time, there are few thin hairs left that help in determining the native hair patterns in the vertex. If a patient does not have any whorl left, it is better to place a single whorl off-center, precisely on the side of the part, with the arc matching the part. If the patient parts his hair from left to right, the whorl should be designed clockwise on the left side of the head so that the upper limb of the vertex arc matches the hair part. Also, matching the same direction of the hair part facilitates hair styling.

Slit Creation in Vertex

Slit creation and implantation are best done with the patient either in a prone position or in a sitting position with the patient reclined approximately 45° and the surgeon standing. This position can be very well maintained on the Thai massage chair, as shown in **Figures 3A and B**. Another option is with the patient lying in the lateral positions.

Vertex can be divided into three subzones **(Figs. 4A to D)**:

1. Upper zone
2. Middle zone
3. Lower zone

The whorl is part of the middle and lower zones.

Angle of Implantation in the Vertex

The natural angle of hair emergence increases from the nape of the neck to the anterior-most area of the upper

BOX 2 **Planning follicular units (FUs) in the subregion of vertex.**

- Center of the whorl: Smaller grafts, 2 FUs/1 FUs
- Upper arc: Stronger multifollicular units, 3 FUs and 4 FUs
- Lower arc: Finer grafts, like 1 FUs and 2 FUs
- Vertex transition zone: 2 FUs/3 FUs

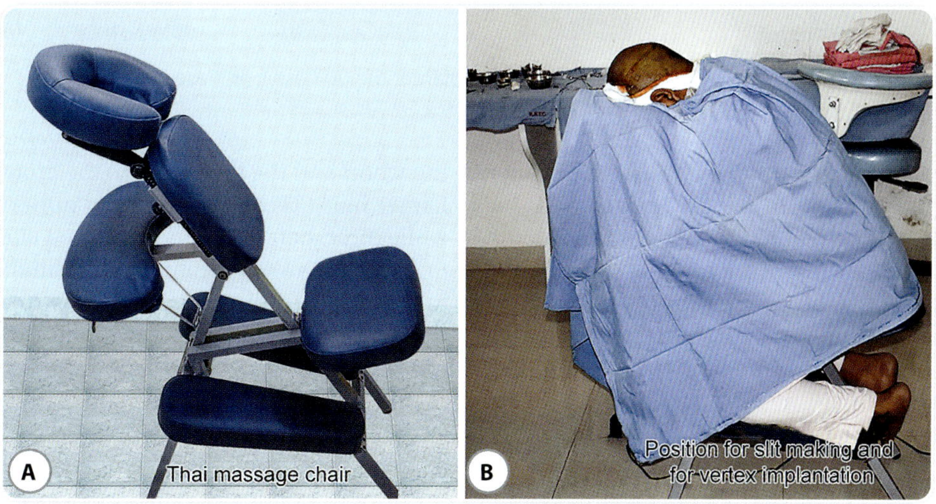

FIGS. 3A AND B: Thai massage chair for slit creation and implantation in vertex area.

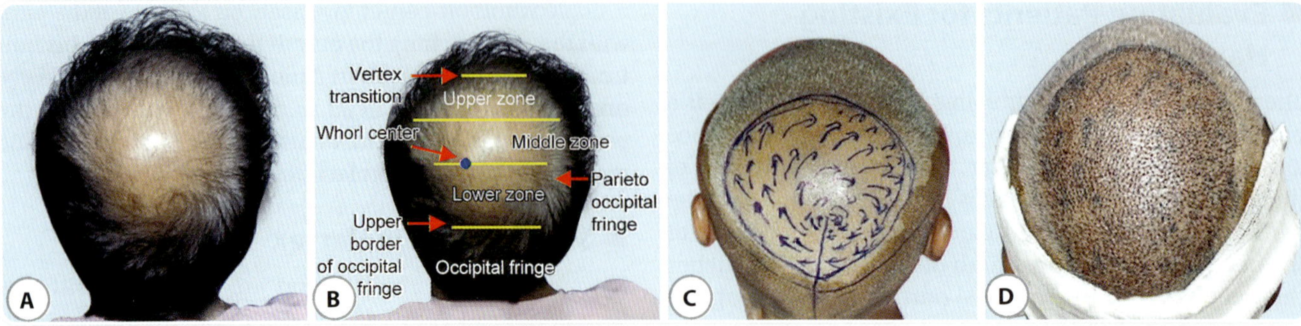

FIGS. 4A TO D: (A) Vertex hair loss; (B) Zones of vertex; (C) Planning of whorl in vertex; and (D) Hair transplant in vertex.

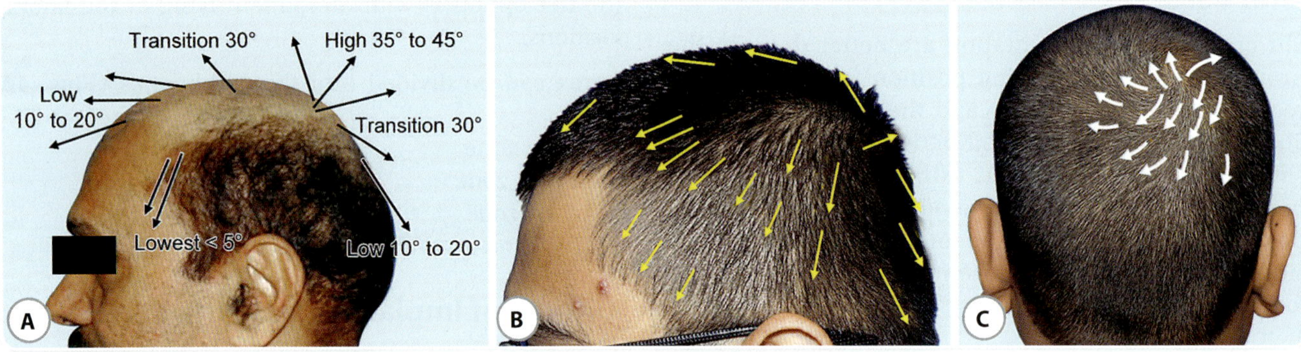

FIGS. 5A TO C: Different angles and directions of implantation in the scalp.

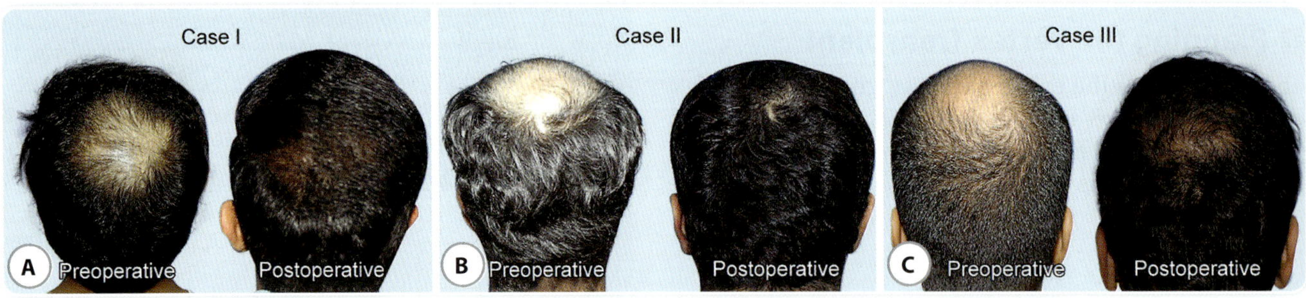

FIG. 6: Preoperative and postoperative photo showing vertex transplantation: (A) Case I; (B) Case II; (C) Case III.

zone of the vertex, at which point the angle of emergence lessens over the mid-scalp, frontal area to the anterior hairline (AHL). This pattern of hair maintains the smooth roundness of the head when we look in a lateral view. During implantation, gradual transition of the angle needs to be maintained to get a good aesthetic outcome **(Figs. 5A to C)**. In the lower zone, it is 10–20°, and near the vertex transition zone, it may go up to 35–45° of implantation **(Figs. 5A to C)**.

It is always advisable to start implanting from the center of the whorl to the periphery, mostly smaller follicular units (FUs) (1 and 2 hair FUs) to the center of the whorl and the lower half of the crown **(Figs. 4 and 5)**. Larger hair FUs are used for the upper arc of the vertex, while three-hair FU grafts are placed laterally to the whorl to create the sweep of hair that transitions from an upward to a downward direction. If reconstruction is needed in the vertex transition zone, two-hair FUs are used to give more density and blend smoothly into the mid-scalp. A mix of single- and two-hair FUs is placed into the circumferential fringe. The upper arc of the vertex needs a higher density grafting. This adds more visual density to the lower vertex area and to the posterior mid-scalp region. **Figure 6** showing few results of vertex transplantation.

SUMMARY

The vertex needs to be approached cautiously, after careful planning and counseling. The adage "undersell and underdeliver" applies more to the vertex than almost any other area.

REFERENCES

1. Ziering C, Krenitsky G. The Ziering whorl classification of scalp hair. Dermatol Surg 2003;29(8):817-21. discussion 821.
2. Garg Anil, Men-Crucial aspects of hair transplant design. In Robert H True, Anil K Garg, Seema Garg, ed. Practical guide to hair transplantation, Ist ed. New Delhi, Thiem 2021:214-18.

CHAPTER 82

Approach to a Patient with Early Hair Loss and Long-term Planning

Sandeep Sattur, Indu S Sattur

Key Messages

- Hair loss at a young age can have a significant impact on the psychosocial behavior of the patient.
- Management of such patients needs a careful approach as the primary aim is to stabilize the hair loss.
- Only in selected cases, hair transplant would be an appropriate option with thorough counseling, proper assessment of donor reserves, and conservative planning.
- Concomitant medical therapy would be necessary.

INTRODUCTION

Male pattern hair loss (MPHL) usually starts after puberty; often, it progresses rapidly and leads to significant hair loss at a very early age.[1-3] This can cause significant adverse effects on psychosocial well-being and lead to demand for transplantation. This chapter deals with issues involved in such patients. The reader is also referred to the chapter 25 on Overview and Approach to Medical Management of Male Pattern Hair Loss.

MANAGEMENT OF MALE PATTERN HAIR LOSS

Management of MPHL depends on the age, grade and pattern of hair loss, expectations, lifestyle, and financial capabilities of the patient. Management can be briefly described as nonsurgical, surgical, and camouflage.

Management of MPHL can be looked at in the manner shown in **Flowchart 1**.

Male pattern hair loss is an age-related problem that gets worse as one gets older. The extent of hair loss as well as the speed with which one loses hair cannot be predicted in all affected individuals. This has to be kept in mind before suggesting treatment options to the patients.

Patients seeking treatment for MPHL fall into one of the following categories:

- Those who wish to know if there is some underlying problem that has led to the hair loss
- Those who wish to maintain their existing hair and stabilize hair loss
- Those who wish to get back some of the hair that was lost
- Those with a body image problem

Based on their expectations, treatment recommendations have to be made. Category 1 needs proper evaluation, appropriate medical treatment, and reassurance; category 2 will need medical treatment; category 3 will need hair transplantation with or without medications (for those patients who do not wish to use long-term medications); and category 4 needs counseling.

Currently, we have limited proven modalities to manage this problem. Topical minoxidil lotion and oral finasteride, an inhibitor of type 2 5α-reductase, are the only medical treatments of proven efficacy in MPHL. They help prevent or delay the progression of hair loss and can stimulate some regrowth of hair in some men. Neither of these drugs will be able to regrow hair on a completely bald scalp, and continued treatment is necessary to maintain the benefits.[4-6]

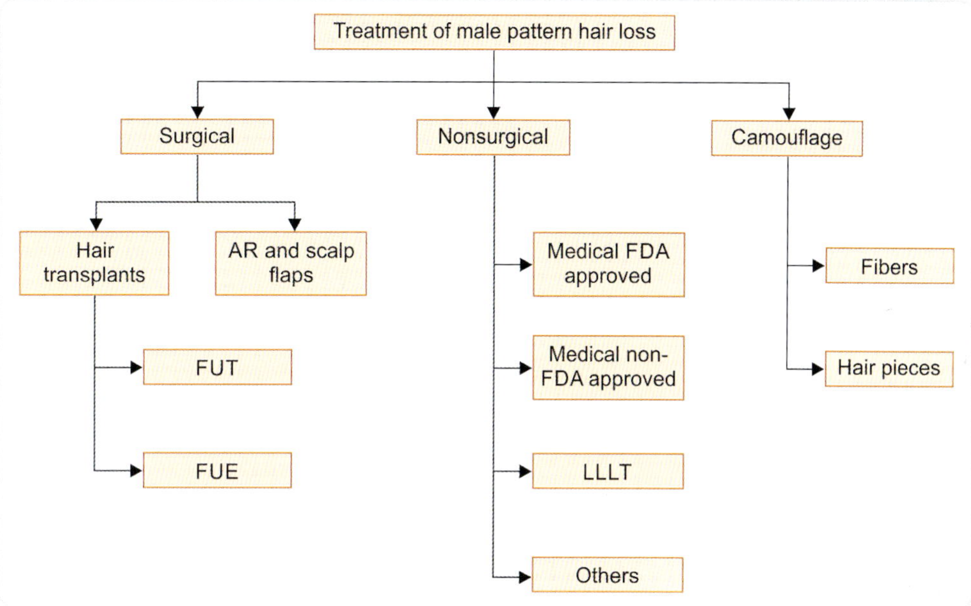

FLOWCHART 1: Management of male pattern hair loss.
(AR: alopecia reduction; FDA: Food and Drug Administration; FUE: follicular unit extraction; FUT: follicular unit transplantation; LLLT: low-level laser therapy)

Today, with refinement in techniques and instrumentation, hair transplantation has evolved into a state-of-the-art therapy. Hair transplantation is the only surgical method that will produce coverage on bald scalp. The most common areas of hair loss that are addressed with hair transplantation are the frontal, temporal, and mid-scalp areas. Moreover, most patients today are more psychologically inclined toward hair transplantation, often demand hair transplant, and this technique remains the primary means by which we address pattern hair loss, providing reasonably satisfying results for the surgeon and recipient alike.

It is equally important to understand that each modality (surgical, nonsurgical, and camouflage) will address different aspect of the hair loss. When we look at a patient with patterned hair loss (PHL), there are two issues that need to be dealt with:

1. The progressive nature of the hair loss
2. The deficit created by receding hairline/baldness

Both of these aspects will have different treatments.

Hair transplantation involves transferring follicles from the permanent zone of the scalp to the areas of baldness.

Hair transplantation will provide permanent follicles where there were none or relatively reduced. But, it has no impact on the progress of hair loss in the other areas of the scalp. So, hair transplantation does not solve the problem completely. On the other hand, when we use minoxidil and/or finasteride, the spectrum of response ranges from keeping the hair loss stabilized to actual regrowth.

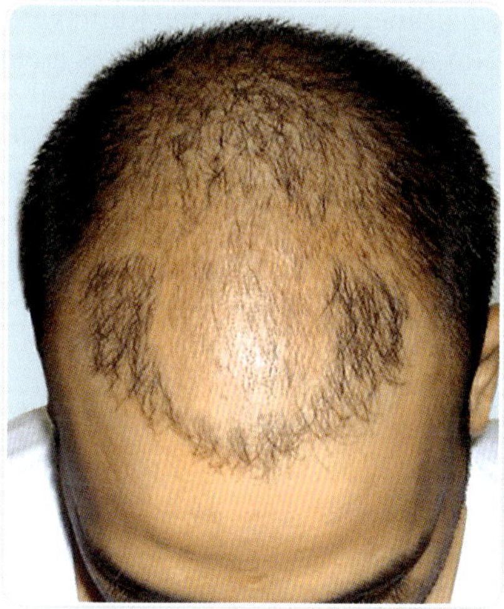

FIG. 1: The result when early hair loss is transplanted in a young patient without starting medical treatment/counseling about the need for multiple transplants.

Note: Evolving nature of hair loss in young males—hair transplantation done prematurely with no supporting medical treatment.

But both these medications will work only in areas of thinning. They do not have any effect on totally bald areas. So, again, the problem is not completely solved.[7,8]

But if we were to combine both forms of treatment, we would be able to achieve more than using the individual treatments. Hence, thorough counseling is of utmost necessity before considering transplantation. Otherwise, it would lead to a situation wherein the young man will return for repeated transplants every 1–2 years **(Fig. 1)**.

Managing MPHL requires the hair transplant surgeon to arrest hair loss and also restore the bald area, partly or completely, depending on the grade of hair loss. For the purpose of arresting the progress of hair loss, only two medical treatments, minoxidil and finasteride, are of proven benefit in male balding. Both are also approved by the United States Food and Drug Administration (USFDA) for treatment in males. Both drugs primarily stop the progress of hair loss but also stimulate some regrowth of hair in some men and hence are better regarded as preventative treatments. Neither will regrow hair on completely bald scalp, and continued treatment is necessary to maintain the response. Both drugs have a good safety record, a consideration of paramount importance when treating hair growth disorders.[9,10]

INDICATION FOR SURGERY IN EARLY BALDNESS

By definition, early baldness could denote frontal or frontotemporal recessions. This would break the hairline and lead to an impression of baldness. Hair transplant is an option when facial aesthetics are altered with respect to receding hairline, thinning in the frontal areas, or frank baldness. Not everyone with hair loss is a candidate for hair transplantation.

Early thinning can occur on the vertex also, but this is generally not an indication for surgery and is dealt with in more detail in the Chapter 80 on Vertex Transplantation.

Criteria to be considered for hair transplantation in early hair loss are as follows:

- Age of the patient
- Degree of frontal and temporal recession with overall impact on facial aesthetics
- Potential areas (presence of anisotrichosis) of future hair loss, possibility of diffuse hair loss
- Patient expectations
- Quality and quantity of the donor area
- Presence of first-degree relatives with advanced hair loss (grades 6 and 7 Norwood)
- Patient's willingness to take drug therapy
- Occupation of the patient; some occupations, such as film acting and visual media, may need special considerations

There is no defined age for hair transplant, but a general preference exists on the minimal requisite age, which is about 25 years. Young patients can be emotionally immature and attribute a greater, often exaggerated importance to minor or very early hair loss. These patients are often very persistent and demand surgical management. A young patient with minimal recession who insists on an adolescent (very low and very dense) hairline should be counseled about the progressive nature of hair loss and finite donor area. However, there is no one age that can be specified as there would be specific issues for each patient. Hence, all aspects need to be taken into consideration during counseling. It is always a good idea to involve parents in very young patients during counseling. It is also good to follow-up with the patient over a period of time to understand his psyche, establish a relationship, and then agree to perform surgery.

When evaluating a young patient, potential future areas of thinning must be looked for. Two ways to do this would be to (1) wet the hair during examination **(Figs. 2A and B)** and (2) trichoscopy **(Fig. 3)**.

Presence of advanced hair loss (grades 6 and 7) in the paternal or maternal ancestry is a definite red flag pointing to possibility of progress of hair loss with age. This has to be factored in while planning young patients, and surgical plans must be altered accordingly. More important than lowering the hairline is to address the watershed areas of thinning. This approach helps to stabilize the progress of thinning in conjunction with medications.

For example, a person with just thinning is a better candidate for medical management as compared to hair transplantation **(Figs. 4A and B)**. Even if this person underwent only hair transplantation to fill in the gaps, in the course of time, the original/native hair may be lost, bringing the thinning to baseline. This might mandate another hair transplant. Considering that the limiting factor in hair transplantation is the donor area, adequate coverage might not be possible.

Young people are often resistant to the idea of taking medicines and push for surgery aggressively, which needs to be resisted. They should be shown photos of medical therapy to convince that drug therapy indeed is helpful.

Addressing these potential areas with surgery or medication forms the major tenets of the treatment plan in early baldness.

The thinning frontal region, as well as the fringe areas surrounding it, has the presence of miniaturized hair. Concomitant medical treatment improves these and adds to the result of the transplant. This helps optimize the use of donor reserves conserving them for future needs. Treatment with oral finasteride and topical minoxidil stops the progress of hair loss, and when they are combined with hair transplantation, this fact helps to increase the interval between two transplants.

Finasteride and to some extent minoxidil are known to increase the anagen hair, and starting these two agents 8–12 weeks before a transplant helps increase anagen hair globally.[11,12] This has two impacts: (1) in the donor area, the increase in anagen hair leads to more visible hair and hence better yield, and (2) in the recipient area

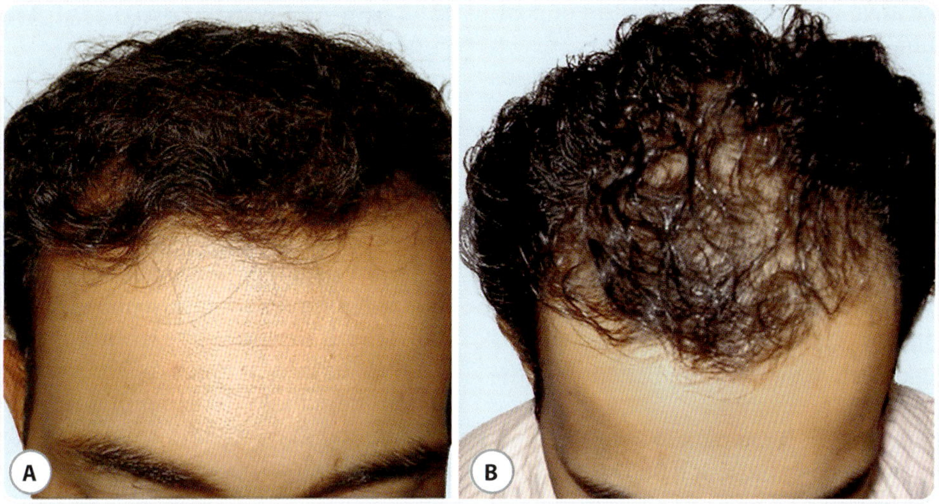

FIGS. 2A AND B: Check for future areas of thinning by wetting the hair. Wetting shows the scalp coverage and the areas of future hair loss.

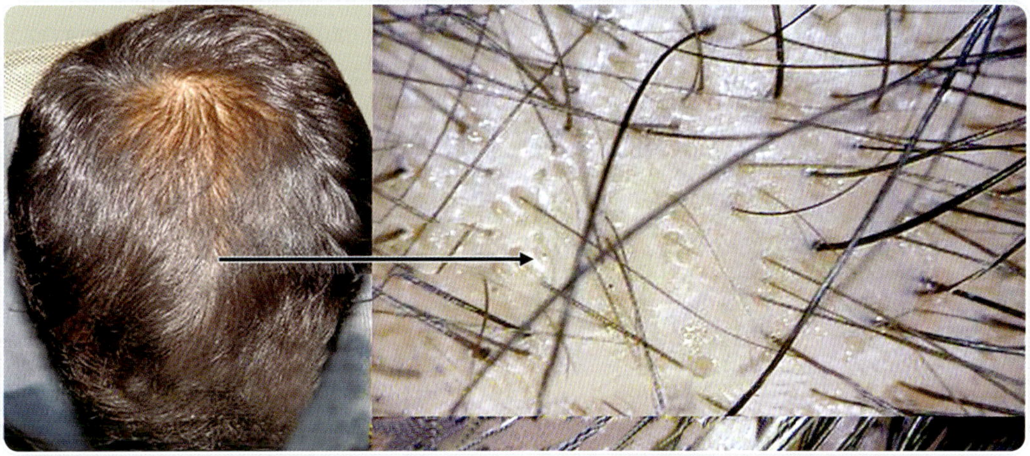

FIG. 3: Trichoscopy. Finding anisotrichosis in the adjoining areas signifies impending hair loss.

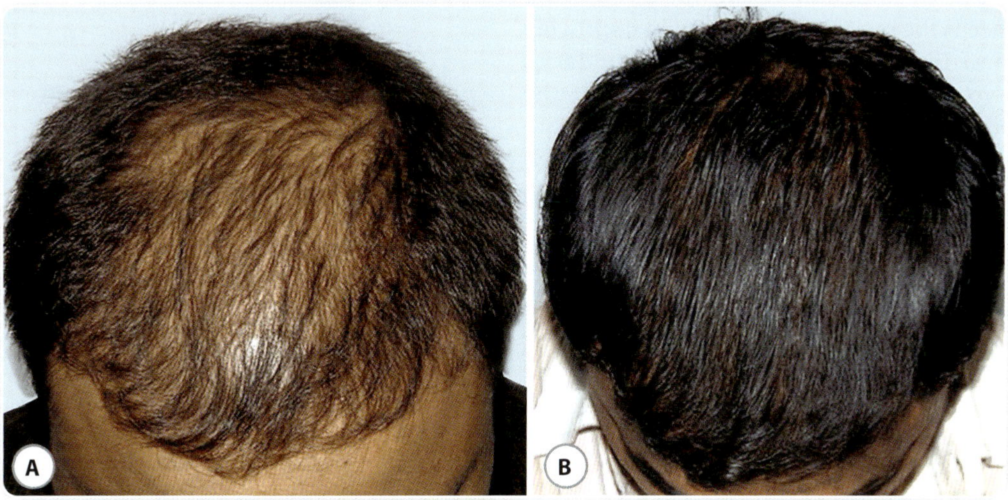

FIGS. 4A AND B: Patients with diffuse thinning but a maintained hairline are ideal for medical therapy (topical minoxidil and oral finasteride). Picture showing the improvement in 8 months.

or nontransplanted area, it reduces the quantum of post-transplant effluvium.

When planning a transplant, these considerations have to be put across to the patient and emphasize the benefits of combination therapy.[13-17]

INDICATIONS FOR HAIR TRANSPLANTATION IN EARLY BALDNESS

- *Loss or break in facial framing*: This is the most important indication. Restoring facial framing is the most satisfying objective for both the patient and the surgeon alike.
- *Professional requirement*: If the patient's professional life is impacted by the early recession and would have a bearing on his self-confidence. This is very true of people in media as well as sales.
- *Social requirement*: Today, the importance placed on appearance cannot be overstated, and matrimonial prospects (Indian perspective) are definitely impacted with early recession in young men.

While transplanting in patients with early baldness, especially very young male patients, one must remember the following:

- Indication to be decided based on individual merits
- Always plan for future hair loss
- Counseling for conservative hairline placement
- Do not exhaust the donor reserves with large sessions
- Moderate sessions (1,500–2,000 follicular unit grafts)

PLANNING IN EARLY BALDNESS

Importance of Intact Frontal Hairline

The face is like a picture frame with the frontal hairline forming the upper border. Loss of the frontal hairline alters the unique facial characteristics of the person. Framing the face is the most important goal in improving facial aesthetics. The hairline is one of the boundaries demarcating youthful proportions of the face. If the hairline recedes, then the aesthetic proportions are distorted giving rise to an age-inappropriate look. Hence, the hairline needs to be the most important landmark to be restored by hair transplantation.

Placement of the Mid-frontal Point

The approach to planning in early hair loss or young patients is discussed here. The placement of the mid-frontal point as well as the apex of the frontotemporal angle has to be conservative, and this will usually be quite contrary to what the patient would be expecting. It is important to convince him about the same.

Apex of Frontotemporal Angle (Figs. 5 and 6)

The apex of the frontotemporal angle should be placed on or medial to the vertical canthal line (VCL) (a line that runs sagittally from the lateral canthus of the eye).

Placing the Apex of Frontotemporal Angle

The most usual request is for this angle to be below and lateral. If the apex is lateral to the VCL, it gives an unnatural look (comb over look). It is with tact that one has to get them to see things from a different perspective. Often, the patient demands a hairline that he remembers from his prepubertal days, which would be totally unnatural as he progresses in age.

Dealing with Watershed Areas (Areas of Thinning Adjoining the Bald Areas)

It is more important to address the adjoining areas, which have early changes of thinning (as evidenced on trichoscopy or by wetting the hair) rather than lowering the hairline. This move helps to mitigate the evolving hair loss to some extent.

Transplanting hair in areas of thinning requires some experience and should not be attempted by the beginner.

While implanting in between existing hairs, a few points have to be noted:

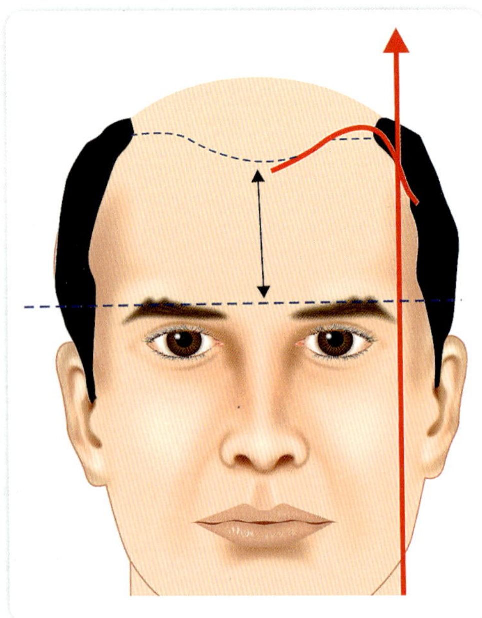

FIG. 5: Location of the apex of frontotemporal angle with reference to the vertical canthal line (VCL). The apex should always be on or medial to the VCL.

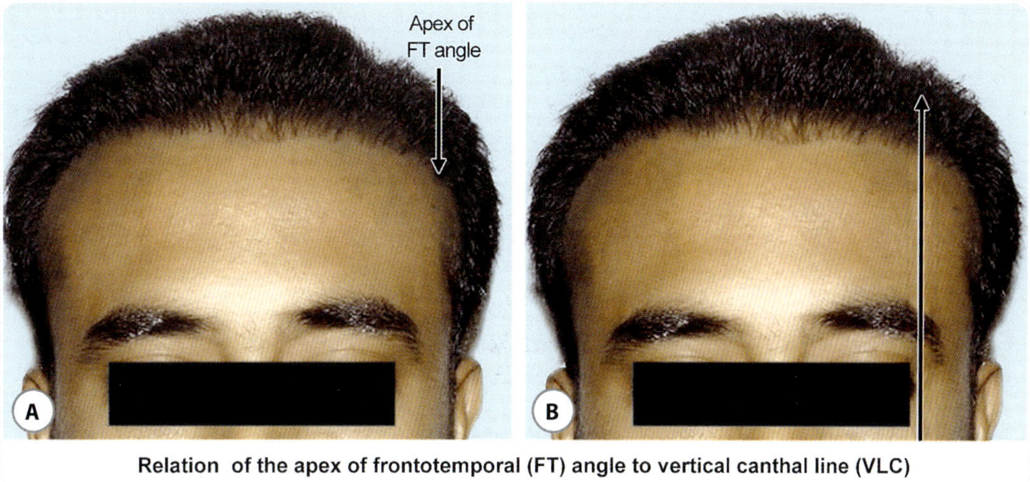

FIGS. 6A AND B: The result when the apex of frontotemporal angle lies lateral to the vertical canthal line, giving an artificial comb over look. This kind of request is quite usual from the patients, and it is up to the surgeon to convince them against it.

- Use of good magnification with a larger field of vision. This improves the accuracy of the implantation. It will be ideal if the patient is willing to trim the area, but many patients are not willing for this as they would be resuming work in a short while, and their professional profile would not permit them to wear a cap or, generally, they would not want the world to know that they have undergone a hair restorative procedure.
- Stick and place is a better method of implantation in areas of thinning. It is slightly more time consuming but more accurate. If premade incisions are used, then they need to be carefully looked for while implanting.
- Wetting the hairs enhances the visibility of the gaps.
- Small possibility of potential damage to existing hair should be discussed with the patient. So, the patient should be informed that transplantation will only be done in such areas that are considered "safe" for the existing neighboring hairs. Hence, not all gaps will be filled.
- *Postoperative effluvium*: Postoperative shock loss is common when transplantation is carried out in areas of thinning. The exact reason is not known but could be due to local stress created by surgery or overenthusiastic use of adrenaline-containing tumescent solution. The author does not tumesced in the recipient area as stick and place technique does not need tumescence.
- *Presence of small miniaturized hair*: Many patients with early hair loss have small miniaturized hairs in the affected areas as well as in the adjoining areas. The approach to these hairs depends on various factors: Level of miniaturization, quality and quantity of donor area, the patient's willingness to adhere to long-term medication schedule, the age of the patient, and the financial condition of the patient. If the donor area is optimal in terms of quality and quantity, the patient does not have any close degree relative with advanced hair loss, and the examination does not reveal the potential for rapid future hair loss—in such cases, one could disregard the presence of these fine hairs, particularly those in advanced miniaturization, and proceed to create the density as desired and planned. However, if the donor area is not optimal and patient could be progressing to advanced hair loss and is willing to use long-term medication, then it would be ideal to work around these fine hairs and not damage them during implantation, so that they can be activated with drugs. In short, it is always preferable to save as much as one can.
- It is best to use the larger follicular unit grafts, where feasible, inside the areas of thinning to improve the illusion of better density.
- It is quite rewarding to see what a combination of medications with a moderate session of hair transplant can achieve **(Figs. 7A and B)**.

DONOR HARVEST TECHNIQUE

With regards to the technique of donor harvest, the author is of the opinion that the decision should be taken after discussing with the patient on the following points:

- *Grade of hair loss and hence the quantum of grafts needed*: For early hair loss, one could opt on using either technique—follicular unit extraction (FUE) or follicular unit transplantation (FUT) strip for donor harvest. If there is evidence by way of examination of

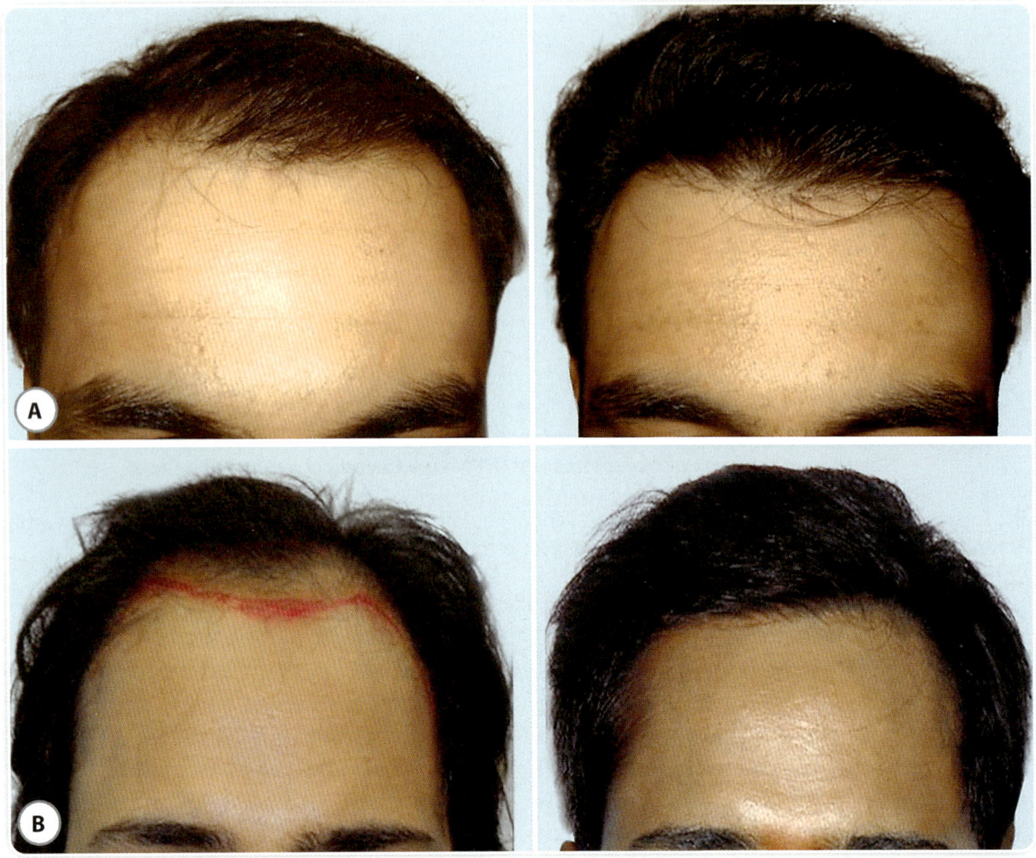

FIGS. 7A AND B: Rather than lowering the hairline significantly, it is better to address the adjoining areas where there is a potential to undergo further hair loss.

future hair loss or family history of advanced grade of hair loss, then it would be fair to go ahead with strip harvest. The logic of this is that after the strip harvest, the donor area above and below the donor scar is untouched and available for either technique of donor harvest, and hence, one can get the most out of the donor area to fulfill the demand of advancing hair loss. While planning in early hair loss or young patient, it is always important to think a decade ahead with respect to future hair loss and optimizing donor yield. The author believes in using both techniques to get the most out of the donor area. When multiple sessions would be deemed necessary, the first session would always be a strip harvest if the patient agrees and is eligible for the same.

- *Scalp laxity*: A tight scalp would mean that one will have to go ahead with FUE.
- *The hairstyle that the patient sports*: If the patient is one who frequently shaves his head or keeps very short hairstyles, then it is best to proceed with FUE.
- *Apprehension about the linear scar or poor pain threshold*: In this scenario where the patient is very apprehensive about a linear scar in the donor area, it is better to choose FUE. Some patients have very low pain thresholds. This information can be gained during history taking, where the patient mentions history of syncopal attacks with painful stimuli or admits to be unable to bear even a little bit of pain. It must be explained that the pain during the surgery (while injecting anesthesia) is the same with either technique of donor harvest, but the postoperative soreness is a little more with strip harvest as compared with FUE. In a motivated patient, this difference is negligible. However, if the patient is apprehensive about the postoperative pain, then it is best to go ahead with FUE.
- *Willingness to shave the entire donor area for the surgery*: For many patients, disclosing that they have undergone a hair restorative procedure to their relatives, friends, colleagues, and the world at large is not an acceptable option. Though the postoperative scabs in the recipient area are the same with either technique, to sport a complete shaved look after surgery is not acceptable for many. Here, the strip

harvest works better as there is limited trimming, and the donor area suture line is completely covered right after the surgery by the hair combed down.

- *Sportsperson*: If the patient is an active sportsperson who has to go back to active physical activity at the earliest, then FUE would be the more suitable option of donor harvest. This is because there is restriction of heavy physical activity for 4–6 weeks post a strip harvest, while a person can resume all of this after 10 days in case of FUE.
- *Financial status*: Hair transplantation using FUE is more expensive than strip harvest. This is true across the world. This would be an important factor for the patient to decide about the type of hair transplant he would choose.
- *Surgeon's skills*: It goes without saying that a hair transplant surgeon should be adept at both techniques of donor harvest. But if one of the techniques clearly has better results in the surgeon's experience, this should be honestly conveyed to the patient so that he can decide.

SUMMARY

As hair transplantation does not influence the progression of MPHL, long-term results in the early stages depend on medical stabilization. Hair transplantation results can be considerably augmented and maintained when combined with topical minoxidil and oral finasteride. Management of MPHL can be rewarding despite the limitations of the treatment modalities, as the current treatments are capable of providing significant benefits provided the patient is fully aware of what can be achieved.

REFERENCES

1. Hamilton JB. Patterned loss of hair in man; types and incidence. Ann N Y Acad Sci. 1951;53(3):708-28.
2. Hamilton JB. Male hormone stimulation is a prerequisite and an incitant in common baldness. Am J Anat. 1942;71:451-80.
3. Price VH. Testosterone metabolism in the skin. A review of its function in androgenetic alopecia, acne vulgaris, and idiopathic hirsutism including recent studies with antiandrogens. Arch Dermatol. 1975;111(11):1496-502.
4. Olsen EA. Androgenetic alopecia. In: Olsen EA (Ed). Disorders of Hair Growth: Diagnosis and Treatment. New York: McGraw-Hill; 1994. pp. 257-83.
5. Leyden J, Dunlap F, Miller B, Winters P, Lebwohl M, Hecker D, et al. Finasteride in the treatment of men with frontal male pattern hair loss. J Am Acad Dermatol. 1999;40(6 Pt 1):930-7.
6. Whiting DA. Advances in the treatment of male androgenetic alopecia: a brief review of finasteride studies. Eur J Dermatol. 2001;11(4):332-4.
7. Ellis JA, Sinclair R, Harrap SB. Androgenetic alopecia: pathogenesis and potential for therapy. Expert Rev Mol Med. 2002;4(22):1-11.
8. Khandpur S, Suman M, Reddy BS. Comparative efficacy of various treatment regimens for androgenetic alopecia in men. J Dermatol. 2002;29(8):489-98.
9. Arca E, Açikgöz G, Taştan HB, Köse O, Kurumlu Z. An open, randomized, comparative study of oral finasteride and 5% topical minoxidil in male androgenetic alopecia. Dermatology. 2004;209(2):117-25.
10. Finasteride Male Pattern Hair Loss Study Group. Long-term (5-year) multinational experience with finasteride 1 mg in the treatment of men with androgenetic alopecia. Eur J Dermatol. 2002;12(1):38-49.
11. Van Neste D, Fuh V, Sanchez-Pedreno P, Lopez-Bran E, Wolff H, Whiting D, et al. Finasteride increases anagen hair in men with androgenetic alopecia. Br J Dermatol. 2000;143(4):804-10.
12. Kassimir JJ. Use of topical minoxidil as a possible adjunct to hair transplant surgery. A pilot study. J Am Acad Dermatol. 1987;16(3 Pt 2):685-7.
13. Bouhanna P. Topical minoxidil used before and after laser hair transplantation. J Dermatol Surg Oncol. 1989;15(1):50-3.
14. Roenigk HH, Berman MD. Topical 2% minoxidil with hair transplantation. Face. 1993;4:213-6.
15. Avram MR, Cole JP, Gandelman M, Haber R, Knudsen R, Leavitt MT, et al. The potential role of minoxidil in the hair transplantation setting. Dermatol Surg. 2002;28(10): 894-900.
16. Leavitt M, Perez-Meza D, Rao NA, Barusco M, Kaufman KD, Ziering C. Effects of finasteride (1 mg) on hair transplant. Dermatol Surg. 2005;31(10):1268-76.
17. Blume-Peytavi U, Blumeyer A, Tosti A, Finner A, Marmol V, Trakatelli M, et al. S1 guideline for diagnostic evaluation in androgenetic alopecia in men, women and adolescents. Br J Dermatol. 2011;164(1):5-15.

CHAPTER 83

Hair Transplantation in Female Pattern Hair Loss

Madura C, Venkataram Mysore, Nitin Barde

Key Messages

- Management of female pattern hair loss needs a multipronged approach.
- Hair transplantation in women is one of the definitive therapies considered along with proper medical management.
- Hair transplantation in women needs technically a well-experienced surgeon and team to deliver optimized results.
- Ensure that patients understand the progressive nature of disease and requires continued use of minoxidil to maintain the result.

INTRODUCTION

Female pattern hair loss, also known as female androgenetic alopecia (FAGA) or female patterned alopecia (FPA), is the most likely cause of hair loss in women presenting to a dermatologist's clinic. Female alopecia with androgen increase is called FAGA and without androgen increase is called female pattern hair loss (FPHL). The clinical picture of a typical case begins with a specific diffuse loss of hair from the parietal or frontovertical areas with an intact frontal hairline **(Figs. 1A to C)**.[1]

Hair transplantation (HT) in women is one of the definitive therapies if concomitantly done along with proper medical treatment. The transplantation in women is infrequent compared to men and also it is not easily accepted by patients and also by surgeons due to various factors: (1) FPHL is multifactorial and progressive. (2) it is more diffuse and not as precisely defined as male pattern hair loss (MPHL), (3) coexistent chronic telogen effluvium and/or alopecia areata incognito may lead to failure of surgery as no hairs are immune to it, (4) expectation level of most of the females is higher as

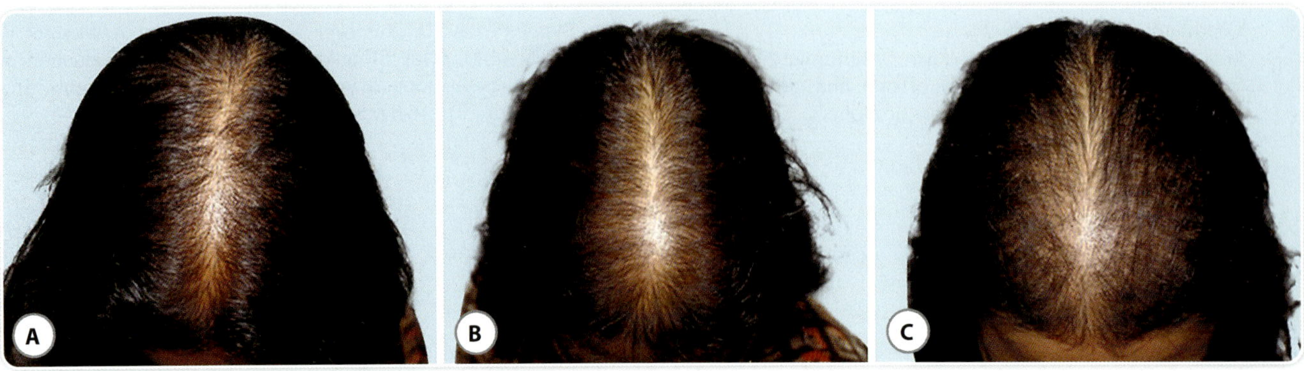

FIGS. 1A TO C: Female pattern hair loss Ludwig grades I, II, and III.
Courtesy: Cutis Academy, Bengaluru, Karnataka, India.[2]

stress and anxiety related to hair loss are high, (5) strip method [follicular unit transplantation (FUT)] was a more popular and well-established way to restore hair in the past, and females seem to be more apprehensive about more invasive surgical procedure and linear visible scar, and (6) the *pattern of baldness is more* diffuse, making it technically more difficult to operate and ensure good results. Several factors contribute to the uncertainties surrounding the success of hair transplant (HT) in women. The technical complexity of performing hair transplant procedures in women and the influence of these factors indirectly affect a surgeon's decision when determining whether to accept a case or not.[3,4]

Over time, this landscape has been transforming. There's a surging demand, heightened awareness of the importance, and a substantial accumulation of expertise, all converging to deliver increasingly satisfactory outcomes. Consequently, hair transplants for women have gained substantial popularity. Hence, HT in women has become increasingly common. In 2014, 15.3% of all hair restoration surgical patients worldwide were female. Since 2006, the proportion of female surgical hair restoration patients worldwide increased by 11%.[5] A number of publications have dealt with this issue.[6-13] This chapter will focus only on the surgical aspects of management, and the reader is referred to the chapters on FPHL and Medical Management for other details.

BOX 1 Special characters of FPHL.[14,15]

- FPHL is diffuse, less defined, and diagnosis is imprecise; there is a lack of clear-cut demarcation separating the affected and unaffected areas
- It is multifactorial, and progression is common
- Many times, other coexisting factors are associated, the most common being chronic telogen effluvium, which may result in diffuse thinning of hair over the entire scalp
- FPHL rarely causes total balding in a localized area, and it usually causes diffuse thinning **(Figs. 1A to C)**
- In FPHL, individual units do not disappear but just the number of hairs in each unit decreases. Hence, we see intact units with single hair, and also there is reduction in the thickness of hair shaft, leading to overall decrease in the hair volume
- DUPA—diffuse pattern hair loss is common in women
- Strip surgery is more daunting for a woman
- Planting in between hairs is more difficult
- Shock loss may be more common
- Results are often more delayed
- Expectations are higher in women

(DUPA: diffuse unpatterned alopecia; FPHL: female pattern hair loss)

SPECIAL CHARACTERS OF FEMALE PATTERN HAIR LOSS

The special characters of FPHL make hair transplant surgery more challenging than in men **(Box 1)**; hence, experience and expertise are needed before venturing into this difficult area.

PREOPERATIVE EVALUATION

History, Examination, and Investigations

Before considering a female as a suitable candidate for surgery, it is mandatory to find out what is causing hair loss and not just conclude it as FPHL. The physician must evaluate the patient's history, physical examination, investigations, and, if needed, even biopsy before considering surgery as an option.

A detailed history and examination will rule out impostors such as chronic telogen effluvium, fibrosing alopecia in patterned distribution, and alopecia areata incognito. A history of trichotillomania should also be elicited. Many women have significant thinning over the occipital area too, and these are not good candidates; hence, donor area examination is important not only to rule out diffuse unpatterned alopecia (DUPA) but also for donor area assessment with respect to density, grouping, and laxity. A thorough scalp examination is mandatory to look for coexisting seborrheic dermatitis, folliculitis, and scars.

TrichoScan is a popular investigation that helps in both diagnosis and evaluating donor area. The assessment is done in all zones to see the possible stable donor zone. Biopsy is indicated in suspected cases of fibrosing alopecia in a pattern distribution (FAPD), frontal fibrosing alopecia (FFA), and other diagnostic dilemmas.

A detailed psychological history is mandatory; often a small amount of thinning may elicit an exaggerated response, and these women may put pressure on the surgeon for early surgery. Expectations should be assessed by leading questions (what will make you happy; what area do you wish to be covered; what is your expectation) and possible results be explained. Preoperative surgical screening and necessary investigations are similar to male HT.

Case Selection

The most important criteria for case selection are to have realistic expectations on results apart from an optimal grade of baldness, completed medical therapy, with good donor asset, and after proper counseling, they clearly

BOX 2 Good candidates for surgery.

- Women who have significant thinning, i.e., >50% thinning in specific area
- Women who have not had improvement in appearance after medical treatment
- Women who agree to take medical treatment to retain existing hair and treat the underlying cause
- Women with good long-term potential donor-to-recipient area ratio
- A motivated woman with realistic expectations
- Scarring alopecia
- Women with high hairline and wide forehead

BOX 3 Poor candidates for surgery.

- Women with diffuse thinning, including occipital area (DUPA)
- Women not willing to undergo medical treatment
- Women with unrealistic expectations
- Women who are not psychologically stable and show evidence of dysmorphophobia

BOX 4 Preoperative counseling.

- *Nature of procedure*: FUT/FUE
- *Purpose of hair transplantation*: To only camouflage and create an illusion to cover the scalp well and hide baldness and visible thinning areas
- *Hair style*: Know their combing style
- *Complications*: To explain both long- and short-term side effects, especially shock loss
- *Sequelae and timeline*: To inform on what is expected postsurgery on day 0, 10, 40, and 90 and about the time taken to see the result
- *Expectations*: Counsel that they can never restore the original density/head full of hair. There will be no much change in girth of ponytail, and results are often delayed in comparison to men's transplantation
- Risk and benefits associated with the procedure
- *Postprocedure care and treatment*: To continue medical treatment after the hair transplant for better outcome

(FUE: follicular unit extraction; FUT: follicular unit transplantation)

understand what is possible and what is not. Most women often need a smaller number of grafts, 1,200–1,500 grafts, to cover a specific area. Since women grow long hair, camouflage with existing hair is easier, and it is possible to give satisfactory results with a small number of grafts. Mega sessions over 3,000 grafts are rarely necessary nor are they advisable **(Boxes 2 and 3)**.

Counseling

A detailed counseling of procedure, anesthesia, sequelae, outcome, side effects, and the need for continued medical treatment must be stressed.

The preferred hairstyle should be noted, and patients should be told clearly which area will be operated on, so if the hairstyle is changed later, another thinning area may get highlighted. The process of counseling should last over more than one consultation; it is never wise to agree for surgery in the first consultation. Medical management should be utilized fully and its response assessed before considering surgery. Serial photographs should be obtained. Possibility of future progression and the need for continuing medical treatment should be stressed. The process of surgery should be explained fully, the need for trimming hair, the need for a longer time in women for the growth, and hence full results to be achieved should be explained. The adage "underpromise and overdeliver" is never perhaps more relevant than in HT for FPHL. Often, women may expect a full head with every area covered; this is never possible and should be conveyed clearly. Pain is another consideration; while women tolerate pain effectively, the apprehension about pain is greater. This needs to be addressed during counseling **(Box 4)**.

Preoperative Medications

Preoperative medication is an important consideration for a female undergoing hair transplant surgery. If a female is undergoing hair loss, then medical therapy will be an important adjuvant to surgery in checking hair loss. Females are more prone to postoperative hair shedding, so it is prudent to start preoperative medication for prevention. The prophylaxis of 6 weeks minoxidil topical solution will prevent such postoperative hair shedding. The minoxidil 5% solution can be used and stopping minoxidil 2–5 days prior and resuming 1 week postoperatively. Also, educating female patients beforehand will also help to avert the trust crisis if hair shedding occurs. Rest of preoperative medication such as prophylactic antibiotics and anxiolytics are the same as for men.

OPERATIVE STEPS

1. Hairline design
2. Calculate area of transplant.
3. Decide the donor area that needs to be trimmed.
4. Anesthesia (can refer to respective chapters for Operative Steps)
5. Donor area harvest and segregation of grafts (can refer to respective chapters for Operative Steps)
6. Recipient site preparation and implantation (can refer to respective chapters for Operative Steps)
7. Postoperative dressing and care

Anesthesia Considerations

The anesthesia technique is the same as we use for males. The only consideration here is to modify the local anesthesia solution to prevent the postoperative shock loss. Though the condition is temporary, sometimes hair may not regrow completely.

Reduction of the epinephrine load to the patient has been thought to limit the risk of shock loss, since it will minimize the excessive vasoconstriction, which, in turn, promotes the postoperative hair loss.

For ring block, the same anesthetic solution can be used for males and females. But for tumescent anesthesia, there should be no epinephrine or half the dose used for men. Also, it is advised not to use tumescent fluid in excess; if used in abundance, it can precipitate postoperative hair shedding. We can also add an additional steroid component to reduce postoperative forehead edema. Anesthesia needs to be administered slowly, and the total dosage should always be cautiously observed as women have less body mass; hence, lignocaine toxicity is a possibility. Rest of the considerations are the same as those in men, and the reader is advised to consult the relevant chapters for details.

Donor Area Considerations

Since women have long hairs, trimming over the donor area is rarely a problem. Therefore, either strip surgery or follicular unit extraction (FUE) can be performed safely. Women also tend to have lax skin (personal observation). Since the number of grafts needed generally does not exceed 1,500–2,000 grafts, a thin long strip can easily be taken. It is therefore possible to ensure a thin scar. For the same reason, FUE can also be performed easily if the woman asks for it. FUE can be undertaken by making a window in the donor area where hairs above the donor area cover the defect till leftover hairs in the donor area regrow **(Figs. 2A to C)**. Nonshaven FUE is another technique wherein FUE is performed without trimming the donor area. This technique demands more skill and preciseness while scoring the graft as the origin of graft on the skin surface is not clearly visible. The wastage in terms of complete and partial transection is more and so is the incidence of buried grafts. Overall, the speed of extraction is reduced greatly, and it is difficult to extract a higher number of grafts by nonshaven FUE due to the abovementioned challenges.

Recipient Area Considerations

There can be variations in recipient site designing. (1) In FPHL, the hairline is intact with loss of density just behind it, making the scalp visible through the hairs. These cases need only to create recipient sites in the areas of low density **(Fig. 3A)**. (2) If the hairline is weakened, then the surgeon can create recipient sites to strengthen existing hairline **(Fig. 3B)**. (3) To camouflage the triangular temporal recession in an M-shaped hairline. (4) Few cases require recreation of new hairline such as women with wide forehead, wear and tear of hairline due to traction **(Fig. 3C)**, FPHL with MPHL, and cases having progressive frontal hair loss "Christmas tree pattern" **(Fig. 3B)**.

For those females having gross mismatch in donor to recipient area and having limited graft numbers, design of hairline can be modified and optimized to get illusion of head full of hairs. Many women wear their hair long, so creative styling can be used to cover those areas where transplant was not done. Three typical designs to make up hairline are as follows: T, L, and reverse L. The objective

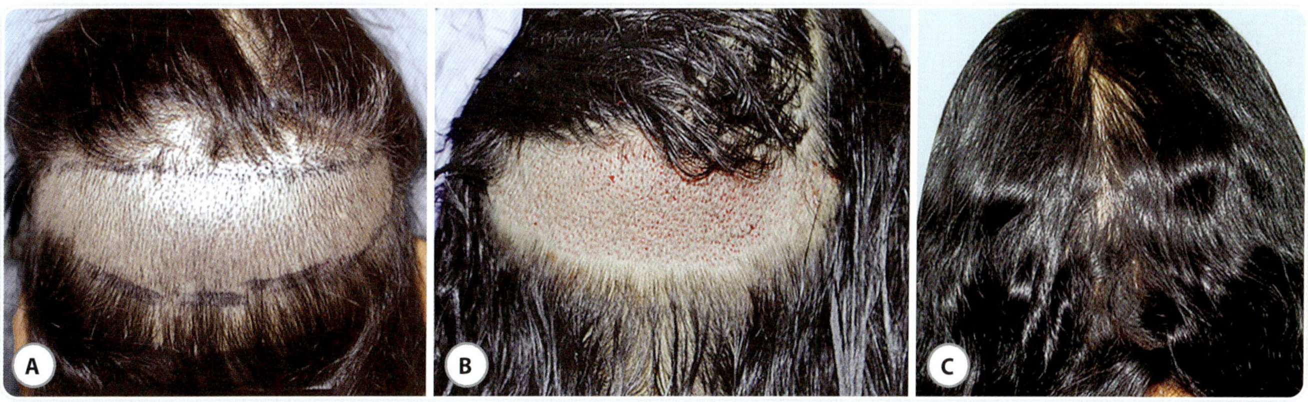

FIGS. 2A TO C: (A) A small window in donor area is trimmed based on the number of grafts required; (B) Donor zone postharvest; (C) Hairs above the donor area cover the defect till leftover hairs in the donor area regrows.

Courtesy: Cutis Academy, Bengaluru, Karnataka, India.

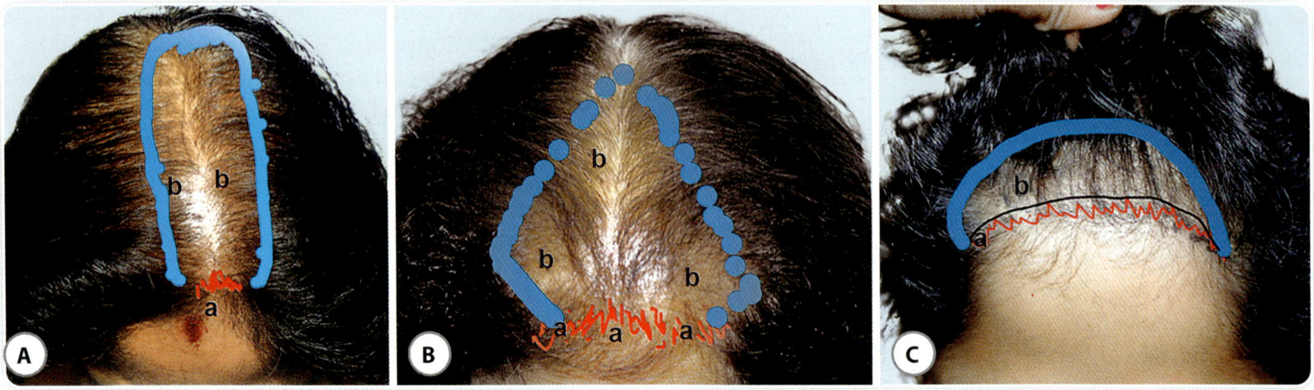

FIGS. 3A TO C: (A) FPHL with intact hairline; (B) FPHL "Christmas tree pattern," with weathered hairline; (C) FPHL that needs recreation of hairline. (a) Single hair grafts for hairline and (b) multigraft units.
(FPHL: female pattern hair loss)
Courtesy: Cutis Academy, Bengaluru, Karnataka, India.

of such design is to restore the hairline, central forelock, and the hair part. If women part hair at center, then design would be T. Similarly, those females opting for left or right part can use L design where the vertical limb of L will be on the part side and the horizontal limb of L will cover the hairline and forelock area. The female should be counseled to adhere to the styling which was opted before surgery.[16]

Hairline Designing[17,18]

The wide forehead is the common indication for lowering hairline. *It is the most important and crucial step in HT*. This needs careful consideration of reconstruction of hairline **(Box 5)**. Precise drawing needs to be made and discussed about the shape and the concavity of the hairline. Women expect a near-perfect result in this area, and hence a higher density needs to be planned, after careful consideration of the hairstyle preferred by the patient. The patient should also be told that if she is not satisfied with the density, a second session can be planned to enhance density.

Direction of Hair[19]

The direction of hair is upward in the center on the vertical part of forehead. Then, hair is directed on one side and slightly forward as we move up in the center and near the junction of vertical and horizontal planes. The direction of hair is more forward with slight inclination toward one side at a completely horizontal plane. On moving laterally, the direction of hair changes rapidly toward the respective side with forward inclination just after crossing the midpupillary line. Near the frontotemporal point, the direction of hair is almost lateral yet slightly forward, and after reaching the temporal part, the hair runs downward and backward **(Fig. 5)**.

BOX 5 Salient features of female hairline.

- Female hairline is less irregular—create microirregularities
- The female hairline begins on the vertical part of forehead, hence making the forehead look smaller
- Hairline runs through the forehead to give an oval to round shape to the female face
- Hairline shows downward concavity as opposite to male hairline, which is "M" shaped or showing the convexity toward the front. As the curvature of this concavity varies greatly among different females, both overall shape of the face and forehead must be considered while giving the curvature to the hairline
- Creating a small peak "widow's peak" in the center can make concave/round hairline to look "heart shape," can be attractive and preferred in few women
- In women with long face, a slightly flat hairline with slight concavity downward and medially at the ends is preferred to make their forehead match with long face
- *There are four kinds of hairline designs*:[21] M, rectangular, oval, and triangular shape **(Figs. 4A and B)**

Reconstructing Hairline

Women with a wide forehead wish to lower their hairline. The hairline needs to be concave downward and should gradually merge with the hairline over the temporal areas. While two to three hair units can be used in the hinder part of the area to be grafted, the anterior hairline should consist of thinner hairs; this is particularly true of lateral areas toward temples. A higher density needs to be planned **(Figs. 6A to C)**.

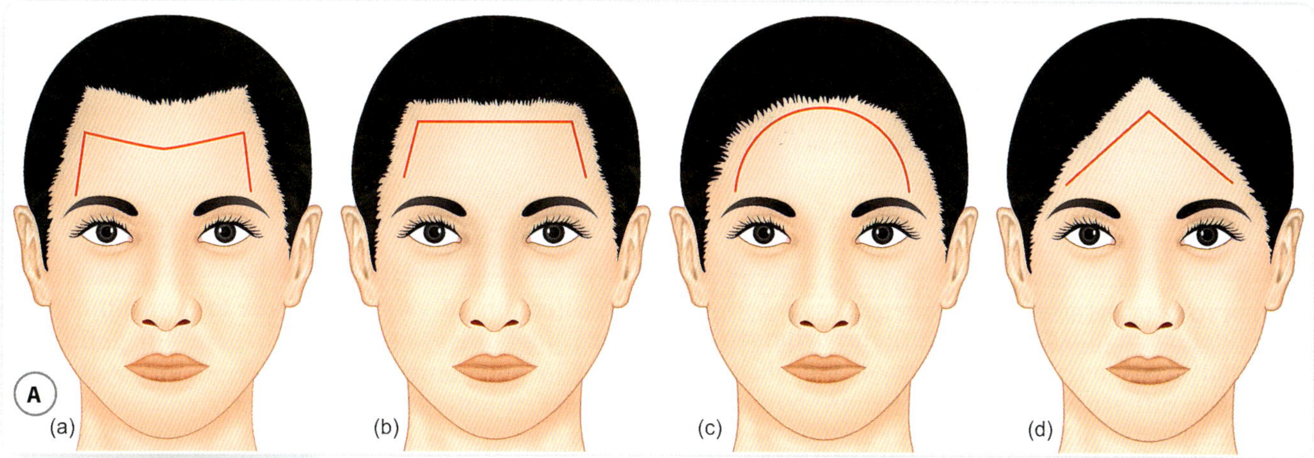

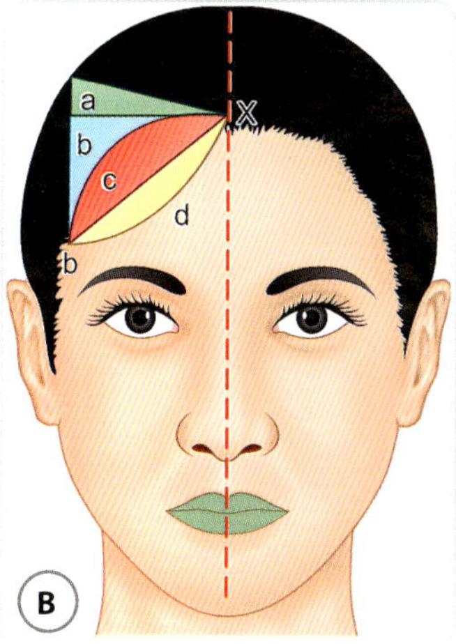

FIGS. 4A AND B: Patterns of hairline: a. M shape, b. rectangular, c. oval, and d. triangular shape.

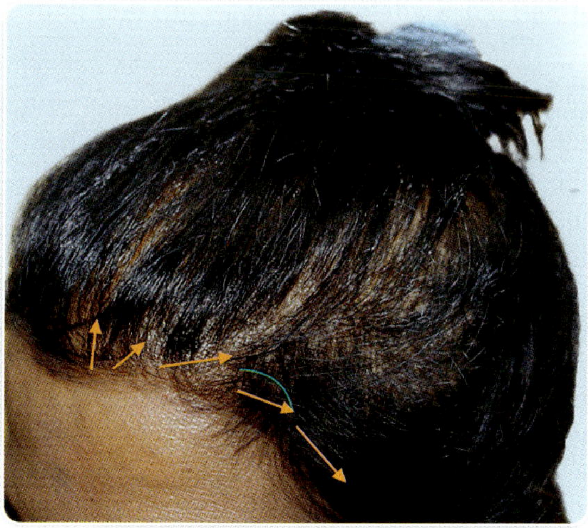

FIG. 5: Direction of hair.

Courtesy: Cutis Academy, Bengaluru, Karnataka, India.

Recipient Area Considerations—Challenges Faced and Remedies[19]

- This is challenging as grafting needs to be performed in between existing hairs, and women usually do not allow shaving of the head **(Fig. 3)**. Women typically have mostly intact units, with single hairs, and complete balding is rare. Small patches of baldness are seen amidst areas with hairs. Therefore, the size of grafts used varies depending on the area, with a mixture of single- and two-hair units predominating, along with a smaller number of three- and four-hair units. Dense packing of areas in female hair transplant should be avoided to prevent postoperative shock loss. Single-hair grafts are suitable for the hairline to make it softer, while the area posterior to the hairline requires two-hair grafts with moderate-to-high density. It is advisable to provide more density along the parting line **(Figs. 7 and 8)**.

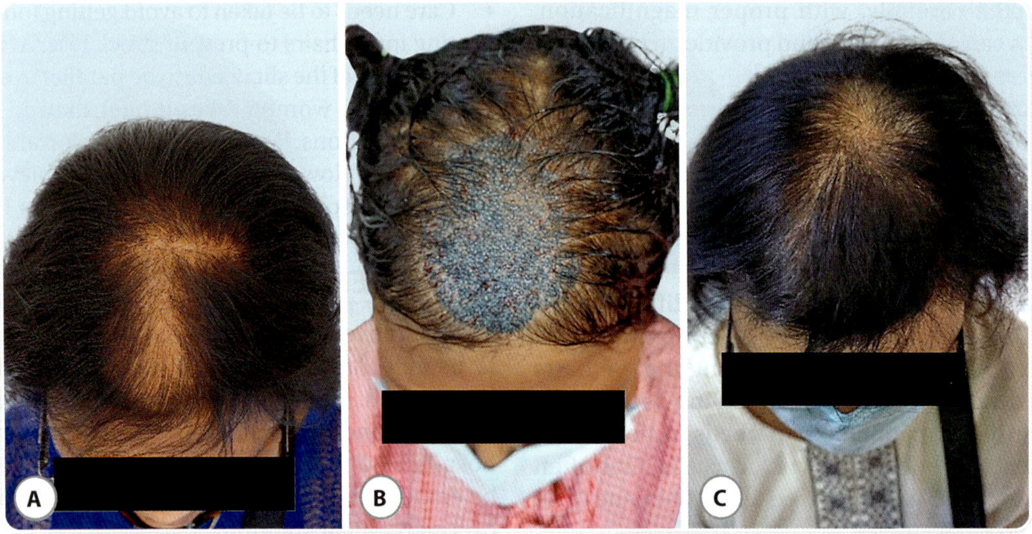

FIGS. 11A TO C: Female hair transplant: (A) Before hair transplant; (B) Immediate after procedure; (C) Post 7 months.
Courtesy: Dr Nitin Barde, Radiance Skin Antiaging and Hair Transplant Clinic, Nagpur, Maharashtra, India.

Postoperative hair shedding can be managed with proper planning. We can start the patient on prophylactic topical minoxidil for 6 weeks and use epinephrine in low doses as discussed in anesthesia considerations are ways to prevent this. If there is mild shedding with some visible patches, hair-fiber camouflage can be considered as a simple and inexpensive solution. Reassurance that hair will regrow within the next few months and preoperative counseling will help. Creative hairstyling is another way to hide the visible patches, if any. Minoxidil needs to be started early, similar to men.

SUMMARY

Despite the many challenges, it is possible to ensure a satisfactory outcome. Careful counseling, planning, and surgical techniques are essential. The following tips are offered to help the beginner:

- Ensure thorough counseling.
- Choose cases carefully.
- Avoid patients with poor donor, extensive baldness, and exaggerated expectations.
- Most cases need up to 2,000 grafts.
- Either strip or FUE can be performed.
- Slit and place and implanters are preferred; if preformed slits are done, then it needs to be combined with the other two techniques.
- Both coronal and sagittal incisions may be needed.
- Wetting the hairs and separation of existing hairs by a comb are useful.
- Slits need to be performed parallel to the direction of existing hairs.

REFERENCES

1. Camacho-Martínez FM. Hair loss in women. Semin Cutan Med Surg. 2009;28(1):19-32.
2. Ludwig E. Classification of the types of androgenetic alopecia (common baldness) occurring in the female sex. Br J Dermatol. 1977;97:247-54.
3. Unger WP, Unger RH. Hair transplanting: an important but often forgotten treatment for female pattern hair loss. J Am Acad Dermatol. 2003;49(5):853-60.
4. Epstein JS. The treatment of female pattern hair loss and other applications of surgical hair restoration in women. Facial Plast Surg Clin North Am. 2004;12(2):241-7.
5. International Society of Hair Restoration Surgery (ISHRS). (2015). Practice Census Facts and Figures [online].
6. Unger RH. Female hair restoration. Facial Plast Surg Clin North Am. 2013;21(3):407-17.
7. Avram MR. Hair transplantation. Cutis. 2012;90(6):317-20.
8. Atanaskova Mesinkovska N, Bergfeld WF. Hair: what is new in diagnosis and management? Female pattern hair loss update: diagnosis and treatment. Dermatol Clin. 2013;31(1):119-27.
9. Sinclair R, Patel M, Dawson TL, Yazdabadi A, Yip L, Perez A, et al. Hair loss in women: medical and cosmetic approaches to increase scalp hair fullness. Br J Dermatol. 2011;165(Suppl. 3): 12-8.
10. Avram MR. Hair transplantation for men and women. Semin Cutan Med Surg. 2006;25(1):60-4.

11. Epstein JS. Hair transplantation in women: treating female pattern baldness and repairing distortion and scarring from prior cosmetic surgery. Arch Facial Plast Surg. 2003;5(1): 121-6.
12. Vogel JE. Hair transplantation in women: a practical new classification system and review of technique. Aesthet Surg J. 2002;22(3):247-59.
13. Halsner UE, Lucas MW. New aspects in hair transplantation for females. Dermatol Surg. 1995;21(7):605-10.
14. Blume-Peytavi U, Blumeyer A, Tosti A, Finner A, Marmol V, Trakatelli M, et al. S1 guideline for diagnostic evaluation in androgenetic alopecia in men, women and adolescents. Br J Dermatol. 2011;164:5-15.
15. Olsen EA. The midline part: an important physical clue to the clinical diagnosis of androgenetic alopecia in women. J Am Acad Dermatol. 1999;40:106-9.
16. Samuel ML. Hair loss and hair restoration in women. Facial Plast Surg Clin North Am. 2020;28:205-23.
17. Jung JH, Rah DK, Yun IS. Classification of the female hairline and refined hairline correction techniques for Asian women. Dermatol Surg. 2011;37:495-500.
18. Nusbaum BP, Fuentefria S. Naturally occurring female hairline patterns. Dermatol Surg. 2009;35:907-13.
19. Kyle KS. Hair transplantation for female hairline in Asian women. In: Pathomvanich D, Imagawa K (Eds). Practical Aspects of Hair Transplantation in Asians. Japan: Springer; 2018. pp. 485-98.

CHAPTER 84

Hair Transplantation in Scarring Alopecia

Syed Mubashir

Key Messages

- Hair transplantation into scarring alopecia can be challenging.
- Proper diagnosis of scarring alopecia entails performing a detailed history and scalp examination.
- Surgical management includes scar revision, tissue expanders, and hair transplantation.
- Reactivation of the inflammatory stage may also occur post-transplant and lead to loss of the transplanted hairs.
- In cases of cicatricial alopecia secondary to disease, stability of the disease needs to be established before considering surgery.
- Skin texture, underlying dermal infrastructure, fat status, and vascularity affect the outcome.

INTRODUCTION

The term "scarring alopecia" *(cicatricial alopecia)* implies permanent destruction of the hair follicle. There is potential for permanent destruction of the hair follicle.[1]

It is caused as a result of irreversible damage to the epithelial hair follicle stem cells. If the stem cells and sebaceous gland are destroyed, there is no possibility for the regeneration of the hair follicle, leading to permanent hair loss.

Cicatricial alopecia has two forms.

1. In the primary form, the target is the destructive process of the hair follicle.
2. In the secondary form, the hair follicle is a bystander, destroyed by another cause. This can be due to a severe burn, an infection, radiation, or a tumor. The aim of the treatment should be to stop the progression of active lesion and correct the bald patch by hair transplantation once stability has been achieved. Cicatricial alopecia can either be a primary process, whereby it directly attacks the hair follicles, or a secondary process, whereby it indirectly attacks the hair follicles.

The actual mechanism that causes scarring alopecia involves the destruction of the isthmus segment of the hair follicle **(Box 1)**.

BOX 1 Proposed working classification of cicatricial alopecia.

- *Primary scarring alopecias: Pathology directed at the hair follicle*
  - Group 1: Lymphocytic—
    - Discoid lesion of lupus erythematosus
    - Lichen planopilaris (LPP)
    - Classic LPP
    - Frontal fibrosing alopecia
    - Classic pseudopelade (Brocq's alopecia)
    - Central centrifugal alopecia
    - Alopecia mucinosa
    - Keratosis follicularis spinulosa decalvans
    - Graft-versus-host reaction
  - Group 2: Neutrophilic—
    - Folliculitis decalvans
    - Dissecting cellulitis
    - Tufted folliculitis
  - Group 3: Mixed—
    - Acne keloidalis
    - Acne necrotica
    - Erosive pustular dermatosis
  - Group 4: Nonspecific—
    - Cicatricial pemphigoid
    - Busulfan-induced alopecia

Continued

Continued

- *Secondary cicatricial alopecias: Pathology nonspecifically affects the hair follicle*
    - Inflammatory/autoimmune:
        - Follicular mucinosis (alopecia mucinosa)
        - Scleroderma/morphea
    - Infectious:
        - Viral
        - Fungal
        - Bacterial
    - Neoplastic:
        - Primary and metastatic carcinoma
        - Granulomas
    - Physical agents:
        - X-ray
        - Burns

TREATMENT OPTIONS

Medical Treatment

In primary scarring alopecias, there is a tendency of progression and recurrence intermittently with time.

Medical therapy should be initiated as soon as possible before irreversible scarring occurs and make the disease stable.

Treatment of lymphocytic cicatricial group involves the use of anti-inflammatory medications such as steroids, cyclosporine, and hydroxychloroquine. In neutrophilic cicatricial alopecias, dapsone, colchicines, and steroids are useful. When hair follicles get destroyed, hair does not grow back. However, in some cases, using minoxidil solution can help to stimulate the growth of some of the remaining hair.

Hair transplantation can be taken only in nonactive and stable primary scarring alopecia, and it is advisable to confirm the disease being stable.[2] The stability means the disease has been inactive for at least 2 years. Hair transplantation can produce better results in certain cases.[3] It can be done using both follicular unit (FU) extraction or via strip technique, depending on the donor.[3,4]

Along with hair restoration surgeries, the following procedures can be performed, especially in large scarred areas of hair loss:

- Scalp repair using tissue expanders
- Serial scalp reduction
- Scalp reduction and the Frechet triple flap repair
- Transposition of scalp flaps
- Repair of wide donor scar, multiple W-plasty along with follicular grafting with micropigmentation

Test sessions should be carried out in these populations:

- Presence of scar tissue that binds to the FUs
- African patients who have a high degree of follicular curvature, which will lead to high transection rates
- Patients with primary scarring alopecia

CHALLENGES FOR HAIR TRANSPLANTATION IN SCARRING ALOPECIA

- The disease should be stable for at least 2 years.
- The blood supply of the scar tissue varies from patient to patient.
- Atrophy, texture variation, and elasticity make things complicated.
- Follicular survival in scar tissue depends upon lot of variables.
- Disease relapse and loss of grafted FUs should be kept in mind.
- In extensive scarring, hair transplantation can be difficult due to poor donor.
- Patient may need multiple sessions to achieve good cosmetic results.
- Male pattern baldness (MPB)/female pattern hair loss (FPHL) can evolve in future, so surgeon should plan surgery accordingly in cicatricial alopecia.
- Wound healing varies widely and remains unpredictable.

PRACTICAL TIPS IN HAIR TRANSPLANTATION

- Packing of the grafts should not be too dense.
- Chubby grafts containing 2–3 follicles are ideal.
- It is highly recommended to perform a small test area before undergoing a larger transplantation session.
- A 1–2 cm^2 area can be transplanted initially. In 9–12 months, depending on the assessment of graft survival in the test area, a larger session can be performed.
- A 10–25 FUs/cm^2 is recommended.
- The patient is counseled that 2–4 sessions may need to be performed every 9–12 months minimum, and that with each session, higher densities can be achieved.
- Candidate for hair transplant must have reasonably good donor area.
- Minoxidil 5% must be started 2–3 months before surgery and after surgery.
- Autologous fat transplantation can also be tried as it enhances graft uptake.
- Prior fractional ablative laser therapy can help improve skin texture and vasculacity.

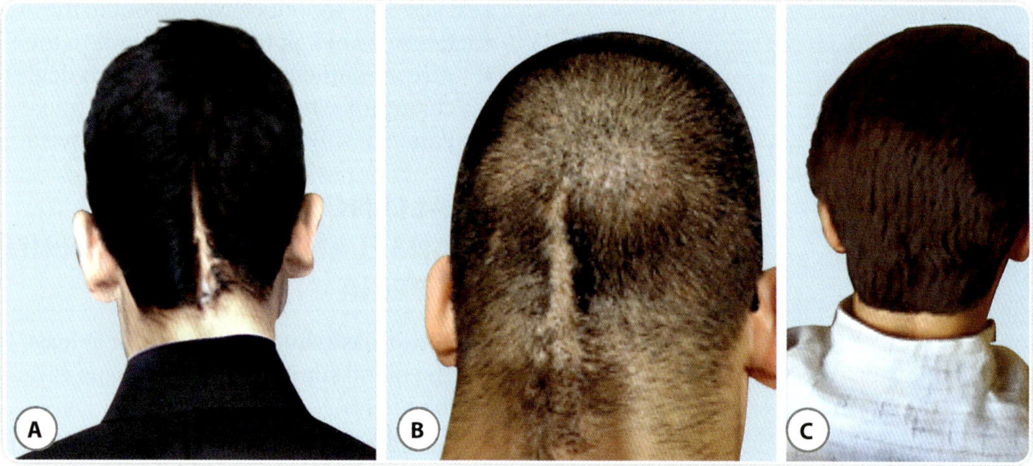

FIGS. 1A TO C: Hair transplant in secondary cicatricial alopecia due to tumor.

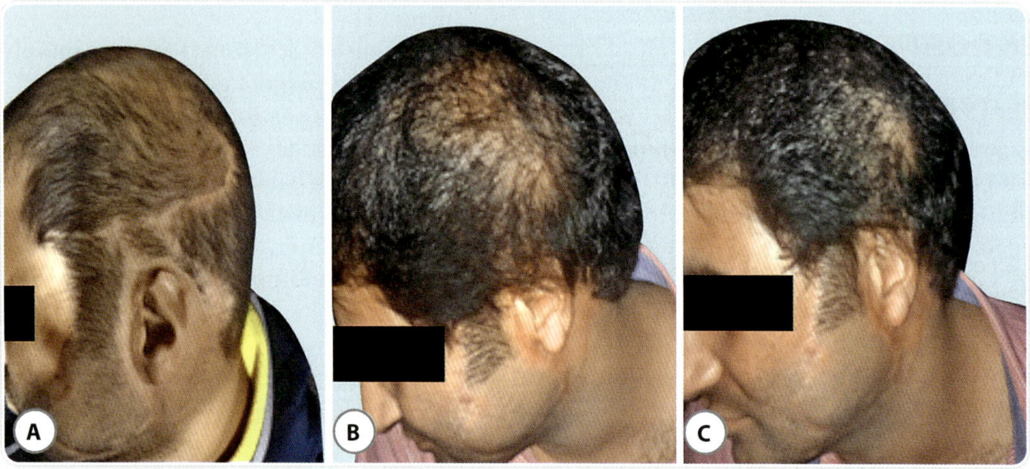

FIGS. 2A TO C: Hair transplantation in secondary cicatricial alopecia due to burn and expanders have been used earlier, to expand the scalp and later for scars, hair transplant was done.

- If possible, try to use plain 1% lidocaine; the use of adrenaline should be limited.
- Using blades or needles for making slits should be better for depth control.

Figures 1 to 4 show results after hair transplantation in patients with scarring alopecia.

PLANNING HAIR TRANSPLANTATION IN CICATRICIAL ALOPECIA

Donor–Recipient Ratio

Donor-recipient ratio is important as far as hair transplantation in cicatricial alopecia is considered. Body reserves should be considered in areas where the donor too is depleted.

Scar Texture

Scar tissue may be atrophic or hypertrophic. In atrophic scars, grafts would get accommodated as the lack of underneath subcutaneous tissue and compromised perfusion to grafts. As far as hypertrophic scars are concerned, implanted follicles may not reach proper alignment and depth. In the same scar, we may find both atrophic and hypertrophic areas.

Location of the Scar

Proper planning is needed as far as hair transplant in cicatricial alopecia is considered. The hairline should be properly designed with planning with a relatively high-density FU (25–35 FU/cm), as 50 these regions have good adjacent vascularity. Shao et al. used a follicular density

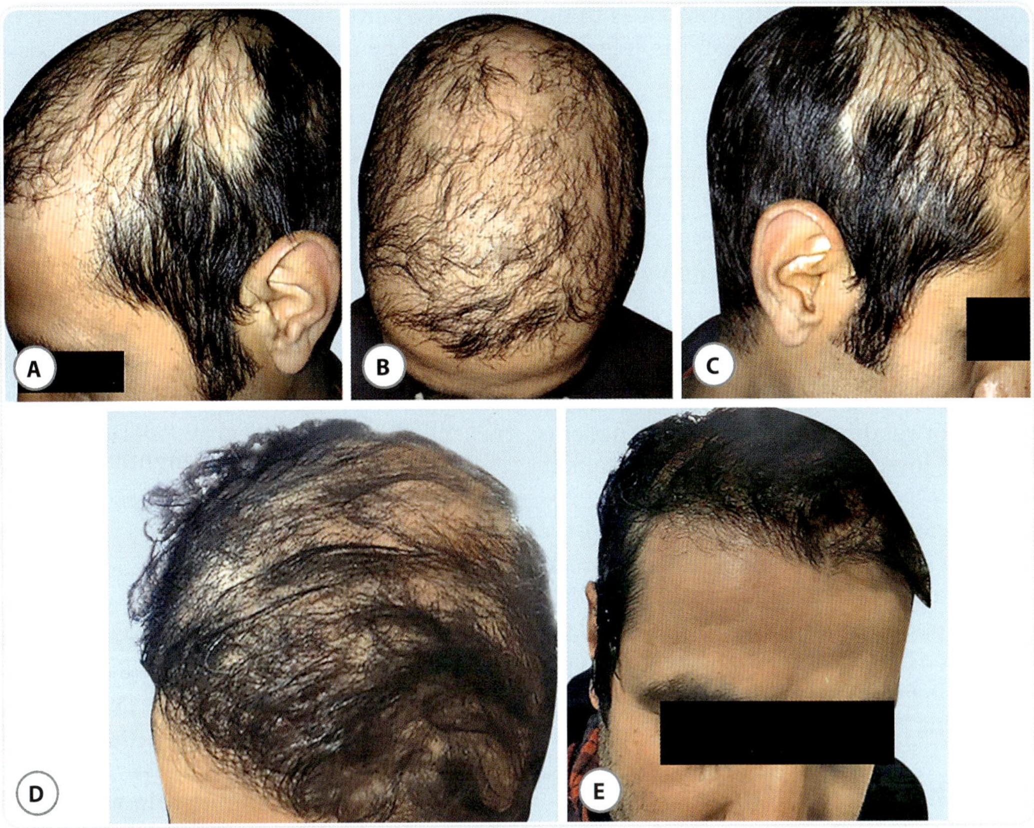

FIGS. 3A TO E: Hair transplantation (HT) in scarring alopecia.

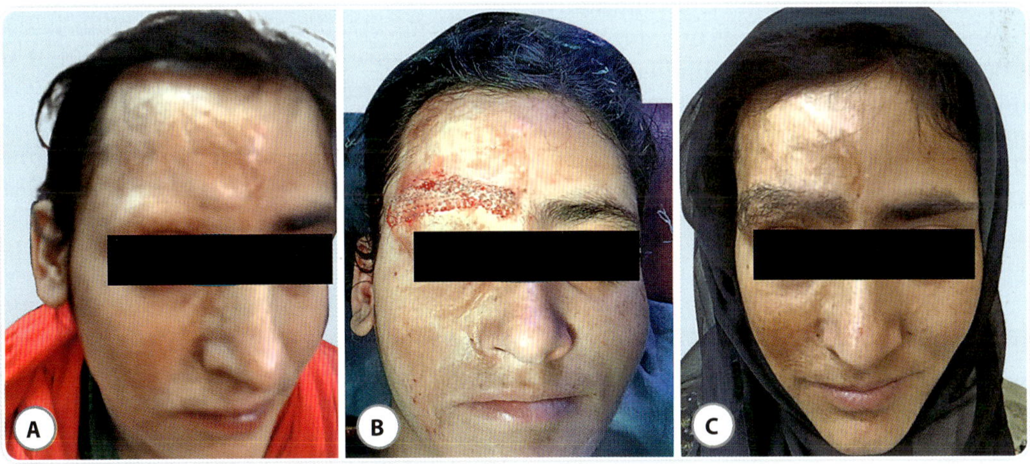

FIGS. 4A TO C: Eyebrow hair transplant due to secondary cicatricial alopecia.

of 20-48 FU/cm^2 in their series. Placing 45-50 FU on the normal-looking skin adjacent to the scars provides good camouflage. Vertical scars are more difficult to conceal than horizontal or oblique scars; vertical scars need long hair to fall over the alopecia in order to provide cover.

Scar Vascularity

Scar vascularity is one of the key components as far as survival of grafts is considered. Placing grafts too tightly can compromise vascularity,[5] and the follicles in the center of the scar have less vascularity compared to the periphery of the scars, which can cause necrosis, infection, and rejection.[6]

Alopecia Reduction versus Hair Transplantation

Hair transplantation has an edge over scar excision/alopecia reduction (AR) in patients having minimal elastic recoil and elasticity.[7]

In scalps where surgical undermining of the tissue is not possible, hair transplantation is preferable.

Hair transplantation is preferred in poor donor reserves (Hamilton-Norwood scale 7), very young patients with evolving hair loss, and those with unrealistic expectations.

Good candidates for AR are those 40 years and above with stable hair loss pattern (Hamilton-Norwood scale 4–6), good donor hair in the occipital region, smaller/solitary cicatricial alopecia lesion, and those who accept hair loss on the incision lines. Scalp flaps can be considered in cases of cicatricial alopecia, where local flaps can be utilized without having a secondary defect to restore.[8]

Factors by Which Aesthetic Results in Hair Transplant can be Increased

It can be assessed by making incisions in scar tissue using needle. If bleeding is present, we can go for hair transplantation; if no bleeding is present, alternative treatment options should be explored. In some cases, the use of carbon dioxide laser, along with platelet-rich plasma therapy, has been tried to increase the vascularity and make hypertrophic scars less and give better results. Adrenaline should be avoided in the recipient area, as vascularity is already compromised due to scarring. The recipient area should be anesthetized with a 2% lidocaine solution without epinephrine.[7]

Follicular Unit Graft Size Selection

Chubby grafts or two closely placed FUs [follicular family (FF)] give better coverage. FF grafts provide a greater number of hair follicles within the same recipient site and reduce the need to make multiple incisions, minimizing vascular damage.[7]

Recipient Area Slit

In atrophic scars, incision should be made at an acute angle and deeper to accommodate the graft.

In hypertrophic scars, fractional carbon dioxide laser can be used to improve texture, remodel the scar, and increase perfusion so that the graft fits properly. Vascularity needs to be checked, and always make incisions parallel to hair follicles.

Test Grafting in Recipient Area

In cicatricial alopecia, a test graft session is a must and should wait for 6 months to assess results. The follicles density per centimeter in cicatricial alopecia varies from patient to patient. In cicatricial alopecia regions with poor blood supply, 15–20 FU/cm^2 are considered optimal for better survival of the FU. In cases with good blood supply, the density of FU can be 20–30 FU/cm^2.[9] In some cases, the surgeon does surgery in two phases, and the second surgery is done after 9–12 months. For better aesthetic results, hair follicle transplantation on the scar may need secondary or more operations.[10]

Adjuvant Treatment

Application of topical minoxidil (2–5%) in the recipient area for 2 weeks before and at least 5 weeks is recommended, as it increases the local blood supply, prolongs the anagen (hair growth) phase, and provides better results.

Oxygenation of the recipient area by using Pentoxifylline, 400 mg, thrice a day with meals, for 2 weeks prior to surgery.

To reduce the scar texture, intralesional steroid injection can be given.

Using fractional carbon dioxide laser on the scar tissue causes collagen remodeling and increases the growth of transplanted hairs due to the promotion of neoangiogenesis. This causes a cascade of various growth factors and cytokines that promote hair growth.[11]

Platelet-rich plasma (PRP) has been used with good success, as it causes wound healing and scar remodeling and helps in FU survival.[12]

Common complications in hair transplantation are:

- Inadequate density
- Delayed healing
- Hypertrophic scars
- Rejection of grafts
- Infection
- Corkscrew hair transplantation
- Damage to occipital artery and nerve
- Bleeding
- Hematoma
- Postsurgical anagen effluvium
- Hypo-/hyperesthesia
- Neuromas
- Neuralgias[13]

SUMMARY

Hair transplantation in cicatricial alopecias can give better aesthetic results if properly evaluated. Secondary cicatricial alopecias need no medical management; however, primary cicatricial alopecias need medical management, and the disease should be quiescent for almost 2 years. Test patch is a must before taking patient for hair transplantation. Vascularity of the recipient area should be good, and donor area should be sufficient.

REFERENCES

1. Unger W, Unger R, Wesley C. The surgical treatment of cicatricial alopecia. Dermatol Ther. 2008;21:295-311.
2. Madura C, Vinay N, Kusuma MR, Harsha S, Chandrashekar BS. The assessment of hair transplantation outcomes in cicatricial alopecia. Int J Trichology. 2020;12(4):164-7.
3. Barrera A. The use of micrografts and minigrafts for the treatment of burn alopecia. Plast Reconstr Surg. 1999;103:581-4.
4. Shao H, Hang H, Yunyun J, Hongfei J, Chunmao H, Zhang J, et al. Follicular unit transplantation for the treatment of secondary cicatricial alopecia. Plast Surg (Oakv). 2014;22(4):249-53.
5. Jung S, Oh SJ, Hoon Koh S. Hair follicle transplantation on scar tissue. J Craniofac Surg. 2013;24:1239-41.
6. Thakur BK, Verma S. Is hair transplantation always successful in secondary cicatricial alopecia? Int J Trichology. 2015;7(1):43-4.
7. Sattur SS. A review of surgical methods (excluding hair transplantation) and their role in hair loss management today. J Cutan Aesthet Surg. 2011;4(02):89-97.
8. Unger MG, Unger WP. Management of alopecia of the scalp by a combination of excisions and transplantations. J Dermatol Surg Oncol. 1978;4(09):670-2.
9. Kutlubay Z, Kucuktas M, Engin B. Hair transplantation in the cicatricial alopecias. Hair Ther Transplant. 2013;3:1-4.
10. Moser K, Hugeneck J, Rohrbacher W, Moser C. The pairing technique of the Moser Medical Group. Hair Transpl Forum Int. 2005;15:41-6.
11. Kwon OS, Kim MH, Park SH, Chung JH, Eun HC, Oh JK. Staged hair transplantation in cicatricial alopecia after carbon dioxide laser-assisted scar tissue remodeling. Arch Dermatol. 2007;143:457-60.
12. Kumar AR, Ishii LE. Hair transplantation for scarring alopecia. Facial Plast Surg Clin North Am. 2020;28(02):177-9.
13. Cooley J. Complications of Hair Transplantation. New York: Marcel Dekker; 2004. p. 573.

CHAPTER 85

Nontransplantation Methods of Hair Transplantation

Sandeep Sattur, Indu S Sattur

Key Messages

- Nonhair transplantation methods of hair restoration were popular at one point of time but now have been replaced by hair transplantation.
- Flaps and scalp reductions are the options that can used in select cases of localized hair loss in cases of cicatricial hair loss caused by injury or burns.

INTRODUCTION

The search for ideal treatment for baldness has been ongoing for a very long time. The constant desire to produce natural-looking results and meet ever-increasing patient expectations has driven this evolution of techniques in the last few decades. Surgical methods to address hair loss were actually based on various scalp reconstruction techniques. They were modified for use in the patient with pattern hair loss. Today, with hair transplantation techniques assuming a preeminent rank in modern hair restoration, the older techniques have taken a back seat. They still have a role to play in selective cases, and a hair restorative surgeon should be well versed in these techniques as well to be able to offer a patient with hair loss all the possible options.

HISTORICAL BACKGROUND

Hunt (1926) was one of the first practitioners who proposed serial excision of small patches of alopecia and advancing hair-bearing scalp to close the defect.[1] Passot, in his classic text published in 1931, mentioned long, narrow, hair-bearing flaps for correction of alopecia.[2] This is considered by many as the precursor of present-day scalp flaps. In 1939, Tauber applied Passot's techniques and described the use of local flaps elevated from lateral and posterior scalp for the replacement of hair.[3] This was followed by Lamont in 1957, who described lateral scalp flaps for the treatment of frontotemporal baldness.[4] Correa-Iturraspe and Arufe, in the same year, attempted several different methods to correct partial alopecia, one of which was excision of full-thickness segments of hairless scalp skin and primary closure of the wound margins.[5] Small pedicle flaps of donor scalp were employed for decades for scar correction on the scalp, but it was only after 1975 that they had a resurgence, largely due to the work of J Juri in Buenos Aires. His long, twice-delayed (delay in a surgical procedure for improving the survival of flap on limited blood supply) temporo-parieto-occipital (TPO) scalp flaps eliminated the curious tufted appearance of a punch graft hairline.[6] But these flaps also did not become very popular because of their high failure rate, and even when successful, the frontal hair growth was frequently unnatural in density and direction. Harii et al. made use of microsurgical techniques in 1974 to transplant hair by free scalp flaps.[7] To some extent, the unnatural direction of hair in the Juri flap was tackled by Ohmori in 1980. He designed a large Juri flap but transferred it using microsurgical techniques. The advantage was to transfer large amounts of hair in one stage and position the flaps in such a way that the direction of hair is natural.[8] In 1976, Blanchard and Blanchard (credited with the first scientific paper on scalp reduction) described the technique of scalp reduction, which they called "obliteration of alopecia by hair lifting".[9] The term "scalp reduction" was first used by Sparkuhl in 1978, and he defined it as the surgical excision of redundant tissue from one or more areas of scalp alopecia.[10] Scalp reduction had a somewhat variable course of success, partly due to its complications. To some extent, these shortcomings were addressed by Manders and his associates, Nordstrom and Devine, and Leonard and Small with the use of tissue expanders[11,12] and later by Fréchet in 1993[13] with the use of an implanted extender. Subsequently, many procedures and devices were proposed to lessen the effects of stretch-back and other associated problems. These included the Seery periosteal flap anchor,[14] the Unger prolonged acute tissue expansion (PATE)[15] procedure, and the Nordstrom silastic suture. Cohen's innovative skin-stretching device was called the Miami suture tension adjustment reel (STAR).[16] Marzola tackled the problem of the unsightly scar from a different approach by using the M-shaped incision.[17]

SURGICAL HAIR RESTORATION

Surgical hair restoration can be classified into the following headings:

- Hair transplantation
- Scalp flaps:
  - Rotation flaps
  - Transposition flaps
  - TPO (pedicled)/Juri flaps (TPO flaps)
  - TPO (free/microvascular/microsurgical) flaps
  - Lateral scalp flaps
  - Temporovertical flaps
  - Other flaps
- Alopecia reduction (AR)/scalp reduction:
  - Simple AR
  - Major AR/scalp lift
  - AR with prior scalp extension (nonvolumetric)
  - AR with prior tissue expansion (volumetric)
  - AR with intraoperative stretching (volumetric and nonvolumetric).

SURGICAL CONSIDERATIONS OF SCALP ANATOMY

The scalp skin is thicker than skin in most places on the body, and the vascular supply of the scalp is centripetal (vessels enter from the periphery and run medially) **(Fig. 1)**; hence, incisions in the peripheral scalp that transect arteries may grossly limit blood supply to areas both adjacent to and remote from the locus of transection.[18] Subcutaneous fat is divided into multiple small compartments by fibrous septa, which bind down the scalp skin firmly to the muscles and aponeurosis **(Fig. 2)**, making dissection in this plane difficult and bloody. The galea is inelastic and limits the extent of scalp reduction, which can be overcome partly with incision of the galea (galeotomy). The subgaleal compartment is largely avascular, containing only a layer of loose areolar tissue. This enables surgical dissection in the subgaleal plane during reconstructive procedures,

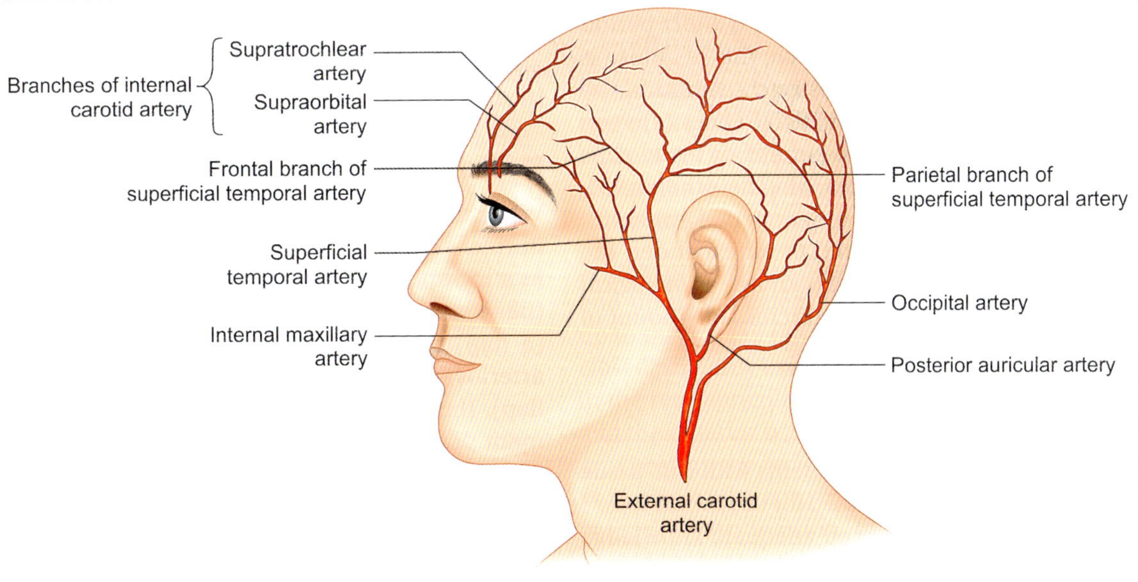

FIG. 1: Arterial supply of scalp: Branches of the internal carotid artery (supratrochlear and supraorbital) and external carotid artery (superficial temporal, posterior auricular, occipital artery).

skin is sutured over this to ensure that the hair grows through the scar (trichophytic).

A second flap from the contralateral side may be raised similarly depending on the extent of frontal hair loss. The Juri (TPO) flap is the only method that can give instant results with an astonishing density compared to the conventional hair transplant, which requires 6–12 months to produce good cosmetic results.

Complications

The potential complications include wide donor scars and partial or complete necrosis of the flap. A common problem seen with most transposition flaps, dog-ear deformity, is seen with TPO flap.

Lateral Scalp Flaps

Technical difficulties and the hassle of delay were overcome when Elliott[26] described the shorter version of the temporo-parietal flap. This flap was **(Fig. 6)** based on the anterior hairline, which curved over the ear and directed posteriorly, having a width averaging 2.5 cm. It was easier to execute given its narrower width and shorter length. The temporo-parietal flap is too short to traverse the entire frontal hairline, and usually, a flap from the opposite side is required to bridge the gap. Unfortunately, this narrow flap often appears unnatural, especially with progress of hair loss, leaving an isolated, narrow strip of hair that serves as the manufactured frontal hairline.

Temporovertical Flaps

Nataf, in 1984, designed a flap based superiorly in the parietal scalp, which extends vertically downward either in pre- or retroauricular areas. This flap was meant primarily for frontal baldness of MPHL and designed in such a way that the hair would be oriented in a forward direction. It can be as long as 25 cm, but more importantly, the quality of hair (retroauricular) it contains is ideal for frontal hairlines. Due to its narrow width and long length, this flap too needs a delay but it leaves the temporal area intact.[27]

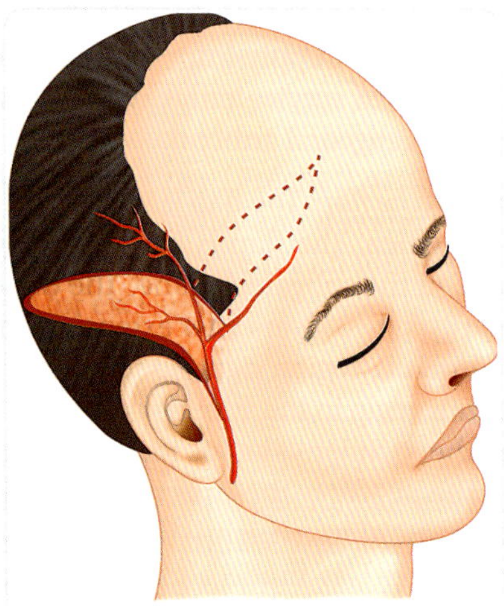

FIG. 6: Elliott flap (lateral scalp flap).

Temporo-parieto-occipital (Free/Microvascular/Microsurgical) Flaps

Due to the fixed attachment of the pedicle, positional adjustment of the flap in the recipient area is somewhat limited in traditional scalp flaps. It is difficult to change the direction of hair, and a redundant fold of skin may occur at the base of the pedicle (dog-ear deformity). Harii et al. overcame these two problems when they made use of microsurgical techniques to transplant hair by free-scalp flaps. By using specialized microsurgical instrumentation and operating microscopes, they could transfer large amounts of hair-bearing tissue in one stage.

In 1980, Ohmori described a free-Juri flap. He transferred the TPO flap in one-stage anastomosing the donor vessels to the contralateral temporal vessels. The advantage of this technique was that the flap could be positioned in such a way so that the hair is oriented in a natural direction, and the dog-ear deformity is avoided. This method is technically demanding and needs the surgeon to be well trained in microvascular surgery.[7,8]

Other Flaps

Bipedicle (visor) flaps from the occipital area, having two pedicles, are rotated over the vertex like a visor to reach the frontal area. These flaps were basically described in cases of cicatricial alopecia. Smaller bipedicle flaps based on temporal areas can be used to cover areas of cicatricial alopecia in the frontal region.[21] The advantage was one-stage transfer and primary closure of the donor defect.

ALOPECIA REDUCTION OR SCALP REDUCTION

Scalp reduction, now appropriately called AR, can be defined as an excision of area of alopecia. ARs are used for MPHL and also for cicatricial alopecia.

The extent of bald scalp that can be excised is limited by:

- Scalp laxity
- Surgical undermining
- Amount of creep (stretching) obtained preoperatively or intraoperatively.

Timing of Alopecia Reduction

Alopecia reduction works best when used in combination with hair transplantation for correcting hair loss. It can be planned before or after the hair transplant **(Fig. 7)**, each sequence having its own advantages and disadvantages. AR performed before hair transplantation has the following advantages:

- It ensures adequate blood supply.
- It avoids distortion of transplanted frontotemporal areas.

Patient Selection for Alopecia Reduction

Dominic Brandy had suggested patient selection criteria for AR. He concluded that the evaluation system should help the hair restoration surgeon determine who is a good candidate for AR and who is a poor candidate.[28] Ideal candidates are males with Norwood grades 4, 5, and 6, who are above the age of 40 years with stable hair loss. These patients should have little or no hair in the scalp that is to be excised but have dense hair on the sides and back of the head (good parietal humps) with good scalp laxity. The occipital fringe should be at least 10 cm wide with no retrograde recession (low-occipital hairline). In addition, patients should be counseled preoperatively on the likely further loss of some hair near the incision line.

Alopecia reduction is contraindicated in the following situations:

- Very tight scalp
- Thinning or poor density on the sides and back of the scalp
- Area for excision has significant hair (better managed with medical treatment)
- Very young patient with evolving hair loss or very high expectations
- Grade 7 Norwood.

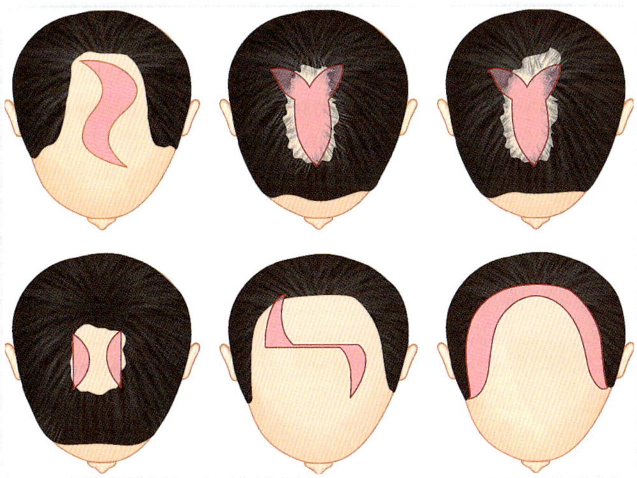

FIG. 7: Different shapes for alopecia reduction (AR).

Preoperative Preparation

Preoperative Scalp Massage

The ability of the scalp skin to stretch over a period of time from prolonged tension (mechanical creep) is utilized preoperatively. To accomplish this, scalp massage is advised at least 4–8 weeks prior to surgery. The amount of laxity that is generated from this can be quite surprising.

Anesthesia for Alopecia Reduction

Simple ARs can be carried out under local anesthesia with sedation. But the major ARs or the ARs with stretching or expansion would need general anesthesia.

Simple Alopecia Reduction

A variety of patterns for AR have been described, and the most common are the ellipse, the inverted Y-shaped or the rocket-ship pattern, the flattened S-shaped, or the M-shaped designs **(Fig. 8)**. The idea is to remove as much bald scalp as possible, preserving the part that contains hair. The choice of design depends upon individual patients and their pattern of hair loss. After the design has been marked, an incision is made on one side, right down to the galea all through its length. Beveling the blade is helpful in preventing injury to the follicles along the margin. After achieving hemostasis, undermining is begun in the subgaleal space. A combination of sharp and blunt dissection helps to create flaps on either side. Bleeding is rare, and coagulation is required only in the occipital areas or the vertex where two or more perforators are usually transected. The amount of excess scalp is

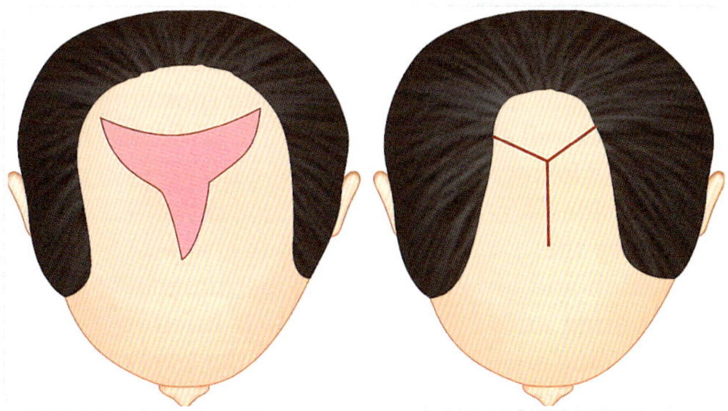

FIG. 8: Excision of bald area by alopecia reduction (AR).

- *Stretch-back*: It is re-expansion of the bald area after reduction (Norwood et al.).[40] There is always some degree of stretch-back in AR, which varies from 10 to 50%.
- *Pain (tight scalp feeling)*: Initially, it is due to tension in the wound, but pain coming after 3–5 days postoperatively could be due to enlarging hematoma or infection.

Cosmetic Complications

- *Distortion of bald area*: It is usually seen at the vertex where the normal round or U-shaped bald area gets converted to an extended oval, triangular area with slot formation, etc. **(Fig. 10)**. This can be avoided to some extent with proper planning. Meeting of both the sutured edges in the midline with hair growing in opposite directions is called a slot deformity.
- *Retraction of frontotemporal hairline*: It can occur in cases of a transverse excision of the bald area.
- *Scars*: They are unavoidable, but poor scars result because of tight closures, improper suturing, and inadequate galeal fixation.
- *Thinning*: It is seen in temporal and occipital areas due to stretching of skin in these areas.
- *Apparent acceleration of MPHL*: It can be attributed to the fact that the area of future baldness is stretched over a wider area in a younger patient; the apparent increase in hair loss will be noted because of geometric reasons. The hairline over the ears can also appear elevated, giving the impression of a recent haircut.
- *Effluvium (anagen as well as telogen)*: It can be observed in some cases, especially near the suture lines.

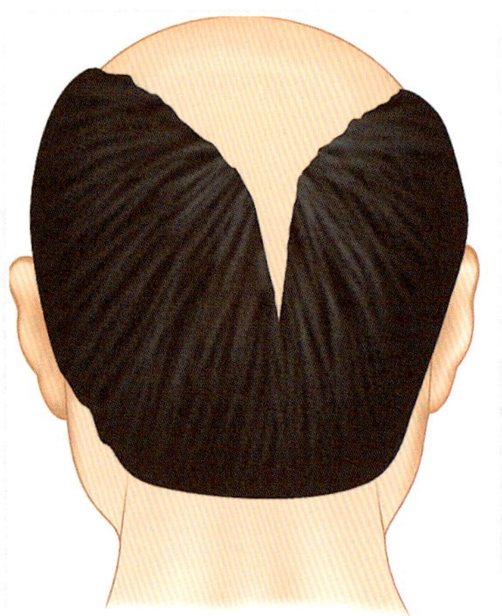

FIG. 10: Slot deformity following alopecia reduction (AR).

PRESENT STATUS OF NONTRANSPLANTATION SURGICAL RESTORATION

Hair restoration was given a major boost by the introduction of hair transplantation by Orentreich.[41] But as time passed, the pluggy look left these patients desiring something better. This along with the inadequacies in treating vertex hair loss were some of the reasons why scalp reduction gained importance. Scalp rotation (flaps) and AR started to wane as more complications and patient dissatisfaction began to get reported. Even if one were to look at the literature being published on hair restoration or papers being presented today, there is very little or practically no mention of ARs and scalp flaps.

One can evaluate their (ARs and scalp flaps) relevance today if one analyzes the patient who requests help for hair loss problem. Today, the average hair loss patient is a person who comes with very high expectations, is relatively younger, does not want invasive/major surgery, and is extremely concerned with postoperative scars, permanence of results, etc. In short, he/she wants a procedure that can boast of a very good risk-to-benefit ratio, i.e., very little risk (morbidity) and lot of benefit. Also, there is help available from the pharmaceutical industry (finasteride and minoxidil), which has, in fact, changed the whole approach to hair restoration in younger patients.

But if one were to look at long-term implications, ARs actually decrease the effective amount of hair that could be moved during subsequent hair transplantation to the front and top of the scalp due to reduced donor density and scalp laxity. As a result, the more cosmetically important frontal area is denied the benefit of transplantation due to reduced donor reserves. Although a scalp reduction may be performed with the best intent, it can place the patient in the precarious position of having more cosmetic problems than he started with and the lack of donor reserves to correct them, due to the progressive nature of hair loss.

In today's hair restoration practice, ARs could be useful in treating small cicatricial alopecia (pathological or traumatic) patches. Reduction of the scarred area (depending on the size and location) could be a better option than transplanting it, especially for smaller areas that do not require undermining. Slightly larger areas could be excised and covered by using tissue expansion principle, and hair restoration surgeons must know how to identify these cases in order to assure patients of the best outcomes. It is important that the person practicing hair restoration has to have a basic knowledge of these techniques and should be familiar with the principles of plastic surgery. Scarred areas oriented in a linear fashion on the crown or vertex areas are better suited for tissue expansion. In the presence of significant scarring or areas where split or full-thickness skin grafts were placed over the cranium (not suitable for hair transplantation), it is best to excise and replace them with healthy skin containing hair.

A patient who desires rapid, dense coverage in the frontotemporal region and who possesses adequate parietal donor hair may be eligible for TPO flap. Even with multiple sessions of hair transplant, one cannot achieve the density seen in TPO flap transfer. But, with the scalp flaps, especially the Juri flap and temporovertical flaps, the density and the direction of the hair are not natural and hence not very acceptable. Moreover, the flaps have a significantly high failure rate, with flap necrosis at the tip and a very visible scar at the anterior hairline. The free flap described by Ohmori did take care of these issues but was technically very demanding and could not justify the means to the result. These procedures require a lot of skill and surgical experience, and even in the best of hands, these procedures are risky and create too many cosmetic problems for the patient in the long run. In the current practice, the routine use of scalp flaps remains restricted for reconstructive measures and not as a first-line choice for cosmetic hair restoration.

Hair transplantation has evolved to state-of-the-art therapy, with notable refinements in instrumentation and approach to the problem of pattern hair loss. Moreover, most patients today are more psychologically inclined toward hair transplantation, and this technique remains the primary means by which pattern hair loss is addressed, providing reasonably satisfying results for surgeon and recipient alike. In contrast, ARs and scalp flaps have a very limited or practically no role in the restoration of patients with pattern hair loss because of invasive nature of these procedures and concerns that surgical outcomes are not commensurate with the perceived added morbidity. Simply put, they do not have a very good risk-to-benefit ratio. ARs could have a very favorable safety profile in selected cases of cicatricial alopecia, which have very small patches of hair loss. Scalp flaps could find favor in small cases of cicatricial alopecia, where local flaps could be used without having a secondary defect to restore.

Presently, most of the surgical hair restoration is hair transplant-based, with little or no contribution from scalp reduction and scalp flap procedures.

REFERENCES

1. Hunt HL. Plastic Surgery of the Head, Face and Neck, 1st edition. Philadelphia, PA, USA: Lea & Febiger; 1926.
2. Passot R. Chirurgie Esthétique Pure: Techniques et Résultats. Paris, France: Gaston Doin et Cie; 1931.
3. Taabor HT. The problem of premature alopecia: its surgical treatment. Minerva Dermatol. 1961;36:214-7.
4. Lamont ES. A plastic surgical transformation; report of a case. West J Surg Obstet Gynecol. 1957;65(3):164-5.
5. Correa-Iturraspe M, Arufe HN. Plastic surgery in certain partial alopecias of the scalp. Bol Trab Soc Cir B Aires. 1957;41(10): 299-317.
6. Juri J. Use of parieto-occipital flaps in the surgical treatment of baldness. Plast Reconstr Surg. 1975;55(4):456-60.
7. Harii K, Omori K, Omori S. Hair transplantation with free scalp flaps. Plast Reconstr Surg. 1974;53(4):410-3.
8. Ohmori K. Free scalp flap. Plast Reconstr Surg. 1980;65(1):42-9.
9. Blanchard G, Blanchard B. Obliteration of alopecia by hair-lifting: a new concept and technique. J Natl Med Assoc. 1977;69(9):639-41.
10. Sparkuhl K. Scalp reduction: serial excision of the scalp with flap advancement. Read before the International Hair Transplant Symposium, Lucerne, Switzerland on February 4, 1978.
11. Manders EK, Graham WP. Alopecia reduction by scalp expansion. J Dermatol Surg Oncol. 1984;10(12):967-9.
12. Nordstrom RE. Tissue Expansion. Oxford, UK: Butterworth-Heinemann; 1996. p. 17.
13. Fréchet P. Scalp extension. J Dermatol Surg Oncol. 1993;19(7): 616-22.
14. Seery GE. Anchor scalp reduction. Dermatol Surg. 1996;22(12): 1009-13.
15. Unger M. Advantages and disadvantages of the Unger PATE procedure. Am J Cosmet Surg. 1997;14(2):155-8.
16. Cohen BH, Cosmetto AJ. The suture tension adjustment reel. A new device for the management of skin closure. J Dermatol Surg Oncol. 1992;18(2):112-23.
17. Marzola M. A new alopecia reduction design, no visible scars, no slots, no Fréchet flaps. Am J Cosmet Surg. 1997;14(2):167-76.
18. Seery GE. Surgical anatomy of the scalp. Dermatol Surg. 2002; 28(7):581-7.
19. Seery GE. Scalp surgery: anatomic and biomechanical considerations. Dermatol Surg. 2001;27(9):827-34.
20. Purslow PP, Wess TJ, Hukins DW. Collagen orientation and molecular spacing during creep and stress-relaxation in soft connective tissues. J Exp Biol. 1998;201(Pt. 1):135-42.
21. Vallis CP. Hair replacement surgery. In: McCarthy JG (Ed). Plastic Surgery (Volume 2: The Face, Part 1), 3rd edition. Philadelphia, PA, USA: WB Saunders; 1990.
22. McGregor IA, McGregor AD. Flaps. Fundamental Techniques of Plastic Surgery and Their Surgical Applications, 10th edition. New York, NY, USA: Churchill Livingstone; 2000.
23. Stough DB, Cates JA, Dean AJ. Updating reduction and flap procedures for baldness. Ann Plast Surg. 1982;8(4):287-95.
24. Fleming RW, Mayer TG. Short vs long scalp flaps in the treatment of male pattern baldness. Arch Otolaryngol. 1981;107(7): 403-8.

25. Fleming RW, Mayer TG. Scalp flaps—reconstruction of the unfavorable result in hair replacement surgery. Head Neck Surg. 1985;7(4):315-31.
26. Elliott RA. Lateral scalp flaps for instant results in male pattern baldness. Plast Reconstr Surg. 1977;60(5):699-703.
27. Nataf J. Surgical treatment for frontal baldness: the long temporal vertical flap. Plast Reconstr Surg. 1984;74(5):628-35.
28. Brandy DA. An evaluation system to enhance patient selection for alopecia-reducing surgery. Dermatol Surg. 2002;28(9): 808-16.
29. Unger WP, Shapiro R, Unger R, Unger M (Eds). Hair Transplantation, 5th edition. Philadelphia, PA, USA: Informa Healthcare; 2011.
30. Swinehart JM, Brandy DA. Scalp lifting. Anatomic and technical considerations. J Dermatol Surg Oncol. 1994;20(9):600-12.
31. Swinehart JM. Color Atlas of Hair Restoration Surgery, 1st edition. California, CA, USA: Appleton & Lange; 1996.
32. Mangubat EA. Preservation of the occipital artery during extensive scalp lifting. Am J Cosmet Surg. 1997;14 (2):161-6.
33. Brandy DA. The effectiveness of occipital artery ligations as a priming procedure for extensive scalp-lifting. J Dermatol Surg Oncol. 1991;17(12):946-9.
34. Fréchet P. A new method for correction of the vertical scar observed following scalp reduction for extensive alopecia. J Dermatol Surg Oncol. 1990;16(7):640-4.
35. Fréchet P. Slot correction by a three hair-bearing transposition flap procedure in combination with scalp reduction. Int J Aesthetic Restor Surg. 1994;2:27-32.
36. Neumann CG. The expansion of an area of skin by progressive distention of a subcutaneous balloon; use of the method for securing skin for subtotal reconstruction of the ear. Plast Reconstr Surg (1946). 1957;19(2):124-30.
37. Nordström R. Tissue expansion and flaps for surgical correction of male pattern baldness. Br J Plast Surg. 1988;41(2):154-9.
38. Epstein JS, Florida M. Scalp reconstruction: the role of tissue expansion. Forum. 2006;16:15371.
39. Norwood OT, Shiell RC, Morrison ID. Complications of scalp reductions. J Dermatol Surg Oncol. 1983;9(10):828-35.
40. Unger MG, Unger WP. Management of alopecia of the scalp by a combination of excisions and transplantations. J Dermatol Surg Oncol. 1978;4(9):670-2.
41. Orentreich N. Autografts in alopecias and other selected dermatological conditions. Ann NY Acad Sci. 1959;83:463-79.

CHAPTER 86

Hair Transplantation and Dermatological Conditions

Ruhi Uttamani-Sangle, Venkataram Mysore

Key Messages

- In the presence of autoimmune disorders, such as vitiligo and alopecia areata, or chronic inflammatory disorders, such as various connective tissue diseases (CTDs) and psoriasis, it is imperative to check for disease stability before planning hair transplantation.
- The possibility of reactivation of the disease post transplant, and even possible damage to the grafts must always be explained to the patient, and consent stating the same must be taken.
- Various disorders affecting the scalp may impact the process of hair transplant (HT) itself, such as excessive bleeding during hair transplantation in the case of scalp psoriasis and fibrotic scalp in the case of chronic folliculitis. The skill of an HT surgeon will be put to the test while dealing with such situations.

INTRODUCTION

Hair loss is a common problem affecting both men and women. It can have an immense effect on one's self-esteem and emotional well-being. In an attempt to treat hair loss more effectively, hair transplant (HT) surgery has become increasingly popular. At some instances, we may come across other coexisting dermatological conditions, which may or may not be related to hair loss directly, but may have implications in planning HT surgery. The relation between hair, scalp diseases, and hair transplantation largely depends on the nature of the disease, whether it may be induced or worsened by the surgical procedure or chances of the condition interfering with the procedural technique. For example, papulosquamous diseases such as psoriasis and seborrheic dermatitis (SD) may flare up because of hair transplantation, while transplanted grafts in patients with any of the primary cicatricial alopecias would most likely shed eventually due to the underlying disease process. We will be discussing a few such conditions in this chapter.

PAPULOSQUAMOUS DISORDERS

Seborrheic Dermatitis

Seborrheic dermatitis is a common condition that presents as chronic, recurrent, mild to moderately erythematous patches with greasy scales mainly over the scalp, beard, nasolabial folds, retroauricular folds, and chest. The scales may be minimal, with mild to absent pruritus. Whereas in moderate to severe SD, there might be extensive scaling associated with severe pruritus. It is recommended to manage this condition before the hair transplantation procedure to lessen the scaling and control the pruritus. Itching post hair transplantation has a detrimental effect on graft uptake. Resolution of lesions would likewise decrease the possibility of significant pruritus over the donor site, which may occur during the healing period post transplant.

Management options include the use of tar-, salicylic acid-, or selenium-based shampoos and/or ketoconazole shampoo as well as a topical antifungal medication (e.g., ketoconazole) and topical calcineurin inhibitor solutions.

Corticosteroid lotions may be used for acute flares. In very severe cases, systemic drugs such as terbinafine (250 mg for 4 weeks) or itraconazole (100 mg/day for 3 weeks) can be used, and for recalcitrant cases, oral steroids and oral isotretinoin (2.5–5 mg/day) can be used.[1] *The possibility of worsening of SD after HT surgery must be kept in mind* because of improper/inadequate washing of scalp by the patient due to the fear of harming the grafts. Ideally, scalp wash on postoperative day 3 and day 10 must be done at the clinic for adequate removal of scabs and scales and also for the demonstration of proper scalp washing technique.

The possibility of misdiagnosing fibrosing alopecia in pattern distribution (FAPD) as androgenetic alopecia (AGA) with concomitant SD should always be kept in mind. FAPD is a primary cicatricial alopecia characterized by thinning of hair on the centroparietal scalp with histopathologic features of AGA as well as lichen planopilaris.[2-4] Diagnostic criteria for FAPD include symmetrical hair loss in androgen-dependent areas with sparing of the occipital scalp **(Fig. 1)** and supporting trichoscopic features including hair shaft diameter variability, perifollicular scaling, and loss of follicular ostia **(Fig. 2)**.[3]

Seborrheic dermatitis is characterized by perifollicular scaling and thin arborizing vessels dermoscopically.[5] Therefore, if SD occurs on a background of AGA, distinction from FAPD may be challenging. It is essential to distinguish FAPD from AGA with concomitant SD before planning hair transplantation, because *patients with FAPD are not suitable candidates for the procedure.* Clues suggesting the possibility of FAPD are the symptoms of pruritus, pain, and burning sensation. A simple method to help distinguish the two conditions is by scraping the scalp and looking for changes in scales.[6] In SD, the perifollicular scale is loosely attached, and the interfollicular skin harbors a "hidden" scale which can be readily lifted by scraping. In FAPD, the perifollicular scales remain unchanged on scraping.

A skin punch biopsy is needed to confirm the diagnosis and to properly exclude such conditions before proceeding with hair transplantation.

Recommendations

- Manage SD before the hair transplantation procedure to lessen the scaling and control the pruritus.
- In cases of AGA with concomitant SD, differential diagnosis of FAPD must be kept in mind. Biopsy for confirmation is recommended as FAPD patient is not a candidate for HT.

Scalp Psoriasis

Scalp psoriasis is characterized by erythematous plaques with thick silvery scales, with mild to no pruritus. Up to 90% of psoriatic patients may have lesions on the scalp at some point during their lifetimes. In about 25% of patients, the unique localization of the disease remains limited to the scalp.[7,8] Clinical patterns include plaque type (erythematous plaques with thick silvery white scales), thin desquamation type, psoriatic cap, pityriasis amiantacea, and relatively rare variants such as cicatricial psoriatic alopecia and pustular psoriasis of the scalp.[8]

The role of microvascular abnormalities and angiogenesis is well known in the pathogenesis of psoriasis.[9,10]

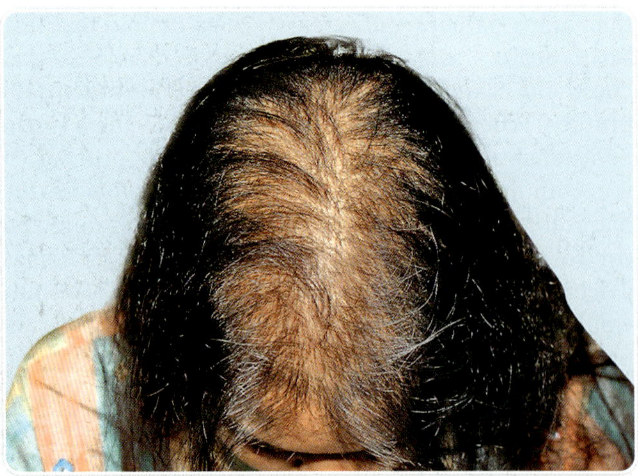

FIG. 1: Clinical presentation of fibrosing alopecia in pattern distribution (FAPD). May be misdiagnosed as female pattern hair loss (FPHL)/androgenetic alopecia (AGA) with seborrheic dermatitis (SD).

Courtesy: Cutis Academy of Cutaneous Sciences, Bengaluru, Karnataka, India.

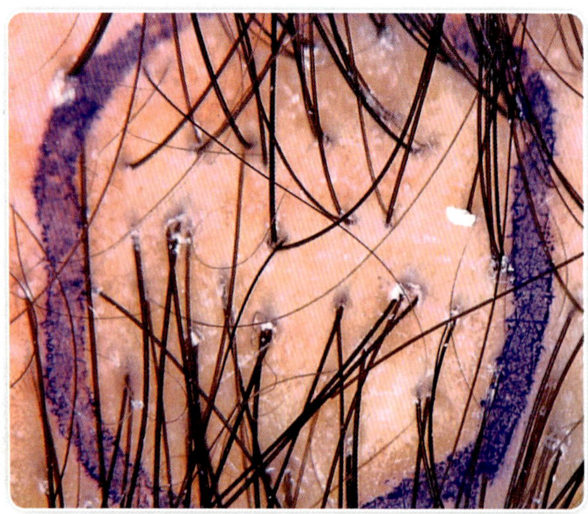

FIG. 2: Trichoscopic image of fibrosing alopecia in pattern distribution (FAPD) showing hair diameter variation with perifollicular scaling.

Courtesy: Cutis Academy of Cutaneous Sciences, Bengaluru, Karnataka, India.

Immunohistochemistry studies have revealed a nearly four-fold increase in the endothelial vascular surface in psoriatic lesional skin in comparison with normal skin.[11,12] Studies on psoriatic skin blood flow measured by Doppler flowmeter have shown that cutaneous blood flow is 9–13 times greater in lesional skin and 2.5–4.5 times greater in perilesional skin compared with normal skin.[12] Hence, the possibility of excessive bleeding during hair transplantation in a patient with scalp psoriasis must be kept in mind. The use of Namazi solution by adding an ampoule of tranexamic acid (TXA) (5 mL, 500 mg) to the tumescent anesthetic solution may be employed during hair transplantation to manage excessive bleeding in order to ease and shorten the procedure.[13]

Due to the inherent nature of psoriatic lesions to arise in areas affected by trauma (Koebner phenomenon), this condition has to be medically controlled before the hair transplantation procedure. *In patients with preexisting lesions, there may be flare-up due to the trauma caused by hair transplantation surgery.* Although there is limited literature regarding hair transplantation in cases of scalp psoriasis, and till date there are no studies reporting any deleterious effects of psoriasis on the eventual transplanted hair growth; the possibility of a flare-up post surgery must be discussed with the patient. It is imperative to procure a written consent stating the same before the surgery.

In a case series reported by Vaggu et al.,[14] seven patients of psoriasis undergoing HT demonstrated excellent growth of transplanted hair at the 9-month follow-up. They reported their findings as follows:

- Only one of the seven patients developed a flare-up of psoriasis post procedure, which was easily treatable with methotrexate and topical corticosteroids.
- Infections did not occur in either the donor or the recipient areas, and normal healing occurred in the donor area in all the patients, even in the patient where the skin incision was placed at the edge of the psoriatic plaque.
- No complications resulting from incorporating the psoriatic lesion in the donor strip were encountered, and also the transplanted grafts prepared from the lesion showed excellent growth.
- They concluded that the risk of koebnerization is very low and any flare-up post procedure would not affect adversely the hair transplantation outcome with the institution of proper dermatological treatment.

In another case report, Shiell stated, anecdotally, that all the lost hair returned back in his psoriasis patient even after a violent reaction with massive encrustation after hair transplantation.[15] Mohebi has concluded in his case series of three patients that transplantation of hair follicular units into psoriatic scalp lesions could be an effective method to alleviate the symptoms of psoriasis and possibly be used as a treatment option for psoriasis.[16] In his study, he did not observe any reactivation of psoriatic lesions and, to the contrary, improvement of long-standing psoriatic plaques was seen. He could not conclude whether the steps in the processes of healing post transplantation were responsible for the therapeutic effect within a psoriatic-laden zone, or the improvement was related with the hair follicles or its stem cells.

It is recommended that if any psoriatic lesion is present in the donor area, it is imperative to treat it at least 2 weeks prior to hair transplantation. Mild to moderate erythema and scaling can be managed with tar-based shampoos and application of a potent corticosteroid solution such as clobetasol scalp solution with or without salicylic acid. For moderate to severe pruritus, antihistamines may help. For severe psoriasis, systemic medications such as methotrexate, cyclosporine, acitretin, or biologics can be administered.

Recommendations

- Hair transplantation must be avoided if the psoriasis process is active due to the risk of koebnerization.
- The possibility of a flare-up of psoriasis post surgery must be discussed with the patient.
- The possibility of excessive bleeding during hair transplantation in a patient with scalp psoriasis must be kept in mind.
- Graft uptake is not affected by psoriasis.

SCALP FOLLICULITIS

Folliculitis is a folliculocentric infection, mainly starting at the infundibular opening of the hair follicles.[17,18] It is most commonly due to *Staphylococcus aureus* and coagulase-negative staphylococci.[19] The erythematous pustular lesions heal in a week but often tend to be chronic. Chronic folliculitis is seen more commonly in males compared to females. Mixed infections and biofilm formation, an oily scalp, excessive sweating, and the use of harsh hair cosmetics aggravate preexisting folliculitis. It is imperative to adequately treat chronic folliculitis before the patient undergoes hair transplantation surgery. Topical antibacterial agents such as mupirocin and fusidic acid form the first-line therapy.[20-23] Extensive lesions require systemic antibiotic therapy with penicillins or cephalosporins (first-line) for 7–10 days; or oral azithromycin or erythromycin. Decolonization regimen with mupirocin nasal ointment application may be advocated in the management of chronic staphylococcal folliculitis to prevent recurrence.[19-22] Prophylactic antibiotics such as doxycycline must be started 5–7 days prior to HT surgery in patients with a known history of chronic folliculitis.

Hair transplantation procedures may be more time consuming and difficult in cases of chronic folliculitis due to the presence of a fibrotic, tight scalp. Rates of follicular transection may be higher, and extraction may be difficult with a higher FOX grade. However, a past history of chronic folliculitis does not usually affect graft survival when done by skilled and experienced HT surgeons.

In case of repeated episodes, it is advisable to rule out tufted folliculitis and folliculitis decalvans. Folliculitis decalvans may also occur over the donor as well as the recipient site post hair transplantation.[24] Otberg et al. described a case of folliculitis decalvans developing in punch grafts 20 years after hair transplantation.[25] Management of this condition is generally difficult due to the waxing and waning course of the disease, which can span a few years. Systemic antibiotics effective toward the eradication of *S. aureus* are recommended. However, relapses are frequent on discontinuation of the drugs.

The reported incidence of postoperative folliculitis in hair transplantation varies from 1.1 to 20%, and the severity ranges from mild superficial inflammation to scattered pustules. It should be treated with topical antibiotics, systemic antibiotics based on culture report, and incision and drainage. Sterile folliculitis in the recipient area is a frequent complication usually seen weeks or months after transplantation. Etiological theories for these include "ingrown" hair, foreign body reactions, epithelium logged into slit sites during recipient site creation, piggybacked grafts, and "idiopathic" intrinsic properties of the host scalp.[26] *Care should be taken to avoid missed grafts in the donor area and piggybacked grafts in the recipient area* to minimize the chances of postoperative folliculitis in both the donor and recipient areas, respectively.

Recommendations

- Prophylactic antibiotics such as doxycycline must be started 5–7 days prior to HT surgery in patients with a known history of folliculitis.
- HT may be difficult and more time consuming in patients with a history of chronic folliculitis.
- Missed grafts in the donor area and piggybacked grafts in the recipient area must be avoided to prevent postoperative folliculitis.

ALOPECIA AREATA

Alopecia areata (AA) is a chronic, noncicatrizing, immune-mediated disease of the hair follicle.[27] The concern with AA and hair transplantation is the possibility that *transplanted follicles might undergo hair shedding postoperatively*. Due to the autoimmune nature of the disease, the occurrence of lesions is unpredictable, and the disease may recur at any point in time; hence, it is important to diagnose this condition in a potential hair transplantation candidate. The common patchy type of AA appears as bald nonscarring patches that can be readily diagnosed clinically and on trichoscopy. *The diffuse variant of AA* is one of the concerns because of *the lack of well-demarcated alopecic lesions* **(Figs. 3 and 4)**. Rather the patient presents with diffuse thinning, which *may even appear similar to pattern hair loss*.[28]

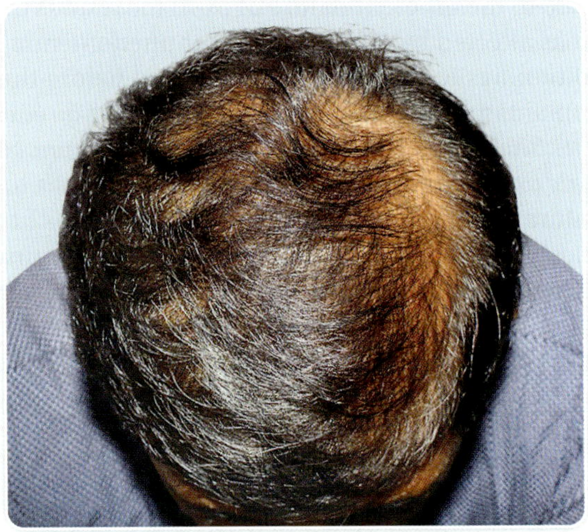

FIG. 3: Clinical picture seen in diffuse alopecia areata—can be easily misdiagnosed as androgenetic alopecia (AGA).
Courtesy: Cutis Academy of Cutaneous Sciences, Bengaluru, Karnataka, India.

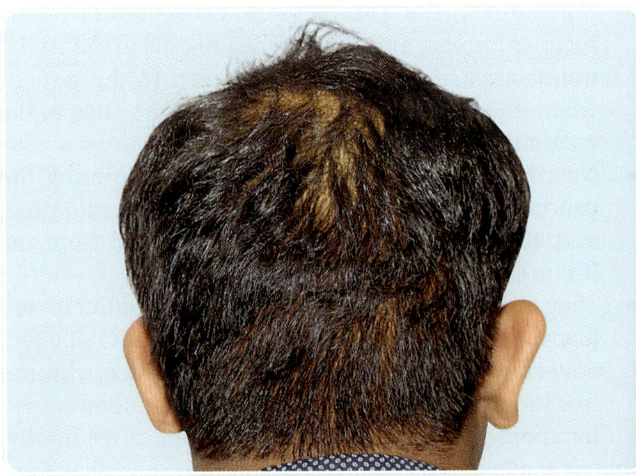

FIG. 4: Clinical picture seen in diffuse alopecia areata—can be easily misdiagnosed as androgenetic alopecia (AGA).
Courtesy: Cutis Academy of Cutaneous Sciences, Bengaluru, Karnataka, India.

Trichoscopy can be helpful in identifying features of diffuse alopecia areata such as exclamation hairs and broken, dystrophic hairs. In contrast, patterned hair loss (PHL) or AGA on dermoscopy shows primarily miniaturized hairs or hairs in varying diameters.[29] In doubtful cases, a punch biopsy from the scalp must be performed to confirm the diagnosis.

Before planning hair transplantation for AGA in a patient with a previous history of AA, it is mandatory that the disease has been inactive for at least 1-year duration. Signs of activity must be actively sought for by detailed trichoscopy of the entire scalp. In case of existing stable/resistant patches, it is better to perform a biopsy and check for signs of active disease before planning hair transplantation. *Reactivation of AA could lead to the loss of all transplanted hair*—and this possibility must be explained in detail to the patient, and consent stating the same must be taken.

Although there is no published data regarding the outcome of HT for AGA in patients with coexisting AA, there is some data on successful HT in areas of scalp AA. Orentreich's original paper on punch grafting in nine patients with AA of the scalp reported that *"only sparse and weak hair growth took place in both the 'hair-to-hair' grafts and the 'hair-to-alopecia' grafts."*[30] In 2005, Barankin et al. presented a case of successful hair transplantation into an area of *a chronic resistant patch of AA affecting the eyebrow.*[31] *The grafts survived, but the disease process became reactivated* after 8 months at the treatment sites, which was responsive to treatment with monthly intralesional steroids.

In 2008, Unger et al. presented a case *of successful hair transplantation for recalcitrant patches of AA as well as areas of hair loss due to AGA.*[32] In their case report, a 64-year-old man with a 4-year history of AA (biopsy proven), treated with multiple drugs over 4 years' duration, had two resistant patches of AA. He also had AGA (Hamilton/Norwood type Va). After a biopsy from recalcitrant AA patches showed no signs of activity, *test grafting* was done for a part of one of the resistant patches and also at the edge of the area affected by AGA. At the time of test grafting, his disease had been stable for approximately 10 months. After 9 months of the test grafting procedure, they found that the transplanted grafts at both areas yielded terminal hairs of a similar caliber as the hairs found in the donor area. In addition, in the AA test site, new hair growth was also noticed surrounding the transplanted hairs, as well as in the areas peripheral to the grafted area. This phenomenon did not occur in the test area of AGA. There were no signs of disease activity and no requirement for any treatment to maintain the growth of the hair in the previously treatment-resistant areas of AA. After 11.5 months of the test grafting, a full-size HT session for his frontal area of AGA, as well as an additional region of resistant, quiescent AA was performed successfully.

In an attempt to explain the reason for the "spontaneous" new growth of hair in the ungrafted area of resistant AA, the authors have provided the following possible explanations:[33]

- The new grafts might improve the skin "quality" in the area, making it more favorable for hair growth due to increasing the blood flow to the area by angiogenesis.
- HT as a surgical procedure includes trauma and irritation to the tissue followed by an inflammatory response, and perhaps the AA responded in a similar way as seen with immunotherapies or irritants.
- Possible repopulation of the area by transplanted cells, in a similar manner as those observed with grafting of healthy melanocytes into areas of vitiligo.
- Because AA has an unpredictable course, this may be just coincidental timing in the regrowth of hair in the area.

The unexpected hair regrowth surrounding the transplanted grafts has not only provided new avenues for investigation in the treatment of AA itself but also for cases of AGA with a history of AA. Before embarking on a possible new treatment plan such as hair transplantation in cases of AA, it is imperative to inform the patient in detail about the nature of the disease, course, and prognosis, and the risk of recurrence that would probably affect the original and transplanted hair. A biopsy to confirm the inactivity of the disease is essential before planning the hair restorative surgery.

Recommendations

- In doubtful cases of PHL or diffuse unpatterned alopecia (DUPA), a biopsy must be done to rule out diffuse AA.
- Disease inactivity must be confirmed histopathologically before planning HT.
- The possibility of reactivation of AA after surgery must be explained to the patient and also documented.
- Test grafting in a small area is recommended before planning HT for a bigger area.

VITILIGO

Vitiligo is an idiopathic, acquired melanocytopenic condition leading to depigmented patches. *As with any other autoimmune disorder, there is a risk of koebnerization if hair transplantation is done in a patient with vitiligo*—be it hair transplantation for other indications in a patient of vitiligo, or hair transplantation for the treatment of vitiligo itself. Stability of the disease has to be established, i.e., a period of *inactivity for 1 year* (no new lesions or no increase in the size of preexisting lesion) and absence of

Koebner phenomenon before planning HT in such cases. A *test graft on a smaller area can be done to assess the stability of the disease* before taking up for HT on a larger area. Vitiligo Disease Activity Score (VIDA) can be used as objective criteria for vitiligo stability before planning HT in such cases, just like planning vitiligo surgeries. It is a six-point scale on which the activity of the disease is evaluated based on the appearance of new vitiligo lesions or the enlargement of the preexisting lesions, assessed during a period ranging from <6 weeks to 1 year. HT, just like vitiligo surgeries, may be performed only in patients with VIDA scores of −1 or 0.[34]

In cases of long-standing vitiligo taking phototherapy for a long duration, there may be thickening of the skin. *Graft uptake and the outcome of surgery are usually unaffected even if vitiligo reactivates post HT.* But the possibility of the reactivation of vitiligo after hair restoration surgery must always be explained to the patient. After hair restoration surgery, when restarting minoxidil for such patients, it may be worthwhile to consider a mixture of melatonin with minoxidil. This will provide antioxidant action additionally.

Recommendations

- Before planning HT for any indication in a known case of vitiligo or before follicular unit extraction (FUE) for vitiliginous patch itself, a stability period of 1 year must be achieved.
- Test patch of HT in a smaller area before an extensive surgery should be considered.

CONNECTIVE TISSUE DISEASES

When planning hair transplantation in patients with a history of connective tissue diseases (CTDs), the possibility of the *transplanted grafts eventually undergoing hair shedding* with the progress of CTD must always be considered. In fact, the grafted hair, just like the natural ones, can undergo scarring alopecia also depending on the nature and progress of CTD. *HT must be done only once the disease is inactive.*[33] Even in inactive disease, the hair transplantation process could be a triggering mechanism that reactivates the disease with the eventual destruction of the hair follicles over the recipient and/or donor area. *Telogen loss, which is expected post HT, may be excessive* in cases of CTD as it is associated with high levels of proinflammatory cytokines, especially during flares, which lead to diffuse "inflammatory shedding."

While performing HT, the surgeon may face difficulty because of *a tight, fibrosed scalp,* due to subclinical involvement of a clinically unaffected scalp. This may lead to higher transection rates during the procedure. In known cases of cicatricial alopecias due to CTDs, repeat biopsy to determine the inactivity of the disease before planning HT should always be undertaken. *The presence of scarred tissue interferes with implantation and also with the uptake of grafts post FUE. Intralesional steroids prior to FUE and postprocedure platelet-rich plasma (PRP) improve the outcome of FUE.* In case of morphea, the atrophic skin is usually very thin. *A lesser depth of implantation* is recommended in such cases.

Due to the long-term use of immunosuppressants in these patients, kidney or liver damage should be investigated prior to surgery, and *the dosage of local anesthesia may have to be modified accordingly.* The risk of infections and sepsis after the surgery must also be kept in mind, due to chronic use of immune-suppressant drugs.

Hair transplantation has also been done as a treatment for scarring alopecias associated with CTDs. Data from as early as the 1970s regarding patients with discoid lupus erythematosus (DLE) undergoing successful hair transplantation is available, wherein an average of 72% graft survival was reported.[35] Recently, Sharkov et al. reported good improvement with the combination of nano lipofilling followed by hair transplantation for correction of the hypotrophic cicatrix and the alopecia in patients with linear scleroderma "en coup de sabre."[36] In the case of extensive disease, camouflage techniques such as scalp micropigmentation should be considered over hair transplantation. Wigs and other permanent sewn-in hairpieces are also options to help patients camouflage scarring hair loss and have a positive impact on the quality of life.[37]

Recommendations

- A biopsy to determine the inactivity of the disease before planning HT is recommended.
- Preoperative steroid injections and postoperative PRP injections may help in enhancing the graft uptake.

PEMPHIGUS

Pemphigus vulgaris (PV) is a rare autoimmune mucocutaneous blistering disease characterized by epidermal acantholysis, flaccid bullae, and erosive lesions in the skin and mucosa. It is characterized by the presence of circulating autoantibodies directed against desmogleins. Scalp involvement is commonly seen in patients of PV because the hair follicles are a rich source of common PV antigens such as Dsg 1 and Dsg 3. Scalp involvement is often an early finding in the course of the disease, and the lesions are often recalcitrant to treatment. Clinical manifestation involves corn flake-like scales and crusted erosions, often on an erythematous base.

Scalp lesions in the course of pemphigus can lead to several types of noncicatricial and cicatricial alopecia. Hair loss has been described both within and around the erosive lesions on the scalp.[38] Hair shafts may detach from the hair follicle as a result of acantholysis, causing anagen hair loss. This phenomenon was described as a Nikolsky sign of the scalp in a subclinically affected area.[39] So, easily extractable anagen hairs could be considered a sign of disease activity. This must be checked for before planning hair transplantation for AGA in known cases of immune-bullous disorders.

Koebner phenomenon is described in several skin disorders, including psoriasis and lichen planus, but it remains questionable in PV.[40] In the literature, reports on Koebner phenomenon occurring in PV patients have included the stimulation of PV lesions by ionizing radiation, surgical procedures,[41,42] burns,[43] and chemical peel.[44] Koebner phenomenon in a patient of PV has been described 2 months after hair transplantation surgery.[45] Mehregan et al. also reported a case of PV appearing in the area of a surgical site after rhinoplasty and hair transplantation.[46] It is imperative to plan hair transplantation only when the disease is inactive. The possibility of Koebner phenomenon must always be explained to the patient, and written consent must be taken accordingly.

Recommendations

- Even though Koebner phenomenon is not well established in pemphigus in comparison with other autoimmune disorders, it must be kept in mind.
- HT must be undertaken only when the disease is inactive.

CUTIS VERTICIS GYRATA

Cutis verticis gyrata (CVG) is a disease condition of the scalp manifested as convoluted folds and furrows formed from thickened skin of the scalp resembling a convoluted cerebriform pattern. Usually, 2–30 folds can exist within 0.5–2.0 cm width, and the depth of furrow is about 1 cm.[47] According to its cause, the disease can be classified as primary (essential or nonessential) or secondary CVG (**Box 1**). Primary CVG is a benign condition characterized by symmetrical longitudinal folds over the vertex and occiput. Secondary CVG presents as variable folds, which do not run longitudinally.

Patients with metabolic syndrome, at times with a background of chronic folliculitis, may have associated secondary CVG. At times, CVG may be an incidental finding after taking up the patient for surgery. Smaller lesions usually do not affect the outcome of HT; graft uptake is unaffected. Larger lesions may have to be treated before planning HT. The real concern for physicians is the possibility of malignant transformation of the lesions rather than aesthetics. Treatment options are usually related to the size of the lesion, but the main objective is removal of the lesion and scalp reconstruction with either excision and primary repair, staged excision, use of skin grafts, local flaps, free flaps, or tissue expansion.[39,48-52] Many of these approaches lead to scars and decreased hair density. Recently, hair transplantation as a part of combination hair restoration techniques in the treatment of severe CVG has been described.[53]

BOX 1 Primary and secondary cutis verticis gyrata.

Primary CVG

- *Nonessential form:*
  - *Associated with disorders*: Neurological (such as microcephaly and epilepsy), ophthalmological (such as cataract, strabismus, blindness), psychiatric (such as mental retardation and schizophrenia)
- *Essential form*: Only skin abnormalities, not associated with any systemic disorder

Secondary CVG/pseudo-CVG

- *Inflammatory*: Psoriasis, acne keloidalis
- *Hamartomas*: Intradermal nevus, lipomatous nevus, sebaceous nevus
- *Benign neoplasms*: Cylindromas, neurofibromas
- *Malignant*: Metastatic disorders
- *Depository disorders*: Amyloidosis, myxedema
- *Miscellaneous*: Acanthosis nigricans, acromegaly, Ehler–Danlos syndrome, pachydermoperiostosis, tuberous sclerosis

An interesting point to be noted is that in CVG, the postsurgical scar is usually not widened. This is due to the redundant, relatively stiff skin which glides freely over the person's scalp and offers the surgeon an abundance of scalp tissue. In comparison with Ehler–Danlos syndrome, wherein defects in elastic tissue result in widened linear scars and difficult extraction. Hence, a patient with Ehler–Danlos syndrome is most likely to have a wide scar after hair transplantation, due to laxity of the skin; whereas CVG yields a good acceptable scar, despite the rugosity.

Recommendation

The postsurgical scar is usually good in CVG.

ALLERGIC CONTACT DERMATITIS TO HAIR DYE

Hair coloring is a common practice in India. Although the scalp is inherently resistant to allergic contact dermatitis (ACD) because of thick skin and high density of sebaceous glands, exposure to various allergens present in hair coloring, hairstyling, and hair cleansing products predisposes the scalp to ACD. ACD to hair dyes and *p*-phenylenediamine (PPD) is quite common in India. The positive patch test for PPD has been demonstrated in 4.4% of patients in Asia, 4.1% in Europe, 6% in North America, and 11.5% in India.[54] The spectrum of ACD signs and symptoms ranges from mild-pruritus, erythema, oozing, to severe - crusting edema of scalp, eyelids, face, or anaphylaxis. Treatment depends on the severity of ACD. Mild reactions can be treated with topical midpotent steroids. In severe cases, oral or parenteral corticosteroids are required.

Most HT surgeons prefer to dye gray hair before the procedure. This facilitates better visualization of hair, making the process less strenuous. It is advised to dye the hair at least 48–72 hours prior to the planned HT procedure. It is recommended to carry out a patch test on the retroauricular area or the inner aspect of the elbow before using hair dye. Avoidance of a longer contact period than recommended and thorough cleansing of hair after the application of hair dye help in reducing the risk of ACD. Patients with ACD to PPD benefit from PPD-free hair dyes containing *para*-toluenediamine sulfate (PTDS). It has been demonstrated that 57% of patients allergic to PPD tolerate PTDS-containing permanent and semi-permanent hair dyes.[55] *In patients with a known history of ACD to hair dye, temporary colors may be used on the day of HT just before the procedure.* These consist of nonoxidative dyes that have a high molecular weight; these get deposited on the hair surface post coloring and do not penetrate the cortex. These get removed easily in the first shampoo wash itself. These are available in powder, shampoo, and crayon formulations. These are easy to use and carry little risk of contact dermatitis.

Recommendations

- It is advised to dye the hair at least 48–72 hours prior to the planned HT procedure, preferably after a patch test on the retroauricular area or the inner aspect of the elbow.
- In patients with a known history of ACD to hair dye, temporary colors may be used on the day of HT just before the procedure. These carry little risk of contact dermatitis.

MISCELLANEOUS COMMON CONDITIONS

Trichilemmal cysts are a common finding on the scalp, more common in females than males. In most cases, they are slow growing with no symptoms; however, some lesions rarely may become inflamed or secondarily infected. When they are found over the recipient or donor area, recipient slit creation or donor harvesting may cause cyst rupture, leading to a foreign-body reaction. Thus, it would be better to excise the lesion before the hair transplantation procedure.

Seborrheic keratoses on the scalp are commonly encountered benign lesions that appear as sharply demarcated brown macules or plaques with uneven surfaces. These lesions can be removed by surgical excision or electrodessication with curettage a few days before, or even during, the hair transplantation procedure. These need to be differentiated from warts.

Warts or verruca are caused due to human papillomavirus (HPV). They may be present as solitary or more commonly, multiple verrucous outgrowths. Ablation using radiofrequency or CO_2 laser is the preferred choice of treatment. This should be planned a few weeks before the hair transplantation procedure. Solitary lesions at times may be an incidental finding on the day of HT after trimming the hair. These can be addressed with radiofrequency ablation or CO_2 laser-assisted ablation before or after the HT procedure. In case ablation is done after HT, it is advisable to keep the area covered with micropore sticking to prevent unintended autoinoculation and spread of viral lesions.

Lesional growths such as *melanocytic nevi or sebaceous nevus* may occur over the donor or recipient area. Small- or medium-sized lesions of melanocytic nevi that are not in a visible location need not be removed. Larger lesions in a prominent location, such as a nevus over a patient's hairline, may require surgical excision and wound healing several weeks before the hair transplantation procedure. In the case of nevus sebaceous, due to the risk of malignancies with an increase in age, surgical removal is recommended at puberty. Excision is followed by grafting or reconstruction, or serial excisions are usually employed. Superficial ablation must be avoided as it may lead to malignant transformation of deeper components.

SUMMARY

- In all autoimmune diseases, it is recommended to do a biopsy to confirm the inactive state of the disease before planning hair transplantation.
- The possibilty of reactivation of the underlying disease must be explained in detail to the patient, and consent stating the same must be taken.
- Whenever possible, a test patch of FUE is recommended before planning a full HT procedure for an extensive area.

REFERENCES

1. Collin C, Hivnor C. Seborrheic dermatitis. In: Goldsmith L, Katz S, Gilchrest B, Paller AS, Leffell DJ, Wolff K (Eds). Fitzpatrick's Dermatology in General Medicine. New York: McGraw-Hill; 2012.
2. Zinkernagel MS, Trueb RM. Fibrosing alopecia in a pattern distribution: patterned lichen planopilaris or androgenetic alopecia with a lichenoid tissue reaction pattern? Arch Dermatol. 2000;136:205-11.
3. Griggs J, Trüeb RM, Gavazzoni Dias MFR, Hordinsky M, Tosti A. Fibrosing alopecia in a pattern distribution. J Am Acad Dermatol. 2021;85:1557-64.
4. Olsen EA. Female pattern hair loss and its relationship to permanent/cicatricial alopecia: a new perspective. J Investig Dermatol Symp Proc. 2005;10:217-21.
5. Kim GW, Jung HJ, Ko HC, Kim MB, Lee WJ, Lee SJ, et al. Dermoscopy can be useful in differentiating scalp psoriasis from seborrhoeic dermatitis. Br J Dermatol. 2011;164:652-6.
6. Bhoyrul B. A simple technique to distinguish fibrosing alopecia in a pattern distribution from androgenetic alopecia and concomitant seborrheic dermatitis. J Am Acad Dermatol. 2022;86(1):163-5.
7. Dopytalska K, Sobolewski P, Błaszczak A, Szymańska E, Walecka I. Psoriasis in special localizations. Reumatologia. 2018;56(6): 392-8.
8. Bruni F, Alessandrini A, Starace M, Orlando G, Piraccini BM. Clinical and trichoscopic features in various forms of scalp psoriasis. J Eur Acad Dermatol Venereol. 2021;35:1830-7.
9. Micali G, Lacarrubba F, Musumeci ML, Massimino D, Nasca MR. Cutaneous vascular patterns in psoriasis. Int J Dermatol. 2010;49(3):249-56.
10. Heidenreich R, Röcken M, Ghoreschi K. Angiogenesis drives psoriasis pathogenesis. Int J Exp Pathol. 2009;90(3):232-48.
11. Creamer D, Allen MH, Sousa A, Poston R, Barker JN. Localization of endothelial proliferation and microvascular expansion in active plaque psoriasis. Br J Dermatol. 1997;136:859-65.
12. Hern S, Stanton AW, Mellor R, Levick JR, Mortimer PS. Control of cutaneous blood vessels in psoriatic plaques. J Invest Dermatol. 1999;113:127-32.
13. Namazi M. Practice pearl: a novel anesthetic solution for decreasing the blood loss at the recipient site of hair transplantation (Namazi solution). Aesth Plast Surg. 2007;31:415.
14. Vaggu AK, Panchaprateep R, Caroli S, Amonpattana K, Pathomvanich O, Pathomvanich D. Should hair transplantation be performed in psoriasis? Hair Transplant Forum Int. 2012;22(4): 124-6.
15. Shiell R. Transplanting in the psoriatic patient. [Cyberspace Chat]. Hair Transplant Forum Int. 2006;16(6):223.
16. Mohebi P. Hair transplant for treatment of psoriasis. Adv Plast Reconstr Surg. 2017.
17. Luelmo-Aguilar J, Sàbat Santandreu M. Folliculitis: recognition and management. Am J Clin Dermatol. 2004;5(5):301-10.
18. Craft N. Superficial cutaneous infection and pyodermas. In: Goldsmith LA, Katz S, Gilchrest B, Paller AS, Leffell DJ, Wolff K (Eds). Fitzpatrick's Dermatology in General Medicine, 8th edition. New York: McGraw-Hill; 2012. pp. 2128-47.
19. Disorders of hair follicles and related disorders. In: Wolff K, Johnson RA, Saavedra A Fitzpatrick TB (Eds). Fitzpatrick's Color Atlas and Synopsis of Clinical Dermatology, 7th edition. New York: McGraw-Hill; 2013.
20. Sladden MJ, Johnston GA. Common skin infections in children. BMJ. 2004;329(7457):95-9.
21. Messenger AG, de Berker DAR, Sinclair RD. Disorders of hair. In: Burns T, Breathnach S, Cox N, (Eds). Rook's Textbook of Dermatology. Volume 4, 8th edition. West Sussex: Blackwell Publishing Ltd; 2010. pp. 66.38-52.
22. Motswaledi MH. Common scalp disorders in general practice. S Afr Fam Pract. 2012;54(1):10-3.
23. Lee AHY, Cho SY, Yam TS, Harris K, Ardern-Jones MR. Staphylococcus aureus and chronic folliculocentric pustuloses of the scalp—cause or association? Br J Dermatol. 2016;175(2): 410-3.
24. Avram M. Managing complications in hair restoration. Hair Transplant. 2014;360(3):364.
25. Otberg N, Wu WY, Kang H, Martinka M, Alzolibani AA, Restrepo I, et al. Folliculitis decalvans developing 20 years after hair restoration surgery in punch grafts: case report. Dermatol Surg. 2009;35(11):1852-6.
26. Vogel JE, Jimenez F, Cole J, Keene SA, Harris JA, Barrera A, et al. Hair restoration surgery: the state of the art. Aesthet Surg J. 2013;33:128-51.
27. Gilhar A, Kalish RS. Alopecia areata: a tissue specific autoimmune disease of the hair follicle. Autoimmun Rev. 2006;5:64-9.
28. Shapiro J. Alopecia areata. In: Shapiro J (Ed). Hair Loss: Principles of Diagnosis and Management of Alopecia. London: Martin Duniz; 2002.
29. Bowling J. Diagnostic Dermoscopy: The Illustrated Guide. Hoboken, NJ: Wiley Blackwell; 2012.
30. Orentreich N. Autografts in alopecias and other selected dermatological conditions. Ann N Y Acad Sci. 1959;83:463-79.
31. Barankin B, Taher M, Wasel N. Successful hair transplant of eyebrow alopecia areata. J Cutan Med Surg. 2005;9:162-4.
32. Unger R, Dawoud T, Albaqami R. Successful hair transplantation of recalcitrant alopecia areata of the scalp. Dermatol Surg. 2008;34(11):1589-93.
33. Altman J, Perry HO. The variations and course of lichen planus. Arch Dermatol. 1961;84:179-91.
34. Khunger N, Kathuria SD, Ramesh V. Tissue grafts in vitiligo surgery—past, present, and future. Indian J Dermatol. 2009;54:150-8.
35. Nordström RE. Hair transplantation. The use of hairbearing compound grafts for correction of alopecia due to chronic discoid lupus erythematosus, traumatic alopecia, and male pattern baldness. Scand J Plast Reconstr Surg Suppl. 1976; 14:1-37.
36. Sharkov E, Todorov RS, Yonkov A, Simeonov D, Stefanov M. Patient with linear scleroderma "En Coup De Sabre"—nano lipofilling followed by hair transplantation. Adv Bioeng Biomed Sci Res. 2021;4(1):29-32.
37. Joseph AK, Abbas LF, Chong BF. Treatments for disease damage in cutaneous lupus erythematosus: a narrative review. Dermatol Ther. 2021;34:e15034.
38. Delmonte S, Semino MT, Parodi A, Rebora A. Normal anagen effluvium: a sign of pemphigus vulgaris. Br J Dermatol. 2000;142:1244-5.

39. Li J, Wang B, Chen M. The evaluation of externalized catheter expander in clinical application. Chin Cosmet Med. 2003;12: 43-4.
40. Weiss G, Shemer A, Trau H. The Koebner phenomenon: review of the literature. J Eur Acad Dermatol Venereol. 2002;16(3): 241-8.
41. Nazik H, Ozturk P, Mulayim M, Koyuncu E. Pemphigus vulgaris and Koebner phenomenon. Med Sci. 2019;8:464-5.
42. Rashid A, Wang J, Fu P, Wang W, Xie H. Pemphigus vulgaris associated with surgery: a rare association. Indian J Dermatol Venereol Leprol. 2015;81:299-301.
43. Daneshpazhooh M, Fatehnejad M, Rahbar Z, Balighi K, Ghandi N, Ghiasi M, et al. Trauma-induced pemphigus: a case series of 36 patients. J Dtsch Dermatol Ges. 2016;14(2):166-71.
44. Kaplan RP, Detwiler SP, Saperstein HW. Physically induced pemphigus after cosmetic procedures. Int J Dermatol. 1993; 32(2):100-3.
45. Balighi K, Daneshpazhooh M, Azizpour A, Lajevardi V, Mohammadi F, Chams-Davatchi C. Koebner phenomenon in pemphigus vulgaris patients. JAAD Case Rep. 2016;2(5):419-21.
46. Mehregan DR, Roenigk RK, Gibson LE. Postsurgical pemphigus. Arch Dermatol. 1992;128(3):414-5.
47. Wang M, Chu Y, Shui Q. Abnormality of cutis verticis gyrata. J Plast Surg. 2007;23:112-4.
48. Radovan C. Tissue expansion in soft tissue reconstruction. Plast Reconstr Surg. 1984;74:482-92.
49. Lei Y, Lu K, Ai Y. Clinical experience of skin expansion. Chin J Aesthet Med. 2003;9:378-9.
50. Hu S, Zhang H, Feng Y. The application of repeated skin expansion in repairing large area cheek skin defects. Chin Aesthet Plast Surg. 2006;17:284-6.
51. Li H, Li Y, Ji Y. Application of excessive dilation of skin in the repair of large facial and neck scar. Chin Cosmet Med. 2007;16:756-8.
52. Zhao D, Li J, Wang K, Guo X, Lang Y, Peng L, et al. Treating cutis verticis gyrata using skin expansion method. Cell Biochem Biophys. 2012;62(2):373-6.
53. Eginli A, McMichael A, Cooley J. Combination hair restoration techniques in the treatment of severe cutis verticis gyrata. Dermatol Surg. 2021;47(6):874-6.
54. Gupta M, Mahajan VK, Mehta KS, Chauhan PS. Hair dye dermatitis and p-phenylenediamine contact sensitivity: a preliminary report. Indian Dermatol Online J. 2015;6:241-6.
55. Scheman A, Cha C, Bhinder M. Alternative hair-dye products for persons allergic to para-phenylenediamine. Dermatitis. 2011;22:189-92.

CHAPTER 87

Hair Transplantation and Medical Conditions

Sandeep Sattur, Indu S Sattur

Key Messages

- The incidence of medical conditions is not uncommon in the younger population.
- Many of these opt for hair transplantation.
- It is important to assess the patient properly before deciding their candidacy for hair transplantation as the medical conditions may influence the procedure as well as the outcome.

INTRODUCTION

Patients interested in aesthetic surgeries, including hair transplantation, may have medical conditions, which may influence the operative plan and surgical outcome.[1] The patient's overall medical health is obviously important to consider before beginning a series of hair restoration procedures that can extend over many years. Hair transplantation may actually be contraindicated in certain conditions such as uncontrolled hypertension unless it is properly optimized for surgery.[2] During the consultation, not only is it important to take a complete history regarding any symptoms, which may allude to the presence of a medical condition but ensure detailed physical examination to confirm or rule out the same. Family history, especially in cases of diabetes, hypothyroidism, hypertension, and coronary artery disease (CAD), is important. Drugs used to treat medical conditions may potentially interact with the anesthetic agents used during hair transplantation, and this must be kept in mind while planning hair transplant surgery. Smoking is known to influence wound healing, and the patient needs to be counseled about cutting down or quitting in the perioperative period. All these factors require proper consideration while planning the hair transplant.

UNIQUE REQUIREMENTS OF HAIR RESTORATION SURGERY

Hair transplant surgery is one of the most sought-after cosmetic surgeries.[3] It is a surgery performed on a healthy patient under local anesthesia and takes about 6–8 hours on an average. The challenge is to ensure that the patient is comfortable and pain free during this period, and the physiology is maintained optimally during the procedure. Preexisting medical conditions can influence this. Hence, preoperative due diligence on part of the hair transplant surgeon with regards to the patient's health is crucial.

A few common red flags of concern for hair transplantation are hypertension, diabetes mellitus, coronary artery or ischemic heart disease, patient on blood thinners, smokers, patients who are human immunodeficiency virus (HIV) positive, etc.

Hypertension

Raised blood pressure during hair transplant surgery can cause excessive bleeding during harvesting as well as during implantations and even after the surgery, resulting in poor results.[2] Moreover, hypertension in the perioperative and postoperative period can potentiate cardiovascular events, cerebrovascular events, bleeding, and mortality[4] and should be controlled prior hair transplant surgery.

The majority of the patients undergoing hair transplantation are in the younger age group.[5] Patients in this age group are generally perceived to be healthy and do not have significant medical issues. Whether it is bad lifestyles or the genes, the authors have found a significant incidence of metabolic disorders in this age group of patient population. The National Family Health Survey-4 data revealed that >1 in 10 young adults (<40 years of age) have hypertension and only half of these were aware of the hypertension.[6]

Many factors influence blood pressure during the hair transplant procedure. The factors which may potentially increase the blood pressure are:

- Anxiety
- Position
- Pain
- Distended bladder

Hair transplant surgery is performed under local anesthesia with or without sedation. It is not unusual for the patients to have slightly elevated blood pressure on the morning of the surgery. Blood pressure elevations due to apprehension regarding the pain associated with the procedure or general anxiety of being in an operation theater are not uncommon.[7,8] Usually, an anxiolytic given preoperatively addresses this problem.[8,9]

Hair transplant surgery involves putting the patient in different positions throughout the surgery, including prone position. The authors have been recording vital parameters throughout the procedure for over a decade and have noted significant increases in blood pressure in the prone position. They have observed a rise of systolic blood pressure by 20–30 mm Hg in the prone position in normotensive individuals. Studies have shown that heart rate, systolic, and diastolic blood pressure are increased in prone position.[10]

The most painful part of hair transplant procedure is the injection of the anesthetic.[9] Pain is an important trigger for raising blood pressure. Due to built-in survival mechanisms, severe acute pain can raise the blood pressure by about 30 mm Hg.[11] To be able to deliver adequate and complete anesthesia which is sustained through the procedure with timely repetition of anesthesia, and use of analgesics intraoperatively, is the key to successful anesthesia. Inadequate and incomplete anesthesia during the procedure tends to increase the blood pressure significantly even in normotensive individuals, and this can interfere with the procedure.

As hair transplantation is a long procedure, patients are prone to develop a full bladder. A distended bladder is also known to raise the systolic and diastolic blood pressure.[12,13] Breaks given at regular intervals help in reducing the possibility of a distended bladder.

With so many potential factors capable of raising the blood pressure, it important to ensure that the patient is normotensive at the start of the surgery.

These facts highlight the need for screening potential candidates for hair transplantation during the first consultation itself. White coat hypertension is a type of labile hypertension where the fear of the procedure or the environment of the operating room can raise the systolic and diastolic blood pressure. The practice of giving the patient an anxiolytic preoperatively is quite effective. Reassurance by the operating surgeon plays an important role. Mostly such patients become normotensive after the start of the procedure. There is no consensus or no universally accepted guidelines stating the level of blood pressure at which elective surgery should be canceled. It has been recommended to cancel elective surgery if the systolic blood pressure is 180 mm Hg or higher or if the diastolic blood pressure is 110 mm Hg or higher.[4,14,15] However, the authors feel that diastolic blood pressure above 100 mm Hg or systolic blood pressure above 160 mm Hg, despite the anxiolytic, in a previously normotensive patient or a hypertensive patient who has taken his/her dose of medications, then it is best to reschedule the surgery and refer the patient to a physician for proper assessment. The authors rationalize that hair transplant surgery being a long surgery with some part being in prone position, an increase in blood pressure by 20–30 mm Hg during the procedure is not uncommon, and hence, the cutoff limit of blood pressure should be 160 mm Hg for systolic and 100 mm Hg for diastolic blood pressure.

It is important to wait for a week or more after starting antihypertensive therapy as it may take up to a week for the effect of the antihypertensive medications to show.[16] Titration of dose may be needed in some patients.

Drug Interactions between Antihypertensives and Local Anesthetics Containing Epinephrine

In hypertensive patients who are on antihypertensive it is important to check the drugs that the patient is taking for hypertension. Antihypertensive medications such as nonselective beta-blockers (propranolol) are known to interact with the anesthetic agents containing epinephrine. If a patient on a nonselective beta-blocker such as propranolol receives a systemic dose of local anesthetic containing epinephrine, the beta-blocker prevents the vasodilation, leaving unopposed alpha vasoconstriction caused by the epinephrine.[17,18] The resulting hypertensive reaction can lead to a hypertensive crisis with systolic blood pressure above 200 mm Hg. If the patient is on nonselective beta-blockers, then a discussion with treating physician is needed for modifying the treatment before proceeding with hair restoration surgery. Other drugs that can raise the blood pressure when used along with epinephrine are the tricyclic antidepressants.[18]

Diabetes Mellitus

Successful outcomes in hair transplantation depend on all stages of wound healing to be executed successfully. The implanted follicle survives for the first couple of days by the process of plasmatic imbibition where the implanted follicle absorbs the wound exudate by capillary action. Revascularization of the grafted follicle is not clearly understood but may occur by anastomosis of the follicle with the vessels of the recipient site or there may neovascularization.[19] The graft derives oxygen from the surrounding vasculature, and compromise of the vasculature may compromise the graft survival due to poor oxygenation.[19,20]

Surgical stress induces hyperglycemia as a physiologic response, and this is further aggravated in diabetes. Activation of the hypothalamic–pituitary–adrenal axis due to surgical stress causes elevation of cortisol and catecholamine levels. Ultimately, insulin sensitivity decreases followed by an increased sympathetic response leading to gluconeogenesis and glycogenolysis due to increased glucagon and growth hormone secretion.[21] The bottom line is hyperglycemia. This hyperglycemia is further compounded in diabetic patients.

Hyperglycemia in the perioperative period is associated with delayed healing and increased incidence of postoperative complications. Almost one-third of people suffering from diabetes are undiagnosed and untreated.[1] Diabetes is known to impact possibly every organ system, and apart from the complications such as heart disease, stroke, high blood pressure, blindness, kidney failure, neuropathy, peripheral vascular disease, it impacts wound healing.[1] Hyperglycemia is associated with likely risks for poorer wound healing and increased susceptibility to infection. The exact mechanism for delayed wound healing is not known, but it could be a combined effect on macro- and microvasculature, impaired phagocytosis, accumulation of advanced glycosylated products leading to tissue hypoxia.[1,19] The degree of microvascular affectation correlates inversely with the glycemic levels.[1] Rat studies have revealed that diabetic wounds have higher levels of inducible nitric oxide synthetase which is responsible for increased inflammation and lower oxygen saturation levels.[22]

Optimal evidence-based perioperative blood glucose control in patients undergoing ambulatory surgical procedures remains controversial. The primary approach to a patient with diabetes undergoing hair transplantation procedure, which is an outpatient procedure, is to ensure that optimal glycemic control is achieved prior to surgery. The clinical practice guidelines from the Endocrine Society published institutional protocols in 2012 for preoperative management of diabetic patients undergoing surgery. Further adaptations to this were published in 2016.[21,23] For diabetic patients, the goal of treatment is to ensure that fasting blood sugar should be below 140 g/dL and random blood sugars below 180 g/dL. Along with fasting and postprandial blood glucose, patients undergoing outpatient procedures should have a documented glycated hemoglobin (HbA1c) value within the last 3 months. The goal is to have an HbA1c <8.0%. If the HbA1c value is >8, then it is best to postpone the surgery and refer the patient to the physician or endocrinologist to improve control prior to proceeding with surgery. However, the authors feel that it is best to have the A1c levels between 6% and 7%, but this will have to be dealt on a case-to-case basis and correlation between fasting and postprandial blood glucose levels and HbA1c levels.[24]

While operating on a diabetic patient, it is important to have glucometer in the operation theater to check the levels before, during, and after the hair transplant surgery.

Coronary Artery Disease/Ischemic Heart Disease

Hair loss patients can have coexisting CAD/ischemic heart disease, and these patients may desire surgical hair restoration. Patients with active heart disease would not be eligible for hair transplant surgery. Patients who have stable CAD and are not symptomatic could be considered for hair transplantation only after they are cleared by their treating cardiologist.[14] When considering noncardiac surgery, cardiovascular morbidity and mortality are decided by two main factors: Patient-related risk and type of surgery or procedure, including the circumstances under which it takes place (experience of institution, elective vs. emergency procedure).[25] Hair restoration surgery is a completely elective surgery done to improve appearance. Hence, it is important that informed consent with respect to risk–benefit ratio should be mandatory in such patients.

Screening tests such as resting electrocardiograph (ECG), two-dimensional (2D) echocardiography, exercise stress testing, or similar, as recommended by the treating cardiologist, should be done. The presence of an anesthetist is mandatory while performing hair transplant surgery in such patients. The operation theater should be well equipped with requisite resuscitative equipment. If possible, hair transplant surgery in patients with coronary heart disease (CHD) should be performed in a hospital setting. The hair transplant clinic should have arrangements for quick and safe transfer of patients in event of them developing symptoms of angina or any unusual symptom. While performing hair transplant surgery on CHD patients, the hair transplant surgeon should be aware of any unusual symptoms and quickly start emergency care such as oxygen, aspirin, nitroglycerine and have no hesitancy in transferring the patient to a hospital.[14]

Patient on Blood Thinners

Patients with medical conditions who are on antithrombotic medications can come up for hair transplant surgery. Perioperative management of antithrombotic therapy in patients on antithrombotics who are undergoing elective noncardiac surgery remains poorly defined. In catch-22-like situation, discontinuation of the antithrombotic medications can potentially precipitate a cardiac event or cerebrovascular incident, and continuing the antithrombotic medications perioperatively can increase the chances of bleeding intraoperatively.[26]

Antithrombotic drugs are divided into anticoagulants and antiplatelet drugs.[27] Anticoagulant drugs reduce fibrin formation and slow down clotting, while antiplatelet drugs prevent platelet aggregation. A combination of anticoagulant and antiplatelet drugs is important to prevent clot formation and growth.[28]

Anticoagulants:

- Vitamin K antagonists, also called coumarins (warfarin is the commonly used coumarin)
- Direct inhibitors of factor Xa, also known as direct oral anticoagulants (DOACs), examples are: Rivaroxaban, apixaban, edoxaban, betrixaban
- Direct inhibitors of thrombin—dabigatran
- Indirect factor Xa inhibitor—fondaparinux
- Heparin

Antiplatelet/antiaggregation agents:

- Aspirin (acetylsalicylic acid), ticlopidine, dipyridamole
- Thienopyridines (clopidogrel and prasugrel)
- Nonthienopyridines (ticagrelor and cangrelor)
- Nonsteroidal anti-inflammatory drugs (NSAIDs)[27]

Risk stratification of the patients on antithrombotic agents who need to undergo noncardiac surgery depends upon the probability of thrombotic events versus the higher chances of bleeding intra- and postoperatively. Generally, patients with atrial fibrillation, mechanical prosthetic valves, deep vein thrombosis, and pulmonary embolism are considered high risk, where discontinuation of anticoagulants puts them at a higher risk of thrombotic episodes. Also, patients with recent interventions such as percutaneous transluminal coronary angioplasty (PTCA), coronary artery bypass graft (CABG) surgery, recent myocardial infarct and cerebral infarct, and unstable angina are considered high risk. On the other hand, patients on prophylactic use of antiplatelet agents, old myocardial infarcts, >2 years post-PTCA or CABG would be considered low risk and would usually be on single or dual antiplatelet (DAP) medications.[27-29] Temporary discontinuation or dose reduction in this group would not pose a big risk to these patients.

Balancing the risk of thrombosis with the risk of bleeding is key to manage patients on antithrombotic needing hair transplantation. Most of the guidelines or protocols have looked at medically necessary surgery, but very few have looked at elective cosmetic procedures such as hair transplantation. Since it is elective and not necessary from a medical or health perspective, one must critically look at risk–benefit ratio while deciding on the plan for antithrombotic medications perioperatively. Clinical judgment is imperative, as there is no score or calculator to determine the classification of the patient in a simple manner. It is up to the hair transplant surgeon and the treating physician to jointly decide on the management of antithrombotics.

Determining the Risk of Procedural Bleeding

When evaluating bleeding risk, it is essential to consider the type of surgery and clinical characteristics of the patient. These characteristics are assessed with the HAS-BLED [Hypertension, Abnormal Liver or Kidney Function, Stroke, Bleeding History or Predisposition, Labile International Normalized Ratio (INR), Elderly, Drugs, Alcohol] score. Each positive item earns 1 point, and a HAS-BLED score >3 indicates a high bleeding risk.[27] Generally, patients who are candidates for hair transplantation are healthy and should have a score <3. The assessment of prothrombin time and international normalized ratio (PT/INR) preoperatively can guide the hair transplant surgeon. In patients who are on antithrombotic medications, a PT/INR of 1.5–1.6 helps to reduce the risk of thrombosis, and the risk of bleeding is also minimal.[28,30]

Bleeding during hair transplantation can occur while harvesting or during creation of recipient sites for implantation. Strategic (intradermal) and conservative use of tumescent solution with very high dilution of epinephrine (1 in 800,000) can be used if permitted by the treating physician. Moreover, simple external pressure with a gauze piece for a few minutes will help reduce the oozing. If the patient is only on a single antiplatelet medication such as aspirin, there may be no need to stop it if the INR is ≤1.5 and the patient's HAS-BLED score is <3. In patients on warfarin, if the PT/INR is between 1 and 5/1.6, hair transplants have been successfully carried out without discontinuing warfarin, and the intraoperative bleeding is well controlled with intradermal tumescence using higher concentration of epinephrine (up to 1:50,000).[18]

The current recommendations after PTCA with newer drug-eluting stents are a combination of P2Y12 inhibitor such as ticagrelor and cangrelor with low-dose aspirin, and this may be followed by monotherapy with P2Y12 inhibitor or aspirin; this is titrated based on the risk of thrombosis or risk of bleeding.[31] Generally, one should wait for 24 months post a PTCA procedure to decide about modifying antithrombotic medications or considering hair transplantation.[27]

Other precautions while operating on patients who are post-PTCA or post-CABG status on antithrombotic medications include:

- Clearance from treating physician regarding fitness of the patient to undergo elective hair transplantation
- Informed consent clearly explaining the risk–benefit ratio with degree of risk as explained by treating physician
- Presence of an anesthetist throughout the procedure
- Intravenous (IV) cannula should be inserted before surgery.
- Blood pressure, oxygen saturation, and ECG monitoring during the procedure
- Adequate analgesia
- Use of dilute epinephrine in tumescent solution
- Emergency preparedness

HIV-positive Patients

The HIV is an enveloped retrovirus that causes the acquired immunodeficiency syndrome (AIDS), which is the last stage of HIV disease. The HIV is classified into HIV-1 (more widespread and virulent) and HIV-2 (mostly localized to Western Africa and less virulent).[32] This virus is sexually transmitted through unprotected sex or use of contaminated IV cannulas/needles in drug addicts, through blood transfusions and vertical transmission.[32] Primary infection usually occurs 2–4 weeks after exposure when HIV enters the body. This is followed by chronic infection, which may last for decades. The culmination is into AIDS characterized by opportunistic infections (OIs) and tumors, which are usually fatal without treatment.

Uncertainty about the advisability of elective procedures for these patients and fears of infection transmission may cause trepidation among hair transplant surgeons. The apprehension is mainly about the eligibility of these patients for hair transplantation (potential risk of infection) and safety for the operating team.[32]

It is important to understand that being HIV positive is not a contraindication for elective surgery provided certain criteria are met. An HIV-positive patient who is virally suppressed does not have any added surgical risk and neither poses a risk to the surgical team.[33]

The introduction of highly active antiretroviral therapy (HAART) helps to suppress the viral activity, improves CD4 counts, and has significantly improved the life expectancy of patients infected with HIV and those diagnosed with AIDS.[34]

The progressive failure of the immune system in patients caused by HIV can increase the possibility of developing surgical site infections (SSIs) after surgery. HIV-infected individuals, even with high CD4+ cell counts, are at a higher risk of developing both common and OIs than the general population. As per the Surgical Wound Classification (SWC) created by the Centers for Disease Control and Prevention, hair transplantation falls in the category of SWC-1—clean wound,[35] and the reported rate of SSIs after hair transplant surgery in non-HIV patients is <1%.[36] There are no published studies which have looked at SSIs in HIV positive hair transplant patients.

Guidelines When Deciding Candidature of HIV Positive Patient for Hair Transplant Surgery

Examination of the patient should include a detailed history of the infection and the treatment taken (HAART), last CD4 count, viral load count (apart from hair loss), and a thorough assessment to rule out the presence of any OIs.

If a patient is taking HAART and has an HIV viral load <200 copies/mL and a CD4 count >200 cells/mm^3 (ideal to have CD4 counts above 400 cells/mm^3), the hair transplant surgeon should proceed with the surgical plan as with a patient who does not have HIV. All standard preoperative assessments should be performed in patients with HIV, including cardiovascular and pulmonary evaluations. Individuals with HIV tend to have earlier and more comorbidities than those without HIV, including CAD, thromboembolic events, and pulmonary complications.[33]

If the HIV viral load is high or if the CD4 count is low, patient should be referred to physician caring for HIV patients for opinion and treatment. If there is possibility of improvement in these parameters with HAART, then there must be a clear discussion with the patient regarding the benefits and any potential risks of delaying elective surgery and engage the patient in shared decision-making regarding whether or when to proceed with hair transplantation.[33]

If HIV-positive patient is to be taken up for hair transplantation, it is important to discuss with the infectious disease specialist regarding antimicrobial prophylaxis for these patients before hair transplantation. Equally important is to check for any drug interactions between the retrovirals used and those drugs used before, during, and after hair transplantation.[33] Drug to drug interactions between some retrovirals (atazanavir, elvitegravir/cobicistat, etc.) and lidocaine can increase lidocaine levels due to CYP3A4 inhibition. Similarly, drug interactions between anxiolytics such as midazolam, NSAIDs, and retrovirals are also known and should be used only after ascertaining the package insert details.[33]

In individuals with controlled HIV and higher CD4 counts, the risk of surgical complications is approximately the same as in individuals without HIV, and reported transmission between HIV patient and healthcare worker is also rare.[33]

Smoking

Cigarette smoking is known to be associated with perioperative pulmonary, cardiovascular, bleeding, and wound healing complications. It is an important cause of preventable death.[1] Over the past decade, there has been a significant increase in the use of electronic cigarettes (e-cigarettes). These e-cigarettes deliver nicotine through inhalation by aerosolization.[37]

Inhaled smoke from cigarettes contains a host of toxins such as acetone, ammonia, benzene, cadmium, carbon monoxide, formaldehyde, hydrogen cyanide, nicotine, lead, tar, and shellac, which have widespread effect on the whole body.[1]

From hair transplant perspective, the impact on cutaneous macro- and microvasculature and wound healing is the most important. Vasoconstriction due to nicotine is caused due to release of catecholamines (also causing tachycardia and rise in blood pressure) from the adrenal medulla and sympathetic ganglia, ultimately causing tissue hypoxia. Vasoconstriction caused by nicotine is so potent that as few as two cigarettes transiently reduce peripheral circulation by 9–55%.[38] Carbon monoxide further contributes to tissue hypoxia by competitive inhibition of oxygen. The above-mentioned chemicals together with by-products cause a cascade of events eventually leading to hypoxia, thrombogenesis, and inactivation of the inflammatory cells imperative for normal wound healing and scar maturation.[1] Nicotine within e-cigarette aerosol will have the same effects on tissue oxygenation. E-cigarettes are associated with similar proinflammatory, cytotoxic effects, and decreased immune cell function, all increasing the risk of perioperative complications. Due to similar physiologic effects, both tobacco use and e-cigarettes would have similar perioperative considerations.[37]

Normal recommendation is to stop smoking/vaping a few weeks before surgery (a minimum of 2 weeks) till 2 weeks after surgery.[38] However, patients who have a long history of heavy smoking find it difficult to completely quit smoking. If they are made to quit completely, it has been found that there is increased intraoperative bleeding.[18] The authors have also found that chronic and heavy tobacco users have a lower pain threshold when they quit smoking preoperatively, and many times, it is actually better to allow them limited use perioperatively. This helps to reduce intraoperative bleeding and pain management.[18] In fact, in chronic smokers, a more pragmatic advice is to reduce smoking/tobacco usage as much as possible. Of course, it goes without saying that the risks of smoking and the potential impact on the final result of the hair transplant should be clearly discussed.

Alcohol

Alcohol consumption is a well-documented determinant of adverse perioperative outcome.[39] Active alcohol consumption, quantified by active alcohol use of at least two drinks per day within 2 weeks of surgery, is known to adversely affect postoperative outcomes in elective surgery and is associated with an increased risk of general postoperative morbidity, general infections, and wound complications.[40] This kind of alcohol consumption has also been shown to prolong the bleeding time and impair platelet function, which takes about 7 days to come back to normal after abstinence.[18] In chronic drinkers, preoperative abstinence of almost 4 weeks is needed to reduce preclinical organ dysfunction and reduce the response to surgical stress.[41] In patients who drink responsibly, the authors recommend an abstinence of 1 week preoperatively and 1 week postoperatively (to reduce interaction with antibiotics and NSAIDs used for analgesia).

Vitamins and Foods

Today, with social media recommendations, many people tend to self-medicate with various multivitamins and herbal supplements. Prolonged use of certain foods such as ginger, flaxseed, nonconventional supplements containing ginkgo biloba, ginseng, saw palmetto, nutritional supplements containing tocopherol (vitamin E), magnesium show increased bleeding intraoperatively. Patients consuming herbal teas should be asked to look at the constituents as many of these contain ingredients that may alter the clotting cascade.[18]

It is best to discontinue all nutritional (conventional and herbal) supplements at least 10 days before their hair transplantation.

ROUTINE PREOPERATIVE ASSESSMENT PRACTICED BY THE AUTHORS

The need to perform general preoperative laboratory testing and screening to evaluate the patient's "fitness" to withstand anesthesia, achieve homeostasis, and tolerate the surgical insult is subject to debate. Ideally, most of this information can be collected from history and physical examination, but keeping in mind patient variability, surgeon's background and training, and medico-legal aspects, it is better to perform and document these before surgery.

The importance of the preoperative tests is not only to ascertain the ability of the patient to heal normally after the surgery but also to make sure the hepatic and the renal systems are functioning optimally.

At times, relatively large amounts or repeated doses of local anesthetics are required for extensive and prolonged procedures. When this occurs, issues regarding hepatic clearance of local anesthetics should be considered. Keep in mind that both liver and renal functions decline by 50% by the age of 65 years.

The authors routinely advise the following assessments before taking up a patient for hair transplant surgery:

- Complete hemogram
- Creatinine
- Liver function tests
- Coagulation studies—bleeding time, prothrombin time/INR, partial thromboplastin time
- HbA1c and fasting and postprandial blood sugar
- HIV 1 and 2, hepatitis B surface antigen (HbsAg), hepatitis C virus (HCV)
- Resting ECG
- Physician assessment for fitness to undergo hair transplantation under local anesthesia

THE NEED FOR PHYSICIAN ASSESSMENT BEFORE HAIR TRANSPLANT SURGERY

It is a good policy to get the patient assessed by an independent physician before performing the procedure. This helps to screen out cardiopulmonary issues or other medical issues, including allergies, psychiatric issues, etc. The healthcare scenario in our country is very different. The average patient consulting for hair loss may not have a regular primary general practitioner (GP). As a result, the patient's medical background is not well documented, and most patients consult physicians only when encountered with some health issue. It is in the interest of the patient as well as from a medicolegal aspect for the surgeon to get a physical assessment of the patient before surgery.

Hair transplantation surgery is categorized as level I surgery, with patients belonging to American Society of Anesthesiologists (ASA) 1 category (normal healthy patient, nonsmoking, no or minimal alcohol use), and performed in class A facility. This basically categorizes a surgery with minimal risk to the patient independent of anesthesia, minimally invasive procedures with little or no blood loss, often done in an office setting with the operating room principally for anesthesia and monitoring. In this scenario, it is the hair transplant surgeon's duty to ensure that optimal physiology is maintained perioperatively with due diligence regarding patient's general health and existing comorbidities.

REFERENCES

1. Ellsworth IV WA, Colon GA. Management of medical morbidities and risk factors before surgery: smoking, diabetes, and other complicating factors. Semin Plast Surg. 2006;20(4):205-13.
2. Unger WP. My personal approach to the consultation. In: Unger WP, Shapiro R, Unger R, Unger M (Eds). Hair Transplantation, 5th edition. New York: Informa Healthcare; 2011.
3. Clark K. Seven most popular procedures men are booking. [online] Available from https://www.plasticsurgery.org/news/articles/seven-most-popular-procedures-men-are-booking. [Last accessed October, 2023].
4. Aronow WS. Management of hypertension in patients undergoing surgery. Ann Transl Med. 2017;5(10):227.
5. International Society of Hair Restoration Surgery: 2022 Practice Census Results. [online] Available from https://ishrs.org/wp-content/uploads/2022/04/Report-2022-ISHRS-Practice-Census_04-19-22-FINAL.pdf. [Last accessed October, 2023].
6. Krishnamoorthy Y, Rajaa S, Sulgante S, Chinnakali P, Jaswal N, Goel S. Prevalence of hypertension and determinants of treatment-seeking behaviour among adolescents and young adults in India: an analysis of NFHS-4. J Public Health (Oxf). 2023;45(1):e48-56.
7. Özyüncü N, Çağlar N. Labile hypertension in the clinic. Turk Kardiyol Dern Ars. 2019;47(8):701-4 [in Turkish].
8. Kohn T, Zari S. Local anesthesia techniques in hair restoration surgery. J Cutan Med Surg. 2016;20(6):610-2.
9. Nusbaum BP. Techniques to reduce pain associated with hair transplantation: optimizing anesthesia and analgesia. Am J Clin Dermatol. 2004;5(1):9-15.
10. Watanabe N, Reece J, Polus BI. Effects of body position on autonomic regulation of cardiovascular function in young, healthy adults. Chiropr Osteopat. 2007;15:19.

11. Pfoh ER, Chaitoff AM, Martinez K, Keenan K, Rothberg MB. Association between pain, blood pressure, and medication intensification in primary care: an observational study. J Gen Intern Med. 2020;35:3549-55.
12. Choi EJ, Jeong DW, Lee JG, Lee S, Kim YJ, Yi YH, et al. The impact of bladder distension on blood pressure in middle aged women. Korean J Fam Med. 2011;32(5):306-10.
13. Scultéty S, Varga B, Szabó D. Effect of bladder distension on blood pressure. Int Urol Nephrol. 1971;3:11-19.
14. Puig CJ, Shapiro R. Emergency intervention in hair restoration surgery. In: Unger WP, Shapiro R, Unger R, Unger M (Eds). Hair Transplantation, 5th edition. New York: Informa Healthcare; 2011.
15. Hartle A, McCormack T, Carlisle J, Anderson S, Pichel A, Beckett N, et al. The measurement of adult blood pressure and management of hypertension before elective surgery: Joint Guidelines from the Association of Anaesthetists of Great Britain and Ireland and the British Hypertension Society. Anaesthesia. 2016;71(3):326-37.
16. Lasserson DS, Buclin T, Glasziou P. How quickly should we titrate antihypertensive medication? Systematic review modelling blood pressure response from trial data. Heart. 2011;97(21):1771-5.
17. Kim Y. Interaction between beta blockers and epinephrine on hemodynamics of spontaneously hypertensive rats. Res Commun Chem Pathol Pharmacol. 1993;80(1):3-19.
18. Unger W. Preoperative preparation and instructions. In: Unger WP, Shapiro R, Unger R, Unger M (Eds). Hair Transplantation, 5th edition. New York: Informa Healthcare; 2011.
19. Terranova A. The effects of diabetes mellitus on wound healing. Plast Surg Nurs. 1991;11(1):20-5.
20. Cooley J. Achieving optimal growth. Hair transplantation in women. In: Haber R, Stough D (Eds). Hair Transplantation. Philadelphia: Elsevier; 2006. pp. 111-6.
21. Dortch JD, Eck DL, Ladlie B, TerKonda SP. Perioperative glycemic control in plastic surgery: review and discussion of an institutional protocol. Aesthet Surg J. 2016;36(7):821-30.
22. Saidian M, Lakey JRT, Ponticorvo A, Rowland R, Baldado M, Williams J, et al. Characterisation of impaired wound healing in a preclinical model of induced diabetes using wide-field imaging and conventional immunohistochemistry assays. Int Wound J. 2019;16:144-52.
23. Umpierrez GE, Hellman R, Korytkowski MT, Kosiborod M, Maynard GA, Montori VM, et al. Management of hyperglycemia in hospitalized patients in non-critical care setting: an endocrine society clinical practice guideline. J Clin Endocrinol Metab. 2012;97(1):16-38.
24. Australian Diabetes Society. Peri-operative Diabetes Management Guidelines. Sydney: ADS; 2012. [online] Available from https://diabetessociety.com.au/documents/PerioperativeDiabetesManagementGuidelinesFINALCleanJuly2012.pdf. [Last accessed October, 2023].
25. Halvorsen S, Mehilli J, Cassese S, Hall TS, Abdelhamid M, Barbato E, et al. 2022 ESC Guidelines on cardiovascular assessment and management of patients undergoing non-cardiac surgery: developed by the task force for cardiovascular assessment and management of patients undergoing non-cardiac surgery of the European Society of Cardiology (ESC) endorsed by the European Society of Anaesthesiology and Intensive Care (ESAIC). Eur Heart J. 2022;43(39):3826-924.
26. Rossini R, Tarantini G, Musumeci G, Masiero G, Barbato E, Calabrò P, et al. A multidisciplinary approach on the perioperative antithrombotic management of patients with coronary stents undergoing surgery: surgery after stenting 2. JACC Cardiovasc Interv. 2018;11(5):417-34.
27. Polania Gutierrez JJ, Rocuts KR. Perioperative Anticoagulation Management. StatPearls. Treasure Island (FL): StatPearls Publishing; 2023. [online] Available from https://www.ncbi.nlm.nih.gov/books/NBK557590/. [Last accessed October, 2023].
28. Yagyu K. Peri-operative antithrombotic therapy in hair transplantation. Hair Transplant Forum Int. 2016;26(6):241-52.
29. Yagyu K. Guidelines for perioperative antithrombotic therapy in hair restoration surgery: management of patients with coronary heart disease, mechanical heart valve, and atrial fibrillation. Hair Transplant Forum Int. 2012;22(2):59-64.
30. Spyropoulos AC, Douketis JD. How I treat anticoagulated patients undergoing an elective procedure or surgery. Blood. 2012;120(15):2954-62.
31. Natsuaki M, Kimura T. Antiplatelet therapy after percutaneous coronary intervention—past, current and future perspectives. Circulation J. 2022;86(5):741-7.
32. Justiz Vaillant AA, Gulick PG. HIV Disease Current Practice. StatPearls. Treasure Island (FL): StatPearls Publishing; 2023. [online] Available from https://www.ncbi.nlm.nih.gov/books/NBK534860/. [Last accessed October, 2023].
33. Yan L, Ellman T, McNairy M, McGowan JP, Fine SM, Vail RM, et al. Perioperative Care in Adults With HIV. Baltimore (MD): Johns Hopkins University; 2021. [online] Available from https://www.ncbi.nlm.nih.gov/books/NBK576018/. [Last accessed October, 2023].
34. Zhang L, Liu BC, Zhang XY, Li L, Xia XJ, Guo RZ. Prevention and treatment of surgical site infection in HIV-infected patients. BMC Infect Dis. 2012;12:115.
35. Onyekwelu I, Yakkanti R, Protzer L, Pinkston CM, Tucker C, Seligson D. Surgical wound classification and surgical site infections in the orthopaedic patient. J Am Acad Orthop Surg Glob Res Rev. 2017;1(3):e022.
36. Zito PM, Raggio BS. Hair Transplantation. StatPearls. Treasure Island (FL): StatPearls Publishing; 2022. [online] Available from https://www.ncbi.nlm.nih.gov/books/NBK547740/. [Last accessed October, 2023].
37. Krishna A, Mathieu W, Mull E, Tobias JD. Perioperative implications of vaping. J Med Cases. 2020;11(5):129-34.
38. Parsley W, Beehner M, Perez-Meza D. Studies on graft hair survival. In: Unger WP, Shapiro R, Unger R, Unger M (Eds). Hair Transplantation, 5th edition. New York: Informa Healthcare; 2011.
39. Nath B, Li Y, Carroll JE, Szabo G, Tseng JF, Shah SA. Alcohol exposure as a risk factor for adverse outcomes in elective surgery. J Gastrointest Surg. 2010;14(11):1732-41.
40. Eliasen M, Grønkjær M, Skov-Ettrup LS, Mikkelsen SS, Becker U, Tolstrup JS, et al. Preoperative alcohol consumption and postoperative complications: a systematic review and meta-analysis. Ann Surg. 2013;258(6):930-42.
41. Tonnesen H, Rosenberg J, Nielsen HJ, Rasmussen V, Hauge C, Pedersen IK, et al. Effect of preoperative abstinence on poor postoperative outcome in alcohol misusers: randomised controlled trial. BMJ. 1999;318(7194):1311-6.

CHAPTER 88

Unconventional Uses of Follicular Unit Extraction

Amit Kerure, Nitika Deshmukh Wagh

INTRODUCTION

Hair transplantation is practically a hair follicle rearrangement procedure in which the follicular grafts are extracted from the donor area and are implanted in the recipient area. Follicular unit transplant (FUT) and follicular unit extraction (FUE) are the methods done popularly for hair transplantation in androgenetic alopecia. The FUT technique involves the extraction of a strip of hair from the occiput (donor area), suturing, graft harvesting using a microscope, slit making, and implantation. Since it involves suturing, it can lead to a linear scar in the donor area. The FUE technique involves the removal of individual follicular grafts by an FUE motor (extraction), graft harvesting, slit making, and implantation as crucial steps in the procedure. It is comparatively scarless as there would not be any linear scar, unlike FUT. So, it has a better aesthetic acceptance as compared to FUT. Also, it has less healing time and does not require a microscope. Technicians need not use microscopes; hence, the learning curve is much easier as compared to FUT.

The FUE is the most popular technique nowadays and is known for its utility in androgenetic alopecia **(Figs. 1A and B)**. FUE can be used for treating androgenetic alopecia not only in men but also in women. In this chapter, the authors aim to highlight not only the conventional indications of FUE but also to elicit the multifaceted and "out-of-the-box" utility of FUE in dermatological indications such as stable vitiligo, traction alopecia, alopecia areata, and hirsutism **(Box 1)**.

BOX 1 **Unconventional uses of follicular unit extraction (FUE) in dermatology.[1-4]**

- Burnt-out alopecia areata
- Stable patches of vitiligo on hairy and nonhairy sites of the body
- White hair hirsutism
- Pubic hair transplant

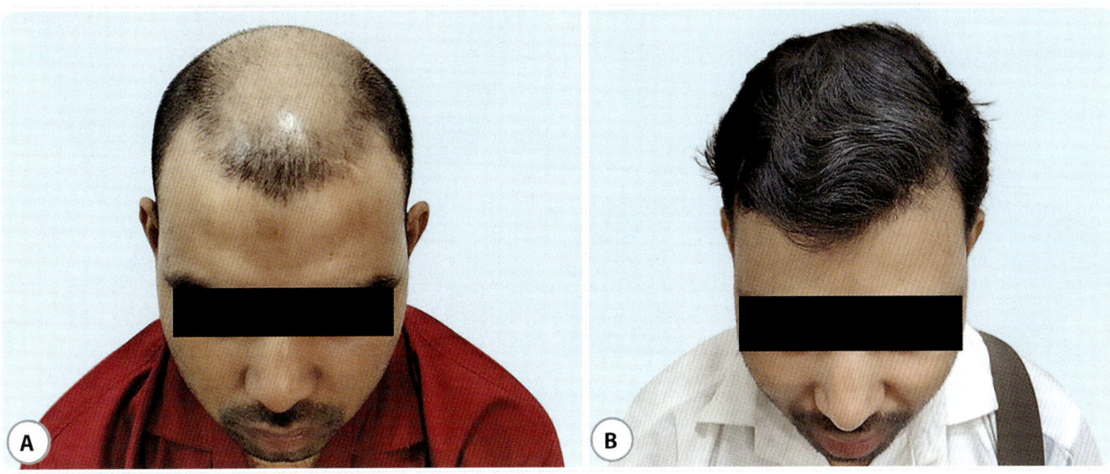

FIGS. 1A AND B: Follicular unit extraction in a case of androgenetic alopecia.

FOLLICULAR UNIT EXTRACTION IN ALOPECIA AREATA

Alopecia areata is a nonscarring and autoimmune type of alopecia. It is a cell-mediated autoimmune inflammatory dermatosis, in which autoreactive cytotoxic T cells destroy the hair follicles leading to hairless bald patches. It usually responds moderately to medical management and is renowned for its recurrence. Medical management of alopecia areata includes systemic steroids, intralesional steroids, and immunomodulators such as azathioprine, tofacitinib, and cyclosporine in severe cases. Hair transplantation in active/unstable forms of alopecia areata is not the treatment of choice as the implanted follicular grafts might be destroyed due to underlying autoimmune pathology; in rare cases, it might cause disease exacerbation. There is very little data on hair transplantation in alopecia areata.

The chances of success of FUE in alopecia areata can be attributed to the following factors:[1-4]

- Phenomenon of "donor dominance" by the extracted hair follicles from the occiput displaying their inherent growth characteristics and immunity to autoimmune activity onto the recipient area.
- Addition of triamcinolone acetonide in the tumescence solution while performing FUE in the recipient area can be done to avoid recurrence.
- Improved angiogenesis in the recipient area post surgery; trauma and irritation over the patch may lead to hair growth in a similar fashion like other sensitization methods; or due to possible repopulation of the area with transplanted cells.
- Inactivity of the underlying disease status in the patch which needs to be proven by histopathology and dermoscopy before selecting such patients of burnt-out alopecia areata for FUE.
- The procedure can be done with a disease-free donor area in the occiput.

Assessment of disease activity by histopathology and dermoscopy forms the crux of patient selection in such situations. FUE, though not routinely performed in alopecia areata, can lead to promising cosmetic outcomes if the disease is inactive in long-standing cases. **Figures 2A and B** demonstrate optimal and sustained hair growth in a case of long-standing alopecia areata over the left side lock area in a 32-year-old male in whom FUE was performed by the authors.

FOLLICULAR UNIT EXTRACTION IN TRACTION ALOPECIA (FIGS. 3A AND B)

Tractional alopecia is noncicatricial in the early stages.[5,7] But in advanced stages, this can lead to scarring hair loss. It is one of the most common causes of cicatricial alopecia in Black women who tie their hair tightly and in Sikhs who tie their scalp and beard hair tightly.[5-7] Persistent pulling forces on the hair follicles from traction induce hair loss. Traction induces inflammation and follicular damage. In the initial phases, it is reversible, but later on, can lead to scarring alopecia. *Dermoscopy* in traction alopecia is reported as traction folliculitis, the fringe sign, hair casts (pseudonits), broken hair, black dots, sparse hair follicles, and reduced follicular ostia. In advanced cases, there is a complete loss of follicular

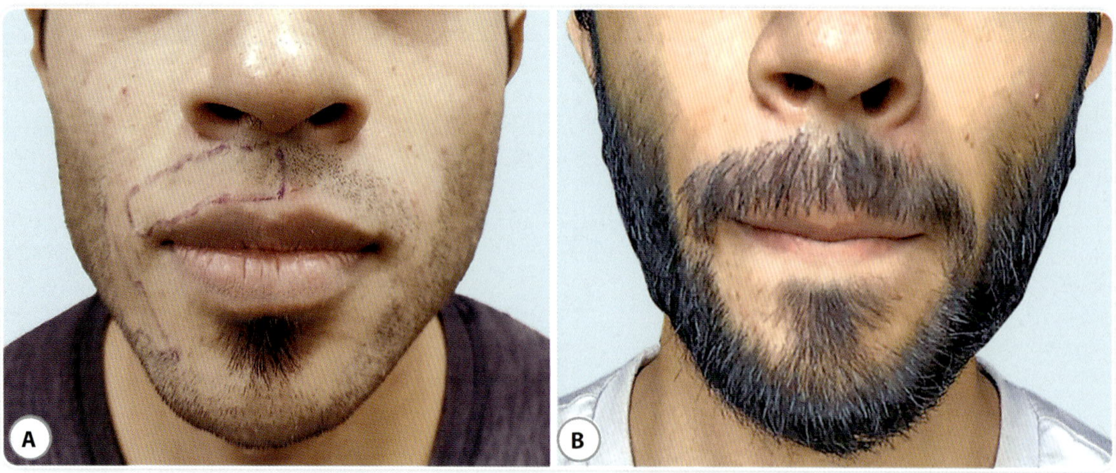

FIGS. 2A AND B: Follicular unit extraction in a case of long standing alopecia areata (A) before and (B) after.

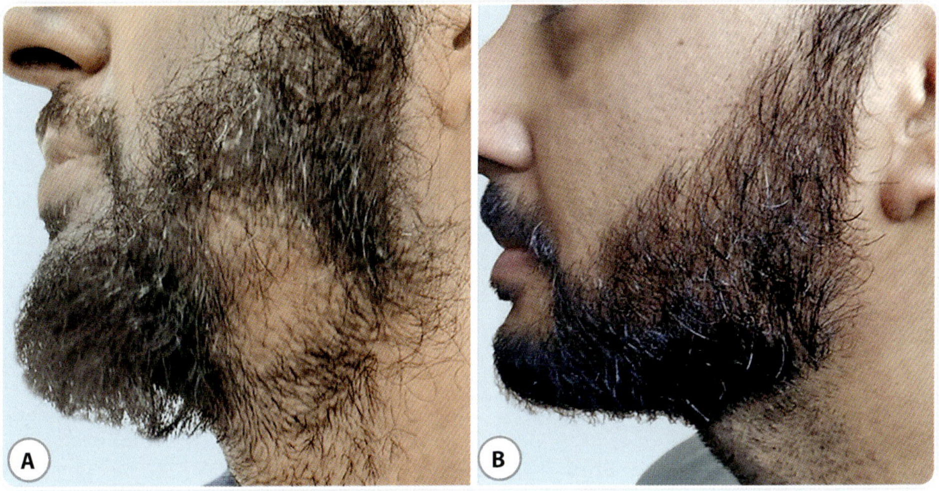

FIGS. 3A AND B: Follicular unit extraction in a case of traction alopecia beard in a Sikh male (A) before and (B) after.

openings. Dermoscopy and histopathological evidence of the absence of inflammatory changes aid in appropriate patient selection for FUE in such long-standing cases of traction alopecia.[7] Reports on medical management in the initial stages are anecdotal. Prompt diagnosis and the identification of causative hairstyle comprise the mainstay of management. But advanced cases require surgical management options like FUE.

For patches of alopecia on the face, a punch size of 0.7–0.8 mm should be used, and nape of the neck or postauricular hair grafts can be selected as their follicular units comprise single hair follicles. For FUE on patches of the scalp, a punch size of 0.9 mm can be taken, with occiput being the donor area. **Figure 3B** elicits a successful case of FUE in traction alopecia in an Indian Sikh male **(Figs. 3A and B)**.

FOLLICULAR UNIT EXTRACTION IN SCARRING ALOPECIA

Scarring Alopecia Secondary to Inflammatory Skin Disease

Cicatricial alopecia means permanent destruction of hair follicles as a result of irreversible damage to hair follicle stem cells due to disease pathology or trauma. Trauma could be chemical, physical, or thermal. Dermoscopic assessment of these lesions helps in differentiating them from scarring and nonscarring alopecias. Factors that impact the final output of FUE in scarring alopecia are the age of the scar, presence of atrophy or hypertrophy, condition of underlying tissue, any underlying pathological disease process, skin texture, area involved, and availability of donor area; all these factors decide graft survival and optimum hair growth following FUE in scarring alopecia.[8,9] In case of cicatricial alopecia secondary to inflammatory dermatological diseases, FUE can be considered as an option only when the disease activity is quiescent or inactive and long standing. If the disease is unstable with plenty of inflammatory infiltrate, the implanted follicular grafts might get destroyed with the same mechanism of the underlying disease pathology.[8,9]

Follicular Unit Extraction in Thermal Burn Scar (Figs. 4A and B)

Burn injuries, whether thermal or chemical, can lead to the complete destruction of hair follicles along with severe scarring of tissue. Dermoscopy and histopathological assessment aid in judging the prognosis of FUE in burn scars. Dermoscopic features such as reduced blood supply and thick underlying tissue with increased collagen make hair transplant challenging in such cases. **Figures 5A and B** demonstrate fair improvement in burn-induced scarring alopecia in a young female. The authors confirmed the cicatricial alopecia prior to FUE by dermoscopy and histopathology. FUE was done using a punch size of 0.9 mm, with occiput being the donor area. A similar case of FUE in burn scar has been reported in the literature by Bushan and Mysore with a successful outcome.

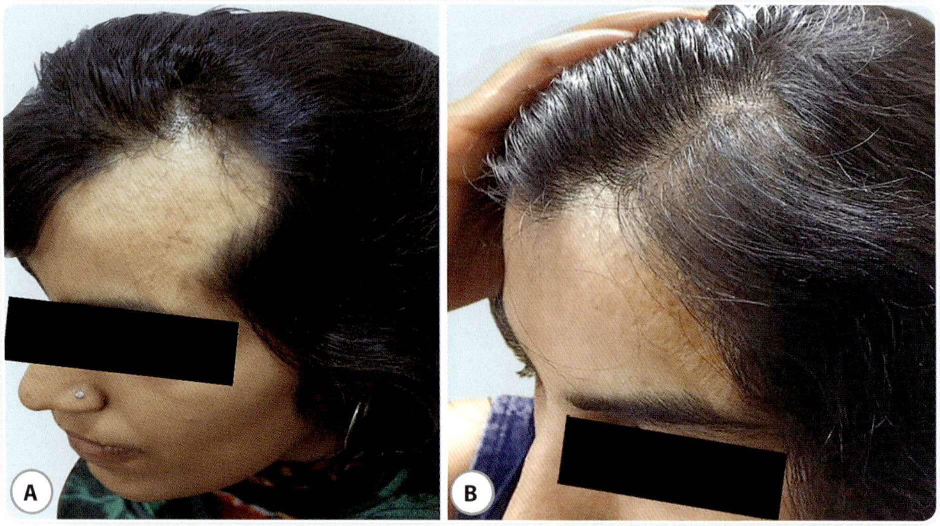

FIGS. 4A AND B: Follicular unit extraction in scarring alopecia due to burn in an Indian female (A) before and (B) after.

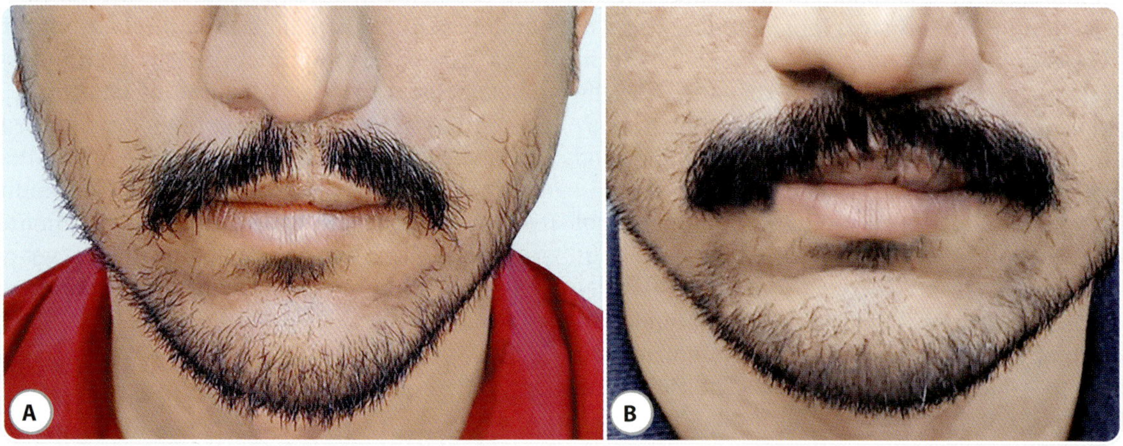

FIGS. 5A AND B: Follicular unit extraction in a scar over upper lip-[healed cleft lip surgery scar] (A) before and (B) after.

Follicular Unit Extraction in Traumatic Scar/Surgical Scar

Scarring alopecia due to trauma or surgery is best treated by FUE.[10] **Figures 5 and 6** demonstrate the effective utility of FUE in improving the appearance of traumatic scars or surgical scars, e.g., scars due to cleft lip/palate surgery **(Figs. 5A and B)** and postcraniotomy scars **(Figs. 6A and B)**. Thus, FUE does not heal the scar per se but helps camouflage it by growing new hair over bald areas on hair-bearing sites of the face and scalp.

Follicular Unit Extraction in Follicular Unit Transplant Scar (Strip Method)

Follicular unit transplant is a method of hair restoration that uses a strip from the back of the scalp as a source of follicular grafts. After healing, it might lead to a visible ugly scar over the occiput, which is inconvenient for adults who prefer to keep their hair short. This FUT-induced scar can be corrected in a similar fashion as any other scar on hair-bearing areas by FUE and implantation. The only condition for doing FUE in such cases is that there should

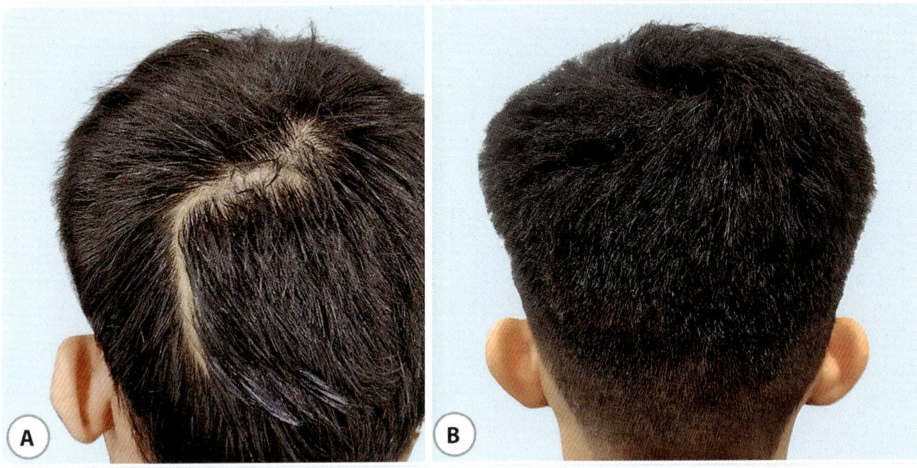

FIGS. 6A AND B: Follicular unit extraction done in a postcraniotomy scar in a young Indian boy (A) before and (B) after.

BOX 2 Key points for follicular unit extraction (FUE) in scarring alopecia (inflammatory type).[7-10]

- Always check for disease activity status while considering FUE in alopecia areata or alopecia due to autoimmune or inflammatory etiology
- Dermoscopic and histopathological evidence for disease inactivity are mandatory before performing FUE in inflammatory causes of alopecia
- Patient counseling for failure rates is crucial
- Appropriate medical management must be completed before considering the patient for surgical intervention

be an availability of donor grafts from safe zones of the scalp.[10] Otherwise, body hair can be used to cover the defect. FUE serves as one of the options for correction of such surgical scars; other modalities include scalp micropigmentation, intralesional steroids (for hypertrophied scars), or simply keeping the hair long to camouflage the defect **(Box 2)**.

FOLLICULAR UNIT EXTRACTION IN STABLE FOCAL VITILIGO (FIGS. 7A AND B)

Vitiligo is a disease with a social stigma with a prevalence rate of 2–5% in the Indian population. The rationale behind using FUE grafts to repigment vitiliginous skin is that the outer hair root sheath of hair follicles has stem cells and a larger number of melanocytes as compared to normally pigmented glabrous skin, which is used for skin grafting procedures. It is proposed that the stem cells and perifollicular melanocytes migrate onto the perifollicular skin and produce melanin giving pigment to the vitiliginous patches.[11-13]

Follicular unit extraction and implantation were first introduced to repigment vitiligo patches in 1998 by Na et al.[12] As per a study conducted on 63 vitiligo patients by Sacchidanand et al., a very good color match in vitiligo patches was reported in 72.1% of patients while a good color match was reported in 26.2% of patients.[13] Ample literature is available demonstrating the effectiveness of FUE as a dermatosurgical procedure for treating stable focal vitiligo.[12-14]

Follicular unit extraction is particularly useful on hairy areas of the body affected by vitiligo associated with leukotrichia.

Figures 7A and B demonstrate a successful outcome in few of our cases of localized vitiligo with coexisting leukotrichia in whom we used FUE as a surgical treatment modality. As these patches were located on hairy areas, FUE managed to recolor and avoid procedure-related scarring and hypo-/hyperpigmentation. Cobblestoning in the recipient area is absent or very minimal as a very small-sized punch is used for extracting grafts as compared to 1.5–3 mm size punches used in mini punch grafting in stable vitiligo. It helps achieve a good color match with the surrounding skin. Dermoscopy of the patch and the surrounding area helped us calculate the approximate number of grafts required in these patients.

FOLLICLE CELL SUSPENSION FOR VITILIGO (FIGS. 8A AND B)

Like melanocyte cell suspension using skin tissue grafts, follicular grafts can also be used for performing melanocyte-keratinocyte cell suspension. The hair follicle outer root sheath is a rich source of dihydroxyphenylalanine (DOPA)-negative inactive melanocytes (stem

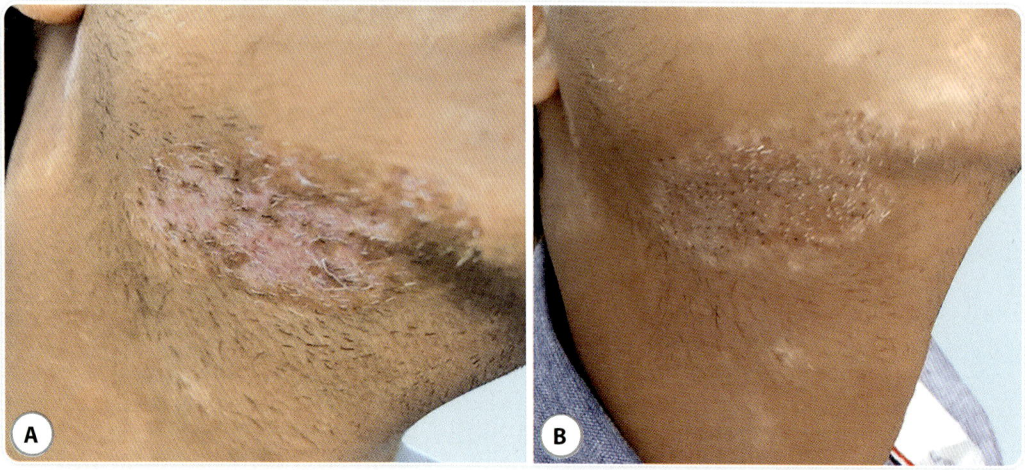

FIGS. 7A AND B: Follicular unit extraction (FUE) done in stable vitiligo in beard area (A) with good repigmentation after FUE (B).

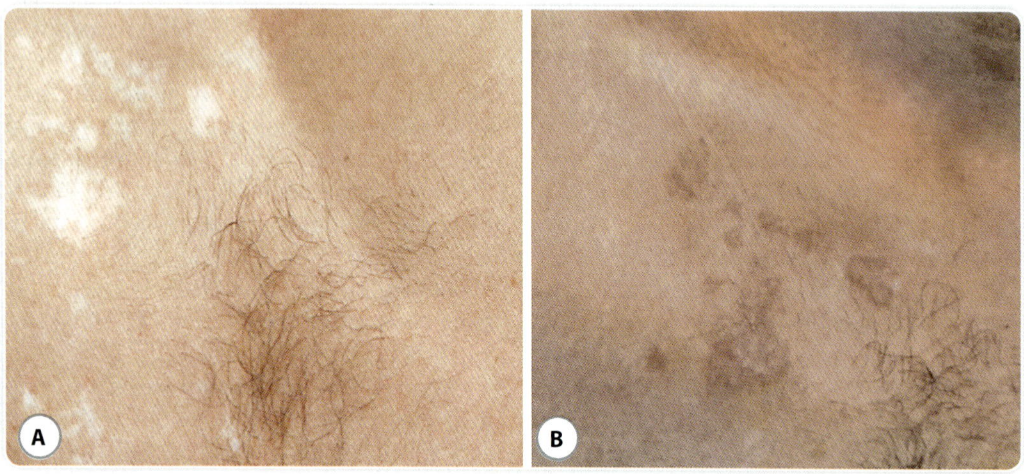

FIGS. 8A AND B: Follicular cell suspension in a stable vitiligo patient (before and after surgery).

cells). These melanocyte stem cells (MelSCs) have the capacity to migrate and enter vacant areas in the epidermis to cause perifollicular repigmentation, which later spreads in a concentric pattern causing diffuse repigmentation. This principle was used by Sawatkar et al. in the melanocyte cell suspension method in a localized case of vitiligo where follicular units were used instead of epidermal grafts as the source of melanin.[15]

Hair follicle melanocytes have some unique properties. A follicular melanin unit is constituted by one melanocyte for every five keratinocytes in the hair bulb as compared to the standard ratio of 1:36 in glabrous skin grafts. Also, hair melanocytes have a very fast and remarkable growing quality, and a relatively small number of melanocytes can potentially produce sufficient melanin to pigment up to 1.5–2 mm of radius around the implanted graft. The hair follicle is a rich source of three different types of stem cells, and it appears that all of them are important in hair growth. These stem cells include MelSCs, keratinocyte stem cells, and mesenchymal stem cells. With all these properties, the hair appears to be a more attractive source of melanocytes than the epidermis for cell-based therapies in vitiligo.[15]

Also, with follicular unit cell suspension, wound creation is smaller as compared to epidermal shave grafts. Hence, the healing period is faster with a smaller wound size. In comparison with the conventional non-culture melanocyte cell suspension, the technique of preparation of follicle cell suspension is simpler as it does not require separation of the epidermis from the dermis and manual breaking of epidermal samples into small pieces. **Figures 8A and B** elicit a repigmentation in stable vitiligo patches achieved by the follicle cell suspension technique **(Box 3)**.

BOX 3 Key points for follicular unit extraction (FUE) in vitiligo.[12-15]

- FUE can be used by two means in stable vitiligo:
  - By putting follicular grafts directly into the recipient area
  - By performing a cell suspension of keratinocytes and melanocytes obtained from follicular grafts
- Option (a) can be used only in hairy areas of the body such as beard, mustache, scalp, eyebrows, and eyelashes
- Option (b) can be performed for glabrous skin vitiligo patches also
- Punch size should be decided (0.7–0.9 mm) based on the local characteristics of the recipient area

FOLLICULAR UNIT EXTRACTION IN HIRSUTISM ASSOCIATED WITH WHITE HAIR (FIGS. 9A AND B)

Hirsutism associated with white or gray hair may not respond to laser hair reduction as the chromophore "melanin" is missing. In white hair in hirsute females, electroepilation is the treatment of choice. However, FUE can also be done on these white hairs using small-sized punches (approximately 7–9 mm in size).[16,17,20]

Many light- and heat-based therapies have been tried for white hair removal, such as the use of radiofrequency, laser after coloring, or the use of melanin-encapsulated liposomes before laser therapy.[18] However, none of them have proven to be an effective therapy, with results varying from 17 to 54%. Electrolysis can sometimes take multiple sessions to get rid of white hair completely as there are chances of regrowth from the hair bulge. Also, there are chances of folliculitis, recurrence, and hyperpigmentation.

Follicular unit extraction serves as a unique substitute for such a tedious process like electrolysis and can prove beneficial by removing the hair bulb as a whole, including its bulge region, thus minimizing the chances of recurrence and repeat sessions.[19] Side effects of minimal scarring and a downtime of 7–10 days must be explained to the patient.[20]

Figures 9A and B show the removal of all hirsute hair over the chin by the FUE method.

PUBIC HAIR RESTORATION (FIGS. 10A AND B)

Pubic atrichosis or hypotrichosis is common in particular races, especially the Mongolian race. The reason could

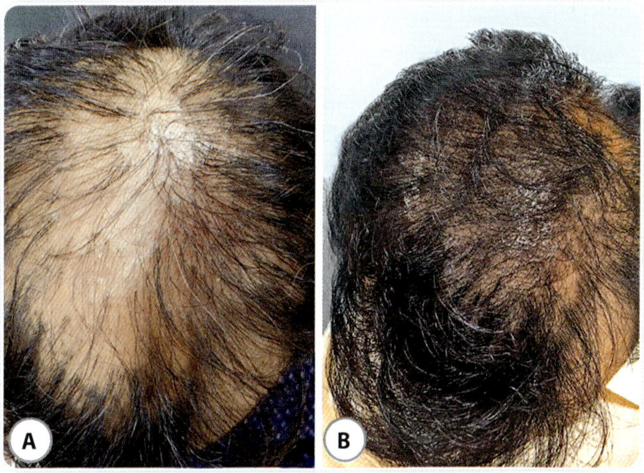

FIGS. 10A AND B: Follicular unit extraction done using pubic hair for a case of Androgenetic alopecia with poor occipital donor area (A) before and (B) after.

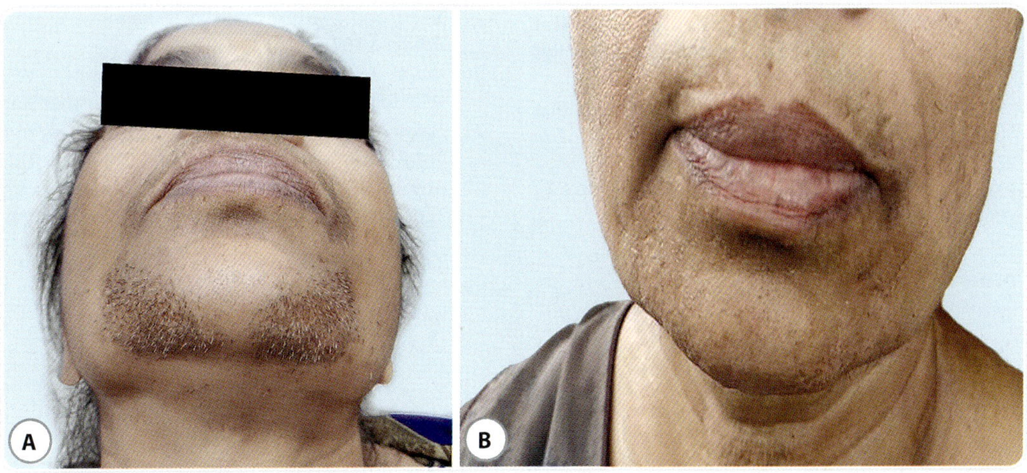

FIGS. 9A AND B: Follicular unit extraction done for white hair for post menopausal female (A) before and (B) after.

be genetic but is mostly idiopathic. It can be associated with lowered self-confidence and consequently can lead to psychiatric changes and social withdrawal. Surgical pubic hair restoration using FUE can help restore their confidence.[21,22]

SUMMARY

Follicular unit extraction is a versatile technique, and its effective utility in various indications is proven. Good clinical knowledge helps in the appropriate selection of patients, and good surgical skill helps achieve optimum results.

Tips and Pearls

- FUE is a unique and multifaceted technique.
- Its use in many dermatological disorders is still unexplored.
- Scarring alopecia due to various etiologies (traumatic or inflammatory) can be managed successfully with FUE.
- Inactivity of underlying disease pathology must be made sure before posting the patient for FUE.
- Some other off-label uses of FUE are stable vitiligo patches in hairy parts of the body, follicular melanocyte and keratinocyte cell suspension in stable vitiligo patches, hirsutism with white hair, and long-standing and burnt-out alopecia areata.

REFERENCES

1. Ito T. Recent advances in the pathogenesis of autoimmune hair loss disease alopecia areata. Clin Dev Immunol. 2013;2013: 348546.
2. Barankin B, Taher M, Wasel N. Successful hair transplant of eyebrow alopecia areata. J Cutan Med Surg. 2005;9:162-4.
3. Unger R, Dawoud T, Albaqami R. Successful hair transplantation of recalcitrant alopecia areata of the scalp. Dermatol Surg. 2008;34:1589-94.
4. Civas E, Aksoy B, Aksoy HM, Eski M. Hair transplantation for therapy-resistant alopecia areata of the eyebrows: is it the right choice? J Dermatol. 2010;37:823-6.
5. James J, Saladi RN, Fox J. Traction alopecia in Sikh male patients. J Am Board Fam Med. 2007;20:497-8.
6. Kanwar AJ, Kaur S, Basak P, Sharma R. Traction alopecia in Sikh males. Arch Dermatol. 1989;125:1587.
7. Akingbola CO, Vyas J. Traction alopecia: a neglected entity in 2017. Indian J Dermatol Venereol Leprol. 2017;83:644-9.
8. Farjo B, Farjo N, Williams G. Hair transplantation in burn scar alopecia. Scar Burns Heal. 2015;1:2059513115607764.
9. Bushan R, Mysore V. Hair transplantation in scarring alopecia. In: Mysore V, Sattur S, Garg AK, Dua K, Patwardhan N (Eds). Hair Transplantation, 1st edition. New Delhi, India: Jaypee Brothers Medical Publishers; 2016. pp. 353-4.
10. Yoo H, Moh J, Park J. Treatment of postsurgical scalp scar deformity using follicular unit hair transplantation. BioMed Res Int. 2019;2019:3423657.
11. Kumar AV, Parthasaradhi A. Follicular unit extraction technique in treating stable vitiligo with leukotrichia. J Dermatol Dermatol Surg. 2018;22:72-4.
12. Na GY, Seo SK, Choi SK. Single hair grafting for the treatment of vitiligo. J Am Acad Dermatol. 1998;38:580-4.
13. Sacchidanand S, Thakur P, Purohit V, Sujaya S N. Follicular unit extraction as a therapeutic option for vitiligo. J Cutan Aesthet Surg. 2013;6:229-31.
14. Menon SM, Sharma YK, Bansal P, Ghadgepatil SS. Restoration of pigmentation by follicular unit extraction transplant in three cases of focal vitiligo recalcitrant to therapy including with previous nonculture melanocyte-keratinocyte transplant. Int J Trichology. 2016;8:87-8.
15. Sawatkar GU, Keshavamurthy V, Dogra S. Follicle cell suspension: a new surgical modality to treat vitiligo. Pigment Int. 2015;2:4-8.
16. Sadick NS, Laughlin SA. Effective epilation of white and blond hair using combined radiofrequency and optical energy. J Cosmet Laser Ther. 2004;6:27-31.
17. Alijanpoor R, Poorsattar BejehMir A, Mokmeli S. Successful white hair removal with combined coloring and intense pulsed light (IPL): a randomized clinical trial. Photomed Laser Surg. 2011;29:773-9.
18. Sand M, Bechara FG, Sand D, Altmeyer P, Hoffmann K. A randomized, controlled, double-blind study evaluating melanin-encapsulated liposomes as a chromophore for laser hair removal of blond, white, and gray hair. Ann Plast Surg. 2007;58:551-4.
19. Richards RN, Meharg GE. Electrolysis: observations from 13 years and 140,000 hours of experience. J Am Acad Dermatol. 1995;33:662-6.
20. Gupta J, Chouhan K, Kumar A, Ariganesh C. White hair removal with follicular unit extraction. J Cutan Aesthet Surg. 2016;9:209-10.
21. Saxena K, Savant SS. Body to scalp: evolving trends in body hair transplantation. Indian Dermatol Online J. 2017;8:167-75.
22. Hwang S. Pubic hair transplant. In: Pathomvanich D, Imagawa K (Eds). Hair Restoration Surgery in Asians. Tokyo: Springer; 2010.

SECTION

4

Management Issues for Hair Transplant Clinic

SECTION OUTLINE

CHAPTER 89

Setting Up Hair Practice

Viral Desai

INTRODUCTION

Hair loss is a prevalent concern that affects a significant proportion of the population, encompassing around 85% of males and 40% of females. Moreover, the likelihood of experiencing hair loss seems to rise with advancing age for individuals of both genders. Hair loss can be attributed to various factors, but the most prevalent cause is androgenic alopecia (AGA), which is a pattern of hair loss that is influenced by androgens and affects both males and females.[1]

There are several nonsurgical techniques available that have the potential to impede the advancement of AGA and facilitate the growth of new hair strands. These modalities encompass minoxidil, finasteride, dutasteride, low-level laser light treatment, platelet-rich plasma (PRP), adenosine, and ketoconazole.[2,3] In addition, current progressions in the field of surgical hair restoration have resulted in hair transplantation (HT) being a progressively efficacious, secure, and dependable method for individuals experiencing distress due to AGA to restore a more youthful and authentic hair appearance.[4]

Hair transplantation surgery is regarded as an outpatient procedure that does not necessitate hospitalization. Nevertheless, like other surgical interventions, it is crucial to uphold standards of care.[5] This chapter elucidates the requisite level of care in constructing a setup for HT surgery, the sterilizing procedure, and related aspects. It serves as a valuable reference for developing a thriving hair practice.

In the event that one intends to establish a hair transplant clinic, it is important to acknowledge the substantial increase in demand within the business in recent years. With only two main transplantation methods available, you will not need to invest a fortune to initiate the business, as limited equipment and a handful of staff members are enough to get started.

However, thoughtful planning is vital for both small-scale and large-scale businesses. This chapter will guide you on the right path toward building a successful hair restoration clinic.

THE SIX STEPS TO START UP A HAIR TRANSPLANT CLINIC

Step 1: Formulate a Realistic Business Plan

Launching a hair restoration clinic requires preliminary planning like any other business. Although your business can only be successful with a formal plan, formulating one enables faster and more tremendous success.

Your business plan should cover the following:

- The investment required (equipment cost, asset value, billing, etc.)
- Insight details of competitors to beat
- Type of treatments offered (surgical and nonsurgical)
- Strong marketing strategies for target clients
- Location and accessibility
- Renting or buying the clinic
- Financial budget and risks

In short, one should consider every tiny detail of the plan carefully. By planning all these details in a methodical way, one can rightly draw up a sound strategy to make a place in the market. You can design the plan using the business templates available or by taking guidance from an experienced business mentor. Engaging in discussions with multiple experts in the field of hair restoration can prove advantageous, as it allows for a comprehensive understanding of the subject matter and facilitates the alignment of one's goals and plans.

Step 2: Secure Finances

Once you are done composing the business plan, you will have a rough idea of how much money is needed. You can start the clinic alone or have a fair share of lenders or partners invest in your dream project.

Securing grants or loans from the government, private sources, crowdfunding, or bringing friends and family into the idea by signing them as creditors are common ways of getting the requisite finance.

Step 3: Setting up the Practice

Location plays the most critical role in making a business successful. Besides, a large proportion of finances are invested in renting or buying a location. The top of the agenda should be following a strict business plan and finding a good location for the establishment.

Below are the three questions you should ask yourself before choosing a location:

- Can the patients access my clinic quickly?
- Is the covered area sufficient for the desired setup?
- Are there any competing clinics nearby? If yes, then what is their service strategy?

If no strong competitors are nearby, keeping the rent-to-revenue ratio low and starting with a small-scale clinic can work out well for you. In case of competition nearby, modify your business plan to include services that are exceptional, different, and a notch above what is offered by others.

Infrastructure

According to the National Medical Commission (NMC) guideline[6] on aesthetic surgery and hair transplant procedures, the following key points are to be noted vis-à-vis setting up of hair practice:

- The ideal establishment would be a medical facility equipped with the necessary amenities to provide care for patients requiring indoor treatment.
- If a clinic exclusively does day care surgeries, it is advisable for it to have a strong affiliation with a neighboring hospital that possesses a fully equipped intensive care unit and critical care resources, should the need arise for emergency intervention. Additionally, prominently displaying a 24-hour emergency hotline number would be beneficial.
- It is imperative to establish a well-structured operation theater (OT) that adheres carefully to all OT rules.
  - Rigorous adherence to aseptic techniques and fumigation protocols
  - The implementation of appropriate protocols for the management of biomedical waste, including the processes of segregation, transfer or transportation, and disposal.
  - The appropriate sanitation of surgical tools, drapes, and other related items.
- The presence of an anesthesiologist, as needed, is essential due to the invasive nature of the operating room operation. It is imperative that a crash cart trolley be equipped with all necessary resuscitative amenities.
- It is imperative to preserve accurate documentation of patients who have undergone surgery, including pre- and postoperative pictures, as well as details of any complications that may have arisen.

General Setup

The ease and efficiency provided to patients by office- or clinic-based surgery have been widely acknowledged. The initiation and sustenance of clinic-based settings incur significant costs. However, when considering the viewpoint of patients, such settings present advantages such as reduced paperwork, enhanced privacy, and diminished psychological intimidation compared to surgery conducted in a hospital-based environment.[7] The utilization of a hair transplant facility, equipped with its own dedicated operating theater, offers superior advantages in terms of scheduling and cost-effectiveness compared to conducting the procedure within a hospital setting.[8]

The strategic positioning of a clinic in close proximity to hospitals and with ample parking space can enhance patients' perception of the clinic and contribute to effective company promotion.[9,10] The typical spatial need for a cosmetic surgery clinic is roughly 1,000 square feet.[8]

Step 4: Install the Right Equipment

Although the right location can attract patients to your clinic, more is needed to convince them to invest hefty sums for treatment. Since the cost of hair treatments is high, the patients generally visit after researching the key points to look for, such as affordability, quality of treatments, and the outlook of the clinic.

Recent market research and trends point toward a surge in follicular unit extraction (FUE) treatment method for transplant versus the traditional follicular unit transplant (FUT). Reasons for this shift include:

- Greater patient acceptance
- Ease of doing the surgery
- Shorter downtime with faster healing and quicker return of function in patients

Therefore, buying FUE or ARTAS (a modified form of FUE done via robotic systems) equipment may attract more potential customers.

We now pay attention to setting up the main surgical center and the guidelines to be followed for the same

Ideally, you may have major and minor OT for transplant surgeries and other routine dermatosurgeries or for nonsurgical hair treatments such as PRP and low level light therapy (LLLT), respectively.

General Safety

It is highly advisable that any medical facility engaging in office-based surgical procedures, irrespective of the type of anesthetic employed, possesses the essential equipment, established protocols, and adequately trained employees to effectively manage any emergent situations arising from the surgical procedure, administration of anesthesia, or other environmental contingencies. In accordance with the Clinical Establishment Act enforced by the relevant state body, it is imperative to adhere to all pertinent safety protocols mandated by local legislation.[5]

As per the NMC guideline,[6] the day care theater ought to be furnished with capabilities to monitor and manage emergency situations, which should include the provision of emergency medications, Boyle's machine, intubation sets, an Ambu bag, and a defibrillator. It is imperative to establish a comprehensive emergency preparedness strategy, ensuring that all nursing and operating staff are well versed in the prescribed protocol.

Setting up the Operation Theater

Despite being a straightforward and less invasive surgical procedure, it is imperative to adhere to all established protocols in order to guarantee sufficient measures of asepsis, sterilization, disinfection, and resuscitation. The significance of the surgery should not be underestimated, and the task group responsible for establishing hair transplant practices strongly opposes the utilization of temporary facilities, such as consultation rooms, minor procedure rooms, spa rooms, and similar spaces, for conducting hair transplant procedures. The special requirements for OTs have been thoroughly examined and explained in a dedicated chapter.[5,11,12]

- *Photography area or preoperative preparation area*:
  - Photography plays a crucial role in hair transplant surgery due to the visual-oriented nature of the field and its numerous applications.
  - The utilization of this tool allows for the documentation of both the severity and distribution of hair loss, facilitating the development of a comprehensive treatment plan. Furthermore, it aids in the educational process, acts as a valuable resource in legal matters, and perhaps contributes to scientific investigations.
  - Prior to capturing any photographs, it is imperative to secure written informed consent from the patient.
  - This location is also well suited for preoperative patient preparation.
- *Head wash area*:
  - The aforementioned component is a vital element of the hair transplant unit; however, it is not located within the operating theater. Instead, it is situated in a distinct chamber.
  - All plumbing supplies must be sufficient to provide the proper functioning of the shower station, including the connection to a water heater to ensure the availability of warm water for shampooing purposes.
  - An excellent option would be a head wash chair that closely resembles the ones found in salons. It is imperative to do a thorough examination of the position to effectively mitigate hyperextension during shampooing, as this has the potential to induce neurological manifestations, such as dizziness.[13]
- *Patient room*: It is recommended that a patient be provided with a room that includes an adjacent washroom to facilitate rest both before and during breaks, as well as following the surgical procedure.[14] It is advisable to strategically schedule it in close proximity to the OT.[15]

Step 5: Hiring Well-skilled Staff

Generally, hair transplant clinics are owned and run by medical professionals. However, if you are an entrepreneur with a vision to handpick and build a skillful team, the idea is a worthy investment. To start up, you will at least need to hire the following members:

- An administrator to manage appointments and oversee other important works at a clinic
- A team of experienced, well-qualified surgeons (if you are not one)[16]
- Surgical assistants
- Nursing staff
- Housekeeping staff

According to the NMC guideline,[6] a surgical operation refers to any method that involves making an incision in the skin with the intention of removing tissue from the scalp or body or preparing the scalp or body to receive tissue. This can include various techniques such as incising FUE grafts, excising the donor strip in FUT, or constructing recipient sites, and may involve the use of robots or other means. These procedures should be carried out by a duly qualified and licensed registered medical practitioner (RMP), specifically a practitioner of contemporary medicine. It is recommended that those with formal surgical training, such as MCh/DNB plastic surgery or MD/DNB dermatology, and sufficient expertise in dermatological surgical operations, should be the preferred candidates for doing hair transplants.[6] The following aspects of hair transplant surgery should only be performed by RMP:

- Preoperative diagnostic assessment
- Surgery planning
- The surgical procedure encompasses several key components, namely the extraction of donor hair, the meticulous planning of the hairline, the development of recipient sites, the handling of any concurrent medical conditions experienced by the patient, and the control of potential adverse responses.[17]
- Postoperative care

Step 6: Get Ready, Set, Go!

Finally, after arranging all the desirable aspects as per the plan, you are all set to start marketing. Try targeting the pain points of your customers and offering validated solutions to address those problems. Clearly convey what makes your clinic innovative plus unique and establish a strong stance about your objective.

However, to sell your idea effectively, hiring a marketing agency is recommended and can be a thoughtful addition to your team. As they are aware of all the recent and latest technicalities, tools, and emerging ways of attracting customers, trusting them for the launching part will be fruitful.

Tips and Pearls

- You will certainly launch a successful business after considering all the details mentioned in this chapter. Moreover, following the same business plan and adding small tweaks to it will keep your clinic updated and ensure its smooth running in the long run.
- As far as the patients are concerned, it is predicted that the market for cosmetology and esthetic medicine is booming and will grow and expand well in the coming years. Hence, if qualified services are provided, your plan can help you build a successful hair practice.

REFERENCES

1. Kanti V, Messenger A, Dobos G, Reygagne P, Finner A, Blumeyer A, et al. Evidence-based (S3) guideline for the treatment of androgenetic alopecia in women and in men—short version. J Eur Acad Dermatol Venereol. 2018;32(1):11-22.
2. Gupta AK, Mays RR, Dotzert MS, Versteeg SG, Shear NH, Piguet V. Efficacy of non-surgical treatments for androgenetic alopecia: a systematic review and network meta-analysis. J Eur Acad Dermatol Venereol. 2018;32(12):2112-25.
3. Manabe M, Tsuboi R, Itami S, Osada SI, Amoh Y, Ito T, et al. Guidelines for the diagnosis and treatment of male-pattern and female-pattern hair loss, 2017 version. J Dermatol. 2018;45(9):1031-43.
4. Rose PT. Advances in hair restoration. Dermatol Clin. 2018;36(1):57-62.
5. Mysore V, Kumaresan M, Garg A, Dua A, Venkatram A, Dua K, et al. Hair Transplant Practice Guidelines. J Cutan Aesthet Surg. 2021;14(3):265-84.
6. Guideline on Aesthetic Surgery and Hair Transplant Procedures. Ethics and Medical Registration Board, National Medical Commission. R-13014/18/2022 – Ethics/. Dated the 20th September, 2022.
7. Hunstad JP, Walk PH. Office-based anesthesia. Semin Plast Surg. 2007;21(2):103-7.
8. Ersek RA. Office-based plastic surgery. Semin Plast Surg. 2007;21(2):115-22.
9. Norman J. What No One Ever Tells You about Marketing Your Own Business: Real-life Advice from 101 Successful Entrepreneurs. Chicago: Dearborn Trade Publishing; 2004.
10. Sachdev M, Britto GR. Essential requirements to setting up an aesthetic practice. J Cutan Aesthet Surg. 2014;7(3):167-9.
11. Malkin J. Ambulatory surgical centers. In: Malkin J (Ed). Medical and Dental Space Planning: A Comprehensive Guide to Design, Equipment and Clinical Procedures, 3rd edition. New York: John Wiley and Sons, Inc; 2002. pp. 352-3.
12. Rajendran SC, Omprakash HM. Standard guidelines for setting up a dermatosurgery theatre. Ind J Dermatol Venerol Leprol. 2009;75:76-82.
13. Endo K, Ichimaru K, Shimura H, Imakiire A. Cervical vertigo after hair shampoo treatment at a hairdressing salon: a case report. Spine. 2000;25(5):632-4.
14. Park MY, Chai CG, Lee HK, Moon H, Noh JS. The effects of natural daylight on length of hospital stay. Environ Health Insights. 2018;12:1178630218812817.
15. Mysore V, Omprakash HM. Setting up a hair transplant unit. In: Mysore V (Ed). Hair Transplant, 1st edition. India: Jaypee Brothers Medical Publishers Pvt. Ltd; 2016. pp. 378-89.
16. Mark U. The surgical suite. In: Unger WP, Shapiro R (Eds). Hair Transplantation, 5th edition. New York: Informa Healthcare; 2011
17. Tsilosani A, Gugava M. Is there a rationale for use of antibiotics in hair transplantation surgery? Georgian Med News. 2005;(122):7-10.

CHAPTER 90

Tips for Beginners Starting a Practice

Madura C, Megha Chandrashekar

Key Messages

- The practice of hair transplant is unique as it emphasizes on attitude, efficient training with intricate learning of details, stamina for sustained effort during long surgeries, and continued passion for learning.
- A long-term approach is needed to ensure success.

INTRODUCTION

This chapter updates the quintessential mantra for beginners.[1] A beginner should pay attention to the following:

- *A*stute learner with the right attitude
- *B*ase—structural, functional standard operating procedure (SOP), build a team
- *C*ounseling/case
- *D*octor—patient, assistant/diagnosis and delivery of results, documentation
- *E*conomy/employee/ergonomics
- *F*itness
- *G*eneration Z marketing

Attaining precision in hair transplant surgery has a long learning curve. You have to be a good disciple with an intense desire and mindset to seek hair transplantation and continue to stay updated in the field. You should be prepared to face obstacles and overcome them without stress when establishing your new practice. The first and foremost step is to gain knowledge.

HOW TO LEARN HAIR TRANSPLANTATION?

Though multiple training centers/institutes are coming up with crash courses, it is advisable to take up a hair transplant course for a minimum of 1 year as the intricacies of the procedure need a longer learning curve **(Table 1)**.

WHY TRAIN UNDER THESE CENTERS?

In addition to avoiding quackery, training in these centers provides an upper edge in your daily practice. It will not only assist in delivering promised results but also help in handling untoward complications, if any. Staying abreast with the current scientific knowledge, including technological upgradation, can keep your practice par excellence.

Training Module for 1 Year

Training depends on preexisting knowledge, skill, and attitude and needs to be tuned to the individual doctor. Plastic surgeons who have extensive training in microsurgery learn hair transplantation skills very quickly. However, dermatologists, particularly those without prior exposure, need a longer exposure. The following module is recommended for novices without any prior exposure to surgeries:

- *1–2 months*: Observation and handling graft counting, graft segregation, hydrating grafts/measuring the length of grafts/trolley preparation/anesthesia preparation/calibrating machines and loading punch and fixing blade length/training on modules the art of slit making and load of grafts
- *3–5 months*: Anesthesia administration/loading implanters/implantation/extraction of grafts as the second assistant

TABLE 1: National and international courses.

Courses			
National	Rajiv Gandhi University of Health Sciences (RGUHS) affiliated courses	Affiliation: Nil	Indian Association of Dermatologists, Venereologists, and Leprologists (IADVL) and Association of Cutaneous Surgeons of India [ACS(I)] affiliated courses
	• Bangalore Medical College and Research Centre, Bengaluru offers fellowship in dermatosurgery (18 months) and trichology (12 months) • Cutis Academy of Cutaneous Sciences, Bengaluru offers fellowship in dermatosurgery (18 months) and trichology (12 months) • Venkat Charmalaya, Bengaluru offers fellowship in trichology (12 months)	• International Institute of Cosmetic Surgery and Aesthetic Medicine, Agra • International Academy of Cosmetic Surgery and Aesthetic Medicine (IACSAM), Pune • DermaClinix, Delhi • Institute of Cosmetology and Aesthetic Medicine (ICAM), Mumbai	• ACS(I) observership program (1 month) at Deenanath Mangeshkar Hospital • Association of Hair Restoration Surgeons India—Adiva Centre for Skin and Hair
International	• Asian Association of Hair Restoration Surgeons (AAHRS) • International Society of Hair Restoration Surgery (ISHRS) • American Board of Hair Restoration Surgery (ABHRS) • Keimyung University School of Medicine, Daegu, South Korea		

- *6–8 months*: Harvesting small numbers and assessing graft quality, gradually increasing in numbers, and making slits on modules
- *8–12 months*: Harvesting grafts at moderate speed, making slits for small areas, and doing all the steps with good stamina as the first assistant and doing small surgeries of <300 grafts independently under the primary surgeon's coverage

WHO IS AN ABHRS CERTIFIED SURGEON?

The American Board of Hair Restoration Surgery (ABHRS) is a rigorous pathway to achieve the designation of *diplomate of the ABHRS*. To become a diplomate of the ABHRS, a physician must demonstrate training, evidence of post-training surgical experience, aesthetic skill, and a comprehensive clinical understanding of hair loss and its treatment modalities. In order to qualify for the annual examination, a candidate must present case logs and operative reports with surgical details, along with before and after photographs providing evidence of high-quality, cosmetic, and aesthetic results. An applicant must successfully complete a comprehensive examination consisting of both an oral and a written component, identifying a thorough knowledge of hair restoration surgical techniques. The ABHRS exam stands as the only psychometrically and statistically validated examination dedicated to the specialty of hair restoration surgery. The ABHRS is the only recognized board certification by the International Society of Hair Restoration Surgery (ISHRS), the largest hair restoration education society in the world. There are four routes of certifications:[2]

1. *Experience route*: An applicant must have 3 years of experience in the private practice of hair restoration surgery, submit 150 case logs in the preceding 3 years, submit 50 documented operative reports with the applicant noted as a primary surgeon, and out of these, 5 full case reports must include before and after photos that demonstrate satisfactory results.
2. *Fellowship route*: An applicant must document proof of 1 year of experience in the private practice of hair restoration surgery, completion of 70 hair restoration surgery cases as an assistant surgeon in a program recognized by the ISHRS, submit 50 case logs in the preceding 1 year, submit 50 documented operative reports with the applicant noted as a primary surgeon, and out of these, 5 full case reports must include before and after photos that demonstrate satisfactory results.
3. *Lifetime achievement route*: An applicant must submit case logs documenting completion of a minimum

of 400 hair restoration cases performed as a primary surgeon in the preceding 8 years of the date of application, submit 50 documented operative reports with the applicant noted as a primary surgeon, and out of these, 5 full case reports must include before and after photos that demonstrate satisfactory results.

4. *Physicians new to the specialty* are applicants who do not meet the criteria in the three routes of certification. They must submit proof of attendance of at least two ISHRS annual meetings, proof of attendance at ISHRS-endorsed programs consisting of a minimum of 16 hours of live surgery workshop, and submit case logs documenting completion of a minimum of 25 hair restoration cases performed as a primary surgeon.

In order to become an ABHRS board-certified diplomate, the applicant must successfully pass both written and oral components of the examination.

COMMON MISTAKES DONE BY BEGINNERS AND TIPS FOR CORRECTION

- *Wrong case selection*:
  - Identifying the red flags during consultation is crucial. This avoids not only compromised results but also possible future litigations, if any. Factors such as unrealistic expectations, diffuse unpatterned alopecia (DUPA), scarring in the donor area, presence of black dots, broken hairs, and body dysmorphic disorder (BDD) patients should be evaluated and considered as relative contraindications for surgery.
  - Each case needs to be individualized with meticulous planning.
  - Select cases with a good donor area with 3–5 grade of androgenetic alopecia (AGA), age 25 years and more, and who have taken complete medical therapy. Have a close friend or relative as a client to start with.
  - Avoid cases associated with comorbidities till you gain experience in handling associated complications.
- *Trying to perform mega sessions during the initial phase*:
  - Beginners must always do small cases and gradually increase the number of grafts based on the efficiency of the team.
  - Start with smaller cases first. Spread the procedure over more stages or days for larger cases.
- *Hiring freelancing and mercenary technician squad*:
  - The results of a hair transplant depend on dedicated teamwork. A well-trained technical staff is the backbone of our practice. A team of five people, one surgeon and four assistants, can be adequate to start with.
  - Committed full-time staff is recommended than part-time. Authors feel that hiring technicians from other institutes/clinics/freelancers on a part-time basis is unethical and not recommended for long-term practice.
  - Multitask technicians are preferred over single task. Periodic promotion should be done based on skill, patience, accuracy, concentration, tissue respect, knowledge, endurance, and speed.
- *Failure to delegate work, multitasking alone, and getting stressed*:
  - *Setting up SOPs* assists in uniform care delivery, organizing functioning, and saving time. Various SOPs can be designed based on the size of the organization/practice. Common ones are *counseling protocol*, providing the patient with baseline investigations, preparation of the patient, pre- and postoperative instructions, anesthesia preparation, and operative steps.
  - Hair transplant, being one of the longest aesthetic surgeries in practice, demands physical and mental fitness for a successful outcome. One should be able to stand for hours and perform procedures without losing hand-to-eye coordination, accuracy, and skill, which is particularly important in follicular unit extraction (FUE). The body should be able to produce what the mind thinks.
- *Pain in between the surgery and faster weaning of anesthesia create anxiety in the patient and panic in the young surgeon*: minimizing pain perception with infiltration of adequate local anesthetic cocktail, proper nerve blocks, and timely topping up of anesthesia.
- *Poor management of the donor area*:[3,4]
  - Harvesting beyond the safe donor area: Beginners tend to harvest beyond the safe donor area to meet the demand of the patient's large area. This could cause early miniaturization and shorter-lasting results. Always limit harvesting to the safe donor area.
  - Overharvesting of grafts to cover a large donor area: Overzealous extraction of grafts in the vicinity and cherry-picking cause moth-eaten alopecia and can damage the donor zone, leading to a visible and see-through scalp. Always make grids in the donor area during your practice to limit overharvesting of the grafts.

    To avoid overharvesting, cherry-pick a maximum of 10–15 grafts/cm^2. Assess the need for the number of single hairs. Limiting to 2 and 3 follicular units for smaller surgeries needing up to 800 grafts, and avoiding harvesting 3 and 4 follicular units in such cases.

- Use of sharp-tip punches to ease the burden of extraction can exceed the permissible limit of the graft transection rate. It is preferable to use blunt-tip punches to avoid transection with a permissible limit of 10% per surgery. Use of powered devices with oscillatory and/or rotatory punches and suction apparatus will facilitate atraumatic extraction. Based on scalp assessment (tight/lax) and test grafts assessment that includes fox grading, transections (partial/complete), capping/burial, the torque and speed of the machine need to be adjusted and also the type of punch must be selected based on the length and size of grafts for optimal harvest. Starting with a 0.9-mm punch minimizes the margin of error. In cases with difficulty in the extraction of grafts, use the assistance of a retractor (skin retractor/Kerure clamp)—this reduces the acute angulation of the hair shaft, minimizing the transection.

- *Recipient area mismanagement*:
  - Placing the hairline too low to match the expectations of the patient can give an unnatural look altogether, making the hair transplant procedure evident.
  - Slit placement: Trying to give maximum density by placing slits close to each other can cause the merger of slits and can cause laceration.
  - Placement of sagittal slits adjacent to one another can have a more see-through appearance.
  - Grafts placed too superficial or too deep can cause either cobbling or dimpling of the transplanted site.
  - Trying to fit in chubby grafts into a smaller channel implanter [e.g., 3–4 hair follicular unit (HFU) in 1.0 implanter] can cause damage to the bulge area while loading.
  - Accidental placement of 2/3 HFU in the anterior hairline results in doll hair appearance.
  - Avoid piggybacking of grafts in the urge to complete the surgery.

  In slit making with a chisel blade/hypodermic needle, needle incisions need to be deeper than chisel blade incisions as they are narrower at the bottom and may not insert completely. Place test grafts to see if they snugly fit in the slits. Assess the bulb; if they are bent, then slits need to be deeper.[5] Semiconical blades are preferred as they cause less collateral damage to the dermis and the vascular plexus as lower depth of penetration is sufficient.[6] Though the possibility of vascular damage is more in coronal slits, the change in angle seldom causes increased length of the slit like in sagittal slits. The artistic use of different sized needles and blades to accommodate different sized needles adds to the natural appearance of the outcome, for example, use a 0.7-mm blade/20G needle for a single follicular unit (FU) and a 1.1–1.2-mm blade/18G needle for 4 FU. To attain higher density in selective areas, dull implanters can safely be used (e.g., KNU, Lion implanters, Choi implanters). Professor Robert True utilizes single-hair grafts to make 0.63-mm premade incisions (23G needle) and places the grafts with 0.74-mm dull needles. For two- to three-haired grafts, Garg et al. use 0.8–0.85-mm premade incisions and 0.96-mm dull needle implanters.[5]
- *Poor handling of grafts can lead to poor results*: Avoid crush and desiccation injury. Hair transplant being a long procedure, the course of the grafts outside the body should be well hydrated to avoid reperfusion injury and desiccation. Graft survival depends on the quality of the transplanted grafts. It is best to avoid the implantation of injured bulb and fractured or paired grafts.[7,8]
- *Slit making and extraction disparity*: It is permitted to make 20% additional slits more than the harvested grafts. If needed, additional grafts can be harvested during the course of the transplant. Making too many slits without a plan can cause scarring in the recipient area.
- *Miscellaneous mistakes*:
  - Inadequate trimming of donor area hair length of 2 mm or more/too short trimming can pose difficulty in extraction.
  - Reusing the punch after sharpening can change its diameter and cause more trauma in the donor zone.

TIPS FOR BEGINNERS

- Prefer to start your practice in your hometown or where you have studied so that you already have a circle of friends and relatives. Freelance with outpatient clinics at a travelable distance, but keep operating at one place only.
- Invest in *precise instruments and equipment*: The magnifying loop of 4–5×, depending on your comfort of accommodation, is mandatory. Use 2.5× for technical assistants.
- Do structured counseling covering the pathology and progression of hair loss, need for a medical line of treatment as maintenance, operative steps, pre- and postoperative measures, and single/multiple sessions.

- Be honest and transparent.
- *Planning the case, documentation, and consent are vital parts of hair restoration surgery.* Maintain a case sheet and a planning sheet to include the examination findings and the plan of surgery, including additional instructions such as dyeing white hair on the day of surgery.

  Select donor area with the scalp as the first option and the rest (chest, beard legs, back, axilla) later. Cover totally bald areas first and later perform dense packing over the selected recipient area.
- The practice of hair transplant seems lucrative. It often projected as an easy way to earn quick money with minimal effort. In reality, nothing in life comes easy. Do not cut corners at the cost of quality. Keep your rates reasonable (not too high, not too low).
- Do not promise more than what you can deliver.
- *Practice training*: Make training models first and have a training program for doctors and technicians. Do not make operation theater a classroom.
- *Be patient*: It takes about 1 year to judge the result of your procedure. Hence, it takes about 2 years for your work to be recognized and to establish practice. So, be patient. Let your results speak for you in the society.
- *Peace and pleasure*: The goal of starting a new venture should be a "stress-free" life. If you do not find peace and pleasure during practice, check on the reasons and rectify them.

SUMMARY

With continued learning, your proficiency will scale up, and so will your practice of hair transplantation. The ultimate aim should be patient and physician gratification and not just economic returns.

Tips and Pearls

For long-term benefit, maintain honest, transparent, ethical, and scientific practice updated with newer technologies.

REFERENCES

1. Sanjiv V. Tips for beginners starting a practice. In: Venkataram M, Sandeep S, Anil Kumar G, Kapil D, Narendra P (Eds). Hair Transplantation. New Delhi: Jaypee Brothers Medical Publishers; 2016. pp. 375-77.
2. ABHRS Certification. [online] Available from https://abhrs.org/certification/. [Last accessed September, 2023].
3. Unger W. The donor site. In: Unger W (Ed). Hair Transplantation, 3rd edition. New York: Marcel Dekker Inc.; 1995. pp. 183-212.
4. Kerure AS, Deshmukh N, Agarwal S. Challenges in hair transplantation practice as a beginner. Indian J Dermatol Venereol Leprol. 2021;87:303-5.
5. True RH, Garg AK, Garg S. Initial treatment plan. In: Practical Guide to Hair Transplantation. Interactive Study for the Beginning Practitioner. New York: Thieme; 2021. pp. 44-51.
6. Atodaria PR, Venkataram A, Mysore V, Atodaria KP. Optimal hair transplant recipient site slit design: minimizing vascular damage. Indian J Plast Surg. 2021;54(4):471-6.
7. Kwack MH, Kim MK, You SH, Kim N, Park JH. Comparative graft survival study of follicular unit excision grafts with or without minor injury. Dermatol Surg. 2021;47(5):e191-4.
8. Mysore V, Kumaresan M, Garg A, Dua A, Venkatram A, Dua K, et al. Hair transplant practice guidelines. J Cutan Aesthet Surg. 2021;14(3):265-84.

CHAPTER 91

Guidelines for Hair Transplantation Operation Unit

Venkataram Mysore, Sukhbir Singh, HM Omprakash

Key Messages

- Hair transplantation theater has certain special requirements that need close attention.
- While hair transplant (HT) is a minor surgery, all protocols for an operation theater, including emergency resuscitation, must be in place.
- A well-equipped, well-designed surgical suite improves the experience for both patients and the surgeon.

INTRODUCTION

Hair transplantation, while being an outpatient procedure, needs to be taken seriously to follow all proper surgical protocols. This is particularly so, as this is a surgery that is performed by doctors of diverse backgrounds and often without prior surgical training, particularly with the advent of follicular unit extraction (FUE), which is seen as noninvasive. Since patient safety is the first concern, it is not only the surgeon's skill that matters but also the infrastructure. A well-equipped, well-designed surgical suite improves the experience for both patients and the surgeon.[1]

NOMENCLATURE

The unit where hair transplantation is performed can have different nomenclatures: The operation theater (OT), the ambulatory surgery facility, and office-based surgery. But in this chapter, it shall be known as *the hair transplant OT.*

Why the Need for Separate Hair Transplant Operation Theater?

Hair transplantation, like any surgery, can be associated with risks. The associated problems include mild scalp infection, anaphylactic reactions, or airway compromise due to the use of topical or infiltration anesthetics. Therefore, we should have a separate hair transplantation theater unit with a clean, if not sterile, environment and backup of advanced life support.

While it may make economic sense to use the existing minor or major OT of an existing hospital, it has definite drawbacks. Hair transplant patients are relatively healthy patients compared to major surgical patients. Dermatologist's clinics usually have heavy outpatient flow, and planning surgery time could be difficult sometimes. If the OT is taken on rent, it would incur an additional cost.[1]

As it is an outpatient procedure, people prefer a hair transplantation unit to a general hospital OT since the environment is soothing there. If the hair transplantation theater unit is in the same premise as the consultation room, patients are already familiar with the surroundings and the personnel, and they prefer this personalized care.[2]

Where should the Hair Transplantation Theater Unit be Located?

The hair transplantation theater unit may be housed in a general hospital, doctor's private clinic, or a form of polyclinic where different doctors work, such as plastic surgeons, general surgeons, or a group of dermatologists.

Requirements for Starting a Hair Transplantation Theater

Each hair transplant surgeon will have their own likes and dislikes. So before embarking on designing, one has to keep in mind the statutory standards and then tailor-make the facility to meet one's requirements.

The Indian standards, National Medical Commission (NMC) guidelines,[3] basic requirements for hospital planning,[4] NMC guidelines,[5] and the Indian Association of Dermatologists, Venereologists, and Leprologists guidelines,[6] are the few national standards to look into.

There are various international guidelines, such as The American Association for Accreditation of Ambulatory Surgery Facilities,[7] Singapore: Directives for Private Ambulatory Surgical Centers Providing Ambulatory Surgery,[8] Netherlands: Building Guidelines for a Surgical Department,[9] World Health Organization guidelines,[10] which are some of the other best resources.

Other publications, such as Savant and Gore[11] and Unger,[12] should also be referred to before starting a hair transplantation theater unit.

HAIR TRANSPLANTATION THEATER UNIT TYPES

There are various dermatological procedures, such as skin biopsies, cryotherapy, toxins, and fillers, which can be performed in an *unrestricted zone* **(Fig. 1)** of the OT. Major anesthesia, such as general anesthesia (GA) and spinal, are not permitted.[13]

But hair transplantation requires a separate theater. This is the *restricted zone* **(Fig. 2)** or the traditional operation room where everyone, including the surgeon, patient, and assistants, changes their dress, wear gowns, caps, masks, and different footwear marked for OT use only.[14] This is for all techniques of hair transplant, particularly for strip dissection. GA and intravenous anesthesia are permitted here.[8]

Location of the Hair Transplantation Theater Unit in the Office or Hospital

The Indian standards for hospital planning[4] clearly define that the traditional OT unit be located in:

- Quiet environment
- Freedom from noise and other disturbances
- Freedom from contamination and possible cross infection
- Maximum protection from solar radiation
- Efficient lift service if located on upper floors
- Miscellaneous things such as proper water and electrical supply with backup, fire extinguishers, fire alarm systems, etc.

Layout of the Hair Transplantation Theater Unit (Fig. 2)

As already stated, the hair transplant theater should be of the restricted type. Depending on cleanliness, there are few well-defined zones. This helps to keep the OT complex free from any bacterial contaminations.

- The first is the *protective zone*, which includes waiting zone, anesthesia examination room, separate changing rooms for staff and patients, and the supply rooms.
- The second is the *clean zone*, which includes theater pack preparation, preoperative room, and recovery room.

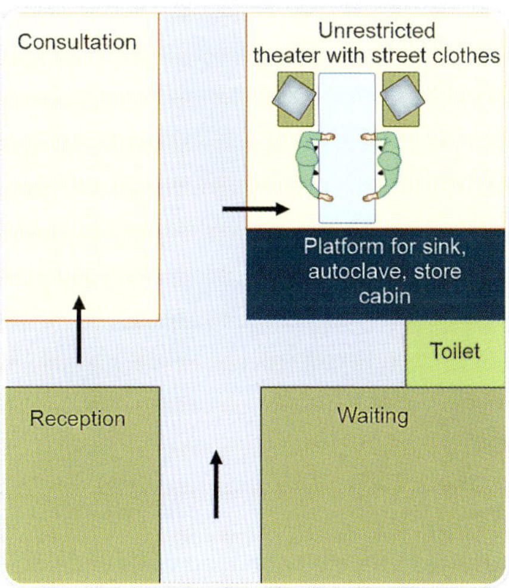

FIG. 1: Unrestricted type of theater unit.

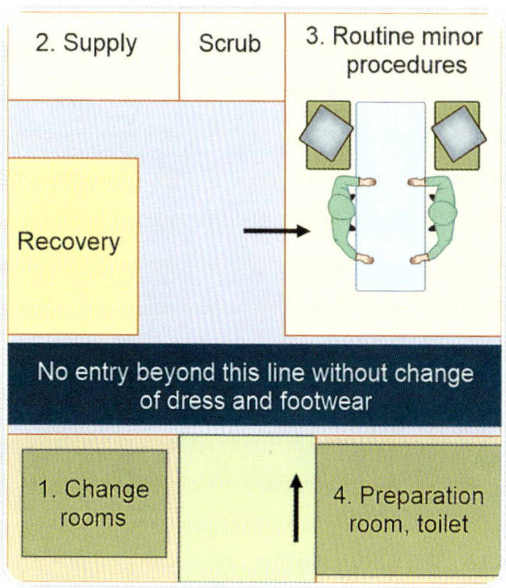

FIG. 2: Restricted zone—hair transplantation theater unit.

- The third is the *asepsis or sterile zone*, which includes the sterilization room and OT.
- The fourth is the *disposal or dirty zone*, which includes dirty instruments, dissected tissues, and dressings that are washed or disposed here.[4]

Guidelines for the Hair Transplantation Theater Unit-complex

- The door of the complex should be two-leaf type with hinge-like doors that close automatically. The theater complex doors should be 1 m wide.
- Tiling is preferred for the floor, and the side of the passage in the OT complex should be tiled so as to avoid washing it repeatedly. As an alternative, the side walls can be just painted with washable, light-colored paint.
- Adequate size of the corridor is important to facilitate easy movement of trolleys. The adequate size may be 2 m.[15]
- Fire extinguishers (powder type) and proper fire alarms should be in place **(Fig. 3)**. For equipment in the theater, carbon dioxide (CO_2) type fire extinguishers are preferred, but foam type and water should not be used on lasers and other type equipment in the theater.[16]
- Changing rooms should have lockers.
- No window curtains or floor mats are permitted on the premises.
- Elbow or foot-operated taps should be available for scrubs, and elbow-operated hand disinfectant dispenser should be provided. Water in the OT complex should be ultraviolet (UV) and heat-treated to prevent the growth of microbes, especially pseudomonas.

Common Features of the Operation Theater of Both Restricted and Unrestricted Type

- The OT should be dust and moisture proof.
- For easy cleaning and to prevent dust accumulation, rounding of the corners and junctions of walls, floor, and ceiling could be done **(Fig. 4)**. Flooring is different for restricted and unrestricted types; in restricted type, seamless is preferred, whereas, in unrestricted type, tiling **(Fig. 5)** or anything concrete is done so that it can tolerate repeated washing.
- All doors should have a width of 1.5 m, and laser signage should be used as and when required.
- Theater dimensions could be a minimum of 3 × 3 m,[11] 4 × 4 m,[17] or 4 × 5 m.[12]
- The wall height should be 2.6 m[15] or 3.0 m.[4]

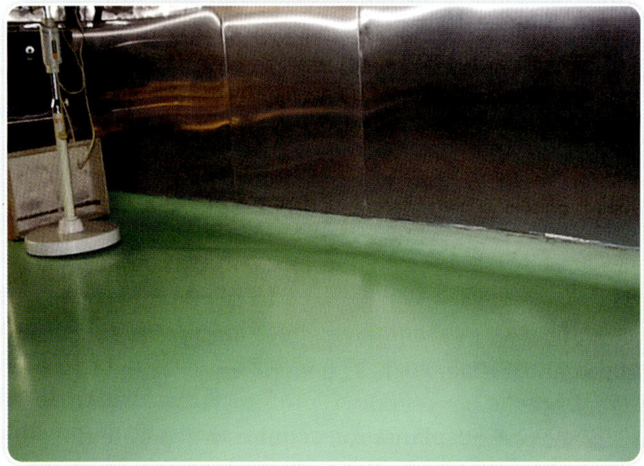

FIG. 4: Theater rounded corners and epoxy seamless flooring.

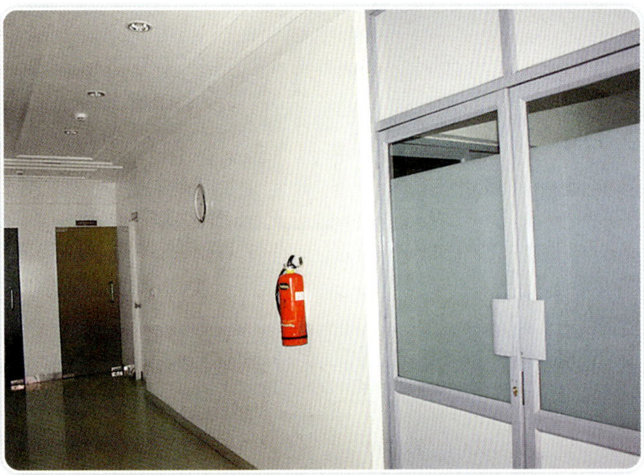

FIG. 3: Note the fire alarms in ceiling, powder-type fire extinguishers, tiled floor, and washable walls.

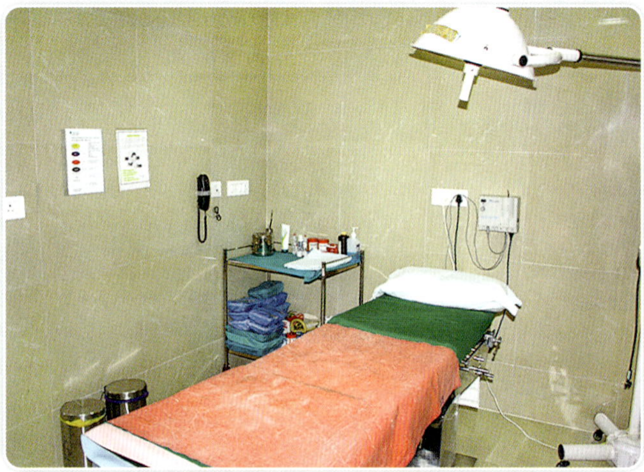

FIG. 5: Unrestricted theater with tiled walls and floors, electrical outlets, phone, operating theater (OT) light, table, trolley, and kick bucket for waste.

Courtesy: Vikram Hospital, Mysuru, Karnataka, India.

Dissecting Room

- For follicular unit transplantation (FUT) surgeries, either an additional dissecting room of equal size should be present, otherwise, a larger OT of 20 × 12 feet can accommodate both OT and dissecting room.
- Adequate space is important in the operating room to help move the OT table in times of emergency and also help in the easy movement of the stretcher or trolley.
- The OT door width should preferably be >24 inches.

Magnification[1]

Magnification is important aspect of any hair transplant procedure, whether it is for strip harvesting, slivering, or for FUE follicle harvesting or implantation. Various magnification devices, such as a stereo microscope, video microscopes, and magnifying loupes, have been routinely used by the surgeons and their team. These details are discussed in a separate chapter.

Lighting of Theater

- OT lights used should be shadowless:[18] Minimum light required is 3,000–8,000 foot candles.
- Nowadays, white light is preferred, which is shadowless and also heat generation is kept to minimum.
- Ceiling lights are usually preferred.
- *The artificial light*, such as fluorescent tubes, compact fluorescent lamps (CFL), or light-emitting diodes (LEDs), should match the color of the objects as they are seen in outdoor natural sunlight.
- CFL and cluster white LED lights can save power. LED lights last 50,000 hours. But for long life, low power consumption, and being mercury free, LED light requires further standardization as of today.

Operation Theater Light

- Before purchasing a light for the surgical field, check for (1) light intensity, (2) illuminated field size, (3) amount of heat and shadows produced, (4) light positioning and ease of change, and (5) ceiling mounted or floor movable.
- Shadowless lighting, delivering 3,000–8,000 foot candles,[19] is the basis of OT light required (i.e., dental chairs have halogen lamp of 50 W power).
- *It is important that the lights do not heat up the area of grafting, as heat is lethal to the grafts.*

Electrical Outlets

- All three-pin outlets should be located about 1.5 m above the floor to prevent wires on the floor. There should be good earthing.
- No extension cords or boards are permitted.
- 5-amp and 15-amp sockets are required. The 5-amp sockets, on an average of 4, should be located on each wall.
- For lasers and OT lights, online uninterruptible power supply (UPS) and servo stabilizers are required.
- Standby generators should be planned.

Air Conditioning

- It is recommended to keep air conditioning of office type with 10 μm dust filter.
- The ambient temperature of the OT should be 21° and humidity 50–55%.
- It is not recommended by the National Accreditation Board for Hospitals (NABH) to use split and window air conditioning for restricted-type OTs.[20]
  Figure 6 shows a restricted type of OT.

Operation Table

- Stainless steel operation table, with adjustable head, foot end, and armrest, is the heart of the theater. This could be preferably electrically powered and controlled with foot or fingertip controls.
- The dimensions of the table should be a minimum of 1 m in length and 30 cm in breadth.[19]
- *While conventional operation tables are preferred by many, other surgeons prefer reclining chair, such as a dental chair or cosmetic chair, for FUE or FUT. For vertex area, a prone chair is used* ***(Fig. 7)***.

Instrument Trolley

The preferred trolley is a Mayo stand with four wheels. To prevent the table from getting soaked, it is advised to use an autoclaved rubber sheet/mackintosh. With the

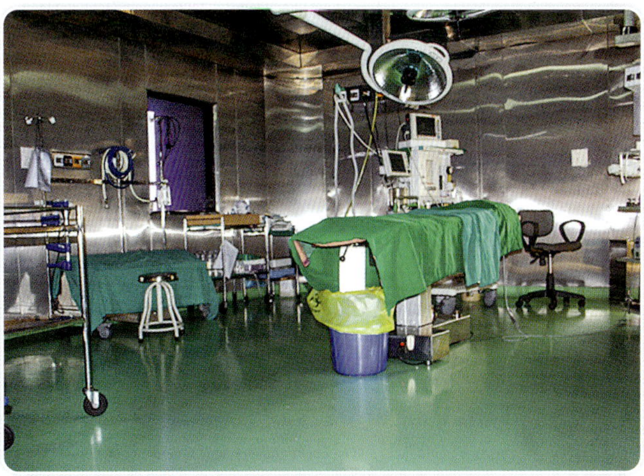

FIG. 6: Restricted theater: Seamless epoxy flooring, natural closed window light, and washable walls.
Courtesy: Vikram Hospital, Mysuru, Karnataka, India.

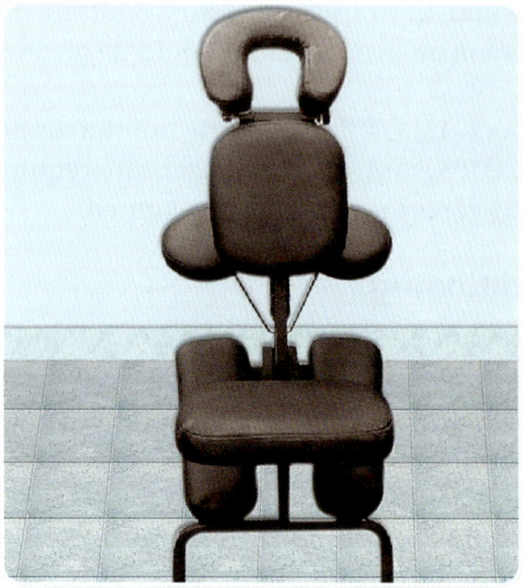

FIG. 7: A chair used by the author for performing follicular unit extraction (FUE).

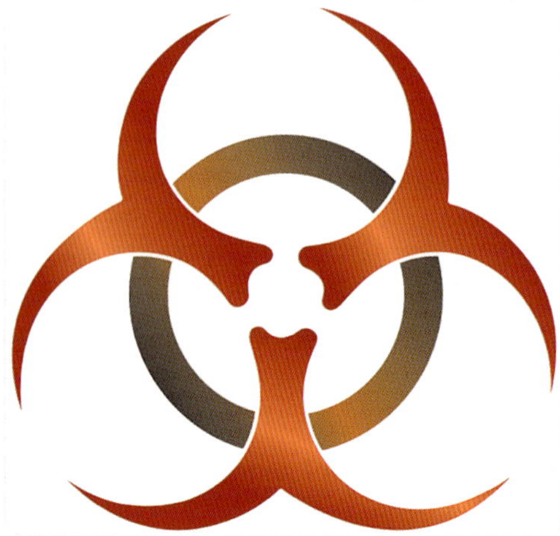

FIG. 8: Biohazard logo.

use of simple cloth, moisture will percolate down and contaminate the instruments.

Surgeon Stool

Surgeon's stool should contain wheels with pneumatic height adjustment, controlled by the foot, is preferred. Backrest, if available, is preferred, and the addition of armrest is even better (*see also* section on ergonomics).

Waste Containers

Four main types of waste are generated in the theater of a dermatologist: (1) Blood-soaked gauze, (2) latex gloves, (3) paper (glove and plastic cover), and (4) sharps, including needle and syringes. These are segregated at source[21] into (1) yellow plastic cover, (2) blue plastic cover, (3) white plastic cover, and (4) biohazard logo to be pasted onto a separate plastic container **(Fig. 8)**.

Surgical Instruments

The surgical instruments **(Figs. 9A to I)** depend upon the type of work and individual surgeon's preference.[11,12] The list below **(Box 1)** is not comprehensive and consists of basic requirements for a functional theater.

Advanced Cardiovascular Life Support

This is dealt with in greater detail in the chapter 43 on Emergencies and Resuscitation in Transplantation. As per the Government of India and the Supreme Court verdict, all personnel in the OT should be familiar with basic and advanced life support.[22,23] Basic life support (BLS) does not require any devices or drugs, but advanced cardiovascular life support (ACLS) does. A standby anesthetist is advisable. Also, it is better to liaison with a local hospital with intensive care unit (ICU) facility and ambulance service.

Advanced life support requires drugs and devices, which are listed in **Tables 1 and 2**.[24]

Operation Room Records

A record containing the following should be maintained:

- Patient identity
- Diagnosis
- Procedures performed
- Persons involved in the procedures
- Complications

Surgical Drapes and Attires

Surgical drapes form an important part of the OT preparation for any procedure. They are available in different materials: Cotton and disposable paper or plastic. The preferred material is cotton, which is porous and comfortable for the patient. But disposable paper and plastic avoid the need for washing and autoclaving.

Mask definitely protects the dermatologist from splash of blood, injectable anesthetics, and spill of viral particles during electrosurgery. It also protects the surgical wound from operators' and assistants' secretions in the event of coughing and sneezing, since the aerosol can travel up to 3 m. Mask should cover both the nose and mouth. Cotton, paper, and gauze masks should not be used. Paper with synthetic material offers effective barrier.[25] The pore size of the mask should be 1 μm.[26]

Surgical cap should cover the hair on the scalp. This prevents contamination of the surgical suit and also the operation site by hair organisms.

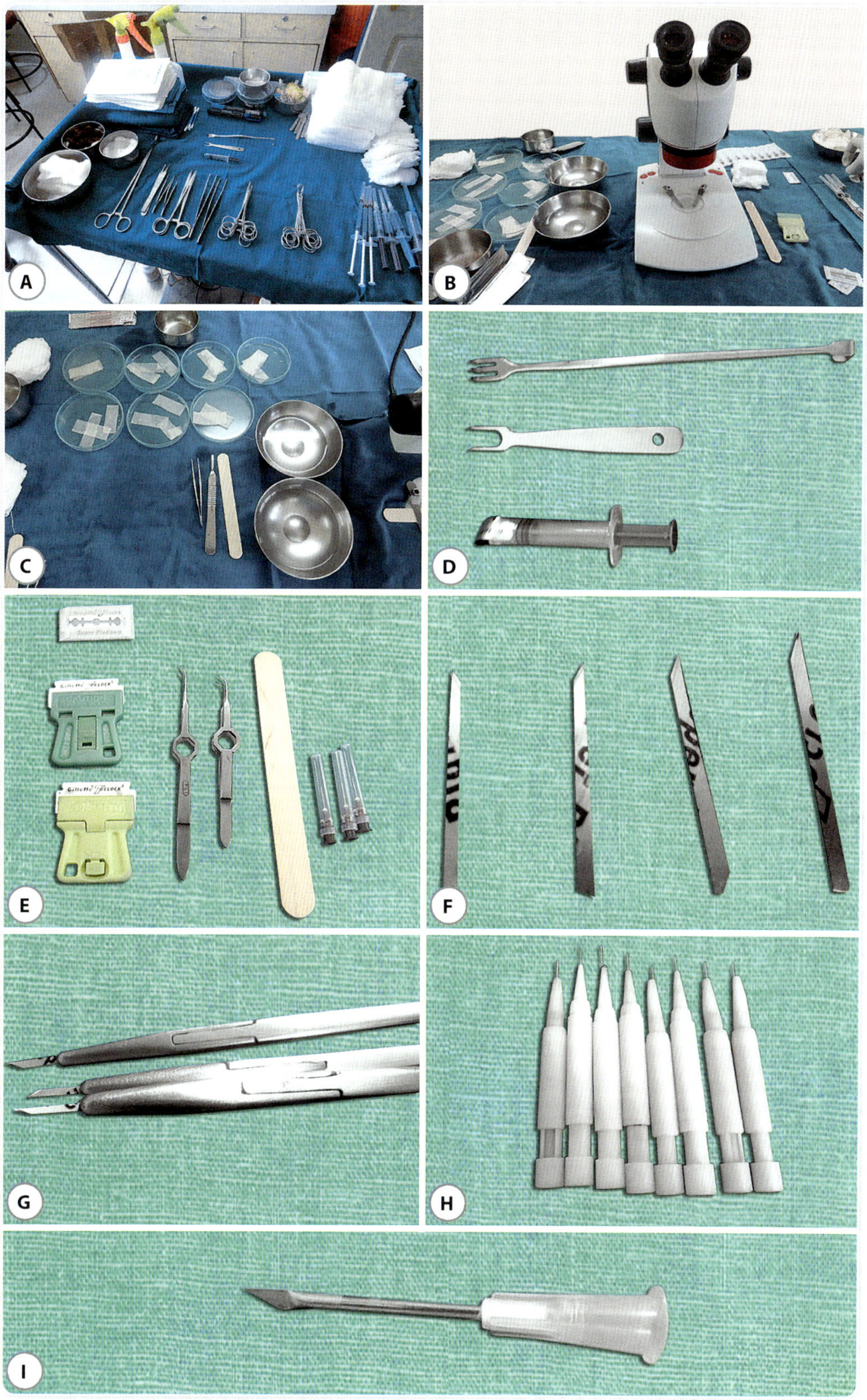

FIGS. 9A TO I: (A to C) Instruments for dissection; (D) skin hooks; (E) dissection blades; (F) custom-made blades for recipient sites; (G) custom-made blades in holders; (H) implanters; (I) Nokor needles for recipient sites.

BOX 1 Basic requirements for a functional theater.

- *Forceps*:
  - Cheatles
  - Sponge holding
  - Adson nontoothed
  - Adson toothed
  - Jewelers
  - Mosquito artery
  - Spencers suture
  - Removal
- *Sharp instruments*:
  - Bard Parker handle numbers 3, 4, and 5
  - Disposable surgical blades number 11 and 15
  - Disposable punches
- *Scissors*:
  - 5-inch blunt and sharp (Lister)
  - Iris scissors
  - Castroviejo
- *Miscellaneous*:
  - Skin hooks
  - Needle-holder: Halsey and box type
- *Specific instruments*:
  - Blades, tissue spreader
  - Counter for grafts
  - Implanters (if used)

TABLE 1: Devices required for advanced life support.

Devices	Quantity
Ambu bag	1
Laryngoscope with different size blades	1
Endotracheal tube of different size (6–8 numbers)	1
Intravenous (IV) cannula: Adult and pediatric	2
Drip set	2
Airway of all sizes	1
Stethoscope	1
Blood pressure (BP) apparatus	1
Cardiac monitor with built-in defibrillator	1
Oxygen cylinder with connectors	1
Suction device	1
Disposable syringes	2

Surgical suits are clothes (pants and shirts) that theater personnel change from street clothes. These must be cotton and clean but not sterile. These are required for restricted zones of the theater.

Gowns are sterile cotton material, full sleeve with knee length attires to prevent contamination.

TABLE 2: Drugs required for advanced life support.

Drugs	Quantity
Adrenaline: 1:1,000	10
Atropine: 0.6 mg	10
Sodium bicarbonate (7.5%) ampoule	12
Chlorpheniramine maleate: 22.75 mg/mL, 2 cc	10
Hydrocortisone: 100 mg/mL	2
Injection furosemide	10
Aminophylline: 250 mg/2 mL ampoule	5
Dopamine: 200 mg/5 mL	2
Normal saline: 500 mL	2
5% dextrose normal saline: 500 mL	2
Mephentermine: 15 mg/mL	5
Dextrose: 25%	2 ampoule

Sterile plastic apron could be donned over a surgical suit during dermabrasion to prevent soiling of the cotton suit.

Patient suits are required to prevent soiling of clothes during surgery. They just have to be clean and not sterile.

Gloves can be either latex or nonlatex type of various sizes. Double-gloving can be practiced when operating on high-risk cases (for hand hygiene and glove donning technique).

Cloth instrument packing is the traditional way of securing the instrument tray. It has to be 270 thread count Pima cotton fabric. The only drawback is that the cloth has to be laundered every time. Hence, nowadays, disposable paper, such as crepe-type or medical-grade plastic paper reels, is available **(Fig. 10)**.[27] The storage shelf life varies from 1 to 12 months depending upon the material **(Figs. 11A and B)** (refer to the manufacturer's guidelines).

Be autoclaved or need not be autoclaved, (c) nondisposable items, (d) to deal with spillages of infectious material.

1. Cleaning removes debris.
2. Disinfection reduces the bacterial and viral load but does not remove debris or sterilize.
3. Sterilization kills microbes.
4. *Sterilization is not a method of cleaning.*[10]

Disinfection and Sterilization of Theater Equipment

Disinfection in the OT refers to (1) cleaning working surfaces and (2) equipment that cannot be autoclaved or need not be autoclaved.

1. *Cleaning working surfaces*:
   a. Before surgery:
      i. Mop the floor using 0.5% chlorine solution **(Box 2)**

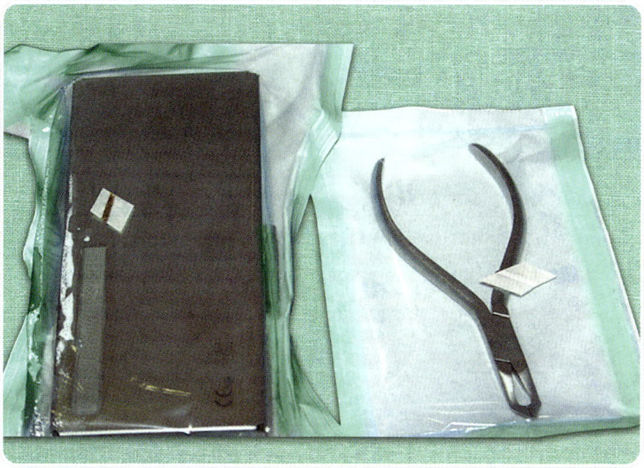

FIG. 10: Medical-grade plastic paper pack with one side transparent and autoclave indicator, left autoclaved with black line and right not autoclaved with white line.

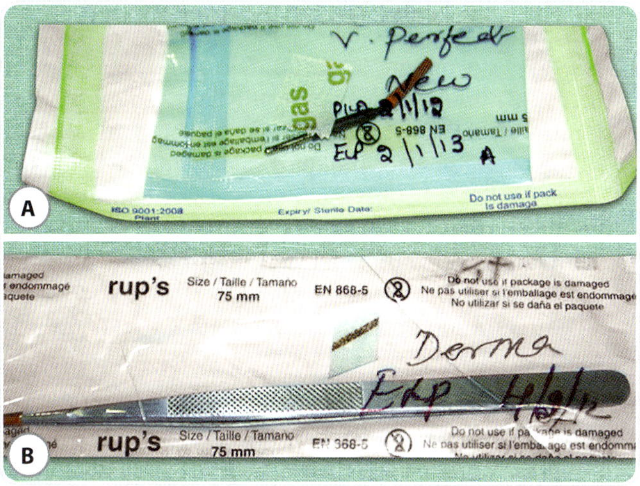

FIGS. 11A AND B: (A) Medical-grade plastic reel used to ETO gas sterilize electrosurgery tip: Expiry date 1 year; (B) forceps autoclaved; expiry 1 month.

   ii. Using cloth, wipe the operation table and trolley with 0.5% chlorine solution
  b. After surgery: Repeat the above steps. Keep it ready for the next case.
2. *Equipment that cannot be autoclaved or need not be autoclaved*, e.g., electrosurgery tips, sharps, gloves, linen, OT dresses.
3. *Nondisposable items*, e.g., stainless steel instruments: Comedone expressor, forceps, gallipots.

Steps for disinfecting category "2" and "3" items:

- Items in category "2" and "3" should be collected in separate plastic buckets, basins, or waste disposal leak-proof plastic containers for sharps.

BOX 2 Preparation of 0.5% chlorine solution.

- Procure commercially available bleaching powder
- Add 150 g in 10 L of tap water (10 tablespoons or 30 teaspoons)
- First, premix the required amount of powder in small quantity of tap water, and later add remaining quantity of water
- Use the same day

- 0.5% chlorine solution should be poured and left in contact for minimum of 10 minutes to maximum of 30 minutes. The instruments and linen should be fully immersed in the solution.
- After the "contact" time and wearing mask and thick rubber gloves, the equipment should be rinsed in tap or lukewarm water. Do not use very hot water because it coagulates blood and makes it hard to clean.
- Using a toothbrush, scrub the instruments or brush the clothes.
- Use commercial detergents to further clean them.
- Do not use soap, as it leaves a precipitate on the steel surface.
- Linen—drapes, suits, gowns, and hand towels—should be washed with household detergent at 71°C for 25 minutes. Later, they can be sterilized or disinfected.[10] *Note*: Drapes, gowns, and hand towels require later autoclaving, but not suits.
- After cleaning and disinfecting, the instruments and clothes must be dried and later sent for sterilization.

Steam Sterilization (Autoclave)

- Dry the equipment or clothes
- Wrap the equipment in cloth, paper, or medical-grade plastic paperback **(Figs. 10 and 11)**
- Lay the instruments in the autoclave so that all surfaces of the device will come in contact with heat
- Before packing, lay the instruments, such as scissors, in an open position
- Refer to the manufacturer's time recommendations for the duration of autoclave
- Also, buy a small autoclave that can be reused many times in a day than a large one once a day. Tabletop autoclave should be considered.
- Generally, it is 121°C for 15 minutes, with a pressure of 2.4 bar in porous stainless steel containers.
- The outside of the packs should not be wet. If that is so, the autoclave process has failed.
- Appropriate color indicators should be used on packs to know the adequacy of autoclaving.
- Date of autoclave should be mentioned. The expiry date varies. If polythene bags are used for biopsy trays

TABLE 3: Methods of high-level disinfection.

Chemical used	Quantity required	Time for disinfection	To be changed	Comment
Formalin in chamber	7 g of formalin for one cubic meter area at 20°C (1 g tablet available)	12 hours	Daily	• For disinfecting electrosurgery electrodes and cables • For disinfecting sharp instruments *Note*: It is an irritant and carcinogen
Glutaraldehyde	2.45% concentration	20 minutes	14 days	For disinfecting sharp instruments
Isopropyl alcohol	70%	2 minutes	Daily	*Caution*: Inflammable near lasers and electrosurgery units

Note: Safer alternatives to formalin chamber and glutaraldehyde should be explored, such as peracetic acid. Formalin chambers may not be effective in cold areas of the country and during cooler nights.

before autoclaving, sterility is ensured for 8 weeks. If double packed and medical-grade plastic paper packs are used, the sterility is valid for 1 year.

Chemical Sterilization[10-12]

- Cleaned, disinfected, and dried instruments should be fully soaked in a steel or plastic container having 2% glutaraldehyde for 8–10 hours.[10] *Note*: For disinfection, the contact time is 20 minutes.
- Instruments, such as scissors, should be in open position when soaked.
- The contact time for high-level disinfection is just 20 minutes compared to the 10 hours required for sterilization.
- Ethylene oxide sterilization is used for follicular unit excision machines and implanters.[11,12]

Newer Agents for High-level Disinfection and Sterilization (Table 3)

For emergency disinfection of equipment within 5 minutes, a combination of glutaraldehyde + dioxahexane + rust inhibitors at 5% concentration is available.[28]

Operation Theater Fumigation and Surface Disinfection

For theater fumigation, three agents are currently available.

- 40% formalin solution[11]—500 mL of 40% formalin in 1,000 mL of water for 1,000 cubic feet of OT area in a fumigator is the ideal concentration. This requires sealing of windows and doors overnight while fumigating. However, formaldehyde is being replaced by other agents.
- Formaldehyde 6%, glutaraldehyde 6%, and benzalkonium chloride 5% can be used by adequately trained personnel wearing appropriate protective devices.
- Glutaraldehyde 5 g, benzalkonium chloride 5 g, alkyl urea 3 g, and 1,6-dihydroxy-2-5-dioxahexane 11.2 g; all the above in 100 g packing. 0.5% spray or mopping daily may be done. To be left on the surface for 20 minutes and later wiped off.
- *Aldehyde-free, quick-acting*: Ethanol 10 g, 2-propanol 9 g, and 1-propanol 6 g solution in 100 g to be sprayed before 5 minutes of surgery on the floor, table, light, and later wiped.[28] During spraying, no electrical switches to be operated since the spark can ignite the fumigant.
- Bacillocid solution (consists of 1.6-dihydroxy-2-5-dioxahexane 11.2 g; glutaraldehyde 5.0 g; benzalkonium chloride IP 5.0 g) can be used for economical and quick disinfection.
- Ideally, fumigation should be done daily or prior to each surgery.

Housekeeping of the Operation Theater

The OT need only be cleaned of dust and organic matter (*see later*).

OPERATION THEATER ETIQUETTES

- The door of the theater should be kept closed always.
- Movement in and out of OT is to be kept minimum.
- People with respiratory or skin infection should stay out.
- Staff must respect and maintain the dignity of the patient.
- Patient's privacy and modesty should be respected by all staff at all times.[29]
- Patient must be explained all details of the diagnosis, anesthesia, etc., including the cost of the therapy involved.
- Use of mobile in the OT should be restricted.[30]

WASTE DISPOSAL

Biomedical waste disposal is mandatory, and one should be registered with the state health authorities.

Two simple methods of waste management include (1) Sharps, plastic syringes, and needles should be shredded, and (2) blood-soaked gauze (to be treated in chlorine bleach for 12 hours) should be incinerated.[31]

ERGONOMICS

Ergon (work) + Nomo's (law) is the study focusing on workers' safety and productivity. The OT staff should concentrate on his/her work at hand rather than anything else.

In the theater during hair transplantation, a surgeon could experience strain in the following four segments:

- Lower limb
- Back
- Neck and shoulder
- Arm, wrist, and hand

But unfortunately, surgical training discourages complaining of stress and fatigue.[32]

What is the Best Posture during Standing or Sitting?

During standing, the head should be upright on the torso. During sitting, the ideal position of hip flexion is 105° with the back supported by the backrest. This puts the least pressure on the intervertebral disc.

Positions during the transplantation: Both sitting and standing positions are needed during hair transplant. Strip dissection is always performed with the surgeon standing, while FUE harvesting is performed with both sitting or standing positions. Recipient area implantation is usually done sitting. During standing position, the pressure on the intervertebral disc is 33% lesser than that of sitting. So, standing in upright posture is more disc-friendly. But sitting requires 20% less energy than standing. During sitting, only a few muscle groups are active, and the large muscles of the lower limbs are inactive. Ergonomically designed chair is, therefore, important to prevent fatigue and backache **(Box 3)**.

Surgeons were still reluctant to have their work habits analyzed or criticized by others.[32]

To reduce the effect of posture on the body, several rules should be kept in mind:

- Change the position frequently
- All procedures require forward bending, putting strain on the neck and back, so position the operation table in a high visual field range to keep the head balanced on the spine.
- Neutral position of the arm to be maintained.
- Proper visualization and arm support are required for precise surgeries.
- Regular breaks are encouraged during prolonged surgeries.
- A short break of 30 seconds is as good as long breaks.[33]

BOX 3 Ergonomically designed chair.

What is an ergonomically designed chair?

- These at height are adjustable with pneumatic pedestal (15–22 inches)
- Good lumbar support
- A seat pan with curved front
- 5-pronged base support to prevent the chair from falling
- A good footrest to prevent the stress of dangling thigh and leg on the hip **(Fig. 12)**

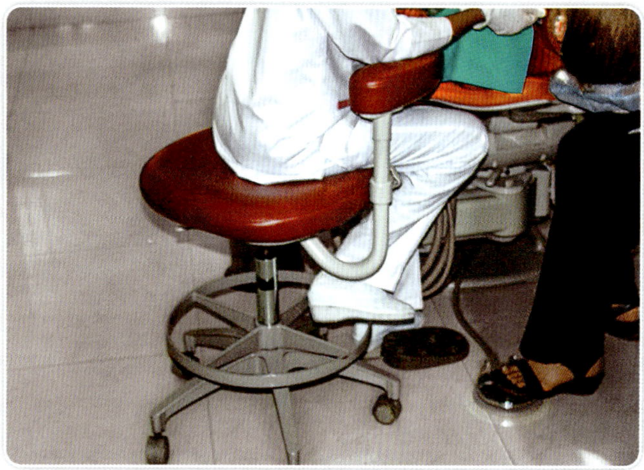

FIG. 12: An ideal chair with good base, footrest, seat pan, lumbar seat that can change to hand support, and adjustable height.

Dressing Room

A separate room for dressing or a room (smaller than the main procedure room or OT) with dressing facilities should be available when patient comes postprocedure for dressing removal or scab cleaning. The room should have a bed, adequate movement space, and ambient lighting to facilitate the dressing or any minor procedure.

Dedicated Area for Photography

Medicolegal issues are on the rise, and proper documentation is a must for all doctors and more so for the surgical field doctors. Photography forms an important aspect for the same. Theater or dressing room can have a dedicated space with preferably black background so that nonreflective proper pics can be taken at the same distance always to help in future comparisons at the end of surgery.

Tips for OT:

- All protocols of surgery are to be followed during hair transplant surgery, though it is a minimally invasive surgery.
- Adequate staff training is a must for increased efficiency.
- Separate changing rooms and washing areas to be there.
- No fans are to be used in the OT to avoid aerosolization of dust.

SUMMARY

Hair transplant procedure is in great demand. It is a minimally invasive procedure where painless aseptic wound healing should occur with minimal blood loss. Properly trained staff, clean environment, surgeon expertise, and good instrumentation are most important to achieve best results with maximum patient comfort. To achieve this, the World Health Organization calls for "sober, down-to-earth planning and design" of the theater. OT should be a place of patient safety with economical use of manpower and other resources.

REFERENCES

1. Geisse JK. The dermatologic surgical suite. Semin Dermatol. 1994;13(1):2-9.
2. Phillips P, Elston DM, Ratner D, Wells MJ, Albertini JG, Crawford GH. (2009). Outpatient surgical suite. [Online] Available from http://emedicine.medscape.com/article/1128609. [Last accessed October, 2023].
3. National Medical Commission. Ethics and Medical Registration Board. (2022). Guideline on Aesthetic Surgery and Hair Transplant Procedures. [Online] Available from https://www.nmc.org.in/MCIRest/open/getDocument?path=/Documents/Public/Portal/LatestNews/20220927051220.pdf. [Last accessed October, 2023].
4. Bureau of Indian Standards. (2001). Indian Standard. Basic requirements for hospital planning. Part 2 up to 100 bedded hospital. Reaffirmed 2006; IS 12433:26-39.
5. Mysore V, Kumaresan M, Garg A, Dua A, Venkatram A, Dua K, et al. Hair transplant practice guidelines. J Cutan Aesthet Surg. 2021;14(3):269.
6. Rajendran SC, Omprakash HM. Standard guidelines for setting up a dermatosurgery theatre. Indian J Dermatol Venereol Leprol. 2009;75(Suppl. 2):76-82.
7. Joint Commission International. Ambulatory care. [Online] Available from http://www.jointcommissioninternational.org/ambulatory-care. [Last accessed March 2016].
8. Ministry of Health, Singapore. Directives for private ambulatory surgical centres providing ambulatory surgery. 2007. pp. 1-6.
9. Netherlands Board for Hospital Facilities. Building guidelines for a surgical department. 2004. pp. 1-16.
10. WHO. Surgical care at the district hospital. 2003. pp. 2-13.
11. Savant SS, Gore D. Instruments, equipment, and universal precautions. In: Savant SS (Ed). Textbook of Hair Transplantation Theatre and Cosmetology. Mumbai, India: Association of Scientific Cosmetologists and Dermatosurgeons; 2005. pp. 26-34.
12. Unger WP. The surgical suite. In: Unger WP, Shapiro R (Eds). Hair Transplantation, 4th edition. New York: Marcel Dekker; 2004. pp. 833-4.
13. Malkin J. Ambulatory surgical centers. In: Malkin J (Ed). Medical and Dental Space Planning: A Comprehensive Guide to Design, Equipment, and Clinical Procedures, 3rd edition. New York: John Wiley and Sons; 2002. pp. 334-6.
14. Malkin J. Ambulatory surgical centers. In: Malkin J (Ed). Medical and Dental Space Planning: A Comprehensive Guide to Design, Equipment, and Clinical Procedures, 3rd edition. New York: John Wiley and Sons; 2002. pp. 352-3.
15. Ministry of Health. Government of South Africa. Regulations governing private hospitals and unattached operating theatre units. 1993. pp. 8-10.
16. Ridley SA, Parry G. Guidelines for fire safety in intensive care units. NHS, UK: Intensive Care Society Publication; 1998. pp. 1-16.
17. Lawrence C. Equipment. In: Lawrence C (Ed). An Introduction to Dermatological Surgery, 2nd edition. London: Churchill Livingstone; 2002. pp. 9-10.
18. Malkin J. Construction methods and building systems. In: Malkin J (Ed). Medical and Dental Space Planning: A Comprehensive Guide to Design, Equipment, and Clinical Procedures, 3rd edition. New York: John Wiley and Sons; 2002. pp. 556-61.
19. Perez M, Lodha R, Nouri K. Surgical equipment and instrumentation. In: Nouri K, Leal-Khouri S (Eds). Techniques in Dermatologic Surgery. Missouri: Mosby; 2003. pp. 25-31.
20. NABH-Air Conditioning OT. Revised guidelines for air conditioning in operation theatres. [Online] Available from www.nabh.com. [Last accessed October, 2023].
21. Ministry of Environment and Forests, India. Bio-Medical Waste Management and Handling Rules. Second Amendment. 2000.
22. Government of India Standards. (2005). Female sterilization operation. Ensuring right to safety, dignity, and informed choice. Order dated 01.03.2005 passed in writ petition {civil} no-209/2003; Ramkant Rai v/s. Union of India and others. [Online] Available from http://www.hrln.org. [Last accessed October, 2023].
23. Field JM, Gonzales L, Hazinski MF, Ruple J. Advanced Cardiovascular Life Support Provider Manual. Texas: American Heart Association; 2006. pp. 1-42.
24. Department of Family Welfare, National Rural Health Mission (India). Emergency drugs for both tubectomy and vasectomy camps. Standard Operating Procedures for Sterilization

Services in Camps. New Delhi: Family Planning Division, Ministry of Health and Family Welfare, Government of India; 2008. pp. 30-1.

25. Pratt RJ, Pellowe C, Loveday HP, Robinson N, Smith GW, Barrett S, et al. The epic project: developing national evidence-based guidelines for preventing healthcare-associated infections. Phase I: guidelines for preventing hospital-acquired infections. Department of Health (England). J Hosp Infect. 2001;47(Suppl):S3-82.
26. Sawchuk WS, Weber PJ, Lowy DR, Dzubow LM. Infectious papillomavirus in the vapor of warts treated with carbon dioxide laser or electrocoagulation: detection and protection. J Am Acad Dermatol. 1989;21(1):41-9.
27. Marra DE, Fincher EF, Moy RL. Surgical preparation, facilities, and monitoring. Roenigk's Dermatologic Surgery. Current Techniques in Procedural Dermatology, 3rd edition. New York: Informa; 2007. pp. 1-9.
28. Korsolex. Baccillol agents. [Online] Available from www.bode-chemie.de. [Last accessed October, 2023].
29. Satyanarayana Rao KH. Informed consent: an ethical obligation or legal compulsion? J Cutan Aesthet Surg. 2008;1(1):33-5.
30. Operation Theatre Standard No. 27. Theatre Etiquette. Royal United Bath Hospital NHS Trust. Theatre practice policy—Reference no. 742 2006. p. 75.
31. Ministry of Environment and Forest, Government of India. Categories of biomedical waste. Schedule I. [Online] Available from http://envfov.nic.in/legis/hsm/biomed.html.
32. Burger R. Surgery and ergonomics. Arch Surg. 1999;134:1011-6.
33. Jacobs K. Ergonomics for Therapists. Missouri: Mosby; 2008. pp. 1-460.

CHAPTER 92

Role of Assistants in Hair Transplantation

Anil Kumar Garg, Seema Garg

Key Messages

- Hair transplantation surgery is a teamwork during all its processes.
- The team should consist of surgeon, assisting surgeon, dissecting assistants, implanting assistants, and counselors.
- The team needs training and working together for adequate length of time to achieve best results.

INTRODUCTION

Hair transplantation (HT) is a surgery that is the end result of multiple procedures done by different staff who are trained for that purpose. So, a team of surgeons with assistants work together to give a successful transplant. There is a great difference between other surgeries, such as hernia, appendectomy, and HT. In appendectomy, the major role is of surgeon, and assistants help the chief surgeon. Responsibility of success of surgery lies on the shoulders of the chief surgeon. On the contrary, HT involves a series of surgical procedures such as strip harvesting, slivering, follicle dissection, slit creation, and implantation of grafts. Each of these procedures is independent and requires skill and precision to give successful HT as end result. So in HT, surgeon and assistants work together, and the ultimate final outcome is sum of skills of all members of team **(Figs. 1 and 2)**.

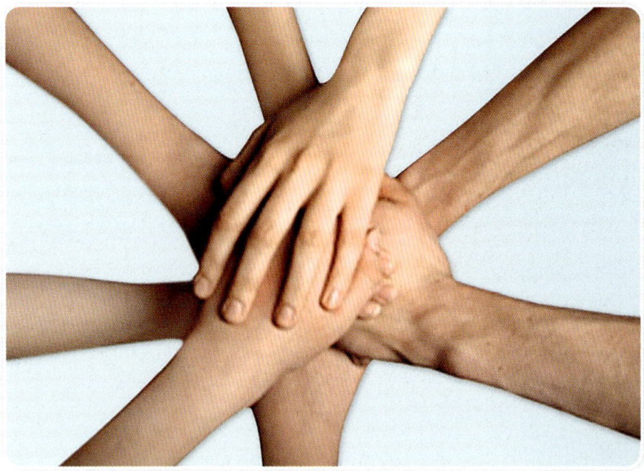

FIG. 1: Assistants are neither assisting nor helping but working together with the chief surgeon.

Usually, there are about eight assistants in a team for strip dissection; four assistants for follicle dissection, two for slivering (for strip harvesting), and two for implantation. With advent of follicular unit extraction (FUE), the number of assistants needed has come down as FUE skips the strip dissection, and grafts are harvested directly and implanted with minimum dissection. FUE therefore can be managed with a team of three to four assistants. However, if FUE mega and giga sessions are planned, a larger team is needed as FUE is an exhaustive and tiring procedure, and teams need to alternate and take rest.

In addition, there can be a couple of counselors. Assistants not only play a role in operation room but they have an important role in office before surgery and after surgery. Patients are more friendly and open up with assistants better than surgeon. Convincing a patient can sometimes be better done by staff than surgeon. The counseling sessions are time-consuming, and hence, counselors are very useful.

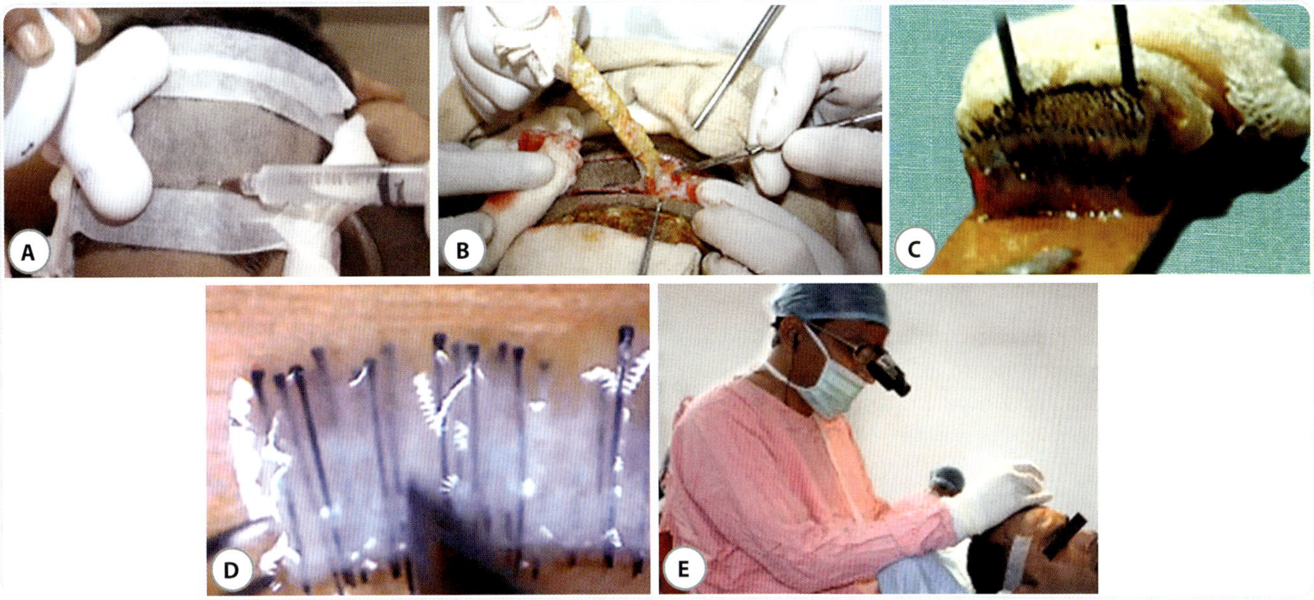

FIGS. 2A TO E: Hair transplant involves anesthesia, strip harvesting, slivering, follicle dissection, and lastly implantation of follicles. All procedures are done independently by different persons. All steps are equally important for the success of hair transplant.

ROLE OF ASSISTANTS

Of late, there has been a debate as to what are the steps of HT that can be performed by assistants.[1] There even have been teams of assistants freelancing and claiming to perform the entire procedure by themselves. This is unacceptable legally and ethically.

In HT, strip harvesting, site creation in FUE, and slit making should only be done by a trained physician. These steps cannot be left to the assistant. Local anesthesia should also be given by physician. Other steps of HT such as slivering, follicle dissection, pulling the units out after FUE site creation, and implantation can be done by nonphysician assistants and/or technicians.

Assistants are also of two types:

1. *Nurses or operation theater (OT) assistants*: These are qualified nurses/paramedical technicians with proper knowledge of nursing, monitoring, fumigation, disinfection, arranging trolley, etc. These staff will also be able to help physician in strip harvesting and resuscitation procedures. They can also be doctors.
2. Another set of surgical assistants[2] can also be called technicians. The technician is a person who is not in direct contact with patient. They are trained to do a particular type of procedure and have knowledge pertaining to only that for which they have been trained. These technicians need not be registered nursing staff. They only perform follicle dissection. They should not be asked to do any other task. However, they should also have some medical background such as OT technician, laboratory assistant. Totally nonmedical staff should not be employed as assistants.

ROLE OF COUNSELOR

Counseling a patient is an important part of management of a disease in medical science. It should be done at multiple levels:

- First is the physicians, who see the patient for diagnosing a disease and writing the treatment.
- Second level of counseling is physician assistant who may be a junior resident doctor or a paramedical person having experience of working with physician. He is the person who understands his role very well and knows what and how things have to be explained to the patients. Patients feel more friendly with assistants and staff, and they feel free in asking all questions with assistants. A poorly understood treatment is always incomplete treatment.
- Then there can be a third-level general counselors who speak about cost, logistics, accommodation, etc., and also do telephonic discussions, follow-up, postsurgery liaison, etc. In the author's office, multiple calls are made after surgery. Transplanted patients get calls from office on first day night, second day afternoon, at 1 week to know any donor and recipient site problems. After this, they are called after a month and 4 months regarding medical management and any problems about hair growth. We should understand patients' psychology. Patients of HT are always in dilemma that

hair are going to come or not. Another worry is normal loss of hair. They need multiple explanations about all the problems.

The author is of the opinion that every office should have counselors. The counselor should be pleasant, soft spoken, and a good listener. He should have good knowledge of medicines and procedures done by his physician. He should know side effects of medicine, procedure, and postoperative measures to be followed by patient. He should be able to convince the patient so that patient follows all treatment prescribed by physician. A good counselor is basically an extension of physician, with more value in terms of convincing a patient. It is better to have a junior physician as a counselor or registered nurse with adequate experience in HT and knowledge of medical treatment.

DONOR HARVESTING ASSISTANT

He is the first assistant who helps physician in harvesting follicles in FUE or in strip harvesting. He should be a trained nursing staff or a junior physician. He anticipates the intraoperative needs of surgeon and should be efficient and senior enough to provide instruments or help to control bleeding or show a clear field for the next surgical step. He should have proper training in sterile technique, handling instruments, and operative room setup.

Assistants for Slivering and Follicle Dissection

This set of technicians does not need to be a registered nurse or persons from medical background. Any person interested in this field with good hand-eye coordination and attention to detail can participate in HT. Assistants need proper training of slivering and follicle dissection using magnification. The subject of training is described in a separate chapter. Assistants should understand how precious and delicate follicles are. Hydration is an important step for follicle survival. Micro trauma during handling of grafts affect the quality of hair and graft dessication is commenest cause of poor out come of hair transplant.

Implantation Assistant

Slits are made by physician, and implantation is done by senior surgical assistant. Surgical assistants need proper training of implantation and should know the delicacy of follicles, working under magnification, depth of implantation, angle and direction of implantation. They should be experienced enough to control bleeding and manage popping of grafts. They also make judgments regarding the size, shape, and caliber of grafts and place those grafts according to the recipient site outlined by the surgeon. As a part of training for implantation, assistant should watch the surgeon while slit making and understand depth, angle, direction, and pattern of implantation. Next, under supervision, they should practice implantation of small number of grafts and gradually increase the numbers. Hydration of grafts and delicate handling under magnification are important aspects of implantation, and they need to be trained on these aspects.

Assistant in Follicular Unit Extraction

Follicular unit extraction, either by manual and/or motorized, is to be done by trained physician. But assistant plays a great role in assisting his physician. In FUE, there are two steps. First, physician scores follicles, and after scoring, follicles come out but remain in place and with loose attachment. An alert, well-trained, efficient assistant can harvest grafts quickly without injuring them. A well-trained assistant can extract the grafts as they emerge after scoring, minimizing the time consumed for extraction **(Figs. 3A and B)**. He/she helps by exerting traction and also irrigates grafts and cleans field for his surgeon to speed

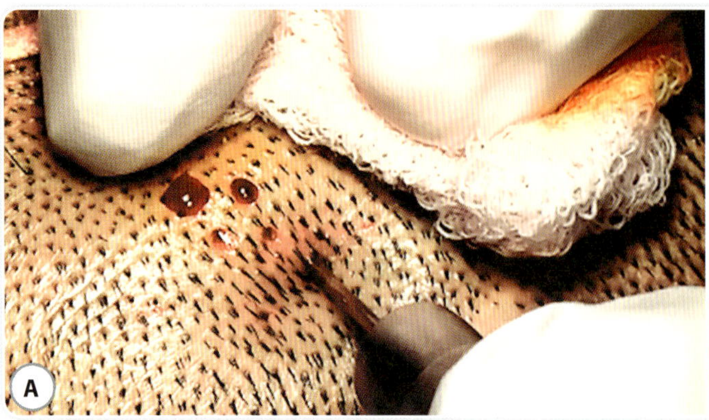

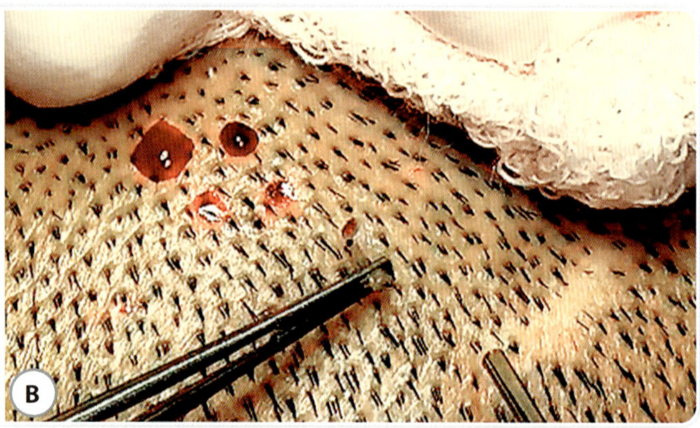

FIGS. 3A AND B: (A) Scoring of grafts by physician; (B) Extraction of grafts by assistant.

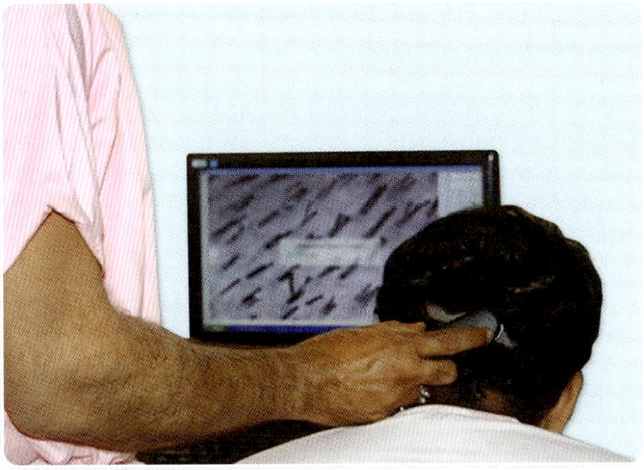

FIG. 4: TrichoScan to calculate donor site density before hair transplant.

up graft scoring and harvesting. *As a rule, nonphysician cannot do FUE scoring by manual or motorized method.*

TRICHOSCAN AND ASSISTANT

Hair analysis is done with two objectives. One is diagnostic, and another is just to know hair density. When TrichoScan is to be done for diagnostic purpose, it should only be done by physician who is trained to recognize different pathological conditions and their scan findings. This way, TrichoScan helps physician in establishing a diagnosis.

Scan done before HT is to know donor site hair density. This scan can be done by a well-trained nonphysician assistant **(Fig. 4)** who otherwise works with someone who does TrichoScan regularly. Mostly TrichoScans are with software that itself calculates density. So, chances of error in calculating hair density are negligible. Physician should regularly check his assistant and guide him. This assistant can also be used for clinical photography.

Managing a Team

Hair transplant is a surgery, and it has all possible complications and risks involved in any surgery. At the same time, it is a combination of science and art. Surgeons face a tough challenge in the restoration process, a condition where there is great gap between recipient area demand and donor area supply. All steps, starting from planning to execution of procedure, require perfection and precision.

Any step in the entire process cannot be underestimated, and if not done properly, it is going to affect the final outcome of hair restoration. Team of assistants plays a vital role. Their attachment with patient, acquaintance with physician, and working area all are important factors. Assistant has to imbibe all the techniques of his surgeon and also predict what is in his mind. For all this, it is necessary that assistant should work regularly with the same physician. The same surgeon-assistant team working together makes synergistic rhythmic actions, which gives best output. Unfortunately, in today's era where commercial aspect is becoming bigger than science, this bond between physician and assistant team is getting violated. A team of assistants working with various surgeons and vice versa certainly affects final outcome of procedure. Proper man management is essential to avoid loss or migration of technicians.

Quality Control

Every step in HT is important, so is every assistant. The success of HT is sum of all the procedures done by all the assistants. Quality of dissection, maintaining cool temperature, avoiding dryness, avoiding transection during FUE, handling grafts properly during implantation, and maintaining good relation with patient all add up to quality care. So, constant monitoring is an important prerequisite to have optimum hair growth.

Structure of a Hair Restoration Team

A hair restoration surgeon is supposed to know all the possible procedures of hair restoration, knowledge of hair science, intensive care management, and should be capable of managing possible complications. When we design a hair restoration center, the vision of surgeon is very important. Making a team is a difficult task and needs human resource management and finance to start with.

First step—establish the goal: What is your requirement in terms of number of assistants, their qualification, and how much you can pay? You have to have a long-term planning. It is preferable to have one or two trained, experienced nurses to start with and a set of new young assistants. Appointing fresh young team members works better rather than hiring all trained assistant from other centers.

Training of team members: It needs minimum 2–3 months to train them. During this period, you have to pay them, which can create a financial pressure, but this is essential and should be planned. When you yourself train them, it develops a strong bond between you and your team, and they morally feel attached to you. Make up your mind that you have to pay staff for 6 months' salary without immediate return. After 2–3 months of training, start taking smaller relatively simple cases. These cases may not give you financial return but will boost up your team, and they will understand that they need more intensive training. Training and updating are an ongoing process and should go on as you grow.

FOLLOW-UP VISITS

Assistant plays important role in follow-up visits. He is the first one to attend to the patient. While operating for long hours, patient develops a bond with the team, and on follow-up, they expect to be received by the same team members with a warm friendly welcome.

The author feels that surgeon should himself remove the dressing and examine the suture line and recipient area in detail. At least few initial sutures removal should be done by surgeon himself and rest can be done by senior assistant. This not only creates impact on patient but surgeon understands patient's healing process and can predict any complication.

ISSUES OF QUACKERY AND BLACK MARKETING

There have been several instances of assistants themselves becoming surgeons, either as freelancing mobile teams or in commercial setups where the doctor is only for appearance. This has led to several medical issues. It is strongly recommended that HT surgeons do not employ such technicians for surgeries. And importantly, surgeons should not delegate steps such as extraction and slit making to technicians.

SUMMARY

Hair restoration team is a vital component of a hair transplant clinic and should consist of:

- One trained surgeon or physician
- Two trained nurses with operating room experience
- A set of four technicians
- A counselor, who can be your senior nurse
- An assistant physician (if possible)

Proper training, quality control, and experience all help in ensuring success of the clinic.

REFERENCES

1. Assistant duties. In: Karamanovski E (Ed). Hair Transplant 360 for Assistants, 2nd edition. New Delhi: Jaypee Brothers Medical Publishers (P) Ltd.; 2016. pp. 47-67.
2. Lardener T, James A. Harries-surgical assistants. In: Unger W, Shapiro R (Eds). Hair Transplantation, 5th edition. New York: Informa Healthcare; 2011. p. 510.

CHAPTER 93

Training Modules in Hair Transplant

Anil Kumar Garg, Seema Garg

Key Messages

- Since hair transplantation requires a team of assistants, training is an ongoing process and is a vital component of a successful team.
- Training of surgeons and assistants in different processes, such as dissection and implantation, needs to be done in a systematic manner, regularly and continuously.
- The training should be done first on models and then on live patients to ensure good quality.

INTRODUCTION

There is a global increase in demand for hair transplants (HTs) as well as an increasing demand for trained assistants and surgeons. It is a fact that permanent donor hair follicles are limited, and any loss during learning is permanent and irreversible. Hence, learning on the patient is not feasible. Therefore, proper training of assistants on in vivo models is vital. Demand for HT is increasing day by day. More and more HT centers are coming up all over the world. There are very few training centers and fellowship programs across the world to fulfill the requirement of trained assistants and technicians. The author has developed a very effective, user-friendly, economical model to learn and practice all steps of HT.[1-3] Materials required for this training model are available around us. Materials such as foam, money plant leaf (thick leaf), simple stitching black thread, needles, wooden spatula, and goat skin are needed for this model.

In this learning module, the materials used are paper, pencil, plant leaf, foam, thread, and goat skin. The module has been divided into multiple steps:

1. The first step is training of a microsurgery position.
2. The second step is training of movement at the wrist using paper and pencil.
3. The third step is strip harvesting and slivering on a foam model.
4. The fourth step is learning of follicle dissection on a leaf model.
5. The fifth step is thread follicle implantation on a leaf bed.
6. After practicing on a nonliving model, lastly, all the steps are practiced on goat skin, starting from slivering, follicle dissection, and implantation of goat follicles on a leaf. It is further clarified that the training module and the materials are the innovations of the author.

MICROSURGERY POSITION

The entire process of HT is a microsurgery. All basic principles of microsurgery should be followed **(Figs. 1A to D)**: Magnification, proper position of surgeon, instrument quality, and range of hand movements.

The position of the surgeon or assistant should be in such a way that all body joints are at a functional position. Feet should rest on the floor and leg to thigh at 90°, spine straight and supported, forearm resting on the dissection table, and all movements should be at the wrist. This position allows the surgeon or assistant to work for a longer period. Wrong posture invites early fatigue and affects the surgeon's performance and efficiency.

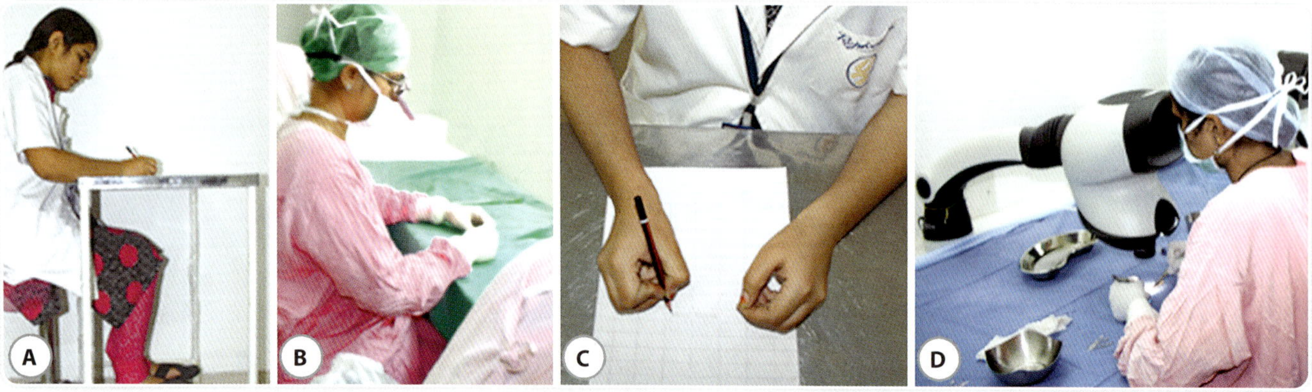

FIGS. 1A TO D: (A and B) Microsurgery position; (C and D) Forearm resting on the dissection table.

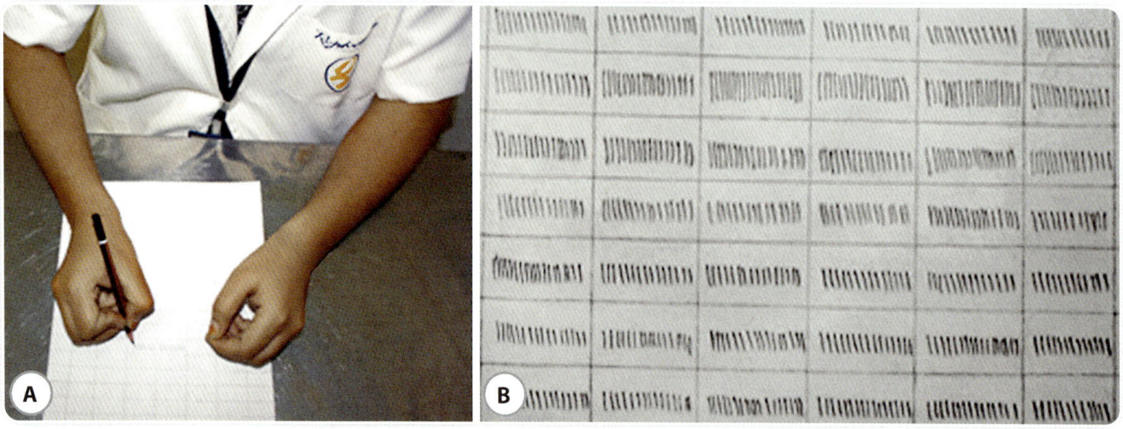

FIGS. 2A AND B: (A) Making straight equidistant parallel lines; (B) Practice sheet.

PAPER MODEL

Training of Movements at the Wrist (Figs. 2A and B)

The microsurgery position enables wrist movements for the surgeon. Follicle dissection involves wrist movements in the forward–backward direction, while slivering and implantation require downward–upward movements. There is no need for side-to-side movements throughout the entire process of hair transplantation. We can learn and practice these movements by drawing straight lines on paper using a pencil or pen.

Materials

The materials required are plain paper and a pencil with suitable magnification.

Method

Make small rectangle/square boxes on paper. Keeping the microsurgery position, ask the assistant to make straight parallel equidistant lines in the box. To start with, he can practice without magnification and then under magnification. He should complete 15 sheets under magnification.

FOAM MODEL (FIGS. 3A TO E)

Strip Harvesting

The foam model is for nonsurgical hands to train how to hold a scalpel, the part of blade to be used in strip harvesting, and how to raise a strip while dissecting in one plane of tissue.

Materials

The materials required are a 1-inch-thick high-density foam piece of size 8 × 10 cm, wooden platform, marking pen, scalpel, and tooth forceps.

Method

Fix the foam on a wooden platform or any table and mark the strip area with a skin marking pen. Hold the scalpel in your dominant hand in a pen-holding position.

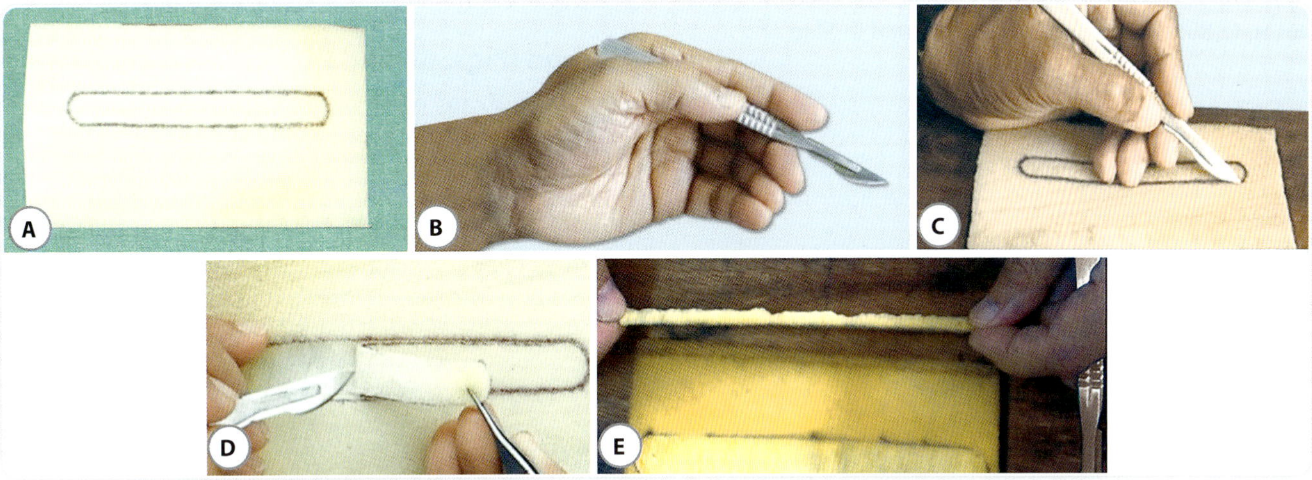

FIGS. 3A TO E: (A) Foam with marking; (B and C) Scalpel in a pen; (C) Holding position; (D) Incision strip harvesting; (E) Harvested strip of uniform thickness.

Keep the sharp edge of the scalpel almost parallel to the surface of the foam and make a partial thickness cut over the marking. Ensure that the depth of the incision is consistent all around, which can be achieved by applying equal pressure on the scalpel. The direction of the incision should be slightly oblique. The reason for this is that the hair direction on the scalp is oblique, so we need to follow the same direction of the hair follicles. Now, using tooth forceps, hold one end of the strip and pull it up while cutting underneath with the scalpel. Be careful to cut in the same plane, harvesting a uniform thickness of the foam strip. Practice this technique multiple times to achieve a uniform thickness and a plane surface of the foam.

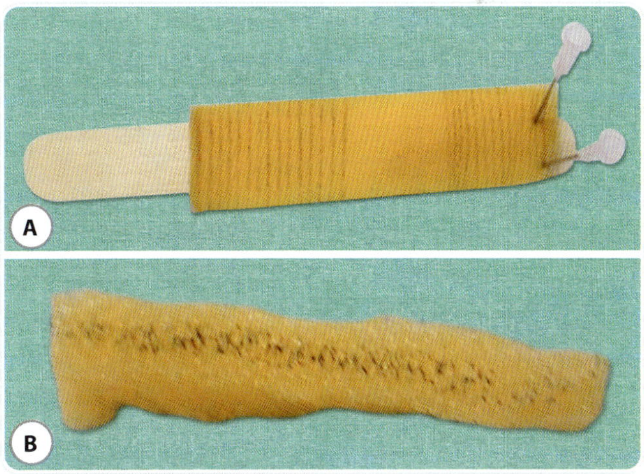

FIGS. 4A AND B: (A) Foam strip. Markings for rows of hair; (B) Foam sliver. Marking indicates rows of hair.

Slivering (Figs. 4A and B)

After strip harvesting, slivering is the second step. This is divided into two steps:

1. In the first step, we learn to move the scalpel in an up-and-down direction while making thin slices of foam.
2. In the second step, we practice slivering on a foam strip woven with thread. Black thread with a knot symbolizes the graft. During this dissection, the thread should not be cut.

Materials

The materials required are 1-inch-thick foam, black stitching thread, sewing needles, and skin marker.

Method

Step 1: Cut small pieces of foam 1 cm thick, 2 cm wide, and 7–10 cm long. Using a skin marker, make multiple straight parallel lines at 2–3 mm distance on the surface of the foam. Now, this foam piece is like a sliver, and marked lines are rows of hair follicles. Fix this foam sliver on a wooden spatula using needles. Start slivering with a fine tooth forceps in the nondominant hand and a scalpel in the dominant hand. Using tooth forceps, catch the upper edge of the foam sliver and cut in between two lines straight from the top surface of the foam to the bottom. While the scalpel is cutting, pull the foam sliver outside and slightly upward so there is an increased gap between two rows. Finally, you must cut very thin, equal, uniform slices of foam.

Step 2: Black stitching thread is used as a symbol of the hair follicle, and a single knot of thread is an indicator of the hair bulb. Using a needle, multiple threads are sewn in rows on a foam strip, with a knot on the underside, leaving small free ends of thread on the other, as shown in **Figures 5A to C**. Slivering is started as explained in *Step 1*.

LEAF MODEL

Follicle Dissection

Materials

A thick plant leaf, such as the leaf of a money plant (*Epipremnum aureum*), is taken. It is thick as well as the texture is similar to normal skin. Lead pen (simple writing pen), scalpel and forceps, magnification is essential.

Method (Figs. 6A and B)

Take a 5 × 2 cm^2 piece of thick leaf. Make markings of size 10 mm long parallel lines in the center of the leaf. These lines symbolize follicles. Start follicle dissection under a microscope or magnification, which you or your assistant is going to use. The assistant makes a cut in between two lines and creates small pieces of the leaf having a line in the center of that piece. The line

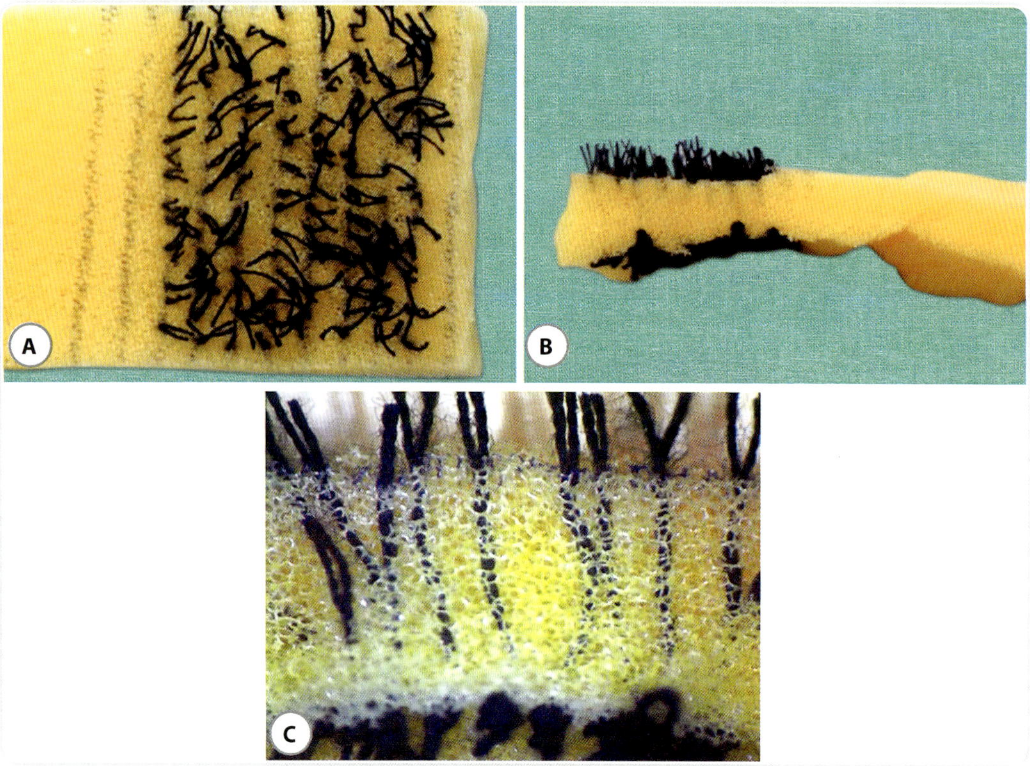

FIGS. 5A TO C: (A and B) Thread woven foam strip; (C) Foam sliver.

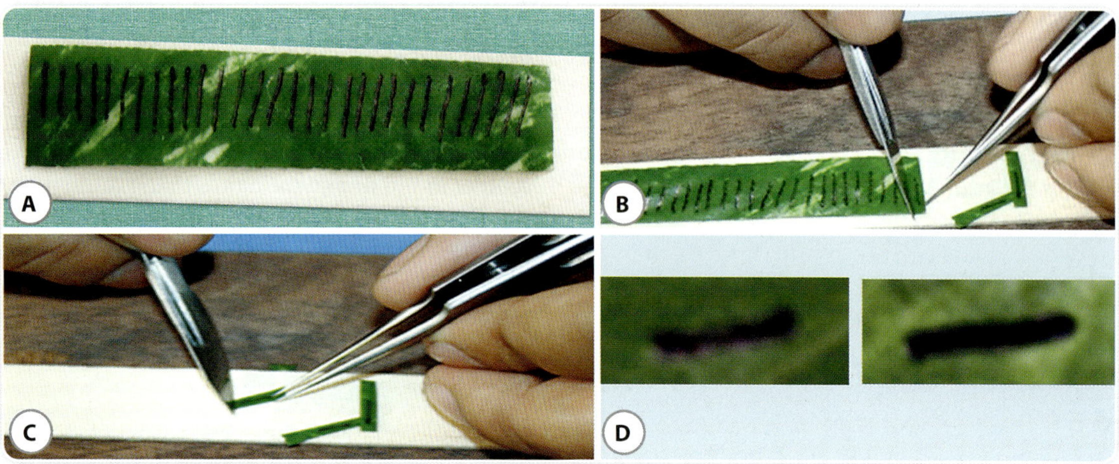

FIGS. 6A TO D: (A) A plant leaf sliver; (B) Follicle dissection; (C) Trimming of the follicle; (D) Follicles.

represents the hair and hair bulb, and the leaf part is the perifollicle tissue **(Figs. 6C and D)**. During this step, he also practices the coordination of the scalpel and forceps. Any indentation of forceps over the leaf surface warns the assistant that his grip on the forceps should be softer to avoid crushing the follicle. He should at least cut around 100 plant slivers.

IMPLANTATION

Both stick-and-place and slit methods of implantation can be practiced.

Materials

The materials required are money plant leaf (or the leaf of any thick and soft plant), wooden spatula, slit-making knife, needles, black thread, and diluted adhesive solution (e.g., Fevicol solution, which is a synthetic resin adhesive).

Method (Figs. 7A to I)

Take multiple pieces of leaf of equal length and width, and put them one over the other so that we have a multiple-layer thick leaf bed; fix them over a wooden spatula.

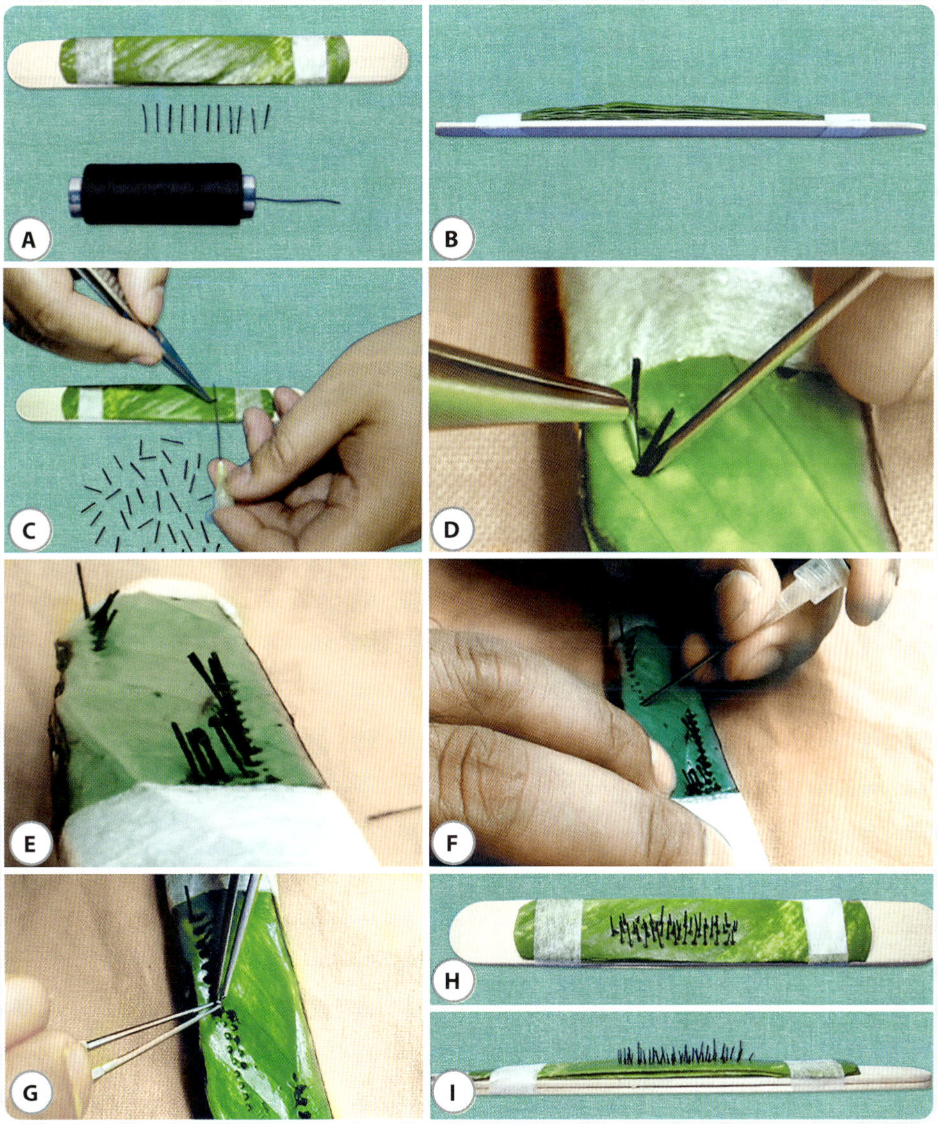

FIGS. 7A TO I: (A to D) Leaf model for implantation. (A to C) Preparing thread follicles and leaf scalp. (E and F) Multiple leaf strips are put over each other to make it as thick as a scalp. (G) Stick-and-place technique. Implantation of thread follicles on the "leaf scalp" using a needle and forceps. (H) Final appearance—premade slits and implantation. Implantation of thread follicles in premade slits using two forceps. Slits made using a needle. (I) Final appearance.

technique of hair transplantation. By using this model, doctors can learn how to correctly engage the hair at the right angle and score the skin before advancing the punch, which helps them to predict the possibility of transection (cutting the hair follicle). This technique also teaches doctors how to stabilize the FUE handle, which allows for precise engagement and advancement of the punch at the correct angle. Overall, this model can be a valuable tool for new doctors who are learning the FUE technique.

MATERIALS FOR FOLLICULAR UNIT EXCISION

The materials required are motorized or manual FUE system, punch, and patient scalp donor area. The technique is called scoring technique.

Scoring Technique

Follicular unit excision aims to achieve zero transections. The scoring technique will develop your hand and eye coordination to minimize hair follicle transections.

The angle of the hair's exit should be the same as the punch's insertion angle. This can be achieved by practicing the "scoring technique." The scoring technique needs magnification. Higher is better, preferably 4× magnification with an excellent quality loupe. Hold the manual punch or motorized hand firmly as you hold a pen. Then stabilize your hand, concentrate on the angle of the hair, and engage the hair, keeping the hair shaft and infundibulum of hair in the center of the circumference of the punch and the punch parallel to the hair shaft **(Fig. 11)**. This is called engagement. Then, gently advance or penetrate the edge of the punch *just enough to score the skin.* Score at least 10 hairs and then check for

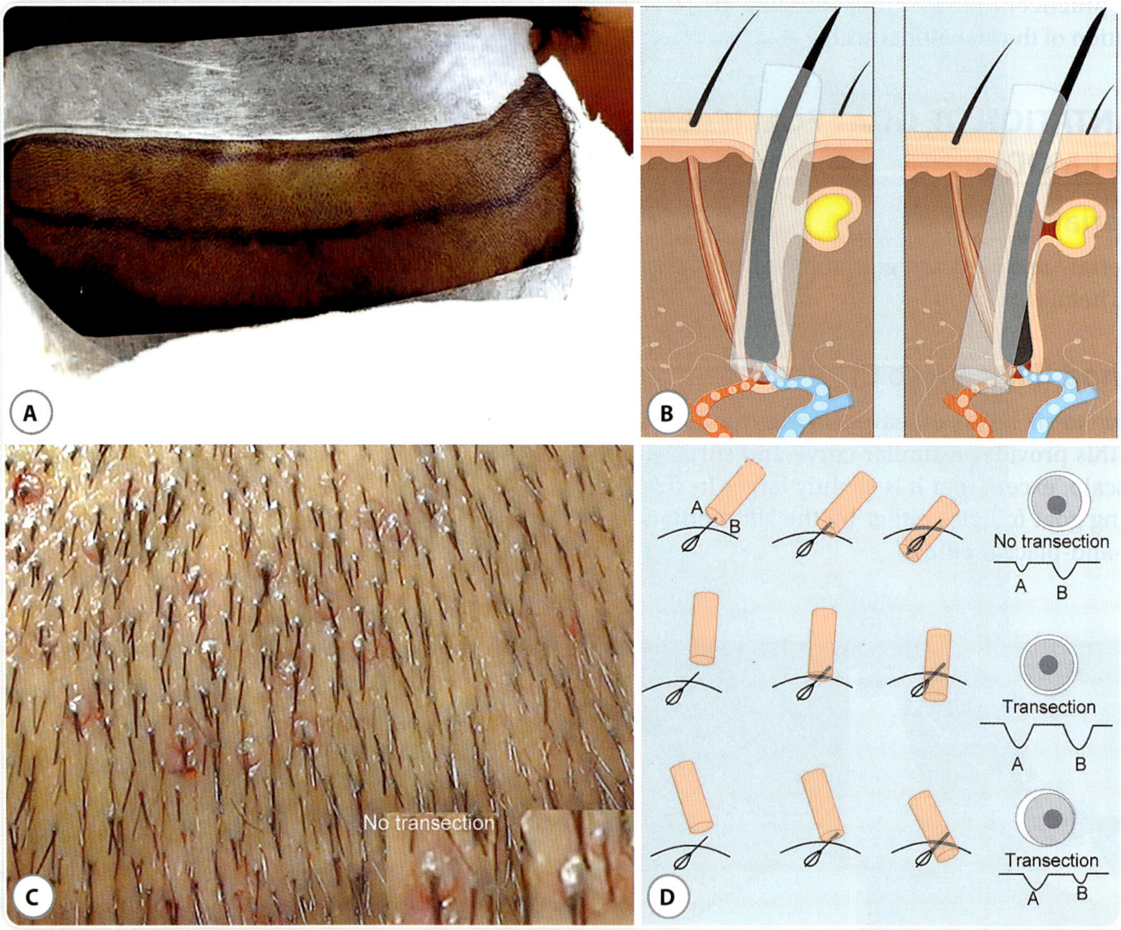

FIGS. 11A TO D: A scoring technique for follicular unit excision (FUE) practice. (A) Strip donor area; (B) Punch alignment to hair follicles. If alignment, engagement and advancement is done same as of hair follicle, there will not be transection, but if deviation then it will transect the follicle; (C) Scoring; (D) Scoring analysis sheet.

centralization of hair and analyze the score characteristic as shown in **Figure 11C**.

Analysis of score: Analyze your scoring as shown in **Figure 11D**. If point B is deeper than point A (as shown in **Fig. 11D)**, the punch is parallel to the hair shaft, and the hair is in the center of the score. So, the follicle has not been transected. Hence, this scoring analysis technique will give an idea of whether there is a transection.

Advices

Surgeons can first start practicing on a limited scalp donor area, preferably before strip harvesting. Finally, they can score and excise a few grafts and slowly increase the number. It is also advised to start with the manual method and then relatively simple motorized FUE machines. We also advise doing this under the guidance of a senior FUE surgeon.

SUMMARY

These learning, training, and practice modules of HT are versatile, user-friendly, and economical. The author has used this to train all his team members. Two hours per day for 3–4 weeks can train a technician in the basic knowledge of the HT procedure, follicle care, and the importance of graft hydration, ischemia, and temperature control. The delicacy of the hair follicle should be repeatedly explained, and we help them realize how important their job is. Hair transplantation requires teamwork, and every step should be performed with the optimum results for the patient in mind.

DISCLAIMER

The methods outlined in this chapter are the original innovations of Dr Anil Kumar Garg.

REFERENCES

1. Garg AK, Garg S. A learning module in hair restoration surgery: A simple and economic method to learn all steps of strip method of hair follicles harvesting and implantation. Indian J Plast Surg. 2017;50(3):230-5.
2. Garg AK, Seema G. Chapter 60. In: Mysore V, Hair Transplantation. 1st ed. New Delhi: Jaypee Brothers. 2016;394-400.
3. Garg AK, Seema G. Chapter 75. In: D. Pathomvanich, ed. Practical Aspects of Hair Transplantation in Asians. Tokyo, Japan: Springer Publication. 2018;719-29

CHAPTER 94

Photography in Hair Patient

Sanjeev Aurangabadkar

Key Messages

- Imaging has become an integral part of electronic medical records and documentation.
- Photodocumentation aids in effective management, counseling, publications, and teaching purposes.
- Mastering the art of clinical photography is fairly easy if some basic rules are followed.
- A DSLR, mirrorless, or bridge camera with adequate lighting, clean background, and fixed distance from the subject ensures good-quality images and consistency.
- *Correct exposure depends on three parameters*: Aperture, shutter speed, and ISO. It is important to understand some basic concepts of photography.
- Always use standardized views while photographing patients.
- Storing, archiving, and securing the images captured are as important as taking the images.
- Processing and manipulation of images should be kept to minimum (within acceptable standards).

INTRODUCTION

Photodocumentation is an important part of dermatology and aesthetic medicine for proper documentation and record keeping. Imaging in medicine helps us in documenting, monitoring, and teaching. The basic concepts of clinical photography still apply to photographing hairy areas, such as the scalp. The critical aspects of medical photography include proper and consistent lighting, standard views, clutter-free background, and fixed camera settings. Hair photography poses certain challenges compared to general clinical photography. Some of these include reflection or shine from the light bouncing off the hairs, maintaining proper angles while taking serial photographs, and dynamic changes in hair loss/regrowth.

ETHICAL ASPECTS IN MEDICAL PHOTOGRAPHY

It is important to take an informed, written consent from the patient before taking a photograph. One must explain why the image is being taken, where it will be stored, and whether it will be used in publications and presentations. A patient's photographs are a part of the electronic health record, and their access must be restricted to physicians and trusted staff. A patient's images should not be shared on social media without their consent. If a mobile phone is used, the image must be transferred to a storage device and the image deleted from phone memory. Ideally, one must avoid using personal phones for medical photography. A dedicated camera or mobile phone should be used in the clinic/hospital. A patient's image belongs to the person and not the photographer, and the patient can withdraw the consent any time.

The devices used for hair photography include:

- A digital camera [point and shoot (PS) type, interchangeable (mirrorless) lens camera, or a DSLR]
- Specialized photography booths or stations for head and face or total body photography (TBP) (FotoFinder, Reveal, etc.)
- Three-dimensional photography
- Smartphone camera and attachments
- Specialized hair photography equipment such as trichoscope and dermatoscope

The common question asked is which camera to get for medical photography. A digital single-lens reflex (SLR) or a mirrorless camera is generally preferred as they have a larger sensor. A larger sensor translates to better image quality (IQ) and less noise (grain) in images. Also, the advantages are that one can use specialized lenses and external flash for better image quality. These cameras have the ability to shoot in RAW (which is the digital negative of a film camera). The downside of these cameras is that they are expensive and have a learning curve. Photo booths or stations are a good option as they are customized for specific types of photography like TBP or facial photography, which aids in standardization. Again, they tend to be expensive. Smartphones are best avoided due to the small sensor size, lens quality, and small flash. Advantages of smartphones are that they are handy and allow quick documentation and easy sharing.

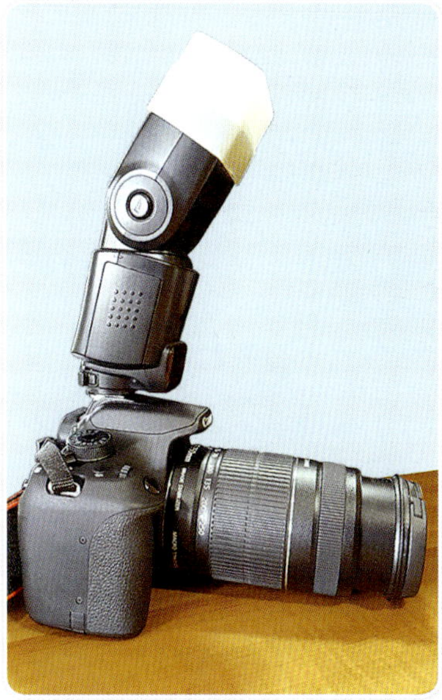

FIG. 1: A DSLR camera with external flash and a diffuser.

ACCESSORIES FOR DIGITAL PHOTOGRAPHY

The accessories include a tripod (to minimize shake/blur), external flash devices with diffusers or softboxes, a fixed screen backdrop (black, gray, light blue, or green), Scotch tape or duct tape to mark the patient's position, and tripod (so that distance remains the same for repeated photographs). Memory cards, hard disk drives, and a laptop/PC to store images are also essential.

BASICS OF PHOTOGRAPHY

Lighting

Lighting is the key element for obtaining good exposures and bringing out detail. As most clinical photography is done indoors, a flash needs to be used to keep the ISO (sensitivity of sensor) low to avoid noise/grain in the photo and also to keep the shutter speed higher to avoid blurring.[1] On-camera flash units are not ideal as the light source is small and gives harsh direct light, thereby whitening out or washing out the area and losing detail. It is best to use an indirect light source such as a bounce-flash (reflected light from the ceiling or a whiteboard or reflector), a ring-flash, or a twin-flash setup to produce even lighting and depth.[2] A ring-flash unit is particularly useful when using macro to take close-ups of the area. An example of bounce flash with diffuser is shown in **Figures 1 to 3**. A typical ring-flash unit mounted on the front of the lens and flash hot-shoe is depicted in **Figure 4**. **Figure 5** shows a twin-flash unit. **Figure 6** shows a compact camera with the ability to tilt and bounce the flash from the ceiling.

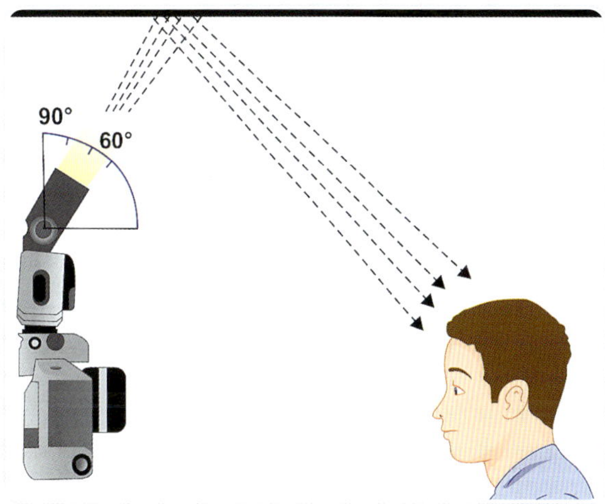

FIG. 2: A diagrammatic representation of the bounce-flash technique.

Background

A consistent, even background is mandatory to minimize distracting elements in the image and yield consistent exposures. A light blue, green, or gray background is ideal. It could be a linen cloth, photography paper, etc.[2] The distance of the subject from the background is also important. If the subject is too close, there will be a shadow cast on the background. It is best to separate them by 60–90 cm to avoid this.

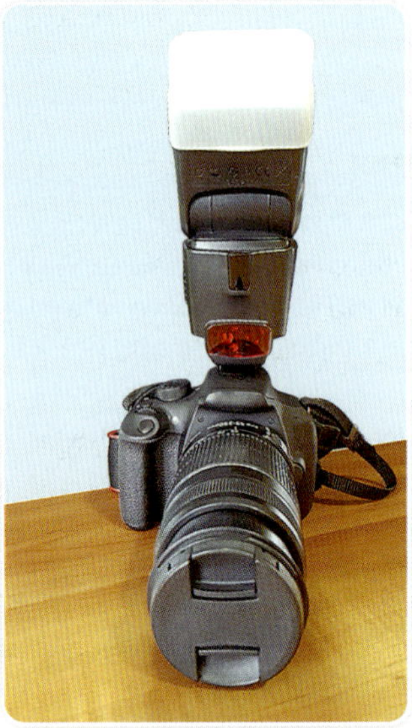

FIG. 3: A front view of DSLR with external flash and a diffuser.

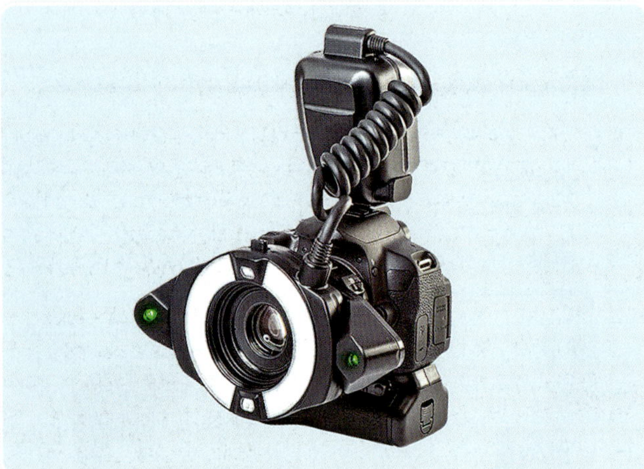

FIG. 4: A DSLR with a ring flash attached to the front of the lens.

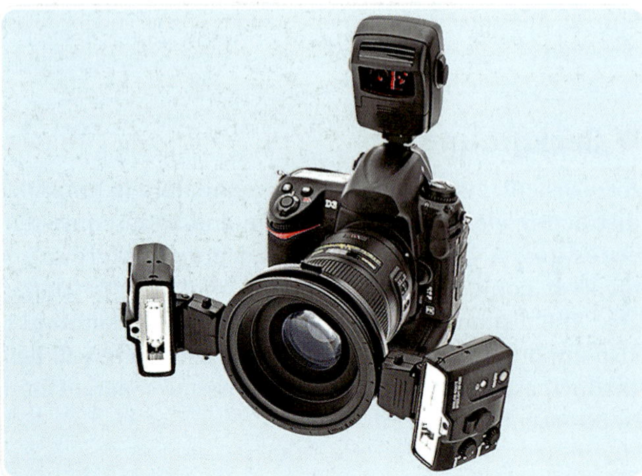

FIG. 5: A DSLR with a twin-flash setup.

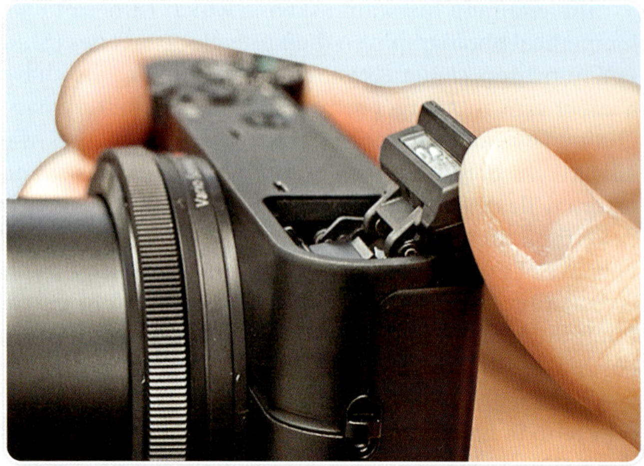

FIG. 6: An advanced compact camera with the ability to tilt and bounce flash from the ceiling.

Preparation of Patient

Make sure the patient is not wearing hairbands, clips, earrings, etc., that can distract from the area in question. Avoid oiled hair; it is best to photograph a patient with clean, dry hair. A tissue can be used to soak and absorb oil if the patient has already oiled his/her hair just before photographing.

Camera Setup

A tripod is helpful to fix the distance and height of the camera from the subject. It also avoids camera shake and gives a sharp image. Always mark the distance between the camera and the subject and use this point for future photographs. A height-adjustable stool for the patient to sit on is ideal. Modern digital cameras have built-in Wi-Fi in them. One can set it up and sync it with the laptop or PC so that the images are transferred wirelessly the moment they are taken. The transferred images can be tagged using the patient's name, diagnosis, and identification number for easy storage and retrieval. It is best to have a master file of each patient where the subsequent images are stored.

Resolution

Resolution is the amount of detail that is captured by a digital camera. It is usually measured in pixels. The higher the resolution, the more the detail is captured. It has been suggested that a resolution of 1.3 megapixels (MP) is sufficient for dermatologic photography.[3] But these days, most digital cameras and smartphones have a resolution upward of 8 MP, going up to 12–20 MP. Practically speaking, a resolution of 8–12 MP is quite adequate, giving very good detail and keeping file size in check. Remember, the higher the resolution, the larger will be the file size.

Framing

It is ideal to fill the frame with the subject and avoid dead space on either side or on top. This will avoid cropping later on and preserve resolution.

Standardization

Standardization is important with regard to pre- and postimages and follow-up photography. The key to this is consistency and involves camera parameters, patient position, background, and lighting.

Commercially available color charts/gray cards can be placed as part of the image for standardization of color and white balance in conditions where the color of the lesion or affected area is key (such as melasma, vitiligo, or vascular lesions).

Standard Views for Hair Photography

There are four standard views, namely vertex, mid-pattern, frontal, and temporal views.[1,4] These views are excellent for documenting global assessment and giving an overview of hair loss. These are also helpful for serial photography to document the progress or worsening of hair loss over time. Generally, a distance of 3 feet is sufficient between the camera and the patient to record these views. For photographing close-ups of localized lesions of scalp/hair disorders, such as alopecia areata and discoid lupus erythematosus, a macro mode (close-up mode) can be used; generally, it is recorded at a distance of <1 foot from the lesion. Most cameras have a macro mode that can be engaged to achieve this. For even closer or higher magnification and for hair shaft defects, a dermascope or videodermascope can be used. These are stand-alone equipment or smartphone attachments that aid in magnification of 10–300× for observing and recording changes in hair shaft and scalp.

It is best to photograph the patient with clean, dry hair and with the same hairstyle if possible. If needed, an assistant can comb and arrange the hair in a set pattern before taking the picture. Always refer to the baseline photograph at subsequent visits to crosscheck the hair and position for maintaining consistency. For global photography of patterned hair loss, it is best to shoot in vertical or portrait orientation of the camera to record maximum detail (as more pixels are utilized).

PHOTOGRAPHING STANDARD VIEWS FOR GLOBAL ASSESSMENT

Vertex View

To photograph the vertex, ask the patient (in sitting position with back toward the camera) to look up to the ceiling. This will give a good view of the vertex. The vertex view is shown in **Figure 7**.

Mid-pattern Position

Ask the seated patient (while facing the camera) to rest the face down on his/her folded hands that are resting on a table. The crown portion of the scalp will be in full view.

Frontal View

The patient should be in a sitting position, facing the camera, which should be at eye level with the patient. The frontal view is shown in **Figure 8**.

Temporal View

Turn the patient's face 45° and take photos of the left and right sides, thus highlighting the temporal regions of the scalp. The temporal view is shown in **Figures 9A and B**.

Standard views in androgenetic alopecia (AGA) and female pattern hair loss (FPHL) for global assessment.

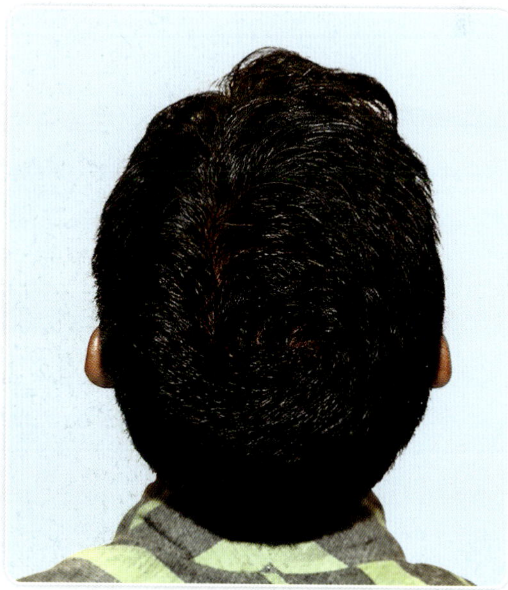

FIG. 7: Vertex view.

For FPHL, the patient can part the hair in the center while photographing so that the parting width and density of hairs can be documented. For scarring alopecias and alopecia areata, it is best to have the hair cut short so that the patches can be visible. For early AGA in males, the patient can be asked to comb the hair back so that the frontotemporal hairline recession can be documented in both frontal view and mid-pattern views.

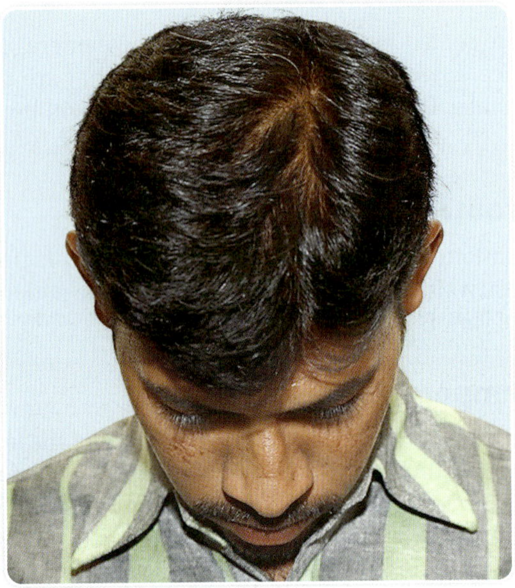

FIG. 8: Frontal view.

CAMERA TYPE

A DSLR generally outscored other camera systems in terms of IQ, responsiveness, manual control, and accessories but tends to be more bulky and cumbersome. PS cameras are smaller and easier to operate but tend to have few manual controls to change aperture, shutter speed, etc. The flash on the PS camera is also not ideal, as it casts harsh light. The newer and high-end PS cameras have impressive IQ and have in-built tilt-flash capability so that light can be bounced off a surface, thus reducing glare/washing out a subject. A third category called interchangeable lens camera (ILC) or mirrorless cameras is available, which is in between DSLR and PS. They are smaller than DSLRs, have interchangeable lenses, and have very good IQ. Any of these systems can be used for hair photography, provided the basic principles are kept in mind.

SMARTPHONES

Mobile phones have come a long way in a short time, and the cameras on them are getting better and better each passing day. They have the single most important advantage that they are handy, portable, and always available. They can be used for hair photography conveniently, but the flash on these units tends to be very small and not ideal. If the flash is turned off, then it is important to take a photo in sufficient ambient light (say near a window) to minimize shake and blur.

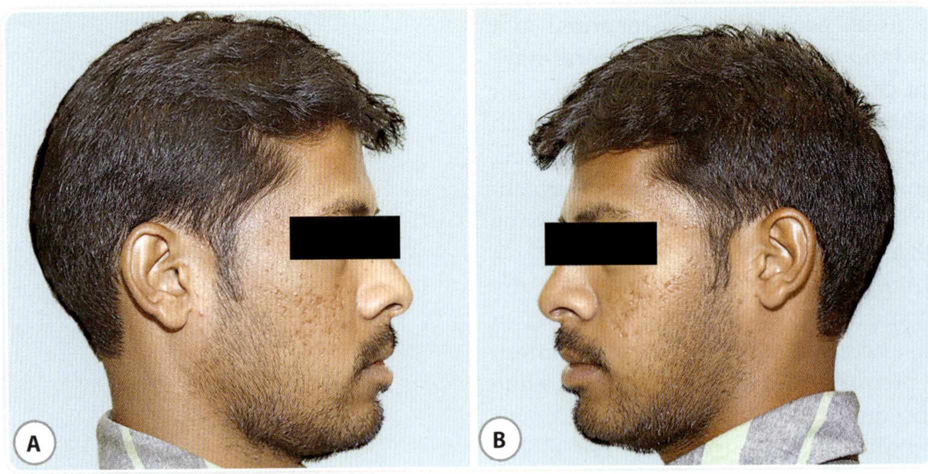

FIGS. 9A AND B: Temporal view.

STORAGE AND SECURITY

Images captured need to be properly stored, both on physical hard drives (preferably solid-state drives) and on the cloud as a backup. Having a cloud backup ensures a double backup, and the images can also be downloaded even while on the move. In the days of cybercrime and cyberattacks, it is a must to have encryption and password protection for both physical drives and cloud backup to avoid unauthorized access to the digital image files.[5]

SUMMARY

Photography of hair disorders is fairly straightforward and relatively easy, provided that some basic rules are kept in mind, and attention is paid to camera setup and patient positioning. Proper photo documentation goes a long way in aiding physicians' global assessment of hair loss and in satisfying the patient.

RECOMMENDATIONS FOR DIGITAL CAMERA

Image quality should be at the top of the mind when choosing a digital camera. A mid or high-end PS or a DSLR from a reputed brand should get the job done. An advantage of a DSLR remains the availability of myriad accessories for better photography. A number of websites that review digital cameras are available, and it is advisable to check the cameras before buying. Some of these include dpreview.com, cameralabs.com, etc.

Due to a sheer number of models and brands available, it is difficult to make specific recommendations.

Some top PS cameras include:

- Sony RX series
- Canon Powershot G series
- Panasonic LX series
- Fujifilm X series

Some top DSLRs and ILCs:

- Canon 650D, 700D, 750D, 760D, 1200D, 1300D, etc.
- Nikon D3200, D5300, D7200
- Sony Alpha series
- Olympus OMD series
- Panasonic G series

If money is not an issue, some of the high-end specialized dermatology imaging equipment, such as those from Canfield or FotoFinder, can be considered. They remain very expensive but have specialized software for analysis.

Tips and Pearls

- Have a dedicated area in the clinic/hospital for digital photography.
- Use a clean background for before and after pictures. Black background works for lighter skin tones, while light blue, gray, or green background works for darker skin tones.
- Avoid oiled hair, gelled hair, and accessories such as clips and bands while photographing.
- Try to use fixed parameters of ISO, aperture, shutter speed, and white balance when possible.
- Use disposable wooden ice-cream sticks or combs to part the hair or position the hairs before photographing.
- Photography is all about light. Make sure it is adequate, consistent, and uniform.
- Store and protect the images on a secure hard drive and on the cloud to have a backup.

REFERENCES

1. Ashique KT, Kaliyadan F. Clinical photography for trichology practice: tips and tricks. Int J Trichol. 2011;3:7-13.
2. Kaliyadan F, Manoj J, Venkitakrishnan S, Dharmaratnam AD. Basic digital photography in dermatology. Indian J Dermatol Venereol Leprol. 2008;74:532-6.
3. Miot HA, Paixyo MP, Paschoal FM. Basics of digital photography in dermatology. An Bras Dermatol. 2006;81:174-80.
4. Canfield D. Photographic documentation of hair growth in androgenetic alopecia. Dermatol Clin. 1996;14:713-21.
5. Pasquali P, Kaliyadan F. Photography in dermatology: basic concepts. Cosmoderma. 2021;1:43.

CHAPTER 95

Role of Marketing

Viral Desai

INTRODUCTION

More and more individuals are turning to hair transplant surgery to fix their thinning hair and receding hairlines. With the growing demand for hair transplant services, it is becoming essential for clinics to market their services to potential clients effectively.[1] In this article, we will discuss how crucial marketing is while launching a hair transplant practice.

THE GROWING DEMAND FOR HAIR TRANSPLANT SERVICES

Millions of individuals all around the globe suffer from hair loss. Therefore, hair transplant surgery has gained popularity as a means to restore the hairline for people who have lost it. With a compound annual growth rate (CAGR) of 25–30%, the Times of India reports that the hair transplant market in India is booming, especially in certain metros and Tier-I cities such as Mumbai, Delhi NCR, and Chennai.[1,2] This indicates a growing demand for hair transplant services, making it a lucrative market for those looking to set up a hair transplant clinic.

THE IMPORTANCE OF MARKETING IN SETTING UP A HAIR TRANSPLANT CLINIC

Marketing is essential for setting up a hair transplant clinic as it helps attract potential clients and build brand awareness.[3] Here are some of the reasons why marketing is essential for a hair transplant clinic:

- *Increased visibility*: A hair transplant clinic's exposure can be increased by strategic marketing efforts, making it simpler for potential patients to locate and contact the clinic.
- *Brand awareness*: Marketing can help build brand awareness for a hair transplant clinic, making it easier for potential clients to remember the clinic and recommend it to others.
- *Differentiation from competitors*: Marketing can help a hair transplant clinic differentiate itself by highlighting unique selling points and showcasing its expertise and experience.
- *Increased trust and credibility*: Marketing can help build trust and credibility for a hair transplant clinic by showcasing client testimonials, before-and-after photos, and other evidence of successful hair transplant procedures.
- *Increased revenue*: Effective marketing can ultimately lead to increased revenue for a hair transplant clinic as more potential clients are attracted to the clinic and choose to undergo hair transplant procedures.

IDENTIFYING YOUR TARGET AUDIENCE

Identifying your target audience is the first step in developing an effective marketing strategy for your hair transplant clinic. Knowing your target audience is important for the effectiveness of your marketing efforts and the acquisition of new patients.

The Significance of Understanding Your Target Audience

The importance of understanding your audience cannot be overstated[4] for the following reasons:

- *Effective communication*: Knowing your target audience allows you to communicate with them in a way that resonates with them, acknowledges their issues, and addresses their specific concerns.
- *Efficient resource allocation*: Identifying your target audience allows you to allocate your resources more

effectively and efficiently as you can focus your marketing efforts on the people who are most likely to become your patients.

- *Better return on investment (ROI)*: A well-defined target audience can lead to a better ROI for your marketing efforts as you target the people most likely to benefit from your services.

Defining Your Target Market

Defining your target market involves identifying the characteristics of the people most likely to benefit from your hair transplant services.[5] Here are some factors to consider for defining your target market:

- *Age and gender*: Hair loss affects both men and women, but the age at which it occurs and the reasons for it can differ. Identifying the age range and gender of your target market can help you tailor your marketing efforts accordingly.
- *Location*: Identifying the location of your target market is essential for developing location-based marketing strategies and identifying areas with the highest demand for hair transplant services.
- *Income and education Level*: The cost of hair transplant surgery is significant for many people. Identifying your target market's income and education level can help you develop pricing strategies that align with their budget.

IDENTIFYING YOUR IDEAL PATIENT

Identifying your ideal patient involves going beyond demographic information and considering the specific needs and concerns of the people most likely to benefit from your hair transplant services.[5] Here are some factors to consider when identifying your ideal patient:

- *Stage of hair loss*: Identifying your ideal patient's hair loss stage can help you tailor your marketing efforts and provide them with the most appropriate treatment options.
- *Motivation for treatment*: Understanding the motivation for treating your ideal patient can help you develop marketing messages that speak to their specific concerns and offer solutions that meet their needs.
- *Preferred communication channels*: Identifying the preferred communication channels of your ideal patient can help you reach them more effectively and increase the chances of converting them into patients.

CRAFTING YOUR BRAND IDENTITY

Crafting your brand identity is essential for developing a successful marketing strategy for your hair transplant clinic in India. A strong brand identity can help you differentiate your clinic from competitors, build trust with potential patients, and establish a memorable and recognizable brand in the minds of your audience.

Creating a Compelling Brand Identity

Creating a compelling brand identity involves developing a unique visual and verbal identity representing your clinic's values, mission, and personality.[6] Here are some factors to consider when creating your brand identity:

- *Logo and visual identity*: Your clinic's logo and visual identity are the most recognizable aspects of your brand. They should be unique, visually appealing, and memorable.
- *Color palette and typography*: The colors and typography used in your branding should reflect your clinic's values and personality. They should be consistent across all marketing materials to establish a recognizable and professional brand.

Defining Your Unique Value Proposition

Defining your unique value proposition is essential for establishing what sets your clinic apart from competitors.[7] Here are some questions to consider when defining your unique value proposition:

- *What makes your clinic unique?* Identify what sets your clinic apart from competitors. It could be your expertise, your approach to patient care, or the technology you use.
- *What value do you offer?* Identify the benefits patients will receive by choosing your clinic over competitors. It could be a better outcome, a more comfortable experience, or more affordable pricing.

Developing a Consistent Brand Voice

Developing a consistent brand voice involves creating a tone and style of communication unique to your clinic.[6] Here are some factors to consider when developing your brand voice:

- *Brand personality*: Your brand personality should reflect your clinic's values, mission, and personality. It should be consistent across all communication channels.
- *The tone of voice*: The tone of voice used in your communication should be appropriate for your target audience and reflect your clinic's personality.
- *Communication channels*: The tone and style of communication should be consistent across all communication channels, including your website, social media, and marketing materials.

INTERNAL MARKETING: CULTIVATING A STRONG ORGANIZATIONAL CULTURE

Fostering a Sense of Purpose

To kickstart the journey of a thriving hair transplant clinic, cultivating a strong organizational culture is paramount. This begins with fostering a sense of purpose among all team members. By clearly communicating the clinic's mission and values, employees are motivated to align their efforts with the overall objectives. A unified sense of purpose creates a cohesive and passionate team, which directly impacts the quality of patient care.[8]

Building a Supportive Environment

An inclusive and supportive environment is the backbone of a successful hair transplant clinic. Employees who feel valued and supported are more likely to demonstrate enthusiasm in their roles, resulting in enhanced patient experiences. Regular team-building activities, open communication channels, and recognition programs are essential in maintaining a positive workplace culture.[8]

Nurturing a Patient-centric Approach among Staff Members

Understanding Patient Needs

In the realm of hair transplant procedures, each patient comes with unique needs and concerns. A patient-centric approach entails going the extra mile to understand these individual requirements. Listening actively to patients' expectations and fears allows the clinic to tailor personalized solutions, fostering trust and rapport.[9]

Empathy and Compassion

Undergoing a hair transplant can be a sensitive and emotional experience for patients. Therefore, it is vital for the clinic's staff members to demonstrate empathy and compassion at every step of the journey. Treating patients with kindness and understanding not only eases their anxieties but also enhances their overall satisfaction with the clinic's services.

Employee Training and Development for Exceptional Customer Service

Specialized Training

Investing in comprehensive training for employees is a crucial element in delivering exceptional customer service. From medical professionals to administrative staff, each team member should receive specialized training to excel in their respective roles. Continuous education on the latest industry advancements ensures that the clinic remains at the forefront of hair transplant technology and methodologies.

Going Above and Beyond

To truly stand out in the competitive healthcare landscape, the hair transplant clinic must go above and beyond standard service expectations. Encouraging staff members to take the initiative in providing personalized care and addressing patient concerns promptly creates a memorable experience that sets the clinic apart from its competitors.[10]

EXTERNAL MARKETING: EXPANDING THE CLINIC'S REACH

In the competitive healthcare industry, reaching out to potential patients is essential for the success and growth of a clinic. External marketing strategies play a crucial role in expanding a clinic's reach and attracting new patients. In this chapter, we will explore various external marketing approaches that can significantly boost your clinic's visibility and credibility.

Print Marketing

Print marketing remains a potent method to connect with the local community and raise awareness about your clinic's services. It allows you to target specific demographics and create a lasting impression. Let us delve into some effective print marketing strategies.

Designing Impactful Print Materials: Brochures, Flyers, and Pamphlets

First impressions matter, and your clinic's printed materials should leave a lasting impact on potential patients. Professionally designed brochures, flyers, and pamphlets can convey your clinic's values, services, and expertise in a visually appealing manner.[11]

Utilize vibrant colors, eye-catching graphics, and concise yet compelling content to entice readers. Highlight the benefits of your clinic's services and showcase testimonials from satisfied patients. Include essential contact information and a call-to-action to encourage readers to take the next step.

Collaborating with Local Publications for Advertisement Opportunities

Partnering with local publications can be a game-changer for your clinic's marketing efforts. Newspapers, magazines, and community newsletters provide an excellent platform to target a specific audience within your locality.

Work with the publication's advertising department to create captivating ads that align with your clinic's branding. Consider offering special promotions or discounts to attract potential patients. Leveraging the readership of these publications can significantly increase your clinic's visibility in the community.

Visual Marketing

In today's digital age, visual content has become an indispensable tool for engaging potential patients. Visual marketing enables clinics to showcase their success stories and services effectively. Let us explore two powerful visual marketing strategies.

Utilizing before-and-after Visuals to Showcase Success Stories

People are drawn to real-life transformations, and before-and-after visuals can be incredibly compelling. Showcase successful patient outcomes through images and videos, highlighting the remarkable improvements they experienced after receiving treatment at your clinic.[12]

Ensure that the visuals are of high quality and clearly demonstrate the positive impact of your services. With patients' consent, feature these visuals on your clinic's website, social media platforms, and print materials to instill trust and confidence in potential patients.

Leveraging Video Marketing for Engaging and Informative Content

Video marketing has witnessed tremendous growth and engagement in recent years. It allows clinics to connect with their audience on a personal level and deliver informative content.

Create short videos that introduce your clinic's team, facilities, and services. Engage in patient interviews, where they share their experiences and success stories. Additionally, consider producing educational videos that address common medical concerns and offer valuable insights to viewers.[13]

Share these videos on your clinic's website, social media channels, and video-sharing platforms such as YouTube to enhance your online presence and attract a broader audience.

Building a Strong Online Presence

In today's digital landscape, having a strong online presence is non-negotiable. Online marketing techniques can significantly impact your clinic's visibility, attracting a larger audience and increasing patient inquiries. Here are two essential online marketing strategies.

Building a Professional and User-friendly Clinic Website

A website is the foundation of your online presence. It provides potential patients with essential information about your clinic, services, and team.[14] Here are some factors to consider when creating a website for your hair transplant clinic:

- *User experience*: Your website should be easy to navigate, visually appealing, and mobile-responsive. It should also have clear calls to action, making it easy for potential patients to contact you.
- *Content*: Your website should have high-quality, informative content that educates potential patients about hair transplant procedures and builds trust.

Search Engine Optimization for Increased Online Visibility

A search engine optimization (SEO) strategy can help your clinic rank higher in search engine results pages (SERPs). Here are some factors to consider when developing an SEO strategy:

- *Keyword research*: Identify relevant keywords that potential patients use to search for hair transplant clinics in India. Use these keywords throughout your website and content to improve your search engine rankings.
- *Link building*: Build backlinks to your website from high-quality, relevant websites. This can help improve your website's authority and search engine rankings.

To enhance SEO, focus on building quality backlinks from reputable healthcare websites, directories, and social media platforms. Engage with your audience through social media, responding to queries, and sharing valuable content regularly.

Social Media Marketing

Social media marketing can help you reach a wider audience and engage with potential patients. Here are some strategies to consider:

- *Identify the right platform*: Identify the social media platforms your target audience uses the most. Focus your efforts on those platforms to maximize your reach and engagement.
- *Create engaging content*: Create engaging content that educates, entertains, and informs your audience. This can include before-and-after photos, patient stories, and educational content about hair transplant procedures.

Google My Business Listing

A Google My Business listing is a free online listing that provides essential information about your clinic, including your address, phone number, and hours of operation. Here are some factors to consider when creating a Google My Business listing:

- *Complete your profile*: Fill out all the essential information on your Google My Business listing, including your address, phone number, and hours of operation.
- *Add photos*: Add high-quality photos of your clinic, team, and before-and-after photos of your patients.

GENERATING LEADS

Generating leads is crucial for the success of your hair transplant clinic in India. Here are some strategies to consider when developing a lead generation strategy.

Developing a Lead Generation Strategy

A lead generation strategy can help you attract potential patients and turn them into paying customers. Here are some factors to consider when developing a lead generation strategy:

- *Targeting*: Identify your target audience and create marketing materials that speak directly to them. This can include social media ads, email marketing, and website content.
- *Offering incentives*: Offer incentives for potential patients to contact your clinic. This can include free consultations, discounts on procedures, and promotional offers.

Utilizing Paid Advertising

Paid advertising can help you reach a wider audience and generate more leads. Here are some platforms to consider:

- *Google Ads*: Google Ads can help you reach potential patients actively searching for hair transplant services in India.
- *Facebook Ads*: Facebook Ads can help you target potential patients based on their demographics, interests, and behaviors.

Developing Referral Programs

Referral programs can help you generate more leads through word-of-mouth marketing. Here are some factors to consider when developing a referral program:

- *Incentivizing referrals*: Offer incentives for patients who refer their friends and family to your clinic. This can include discounts on procedures, free consultations, and promotional offers.
- *Making it easy*: Make it easy for patients to refer their friends and family by providing them with referral cards, email templates, and social media posts.

Organizing Promotional Events

Promotional events can generate more leads and attract potential patients to your clinic. Here are some events to consider:

- *Open houses*: Organize an open house event where potential patients can tour your clinic, meet your team, and learn about hair transplant procedures.
- *Educational seminars*: Host seminars about hair transplant procedures and the latest trends in the industry.

NURTURING LEADS INTO PATIENTS

Nurturing leads is essential for converting potential patients into paying customers. Here are some strategies to consider when nurturing leads into patients.

Understanding the Patient Journey

Understanding the patient journey can help you identify potential roadblocks and opportunities for improvement. Here are the three stages of the patient journey:

1. *Awareness*: At this stage, potential patients become aware of your clinic and services.
2. *Consideration*: At this stage, potential patients are considering your clinic and comparing it to other options.
3. *Decision*: At this stage, potential patients choose your clinic over others.

Creating a Positive Patient Experience

Creating a positive patient experience can help you build trust and credibility with potential patients.[15] Here are some factors to consider when creating a positive patient experience:

- *Communication*: Communicate clearly and promptly with potential patients. This can include responding to inquiries, providing detailed information about procedures, and addressing concerns.
- *Comfort*: Create a comfortable and welcoming environment for patients visiting your clinic.
- *Follow-up*: Follow-up with patients after their procedures to ensure they are satisfied with the results and to address any concerns.

Creating Educational Content

Creating educational content can help you establish your clinic as a thought leader and educate potential patients about hair transplant procedures.[16] Here are some types of educational content to consider:

- *Blog posts*: Write blog posts about hair transplant procedures, the latest trends in the industry, and patient success stories.
- *Videos*: Create videos that demonstrate hair transplant procedures, answer frequently asked questions, and provide tips for postprocedure care.
- *Social media posts*: Share educational content on social media platforms such as Facebook and Instagram to reach a wider audience.

RETAINING PATIENTS

Retaining patients is essential for the long-term success of your hair transplant clinic in India. Here are some strategies to consider when retaining patients.

The Importance of Patient Retention

Patient retention is critical for the following reasons:

- *Cost-effective*: Retaining existing patients is more cost-effective than acquiring new ones.
- *Referrals*: Satisfied patients are more likely to refer friends and family to your clinic.
- *Trust*: Building long-term patient relationships can help establish trust and credibility with your clinic.

Developing a Patient Retention Strategy

Developing a patient retention strategy can help keep patients returning to your clinic.[17] Here are some factors to consider when developing a patient retention strategy.

- *Communication*: Communicate regularly with patients through email newsletters, social media, or other channels.
- *Education*: Continue to educate patients about hair transplant procedures, postprocedure care, and the latest trends in the industry.
- *Offer incentives*: Offer incentives, such as discounts on future procedures or referral bonuses, to encourage patients to return to your clinic.

Creating a Loyalty Program

Creating a loyalty program can help you reward patients for their loyalty to your clinic.[18] Here are some elements to consider when creating a loyalty program.

- *Rewards*: Offer rewards for returning patients, such as discounts, free procedures, or exclusive access to events.
- *Tiered system*: Consider creating a tiered system where patients can unlock additional rewards based on their loyalty to your clinic.
- *Ease of use*: Make the loyalty program easy to understand and use so patients are more likely to participate.

Implementing Patient Feedback

Implementing patient feedback can help you improve the patient experience and address any concerns or issues that patients may have.[19] Here are some ways to implement patient feedback:

- *Surveys*: Conduct patient satisfaction surveys to collect feedback on the patient experience and identify areas for improvement.
- *Follow-up*: Follow-up with patients after their procedures to ask for feedback on their experience and any concerns they may have.
- *Address concerns*: Address any concerns or issues patients may have promptly and professionally.

BUILDING PARTNERSHIPS

To increase the reach and credibility of your hair transplant clinic, it is essential to build partnerships with other healthcare providers and influential individuals. This can help you tap into their existing networks and build trust with potential patients. Here are a few ways you can build partnerships:

- Network with other healthcare providers, such as dermatologists and plastic surgeons, and offer hair transplant services for their patients.
- Collaborate with medical tourism agencies and travel companies to offer hair transplant packages to patients from other countries.
- Partner with local businesses, such as gyms and spas, to offer discounts or promotions to their clients.

Developing Partnerships with Other Healthcare Providers

One effective way to build partnerships with other healthcare providers is to offer complementary services. For example, you could partner with a dermatologist or an aesthetician to offer a complete package of services for patients looking to improve the appearance of their hair and skin. You could also partner with a plastic surgeon to offer a comprehensive approach to facial rejuvenation.

Utilizing Influencer Marketing

Influencer marketing is another effective way to reach your target audience and increase brand awareness.[14] Here are a few ways you can utilize influencer marketing:

- Identify influencers in the beauty and wellness industry who have a significant following on social media and collaborate with them to promote your clinic.
- Sponsor beauty and wellness events and invite influencers to attend and promote your clinic on their social media channels.
- Offer discounts or complimentary services to influencers in exchange for promoting your clinic to their followers.[20]

ANALYZING YOUR MARKETING EFFORTS

Analyzing your marketing efforts is the first step in understanding the effectiveness of your marketing strategies. Here are a few ways you can analyze your marketing efforts:

- Track the number of leads generated from each marketing campaign.
- Monitor the conversion rate of leads into actual customers.
- Keep an eye on your website traffic and engagement metrics.
- Analyze your social media engagement and follower growth.

The Importance of Tracking Your Marketing Efforts

Tracking your marketing efforts is essential to determine the effectiveness of your marketing campaigns. It helps you identify which marketing tactics are working and which ones are not.[21] This information can be used to optimize your marketing strategies and ensure you get the best ROI for your marketing spend.

Utilizing Analytics Tools

Analytics tools can help you analyze your marketing efforts and provide valuable insights into your target audience's behavior. Here are a few analytics tools you can use:

- *Google Analytics*: It tracks website traffic and engagement metrics.
- *Facebook Insights*: It provides insights into your Facebook page's performance.
- *Hootsuite Analytics*: It provides social media analytics for multiple platforms.

Adapting Your Marketing Strategy

Adapting your marketing strategy based on your analysis is crucial to ensure that your marketing efforts are practical.[21] Here are a few ways you can adapt your marketing strategy:

- Optimize your website for search engines.
- Focus on social media marketing to reach your target audience.
- Use targeted advertising to reach specific audiences.
- Engage with your customers through email marketing.

COMPLIANCE WITH ADVERTISING REGULATIONS

Understanding advertising regulations is critical to ensuring your marketing efforts are legal and ethical. Here are a few things to keep in mind:

- The Advertising Standards Council of India (ASCI) governs advertising regulations in India.[22]
- ASCI guidelines require that advertising is honest, truthful, and not misleading.
- ASCI guidelines also prohibit offensive, inappropriate, or harmful advertising to minors.

Understanding Advertising Guidelines

Complying with advertising guidelines in India is crucial to avoid any legal issues or negative consequences. Here are a few guidelines to keep in mind:

- Hair transplant clinics cannot advertise hair transplantation as a guaranteed or permanent solution to hair loss.
- Hair transplant clinics must use actual, unedited photographs of their patients in their advertisements.
- Hair transplant clinics must include disclaimers in their advertisements stating that the results of hair transplantation may vary from person to person.

Avoiding False or Misleading Claims

Making false or misleading advertising claims can result in legal consequences and damage your clinic's reputation. Here are a few things to keep in mind:

- Do not promise immediate or guaranteed results from hair transplantation.
- Do not make claims that cannot be substantiated with evidence.
- Do not use before-and-after photos that have been digitally altered or edited.

SUMMARY

Marketing is essential to establish a successful hair transplant clinic in India. You may expand your customer base, advertise to the right people, and receive more exposure for your business as a result. A well-designed marketing strategy can help you differentiate your clinic from your competitors and position yourself as a trusted and reliable provider of hair transplantation services.

In conclusion, marketing is crucial to establish a successful hair transplant clinic in India. By analyzing your marketing efforts, building partnerships, complying with advertising regulations, and utilizing influencer marketing, you can reach your target audience effectively and attract new patients to your clinic. Investing in marketing can help you grow your clinic and establish a strong presence in the hair transplantation industry in India.

REFERENCES

1. Hair transplant industry is witnessing a rise in demand despite challenges. Times of India. [online] Available from https://timesofindia.indiatimes.com/blogs/voices/hair-transplant-industry-is-witnessing-a-rise-in-demand-despite-challenges/. [Last accessed October, 2023].
2. The growing demand and advancements in hair transplant market: a comprehensive overview. [online] Available from https://www.openpr.com/news/3050676/the-growing-demand-and-advancements-in-hair-transplant-market. [Last accessed October, 2023].
3. Redmond WH. Marketing fundamentals. Occup Med. 2001; 16(3):471-81, iv.
4. Devonshire E, Dodds S, Costa D, Denham R, Fitzgerald K, Schneider CR. Educating and engaging a new target audience about the problem of pain for society. Br J Pain. 2022;16(6):641-50.
5. Santiago S, Talbert EC, Benoza G. Finding Pete and Nikki: defining the target audience for "The Real Cost" campaign. Am J Prev Med. 2019;56(2 Suppl. 1):S9-15.
6. Sammut-Bonnici T. Brand and branding. In: Cooper CL, McGee J, Sammut-Bonnici T (Eds). Wiley Encyclopedia of Management. Hoboken, NJ: Wiley; 2015.
7. Farrell A, Lee N. Unique selling proposition. In: Cooper CL, McGee J, Sammut-Bonnici T (Eds). Wiley Encyclopedia of Management. Hoboken, NJ: Wiley; 2015.
8. Rusu ML. The military organization—a culture of innovation. Land Forces Acad Rev. 2023;28:126-35.
9. Scheepers RA, Boerebach BC, Arah OA, Heineman MJ, Lombarts KM. A systematic review of the impact of physicians' occupational well-being on the quality of patient care. Int J Behav Med. 2015;22(6):683-98.
10. Mysore V, Kumaresan M, Garg A, Dua A, Venkatram A, Dua K, et al. Hair transplant practice guidelines. J Cutan Aesthet Surg. 2021;14(3):265-84.
11. Legge GE, Bigelow CA. Does print size matter for reading? A review of findings from vision science and typography. J Vis. 2011;11(5):10.1167/11.5.8 8.
12. Chen X, Hay JL, Waters EA, Kiviniemi MT, Biddle C, Schofield E, et al. Health literacy and use and trust in health information. J Health Commun. 2018;23(8):724-34.
13. Pu J, Hou J, Wei L, Sun Y. The analysis of marketing strategy of short video platforms—taking Douyin as example. Adv Econ Manage Political Sci. 2023;9:355-60.
14. Garett R, Chiu J, Zhang L, Young SD. A literature review: website design and user engagement. Online J Commun Media Technol. 2016;6(3):1-14.
15. Georgieva G. Effective doctor-patient communication a key factor for assessing patient satisfaction with dental services provided. MEDIS Int J Med Sci Res. 2023;2:45-51.
16. Maharyawan I, Swarjana I, Rismawan I, Pranata Gst. The experience of nurse anesthetists in educating patients and families: a qualitative study. Nurse Health J Keperawatan. 2023;12:54-63.
17. Arora A, Siddhey PK. Retaining sustainable customers through online marketing. In: Gupta N, Shinde R, Malviya RK, Gupta A (Eds). Industry 5.0 and Paradigm Shift: Emerging Challenges. Mumbai, Maharashtra: Allied Publishers Private Limited; 2023.
18. Güzel R, Oktay K, Orynbaeva U. Guest loyalty programs of chain hotels: the case of Turkey. Eurasian J Econ Bus Stud. 2023;67: 69-78.
19. Al-Jabr H, Twigg MJ, Katangwe-Chigamba T, Saadvandi R, Desborough JA. Patient feedback on hospital pharmacists' consultation skills: a feasibility study using the Interpersonal Skills Questionnaire (ISQ). PLoS One. 2022;17(7):e0268544.
20. Mundkur J. Qoruz: riding the influencer marketing wave. Emerald Emerg Markets Case Stud. 2023;13:1-20.
21. Kabiraj S, Joghee S. Improving marketing performance: how business analytics contribute to digital marketing. Int J Technol Innov Manage. 2023;3:9-18.
22. https://www.ascionline.in/

CHAPTER 96

Website and Search Engine Optimization

Aniketh Venkataram

Key Messages

- Your website is your identity on the internet. It is the only online domain you have total control over.
- A website must be functional, user friendly, and mobile friendly.
- Consistency and relevance are crucial for search engine optimization (SEO).
- Constant effort and long-term planning give better outcomes than short-term hacks.

INTRODUCTION

There was a time not too long ago when having a website was not considered a necessity. In today's mobile world, however, it is essential. Doctors are traditionally not very tech-savvy and often have difficulty figuring out the online world. This chapter aims to provide some basic information on how to have a good performing website.

WHY DO I NEED A WEBSITE?

This question is similar to asking why do I need a clinic? Your clinic is a location where people can find, meet, and interact with you. A website accomplishes the same thing in the virtual world. It is your identity, your brand, and your persona on the internet. With the advent of smartphones, the amount of time an individual spends on the internet has skyrocketed. Nowadays, people are becoming habituated to looking up any place or product online before physically going there. If you do not have a good website, you might not have people coming at your door.

HOW DO I BUILD A WEBSITE?

There are basically four steps:

1. Choosing your website platform
2. Choosing a domain name and host
3. Planning your content
4. Building your website

Choosing Your Website Platform

There are basically two ways to build a website: (i) Using a content management system (CMS) or (ii) building a custom website.

A CMS is a system that uses a program or framework to build a website in a certain set manner. This is something that anyone with decent computer skills would be able to understand. Some examples of CMS include WordPress and Wix. WordPress is the most popular CMS and accounts for 30% of all websites. The advantage of using a CMS is that it is easier to use, cheaper, faster to set up, and easier to update. On the downside, there is a limit to how much you can customize it.

A custom website is one that is built for you specifically using a programming language such as PHP. This is something that needs coding knowledge and needs professional IT individuals. It is highly customizable but needs more time and effort and would cost more.

Choosing a Domain Name and Host

Once your platform is chosen, you choose and register a domain name (www.yourdomainname.com) and host for your website. With CMS, this may be built in. A host is basically a server that stores your website. Based on your domain name and host, you would have to pay regular fees to keep renewing this.

Planning Your Content

The next step is to decide what you want on your website, organizing it, and actually building the website itself. With CMS, this is fairly easy to do or supervise if you are not doing it yourself. With a custom website, you would have to rely entirely on your web developer to do this, even for minor updates.

Building Your Website

Once you have planned your content, the next part is to actually build the website. Since there are so many websites nowadays, it is no longer enough to just have a website, but it is essential you have a well-performing one. Performance means your website should be easy to find in a search engine. So, in order to build your website effectively, it is important to understand how search engines work.

WHAT ARE SEARCH ENGINES?

Because there are so many websites, it became essential to have a means to navigate and find what you are looking for. This led to the birth of search engines. Search engines go through all available websites on the internet and build a catalog of them so that when you search for something, it provides you with what it thinks are the best options for what you are looking.

WHAT IS SEARCH ENGINE OPTIMIZATION?

In simple terms, it is the process of trying to get your website to rank as highly as possible on a search engine. Because there are so many websites for any given topic, if you want your website to be seen, it is important you rank highly, preferably on the first page of a search engine. Studies have shown that most users do not go past the first page of Google. The higher you rank on a search engine, the more visitors you get. The more the visitors to your site, the more they interact with you.[1]

It is important to distinguish search engine optimization (SEO) from search engine marketing (SEM). SEO refers to improving the ranking of *unpaid* results, that is, you do not pay any money to the search engine to increase your site's visibility. SEM refers to the process of placing ads with search engines for them to be visible easily.

HOW DO SEARCH ENGINES WORK?

Search engines are programmed to analyze a website's content and understand what that site is about. It does this by using programs called spiders, which scan and analyze websites. These spiders pick up keywords and catalog the website under that keyword.

A keyword is any word or phrase that the search engine considers relevant. A single website can be ranked under more than one keyword. The more relevant a website is considered for a particular keyword, the higher it ranks.

Apart from keywords, the spiders also recognize other factors such as website loading time and content such as photos and videos and links. All of this information is fed into the search engines algorithm. This algorithm is a complex formula (that is proprietary and unique to each search engine). The algorithm then decides what ranking to assign each website for that keyword.

While keywords are important, they are not the end-all to your website's ranking. Earlier search engines relied on them exclusively, which meant that they could be manipulated. Modern search engine algorithms employ a much more holistic approach to calculating your ranking.[2]

WHY IS GOOGLE THE BIGGEST SEARCH ENGINE AND HOW DOES IT WORK?

Initially, there were many competing search engines. Google, however, quickly overtook all of them. This is because it built a huge index of websites and was much faster than others. It gave incredibly relevant results and used the most advanced technology.[3]

No one can claim to know exactly how the Google algorithm works. One key change that Google made was to introduce personalized results for searches. This means that Google keeps a record of your prior internet activity and searches. It then tailors the results of a particular search for you. In essence, if two different people perform the same search, they can get two different lists of websites with different rankings.

WHAT ARE THE FUNDAMENTALS OF SEARCH ENGINE OPTIMIZATION?

The Google algorithm is constantly being updated and modified. What this means is that there is no "hack" or quick way to rank highly on Google. Your website should be built on strong fundamentals to provide the best user experience and Google will reward you accordingly. The following are the principles to keep in mind:

- *Relevance*: The most important thing to remember while building your website is to make it relevant. Your website should be focused on plastic surgery and aim to provide as much useful information on the topic as possible. Search engines keep a track of how much time a person spends on a website. If someone reaches your website for a particular search but then leaves your site quickly, Google downgrades your ranking for the search the next time in favor of a website that keeps the user engaged for a longer time.

- *Consistency*: Your website should be easy to understand both for a user and for a search engine. To achieve this, keep your website well organized and consistent, in terms of both design and content.
- *Build for the long-term*: As mentioned before, you should look at building a strong website for the long term. Try to avoid hacks which might work in the short term but would ultimately be punished by Google.
- *Remember your aim*: The aim of your website is to get the most conversions. There is no point in having a high ranking and high traffic of people visiting your website if they do not like what they see and call you.

HOW TO BUILD YOUR WEBSITE FOR SEARCH ENGINE OPTIMIZATION?

The most important thing to keep in mind while building your website is to keep it user oriented. That should be your first and last concern.

Organization

Keep your website organized. If you have a lot of pages on a lot of topics, organize them into groups (or silos) and have a separate landing page for each silo. This makes it easier for a user to navigate your site and also for a search engine to index your site. Try to make it as intuitive as possible.

Design

While your design should be eye-catching, it should not slow down your website or make it difficult to use. Choose a simple functional design that works for you and make it consistent across the website.

Content

Search engines love a variety of content. Apart from text, use pictures and videos to your advantage. Remember that images can come up separately in Google's image search. Videos can drive traffic from YouTube. Having different types of content caters to different audiences. It is important to create your unique content and not copy from other sites. Google punishes plagiarism.[4]

Mobile Friendly

It is *imperative* that your website be mobile friendly. Two-thirds of all internet use today is done on mobile devices. Mobiles overtook desktops in 2015.[5] This is a fact that can be missed as the website is usually made on a desktop. Do not forget to see how your website performs on a mobile phone.

Updates

Once your website is up and running, the work does not end there. It is important to keep updating your website with news and information. Search engines give a higher preference to websites that keep adding new information rather than remaining static.

HOW DO I USE KEYWORDS EFFECTIVELY?

You might have surmised by now that keywords are very important toward your website's SEO. In order to use keywords effectively, you must first decide which ones to use. Do some research to decide which keywords you want to use for which pages on your website. Choose the most relevant keywords. As mentioned before, there is no point using keywords which drive a lot of traffic to your site if that does not lead to conversions. Apart from basic general keywords, do not ignore more specific ones. While these might not lead to as much traffic as more general ones, the traffic they do generate is more likely to convert.[6]

Once you have decided your keywords, distribute them effectively in your website. Some places you can use them include headings, image titles, captions, and judiciously in the body of your matter. Be careful to avoid stuffing them in your site. This can be downranked by Google as it will deem it to be spam.[7]

SUMMARY

There are a lot more advanced techniques to website building and SEO. The aim of this chapter is to provide a basic understanding and fundamentals for you to start with. It is important to understand that SEO is not a one-time job, and there is no shortcut to it. Search engine algorithms are constantly being changed. Rather than trying to understand the algorithm and manipulate it, the best course is to use basic principles to provide a relevant, useful website that adequately represents you and your practice.

REFERENCES

1. Ortiz-Cordova A, Jansen BJ. Classifying web search queries to identify high revenue generating customers. J Am Soc Inform Sci Technol. 2012;63(7):1426-41.
2. *Demers J.* Is Keyword Density Still Important for SEO. *Forbes*. 2016. Retrieved August 15, 2016. https://ahrefs.com/seo/glossary/keyword-density#:~:text=Is%20keyword%20density%20important%20for,search%20intent%20in%20other%20ways.
3. Jarboe G. (2007). Stats Show Google Dominates the International Search Landscape. Search Engine Watch. [online] Available from https://www.searchenginewatch.com/2007/02/22/stats-show-google-dominates-the-international-search-landscape/ [Last accessed September, 2023].
4. Google Search Quality Updates. Google Blog. https://developers.google.com/search/updates/core-updates.
5. Inside AdWords: Building for the next moment. Google Inside Adwords. Retrieved May 15, 2015. https://adwords.googleblog.com/2015/05/building-for-next-moment.html.
6. The Most Important SEO Strategy. *clickz.com. ClickZ*. Retrieved April 18, 2010. https://www.clickz.com/maximize-your-video-seo-in-2023-proven-strategies-for-success/.
7. Kesmodel D. (2005). Sites get dropped by search engines after trying to 'optimize' rankings. Wall Street Journal. [online] Available from https://www.wsj.com/articles/SB112714166978744925 [Last accessed September, 2023].

CHAPTER 97

YouTube

Suneet Soni

INTRODUCTION

In today's digital age, YouTube has become a powerful platform for education and information dissemination. As a hair transplant surgeon, utilizing YouTube to educate people about the hair transplant procedure and related topics can be an effective way to reach a broader audience and establish yourself as an authoritative source in the field. In this chapter, we will explore the steps to create informative and engaging content on YouTube to educate people about hair transplants.

ETHICAL ISSUES

The following issues should be kept in mind:

- Doctors are not legally allowed to advertise; only educational videos can be produced.
- Informed and written consent from patients is mandatory before publishing their videos or pictures in public or on any social media platform.

CREATING AND CUSTOMIZING YOUR YOUTUBE CHANNEL

This is done through the following steps:

1. *Sign in or create an account*: Use your Gmail credentials to sign in or create a Google account.
2. *Access YouTube Studio*: Click your profile picture and then select "YouTube Studio."
3. *Create your channel*: Click "Create a channel" and choose between a personal and brand account.
4. *Customize*: Upload a profile picture and banner and write a description to reflect your branding.
5. *Add channel art*: Design eye-catching channel art for your page **(Fig. 1)**.
6. *Upload your first video*: Click "Upload" to add your video, provide details, and set it to public.

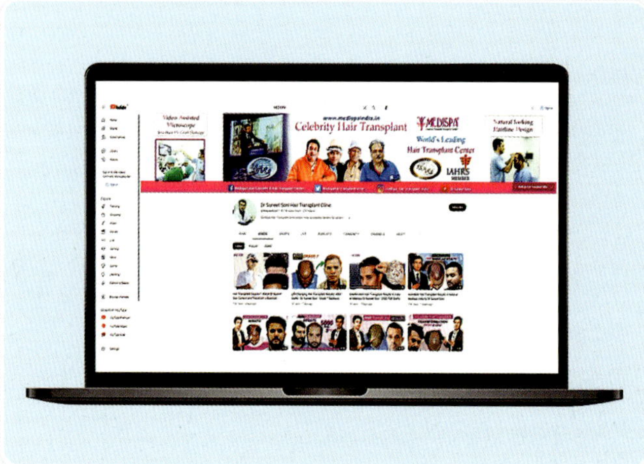

FIG. 1: Example of YouTube channel page.

7. *Optimize*: Use relevant keywords in the title, description, and tags for better search visibility.
8. *Create playlists*: Organize your videos into playlists based on topics such as "hair transplant procedure," "patient testimonials," and "before and after results." This makes it easier for viewers to navigate your content and find what they are interested in.

EDUCATING PEOPLE THROUGH YOUTUBE

YouTube offers an excellent platform to disseminate knowledge about hair transplants. Create well-structured, informative videos that cater to the needs of your target audience. Address frequently asked questions, explain the procedure, and provide insights into the benefits and considerations of hair transplantation. Present the information in a clear, concise, and engaging manner to capture viewers' attention.

- *Know your audience*: Understanding your target audience is vital for creating content that resonates with viewers. Conduct research to identify common demographics and concerns among people seeking information about hair transplants. This knowledge will help you tailor your videos to meet their specific needs.

- *Plan and organize*: Create a content plan that outlines the topics you want to cover and how you will structure each video. A well-organized video will help viewers follow the information easily and keep them engaged throughout the video.
- *Keep it clear and concise*: While in-depth information is crucial, it is essential to present it in a clear and concise manner. Avoid using excessive medical jargon that might confuse viewers. Instead, use simple language to explain complex concepts, making the information more accessible to a broader audience.
- *Use visuals*: Visuals play a crucial role in educating viewers about hair transplants. Incorporate images, animations, and diagrams to illustrate the process, show before-and-after results, and provide a visual representation of the information you are conveying.
- *Address common concerns*: People considering hair transplants often have concerns about the procedure. Address these common concerns in separate videos to give viewers accurate information and help them make informed decisions about their potential treatment.
- *Demonstrate the procedure*: Consider creating educational videos that visually demonstrate the hair transplant procedure. These videos can be a powerful tool to show potential patients what to expect, step by step, during the surgery. It can also help alleviate fears and uncertainties associated with the procedure.
- *Showcase patient testimonials*: Patient testimonials are powerful tools for building trust and credibility. With their consent, feature video interviews or testimonials of satisfied patients who have undergone successful hair transplant procedures. Real-life success stories can inspire and reassure potential patients.
- *Incorporate Q&A sessions*: Regularly host Q&A sessions or "Ask the Surgeon" segments where you answer questions submitted by viewers. This interactive approach fosters a sense of community and encourages engagement with your content. Addressing viewers' specific concerns can help establish you as a reliable authority on the subject.
- *Different aspects of hair transplant*: Diversify your content by creating separate videos that cover different aspects of hair transplantation. Explore topics such as the different techniques [follicular unit extraction (FUE), follicular unit transplantation (FUT)], anesthesia and pain management, preoperative preparation, postoperative care, potential risks, expected outcomes, and the role of genetics in hair loss.
- *Collaborate with industry experts*: Partner with other experts in the field, such as dermatologists, trichologists, and plastic surgeons, to create collaborative videos. This cross-promotion can expand your reach and bring diverse perspectives to your content.
- *Stay updated on advancements*: Keep yourself informed about the latest advancements in hair transplant technology and techniques. Create videos discussing new treatments and their effectiveness, helping your audience stay up to date with the latest developments in the field.
- *Addressing misconceptions*: There are often misconceptions and myths surrounding hair transplants. Use your YouTube channel to debunk these myths and provide evidence-based information to correct misinformation.

UTILIZING KEYWORDS IN YOUTUBE TITLES AND DESCRIPTIONS

Optimize your video titles and descriptions by incorporating relevant keywords related to hair transplants and your expertise. This will improve your videos' visibility in search results, making it easier for potential patients to find your content when seeking information about hair transplants.

INTERACT WITH YOUR COMMUNITY

Engage with your audience beyond videos. Respond to comments on your videos promptly and encourage viewers to share their experiences. Host live Q&A sessions or webinars to create a sense of community and provide personalized responses to their queries.

TECHNICAL SETUP FOR HIGH-QUALITY VIDEOS

- *Camera equipment*: Choosing the right camera
  - Selecting a suitable camera to ensure clear and sharp video footage
  - Considering options such as DSLR or mirrorless cameras with good video capabilities
- *Lighting setup*: Creating a well-lit environment
  - Importance of proper lighting to achieve high-quality visuals
  - Using diffused light sources to minimize harsh shadows and create a professional look
- *Audio quality*: Selecting the right microphone
  - The significance of good audio quality for clear and crisp sound
  - Exploring microphone options such as lapel mics or shotgun mics to capture clear audio

- *Editing software*: Enhancing your videos
  - Utilizing video editing software to enhance the overall quality of the content
  - Editing techniques to improve visuals and audio and create a polished final video

CAPTURING PROPER PRE- AND POSTOPERATIVE IMAGES

Documenting patients' hair conditions before and after the surgery is vital for showing the effectiveness of hair transplants. Ensure consistent lighting, angles, and background for each set of images. Display these images in your videos to demonstrate the transformative impact of the procedure.

SHOOTING THE PROCEDURE

When filming the hair transplant procedure, prioritize patient comfort, safety, and privacy. Obtain explicit consent from patients before recording any part of their treatment. Utilize multiple camera angles to capture various aspects of the surgery. Narrate the procedure step by step, explaining each phase to educate viewers on the intricacies and techniques involved in hair transplantation.

CAMERA AND LIGHTING SETUP

Use high-quality cameras capable of capturing clear and sharp images. DSLR cameras or mirrorless cameras with good video capabilities are popular choices. Ensure adequate lighting to achieve well-lit and detailed footage. Consider using diffused light sources to minimize harsh shadows.

UTILIZING CROMA SHOOTS FOR EDUCATIONAL VIDEOS

Croma shoots can add an extra layer of professionalism and creativity to your educational videos. By using relevant backgrounds, you can visually demonstrate concepts, show images, or add context to your content. Whether you are explaining the hair transplant procedure or discussing advancements in the field, croma shoots can make your videos more visually engaging and captivating for viewers. Remember to maintain a professional appearance while shooting in front of the green/blue screen. Dress appropriately and ensure good lighting and audio quality to deliver a compelling educational experience to your audience.

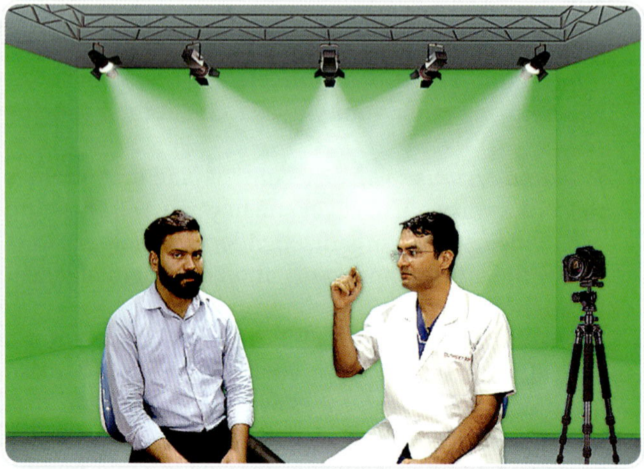

FIG. 2: Croma shoot (green screen).

CROMA SHOOTS

Croma shoots refer to the use of green screen **(Fig. 2)** or blue screen technology to create visually appealing backgrounds in your videos. By shooting in front of a solid-colored backdrop, you can replace the background with relevant visuals, making your content more engaging and professional.

STEPS FOR CROMA SHOOTS

1. *Set up the green/blue screen*: Hang a green or blue screen behind you, ensuring that it covers the entire frame. Ensure the screen is wrinkle-free for a seamless look **(Fig. 2)**.
2. *Proper lighting*: Use well-diffused lighting to eliminate shadows and ensure even illumination on the screen. Proper lighting is essential for a clean keying process.
3. *Camera setup*: Use a high-quality camera with good video capabilities to capture the footage **(Fig. 3)**. Ensure the camera settings are optimized for the best results.
4. *Record the video*: Stand in front of the green/blue screen and deliver your content. Speak clearly and confidently to engage your audience.
5. *Postproduction editing*: Use video editing software with chroma keying capabilities to replace the green/blue background with the desired visuals. Choose relevant backgrounds that enhance your content.
6. *Review and polish*: Watch the edited video to ensure the chroma keying is seamless. Make any necessary adjustments to create a professional-looking final video.

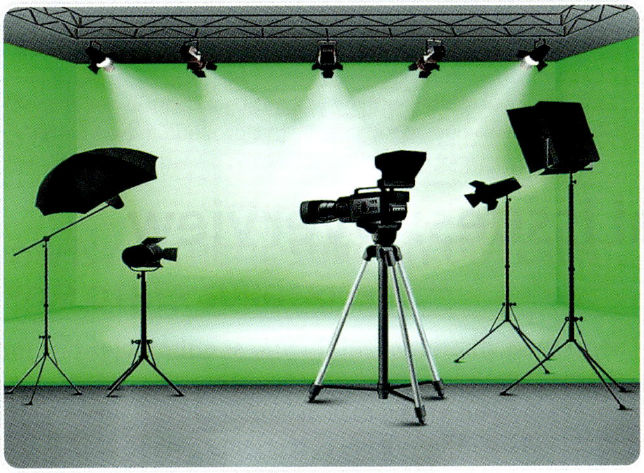

FIG. 3: Camera lighting with green screen.

SUMMARY

Embracing YouTube as an educational platform empowers hair transplant surgeons to positively impact lives worldwide. By delivering informative, engaging, and ethical content, surgeons can foster trust, build a loyal following, and play a vital role in educating individuals seeking hair restoration solutions.

As pioneers in the digital era, hair transplant surgeons have the unique opportunity to connect with their audience, establish authority, and redefine the boundaries of knowledge dissemination in the medical field. Always remember that with great influence comes great responsibility, so prioritize patient care, accuracy, and transparency to make a meaningful difference in people's lives.

ई-मेल/E-mail: ethics@nmc.org.in
वेबसाईट/Website :www.nmc.org.in

110077Pocket- 14, Sector- 8,Dwarka,
Phase – 1, New Delhi-110077

राष्ट्रीय आयुर्विज्ञान आयोग
NATIONAL MEDICAL COMMISSION
आचार और चिकित्सा पंजीकरण बोर्ड
ETHICS & MEDICAL REGISTRATION BOARD

R- 13014/18/2022- Ethics/ Dated the 20th September, 2022

Guideline on Aesthetic Surgery and Hair Transplant Procedures

Hair transplantation:

Any procedure involving a skin incision for the purpose of tissue removal from the scalp or body, or to prepare the scalp or body to receive tissue, (e.g., incising the FUE graft, excising the donor strip, creating recipient sites) by any means, including robotics, is a surgical procedure. Such procedures must be performed by a properly trained and licensed Registered Medical Practitioner (RMP) i.e practitioner of Modern Medicine. RMPs who perform hair restoration surgery must possess the education, training and current competency in the field of hair restoration surgery like adequate knowledge in hair physiology, pathogenesis of scarring and non-scarring alopecia, anatomy and physiology of scalp including scalp vasculature and nerve supply, adequate clinical skill to identify patients who are candidates for hair transplant surgery and contraindications for hair transplant including active scarring alopecia, adequate knowledge and clinical skill pertaining to the medical treatment of alopecia and pre and post-transplant medical care, acquired basic knowledge and skill base in surgeries pertaining to skin and its appendages, adequate training and knowledge pertaining to medical issues and possible adverse reactions that can arise during the hair transplant surgery including basic life support and resuscitation measures.

The hair transplant should preferably be undertaken only by those who have surgical grooming like formal surgical training such as MCh/DNB Plastic surgery, MD/DNB Dermatology with adequate grooming in dermatological surgical procedures. It is also noted that the above-named specialties have Hair transplantation as a core topic in their curriculum.

The following aspects of hair restoration surgery should only be performed by a RMP:

- Preoperative diagnostic evaluation
- Surgery planning
- Surgery execution including: Donor hair harvesting, Hairline design, Recipient site creation and Management of other patient medical issues and possible adverse reactions
- Post-operative care

It is unethical for a RMP to train an individual to perform/assist surgery who is not an accredited health professional licensed to do so.

FIG. 1: National Medical Commission (NMC) notification.

from surgeons for doing multiple procedures while failing to diagnose BDD.[27]

Counseling

Before subjecting a patient to the procedure, the patient should be counseled and given adequate information to enable him/her to take a proper decision. How much information is to be given depends upon what a "prudent client" would expect or demand to know. This should include the type and severity of hair loss that the client has, modes of possible treatment, the procedure proposed, number of sittings, duration and approximate cost of treatment, expected results, need to follow instructions before and after the procedure, possible side effects or complications, etc.[28]

All surgeries have risks.[29-32] Generally, in the surgical field, it is felt that very low risk need not be communicated, but it cannot be so in the case of HT surgery; moreover, even if a specific risk is remote, it may be highly relevant and important in respect of a particular client. For example, an improper hairline may be of more concern to a television newsreader than to a small shop owner in a village.

Good communication skills of the surgeon go a long way in making the client understand things in the proper perspective before they actually decide to undergo the aesthetic procedure and have realistic expectations out of it.[33]

Younger patients need particularly careful handling—repeated sessions of counseling may be needed, and parents may need to be counseled too.[34]

WHAT IS CONSENT?

Under the Indian law, consent has not been defined.[35] Consent generally means permission, but legally it is a contract. As per the Indian Contract Act, "two or more persons are said to consent when they agree upon the same thing in the same sense."

In the medical field, it can be defined as an instrument of mutual communication between the doctor and the patient with an expression of authorization/permission/choice by the latter for the doctor to act/not act in a particular way.[36]

Why Should One Take Consent?

In addition to the ethical need to respect the principle of an "individual's autonomy,"[34-37] there is the legal concept that no one has the right to even touch, let alone treat or operate on a person without obtaining permission. Such an unlawful act would be termed "battery" or physical assault and is punishable. Hence, obtaining consent is a must for doing hair transplantation.

What Constitutes a Valid Consent?

There are three important criteria for consent[38] to be valid:

1. It should be given by an adult or in the case of minors, by one parent. For those aged between 12 and 18 years, the law is not very clear.[39] Therefore, it is better to take assent of the teenager and consent of one parent.
2. It should be fully voluntary and free from any kind of coercion, fraud, pressure, inducement, influence, misrepresentation of facts, or mistake.
3. The consenting person must be of sound mind and in the right state of mind at the time of giving consent.

What is an Appropriate Consent for Hair Transplant Surgery?

- It should be a written consent signed by both the client and the doctor.
- It should be signed by a witness, who is preferably an uninterested third party, which does not include a relative or a friend.
- Consent should be an informed consent, which means it should be preceded by adequate disclosure of relevant information as mentioned earlier. Opportunity and time should be given to the client to clarify any doubt.
- Consent should be obtained a day or two earlier and preferably not on the day of the HT surgery. Likewise, it should not be an "old" consent; if it has been obtained months earlier, a fresh consent needs to be obtained.
- Consent form should preferably be in patient's own language and without the use of technical jargon so that it is understood properly.
- Consent is procedure specific. Therefore, consent for one procedure does not mean permission to do anything more in addition or in lieu of. So, there should be a separate consent form for each technique [follicular unit transplantation (FUT)/follicular unit extraction (FUE)] and each area (scalp/eyebrow).
- Consent is person specific. So, if consent is taken by Dr A, surgery cannot be done by Dr B or by Dr A's assistant.
- Consent is necessary for photographing the patient for scientific/educational/research purposes or for follow-up. Specific consent must be taken if the identity of the patient is likely to be revealed while publishing.
- Specific mention in the consent form is a must if a new procedure or equipment is being tried out.
- There is no prescribed or standard format for a consent form. It should be customized or even handwritten by the client.

Lack of informed consent is a frequent cause of allegations of medical negligence.[40]

A mnemonic—PARCODE can help to remember the important components of an informed consent to be taken before performing HT surgery:

- *P*rocedural details
- *A*lternatives available
- *R*isks involved
- *C*omplications that can arise
- *O*utcome expected
- *D*uration of treatment (average)
- *E*xpenses involved (approximate)

Client's signature on a dotted line obtained casually by a staff cannot constitute a proper consent and can be contested legally by the client.

Should Consent Process be Video Recorded?

It has become the practice in many hospitals to record the consent process by video, though it is not mandatory. This has the advantage over written consent, which obviously cannot include everything that is spoken. Also, it would be difficult for a client to deny what is recorded. It may be useful when the patient is not able to read or write.

IMPORTANCE OF DOCUMENTATION

The medical record is admissible as documentary evidence in a legal suit. So, it is important to maintain meticulous record,[40] clinical details of the client, counseling process, consent taking, detailed preoperative, operative, and postoperative notes (including number of grafts, type of grafts, and donor area) and instructions, follow-up visits, etc.

Photographs taken before and after the procedure provide adequate proof of the outcome of the procedure. The client will not be in a position to claim a lack of improvement later. The patient's failure to adhere to postprocedure consultations, neglect of precautions, and noncompliance of instructions, if any, should also find a place in the record.

Manual records carry greater evidentiary value, but computerized data helps in standardization, storage, and easy retrieval of records.[41]

Medical records of hair transplantation must be preserved for 3 years, but those pertaining to malpractice suits must be preserved until the final settlement of the case. But it must be noted that under CPA, the consumer forums have the power to condone delay in filing a case of negligence beyond the prescribed limitation period of 2 years from the date of occurrence of the alleged negligent act.[42]

Custodial ownership of medical records vests with the HT surgeon or the hospital. But on request by the client or an authorized representative, a copy has to be provided within 72 hours.[43]

Erased entries and overwritings are always viewed with suspicion by the courts. Therefore, all corrections must be done by scoring so that the previous entry is still visible, and the rewriting is done under signature with date and time.

Missing consent papers,[44] tampered medical records, and failure to record the name of the anesthetist[45] may be interpreted as medical negligence.

Medical record is the doctor's best defense against charges of medical negligence.

Confidentiality of Medical Data

The client has the right to confidentiality of medical information. It flows from the right to privacy and autonomy, which, in turn, emanates from the *Right to Life and Liberty* enshrined in *Article 21* of the Indian Constitution.[38] When medical data is computerized, there is a risk of unauthorized access and a breach of confidentiality of clients' sensitive information.

Failure to protect the confidential medical data of a patient could lead to civil liability for invasion of privacy and intentional or negligent infliction of emotional distress.

Inadvertent disclosure of human immunodeficiency virus (HIV) positive status of a patient may be held negligent.[46]

The Delhi High Court has held that medical information is of a personal nature and does not come under the purview of the Right to Information Act unless public interest is involved.[47]

NEGLIGENCE

Negligence per se is defined as "conduct, whether of action or omission, which may be declared and treated as negligence without any argument or proof as to the particular surrounding circumstances, either because it is in violation of statute or because it is so palpably opposed to the dictates of common prudence that it can be said without hesitation or doubt that no careful person would have been guilty of it."

Negligence is the omission to do something which a reasonable man would do or doing something which a prudent and reasonable man would not do. Negligence is culpable rashness and carelessness.

Medical Negligence[42]

Under the Indian legal system, there is no separate law to deal with medical negligence.

Legally, medical negligence is the lack of reasonable care and skill, or willful negligence on the part of the doctor in respect of acceptance of a patient, history taking, examination, diagnosis, investigation, and treatment—medical or surgical, resulting in injury or damage to the patient. Damage may be a physical, mental, or functional injury.

Negligence of a Hair Transplant Surgeon

Medical negligence arises from an act of commission or omission by the HT surgeon, which no reasonably competent and careful HT surgeon would have committed.

What is expected of the surgeon is reasonable skill and care expected from any other similarly qualified surgeon acting in similar circumstance and geographic location. The skill need not be of the highest level.[42] When the standard of care falls below the reasonable standard expected, it is liable to be declared deficient service.

Delegation of some important steps in HT surgery, such as harvesting of grafts to technicians, may be held as medical malpractice.[48]

WHAT IS STANDARD CARE IN HAIR TRANSPLANT SURGERY?[42,49-53]

There is no set standard of care that is universally applicable or acceptable. One of the yardsticks useful in this regard is the standards established by a professional body of similarly qualified aesthetic surgeons in a country or region. Of course, other resources are also helpful—textbooks, peer-reviewed journals, evidence-based guidelines, etc.

Generally, when the medical care is alleged to be substandard by a client, courts take the opinion of expert aesthetic surgeons appearing for both sides to come to a conclusion. But, the stand taken by such an expert witness is not binding on the court. The court will take into consideration whether the deposition of the expert in enunciating what is the standard practice is logical, reasonable, and responsible before taking its own decision as to its acceptability.[42]

The standard of care as existent at the time the aesthetic surgery was carried out is taken into consideration and not that at the time of hearing of the case. For example, trichophytic closure is the most preferred choice now, but was not available earlier and the surgeon cannot be held negligent for not performing the trichophytic closure earlier.

LEGAL LIABILITY OF A HAIR TRANSPLANT SURGEON

A surgeon's liability[54] arises from negligent acts of omission or commission on three fronts—civil liability to pay damages, criminal liability to be punished when the degree of recklessness and negligence is so gross that it is considered a wrong against the society at large, and professional liability to be penalized by the apex medical professional body, i.e., NMC. A single act of negligence can lead to independent liabilities on all the three fronts.

Consumer forums provide a speedier, simpler, and cheaper pathway for aggrieved clients to claim compensation for deficient service in place of prolonged, cumbersome, and expensive civil court procedures. Different liabilities and the consequent actions have been summarized in **Table 1**.

TABLE 1: Different liabilities and the consequent actions.

Law	Forum	Wrong committed	Action
Law of Torts	Civil courts	Injury or damage	Compensation
Criminal Law	Magistrate courts	Death, injury, or risk of injury	Punishment—imprisonment/fine/both
MCI Ethical Code	State Council/MCI	Misconduct	Warning/cancellation of license—temporary or permanent
CPA	Consumer forums	Deficiency of service	Compensation

(CPA: Consumer Protection Act; MCI: Medical Council of India)

MEDICAL MALPRACTICE CASE AGAINST HAIR TRANSPLANT SURGEON

The client who comes up with a case of negligence has the burden to prove the following points to establish negligence of the aesthetic surgeon:

- Duty of the HT surgeon to provide standard care
- Breach of this duty
- Consequent injury or damage
- Direct cause-and-effect relation between the breach of duty and injury/damage

A doctor is not guilty of negligence if he has acted in accordance with a practice accepted as proper by a responsible body of medical men skilled in that particular art. A doctor is not guilty if he is acting in accordance with such a practice, merely because there is a body of opinion that takes a contrary view (Bolam Test).[42,55]

An HT surgeon may be held negligent when he departs from accepted practice. But departure from approved practice per se may not be held negligent if the surgeon is able to justify his actions on the basis of scientific evidence or professional experience. Otherwise, there will be no place for innovations, improvements, and refinement of procedures.

Error in judgment per se is not negligence.[55] The Supreme Court of India has said "It is wrong to assume negligence on the part of the doctor merely because something went wrong with the patient."

Res Ipsa Loquitur[42]

Res ipsa loquitur is a legal concept that literally means "The thing speaks for itself." Suppose a surgeon has operated on the wrong client, wrong part, or wrong side of the body, it will be evident to even a common man that it could have happened only because of negligence. In such a situation, negligence is presumed and the surgeon will have the burden to prove that there was no negligence on his part.

Examples of other situations that may fit into such a legal stand are as follows:
- Not giving a test dose of a drug which has allergic potential such as penicillin and procaine.
- The client experienced an electric shock from equipment during treatment.

Liability of the Healthcare Institution[42,56,57]

The institution is vicariously liable for the negligent acts of medical staff employed by it as the responsibility to appoint competent persons lies with the institution. In addition, the institution is also directly liable for acts of negligence such as not keeping equipment in good working condition and nonavailability of oxygen at times of emergency.

Contributory Negligence[42,58,59]

A patient has certain duties to adhere to. He is expected to act like a reasonable patient. Society expects a patient to conduct in such a way that it would not adversely affect his own safety. If he fails in this duty and it leads to injuries, then it is said to be contributory negligence of the patient. In such a case, damages payable as compensation by the surgeon get reduced in proportion to the degree of the patient's negligence contributing to the injury.

Examples of a patient's conduct which may fall into this category are as follows:
- Not giving a proper past medical history
- Failure to disclose important information such as drug allergy in the past
- Not cooperating during the administration of treatment
- Not adhering to postoperative advice
- Not coming for follow-up, etc.
- A specific example in the case of hair transplantation is noncompliance with taking drug therapy to preserve existing hairs.

Criminal Liability[42]

To fix criminal liability on a surgeon, the standard of negligence required to be proved should be so high that it can be described as "gross negligence" or "recklessness," not merely a lack of necessary care.

Section 304A of the Indian Penal Code (IPC) states "Whoever causes the death of any person by a rash or negligent act not amounting to culpable homicide shall be punished by imprisonment for up to 2 years, or by fine, or both."

The Supreme Court has given the guideline that unless arrest is necessary for furthering the investigation or for collecting evidence or unless the investigating officer feels satisfied that the doctor proceeded against would not make himself available to face the prosecution unless arrested, the arrest may be withheld.[58]

There are two sections in IPC that are helpful. According to Section 80, "Nothing is an offence which is done by accident or misfortune, and without any criminal intention or knowledge in the doing of a lawful act, in a lawful manner, by lawful means and with proper care and caution" and as per Section 88, "Nothing, which is not intended to cause death, is an offence by reason of any harm which it may cause, or be intended by the doer to cause, or be known by the doer to be likely to cause, to any person for whose benefit it is done in good faith, and who has given a consent, whether express or implied, to suffer that harm, or to take the risk of that harm."

- *Taking informed consent for aesthetic surgery is a preventive step.*
- *Proving that the alleged injury or damage was due to accident is a legal defense.*

LEGAL DEFENSE FOR HAIR TRANSPLANT SURGEON[42,60,61]

Professional indemnity insurance that covers cosmetic surgery may be a prudent step to take. Maintaining a cordial relationship with the client and skillful communication go a long way in preventing litigations. In spite of sincere professional job being done and all possible precautions, things can go wrong at times. Many times, frank and truthful discussion with the client can prevent unnecessary litigation. A dissatisfied client may still come up with a case of negligence. At such times, the surgeon should keep his cool and take legal opinion and assistance. Possible defenses available to HT surgeons are described here.

Technical Defenses

- No territorial jurisdiction, for example, District Forums and State Commissions, has fixed jurisdictions.
- No pecuniary jurisdiction, for example, District Forum, can entertain cases claiming damages up to 1 crore rupees, whereas for State Commission, it is up to 10 crore rupees. Only the National Commission can handle damages beyond 10 crore rupees.[62]
- Time-barred—normally a case can be filed within 2 years of the occurrence of the incident.
- If all patients attending a hospital are seen free of cost, the client cannot be considered as a consumer, and hence, CPA will not be applicable. But, liability under civil law of torts still remains.
- Frivolous and vexatious complaint: To extract money or spoil reputation. Unfortunately, there is no scope of imposing a penalty on the complainant.
- Complicated case: To be handled by the Civil Court and not by the consumer forum

Factual Defenses

- Suppression of material facts by the patient, for example, duration of illness, previous illness/treatment, and known drug allergy
- *Contributory negligence:* Patients' or attendants' action has resulted in the damage—lack of follow-up, not following instructions, self-medication, etc.
- *Novus actus interveniens*: A new act in the chain of events between the alleged act of negligence and the resultant damage. For example, simultaneous treatment by another doctor and the use of an alternative system of medicine.

SUMMARY

The increasing popularity of HT surgery has been a global phenomenon. Unlike patients undergoing regular surgery, clients going in for transplant procedures expect perfect results and have zero tolerance for complications. Taking informed consent with full disclosure of all relevant information is of paramount importance. Being competent, following standard procedures, and carrying out HT surgeries with due care in a well-equipped surgical facility go a long way in avoiding mishaps. Good communication skills come in handy to make the client understand the realistic outcomes that can be expected out of the HT surgery and thereby avoid dissatisfaction and consequent litigation.

REFERENCES

1. International Society of Aesthetic Plastic Surgery. ISAPS International Survey on Aesthetic/Cosmetic Procedures performed in 2021. [online] Available from https://www.isaps.org/media/vdpdanke/isaps-global-survey_2021.pdf. [Last accessed October, 2023].
2. Neville JA, Housman TS, Letsinger JA, Fleischer AB, Feldman SR, Williford PM. Increase in procedures performed at dermatology office visits from 1995 to 2001. Dermatol Surg. 2006;32(5):771.
3. Cassetta M. Ethics in aesthetic nursing…avoiding the ugly side of beauty. Plast Surg Nurs. 2008;28(3):117-20.
4. Piras M, Delbon P, Conti A, Graziano V, Capasso E, Niola M, et al. Cosmetic surgery: medicolegal considerations. Open Med (Wars). 2016;11(1):327-9.
5. British Association of Aesthetic Plastic Surgeons. Cosmetic surgery tourists in breast implant risk. [online] Available from https://baaps.org.uk/media/press_releases/1324/cosmetic_surgery_tourists_in_breast_implant_risk/. [Last accessed October, 2023].
6. British Association of Aesthetic Plastic Surgeons. BAAPS consumer safety guidelines. [online] Available from https://baaps.org.uk/patients/safety_in_surgery/consumer_safety_guidelines.aspx. [Last accessed October, 2023].
7. Byrd HS, Barton FE, Orenstein HH, Rohrich RJ, Burns AJ, Hobar PC, et al. Safety and efficacy in an accredited outpatient plastic surgery facility: a review of 5316 consecutive cases. Plast Reconstr Surg. 2003;112:636-41.
8. Stafford BM, La Puma J, Schiedermayer DL. One face of beauty, one picture of health: the hidden aesthetic of medical practice. J Med Philos. 1989;14(2):213-30.
9. Hinderer UT. Indications and significance of esthetic plastic surgery. Handchir Mikrochir Plast Chir. 1984;16(3):145-50.
10. Alam M, Dover JS. On beauty: evolution, psychosocial considerations, and surgical enhancement. Arch Dermatol. 2001; 137(6):795-807.
11. Government of India. The Consumer Protection Act, 1986, published in Gazette of India, Extraordinary, Part II Section I dated 26.12.1986 amended by Act No. 34 of 1991 and 50 of 1993.
12. Indian Medical Association v VP Shantha, AIR 1996 SC 550 (SC 1996).
13. Kunal Saha vs. AMRI. [online] Available from https://lawfoyer.in/kunal-saha-vs-amri/. [Last accessed October, 2023].
14. Botched facial surgery: rare disfiguring result brings record $10 million award. [online] Available from https://abcnews.go.com/

Health/Cosmetic/botched-facelift-surgery-record-10-million-court-award/story?id=13675986. [Last accessed October, 2023].
15. De Sousa A. Concerns about cosmetic surgery. [online] Available from https://www.issuesinmedicalethics.org/articles/concerns-about-cosmetic-surgery/. [Last accessed October, 2023].
16. Kita N. The history of plastic surgery. [online] Available from https://www.verywellhealth.com/the-history-of-plastic-surgery-2710193. [Last accessed October, 2023].
17. Dogra S. Fate of medical dermatology in the era of cosmetic dermatology and dermatosurgery. Indian J Dermatol Venereol Leprol. 2009;75:4-7.
18. Buppert C. Misadventures in cosmetic dermatology. [online] Available from https://www.medscape.com/viewarticle/708186. [Last accessed October, 2023].
19. Mody B. Scar revision is a useless operation. Indian J Plast Surg. 2004;37:23-4.
20. Agarwal P. Perception of plastic surgery in the society. Indian J Plast Surg. 2004;37:110-4.
21. National Medical Commission, Ethics & Medical Registration Board. Guideline on aesthetic surgery and hair transplant procedures. [online] Available from https://www.nmc.org.in/MCIRest/open/getDocument?path=/Documents/Public/Portal/LatestNews/20220927051220.pdf. [Last accessed October, 2023].
22. Goh CL. The need for evidence-based aesthetic dermatology practice. J Cutan Aesthet Surg. 2009;2:65-71.
23. Expert Group on the Regulation of Cosmetic Surgery: Report to the Chief Medical Officer. UK: Department of Health; 2005.
24. Patwardhan N, Mysore V. Hair transplantation: standard guidelines of care. Indian J Dermatol Venereol Leprol. 2008; 74:S46-53.
25. Mysore V, Kumaresan M, Garg A, Dua A, Venkatram A, Dua K, et al. Hair transplant practice guidelines. J Cutan Aesthet Surg. 2021;14(3):265-84.
26. Ritvo E. Never-ending cosmetic surgeries—the patient with body dysmorphic disorder: an expert interview with Eva Ritvo, MD. [online] Available from http://www.medscape.com/viewarticle/725216. [Last accessed October, 2023].
27. Lynn G. et al., Respondents, v. Norman Hugo, M.D., Appellant. 96 N.Y. 2d 306, 752 N.E. 2d 250, 728 N.Y.S. 2d 121 (2001).
28. Rao KHS. Safer practice of dermatosurgery. Indian J Dermatol Venereol Leprol. 2008;74 Suppl.:S75-7.
29. American Society of Plastic Surgeons. Nonsurgical fat reduction. Minimally invasive procedures. [online] Available from https://www.plasticsurgery.org/cosmetic-procedures/nonsurgical-fat-reduction/injection-lipolysis. [Last accessed October, 2023].
30. Whitlock J. Understanding the risks of plastic surgery. [online] Available from https://www.verywellhealth.com/what-are-the-risks-of-plastic-surgery-3156954. [Last accessed October, 2023].
31. Bradbury E. Clinical risk in cosmetic surgery. Clin Risk. 2009; 15:227-31.
32. Nahai F. Minimizing risk in aesthetic surgery. Clin Risk. 2009; 15:232-6.
33. Khoo C. Risk reduction in cosmetic surgery. Clin Risk. 2009; 15:237-40.
34. De U. Genesis and mechanics of malpractice suits—minimizing the risks. Indian J Surg. 2004;66:301-3.
35. Mousavi SR. The ethics of aesthetic surgery. J Cutan Aesthet Surg. 2010;3:38-40.
36. Bastia BK, Kuruvilla A, Saralaya KM. Validity of consent—a review of statutes. Indian J Med Sci. 2005;59:74-8.
37. Satyanarayana Rao KH. Informed consent: an ethical obligation or legal compulsion? J Cutan Aesthet Surg. 2008;1:33-5.
38. Beauchamp TL, Childress JF. Principles of Biomedical Ethics, 5th edition. Oxford: Oxford University Press; 2001.
39. Trehan SP, Sankhari D. Medical Professional, Patient, and the Law: The Institute of Law and Ethics in Medicine, 2nd edition. Bengaluru: National Law School of India University; 2002.
40. Kohli A. Medical consent in India—ethical and legal issues. Anil Aggrawals Internet J Forensic Med Toxicol. 2007;8(2).
41. Government of India, Ministry of Health and Family Welfare, eHealth Section. Notification of electronic health record (EHR) standards—2016 for India. [online] Available from https://main.mohfw.gov.in/sites/default/files/17739294021483341357.pdf. [Last accessed October, 2023].
42. Satish M, Menon R, Rao KV. Professional Accountability and Patients' Rights, 2nd edition. Bengaluru: The Institute of Law and Ethics in Medicine, National Law School of India University; 2002.
43. Indian Medical Council. Indian Medical Council (Professional Conduct, Etiquette and Ethics) Regulations, 2002 (published in Gazette of India, No.14, Part III, Section 4 dated 6.4.2002). New Delhi: Indian Medical Council; 2002.
44. Force vs M Ganeswara Rao. 1998(3) CPR 251; 1998(1) CPJ 413 (APSCDRC 1998).
45. Meenakshi Mission Hospital and Research Centre vs Samuraj and ANR I (2005) CPJ 33 (NC 2005).
46. Dr. Tokugha Yepthomi vs. Appollo Hospital Enterprises Ltd. and ANR III (1998) CPJ 132 (SC 1998).
47. Doctors and Law. Medical records not under RTI: court. [online] Available from https://www.doctorsandlaw.com/2010/02/medical-records-not-under-rti-court.html. [Last accessed October, 2023].
48. Sattur SS, Sattur IS. Patient counselling and medicolegal aspects of hair transplant surgery. Indian J Plast Surg. 2021; 54(4):441-5.
49. Dogra T, Gupta S. Article-10: medico-legal aspect of health care delivery. [online] Available from https://www.ahaindia.org/node/447. [Last accessed October, 2023].
50. Goldberg DJ. Cosmetic dermatology: legal issues. Dermatol Clin. 2009;27:501-5.
51. Goldberg DJ. Medicolegal issues for the dermatologist. Semin Cutan Med Surg. 2000;19(3):181-8.
52. Goldberg DJ. Legal issues in dermatology: informed consent, complications, and medical malpractice. Semin Cutan Med Surg. 2007;26:2-5.
53. Goldberg DJ. Legal issues in laser operation. Clin Dermatol. 2006;24:56-9.
54. Singhal A. The veracity of laws relating to medical malpractice in India. [online] Available from www.ijsrp.org/monograph/Veracity_of_laws_relating_to_medical_malpractice_in_India.pdf. [Last accessed October, 2023].
55. Queen's Bench Division, England. (1957). Bolam versus Friern Hospital Management Committee. [online] Available from https://imlindia.com/downloads/Bolam.v.Friern.Hospital.Management.Committee.pdf. [Last accessed October, 2023].
56. Dr. Kunal Saha vs Dr. Sukumar Mukherjee and Ors. III (2006) CPJ 142 (NC 2006).

57. Shukla R. Medical negligence liability of hospitals. [online] Available from https://www.legalservicesindia.com/article/1741/Medical-Negligence-Liability-of-Hospitals.html#:~:text=Hospitals%20liability%20with%20respect%20to,environment%20for%20treatment%20as%20promised. [Last accessed October, 2023].
58. Satyanarayana Rao KH. Ethics, etiquettes and legal issues. In: Sacchidanand S, Prakash B (Eds). Management Issues for a Dermatologist, 1st edition. New Delhi: Jaypee Brothers Medical Publishers; 2009.
59. Jacob Mathew vs State of Punjab. AIR 2005 SC 3180 (SC 2005).
60. Srinivas P. Consumer Protection Act and Dermatological Practice, A Dermatologist's Perspective of Medical Ethics and Consumer Protection Act: An IADVL Book, 1st edition. Mumbai: Bhalani Medical Book House; 2007.
61. Mathiharan K. Landmark case. [online] Available from https://www.medindia.net/doctors/cpa/case-1_print.asp. [Last accessed October, 2023].
62. Consumer Protection Act, 2019. [online] Available from https://egazette.gov.in/WriteReadData/2019/210422.pdf. [Last accessed October, 2023].

CHAPTER 99

Some Medical–Legal Cases in Hair Transplantation

Anuradha Jindal, Manjot Marwah, Venkataram Mysore

Key Messages

- The rise in the demand for hair transplantation has led to an increase in complications and litigations in the field.
- The legal liabilities include civil liability, criminal liability, and professional liability.
- It is crucial to understand the difference between medical negligence and medical malpractice in legal cases.
- Doctors can be charged under various laws, including Tort law, in India.
- Avoiding false advertisements, ensuring proper qualifications and licenses, and maintaining detailed medical records with consent form are absolutely essential.

INTRODUCTION

There is a constant rise in the demand for hair transplantation with a compound annual growth rate of 25–30% in selected metro and tier-1 cities in India.[1] With the rise in the demand for hair restoration surgery, there is also a rise in the incidence of complications and mishaps during and postsurgery.

Hair transplantation, being an elective cosmetic surgery, the complications—minor or major—or even unsatisfactory results are often taken to courts.

The major change in the Consumer Protection Act (CPA) formulated in 1986, to include the medical profession in the act in 1995 has made a tremendous impact on the relation between the doctor and the patient. The fear of litigation has led hair transplant surgeons to put their guard up and practice more defensively.[2]

Apart from increasing awareness about one's own bodily image, social pressure, increased expectations, circulation of false information over social media platforms with unrealistic results, and tons of quacks and technicians performing hair restoration surgeries have led to a swift rise in lawsuits against doctors and/or clinics.

All the factors that can lead to litigations are included in **Box 1**.

The legal liabilities in case of litigation on a hair transplant surgeon are mentioned below:

If the hair transplantation surgeon is found guilty of unfair/unethical practice and medical negligence, it might lead to one of the following consequences:

- *Civil liability* to pay the damages
- *Criminal liability*—punishment depends on the degree of recklessness and negligence
- *Professional liability*—penalized by the apex medical professional body, i.e., the Medical Council of India

A single act of negligence can lead to independent liabilities from all the other fronts.

The terms medical negligence and malpractice, often used interchangeably, have a different intent and inference as understood by the law and should be well differentiated and understood.

Medical negligence happens when a doctor causes harm to the patient unknowingly, and he/she does not have an intent to do so. It is either a simple ignorance or failing to take action when it was required. While the act of omission is definitely considered as negligence, it is not malpractice as the doctor did not have any intention of harming the patient.

Medical negligence arises in cases such as increased scarring in the donor area, inadequate density of the transplanted site, bald patches, and unaesthetic hairline,[3] whereas *medical malpractice* is when the medical professional is aware of the potential consequences of his/her actions (or nonactions) and proceeds anyway.

BOX 1 Cause of increasing lawsuits.

- *Unrealistic expectations derived from*:
  - Misleading/false advertisements
  - Social media
- *Consultations taken over emails, phone, or teleconsultations lead to*:
  - Communication gap
  - Wrong information about the number of grafts
  - Incomplete discussion about the complications and expected outcome
- *Counselor belonging to a nonmedical field*:
  - Considered as medical negligence

The entire surgery is not done by the doctor alone as HT is a long surgery and most of it is teamwork

- *Lack of follow-up by the patient*:
  - Patients attained via medical tourism
  - Patients working in a different city or country
- Surgeons trying out newer techniques or methods, which are not evidence-based, in research, or not proven to have high efficacy yet
- Progressing androgenetic alopecia (AGA) leading to loss of hair
- *Medical issues*:
  - Patient on blood thinners
  - Keloid formation
  - Scarring
  - Koebnerization—progression or occurrence of vitiligo, psoriasis, or other inflammatory conditions at the site of surgery
  - Reaction to local anesthesia

This may include delegating the surgery to untrained staff, which might result in hairline deformity, scarring, growth failure, and even psychological trauma to the patient. The patient can claim in the court that "the surgery was performed below the acceptable standards of medical practice."[4]

Doctors can be charged under various laws in India, and legal liability in many of the cases may arise out of *Tort law*. Tort law is a branch of law that is primarily developed as "judge-made law" and relies mainly on the principles set on previous judgments.[5,6]

Below, we have cited some examples of such medico-legal cases, judgments made, and discussion on each case to understand practically what can be or should be done in practice to avoid such circumstances.

CASE 1: UNMET ADVERTISED RESULTS

This is a case of a student who was being treated for hair fall at Dr ABC Chandigarh Center of the XYZ clinic in 2007. The student had taken "gold plan for one year" for ₹5,900 thinking that as advertised and assured by the doctor and his team, he would be able to get rid of his hair fall issue. However, after completion of the gold plan, the hair fall persisted, which forced the patient to approach the consumer's forum.

During the appeal in the court, Dr ABC mentioned that it is clearly stated in the terms and conditions that the charges are not refundable or adjustable and the clinic or the doctor does not guarantee anything about the results or the total duration of the treatment.

Outcome

The court found the clinic "indulging in unfair trade practice." The District Consumer Dispute Redressal Forum directed the clinic to refund the money paid by the patient plus a compensation of ₹25,000 for mental harassment. The consumer forum observed that Dr XYZ's clinic had not given any evidence showing that the treatment was carried out with due care and diligence and that they took all necessary steps for the treatment for which they had taken the payment.[7]

Lessons Learned from the Case

- *Avoid false advertisements*—using words such as "*permanent*," "*cure*," or "*guarantee*" in the advertisement.
- Explain the terms and conditions to the patient in detail. Ideally, the patient should be given a time of a day or two and then followed up afterward to start the treatment.
- All treatments given as a package should have a consent, informing in detail about each type of medicine and procedure, so as to avoid any conflict in the future.
- Medical records of all patients should be preserved for at least 3 years by law and if the case is in a lawsuit, till the case settles. However, the CPA provides the power to allow the consumer to file a case even after several years in special cases.
- The Ministry of Health and Family Welfare, Government of India, has published standards for electronic medical records.[8,9]
- Before and after photographs should always be taken and preserved as a proof in such cases.

CASE 2: ALLERGIC REACTION AND FOLLICULITIS AS A COMPLICATION POST HAIR TRANSPLANTATION

A television scriptwriter filed a case in a civil court claiming that his hair transplantation went "horribly wrong," stating that he has started getting frequent allergic reactions and folliculitis on his face and beard area postsurgery. The folliculitis is not controlled with antibiotics and he is forced to take steroids for the same. He alleged a case of fraud, cheating, and criminal breach of trust under the Indian Penal Code (Section 405) and offenses under the Drugs and Magic Remedies (Objectionable Advertisements) Act and the Maharashtra Medical Practitioners Act.

In his complaint, he stated that he approached the clinic after he came across their advertisements and underwent a hair transplant surgery. According to his complaint, Dr XYZ assured that the surgery would be carried out by highly skilled and learned medical practitioners and surgeons, but the entire procedure was done by assistants and a nurse, and there were no certified doctors in the operation theater (OT) during the surgery. The Metropolitan Magistrate directed the police to carry out a preliminary inquiry into the complaint.[10]

The accused doctor claimed that the patient already had allergic tendencies before surgery and was advised to get it checked, but the patient refused to do so. He also stated that they always perform such surgeries in the presence of a plastic surgeon and a dermatologist.

Outcome

The proceedings of the case are unknown; there is no police report or outcome of the case available from any source. It is not known if the case was settled out of court.

Lessons Learned from the Case

- Always take *informed consent mentioning all the common side effects* in detail and explain them to the patient in detail.
- Folliculitis is common after hair transplantation, but an aggressive form of folliculitis can occur due to errors in surgery such as high transection rate, burrowing of grafts, deep implantation, and incorrect slits.
- It is important to put a CCTV in the OT to avoid such false claims.
- Anesthesia, extraction, designing hairline, and making slits are the surgeon's duties, whereas technicians are supposed to do implantation.
- A consent form should mention the role of the doctor and the technician.
- If negligence occurs on behalf of staff or technicians, the doctor will be held responsible for it. Hence, only reliable and experienced staff must be trusted with surgeries.

CASE 3: ANAPHYLACTIC SHOCK LEADING TO DEATH POST HAIR TRANSPLANTATION

Case 3A

A medical student underwent hair transplantation surgery at a clinic in Chennai on May, 17 2016, and died 2 days postsurgery. The family did not file a police complaint, but the case came to light after 1 week when the batchmates urged the Directorate of Medical Education to look into the death of their young friend. The case was forwarded to the Director of Medical Services, and the center was sealed. The body was exhumed, and after a postmortem analysis, it was concluded that he could have died of toxic shock syndrome/septic shock/anaphylactic shock.[11]

Major issue 1: It was discovered that the operating clinic was actually registered as a salon and did not have a license to perform the surgery. One of the persons running the clinic was an MBBS doctor who graduated from China and the other was an anesthetist who was present only for a part of the surgery and not the entire surgery.

Major issue 2: There was no infrastructure to deal with an emergency in the clinic.

The patient had started developing discomfort during the evening of the surgery and he was taken to the operating anesthetist, who examined him and reported it to be a routine case and was dismissed after giving symptomatic care. After this, the patient returned to his village and was brought to a tertiary care medical center intensive care unit (ICU) on the 2nd day with multisystem failure, where he passed away.

Outcome

One year after the case commenced, the Tamil Nadu Medical Council debarred three doctors from practice for misconduct, including attempt to murder and gross negligence that led to the death of the boy.

Lessons Learned from the Case

This was one of the heart-wrenching cases with so many factors being wrong:

- *The license of the premises and adequate qualification of the doctors* performing surgery are a must before proceeding. Adequate sterilization and crash cart preparation before every single surgery should be done.

- A registered doctor has to be present throughout the surgery.
- *A test dose must be done prior* and documented for the anesthetic agent and for any intravenous medications well before the administration of the same.
- If a patient complains of discomfort during the surgery, it is better to record all the findings and tests and try to address the cause of discomfort.
- Continuous monitoring is a must during the surgery. It is the duty of the anesthetist doctor to examine the patient during the discomfort: In this case, the presentation to the anesthetist *was the window of opportunity* where the initial signs of anaphylactic shock could have been picked up.
- Patients residing far from the operating center should be informed about the importance of visiting the clinic on the next day of the surgery. The well-being of the patient postsurgery days also should be documented in the records.

Case 3B

This is a case of a 35-year-old boy from Delhi who underwent hair transplantation at a hair studio. The patient had severe shooting pain over the scalp after the surgery, followed by swelling all over the face and shoulder and labored breathing. The patient's family members tried to contact the center where the surgery was performed, but no one responded, and the technicians fled away. The patient was admitted to a tertiary care center, where he was diagnosed with Stevens–Johnson syndrome with septic shock and multiorgan failure. The young man passed away in the treating hospital.

Major issue 1: The surgery was performed by technicians.

Major issue 2: The clinic had no license and the surgery was performed at a salon.

Lessons Learned from the Case

Apart from the lessons mentioned above:

- Patients should always be provided with a telephone number where they can approach the medical professional postsurgery in case of emergencies, and this should be mentioned in the informed consent as well.
- We need more rules and regulations in place as to who are authorized to perform hair transplantation surgeries.
- Stevens–Johnson syndrome can occur to anyone, with any drug; proper follow-up, early detection, and management will help in preventing such tragedies.
- A test dose of antibiotics must be performed always and documented before administering them intravenously.
- No symptom or sign presented by the patient should be neglected and requires complete evaluation, even if the evaluation might seem unnecessary at that point of time. This can help in justifying that the doctor did what was possible in his reach to prevent or manage the side effects.

CASE 4: "BAD JOB" OF HAIR TRANSPLANTATION

This is a case of a diabetic man who made an agreement with the clinic to undergo a transplant with 6,000 strands of hair for a total of ₹1,40,000. While in the OT, following the implantation of 500 hair strands, the patient had giddiness, headache, diarrhea, and wanted to discontinue the surgery. However, as he had already paid for the procedure, he, at a later date, underwent surgery again. He developed pustules on his scalp postsurgery. He later approached the consumer forum seeking redressal and demanding compensation and refund.

Outcome

The forum observed that the consumer had suffered and had had unnecessary expenditure, which was entirely due to the medical negligence and gross deficiency in service. They stated that the clinic's conduct has been "unethical, unprofessional, highly casual, unconcerned and regardless towards complainant and his health."

The Directorate of Health Services informed that the clinic has not taken any license under the State Medical Practitioner's Act, 2004 and Rules 2011 to operate as a health clinic. The forum directed the clinic to pay a compensation of ₹1 lakh for harming the consumer for "illegal activities of hair transplant." They were also asked to refund ₹95,000 for the remaining 5,000 hair strands that were not implanted and ₹20,000 toward the cost of litigation.[12]

Lessons from the Case

- There is no definition of "standard of care" which is universally acceptable or applicable. In such situations, the standards established by a professional body of similarly qualified aesthetic surgeons in the country or region are regarded as standard of care.
- Other useful resources such as textbooks, peer-reviewed journals, and evidence-based guidelines are also helpful.

- Generally, in court, when medical care is said to be substandard, the court takes the opinion of the expert aesthetic surgeons in the field. But the stand taken by such an expert is not binding on the court. The court will see if the deposition of the expert is reasonable and responsible enough before taking a decision.[13]

CASE 5: INFECTION LEADING TO A WIDE SCAR POST FOLLICULAR UNIT TRANSPLANTATION SURGERY

This is a case of a 25-year-old male who underwent hair transplantation in Seoul in 2012. After the surgery, the patient developed a skin infection that left a 22 × 3 cm scar on his scalp.

Outcome

The Seoul court ruled that the hospital was responsible as the patient lost so much of hair due to faulty hair transplantation. The Seoul Central District Court ordered the two doctors who performed the surgery to pay 54 million won ($65,000) in compensation to the patient.

According to the court, the hospital had excessively cut the scalp during the surgery and did not give proper treatment postsurgery. Scalp incision requires extra care as it can easily get infected.

The court also said in its ruling that the hospital was responsible for paying for the new plastic surgery so that the patient can recover.[14]

Discussion

- A large follicular unit transplantation (FUT) scar with improper closure can occur in cases where surgery is done by an untrained staff/doctor.
- There is no proper law regarding who can do hair transplantation, but proper training to the staff can be provided.
- If a staff member is being trained on a patient, it is important to mention that in the consent form and inform the patient.
- Better to avoid overzealous extraction. Overextraction and dense packing of grafts are common scenarios since the advent of follicular unit extraction (FUE), which can lead to necrosis.
- Many patients travel postsurgery and do not follow up with the surgeon. These cases usually lead to litigation. The documentation of the patient's lack of follow-up and noncompliance to postsurgery instructions should be documented if any.

WHAT CAN BE DONE TO PREVENT LAWSUITS?

Three important things that can prevent lawsuits apart from getting properly trained in the procedure are as follows:

- *Patient selection and counseling*: Identify red flags during the consultation. These should be considered as relative contraindications to avoid future complications.
- *Informed consent*: Not taking consent is considered as medical negligence. The consent form should be complete, should cover all aspects of the surgery, and should be in patient's language, and it should be ensured that the patient reads and understands it. The important components to be covered in the informed consent are given in **Box 2**.
- *Documentation of photos and videos (including video consent)* is especially useful if the patient is not able to read and write.[15,16]

BOX 2 Informed consent.

- Nature and prognosis of hair loss
- Nature of the proposed treatment or procedure and necessary adjuvant treatments needed
- Alternative treatments or procedures that are available for the condition
- Risks of the proposed treatment and alternative treatments or procedures
- Probable outcome and chances of success or failure of the treatment
- Timeline of the events, starting from duration of the surgery, postoperative period, and the final outcome
- Mention all the sequelae to hair transplant—swelling, scabbing, pain, etc.
- Estimated cost of the procedure including pre- and postoperative services
- Full name of the doctor performing the surgery; the form should be duly signed by the doctor
- Consent form to be signed by the patient in addition to a third party (witness)
- The last part of the consent form should include "I acknowledge that I have read this form and have understood the contents. I have been given the opportunity to ask questions, and my questions have been answered to my satisfaction. The risk and benefit of this treatment have been explained to me including the other options available for my condition. I choose to go ahead with hair transplantation"

TABLE 1: Factors causing increased litigations and how these situations can be avoided.

Cause of increasing lawsuits	What can be done to avoid this situation
Unrealistic expectations derived from: • Misleading/false advertisements • Social media	• In-depth counseling • Asking the patient what are his/her expectations and explaining how much of that is achievable • Showing own clinic's result images to set real expectations in the patient's mind • Informed consent regarding filling the number of grafts done and the desired outcome explained to the patient
Consultations taken over emails, phone, or teleconsultations lead to: • Communication gap • Wrong information about the number of grafts • Incomplete discussion about complications and expected outcome	Follow-up in person consultation with the doctor: • Recording everything in the informed consent form • Writing discussed matter in the prescription
Counselor belonging to nonmedical field: • Considered as medical negligence	• Employ medical personnel • Final counseling should be done by the operating surgeon or a qualified doctor
The entire surgery is not done by the doctor as hair transplantation (HT) is a long surgery and most of it is teamwork	• Assign technicians with designated work—extraction of grafts is not acceptable • Refer to Chapter 92 (Role of Assistants in Hair Transplantation)
Lack of follow-up with the patient: • Patients attained via medical tourism • Patients working in a different city or country	• Advise the patient to follow up after the surgery • Provide a timeline for the same—follow up on a weekly basis • Mention the same in informed consent with the contact number (given to the patient) • Make sure the patient reads the consent form and duly signs on every page
Surgeons trying out newer techniques or methods, which are not evidence-based, in research, or not proven to have high efficacy yet	All the practices during and postsurgery should be evidence-derived with proper documentation in textbooks and journals • Follow guidelines laid down by the National Medical Commission (added at the end of the chapter)[17]
Progressing androgenetic alopecia (AGA) leading to loss of hair	• Check for the rate of progression • Inform the patient about the outcome of performing the surgery now • Post-HT treatment with medial therapy—minoxidil, finasteride, and all other measures to suppress the progression of AGA
Medical issues: • Patient on blood thinners • Keloid formation • Scarring • Vitiligo formation • Psoriasis progression • Reaction to local anesthesia	• Complete and detailed medical history • Make a presurgery form mentioning all important questions and ask the patient to fill the form (this avoids missing any important information and also acts as a document for future use if required) • Always do test dose for all intravenous (IV) medicines being used • Keep emergency tray, oxygen cylinder, and defibrillator ready and recheck them routinely • Keep in touch with the anesthetist • Display the contact number of the anesthetist in the operation theater • Keep contact numbers of emergency rooms and hospitals nearby • Avoid long cases post evening

A compilation of the factors leading to litigations and how these can be prevented are given in **Table 1**.

Professional indemnity insurance covering all forms of cosmetic procedures, including hair transplantation, is a must-have for all hair transplant surgeons. The financial liability is huge in the event of a lawsuit. Additional insurance covering the staff is also necessary.

SUMMARY

- Patient selection, proper counseling, and informed consent are the pillars of a conflict-free practice, especially hair transplantation.
- Crystal-clear communication with the patient, along with documentation of each step and storing proofs in

the form of photos and videos, helps in preventing or fighting lawsuits.

- It is important to update yourself from time to time with current guidelines laid down by higher authorities to follow standard care practices during surgery.

GUIDELINES LAID DOWN BY NATIONAL MEDICAL COMMISSION

Guideline on Aesthetic Surgery and Hair Transplant Procedures

Hair Transplantation

Any procedure involving a skin incision for the purpose of tissue removal from the scalp or body, or to prepare the scalp or body to receive tissue (e.g., incising the FUE graft, excising the donor strip, creating recipient sites) by any means, including robotics, is a surgical procedure. Such procedures must be performed by a properly trained and licensed Registered Medical Practitioner (RMP), i.e., practitioner of Modern Medicine. RMPs who perform hair restoration surgery must possess the education, training, and current competency in the field of hair restoration surgery including adequate knowledge of hair physiology; pathogenesis of scarring and non-scarring alopecia; anatomy and physiology of the scalp including scalp vasculature and nerve supply; adequate clinical skill to identify patients who are candidates for hair transplant surgery; contraindications for hair transplant including active scarring alopecia, adequate knowledge and clinical skill pertaining to the medical treatment of alopecia, and pre- and post-transplant medical care; acquired basic knowledge and skill base in surgeries pertaining to skin and its appendages; and adequate training and knowledge pertaining to medical issues and possible adverse reactions that can arise during hair transplant surgery including basic life support and resuscitation measures.

The hair transplant should preferably be undertaken only by those who have surgical grooming like formal surgical training, such as MCh/DNB Plastic Surgery or MD/DNB Dermatology, with adequate grooming in dermatological surgical procedures. It is also noted that the above-named specialties have hair transplantation as a core topic in their curriculum.

The following aspects of hair restoration surgery should only be performed by an RMP:

- Preoperative diagnostic evaluation
- Surgery planning
- Surgery execution including donor hair harvesting, hairline design, recipient site creation, and management of other patient medical issues and possible adverse reactions
- Postoperative care

It is unethical for an RMP to train an individual to perform/assist surgery who is not an accredited health professional licensed to do so.

Minimum requirements in a hospital or a clinic performing hair transplant surgery:

The daycare theater should be equipped with facilities for monitoring and handling emergencies including stocking of emergency drugs, Boyle's machine, intubation sets, and Ambu bags. A plan for handling emergencies should be in place, and all nursing staff should be familiar with the emergency plan. It is ideal to have a standby anesthetist.

Aesthetic Procedures

Aesthetic procedures should be undertaken only by those RMPs who have adequate training to do these procedures as per their curriculum.

The curriculum of various specialties should be the guiding principle for all RMPs while undertaking any procedure including aesthetics and hair transplant procedures.

Aesthetic Procedures including Hair Transplant

Aesthetic procedures including hair transplant, as with any other surgical procedure, may have complications and require skills and training in appropriate patient selection, differential diagnoses, surgical techniques, and appropriate postprocedure care to optimize outcomes. It is suggested that anyone who wishes to perform these procedures should be adequately knowledgeable and trained and should ensure that they have adequate infrastructure and manpower to manage any issues that may arise due to the procedure performed.

Aesthetic procedures including hair transplant are not an emergency surgery, and hence there is no case for allowing any untrained person to do it under the pretext of "Exceptional Circumstances." Para 6 of the Judgment mentions "Hair transplantation being an aesthetic surgery needs to be performed by RMPs like qualified dermatologists or trained surgeons."

- It may be noted that watching in workshops or on YouTube or similar platforms is not the adequate training to start aesthetic surgeries including hair transplant.
- Assistants or OT technicians should be from a medical background, such as nurses, lab technicians, and pharmacists. However, they need to be provided

structured, systematic, and proper training (responsibility will lie with the RMP) in all aspects of both aesthetic surgery and disinfection, sterilization, patient communication, etc.

- Surgical assistants/technicians should perform tasks only under the supervision of an RMP.

The RMP should have an anesthesia backup in the form of the presence of the anesthetist in the operation room area with all the requisite resuscitative equipment and drugs in place.

The RMP should ensure that the patient undergoing such surgery should have adequate preoperative clearances from the medical specialists and the anesthetist.

The RMP should have a well-equipped postoperative recovery room with facilities for monitoring of vitals and adequate record keeping.

Manpower and Infrastructure Required at Place of Such Procedure

Manpower

Apart from the surgeon performing hair transplantation and aesthetic surgery, the center should also have trained NIT personnel such as staff nurses, technicians, and OT masters.

Infrastructure

- It should be a hospital with facilities for treating indoor patients.
- The OT should be properly set up with all protocols being followed or implemented strictly, such as:
    - Strict asepsis and fumigation protocols
    - Proper biomedical waste management such as separation, transfer/transport, and disposal
    - Proper sterilization of OT instruments, drapes, etc.
- Availability of anesthetist as it is an invasive OT procedure. A crash cart trolley should be available with all resuscitative facilities.
- If it is a clinic doing daycare surgeries only, then it should be well connected with any nearby hospital with proper ICU and critical care facilities, if needed in case of any emergency, and with a display of 24-hour emergency number for help.
- Proper records of operated patients with pre- and postoperative photographs, records, or any complication need to be maintained.[17]

REFERENCES

1. Shah S. Hair transplant industry is witnessing a rise in demand despite challenges. The Times of India: Opinion. [online] Available from https://timesofindia.indiatimes.com/blogs/voices/hair-transplant-industry-is-witnessing-a-rise-in-demand-despite-challenges/. [Last accessed September, 2023].
2. Kessler D, McClellan M. Do doctors practice defensive medicine? Q J Econ. 1996;111(2):353-90.
3. Bal BS. An introduction to medical malpractice in the United States. Clin Orthop Relat Res. 2009;467(2):339-47.
4. Sohn DH. Negligence, genuine error, and litigation. Int J Gen Med. 2013;6:49-56.
5. Jacob Mathew v. State of Punjab. 2005. 6 SCC 1. [online] Available from https://indiankanoon.org/doc/871062/ [Last accessed October, 2023].
6. Shah AK. Newer implications of medico-legal and consent issues in plastic surgery. Indian J Plast Surg. 2014;47(2):199-202.
7. Dr. Batra vs Harjot Singh on June 8, 2023. [online] Available from https://indiankanoon.org/doc/157599954. [Last accessed September, 2023].
8. Nanda L. The need for a computerized patient-record system for the public hospitals in Andhra Pradesh. J Acad Hosp Adm. 2000;12(1):1-6.
9. Pai MMM, Ganiga R, Pai RM, Sinha RK. Standard electronic health record (EHR) framework for Indian healthcare system. Health Serv Outcomes Res Method. 2021;21:339-62.
10. Hair transplant gone wrong, court asks police to probe. [online] Available from https://indianexpress.com/article/cities/mumbai/hair-transplant-gone-wrong-court-asks-police-to-probe/. [Last accessed September, 2023].
11. Chennai medical student dies after hair transplant surgery. [online] Available from https://www.ndtv.com/chennai-news/chennai-medical-student-dies-after-hair-transplant-surgery-1416981. [Last accessed September, 2023].
12. Court orders cosmetic clinic to pay client ₹1L for bad job. [online] Available from https://timesofindia.indiatimes.com/city/goa/court-orders-cosmetic-clinic-to-pay-client-rs-1l-for-bad-job/articleshow/59922279.cms. [Last accessed September, 2023].
13. Dogra TD, Gupta S. Medico-legal aspect of health care delivery. [online] Available from https://www.ahaindia.org/node/447. [Last accessed October, 2023].
14. Korean hospital responsible for faulty hair transplant: court. [online] Available from http://www.asiaone.com/health/korean-hospital-responsible-faulty-hair-transplant-court. [Last accessed September, 2023].
15. Sattur SS, Sattur IS. Patient counselling and medicolegal aspects of hair transplant surgery. Indian J Plast Surg. 2021;54(4):441-5.
16. Mysore V, Kumaresan M, Garg A, Dua A, Venkatram A, Dua K, et al. Hair transplant practice guidelines. J Cutan Aesthet Surg. 2021;14(3):265-84.
17. Guideline on aesthetic surgery and hair transplant procedures. [online] Available from https://www.nmc.org.in/MCIRest/open/getDocument?path=/Documents/Public/Portal/LatestNews/20220927051220.pdf. [Last accessed September, 2023].

CHAPTER 100

Ergonomics and Hair Transplantation

Vaishalee Kirane

Key Messages

- Hair restoration surgery involves long hours of work, and its nature of focused working using a microscope or lens in one posture can cause stress and strain on the muscles and joints, especially the back. This can increase the risk of spine problems and neurological sequelae.
- Preserving the normal curvature of the spine by adhering to the basic principles of proper posture and helped by regular exercise and good nutrition will go a long way in preventing such problems.
- We should thus pay attention to the ergonomics involved in all the steps of hair transplant surgery, namely donor harvesting, dissection of grafts, and implantation process.

INTRODUCTION

Hair transplantation (HT) is no less than a microsurgery, that too of long hours, done under local anesthesia leading to various challenges for the surgeon, his assistants, and the patient as well. The prerequisite for the success of microsurgery, other than the technical aspect, is the physical comfort of the surgeon, his team, and also the patient as surgery is done under local anesthesia.

This write-up on the ergonomics in HT surgery may be a slight deviation from the usual topic of trichology or hair restoration surgery, but the long hours of back-bending work involved during HT surgery can surely take a toll on our back.

Along with long hours, focused working behind a microscope or using a lens during graft harvesting, the meticulous dissection of the grafts, and also the implantation process of grafts one by one surely cause a lot of stress and strain on the body, especially on the joints of the spine and the supporting muscles and tendons. This can pose a risk of suffering from spinal problems such as chronic nagging backache, slipped intervertebral disk, or even debilitating neurological sequelae.

One, thus, cannot understate the importance of having a strong healthy spine, which will support us for a good, long career as HT surgeons.

Having a healthy body and mind is an asset of our life, and, thus, it is very important to nurture and strengthen them. Maintaining a healthy lifestyle with discipline and consistency is the mainstay and should become a way of life, rather than sporadic bursts lasting just for a few days or weeks. Eating a nutrient-rich diet including all the macro- and micronutrients in appropriate proportions, keeping in line with every individual's health status, takes the role of priority. An optimal exercise program made after proper consultation with a fitness professional goes a long way toward good fitness and avoiding injuries. Rest between exercise regimens, as well as having a good sound deep sleep, is as important for good recovery of the body. Investing time for a balanced and good emotional quotient and mental health always remains a major part of our fitness journey. This will be the foundation to become more creative and productive in our daily activities and in our work and to make life more efficient and successful.

ANATOMY OF THE SPINE

With this introduction, let us first refresh our knowledge about the anatomy of the spine, in order to appreciate and motivate us to preserve it.

A normal spinal curvature consists of three natural curves as in the shape of "S," resulting in an even distribution of body weight and due to which the spine can thus withstand a great amount of stress.

The cervical spine shows a lordotic curve, the thoracic spine a kyphotic curve, and the lumbar spine follows a lordotic curve again **(Fig. 1)**.

The vertebral bones have between them the intervertebral disks, which serve as cushions to help absorb any shock or load. The spinal cord, placed in the spinal canal, gives out the nerve roots which exit through the neural foramen. The soft tissues of tendons, ligaments, and muscles of the spine help to add strength and movement and maintain position against gravity **(Fig. 2)**.

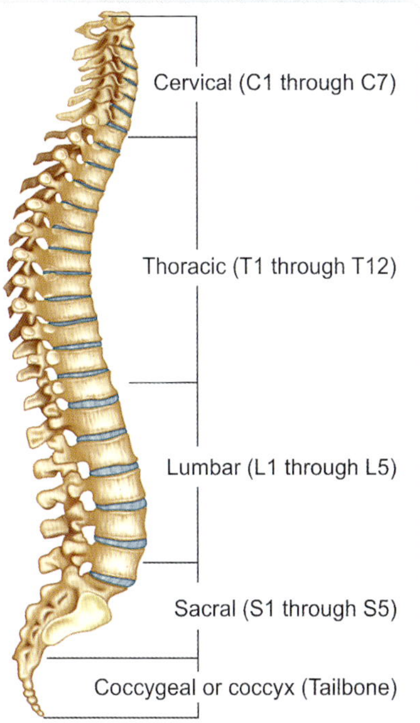

FIG. 1: Normal curvature of the spine.

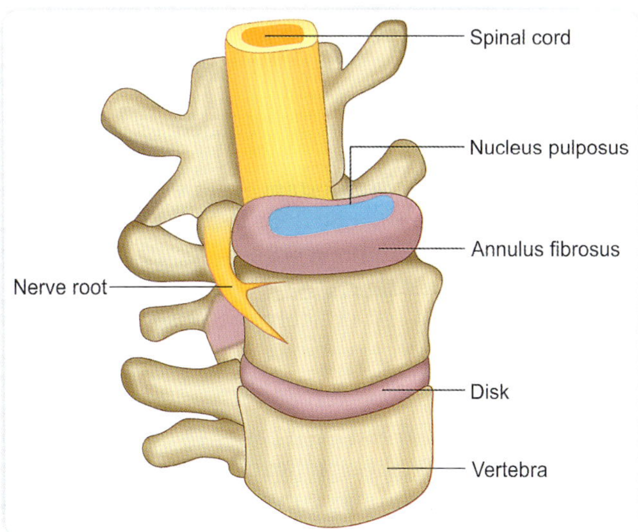

FIG. 2: Anatomy of the spine.

POSTURE

A good posture is a position in which you hold your body upright against gravity while standing or sitting, where the least strain is placed on supporting muscles and ligaments during movement or weight-bearing activities **(Fig. 3)**. It keeps the bones and joints in the correct alignment, prevents abnormal wearing of the joint surfaces, and prevents the spine from becoming fixed in abnormal positions.

In accordance with the three normal curves of the spine, the correct posture one needs to have while sitting is to sit up with the back straight, the shoulders retracted back, and the buttocks touching the lower back of the chair. A small, rolled-up towel or a lumbar roll helps additionally. Knees are to be kept at a level slightly higher than the hips by keeping the feet on a footrest high above the floor. One should sit up close to the workstation and not at a far distance, which will strain the back. Elbows and arms should be supported by resting them on the armrests of the chair or desk, keeping the shoulders relaxed, instead of keeping them hanging in midair. When sitting in a pivot chair, one should not twist at the waist. Instead, the whole body should be turned.

Improper posture, among many other causes, can lead to certain spinal problems, such as:

- Loss of normal curvature of the spine
- Straightening of the spine
- Intervertebral disk prolapse (herniation)
- Nerve compression and neuralgia
- *Cervical spine*: Brachial neuralgia
- *Lumbar spine*: Lower back pain, sciatica, bowel/ bladder problem

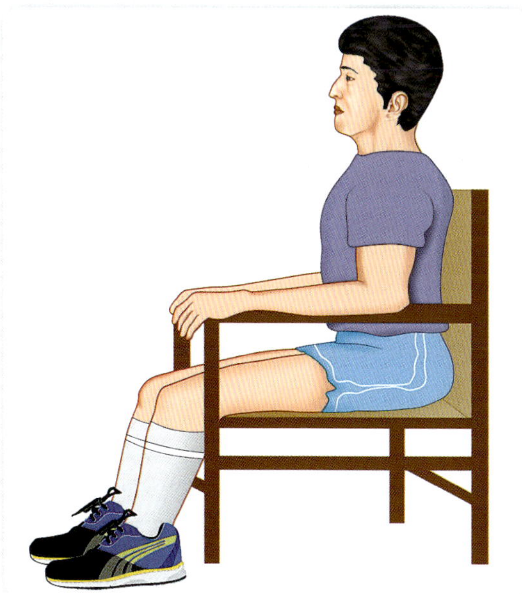

FIG. 3: Proper posture while sitting.

MANAGEMENT OF SPINAL PROBLEMS

- There is no "quick fix" and one most probably needs to wait for natural recovery to take place, mostly by 6 weeks. Medications such as painkillers or those needed for any neurological sequelae need to be taken only after consultation with the respective specialist, avoiding self-medication and overuse or misuse. Other therapies involve spine exercises and physiotherapy, staying active, avoiding being overprotective, and leading as normal a life as possible. Loss of bowel/bladder control or severe neuralgia may indicate surgery.
- Joint bracing and taping to support an injured area
- *Corrective or rehabilitative exercises*: Improve muscle endurance and function and alleviate discomfort while the body heals itself naturally.
- *Nutrition recommendations*: To reduce weight, relieve joint pain, and address posture problems

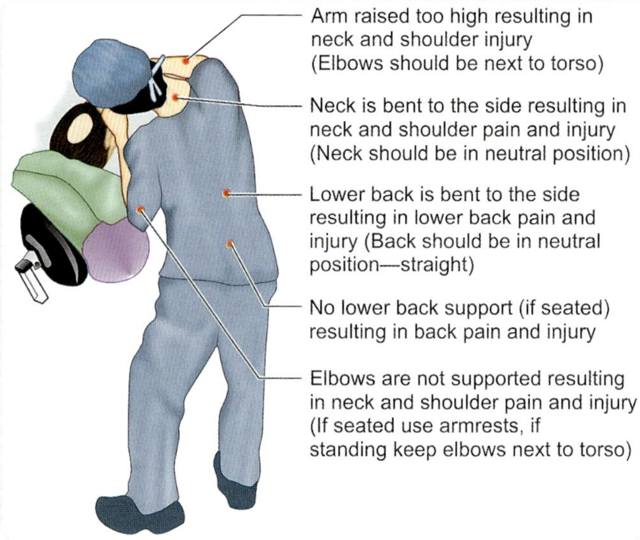

FIG. 4: Improper standing posture during hair transplantation (HT) surgery.

DIFFERENT POSITIONS AND POSTURES DURING STEPS OF HAIR RESTORATION SURGERY

Different positions involved during the various steps of hair restoration surgery are as follows:

- Donor graft harvesting, either strip excision or follicular unit extraction, involves the surgeon to stand or sit at the side or behind the patient's head.
- Graft insertion also requires similar positions. Usually, there are more than one surgeon or assistant performing the procedure, both at either side and from behind the patient's head. They have to adjust their positions to enable working on the small surface area of the patient's scalp and many a time, it becomes difficult to work by attaining proper posture **(Fig. 4)**.
- Graft dissection **(Fig. 5)** involves sitting for long hours in one place and one position with an intent focus on the microscopic dissection **(Figs. 6A and B)**.
- Thus, appropriate posture during all the steps of hair transplant surgery assumes great importance to prevent spinal problems.

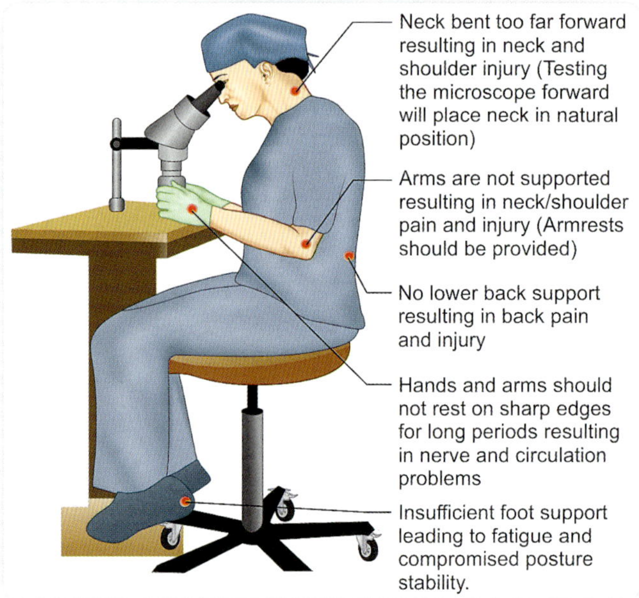

FIG. 5: Improper sitting posture during graft dissection.

ERGONOMICS DURING HAIR TRANSPLANTATION SURGERY

In order to maintain a proper posture, an ergonomically designed chair with good back support, adjustable height, and seat angle is very essential during hair restoration surgery. Armrests to support the forearms, footrests to keep knees at an equal height with hips, and enough room under the working surface to move the chair close to the microscope are other important features. The location and angle of the microscope need to be adjusted to have a comfortable and unstrained position for the many hours involved during the surgery.

Frequent breaks and stretching exercises are also very important.

EXERCISE

Exercise assumes great significance to improve fitness and maintain the normal curvature of the spine and functioning. A disciplined, regular, and consistent exercise

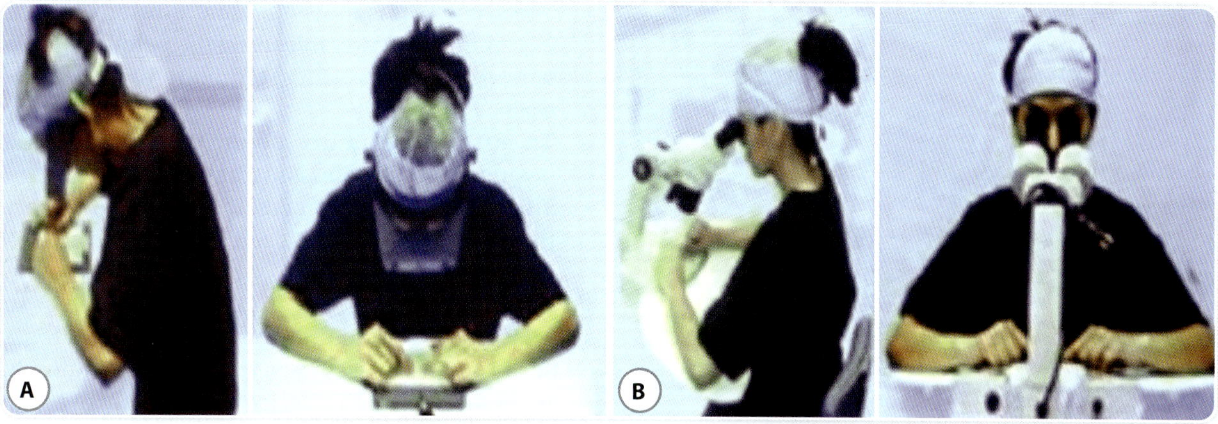

FIGS. 6A AND B: Position during graft dissection; dissecting with (A) loupes: Neck and back bent forward, discomfort and injurie and; (B) binocular microscope: Neck and back supported, in neutral position and elbows supported too.

program is definitely important. One can categorize exercise into three basic groups, namely (i) strengthening, (ii) stretching or flexibility, and (iii) aerobic.

Aerobics

Aerobics involves steady exercises using large muscle groups and engaging in cardiovascular activities, such as walking, jogging, running, cycling, various sports, or swimming, being the gentler option on the joints. It improves stamina, strengthens the heart and lung functioning, and improves the body's ability to use oxygen. The benefits are multifold with increased energy levels, improved mood and mental health, better sleep habits, and, additionally, helping with fat loss. But if such cardiovascular activity is not accompanied by strength training of the muscles, then there is a risk of increased wear and tear of the body, injuries, joint issues, and not just fat but muscle loss too.

Strengthening Exercises

Strengthening exercises require you to tax your muscles with maximum effort in minimum time. It is also important to choose the proper exercises to be done with proper posture and proper breathing technique of inhalation and exhalation.

A simple point to remember is that, since the aim is to be functionally fit in our daily activities and work, it is necessary that you use functional movements while exercising, such as pulling and pushing for strengthening the upper body and squats, lunges, and lifts for the legs and back muscles. Core strengthening is also extremely crucial. Choose exercises that are compound, using more than one muscle and joint at a time. This helps to focus on more surface area of the body, which is the case in real-life movements. Exercises such as squats, deadlifts, and pushing movements, which are called presses, use some muscles of the body isotonically and some muscles isometrically. This helps the body to get stronger as a single unit, which is important for core strengthening as it helps to stabilize the spine, allow proper spinal movement, and make it easier to maintain correct posture. Having a strong core is very important for our profession. It is not advisable for a microsurgeon to do heavy weightlifting and hard workout, especially before surgery.

Stretching and Flexibility

Muscle-strengthening exercises involve a slow and sustained lengthening of the muscle fibers, helping to improve agility, avoid muscle strain, and decrease the possibility of injury. They are done before and after each workout as a part of warmup and cooldown. They are also important for us, considering the long hours of standing required in our surgical work.

Scalp Laxity Exercises

Along with the entire body, let us also see about these exercises which are needed in HT surgery. Certain exercises are advised about 1 month before surgery to increase the laxity of the skin of the posterior scalp from where the donor strip is excised. A loose scalp enables the harvesting of a longer donor strip and thus more number of grafts. The lesser wound tension would, in addition, help to give a better cosmetic scar. Scalp laxity exercises include massaging the back and sides of the scalp.

Methods

- The palm of the hands is placed on the back/sides of the head with the fingers pointing upward and thumbs pointing toward each other **(Figs. 7 to 9)**.

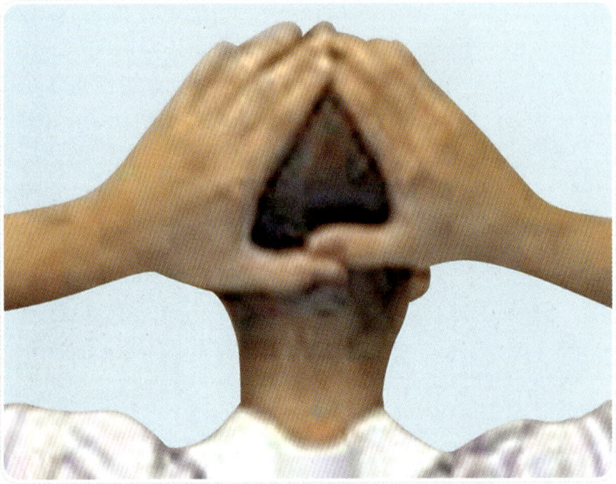

FIG. 7: Position 1: Palms in the back of the scalp with thumbs overlapping.

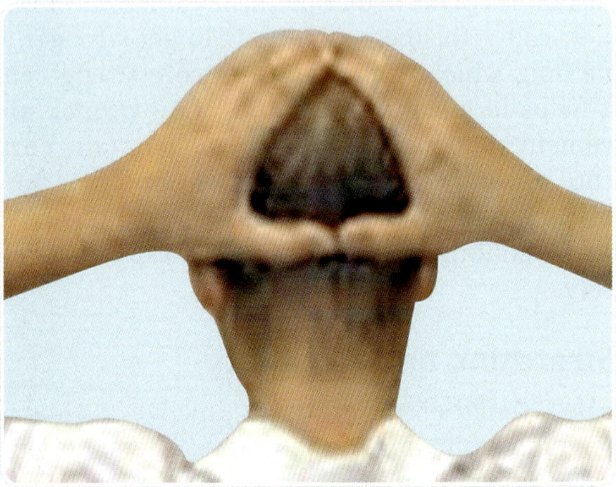

FIG. 8: Position 2: Palms on the sides of the scalp with thumbs touching on the back of the head.

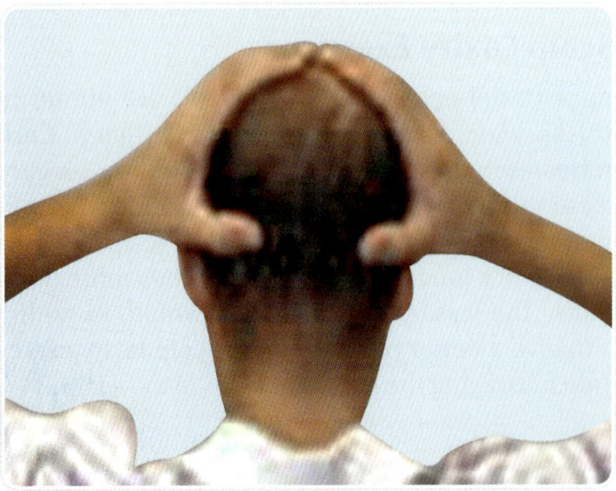

FIG. 9: Position 3: Palms and thumbs on the sides of the scalp.

- The scalp skin is moved up and down over the bone as vigorously as possible using the palms and thumbs, with the fingers resting stationary on the top of the scalp.
- To stretch the entire donor area, three different positions for the palm and thumbs are used.
- This exercise is performed for 5 minutes at each of the three positions (for a total of 15 minutes) every evening at bedtime.

Brandy DA demonstrates an innovative scalp-stretching device that improves scalp laxity and improves on the former use of vigorous, manual preoperative scalp-stretching exercises. This device is in the form of a garment which is simply applied by patients at home for 30 min/day starting 30 days before.

NUTRITION

A healthy, nutrient-rich diet and consumption of enough amount of water and fluids per day are of paramount importance in order to have a healthy body composition with less fat and more muscle, thus reducing unwanted stress on the joints. Consuming more whole foods and less or no processed foods surely helps. The ratio of carbohydrates, fats, and protein in a person's diet should depend on his basal metabolic rate (BMR), lifestyle, and energy requirements. Pay more attention to the macro- and micronutrients you get from a particular food and then decide whether you need to consume it, when to consume it, and how much to consume.

YOGA AND MEDITATION

Let us also enumerate aspects about yoga and meditation as they work both on our body and on our mind, create a sense of persistence, and help to develop patience and mental strength and stability. It is very well said that meditation has to be experienced and silence cannot be talked about. Spiritual practice is not just about busting stress and calming the mind but also about the aspect of "*Seva*," of caring and being there for our patients.

Asanas provide stability and strength to maintain a particular posture for longer duration.

Pranayama (breathing techniques—*Anulom Vilom* and breath holding) reduces stress and relaxes the entire body and mind.

Pratyahara and *Dharna* increase concentration and mental stability.

Yoga and meditation are also beneficial to relax the muscles of the forehead and hands, which also get fatigued due to the long hours of focused work involved in HT surgery.

Some important *asanas* are as follows:

Various micro-*asanas* provide strength, stability, and flexibility of small joints involved during microsurgery. Eyeball exercises strengthen the ocular muscles.

- The sphinx pose and *Dhanurasana* involve lying on the stomach and lifting and extending the back. This helps to strengthen the back muscles of latissimus dorsi and rhomboids.
- The *Yogasanas* of bridge pose and *Matsyasana* work on the muscles and maintain the curvature of the spine.
- The spine twist (*Vakrasana* and *Merudandasana*) pose works on the flexibility of the spine.
- *Surya Namaskar* involves stretching our body into 12 positions and is considered a complete *sadhana* **(Figs. 10A to G)**.

One can thus see how very important it is to invest our time and energy in incorporating into our life proper diet, exercise, and rest in a disciplined and consistent manner so as to maintain and achieve a healthy body and mind and a strong spine in our work as hair transplant surgeons.

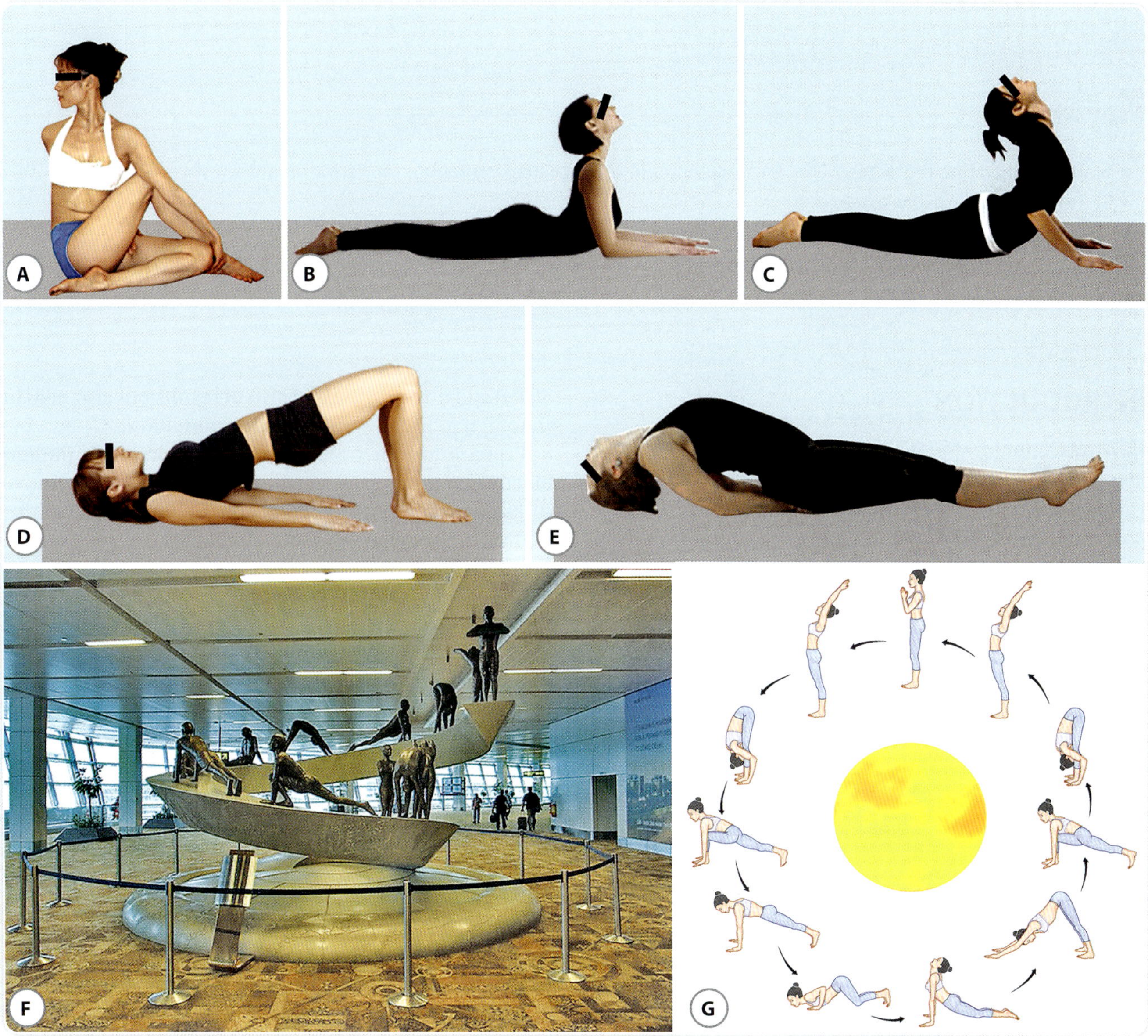

FIGS. 10A TO G: *Yogasanas*: (A) Spine twist pose (*Ardha Matsyendrasana*); (B) *Dhanurasana*; (C) *Matsyasana*; (D) bridge pose; (E) Sphinx pose; (F and G) *Surya Namaskar*: Salutation to the sun (complete *Sadhana*: *Asana*, *Pranayama*, meditation technique).

CHAPTER 101

Standard Operating Protocols for Running Hair Transplantation Practice

Madura C, Ruhi Uttamani-Sangle

Key Messages

- Standard operating protocols (SOPs) are documented step-by-step instructions for performing the tasks.
- They help to achieve consistency.
- They improve quality and safety.
- They save time and avoid missing any steps and knowledge loss.
- They enhance autonomy.

INTRODUCTION

Hair transplantation (HT) is a long surgical procedure involving a team of doctors, nurses, and technicians. There can be constant changes in team members, which can pose challenges to the operating surgeon. Standardization of techniques by following standard operating protocols (SOPs) will not only give consistent results but also help in smooth, hassle-free surgery with automation.

Preparation for transplantation begins with patient selection and counseling and continues to preoperative workup, intraoperative period, and, finally, postoperative (PO) care. This chapter shares the SOPs followed by the author **(Flowchart 1)**.

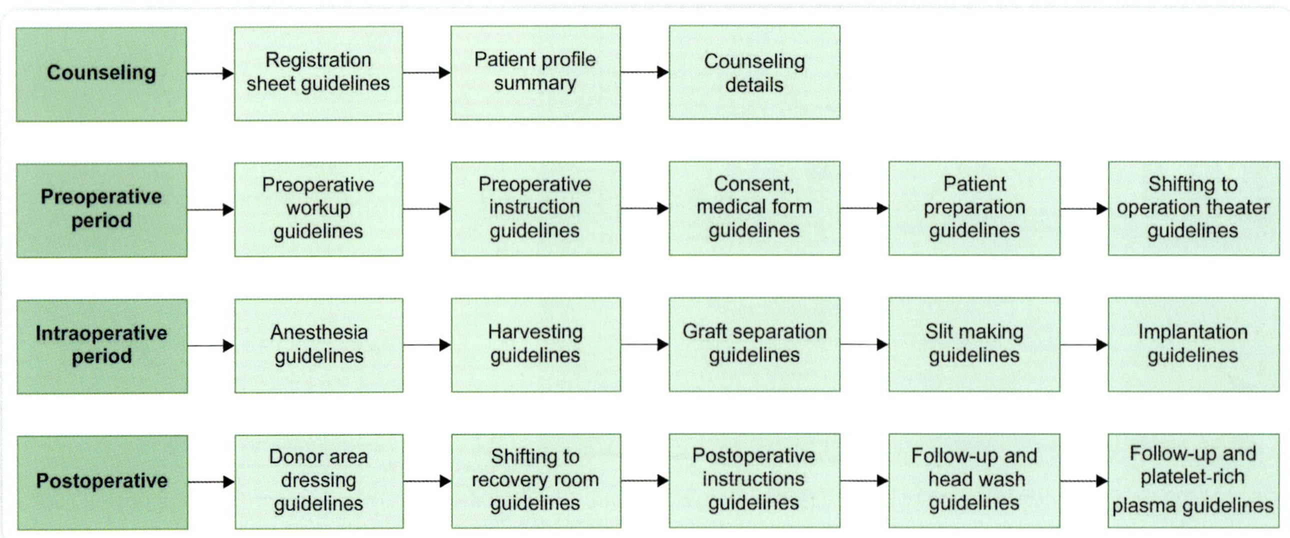

FLOWCHART 1: Flow of events in hair transplantation. The authors follow these guidelines as standard operating protocols.

STANDARD OPERATING PROTOCOL FOR REGISTRATION, HISTORY TAKING, AND EXAMINATION

- *Patient details*: Name, age, sex, residence address, occupation, referring doctor
- Medical history, associated scalp diseases if any, comorbidities, allergies
- Treatment history, including if the patient is using minoxidil lotion currently (advised to stop at least 2 weeks prior to surgery)
- Any previous procedures done for the treatment of androgenetic alopecia (AGA)
- Diagnosis with AGA grade, recipient area (sites that concern the patient)
- *Donor area*: To check for shrinkage of the donor area/ diffuse unpatterned alopecia (DUPA)/*reverse AGA pattern*, density, average thickness of hair in the donor area
- Examining the scalp for the presence of scaling, folliculitis, tight scalp—glidability and laxity
- To understand and set right his/her realistic expectations
- Habits—smoking, alcohol consumption
- Any medications that the patient is taking—aspirin, anticoagulants, etc.
- Stop supplements such as fish oil, ginger, garlic, saw palmetto preparation, vitamin supplements
- Tentative surgery date

Registration Sheet

Patients can be given predesigned questionnaire sheets by the receptionist during the waiting period prior to counseling, which include knowledge about the surgery, level of motivation, any fear factor, language preference, and expectation. This will assist the counselor for patient-oriented counseling.

COUNSELING GUIDELINES

The objective of counseling is to inform the patient about HT, in simple words, to clear all doubts and misconceptions regarding HT and to utilize minimum time duration to deliver appropriate details.

- Explain about the need for HT.
- Details about the procedure are to be explained using a PowerPoint presentation with photographs that explain the technique of HT, time duration of the procedure, donor-recipient area, delivery of local anesthesia, position while extracting and implanting, and sequence of events in HT (pictures of marking/shaving of hair/post HT with dressing/day 3 and day 10/post 1 month/post 2–3 months).
- Draw the planned hairline and discuss the plan with the patient along with the grafts needed and the area to be covered.
- *PO sequence of events*: Immediate PO care, day 3 care, and day 10—till expected results
- Emphasize the importance of continuing the medical line of treatment.

  Preoperative instructions:
  - Advise the patient to stop using minoxidil 10–15 days prior to surgery.
  - Advise the patient to stop smoking and alcohol consumption 1 week prior to and 2 weeks post-transplant.
  - Instructions about preoperative medications (prophylactic antibiotics, anxiolytic 1 night prior, medicine for gastritis)—which tablets, when, and how
  - Hair dye application is to be done 1 day prior to surgery if the patient has gray hair (after a test patch with the dye). Haircut, if required, is to be done 2–3 weeks prior.
  - Less spicy and oily food is to be taken from the previous day.
  - The patient should wear a front buttoned dark-colored shirt, not a pullover T-shirt, and bring an extra pair of dress.
  - One attender should accompany the patient before and after surgery wherever possible. Where it is not possible, contact the number of a friend/ relative.
  - For outstation patients, ascertain where the patient will stay and arrange hospital accommodation for outstation patients with comorbidities.
  - In order to minimize bleeding, avoid the following before surgery: Aspirin or other anti-inflammatory medications (1–2 weeks), vitamin B or vitamin E (1 week), and alcoholic beverages (3 days).
  - Do not drink coffee or any other caffeinated beverages on the day of the procedure.
  - Do not smoke tobacco products for at least 24 hours before the procedure and at least 1–2 weeks after HT.
  - Eat breakfast in the morning before surgery. If the surgery is scheduled in the afternoon, have a light lunch before arrival.
- Provide a list of investigations and a reference letter for fitness from a physician/anesthetist.
- *Patient booked by e-mail*: All instructions are to be sent by e-mail prior to booking.
- The questionnaire is to be signed by the patient.

PREOPERATIVE EVALUATION

- Fill history form.
- Record examination findings.
- Document vital records along with weight.
- *Conduct investigations*: Complete blood count (CBC), liver function tests (LFT), renal function tests (RFT), lipid profile, random blood sugar (RBS), glycated hemoglobin (HbA1c) viral markers, thyroid-stimulating hormone (TSH), electrocardiogram (ECG), hepatitis B and C, and human immunodeficiency virus (HIV) preferably to be done at least 2 weeks prior to surgery
- Check physician's fitness for the procedure—for all patients above 40 years, obese patients, patients with comorbidities.

PREOPERATIVE AND INTRAOPERATIVE PATIENT PREPARATION

- The patient file tag must be ready.
- Allot a bed in the preoperative room, secure the patient tag, and provide a locker to the patient to keep all valuables.
- Confirm if the patient has eaten and taken all preoperative medications.
- Explain the entire procedure briefly.
- Fill the consent form, take patient's and attender's signatures
- Check vitals.
- Secure intravenous (IV) cannula.
- Administer preoperative medication [tetanus toxoid (TT) injection].
- Administer test dose for lignocaine and also if any intravenous antibiotics are advised.
- Photo documentations (before and after marking) **(Figs. 1A to C)**

Team introduction to the patient:

- Introduce the team of doctors, staff nurses, and technicians to the patient.
- Provide an approximate duration of the surgery, breaks between surgery, and washroom and water breaks as and when needed.
- Reassure the patient about the pain of surgery and also the use of pain-distracting devices such as a vibrator and also inform that music of the patient's choice will be played in the operation theater (OT).
- Inform about the position that patient will be in during various phases of the surgery and to keep moving their lower limbs.
- Keep the patient's attender informed about the surgery's progress.

Trimming

- Confirm if marking photographs are done.
- Technician to confirm the trimming site and trimmer length before trimming the area
- Wash the scalp thoroughly using a surgical scrub and reinforce the markings with a marker.
- Post-trimming photographs are to be taken.
- Consent is to be signed after marking that the patient has approved the hairline design.

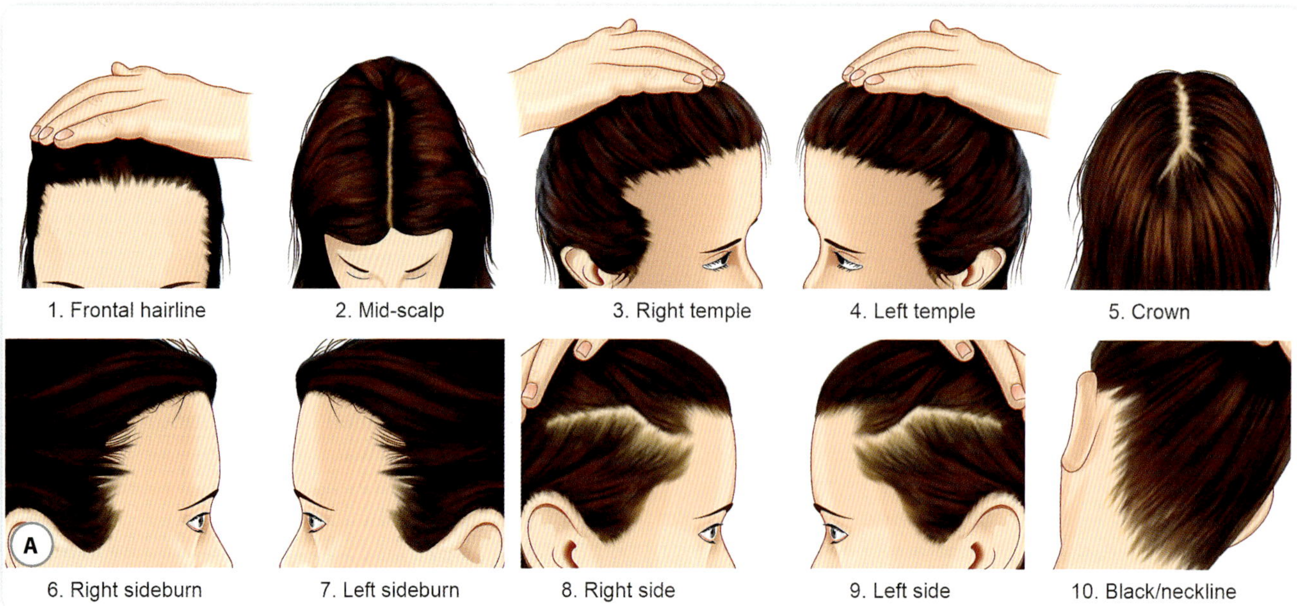

FIGS. 1A TO C: *Continued*

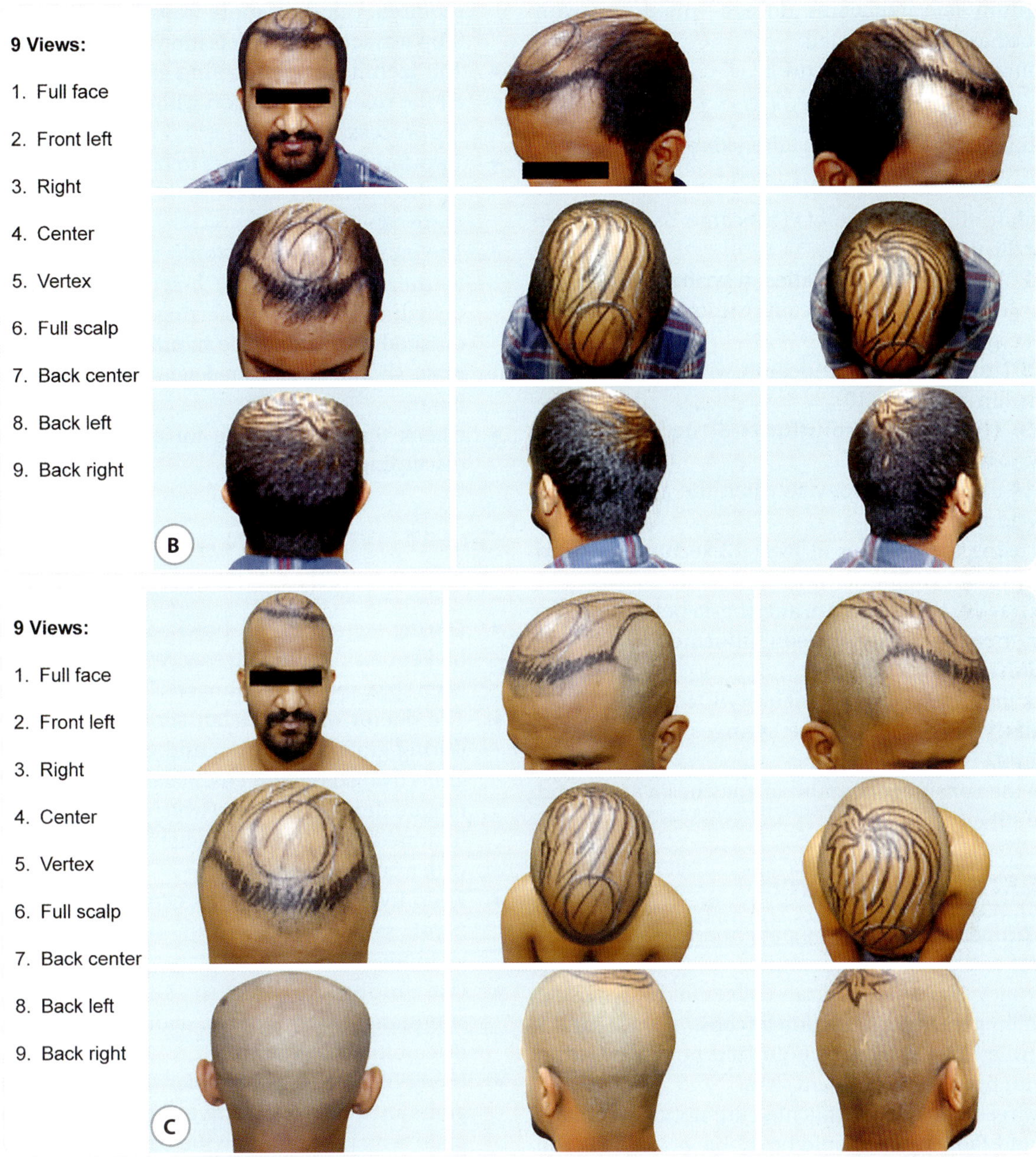

FIGS. 1A TO C: Photo documentation. (A) Photographs; (B) Postmarking photographs; (C) Post-trimming photographs.

- Document any additional points in the consent form by hand writing by the patient himself.
- Don the gown, mask, and foot cover before shifting into the OT.

PAINTING AND DRAPING THE AREA

After the patient is shifted to the OT couch, the staff nurse is to paint the scalp and face area with betadine, with a sponge holder in one hand and a gauze piece to wipe off excess betadine if there is dripping. Inform the patient that the betadine application will be cold to touch. While painting, the marking area should be intact. Do not rub, just tap the area. Inform the patient not to touch the area as it is sterile. The patient's ears should be covered with cotton swabs and gauze while painting the occipital area.

ANESTHESIA GUIDELINES

Anesthesia administration chart: Name of the patient, hospital ID number, age/sex, weight, number of grafts planned, donor and recipient areas have to be documented.

Maximum safe lignocaine dosage—plain and with adrenaline has to be calculated.

- Formula for lignocaine (in mL):

$$\text{Weight (kg)} \times 4.5/21.3$$

- Formula for lignocaine with adrenaline (in mL):

$$\text{Weight (kg)} \times 7/21.3$$

Calculate the safe dose of lignocaine based on the weight of the patient.

- A1/A2/A3 are separately loaded in syringes:
  - A1 (nerve block)—lignocaine without adrenaline—2 cc syringe—2
  - A2 (infiltration)—lignocaine with adrenaline—insulin syringes—10
  - A3 (tumescent solution)—3 cc Luer lock syringes—4
- Always use a vibrator device when the anesthesia is being administered.
- Start using the vibrator at least 12 seconds prior to administration of the anesthesia.
- Keep track of the amount of anesthesia being used.
- Keep the operating surgeon informed when the solution is about to finish.
- Check the vitals of the patient every 10 minutes.
- Regularly keep refilling the syringes as and when required.
- Write the consumed amount of anesthesia at the end of the surgery.

HARVESTING GUIDELINES

- Give proper position to the patient and also look for doctors and assistant ergonomics.
  - Trolley 1 to hold the graft collection bowl on the chilling tray and extraction forceps.
  - Trolley 2 to hold only motorized punch machine with punches of different sizes.

  The wires of the punch machine are not to be entangled and foot switch should be in the vicinity. Fix the wire to the green drape with a towel clip after securing the punch.
- Scoring is to be done from distal to proximal row by row, and alternate units are extracted.
- Use a wet mop to gently wipe the bleeding. In case of excess bleeding, keep tumescent ready. Keep extra wet mops and tumescent-filled syringes ready.
- Few of the first extracted grafts should be measured for follicular length and assessed for thickness. First harvest 100 grafts and assess FOX grade and also any missed grafts. In case of transection or capping, inform the operating surgeon so that depth, sharpness, speed, and torque can be adjusted accordingly.
- Extraction is to be done using traction on one side; in case of a tight scalp, countertraction may also be required. Inform if more transection/capping occurs. Stop extraction if there is more capping.
- The technician performing extraction should follow all the rules of extraction without disturbing the scoring process.
- Two-forceps extraction is to be used, only if approved by the operating surgeon. Stop extraction if there is more capping.
- The extracted grafts should be immediately shifted to the Ringer's lactate bowl without letting them dehydrate. While transferring, follicles should not be crushed and should be handled carefully. Extracted grafts should be collected gently in the bowl, not in the hand.
- Check the mops/gauze for entangled grafts before discarding them.

GRAFT HYDRATION AND SEGREGATION GUIDELINES

- *During segregation*: A bowl containing grafts should be kept on the chilling tray. While segregating grafts, keep spraying chilled Ringer's lactate on the grafts.
- The doctor or technician should *always use loupes* during graft segregation and counting. Take only 10 grafts using blunt forceps. Place the grafts on the sterile tongue depressor/cloth (which is placed over a mop) hydrated with Ringer's lactate using a 2-mL syringe with a cut needle.
- Keep hydrating the grafts every 30 seconds using a 2 mL syringe with a cut needle by saline drop technique.
- Use blunt forceps to segregate and count simultaneously—this can avoid too much handling. Be careful with gray hair.
- Using blunt forceps, transfer the grafts and trimmed grafts into their respective chambers of the holding plate, which is placed on the chilling tray, according to the time of harvest.
- Enter the count on the sterile sheet (can be a sterile glove cover) using a sterile pen; counting is to be updated at the end of the 1-hour harvest.
- *During implantation*:
  - Use continuous spray technique—while grafts are being placed, when there is active bleeding obscuring the field, while fixing the grafts, and on implanted areas. Implanters should always be dipped in Ringer's lactate.
  - Pick the grafts from the bowl while loading implanters.
  - Do not keep more than 25 grafts in your hand. After arranging grafts in your hand, spray every 30 seconds.

RECIPIENT SITE GUIDELINES

Standard Operating Protocol for Slit Making

- Mark the recipient area. Give anesthesia and wait for 7 minutes.
- Meanwhile, check the graft length and fix the blade according to the length of the grafts.
- Inject tumescent solution before slit making.
- A dry mop should be used while making slits in the hairline. A wet mop is to be used later to keep the area bloodless.
- The assistant documenting the slits must update the operating surgeon after every 500 slits.
- Appropriate density, depth, and direction of slits as per different zones of the recipient area must always be kept in mind. Overcrowding of slits may lead to poor wound healing and necrosis.
- After slits are made, stain with methylene blue/gentian violet and clean with a wet mop. Shave the recipient area. Finally, flush with saline.

Standard Operating Protocol for Implantation

Spraying Guidelines

- Use a 20-mL syringe with chilled saline loaded with a 26-gauge amputed needle.
- There are five areas to spray:
  i. Grafts to implant
  ii. Area of implantation
  iii. Oozing area
  iv. Implanted grafts
  v. Arranged grafts on hands
- Do not chase the grafts/change the direction of arranged grafts while spraying.

Implanters Guidelines

- Handle the grafts by holding only epidermis with forceps.
- Grafts within the implanters are to be immersed in chilled normal saline (NS).
- Bulky grafts are not to be loaded in the implanters.
- Grafts should not pop out from the side slit of the implanter.
- Grafts must not be crushed and not allowed to dehydrate.

Implantation Guidelines

- Arrange up to 20 grafts on the hand at a time to supply for forceps implantation.
- Do not let the grafts dry.
- Spray chilled NS on the grafts once placed on the scalp for implantation.
- Follow the plan of implantation on the chart placed in OT.
- Place the grafts one by one without skipping the slits.
- Do not piggyback the grafts.
- Remove the buried grafts immediately and position the graft.
- Grafts should be fixed at the implanted site at the end of implantation. Only implantation forceps are to be used for the fixing of grafts. While fixing, care should be taken not to bury/push the graft inside.

DRESSING GUIDELINES

Recipient Site

- Cold NS spray should be used for spraying in case of any bleeding during the fixation of grafts.
- After fixing, spray the implanted area with betadine solution (2 mL of betadine in 8 mL of NS) and then spray with NS.
- At the end of fixation, the implanted area should be gently pressed with wet mop/gauze.
- Gentle pressure with wet gauze will stop bleeding points.

Donor Area

- Clean blood stains present over the surgical site and povidone-iodine stains on the painted area.
- Post procedure photograph of the donor area.
- Apply povidone-iodine ointment over the donor area or cuticell dressing.
- Use steri pad/dry mop for dressing of the donor site and fix it with micropore tape.
- Provide a surgical cap for the patient (care to be taken that the cap is not touching the grafts).
- Shift the patient to the recovery room, accompanied by a technician and a doctor.

MISCELLANEOUS

Vital Monitoring Guidelines

- When connecting the BP cuff and pulse oximeter, explain about the periodic inflation and deflation of the BP cuff to the patient and also the beep sound.
- Record the baseline reading every 1 hourly in the case sheet. Monitor the reading every 10 minutes and also when there is a beep sound.
- An anesthetist is to be called over when mean arterial pressure (MAP) falls below 65 mm Hg OR

above 100 mm Hg OR BP falls >20% of the baseline reading.

- Do not disconnect the connector until the patient sits for a while.
- A transient rise in heart rate is expected because of the adrenaline in local anesthesia injection.

Break Guidelines

- Inform the patient about planned break times. Inform the patient to alert doctors if there is a need for restroom break or water break.
- All blood-stained mops are to be removed from the patient's visual field.
- Once the patient sits upright, clean all blood stains from the face.
- Whenever taking a break in the middle of surgery, switch off the OT lights, make the patient sit, and enquire whether he is comfortable before he stands up. Keep a record of the vitals and ask the patient if he/she is experiencing any dizziness. Offer him/her water/juice/chocolate. Remove the BP cuff and pulse oximeter only once the patient is stable.
- Stand behind/support the patient throughout, in anticipation of any syncopal episode.
- Instruct them not to lock the washroom, not to look in the mirror, and not to touch the area of surgery. Be in constant communication with the patient while he/she is using the washroom.
- The in-charge technician should mandatorily accompany the patient. If the patient is uncomfortable, the doctor should be called immediately and put the patient in a comfortable position.
- Once you shift the patient back, position the patient, connect the BP monitoring cuff, and ask the patient if he/she is comfortable.

Similarly, authors follow the guidelines designed for managing emergencies such as syncope, bleeding, convulsions, sterilization protocols, trolley preparation, position and ergonomics, cleaning protocols, and managing equipment.

POSTOPERATIVE INSTRUCTIONS

- A brief discharge slip is to be given to the patient documenting the procedure, duration, type of anesthesia, PO medication and instructions, and contact number of the doctor.
- Travel arrangements for the patient should be made.
- The patient is to be admitted to the hospital if the patient has had any issues during surgery meriting monitoring in the opinion of the treating surgeon.
- Clear instructions about the follow-up date and time must be given. Your follow-up visit after surgery is .... at ....
- Reinforce to the patient that hair restoration is a delicate procedure and their adherence to the PO instructions is essential for optimal results.
- Postoperative medications, special instructions on saline sprays, diet instructions, position of sleeping, what to avoid, and to be mindful of surgical site specially when boarding and deboarding a vehicle.
- *Emergency contact*: For any query/emergency, please call Dr .... Phone no. .... Please visit the hospital immediately in case of pain/bleeding/itching/irritation/burning in the operated site.

Shampoo and Cleaning

Transplant area: Hair should be washed 24–48 hours after surgery. Inform the patient that we want the graft to adhere solidly during this time.

- Wet your head with a bowl of room temperature water or with a gentle stream of water from the shower. If you use the shower, block the stream with your hand so that the water pressure is not too strong.
- Lather up the shampoo in a mug of little water and then *with the palm of your hand*, pat this shampoo on the area gently (*do not rub*) and wait for 1–2 minutes.
- Gently rinse off with a bowl of water or a gentle stream of water from the shower.
- Pat dry gently with a towel. *Do not rub the grafts to dry them.*
- After 7 days, you can begin to *gently* rub the grafts to help remove crusts.
- After 10 days, you should be able to shampoo normally. However, scratching with nails should be avoided.
- You can use any good-quality shampoo for hair washing.
- A conditioner can be added to help in breaking down crusts.

SUMMARY

- Standardization leads to consistent results; it becomes easy to train new staff to overcome frequent attrition.
- Avoid medicolegal hassles.
- Good quality of work stimulates.
- It is easy to train junior doctors, and the learning curve becomes short.
- The margin of error gets narrowed.
- Good work should not vanish; it must be transferred, transformed, and automated with multiplied ethical practice of HT.

CHAPTER 102

List of Instrument Manufacturers

Amit Kerure, Sonia Sabhandasani Nanavati

Key Messages

- Types of instruments and their uses.
- Where to procure these instruments from.

INTRODUCTION

Tools to a surgeon are what *"Astras"* are to God, and therefore, using the right surgical instrument is just as crucial as the end result of the surgery. Here is a list of suppliers of all the tools required for follicular unit extraction (FUE). This may not be a complete list; however, it will serve as a guideline for obtaining instruments required for the surgery.

INTERNATIONAL SUPPLIERS OF HAIR TRANSPLANT INSTRUMENTS

- Cole Instruments, USA
- Trivellini Tech, USA
- Magna Surgical Center, USA
- ERTIP Medical, Turkey
- Harris & Harrison, UK
- Prograft Medical, Turkey
- Robbins Instruments, USA
- Mediquip Surgical, USA
- Scharf CE, Turkey
- KLS Martin Group, UK

INDIAN SUPPLIERS OF HAIR TRANSPLANT INSTRUMENTS

Forceps and Hooks

- Plain curved forceps is used to extract the harvested follicles from the donor site.
- Implanter forceps are specifically designed in a Z-shape angle or an angular shape with a fine tip that helps in placing or implanting the follicular unit in the premade slits at the recipient area without damaging the hair follicle.[1]
- Skin hook or skin retractor is an instrument used to give traction at the donor area, which makes it easy to extract the follicular units without damaging the underlying skin.[2]

Suppliers

- Medsor Impex, New Delhi
- Alpha Surgicals, Surat
- Medono India, Alipur
- Innovation Surgicals, Mumbai
- Chadda Surgical, Mumbai
- Staan Bio-med Engineering Pvt Ltd, Coimbatore
- Bardia Devices, Kolkata
- Golden India Surgicals, Jalandhar
- Arora Surgicals, Ghaziabad
- E-Mold Techniques, Ahmedabad
- J. K. Enterprises, Raigad
- S. K. Surgicals, Pune

International Suppliers

- ERTIP Medical, Turkey
- Harris & Harrison, UK
- Prograft Medical, Turkey
- Robbins Instruments, USA
- Mediquip Surgical, USA

- Scharf CE, Turkey
- KLS Martin Group, Germany
- Omega Surgical Instruments, UK

Follicular Unit Extraction Punches

Harvesting the hair follicles from the donor area is done with the help of FUE punch. This circular instrument, ranging from 0.7 to 1.2 mm in diameter, is mounted on a motorized hand device, which with a rotatory movement helps in extracting the hair follicles.[3]

Suppliers

- Innovation Surgicals, Mumbai
- KSK Surgicals, New Delhi
- J. K. Enterprises, Raigad
- Alpha Surgicals, Surat
- Paul Medical Systems, Chennai
- Sabharwal Surgical Store, New Delhi
- Chadda Surgicals, Mumbai
- Med Morphosis LLP, Villupuram
- R. N. Surgicals, Thane
- Tejco Vision, Mumbai
- Healkeren Medtronics Pvt Ltd, Bengaluru
- M/s Kalp Life Care Equipments Industry, Gurugram
- Mcos Solutions, Jaipur

International Suppliers

- Cole Instruments, USA
- Trivellini Tech, USA
- Magna Medical, Turkey
- ERTIP Medical, Turkey
- Harris & Harrison, UK
- Prograft Medical, Turkey
- Robbins Instruments, USA
- Mediquip Surgical, USA
- Scharf CE, Turkey

Needles and Blades

Needles and blades are used to make slits on the recipient area for the hair follicles to be implanted. The most commonly used are:

- 18, 19, and 20 gauge needles
- Designer blades of various sizes
- Self-made blades from razor blades (of varying sizes depending on the thickness of hair follicles) are mounted on a slit blade holder or needle holder.

Suppliers

- J. K. Enterprises, Raigad
- R. N. Surgicals, Thane
- Alpha Surgicals, Surat
- Madhu Instruments Pvt Ltd, New Delhi
- Tejco Vision, Mumbai
- Innovation Surgicals, Mumbai
- Neeta Enterprise, Vapi
- Anand Agency, Pune
- Kashika Enterprise, Indore
- Om Tarang Enterprise, Hyderabad
- Surgifact India, Jalandhar

International Suppliers

- Magna Medical, Turkey
- ERTIP Medical, Turkey
- Harris & Harrison, UK
- Prograft Medical, Turkey
- Robbins Instruments, USA

Surgical Loupes

Two important reasons for using loupes are: (1) To have a bigger and clearer vision of the tiny hair follicles on the scalp, thereby minimizing eye strain and (2) To maintain a proper physiologic body posture while working for long hours in the surgery.

Suppliers

- R. N. Surgicals, Mumbai
- Madhav International, Haryana
- Kawachi Group, Maharashtra
- New India Works, Mumbai
- V Smart Health Care, Bengaluru
- Matronix India Corporation, New Delhi
- Max Optics, Ambala
- Sri Shankar Enterprise, Bengaluru
- Basco India, Chennai
- Visionary Medtech Solutions, Ahmedabad
- Sai Scientific Solutions, Ambala
- Karvy Medical Systems (Pvt) Ltd, New Delhi

Micromotor

An electric micromotor set consists of a motor handpiece, control box, and a foot pad.

Suppliers

- Chadda Surgicals, Mumbai
- Basco India, Chennai
- Netcare Surgicals Corporation, New Delhi
- Golden Nimbus International, Mumbai
- Innovation Surgicals, Mumbai
- Guru Hair Instruments, Jaipur
- Eklavya Surgicals, Jaipur

- Matronix India Corporation, New Delhi
- Ozeki Distributors, Nagpur
- Jullundur Enterprises, Jalandhar

International Suppliers

- Cole Instruments, USA
- Trivellini Tech, USA
- Robbins Instruments, USA

Follicular Unit Extraction Grafts Chilling Machine

Controlled cooling at 12° protects the harvest follicles during the storage period by reducing cell metabolism and promoting better graft survival.

Suppliers

- Guru Hair Instruments, Jaipur
- Alpha Surgicals, Surat
- Adarsh Surgicals, Mumbai
- Innovation Surgicals, Mumbai

International Supplier

- ERTIP Medical, Turkey

Implanters

The Choi implanter consists of a needle with a bevel where the graft is placed, a body, and a plunger, which pushes the graft into the slit.[1] Some studies observed that use of Choi implanters for implantation without premade slits decreased the chances of follicle damage.[3]

Suppliers

- Chadda Surgicals, Mumbai
- Alpha Surgicals, Surat
- Jullundur Enterprises, New Delhi
- Medono India, Alipur
- Medsor Impex, New Delhi
- Innovation Surgicals, Mumbai
- Tejco Vision, Mumbai
- S. P. Enterprise, Kolkata
- Med-Special Devices, Ghaziabad
- Bright Shine, Kolkata
- Namo Pharma, Pune
- Mcos Solutions, Jaipur
- Med Morphosis LLP, Villupuram
- Paul Medical Systems, Chennai

International Suppliers

- Zavimed Medical Equipment, Netherlands
- Scharf CE, Turkey
- Magna Medical, Turkey

Operating Theater Table Suppliers

- KSK Surgicals, New Delhi
- Sharma Surgicals, Haryana
- Sai Mediquip, Mumbai
- Labmicro Meditech India, Satara
- Creative Medical System, Chandigarh
- Hospitech Industries, New Delhi
- Rumax International Private Limited, New Delhi
- Daksh Healthcare, Chhattisgarh
- NM Surgical & Biotech Medicare, Lucknow
- Aryan Industries, Hyderabad
- Akshara Medical Equipments, Chennai
- Science & Surgicals, Kolkata

Operating Theater Lights Suppliers

- Senco Hospital Supply & Company, Kolkata
- VVM BioTech Infra Pvt. Ltd., Thane
- Safex Inc, New Delhi
- KSK Surgicals, New Delhi
- Sharma Scientific Industry, Haryana
- Silicon MedTech Pvt Ltd, Surat
- A. R. Healthcare, Ghaziabad
- Dynamin Kare, Indore
- Aesthetic Surgi Med India, New Delhi
- M/s Limra Healthcare, Lucknow
- O2 Medical Systems, Hyderabad
- Medvalley, Chennai
- Kalki Surgical Supplies, Patna

Other Instruments

Other instruments to be kept in place include Doyen's cross-section towel clips, kidney tray, bowls, etri dishes, etc.

Suppliers

- All India Surgicals, Mumbai
- Indwell Enterprises, New Delhi
- Medinova, Bengaluru
- Sri Sai Enterprises, Lucknow
- Deluxe Scientific Surgico Private Limited, New Delhi
- Jd Medical Systems, Mumbai
- VN Medical Services, Chennai
- Meditech Global, Kolkata

- Super Scientific Industry, Ambala
- Eternal Surgical Solutions, Jaipur
- Hindustan Traders, Jalandhar
- Help Care Meditech, Surat
- Sai Pharma, Ahmedabad

Microblading

Microblading is a cosmetic procedure for eyebrow restoration.[4]

The instruments needed are as follows:

- Golden Mean Brow Caliper—for eyebrow assessment
- Microblading pen—this pen-like instrument is used to hold the microblading needle.
- Blades—microblading blades consist of multiple needles arranged in a row. Blades are available in different numbers ranging from 7 to 21, depending on the number of needles in the blade.
- Ink holder—a plastic or metal ring container used to keep the microblading ink.
- Inks—there are two main types of medical tattooing inks, one made of iron oxide and the other is synthetic. Microblading pigments are synthetic in nature.

Suppliers

- Tekno Midas Aesthetics, New Delhi
- Reelay Ecommerce India Private Limited, New Delhi
- Innovation Surgicals, Mumbai
- Tejco Vision, Mumbai
- Ibrow Academy, Ahmedabad

Scalp Micropigmentation

Scalp micropigmentation is a method of concealing alopecia by depositing permanent pigment in a tattoo-like manner.

Suppliers

- Maquillage Skin Care, Mumbai
- Innovation Surgicals, Mumbai
- Tejco Vision, Mumbai

REFERENCES

1. Marwah MK, Mysore V. Recipient area. J Cutan Aesthet Surg. 2018;11(4):202-10.
2. Kerure A, Rohatgi S, Patwardhan N. Kerure clamp: a new age tool to improve extraction technique in follicular unit extraction. J Cutan Aesthet Surg. 2019;12(2):141-4.
3. Garg AK, Garg S. Donor harvesting: follicular unit excision. J Cutan Aesthet Surg. 2018;11(4):195-201.
4. Marwah MK, Kerure AS, Marwah GS. Microblading and the science behind it. Indian Dermatol Online J. 2021;12(1):6-11.

CHAPTER 103

Hair Transplant Practice Guidelines*

Venkatram Mysore, Kumaresan M, Anil Kumar Garg, Aman Dua, Aniketh Venkataram, Kapil Dua, Mayank Singh, Madura C, Ram Chandran, Rajesh Rajput, Sandeep Sattur, Sukhbir Singh

INTRODUCTION

The field of hair transplant (HT) has grown exponentially in the past decade, especially after the introduction of follicular unit excision (FUE). There is much variation in criteria for case selection, the technique, pre- and post-procedure protocols, by different surgeons. Techniques continue to evolve and evidence in the form of controlled data is not available for all techniques and protocols being used; there is also a debate as to who can do what, what should be the training for staff, role of technicians. This has led to a situation wherein medico legal issues have cropped up as to what is minimum acceptable. An attempt is made to summarize standard protocols with the available evidence. It is emphasized that the objective of these guidelines is to recommend minimum standards for practice of hair transplantation. The principles outlined in these guidelines are of a general nature only, minimal in their level and are not meant to cover all situations. It should be understood that these recommendations are by no means binding and universal, represent minimum standards only and as in all surgical techniques, variations in techniques are possible. It is also further clarified that these are based on current literature, and as science evolves, these guidelines could also change in future. Where published evidence is not available, consensus expert opinion is presented. The task force emphasizes that each patient has to be treated on his/her own merit and that these guidelines do not limit the physician from making an appropriate choice or the necessary innovation for a given patient. The task force recognizes that the treating surgeon is best suited to decide what is needed for a given patient in a given situation. Innovations in medicine need flexibility in approach and these guidelines do not limit the surgeon from undertaking innovative research.

Financial Support and Sponsorship

Association of Hair Restoration Surgeons of India.

Conflicts of Interest

There are no conflicts of interest.

HAIR TRANSPLANT PRACTICE GUIDELINES: PART 1

Introduction, Rationale, and Scope for the Guidelines

The field of hair transplant (HT) has grown exponentially in the past decade, especially after the introduction of follicular unit excision. There is much variation in criteria for case selection, the technique, and pre-procedure and post-procedure protocols, by different surgeons. Techniques continue to evolve and evidence in the form of controlled data is not available for all techniques and protocols being used; there is also a debate as to who can do what, what should be the training for staff, and the role of technicians. This has led to a situation wherein medicolegal issues have cropped up as to what is minimum acceptable. An attempt is made here to summarize standard protocols with the available evidence. It is emphasized that the objective of these guidelines is to recommend minimum standards for

*The following article was published as a CME article: "Mysore V, Kumaresan M, Garg A, Dua A, Venkatram A, Dua K, et al. Hair transplant practice guidelines. J Cutan Aesthet Surg. 2021;14:265-84." It is reproduced with the permission from Journal of Cutaneous and Aesthetic Surgery.

practice of HT. The principles outlined in these guidelines are of a general nature only, minimal in their level and are not meant to cover all situations. It should be understood that these recommendations are by no means binding and universal, represent minimum standards only and as in all surgical techniques, variations in techniques are possible. It is also further clarified that these are based on current literature, and as science evolves, these guidelines could also change in future. Where published evidence is not available, consensus expert opinion is presented.

The taskforce emphasizes that each patient has to be treated on his/her own merit and that these guidelines do not limit the physician from making an appropriate choice or the necessary innovation for a given patient. The taskforce recognizes that the treating surgeon is best suited to decide what is needed for a given patient in a given situation. Innovations in medicine need flexibility in approach and these guidelines do not limit the surgeon from undertaking innovative research.

Evidence Levels and Levels of Recommendation

The taskforce used a modified Harbour and Miller's revised grading system for recommendations in formulating these guidelines.

Levels of Evidence

1. Meta-analyses, systematic reviews of randomized control trials (RCTs)
2. One or more case-control or cohort studies of high quality
3. Nonanalytic studies, for example, case reports and case series
4. Expert opinion

Grades of Recommendations

A. Strongly recommended on the basis of at least one meta-analysis, systematic review, or RCT rated as 1 and likely to be relevant in future also

B. Recommended on the basis of studies rated as 2 and demonstrating overall consistency of results or extrapolated evidence from studies rated as 1; and may change in future subject to future developments

C. Recommended for use based on current use, not sufficiently corroborated, based on evidence rated as 2 or 3, and likely for subsequent change

D. Based on insufficient evidence rated as level 3 or 4 and needs further evidence.

REFERENCE

1. Harbour R, Miller J. A new system for grading recommendations in evidence based guidelines. BMJ. 2001;323:334-6.

PHYSICIAN QUALIFICATIONS, ROLE OF TECHNICIANS, AND TRAINING OF DOCTORS AND STAFF

Hair Transplant Surgeons

There is no uniform opinion as to which specialties can perform HT. Even medical councils have not categorically resolved this issue, and different associations have different criteria for membership.

In October 2015, the Association of Hair Restoration Surgeons – India (AHRS-I) resolved that the only specialties eligible to become members of AHRS-I and practice HT surgery would be,

- The Master of Plastic Surgery (MCh)/DNB Plastic Surgery
- Doctor of Medicine or postgraduate in Dermatology
- Master of Surgery (MS) or postgraduate in Ear, Nose, and Throat (ENT) surgery
- MS General Surgery (MS)
- Modern medical practitioners (MBBS doctors/specialists not included in the qualifications just cited) who have passed the American Board of Hair Restoration Surgery (ABHRS) exam are also eligible to perform HT surgery.

Disclaimer

The eligibility to do HT should be governed by the regulations of the state and/or national medical council.

This taskforce is of the opinion that Ayurvedic doctors, homeopathic doctors, and dentists are not qualified to perform HT surgery.

Any procedure that involves tissue removal from the scalp or body, by any means, should be performed by a licensed physician in the field of medicine. The taskforce recommends that the following aspects of hair restoration surgery should only be performed by a qualified HT surgeon and not by technicians:

- Preoperative diagnostic evaluation and consultation
- Surgery planning
- Surgery execution, including:
  - Donor hair harvesting
  - Hairline design
  - Recipient site creation

- Management of other patient medical issues and possible adverse reactions
- Postoperative care

The concept of nonphysicians removing human tissue and primarily performing HT surgery is improper and not acceptable. It is not consistent with the standard of care in the medical community.

ROLE OF ASSISTANTS (TECHNICIANS)

Hair transplant practice needs assistants, who are also called HT technicians; it is both ethical and necessary that such assistants are from a medical background, such as nurses, lab technicians, pharmacists, and MBBS doctors. However, they need to be provided structured, systematic, and proper training in aspects of both HT and disinfection, sterilization, patient communication etc. However, unrelated nonmedical personnel such as arts graduates, industrial training institute technicians should not be used as they have little understanding of sterilization and cannot handle any medical emergency that may arise during the procedure.

Technicians can be involved only in the following steps of the HT surgery:

1. Picking up the grafts (extraction) after scoring
2. Arranging the grafts
3. Implantation into premade slits
4. Postoperative dressings

Surgical assistants/technicians should perform tasks only under the supervision of a physician and they are allowed to perform only those steps that do not involve an incision of the body. Hence, they should not perform scoring (incision), slit making, and suturing. The assistants should be offered training on models initially, then placed as observers for the surgical process, and finally be deputed for the HT surgery. At least one of the assistants should be a paramedical staff and trained in Basic Life Support/advanced cardiac life support.

Level of Evidence: 4

Grades of Recommendation: D

REFERENCES

1. Kumaresan M, Mysore V. Controversies in hair transplantation. J Cutan Aesthet Surg. 2018;11:173-81.
2. ISHRS.org [Internet]. Geneva, IL, USA: International Society of Hair Restoration Surgery, Inc.; c1993 [updated 2019 March19]. Available from: http://www.ishrs.org/. [Last accessed on 2019 Aug 18].
3. AHRSINDIA.orgcapitalspls (Internet) Ludhiana Association of Hair Restoration Surgeons - India. Inc; c2011 (updated 2015 March 10). Available from: http://www.ahrsindia.org/. [Last accessed on 2019 Aug 18].
4. Williams KL Jr. Current practices and controversies in cosmetic hair restoration. Dermatol Surg. 2013;39:797-801.

TRAINING

Physicians who perform HT surgery must possess the education, training, and current competency in the field of hair restoration surgery. Membership in the national hair restoration society/global society and regular attendance at annual conferences and workshops facilitate the education and training. Fellowship courses from the International Society of Hair Restoration Surgery (ISHRS) would be an added qualification.

It is further observed that HT is not taught as a subject in any of the earlier cited courses that were listed as the eligibility criteria for an HT surgeon. Although the surgical specialties such as Mch/DNB plastic surgery, MS general surgery, and MS ENT provide an adequate surgical background, training in trichology is lacking. Likewise, MD/DNB/Diploma in Dermatology provides adequate training in trichology, but surgical training is lacking.

In view of this, this taskforce recommends that:

1. Mch/DNB plastic surgery, MS general surgery, and MS ENT doctors should undergo further training in trichology in a clinic that provides such training under a dermatologist/HT surgeon, preferably for three months, but at least for a period of 1 month.
2. Likewise, MD/DNB/Diploma in Dermatology doctors should undergo adequate training (both hands on and observational) under the supervision of an experienced HT surgeon. Although no legal guideline exists to define how much observation and supervision is needed, this taskforce recommends that at least 50 surgeries be observed and 25 surgeries be performed under supervision before starting independent practice. This training should also include training in basic surgical practices, sterilization, disinfection, and emergency resuscitation.

The taskforce is of the firm opinion that watching in workshops or on YouTube is not adequate training to start HT practice and strongly condemns and discourages such training.

Level of Evidence: 4

Grades of Recommendation: D

REFERENCE

1. ISHRS.org [Internet]. Geneva, IL, USA: International Society of Hair Restoration Surgery, Inc.; c1993 [updated 2019 March19; cited 2019 August 18]. Available from: http://www.ishrs.org/.

ETHICAL ISSUES

The use of trademarks or service marks as commercial names for a hair restoration procedure, without disclosing the scientific basis for the procedure, its complications and side effects is not in the public interest. Nor is it in the public interest to use a commercial name to market a procedure that is described under a commonly accepted name in the medical literature, without revealing the name used in the medical literature. Professional disagreements should be aired in a forum of peers. Denigration that aims at destroying another physician's practice is morally reprehensible. Physicians who market their services have a responsibility for "truth in advertising."

The following advertisements are considered to be misleading the public:

1. Inaccurate Credentials. Incorrectly claiming to be certified by the AHRS-I, ABHRS or claiming to be a member or Fellow of the ISHRS, and otherwise stating or suggesting any expertise in hair restoration surgery that is false.
2. Misrepresenting Board Certification. Physicians should identify their specific medical specialty certifying board when marketing their board certification in the public domain language, such as "board certified hair restoration surgeon" is not acceptable.
3. Misrepresenting Photographs. Publishing photographs of other physicians' patients in any manner that states or suggests that they are patients of the publishing practice.
4. Copyright/Trademark Violations in General. Republishing or otherwise representing the photographs, publications, trade names, logos, or other trademarks of another practitioner without permission in violation of the owner's copyrights and/ or trademarks.
5. Misleading Language. Use of the following terms and phrases in marketing by a hair restoration surgeon may mislead the public:
    - "Scarless surgery"
    - "No incision"
    - "No touch"
    - "No cutting"
    - "Cloning"
    - "Hair multiplication"
    - "Noninvasive"
    - "Eliminates the need for additional procedures"
    - "Pain free or no pain"
    - "Unlimited grafts"
    - "Guaranteed results"

Level of Evidence: 4

Grades of Recommendation: D

REFERENCE

1. ISHRS.org [Internet]. Geneva, IL, USA: International Society of Hair Restoration Surgery, Inc.; c1993 [updated 2019 March19; cited 2019 August 18]. Available from: http://www.ishrs.org/.

CHARGES FOR THE SURGERY

The surgery cost should be based on the number of follicular units/follicles/package for a particular surface area as per the surgeon's routine pricing practice. However, each term unit/graft/follicle should be explained and the patient should be familiar with the terminology.

Costs should be informed beforehand to the patient and documented in the consent form.

Transparency

Transparency in the HT surgery should be followed in the following aspects:

- The physician who will be performing the surgery and the role of assistants should be informed to the patient prior to the surgery.
- The role of the surgeon and the role of assistants should be documented—who does what
- Hairline design, once accepted by the patient and the surgeon, should be documented with an image.
- Number of grafts/ follicles/ area to be covered initially planned and actually performed should be disclosed to the patient and documented with images. The discharge slips should document the number of units of each type, 1/2/3/4 hairs total; number of units; and total number of hair separately.
- Provision of counting the grafts can be explained to the patient.
- The need for the medical management/chances of inadequate growth/ thinning of grafted follicles with time post-HT should be discussed with the patient and documented.
- Charging for the surgery should be only for viable follicles that are transplanted.

Level of Evidence: 4

Grades of Recommendation: D

DOCUMENTATION AND CONSENT

A medical record is admissible as documentary evidence in a legal suit. So it is important to maintain a meticulous record of clinical details of the patient, the counseling process, consent taking, detailed preoperative, operative, and postoperative notes and instructions, and follow-up visits.

Preoperative documentation should include the details about any preexisting health issues, drug allergy, photograph id lignocaine test dose, baseline vital parameters, hairline design planned, planned number of grafts to be harvested, expected results with duration, donor adequacy, continuation of medical management if required, and the possibility of a second surgery after a particular period.

Intraoperative records should include the vital parameters, drugs administered and their dosage, complications if any and the remedial measures that were carried out, number of grafts planted, the area of scalp covered the details of the surgical team, and the duration of the surgery with the timings of the beginning and the end of each stage of the surgery. Immediate postoperative records should have the following details: vital parameters after the surgery, duration of observation post-surgery, complications if any at the end of the surgery, remedial measures taken, postoperative prescription and advice, emergency contact number for communication, and the details of the follow-up visit.

The patient's failure to adhere to post-procedure consultations, neglect of precautions, and noncompliance of instructions, if any, should also find place in the record.

Both manual signed records and computerized data help in the standardization, storage, and easy retrieval of records.

Photographs taken before, during, and after the procedure provide adequate proof of the outcome of the procedure.

Medical records of HT must be preserved for five years, but those pertaining to malpractice suits must be preserved till the final settlement of the case.

The aesthetic surgeon or the hospital is vested with the custodial ownership of records. However, on request, these should be provided to the patient within 72 hours.

The Consumer Protection Act can condone a delay in filing a case of negligence beyond the prescribed limitation of 2 years from the date of occurrence.

Consent in the medical field can be defined as an instrument of mutual communication between a doctor and a patient with an expression of authorization/permission/choice by the latter for the doctor to act/not act in a particular way.

Lack of informed consent is a frequent cause of allegations of medical negligence.

Consent should have the following details:

- Procedure details in a language that the patient understands
- Risks involved
- Complications that can arise
- Outcome expected
- Duration of treatment (average)
- Expenses involved (approximate)

Evidence Level: 3

Category of recommendation: C

REFERENCES

1. Akshay GN, Aparna S. Clinical photography for periorbital and facial aesthetic practice. J Cutan Aesthet Surg. 2016;9:115-21.
2. Khavkin J, Ellis DA. Standardized photography for skin surface. Facial Plast Surg Clin North Am. 2011;19:241-6.
3. Galdino GM, DaSilva And D, Gunter JP. Digital photography for rhinoplasty. Plast Reconstr Surg. 2002;109:1421-34.
4. Shah AR, Dayan SH, Hamilton GS 3rd. Pitfalls of photography for facial resurfacing and rejuvenation procedures. Facial Plast Surg. 2005;21:154-61.
5. Satish M, Menon R, Rao KV. Professional accountability and patients' rights, 2nd ed. Bengaluru: The Institute of Law and Ethics in Medicine, National Law School of India University; 2002. pp. 57-68.
6. Indian Medical Council. Regulations, 2002 (published in Gazette of India, o.14, part III section 4 dated 6.4.2002). New Delhi: Indian Medical Council; 2002.
7. Mousavi SR. The ethics of aesthetic surgery. J Cutan Aesthet Surg. 2010;3:38-40.
8. Bastia BK, Kuruvilla A, Saralaya KM. Validity of consent – A review of statutes. Indian J Med Sci. 2005;59:74-8.
9. Satyanarayana Rao KH. Informed consent: An ethical obligation or legal compulsion? J Cutan Aesthet Surg. 2008;1:33-5.
10. Beauchamp TL, Childress JF. Fair opportunity. In: Haker H, Beyleveld D, (Eds). Principle of biomedical ethics. 5th ed. Oxford: Ashgate Publishing Co; Oxford University Press; 2001. pp. 335.
11. Trehan SP, Sankhari D. Medical professional, patient and the law: the institute of law and ethics in medicine. 2nd ed. Bangalore: National Law School of India University; 2002. pp. 57-68.
12. Kohli A. Medical consent in India – Ethical and legal issues. Anil Aggrawal's Internet Journal of Forensic Medicine and Toxicity. 2007;8:8-9.
13. Mavroforou A, Giannoukas A, Michalodimitrakis E. Medical litigation in cosmetic plastic surgery. Med Law. 2004;23:479-88.

COUNSELING FOR THE MEDICAL MANAGEMENT

HT surgery should not be considered as a single-step permanent solution for androgenetic alopecia (AGA), since the hair loss in AGA is a continuous process. The taskforce recommends that every patient should be educated about the importance of continuing the medical management even after the HT surgery. Topical minoxidil 2–5% and oral finasteride at a dosage of 1mg/day are the approved medications for AGA. Dosage and duration should be individualized according to the degree of hair loss.

Level of Evidence: 1

Grades of Recommendation: A

REFERENCES

1. Mysore V, Parthasaradhi A, Kharkar RD, Ghoshal AK, Ganjoo A, Ravichandran G, et al. Expert consensus on the management of androgenetic alopecia in India. Int J Trichology. 2019;11:101-6.
2. Blumeyer A, Tosti A, Messenger A, Reygagne P, Del Marmol V, Spuls PI, et al.; European Dermatology Forum (EDF). Evidence-based (S3) guideline for the treatment of androgenetic alopecia in women and in men. J Dtsch Dermatol Ges. 2011;9(Suppl 6): S1-57.

HT PRACTICE GUIDELINES: PART 2

Introduction

HT surgery is considered as a daycare surgery that does not require in-hospital admission. However, similar to all surgical treatments, maintaining standards of care is of utmost importance. This part of the guidelines describes the minimum standard of care in establishing a setup for HT surgery, sterilization process, preoperative workup, case selection, and antimicrobial prophylaxis.

General Safety

It is recommended that any practice performing office-based surgery regardless of anesthesia will have the necessary equipment, protocol, and personnel to handle emergencies resulting from the procedure, anesthesia, and the other environmental emergencies. As per the Clinical Establishment Act of the respective state authority, all applicable safety measures as per local law should be adopted.

Operating Room

Although HT is a simple minimally invasive surgery, all protocols should be followed to see that adequate asepsis, sterilization, disinfection, and resuscitation are in place. The surgery should not be taken lightly and the taskforce strongly disapproves the usage of temporary theaters such as consultation rooms, minor procedure rooms, spa rooms, etc. for performing HT. At least one of the nurses should be an operation theater (OT) trained nurse.

The HT operating room can be located in a multispecialty hospital, a private clinic, or in shared spaces of polyclinics. The operating room should be located in a restricted zone where hair cover, face mask, surgical attire, and slippers for both patient and doctor are required.

The taskforce would like to recommend the minimum size of the HT operating room to be 12 × 12 feet with a height of the room to be a minimum of 10 feet. An additional dissecting room of equal size is needed, particularly for FUT surgeries. Alternately, a larger OT of 20 × 12 feet can include both OT and dissecting room. This criterion of minimum space in the operating room includes the space to move around the operating table in case of emergency resuscitation. The door should be preferably of width more than 24 inches and should lead to adequate space for the trolley/stretcher to be taken out, in case of emergencies. The floors should be impervious to moisture, easy to clean, stain resistant, and suitable for wheeled traffic. Windows, if present, should be sealed and protected to maintain strict asepsis.

Provision for a preparatory room to change slippers and a dress change room, for both patient and staff, should be planned. A dressing/washing area should include a washbasin provided with a hand disinfectant dispenser and a tap with a long handle.

Level of Evidence: 2

Grade of Recommendation: B

REFERENCES

1. Malkin J. Ambulatory surgical centers. In: Malkin J, (Ed). Medical and Dental Space planning, A comprehensive guide to design, equipment and clinical procedures. 3rd ed. New York: John Wiley and Sons; 2002. pp. 334-6.
2. Asadi KA, Goldberg LH, Peterson SR, Silapint S, Jih MH. The incidence of major complications from Mohs micrographic surgery performed in office-based and hospital based settings. J Am Acad Dermatol. 2005;53:628-34.
3. Malkin J. Ambulatory surgical centers. In: Malkin J, (Ed). Medical and Dental Space planning, A comprehensive guide to design, equipment and clinical procedures. 3rd ed. New York: John Wiley and sons, Inc; 2002. pp. 352-3.
4. Drake LA, Ceilley RI, Cornelison RL, Dinehart SM, Dorner W, Goltz RW, et al. Guidelines of care for office surgical facilities. J Am Acad Dermatol. 1992;26:763-5.
5. Savant SS, Gore D. Instruments, equipment and universal precautions. In: Savant SS, (Ed). Textbook of dermatosurgery

and cosmetology. 2nd ed. Mumbai: Association of Scientific Cosmetologists and Dermatosurgeons; 2005. pp. 26-34.
6. Lawrence C. Equipment. In: Lawrence C, (Ed). An introduction to dermatological surgery. 2nd ed. London: Churchill Livingstone; 2002. pp. 5-6.
7. Rajendran SC, Omprakash HM. Standard guidelines for setting up a dermatosurgery theatre. Indian J Dermatol Venerolleprol. 2009;75:76-82.

LIGHTING

General lighting in the theater by a fluorescent lamp-mounted flush with the ceiling is adequate.

- Fluorescent lamp: at the rate of 1W per square foot (i.e., for 120 square feet - 120W - three tubes of 40W). Ceiling or pedestal lighting of the operation field.
- Shadowless lighting delivering 3,000–8,000 foot candles (i.e., the dental chairs have a halogen lamp of 50W power. Each Watt of power will give 50 foot candles of illumination at the site of surgery. So 50W of a halogen bulb can roughly give 2,500 foot candles of illumination at the site of surgery)
- It is important that heat generation by the lighting system is kept to minimum.

REFERENCES

1. Rajendran SC, Omprakash HM. Standard guidelines for setting up a dermatosurgery theatre. Ind J Dermatol Venerolleprol. 2009;75:76-82.
2. Malkin J. Ambulatory surgical centers. In: Malkin J, (Ed). Medical and Dental Space planning, A comprehensive guide to design, equipment and clinical procedures. 3rd ed. New York: John Wiley and Sons; 2002. pp. 334-67.

Alternately, surgeons have used lights attached to loupes, which is also adequate.

Level of Evidence: 3

Grade of recommendation: C

STERILIZATION AND DISINFECTION OF OPERATION THEATER AND INSTRUMENTS

- The operation table, chair, light, shelves, and sink should be wet mopped daily free of dust, with water and the use of a broom should be avoided. Chemical disinfectant is recommended for the floor. The wet mop used should be left in a proper place to dry.
- The OT trolley should be mopped with a chemical disinfectant or isopropyl alcohol before surgery and between two surgeries.
- The floor and other areas of blood spillage should be mopped with a chemical disinfectant. The operating room wall and ceiling need to be cleaned periodically.
- The use of a fan in the OT should be avoided, as it causes aerosolization of dust.
- Regular maintenance of the air conditioner is necessary. The tonnage of air conditioner depends on the size of the room to ensure adequate cooling.
- After an HT surgery, the instruments should be rinsed in 0.5% chlorine for 10 minutes and then should be washed in water and scrubbed with a brush before sending them for sterilization.
- Linen, draped, gowns: Should be washed with a detergent at 71 degrees for 25 minutes, and then sent for sterilization.

FUMIGATION

Formaldehyde fumigation can be done initially during a start-up of the theater or after an overhaul cleaning process. Formaldehyde 6%, glutaraldehyde 6%, and benzalkonium chloride 5% can be used by adequate trained personnel wearing appropriate protective devices. A combination of stabilized hydrogen peroxide 11% w/v and diluted silver nitrate solution 0.01% w/v is an ideal aerial disinfectant and OT fumigant acting as a sterilant at a recommended concentration of 20% at 1 hour contact time. Fumigation should be done daily or prior to each surgery.

In between two operative procedures on the same day, spot cleaning of operation tables, theater equipment with disinfectant solution is recommended. In case of spillage of blood/body fluids, decontamination with bleaching powder/chlorine solution should be done. Fumigation should be repeated prior to the second surgery, if performed on the same day.

AUTOCLAVE

- All material should be dried and wrapped in cloth or medical grade paper.
- The instruments should be laid so that all surfaces come in contact with heat.
- Time depends on individual recommendations, but it is usually 121 degrees for 15 minutes.

Chemical sterilization of instruments:

- Cleaned, disinfected, and dried instruments should be fully soaked in a steel or plastic container having 2% glutaraldehyde for 8–10 hours.
- After 10 hours, using autoclaved water (100 mL of water autoclaved for 20 minutes and not boiled water) the instruments should be washed, dried, packed, and

stored in a sterile tray. Note that the contact time for high-level disinfection is just 20 minutes compared with the 10 hours required for sterilization.

- Sterilization of follicular unit excision machines and implanters:
- Heat- and moisture-sensitive electronic goods and other implanters are sterilized using ethylene oxide sterilization.

REFERENCES

1. Patwardhan N, Kelkar U. Disinfection, sterilization and operation theater guidelines for dermatosurgical practitioners. Indian J Dermatol Venereol Leprol. 2011;77:83-93.
2. Mysore V, Anitha B. Checklists for surgical safety in dermatosurgery. J Cutan Aesthet Surg. 2009;2:1-3.
3. Rutala WA, Weber DJ. Chemical disinfection of medical and surgical materials. In: Block SS, (Ed). Disinfection, sterilization and preservation. 3rd ed. Philadelphia: Lea and Febiger; 1983. pp. 469-92.
4. Kelkar U, Bal AM, Kulkarni S. Monitoring of steam sterilization process by biologic indicators – a necessary surveillance tool. Am J Infect Control. 2004;32:512-3.
5. Simpson RA, Slack RC. Sterilization and disinfection. In: Greenwood D, Slack RC, Peutherer JF, (Eds). Medical Microbiology. 16 th ed. London: Churchill Livingstone; 2002. pp. 73-82.
6. Govindaraj S, Muthuraman MS. Systematic review on sterilization methods of implants and medical devices. Int J Chem Tech Res. 2015;8:897-911.
7. Gupta C, Vanathi M, Tandon R. Current concepts in operative room sterilisation. J Ophthalmol. 2015;25:190-4.

Level of Evidence: 3

Grade of recommendation: C

BIOMEDICAL WASTE MANAGEMENT

- Segregation, collection, transportation, storage, and disposal of biomedical waste should be as per biomedical waste handling rules, and that of general waste should be as per applicable local laws.

Level of Evidence: 4

Grade of recommendation: D

PREOPERATIVE CONSIDERATIONS

A detailed preoperative evaluation of the patient's medical status is essential. It is recommended to get the patient assessed opined upon by a treating doctor or an independent physician regarding the patient's eligibility to undergo HT.

REFERENCES

1. Ellsworth WA, Basu B, Iverson RE. Perioperative considerations for patient safety during cosmetic surgery - preventing complications. Can J Plast Surg. 2009;17:9-16.
2. Unger WP. The initial interview and evaluation. In: Unger WP, Shapiro R, Unger R, Unger M, (Eds). Hair transplantation. 5th ed. Boca Raton, FL: CRC Press; 2011.
3. Unger WP. The preoperative phase. In: Unger WP, Shapiro R, Unger R, Unger M, (Eds). Hair transplantation. 5th ed. Boca Raton, FL: CRC Press; 2011.

CASE SELECTION WITH RESPECT TO AGE

Age is an important, but not the only consideration for case selection. Since AGA is a continuous and progressive condition, early surgery would lead to future hairloss negating the results of surgery and causing an ugly recession that can affect the patient psychologically. Further, younger individuals cannot be relied upon to adhere to long-term drug therapy. Younger individuals are also likely to have unrealistic expectations and often expect a cure of AGA by HT. For these reasons, HT in the early age group is not recommended and it is preferable to wait till at least 23–25 years of age. It is also preferable to treat such patients with medical management for a few months, develop rapport, and then decide for surgery.

However, there are some special situations where early surgery may be necessary in patients who are between 21 and 23 years of age:

1. Advanced hair loss Hamilton–Norwood stages 4–6, which causes severe psychological issues and where drug therapy is unlikely to be beneficial.
2. Young patients in special professions such as acting, media, modeling, etc, whose career gets affected by postponing surgery.
3. Patients who are severely psychologically affected by their baldness.
4. In cases of tractional alopecia, secondary cicatricialalopecias (burns, trauma, surgical scars over hair-bearing regions).

In all these cases, extensive counseling over several sessions, preferably in the presence of their parents, is advocated. This taskforce does not recommend surgery in those younger than 21 years of age.

Level of Evidence: 4

Grades of Recommendation: D

REFERENCE

1. Unger WP. Preoperative preparations and instructions. In: Unger WP, Shapiro R, Unger R, Unger M, (Eds). Hair transplantation. 5th ed. New York: Informa Health Care; 2011. pp. 198-226.

2. Patwardhan N, Kirane V. Case selection, counseling and planning for the surgery. In: Mysore V, (Ed). Hair transplantation. 1st ed. New Delhi: Jaypee Brothers Medical Publishers (p) Ltd; 2016. pp. 119-24.

PREOPERATIVE INSTRUCTIONS

The expert committee recommends the following instructions before the HT surgery: Allergies to any medications in the past, history of previous surgeries, complications if any, and the medications currently being consumed by the patient should be documented in the case sheet. Medications for hypertension, epilepsy, thyroid, and diabetes should be continued, if any, as per the treating physician's recommendation and medical clearance from the physician is recommended for those with history of any cardiac surgeries or cardiac procedures. Specific instructions as per the operating surgeon need to be followed.

Preoperative checklist:

1. Minoxidil to be stopped one week prior to the procedure, as it may increase bleeding.
2. Alcohol to be avoided seven days before and after the procedure.
3. Smoking should be reduced as much as possible before the surgery and it would be safe to stop it entirely.
4. Preoperative tranquilizer in an anxious patient.
5. NSAIDS to be restricted 12–24 hours before the surgery.
6. Antihypertensives to be continued on the day of the surgery. Beta-blockers to be avoided on the day of the surgery.
7. Vitamin supplements and herbal preparations to be avoided for three weeks before the surgery.
8. Lignocaine test dose for sensitivity, preferably one day prior to the surgery to account for delayed allergic reaction to the local anesthetics.
9. Preoperative photographs: standard positions.

Front facial, chin to chest, right oblique, left oblique, and vertex view

Level of Evidence: 4

Grades of Recommendation: D

REFERENCES

1. Patwardhan N, Mysore V; IADVL Dermatosurgery Task Force. Hair transplantation: Standard guidelines of care. Indian J Dermatol Venereol Leprol. 2008;74 Suppl:S46-53.
2. Unger WP. Preoperative preparations and instructions. In: Unger WP, Shapiro R, Unger R, Unger M, (Eds). Hair transplantation. 5th ed. New York: Informa Health Care; 2011. pp. 198-226.

PREOPERATIVE LABORATORY WORKUP

Preoperative laboratory studies to be performed in all age groups include Hb%, blood counts including platelet count, bleeding and clotting time (or prothrombin time and activated partial thromboplastin time), venereal disease research laboratory, ECG, fasting blood sugar, antibodies for hepatitis B and C surface antigen, and HIV screening tests.

INVESTIGATIONS IN SPECIAL SITUATIONS

Electrocardiography

Routine electrocardiography is not recommended routinely before HT surgery; however, it is advisable to perform it in the following circumstances:

- In a patient with any present or past cardiac symptom (including breathlessness, pre-syncope, syncope, or chest pain) or history of cardiac disease or obesity or metabolic syndrome.
- Patients with abnormal ECG are recommended to get a cardiologist's opinion before the surgery.

PREOPERATIVE EVALUATION IN HYPERTENSIVES

In patients with hypertension undergoing surgery, it is recommended to continue most antihypertensive medications until surgery, including the morning of the surgery. Medical fitness for HT surgery should be obtained from the physician. Intraoperative management of hypertension should be done in association with the anesthetist.

EVALUATION IN DIABETICS

A preoperative assessment should be done with support from a diabetologist/endocrinologist. It should occur sufficiently in advance of the planned surgery to ensure optimization of glycemic control as per the recommendation of the treating physician for the particular patient, before the date of the proposed surgery. People with diabetes should have their most recent HbA1c test results analyzed. HbA1c testing should be offered to people with diabetes having surgery if they have not been tested in the past three months. With appropriate guidance, patients with diabetes should be allowed to retain control and possession of, and continue to self-administer, their medication. The aim is to avoid hypoglycemia or hyperglycemia during the period of fasting and the time during and after the procedure, until the patient is eating and drinking normally.

Routine HbA1c testing before surgery to people without diagnosed diabetes is not essential.

Level of Evidence: 4

Grades of Recommendation: D

REFERENCES

1. Patwardhan N, Mysore V; IADVL Dermatosurgery Task Force. Hair transplantation: Standard guidelines of care. Indian J Dermatol Venereol Leprol. 2008;74 Suppl:S46-53.
2. Unger WP. Preoperative preparations and instructions. In: Unger WP, Shapiro R, Unger R, Unger M, (Eds). Hair transplantation. 5th ed. New York: Informa Health Care; 2011. pp. 198-226.
3. National Guideline Centre (UK). Preoperative tests (update): Routine preoperative tests for elective surgery. London: National Institute for Health and Care Excellence (UK); 2016.
4. Hazzi R, Mayock R. Perioperative management of hypertension. J Xiangya Med. 2018;3:25-35.
5. Membership of the Working Party, Barker P, Creasey PE, Dhatariya K, Levy N, Lipp A, Nathanson MH, et al. Peri-operative management of the surgical patient with diabetes 2015. Anaesthesia: Association of Anaesthetists of Great Britain and Ireland. Anaesthesia. 2015;70(12):1427-40.

PRE-OP DRUG THERAPY BLOOD THINNERS

HT surgery is a cosmetic surgery and those patients who are on blood thinners and undergoing HT surgery might have the following issues:

1. Issues in donor area: Increased bleeding during and after surgery.
2. Issues in recipient area: Bleeding during implantation and postoperatively leading to poping, displacement, and poor results affecting the outcome.

These patients also may have underlying cardiac conditions that may necessitate avoidance of adrenaline. This will be an additional challenge as it increases bleeding and also leads to shorter action of lignocaine, needing additional doses of lignocaine, with the possibility of cardiac side effects by lignocaine overdosage. Bupivacaine also needs careful consideration in such patients because of its cardiac effects.

However, blood thinners are lifesaving and hence cannot be stopped casually, that too for a cosmetic surgery. Any decision to perform surgery in such patients, therefore, needs a careful assessment of risk versus benefit and is subject to clearance by a cardiologist/physician. Management of the antiplatelets and anticoagulants should be carried out as per the advice of the concerned physician. The presence of an anesthetist is mandatory during the procedure in such patients.

Level of Evidence: 4

Grades of Recommendation: D

REFERENCES

1. Unger WP. Preoperative preparations and instructions. In: Unger WP, Shapiro R, Unger R, Unger M, (Eds). Hair transplantation. 5th ed. New York: Informa Health Care; 2011. pp. 198-226.
2. Practice Guidelines for Perioperative Blood Management. An updated report by the American Society of Anesthesiologists Task Force on Perioperative Blood Management. Anaesthesiology. 2015;122:241-75.
3. Yagyu K. Guidelines for perioperative antithrombotic therapy in hair restoration surgery: Management of patients with coronary heart disease, mechanical heart valve, and atrial fibrillation. Hair Transplant Forum Int. 2012;22:59-6.
4. Vaishalee K, Aniketh V. Antithrombotic therapy. In: Mysore V, (Ed). Hair transplantation. 1st ed. New Delhi, India: Jaypee; 2016. pp. 132-34.

PREMEDICATION

The primary aim of premedication is to relieve the patient's anxiety/restlessness before anesthesia and to ensure optimum quantity and quality of sleep on the night preceding surgery. With these objectives in mind, oral benzodiazepines are the preferred choice. The taskforce recommends the use of Alprazolam at a dose of 0.5 mg.

Level of Evidence: 3

Category of Recommendation: C

REFERENCES

1. Unger WP. The initial interview and evaluation. In: Unger WP, Shapiro R, Unger R, Unger M, (Eds). Hair transplantation. 5th ed. Boca Raton, FL: CRC Press; 2011.
2. Unger WP. The Preoperative phase. In: Unger WP, Shapiro R, Unger R, Unger M, (Eds). Hair transplantation.5th ed. 2011.
3. Kim D, Lee S, Pyeon T, Jeong S. Use of triazolam and alprazolam as premedication for general anesthesia. Korean J Anesthesiol. 2015;68:346-51.
4. De Witte JL, Alegret C, Sessler DI, Cammu G. Preoperative alprazolam reduces anxiety in ambulatory surgery patients: A comparison with oral midazolam. Anesth Analg. 2002;95: 1601-6.

ANTIMICROBIAL PROPHYLAXIS

HT is categorized as a clean procedure; the taskforce recommends the administration of antimicrobial prophylaxis with cephalosporins since cephalosporins 1h preoperative administration is the most commonly used antibiotic for prophylaxis, apart from Cephadroxil 500 mg one tablet during the night before the surgery, one tablet on the morning of the surgery (before the surgery), and one tablet during the night after the surgery. A full course of five days of antibiotics should be administered in cases of surgery over the facial region. If the patient gives a history of sensitivity to penicillin, then an antibiotic from the macrolide group or Clindamycin can be used. Optimum serum and tissue levels must be reached prior to incision and maintained throughout the procedure and only for a few hours post-op.

Level of Evidence: 3

Category of Recommendation: C

REFERENCES

1. Tsilosani A, Gugava M. Is there a rationale for use of antibiotics in hair transplantation surgery? Georgian Med News. 2005;122: 7-10.
2. Farjo N. Infection control and policy development in hair restoration. Hair Transplant Forum Int. 2008;18:141-4.
3. Unger WP. Hair transplantation. 4th ed. New York: Marcel Dekker; 1995. pp. 363-74.
4. Mangram AJ, Horan TC, Pearson ML, Silver LC, Jarvis WR. Guideline for prevention of surgical site infection, 1999. Hospital infection control practices advisory committee. Infect Control Hosp Epidemiol. 1999;20:250-78; quiz 279-80.
5. Khichy S, Singh B, Singh M, Singh S. To compare the effectiveness of short-term three dose perioperative antibiotic coverage during decisive period with conventional prolonged postoperative antibiotic usage in clean elective surgical cases: An Indian perspective. Niger J Surg. 2017;23:92-7.
6. Lamont P. Surgical infection. In: Williams NS, Bulstrode CJ, O'Connell PR, (Eds). Bailey and Love's short practice of surgery. 26th ed. Boca Raton, FL: CRC Press; 2013. pp. 50-67.
7. Kerk SK, Lai HY, Sze SK, Ng KW, Schmidtchen A, Adav SS. Bacteria display differential growth and adhesion characteristics on human hair shafts. Front Microbiol. 2018;9:2145.

ANTISEPTIC PROPHYLAXIS

Proper cleansing of the surgical areas (scalp, beard, torso, etc.) before surgery helps in reducing colony counts of the local bacteria. It is recommended to advise the patients to shower or bathe (full body) with soap (antimicrobial or non-antimicrobial) or an antiseptic agent plus shampoo (Povidone iodine + Shampoo) on the night before and on the morning of the operative day.

Level of Evidence: 4

Category of Recommendation: D

REFERENCES

1. Unger WP. The Preoperative phase. In: Unger WP, Shapiro R, Unger R, Unger M, (Eds). Hair transplantation. 5th ed. 2011.
2. Farjo N. Infection control and policy development in hair restoration. Hair Transplant Forum Int. 2008;18.

HT PRACTICE GUIDELINES: PART 3

Anesthesia, Resuscitation, and Emergency Preparedness

Introduction

HT surgery is a daycare surgery that is performed under local anesthesia (LA). An emergency situation in HT surgery, although rare, may arise. This part of the guidelines recommends the minimum standard of care in LA administration, emergency preparedness, and treatment of an emergency situation.

Anesthesia for Hair Transplantation

It is recommended that the medications and solution be labeled, and the labels should include the following: medication or solution name - strength, diluent name, and volume (if not apparent from the container) that have been verified both verbally and visually by two individuals of the HT team.

As the procedure involves anesthesia being delivered in a stepwise manner and not at one time, the dosage of the medication and the time of administration should be documented and the details can be displayed on a board nearby and visible to the surgeon.

Allergy Testing for Local Anesthesia

In preoperative screening, it is recommended to ask the patient whether there has been any exposure to local anesthetic (dental procedures, etc.), or whether the patient has ever had an adverse reaction or side effect from an anesthetic or any other drug. Sensitivity to local anesthetics may be either due to the anesthetic itself or due to the preservatives.

Skin tests (prick/puncture and intracutaneous) have evolved as a reliable technique for the diagnosis of IgE-mediated drug reactions. The peak reactivity of prick/puncture tests is 15–20 minutes, at which time both wheal and erythema diameters (or areas) should be recorded in millimeters and compared with positive and negative controls. It should be recognized that prick testing will detect only the immediate type of hypersensitivitiy reactions: It may not detect delayed reactions and, hence, is not foolproof.

Delayed Allergic Reactions to Local Anesthetics

Cutaneous symptoms and systemic complaints occurring between 1h and several days after LA injections may be encountered in some patients. Inflammatory reactions confined to the injection site represent the most common, if not the only, clinical manifestation of late-type LA allergy. Delayed anaphylaxis to LA should be diagnosed by excluding the other causes of systemic symptoms.

Allergic Reactions to Lignocaine

Patients with true allergy to amide local anesthetics present a challenge in HT surgery for providing adequate care with appropriate intraoperative pain management. In case of allergic reactions to amide group anesthetics, ester-type anesthetics can be considered. Cross-reactivity between the amide and ester groups, although rare, had been reported to occur. The taskforce recommends that the patients with proven LA allergy should be referred to specialized allergy clinics for further evaluation with a skin prick test and they should be challenged with an unrelated LA to predict future safety.

Level of Evidence: 3

Category of Recommendation: C

REFERENCES

1. Mysore V, Nischal KC. Guidelines for administration of local anesthesia for dermatosurgery and cosmetic dermatology procedures. Ind J Dermatol Vemerol Leprol. 2009;75:68-75.
2. Jenerowicz D, Polańska A, Glińska O, Czarnecka-Operacz M, Schwartz RA. Allergy to lidocaine injections: Comparison of patient history with skin testing in five patients. Postepy Dermatol Alergol. 2014;31:134-8.
3. Fuzier R, Lapeyre-Mestre M, Mertes PM, Nicolas JF, Benoit Y, Didier A, et al.; French Association of Regional Pharmacovigilance Centers. Immediate- and delayed-type allergic reactions to amide local anesthetics: Clinical features and skin testing. Pharmacoepidemiol Drug Saf. 2009;18:595-601.
4. Trautmann A, Stoevesandt J. Differential diagnosis of late-type reactions to injected local anaesthetics: Inflammation at the injection site is the only indicator of allergic hypersensitivity. Contact Dermatitis. 2019;80:118-24.
5. Cherobin ACFP, Tavares GT. Safety of local anesthetics. An Bras Dermatol. 2020;95:82-90.
6. Bhole MV, Manson AL, Seneviratne SL, Misbah SA. IgE-mediated allergy to local anaesthetics: Separating fact from perception: A UK perspective. Bri J Anaesth. 2012;108:903-11.

TECHNIQUES TO REDUCE PAIN OF ANESTHESIA INJECTION

Most of the pain associated with a HT is during the local anesthesia (LA) injection. There are many techniques to reduce the perception of this pain. They could be used singly or in combination:

1. Topical anesthesia: Eutectic mixtures help in reducing the initial pricking pain felt on piercing the skin with a needle. These mixtures need to be applied at least an hour before the injection of the anesthetic. Common mixtures used contain lignocaine with tetracaine or prilocaine.
2. Warming the local anesthetic solution.

   The simple procedure of warming to 37°C reduced the pain associated with a subcutaneous injection of lignocaine.
3. Buffering the LA solution (Carbonation and pH adjustments).

   The addition of sodium bicarbonate to the LA in order to raise the pH (known as buffering) decreases patient pain during drug delivery via subcutaneous or intradermal infiltration.

   Most solutions were prepared by mixing 8.4% sodium bicarbonate and 1% lidocaine with epinephrine in a 1:9 or 1:10 ratio by volume; both proportions are effective in practice.
5. Slow rate of injection.

   Reducing the rate of administration of LA reduces pain and may have a greater impact on pain than buffering.
6. Simultaneous stimulation of the surrounding skin

   Based on the gate control theory, concomitant physical stimulation (non-painful input) closes the "gates" to painful input, which prevents pain sensation from traveling to the central nervous system. Stimulation of the skin using a vibrating device in the same dermatome results reduced perception of painful stimuli.

Level of Evidence: 2

Category of Recommendation: B

REFERENCES

1. Hogan ME, vanderVaart S, Perampaladas K, Machado M, Einarson TR, Taddio A. Systematic review and meta-analysis of the effect of warming local anesthetics on injection pain. Ann Emerg Med. 2011;58:86-98.e1.

2. Strazar AR, Leynes PG, Lalonde DH. Minimizing the pain of local anesthesia injection. Plast Reconstr Surg. 2013;132:675-84.
3. Gostimir M, Hussain A. A systematic review and meta-analysis of methods for reducing local anesthetic injection pain among patients undergoing periocularsurgery. Ophthalmic Plast Reconstr Surg. 2019;35:113-25.

LOCAL ANESTHETICS

The common anesthetics used for local anesthesia (LA) in HT are Lignocaine (with or without adrenaline), Bupivacaine, Levobupivacaine, and Ropivacaine.

Lignocaine is the most common LA used in HT surgery. The generally recommended maximum dose (Total Daily Dose) for local infiltration is 300 mg or 4.5 mg/kg of body weight. This can be increased to 500 mg or 7 mg/kg after adding adrenaline.

However, it is well recognized that the routine recommendations for infiltration anesthesia are not fully relevant in HT for the following reasons:

1. Tumsecentanesthesia is practiced in HT and tumescent anesthesia allows higher doses to be administered.
2. Since multiple holes are made in the skin, in both donor and recipient area, much of the anesthetic oozes out and is not absorbed.
3. Anesthesia is administered in a graded fashion several times during the long surgery, and, hence, peak values may not be achieved.

However, it is advised that a careful watch is maintained on the amount of anesthetics administered, the quantity given be recorded and documented, and every effort made not to administer excess of anesthetic.

BUPIVACAINE

Bupivacaine is the most commonly used long-acting LA for HT surgery. The maximum daily dose is 175 mg. The use of bupivacaine is limited because of its potential cardiac toxicity. Bupivacaine produces a significantly greater depression of LV pressure than ropivacaine, mepivacaine, or lidocaine. Though these effects are rare with safe dosages, nevertheless there is potential for catastrophic events to occur.

LEVOBUPIVACAINE

Levobupivacaine is the pure S (–) enantiomer of bupivacaine and has emerged as a safer alternative for regional anesthesia than its racemic parent Bupivacaine. The maximum dose for levobupivacaine is 2 mg/kg and the maximum one-time dose is 200 mg. It is a viable alternative to bupivacaine as it is less cardiotoxic but the duration of action is less than bupivacaine but more than ropivacaine and ligocaine. Most of the clinical studies suggest that levobupivacaine is relatively less potent than bupivacaine, but it is more potent than ropivacaine.

ROPIVACAINE

Ropivacaine is a long-acting, enantiomerically pure (S-enantiomer) amide LA and regional anesthetic with an efficacy that is broadly similar to that of bupivacaine. In concentrations of 0.5% and higher, it produces dense blockade with a slightly shorter duration than that of bupivacaine. Various clinical trials have evaluated the safety profile of ropivacaine and found it to be safe. The maximum dose is 3 mg/kg and the maximum one-time dose is 200 mg.

MIXING LOCAL ANESTHETICS

It is unclear whether mixing multiple anesthetics for local infiltration poses further beneficial overuse of a single agent. The systemic effects produced by combinations of LA follow the principles of summation. When adhering to dosage limits, guidelines for various agents should be regarded as additive.

COMBINING LOCAL ANESTHETICS AND ADRENALINE

Use of the lowest effective concentration of adrenaline to provide pain control and vasoconstriction in local infiltrative anesthesia is recommended. The safe dosage of adrenaline is 0.01 mg/kg body weight. It is contraindicated in patients using the nonselective beta-blockers such as propranolol, since concomitant LA administration results in unopposed alpha-receptor mediated vasoconstriction, which can theoretically produce a hypertensive emergency and a profound vagally mediated reflexive bradycardia. Local infiltrative anesthesia with adrenaline may be administered to patients with stable cardiac disease.

Level of Evidence: 3

Category of Recommendation: C

REFERENCES

1. Lam SM. Hair transplant and local anesthetics. Clin Plast Surg. 2013;40:615-25.
2. Patwardhan N, Mysore V; IADVL Dermatosurgery Task Force. Hair transplantation: Standard guidelines of care. Indian J Dermatol Venereol Leprol. 2008;74 Suppl:S46-53.
3. Swinehart JM. Local anesthesia in hair transplant surgery. Dermatol Surg 2002;28:1189.

4. Nusbaum BP. Techniques to reduce pain associated with hair transplantation: Optimizing anesthesia and analgesia. Am J Clin Dermatol. 2004;5:9-15.
5. Bagatin T, Bagatin D, ŠakićL, ŠakićK. Impact of local infiltration anaesthesia on post operative pain management after rhinoplasty in day care surgery. Acta Clin Croat. 2019;58:62-6.
6. Kim H, Hwang K, Yun SM, Kim DJ. Usage of epinephrine mixed with lidocaine in plastic surgery. J Craniofac Surg. 2020;31:791-3.
7. Parekh SB, Parikh SS, Patel H, Mehta M. A prospective comparative observational study of clinical efficacy of isobaric ropivacaine 0.75% with of isobaric bupivacaine 0.5% intrathecally in elective inguinal hernia repair surgeries. Anesth Essays Res. 2017;11:561-6.
9. Heppolette CAA, Brunnen D, Bampoe S, Odor PM. Clinical pharmacokinetics and pharmacodynamics of levobupivacaine. Clin Pharmacokinet. 2020;59:715-45.

SYSTEMIC TOXICITY OF LOCAL ANESTHETICS

Local anesthetic systemic toxicity (LAST) is a life-threatening adverse event that may occur after the administration of local anesthesia (LA) drugs through a variety of routes. In event of the overdose of LA toxicity, immediate management involves the general safety and resuscitation measures that are essential in any emergency. The taskforce recommends the following actions in case of LAST: The LA injection should be stopped; immediate priority is to manage the airway, breathing, and circulation; and the transfer of the patient to a tertiary care hospital should be planned. Early administration of 20% intravenous lipid emulsion therapy is recommended. An initial bolus of 100 mL should be administered over 2–3 minutes (1.5 mL/kg if the lean body weight is <70 kg). This is then to be followed by a 20% lipid emulsion infusion of 200–250 mL over 15–20 minutes (0.25 mL/kg/min if the lean body weight is <70 kg). If circulatory stability is not attained, re-bolusing up to two further times or increasing the infusion to 0.5 mL/kg/ min is suggested. The maximum recommended dose of 20% lipid emulsion is 12 mL/kg.

Seizure activity may exacerbate metabolic acidosis, and prompt prevention and termination is crucial. Due to their cardiostable profile, benzodiazepines are the first-line therapy.

Advanced Cardiac Life Support algorithms for cardiopulmonary resuscitation must be followed should cardiac arrest occur. Chest compressions should be initiated immediately and continued until return of spontaneous circulation. If epinephrine is used, small initial doses of ≤1 μg/kg are preferred to avoid impaired pulmonary gas exchange and increased afterload.

Level of Evidence: 3

Category of Recommendation: C

REFERENCES

1. Kubo A, Shimizu K, Kuroda K, Kanazawa T, Kobayashi M, Morimatsu H. Local anesthetic systemic toxicity following general and epidural anesthesia in a patient with a history of muscle relaxant-induced anaphylaxis. Acta Med Okayama. 2019;73:543-6.
2. Hoegberg LC, Bania TC, Lavergne V, Bailey B, Turgeon AF, Thomas SH, et al.; Lipid Emulsion Workgroup. Systematic review of the effect of intravenous lipid emulsion therapy for local anesthetic toxicity. Clin Toxicol (Phila). 2016;54:167-93.
3. Cao D, Heard K, Foran M, Koyfman A. Intravenous lipid emulsion in the emergency department: A systematic review of recent literature. J Emerg Med. 2015;48:387-97.
4. Sepulveda EA, Pak A. StatPearls [Internet]. Treasure Island (FL): StatPearls Publishing; 2020 Jan-2019 Nov 13.
5. Gitman M, Fettiplace MR, Weinberg GL, Neal JM, Barrington MJ. Local anesthetic systemic toxicity: A narrative literature review and clinical update on prevention, diagnosis, and management. Plast Reconstr Surg. 2019;144:783-95.

EMERGENCY PREPAREDNESS IN HAIR TRANSPLANTATION

Plastic surgeries are classified into three types by the American Association for Accreditation of Ambulatory Surgery Facilities: Class A, minor plastic surgery procedures performed under local, regional, or topical anesthesia; Class A/B, minor or major plastic surgeries performed under intravenous or parenteral sedation, analgesia, or dissociative drugs; and Class A/B/C, major plastic surgeries performed under general anesthesia requiring external support of vital body functions. Surgeries are classified into three types based on the levels of Surgical Complexity: Level 1

- Minimal risk to the patient independent of anesthesia
- Minimally invasive procedures with little or no blood loss
- Often done in an office setting with the operating room principally for anesthesia and monitoring. HT surgery is categorized as Level I surgery and the facility it is performed in is Class A.

Monitoring the following equipment is mandatory for an HT OT:

1. Non-mercury/digital blood pressure apparatus
2. Stethoscope
3. Pulse oximeter
4. Glucometer
5. Digital thermometer
6. Weighing scale

RESUSCITATIVE EQUIPMENT NECESSARY FOR HAIR TRANSPLANT OPERATION THEATER

Resuscitation equipment should be located either in the room or within the premises, to allow basic cardiopulmonary resuscitation. Although there is some medico-legal responsibility, the major concern should be patient safety.

1. Intravenous access cannulas and IV sets
2. Laryngoscope
3. Endotracheal tubes
4. Suction equipment
5. Xylocaine spray
6. Airways: Oropharyngeal and nasopharyngeal
7. Ambu Bag: Adult
8. Oxygen cylinders with flow meter/tubing/catheter/face mask/nasal prongs
9. Defibrillator with accessories (AED preferable)
10. Equipment for dressing/bandaging/suturing
11. ECG Machine

EMERGENCY DRUGS NECESSARY FOR HAIR TRANSPLANT OPERATION THEATER

1. Inj. Adrenaline 1 mg
2. Inj. Hydrocortisone 100 mg
3. Inj. Atropine 1 mL
4. Inj. Pheniramine maleate 10 mL
5. Inj. Promethazine 1 mL
6. Inj. Deryphyline 2 mL
7. Inj. Frusemide 4 mL
8. Inj. Metoclopramide 2 mL
9. Inj. Dexamethasone 2 mL
10. Inj. Diazepam 10 mL
11. Inj. Dicyclomine Hydrochloride 2 mL
12. Inj. Ligocaine without preservative 30 mL
13. Inj. Intralipid 20% 500 mL
14. Inj. 5% dextrose infusion 100 mL
15. Inj. Normal saline 500 mL

Regular inspection of the drugs just mentioned to check their expiry dates should be done periodically.

LIFE SUPPORT TRAINING

Though rare, an HT surgeon may encounter an unresponsive patient or a sudden collapse in a patient. Preventing hypoxic brain damage is the most important task for the surgeon. The surgeon should have been trained in emergency resuscitation skills. If not, an anesthetist should be available for care in such situations. In addition, at least another member of the HT team should be trained in Basic Life Support.

Level of Evidence: 4

Category of Recommendation: D

REFERENCES

1. Singer Robert, Keyes Geoffrey, Nahai Foad. (2019). American Association for Accreditation of Ambulatory Plastic Facilities (AAAASF) History: Its role in plastic surgery safety. Aesthetic Surgery Journal Open Forum. 1. 10.1093/asjof/ojz008.
2. Pasternak LR. Screening Patients – Strategies and Studies. In: By Kathryn McGoldrick, editor. Ambulatory Anesthesiology – A problem-oriented approach. Philadelphia, PA: Williams and Wilkins; 1995. pp. 243.
3. Chakravarthy M. Complications of hair restoration surgery: An overview. In: Mysore V, editor. Hair transplantation. 1st ed. New Delhi: Jaypee Brothers Medical Publishers (p) Ltd; 2016. pp. 149-56.

TRANSFER ARRANGEMENTS

An arrangement should exist with a nearby hospital for the transfer of patients in the event of unexpected serious or potentially serious developments. Surgeons performing office-based HT surgery must have admitting privileges at a nearby hospital or maintain an emergency transfer agreement with a nearby hospital. Ambulance or patient transport services, if provided, should be organized through defined policies and procedures for efficient and effective services. Ambulance or patient transport services, if provided, should comply with the legal and regulatory requirements. Relevant telephone numbers should be displayed prominently, and all staff should be familiar with the telephone numbers.

PRESENCE OF ANESTHETIST DURING HAIR TRANSPLANT PROCEDURE

Typically, patients of HT belong to ASA 1 category (normal healthy patient, nonsmoking, no or minimal alcohol use) and hence the presence of an anesthetist is not routinely necessary. The presence of an anesthetist is not necessary if:

1. The surgeon is well versed with advanced cardiac life support skills
2. The team is Basic Life Support certified
3. All the necessary monitoring and resuscitative equipment is handy
4. Anesthetist services can be accessed easily and quickly
5. The anesthetist services have transfer arrangements with a nearby hospital

When dealing with ASA II (patient with mild systemic disease without substantive functional limitations): Examples include (but not limited to): current smoker, social alcohol drinker, obesity (30 < BMI < 40), well-controlled diabetes mellitus/hypertension, mild lung disease, elderly patient, etc. In such cases, the presence of an anesthetist is advised by the taskforce. Some hair restoration surgeons use parenteral sedatives to create a state of conscious sedation during local anesthesia administration. In this scenario also, the taskforce recommends that the presence of a qualified anesthetist is necessary, not only to monitor the patient but also to manage the patient in case the level of sedation becomes deeper.

The taskforce recommends routine periodic recording and documentation of the vital parameters during the course of surgery. It would be optional for ASA grade 1 but mandatory for ASA grade 2 (hypertension, mild cardiac disease, etc.).

Level of Evidence: 4

Category of Recommendation: D

HT PRACTICE GUIDELINE: PART 4

Surgical Aspects of Hair Transplantation

Introduction

A wide variation exists in the techniques of HT surgery. This part of the guidelines recommends the minimum standard of care in assessing the donor area, surgical steps in follicular unit excision/FUT surgery, recommendations for the magnification, hairline design, duration of the surgery, and the role of platelet rich plasma (PRP) in HT surgery.

Donor Area Issues

Safe Donor Area

Donor harvesting should be from a safe donor area only, and the taskforce discourages harvesting from a nonsafe area, as such hairs would be lost over time. Detailed physical examination and trichoscopic hair analysis should be done to determine donor hair quality (curly or straight), density (must be checked at multiple points, including occipital and temporal), hair caliber, ethnicity, etc.; determination of the safe donor area (SDA) with a focus on areas of hair thinning or retrograde alopecia, if any, should be documented and explained to the patient. Non-scalp donor areas (body hairs) should also be evaluated since too much extraction from SDA might destroy the donor area aesthetics. It is recommended that the surgeon should stay within the SDA while performing excisions, which is a 189–203 cm^2 depending on individual and ethnic variations. There can never be one valid, totally SDA for all patients. The SDA was first suggested by Unger et al. in 1994 and this continues to be the global standard. Other SDA definitions by Cole, Alt, Bernstein, and Rasmann can be considered for demarcating the SDA. A family history, assessment of the future progression of the AGA, and clinical examination would be necessary to confirm the boundaries of SDA. One should always err on the side of caution.

Level of Evidence: 3

Grade of Recommendation: C

REFERENCES

1. Unger W, Solish N, Giguere D. Delineating the "Safe" donor area for hair transplanting. Am J Cosmet Surg. 1994;11:239-43.
2. Devroye J. An overview of the donor area: Basic principles. In: Unger WP, Shapiro R, Unger R, Unger M, editors. Hair transplantation. 5th ed. New York: Informa Health Care; 2011. pp. 247-62.
3. Kumaresan M, Mysore V. Controversies in hair transplantation. J Cutan Aesthet Surg. 2018;11:173-81.
4. Yepuri V, Mysore V. Effects of hormones on hair. In: Mysore V, editor. Hair transplantation. 1st ed. New Delhi, India: Jaypee; 2016. pp. 21-3.
5. Devroye J. An overview of the donor area: Basic principles. In: Unger WP, Shapiro R, Unger R, Unger M, editors. Hair transplantation. 5th ed. New York: Informa Health Care; 2011. pp. 247-62.
6. Bernstein RM, Rassman WR. Follicular transplantation. Patient evaluation and surgical planning. Dermatol Surg. 1997;23:771-84; discussion 801-5.
7. Park JH, Na YC, Moh JS, Lee SY, You SH. Predicting the permanent safe donor area for hair transplantation in Koreans with male pattern baldness according to the position of the parietal whorl. Arch Plast Surg. 2014;41:277-84.

MINIATURIZATION IN THE DONOR AREA

A safe donor area should be evaluated for miniaturization and if present, this should be informed to the patient; excision of grafts should be done carefully to avoid miniaturized hairs since this might hamper the HT result and overharvesting might leave visible depletion of the donor zone. Diffuse type of AGA should always be considered in such cases. Medical treatment and body hair harvesting should be considered in these types of patients.

Level of Evidence: 3

Grade of Recommendation: D

REFERENCES

1. Bernstein RM, Rassman WR. Hair Transplant Forum International March/April 2007;17:201-3.
2. Tobin DJ, Gunin A, Magerl M, Handijski B, Paus R. Plasticity and cytokinetic dynamics of the hair follicle mesenchyme: Implications for hair growth control. J Invest Dermatol. 2003;120:895-904.
3. Garza LA, Yang CC, Zhao T, Blatt HB, Lee M, He H, et al. Bald scalp in men with androgenetic alopecia retains hair follicle stem cells but lacks CD200-rich and CD34-positive hair follicle progenitor cells. J Clin Invest. 2011;121:613-22.

MAXIMUM GRAFTS THAT CAN BE SAFELY HARVESTED FROM SDA

This would depend on:

1. Safe donor area
2. Donor density of both hairs and units
3. Size of head
4. Techniques used
5. Donor skin properties such as elasticity
6. Age of patient and possibility of future sessions

Hence, individual variations may occur. The range of safe upper limit can vary from 4000 to 6500 scalp grafts over a lifetime over multiple sessions and different techniques. Without causing visible depletion of the donor area in one session, an average of 2500–3000 grafts per session is considered as the optimum upper limit of graft harvesting.

Level of Evidence: 3

Grade of Recommendation: D

REFERENCES

1. Bernstein RM, Rassman WR. Follicular transplantation. Patient evaluation and surgical planning. DermatolSurg 1997;23:771-84; discussion 801-5.
2. Harris JA. Application of the Hair Diameter Index (HDI) in Obtaining a Target Hair Density Poster Presentation, International Society of Hair Restoration, 11th Annual Meeting, New York, NY, October 2003.
3. Harris JA. Introduction of the Hair Volume Index (HVI) and Its Correlation to Subjective Visual Hair Density". Scientific Session Presentation and Poster Presentation, International Society of Hair Restoration Surgery 11th Annual Meeting. New York, NY, October 2003.

FOLLICULAR UNIT EXCISION

Follicular unit excision (FUE) involves harvesting hairs from the donor area, under local anesthesia, which is most commonly the scalp but occasionally the beard, chest, and other parts of the body, using circular punches of less than 1 mm diameter, mounted on a manual handle or a motorized hand device or, more recently, a robotic device. There are several options for the punches available. The taskforce recommends that the choice of the punch depends on the individual surgeon's comfort level in reducing the transection of the follicles and to provide optimum outcome and the diameter of the punch to be preferably less than 1 mm. Punches larger than 1 mm are not recommended. Patients' skin characteristics such as variations in the thickness of epidermis, dermal-epidermal junction, and subcutaneous tissue contribute to the challenges of donor harvesting and for obtaining low follicular transection rates. Overharvesting should be avoided, as it may lead to scarring and depigmentation, particularly in patients with darker skin. It is preferable to excise 1 unit out of four follicular units, leaving one intact all around. A general recommendation is to harvest 10–15 excisions/cm^2 as a safe single-pass density in a person with a baseline average density of 65–75 follicles/cm^2. A good magnification device is recommended for the FUE procedure to orient for the follicular unit angle of exit and better excision without transection.

Level of Evidence: 3

Category of Recommendation: C

REFERENCES

1. Devroye J. Donor area harvesting. In: Unger, editor. Hair transplantation. 5th ed. London, UK: Informa Health Care; 2011. pp. 247-8.
2. Garg AK, Garg S. Donor harvesting: Follicular unit excision. J Cutan Aesthet Surg. 2018;11:195-201.

STRIP EXCISION

The size of the strip depends on the demand of number of grafts at recipient site, donor zone elasticity and the donor hair density. Preoperative estimation of scalp laxity and glidability will aid in determining the optimal width to be harvested and also in preventing wound dehiscence postoperatively. The width of the scar is directly proportionate to the width of the strip removed and tension on the wound margins. The width should be preferably less than 1.3 cm. It may be necessary to alter the width of the strip in some areas of increased tension or due to the presence of a preexisting scar.

Evidence level: 3

Grade of Recommendation: C

REFERENCES

1. Marzola M. Single-scar harvesting technique. In: Haber R, Stough D, editors. Hair transplantation. Philadelphia (PA): Elsevier Saunders; 2005. pp. 83-7.
2. Mayer ML. Evaluation of scalp elasticity. In: Unger W, Shapiro R, Unger R, Unger M, editors. Hair transplantation. 5th ed. London, United Kingdom: Informa Healthcare; 2011. pp. 267-70.
3. Huang YL, Chang SL, Lee MC, Chang CH, Hu S, Gold MH. Measuring occipital scalp laxity before donor strip harvesting in hair transplantation. J Drugs Dermatol. 2014;13:1248-52.
4. Park JH. Association between scalp laxity, elasticity, and glidability and donor strip scar width in hair transplantation and a new elasticity measuring method. Dermatol Surg. 2017;43:574-81.

STRIP HARVEST

A single-strip elliptical excision is the gold standard technique with a strip centeredaround occipital protuberance. More superficial scoring incision, angle of the blade parallel to the hair shaft, blunt dissection for separating the scored tissue, and working under good magnification result in lesser transection rates during the strip excision. It is advisable to wait for a minimum of 9–12 months before taking a revision strip surgery.

REFERENCES

1. Tan TY, Pathomvanich D, Castillejes D, Thienthaworn P, Manochai S, Lu N. Follicular transection rate in FUT in Asians: 15 years later. Hair Transpl Forum Intl. 2017;27:1-4.
2. Ahmad M. Comparison of three strip harvesting techniques (Haber's, Pathomvanich's and Ahmad's techniques). J Cosmet Dermatol. 2019;18:589-93.
3. Pathomvanich D. Donor harvesting: A new approach to minimize transection of hair follicles. Dermatol Surg. 2000;26:345-8.

Evidence level: 3

Grade of recommendation: C

WOUND CLOSURE

Depth of dissection and undermining of the edges has been the subject of much debate and at present no uniform recommendations can be made. However, deeper dissection and undermining is associated with a greater risk of injury to vessels and therefore bleeding, needing greater surgical skills. Excessive inadvertent coagulation should be avoided, as it can damage the surrounding follicle and eventually delay healing and might lead to a bad scar.

SUTURING AND SUTURE MATERIAL

- Closure of the strip wound may be performed with sutures (either continuous or intermittent) or with staples, as each of these has its own advantages. The running suture can strangulate the follicles if wound tension is more or if there is significant post-op edema, and it can result in localized hair loss around the suture line and a bad scar unlike staples.
- The quality of the scar is dependent on the amount of width of the strip that is removed during the surgery. Though single-layer closure has been reported to be much faster and cost-effective than double-layer closure, taskforce recommends that strips less than 1.2 cm can be closed in a single layer and that strips more than 1.2 cm must be closed in a double layer.
- Trichophytic closure results in minimizing scarring by regrowing hair through the scar tissue and hence camouflages donor scars. Deepithelialization of the inferior edge of the scalp wound margin is recommended, as the upper edge will slide over the deepithelialized lower edge during the wound closure during the trichophytic closure technique.
- To minimize the reaction from the absorbable sutures, it has been suggested that the use of nonabsorbable sutures such as 3 "0" Nylon interrupted sutures, for the deeper layer to reduce tension on the suture line. The skin can be approximated with 4"0" polyglactin 910.

Evidence level: 3

Grade of recommendation: C

REFERENCES

1. Dua K, Uprety S, Dua A. Donor harvesting: Strip dissection. J Cutan Aesthet Surg. 2018;11:190-4.
2. Ghamdi WA. Vertical harvesting in hair transplantation. Dermatol Surg. 2001;27:597-600.
3. Sam LM. Hair Transplant Operative 360. In: Sam LM, editor. Hair transplant 360 for physicians. New Delhi, India: Jaypee Brothers Medical Publisher; 2011. pp. 47-126.
4. Ahmad M. Single-layer vs. double-layer donor scalp wound closure in strip harvest. Arch Aesthetic PlastSurg. 2017;23:36-40.
5. Adeolu AA, Olabanji JK, Komolafe EO, Ademuyiwa AO, Awe AO, Oladele AO. A prospective study of two methods of closing surgical scalp wounds. Br J Neurosurg. 2012;26:75-7.
6. Bezwada RS, Jamiolkowski DD, Lee IY, Agarwal V, Persivale J, Trenka-Benthin S, et al. Monocryl suture, a new ultra-pliable absorbable monofilament suture. Biomaterials. 1995;16:1141-8.
7. Bernstein RM, Rassman WR, Rashid N. A new suture for hair transplantation: Poliglecaprone 25. Dermatol Surg. 2001;27:5-11.
8. 17 STAPLES REVISITED, Bernstein RM, Hair Transplant Forum International. 2008;18:10–11.

9. Muthuvel K, Lakshmikanthan S, Subburathinam D. Outcomes of staple closure of the donor area during hair transplant by follicular unit transfer. J Cutan Aesthet Surg. 2014;7:103-6.
10. Mubashir S, Sajad P, Rasool F, Hasan I, Bhat YJ. Conventional suture material versus staplers in the closure of donor area in hair transplant. Which is better? Hair Ther Transplant. 2015;5:1000139.
11. Yamamoto K. Double trichophytic closure with wavy two-layered closure for optimal hair transplantation scar. Dermatol Surg. 2012;38:664-9.
12. Yamamoto K. Trichophytic closure of both wound edges after strip excision for hair transplantation. Hair Transplant Forum Int. 2009;19:185,190-1.

MAGNIFICATION FOR THE WORKING FIELD

Magnification for the working field and a clear visualization of the follicles is essential to avoid transection during the process of strip harvesting, slivering, and dissection of follicular units. Various magnification devices such as a stereo microscopes, video microscopes, and magnifying loupes have been routinely used by the surgeons and their team. It is recommended that stereomicroscopic dissection be done for proper identification and dissection to minimize transection during the slivering process. Though stereomicroscopic dissection at magnification of 10–25× gives a good clarity, magnification of 2.5 to 4× can be used to dissect the slivers into follicular grafts.

Evidence level: 3

Grade of recommendation: D

RECIPIENT AREA

Male Hairline Design

The design of the anterior hairline (AHL) is the biggest challenge and most demanding step in hair restoration surgery. It should be designed in such a way so that it not only fulfills present demand but also looks natural for future facial changes, and it should have an undetectable grafty look and be reasonably dense.

The Problems with Hairline Design

1. Most patients ask for a hairline that they had during their teenage years. Making such a lower hairline does not match with facial changes as age advances and, hence, may look unnatural with time. Providing a lower hairline usually consumes a greater number of grafts.
2. Another demand from the patients is to make the frontotemporal angle obtuse and at a low level. The round or obtuse frontotemporal angles are present in the female hairline and may look unnatural when created for men.

Factors for AHL Design

1. Age, hair characteristics, facial features, sex, and ethnicity of the patients should be considered.
2. The placement of AHL should be done preferably higher on the forehead rather than at a lower level. A hairline that is placed higher can be lowered down in future, but the opposite is not possible.
3. A reconstructed hair line should look natural, aesthetically appealing and future hair loss and facial changes with aging should be considered before concluding the final AHL placement.
4. Active involvement of the patient with detailed explanation of the aesthetic concept of the hairline should be done prior to the surgery.
5. Frontotemporal point of the AHL should be at the same level or higher than the midfrontal point.
6. Frontotemporal angle should be in line with the vertical canthal line. The hairline should be aligned so that the receding of the midfrontal point and the frontotemporal angle should be in the same proportion.
7. The distance between the midfrontal and temporal point in the lateral facial profile should not be more than 3cm.
8. For a severe degree of hair loss where the parietal hump has fallen down, it should be reconstructed to meet the new AHL.
9. In a severe degree of temporal recession, temporal fringe reconstruction should be planned to improve the aesthetics of the face in lateral profile.
10. The AHL should have the following components: micro- and macro-irregularities, transition zone, defined zone, and central tuft.
11. The final placement of AHL is to be individualized depending on size and shape of the head, degree of alopecia, and sometimes the patient's wish. The patient's desire for a low hairline can be fulfilled by a properly constructed "widows peak."

Level of Evidence: 4

Category of Recommendation: D

Temporal Triangle Reconstruction

This is an important area of reconstruction for complete aesthetic restoration of the face. The temporal triangle plays an important role in side framing of the face. If enough donor grafts are available, the surgeon will reconstruct this area.

Level of Evidence: 4

Category of Recommendation: D

Vertex Transplant

Vertex area reimplant is a challenge for every HT surgeon. As compared with the front area of the head, the vertex consumes more number of grafts. It is very commonly called as "black hole." Vertex reconstruction is better avoided in young individuals.

Level of Evidence: 4

Category of Recommendation: D

REFERENCES

1. Ronald Shapiro - Principles of creating a natural Hairline. In: avenger W, shapiro R, editorsr. Hair transplantation. 5th ed. Inform healthcare, 2011: 374.
2. Ronald Shapiro Principles & Techniques used to create a Natural Hairline surgical Hair Restoration. Facial Plast Surg Clin North Am. 2004;12:201-18.
3. Paul T. Rose, William M. Parsley. Science of hairline design. In: Robert s Haber, Dowling B stough, editors. Procedures in dermatology – hair transplanting. 1st ed. Elsevier; 2006. pp. 55.
4. Simons C. Five old lines and these new lines that can help when designing a male temporal. Hairline or when transplanting the front temporal apex. Hair Transpl Forum Int. 2004;14:201-3.
5. Ziering C, Krenitsky G. The Ziering Whorl classification of scalp hair. Dermatol Surg. 2003;29:817-21; discussion 821.
6. Mayer ML, Perez-Meza D. Temporal Points: Classification and surgical Techniques for Aesthetic results. Hair Transplant Forum International. 2002;12:147-58.
7. Beehner M. Where is thy crown, your Majesty? HT Forum International. 1998;8:18-9.
8. Rose PT. Consideration in establishing the hairline. Int J Aesth Rest Surg. 1998;1:24-6.
9. Garg AK, Garg S. Decoding facial esthetics to recreate an esthetic hairline: A method which includes forehead curvature. J Cutan Aesthet Surg. 2017;10:195-9.

Female Hair Transplant and Planning and Designing Anterior Hairline

Detailed counseling is necessary in women who have an unrealistic expectation of achieving a full head of hair after the HT. Even when surgical technique and hair survival is excellent, the patient may be very dissatisfied because of poor communication and/or mismatched expectations.

A detailed examination of the recipient area and the donor area to look for diffuse thinning is necessary. General physical examination to look for underlying medical conditions, nutritional deficiencies, and other systemic diseases should be done in all the female patients. These women need to be counseled to seek alternative treatments, including medical treatments, scalp-coloring agents, improved hairstyling, or hairpieces.

Commonly, the areas treated in women include one or more of the following: the hairline, the midline frontal zone just posterior to the hairline, a desired part-line, the center of the vertex, the frontotemporal recessions, and the central caudal region.

Planning of Anterior Hairline in Females

1. Hairline is at a lower level on the vertical portion of the forehead.
2. Frontotemporal angle is obtuse and rounded.
3. A widow's peak or cowlick is usually located in the center of the AHL; the central peak is generally associated with later smaller peaks or mounds.

Level of Evidence: 4

Category of Recommendation: D

REFERENCES

1. Unger WP. Hair transplantation in females. In: Unger WP, Nordstrom RE, editors. Hair transplantation. 2nd ed. New York: Marcel Dekker; 1988. pp. 295-300.
2. Unger WP, Unger RH. Hair transplantation: An important but often forgotten treatment option for female pattern hair. J Am Acad Dermatol. 2003;49:853-60.
3. Shapiro J. Clinical practice. Hair loss in women. N Engl J Med. 2007;357:1620-30.
4. Nussbaum BP, Fuentesfria S. Naturally occurring female hairline patterns. Dermatol Surg. 2009;35:907-14.

SOME IMPORTANT SPECIFIC ISSUES

Maximum Duration of Surgery and Graft Survival Rate

There is no specific recommendation of the duration of surgery. However, out-of-body time for grafts, patients' safety, comfort, physician fatigue, assistants' fatigue, amount of anesthesia and its duration, and patients' state of health need to be taken into account. It must always be remembered that HT is a cosmetic surgery and it is preferable, when a large number of grafts are needed to repeat the surgery than perform prolonged surgeries in one session. Although graft survival has been seen up to 6h of outside body time, it is preferred to insert the grafts within the first 2–4h itself to maximize the graft survival and hence the overall result.

Level of Evidence: 3

Grade of Recommendation: D

REFERENCES

1. Unger W. Effect of rapid transfer of grafts from the donor area to the recipient site. In: Unger W, Shapiro R, editors. Hair transplantation. 4 th ed. New York: Marcel Dekker; 2004. pp. 295.
2. Limmer R. Micrograft survival. In: Stough D, Haber R, editors. Hair replacement. St Louis, MO: Mosby press; 1996. pp. 147-9.
3. Raposio E, Cella A, Panarese P. Effects of cooling micrografts in hair restoration surgery. Dermatol Surg. 1999;25:705-07.
4. Hwang SJ. The effects of dehydration, preservation temperature and time on the hair grafts. Ann Dermatol. 2002;14:149-52.

COMBINATION SURGERIES

In several situations, a combination of techniques (FUT and follicular unit excision) or harvesting from multiple areas (scalp, beard, body) may be needed. These include: advanced grades of alopecia, to maximize the output of the donor grafts, during revision surgeries, second session, diffuse pattern hair loss, and in those with limited donor area combination. Such combination surgeries require expertise in view of longer operating hours, increased anesthetic dose, and patient tolerance. Such combinations can be done either on the same day, after proper assessment by the treating surgeon, or on separate days, depending on the given situation in each case.

Level of Evidence: 3

Grade of Recommendation: D

REFERENCES

1. True R. Combining FUE and Strip Harvesting in the same procedure. Presenting at Seventeenth Annual of the ISHRS, Amsterdam, July 2009;
2. Tsilosani A. Expanding graft numbers combining strip and FUE in the same session. Hair Transplant Forum Int 2010;20:121-3.

PRP IN ANDROGENETIC ALOPECIA AND HT

The available literature suggests that PRP may be effective in treating AGA and may act to reduce hair loss, increase hair diameter and density. However, there exist large variations in optimal PRP preparation method, the optimal frequency, treatment interval, and the long-term efficacy of PRP treatment.

To validate the efficacy and safety of PRP in treating hair loss, more RCTs are required, with standard protocols concerning more objective evaluation of hair loss, the number and interval of treatment sessions, the number of platelets, the method of activation, and the long-term follow-up outcomes.

It is also true that an increasing number of publications have been produced over the past two years, though of lower quality, and the treatment is easy, safe, and cheap. Hence, the taskforce recommends its use as an adjuvant along with other modifications and not as a monotherapy or first-line treatment. The recommendation can be renewed as further evidence becomes available.

The PRP is also used in various steps of the HT procedure intraoperatively to augment the result of HT. The studies reported so far, though small, have documented the reduction in postoperative hair loss after HT and early regrowth of implanted hair. PRP treatment is safe during HT and has strong logic, but it needs validation through proper controlled trials. It is also true that there is no other ideal holding solution. Taskforce recommends its use during the procedure with proper informed consent.

Level of Evidence: 2

Category of Recommendation: B

REFERENCES

1. Li ZJ, Choi HI, Choi DK, Sohn KC, Im M, Seo YJ, et al. Autologous platelet-rich plasma: A potential therapeutic tool for promoting hair growth. Dermatol Surg. 2012;38:1040-6.
2. Dhurat R, Sukesh M. Principles and methods of preparation of platelet-rich plasma: A review and author's perspective. J Cutan Aesthet Surg. 2014;7:189-97.
3. Miao Y, Sun YB, Sun XJ, Du BJ, Jiang JD, Hu ZQ. Promotional effect of platelet-rich plasma on hair follicle reconstitution in vivo. Dermatol Surg. 2013;39:1868-76.
4. Schiavone G, Raskovic D, Greco J, Abeni D. Platelet-rich plasma for androgenetic alopecia: A pilot study. Dermatol Surg. 2014;40: 1010-9.
5. Cervelli V, Garcovich S, Bielli A, Cervelli G, Curcio BC, Scioli MG, et al. The effect of autologous activated platelet rich plasma (AA-PRP) injection on pattern hair loss: Clinical and histomorphometric evaluation. Biomed Res Int. 2014;2014:760709.
6. Khatu SS, More YE, Gokhale NR, Chavhan DC, Bendsure N. Platelets-rich plasma in androgenic alopecia: Myth or an effective tool. J Cutan Aesthet Surg. 2014;7:107-10.
7. Greco J, Brandt R. The effects of autologous platelet crich plasma and various growth factors on non-transplanted miniaturized hair. Hair Transplan Forum Int. 2009;19:49-50.
8. Lopez V, Vaya A, Bautista D, Ricart JM. Autologous platelet-rich plasma as a potential therapeutic tool in androgenetic alopecia. J Am Acad Dermatol. 2013;68:SAB103.
9. Gkini MA, Kouskoukis AE, Tripsianis G, Rigopoulos D, Kouskoukis K. Study of platelet-rich plasma injections in the treatment of androgenetic alopecia through an one-year period. J Cutan Aesthet Surg. 2014;7:213-9.
10. Qu Q, Shi P, Yi Y, Fan Z, Liu X, Zhu D, et al. Efficacy of platelet-rich plasma for treating androgenic alopecia of varying grades. Clin Drug Investig. 2019;39:865-72.
11. Hesseler MJ, Shyam N. Platelet-rich plasma and its utilities in alopecia: A systematic review. Dermatol Surg. 2019;17:93-102.

12. Mao G, Zhang G, Fan W. Platelet-rich plasma for treating androgenic alopecia: A systematic review. Aesthetic Plast Surg. 2019;43:1326-36.
13. Verma K, Tegta GR, Verma G, Gupta M, Negi A, Sharma R. A study to compare the efficacy of platelet rich plasma and minoxidil therapy for the treatment of androgenetic alopecia. Ind J Tricology. 2019;11:68-79.
14. Bayat M, Yazdanpanah MJ, HamidiAlamdari D, Banihashemi M, Salehi M. The effect of platelet-rich plasma injection in the treatment of androgeneticalopecia. J Cosmet Dermatol. 2019;18:1624-8.
15. Stevens J, Khetarpal S. Platelet-rich plasma for androgenetic alopecia: A review of the literature and proposed treatment protocol. Int J Womens Dermatol. 2019;5:46-51.
16. Shetty VH, Goel S. Dermoscopic pre- and posttreatment evaluation in patients with androgenetic alopecia on platelet-rich plasma-A prospective study. J Cosmet Dermatol. 2018;8:1380-8.
17. Butt G, Hussain I, Ahmed FJ, Choudhery MS. Efficacy of platelet-rich plasma in androgenetic alopecia patients. J Cosmet Dermatol. 2019;18:996-1001.
18. Rodrigues BL, Montalvão SAL, Cancela RBB, Silva FAR, Urban A, Huber SC, et al. Treatment of male pattern alopecia with platelet-rich plasma: A double-blind controlled study with analysis of platelet number and growth factor levels. J Am Acad Dermatol. 2019;80:694-700.
19. Hausauer AK, Jones DH. Evaluating the efficacy of different platelet-rich plasma regimens for management of androgenetic alopecia: A single-center, blinded, randomized clinical trial. Dermatol Surg. 2018;44:1191-200.
20. Chen JX, Justicz N, Lee LN. Platelet-rich plasma for the treatment of androgenic alopecia: A systematic review. Facial Plast Surg. 2018;34:631-40.
21. Cervantes J, Perper M, Wong LL, Eber AE, Villasante Fricke AC, Wikramanayake TC, et al. Effectiveness of platelet-rich plasma for androgenetic alopecia: A review of the literature. Skin Appendage Disord. 2018;4:1-11.
22. Giordano S, Romeo M, di Summa P, Salval A, Lankinen P. A meta-analysis on evidence of platelet-rich plasma for androgenetic alopecia. Int J Trichology. 2018;10:1-10.
23. Gupta AK, Versteeg SG, Rapaport J, Hausauer AK, Shear NH, Piguet V. The efficacy of platelet rich plasma in the field of hair restoration and facial aesthetics – A systematic review and meta-analysis. J Cutaneous and Med Surg. 2019;23: 185-203.
24. Puig CJ, Reese R, Peters M. Double-blind, placebo-controlled pilot study on the use of platelet-rich plasma in women with female androgenetic alopecia. Dermatol Surg. 2016;42:1243-7.
25. Garg AK, Garg S. A histological and clinical evaluation of plasma as a graft holding solution and its efficacy in terms of hair growth and graft survival. Hair Transplant Forum Int. 2018;28: 89,94-6.
26. Uebel CO, da Silva JB, Cantarelli D, Martins P. The role of platelet plasma growth factors in male pattern baldness surgery. Plast Reconstr Surg. 2006;118:1458-66.
27. Garg S. Outcome of intra-operative injected platelet-rich plasma therapy during follicular unit extraction hair transplant: A prospective randomised study in forty patients. J Cutan Aesthet Surg. 2016;9:157-64.

SUMMARY

The objective of these guidelines is to recommend minimum standards for practice of HT. The principles outlined in these guidelines are of a general nature only and are not meant to cover all situations. The taskforce emphasizes that each patient has to be treated on his/her own merit and that these guidelines do not limit the physician from making an appropriate choice or the necessary innovation for a given patient.

Index

Page numbers followed by *b* refer to box, *f* refer to figure, *fc* refer to flowchart, and *t* refer to table.

B

C

D

E

N

O

T

U

V